# Genital Dermatology Manual

FOURTH EDITION

# Genital Dermatology Manual

FOURTH EDITION

**Libby Edwards, MD**
Chief of Dermatology
Atrium Health Carolinas Medical Center
Charlotte, North Carolina

**Peter J. Lynch, MD**
Emeritus Professor of Dermatology
Department of Dermatology
University of California
Davis Sacramento, California

Wolters Kluwer

Philadelphia • Baltimore • New York • London
Buenos Aires • Hong Kong • Sydney • Tokyo

*Acquisitions Editor*: James Sherman
*Development Editor*: Eric McDermott
*Editorial Coordinator*: Oliver Raj
*Marketing Manager*: Kirsten Watrud
*Production Project Manager*: Bridgett Dougherty
*Manager, Graphic Arts & Design*: Stephen Druding
*Manufacturing Coordinator*: Beth Welsh
*Prepress Vendor*: Straive



9 8 7 6 5 4 3 2 1

Printed in Mexico

**Cataloging-in-Publication Data available on request from the Publisher**

**ISBN: 978-1-9751-6145-3**



shop.lww.com

QUADM1022

*To Pat and Sue, two people of my heart,*
*who keep my life together and make not only my life,*
*but the world, a better place.*

*To Libby: without her clinical expertise and photographic*
*skills this book would not be possible.*
*In addition, she has been my consummate colleague,*
*collaborator and friend for more than 40 years.*

# Preface

We have made substantial changes for the fourth edition of this book. These include hundreds of new and/or replacement photos; additional pages of disease discussion; revision and update for each chapter; inclusion of recent references; patient handouts in Spanish as well as English; and added additional topics such as special issues relating to transgender individuals.

We have indicated in the preface of previous editions that men and women with disorders of the genitalia are cared for by clinicians with many different backgrounds. These include, but are not limited to, dermatologists, gynecologists, urologists, primary care physicians, nurse practitioners, physician assistants, and midwives. Unfortunately, the training programs for all of these individuals rarely incorporate the information and experience needed to offer the high level of care these patients expect, need, and deserve. In an attempt to improve this situation, we have written this book based on our more than 90 years of combined experience in practices largely devoted to genital disorders. While we hope that the use of this book will help in this regard, we would also encourage our readers to participate in continuing education courses and clinical meetings of the multiple organizations devoted to this subject.

Making the correct diagnosis is the *sine qua non* of assisting patients with all medical problems. After all, how can you find additional helpful information in various reference sources, if the diagnosis is unknown or is incorrect? Conventional textbooks almost always arrange and sort disorders according to etiology (eg, infections) and/or pathophysiology (eg, autoimmune diseases). Such an arrangement may be intellectually satisfying, but it is of little help to a clinician dealing with an unrecognized disorder. For this reason, we have taken a less often used approach and have arranged the genital dermatological disorders on the basis of clinical morphology. Doing so allows the clinician to turn to the appropriate chapter, then form a list of differential diagnoses, match the photos, review the related narrative material, and in nearly all instances allow for establishment of the most likely diagnosis. This approach even has the advantage of allowing one to arrive at a correct diagnosis for a condition that has never before been encountered!

The problem of establishing a correct diagnosis seems to be particularly common in patients with genital disorders. This happens not only because of the lack of training and experience in this area but also because of the warm, moist environment that naturally occurs in the genital region. This environment can obscure even common, readily recognizable conditions and thus cause them to be misdiagnosed. We deal with this problem by including the various morphologies of these disorders in multiple places throughout the book. Doing so converts what might at first appear to be redundancy and allows for making a correct morphological diagnosis even in the situation of an unusual, or atypical, presentation.

In addition, we have included chapters relating to symptoms (such as itching and pain) as well as chapters on special issues such as psychological problems, vaginitis, balanitis, geriatric and pediatric disorders, transgender issues, and conditions that occur in immunosuppressed individuals. We have added dermatoscopic findings for appropriate diseases and more photomicrographs. Finally, as noted above, there are handouts in both English and Spanish, which may be copied and given to patients so that they may better understand the nature and treatment of their disorders.

*Libby Edwards, MD*
*Peter J. Lynch, MD*

# Contents

# Genital Anatomy 1

LIBBY EDWARDS

A knowledge of anatomy and the various normal appearances of the genitalia helps with the recognition of both normal structures and pathologic findings.

Anogenital skin of both genders is composed of different structures and types of skin, each of which is predisposed to different diseases. An understanding of the location and appearance of different types of epithelium is useful in the diagnosis of genital skin diseases. Both male and female genitalia contain dry, keratinized skin with hair follicles (mons, scrotum, lateral labia majora) and modified mucous membranes that are partially keratinized with vestigial follicles and appendages (eg, labia minora, clitoral hood, glans penis), and the female vestibule is composed of a true mucous membrane, which is nonkeratinized and has no hair follicles or appendages.

A familiarity of the location of these different skin types is useful in the diagnosis of anogenital skin disease. Some dermatoses, such as psoriasis, prefer keratinized skin, some dermatoses, such as lichen planus, preferentially affect mucous membranes and modified mucous membranes while sparing keratinized skin, and some dermatoses, such as lichen sclerosus, most often affect modified mucous membranes and spare mucous membranes.

The normal appearance of anogenital skin varies as much from one individual to another as does the face. Most clinicians, despite substantial experience in the evaluation of patients, tend to not "see" an asymptomatic area. Puffiness, erythema, papillomatosis, and asymmetry generally are not noted if a patient has no complaints. However, if a patient reports pain or itching, these normal variants take on the stature of abnormalities. Similarly, patients do not notice these changes if they are comfortable, but they are certain that redness is new as soon as symptoms occur.

This is true of all body surfaces, but especially true of anogenital skin, which is often more difficult than the face or hands for the patient to see on a regular basis. Practitioners, as taught in training, are predisposed to listen to their patients, so that an individual who reports pain and redness is likely to exhibit an examination described by the provider as red. Therefore, it is important for an examiner to be familiar with the normal variation of the genitalia and to make judgments based on the objective findings without being unduly influenced by the patients' perceptions.

A confident patient cannot be dissuaded from their descriptions of abnormalities, and reassurances are generally useless. Sometimes, interpretation of the abnormality can be useful, such as telling a patient that redness can occur with pain syndromes, such as vulvodynia or scrotodynia, but that the redness is not a sign of inflammation or infection in that case.

## Female Genitalia

### Vulva

The periphery of the vulva encompasses the mons anteriorly, the labia majora laterally, and the perineum posteriorly, extending centrally to the hymen, which marks the entrance to the vagina (Fig. 1-1). These structures compose the external genitalia.

The labia majora (singular = labium majus) are two fatty folds of skin that are derived from ectodermal tissues. The lateral aspect of the labia majora is covered with dry, keratinized, conspicuously hair-bearing skin. Each hair follicle is part of a pilosebaceous unit comprising

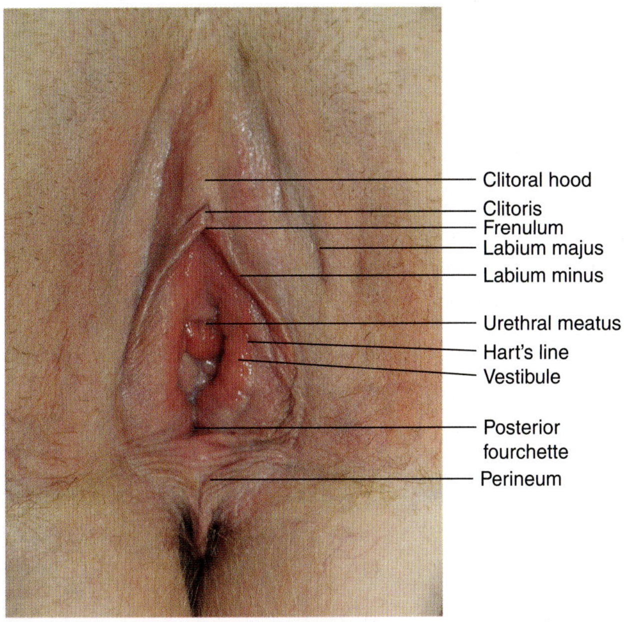


Fig. 1-1. Normal vulva.

the follicle itself, its hair shaft, sebaceous gland, and the erector pili apparatus—a smooth muscle that contracts to form gooseflesh.

The labia minora (singular = labium minus) are much thinner folds of connective tissue and squamous epithelium located medial to the labia majora. This area as well as the medial labia majora, the clitoral hood, and the clitoris are covered with the partially keratinized modified mucous membrane epithelium. The vestibule, or introitus, is mucous membrane that extends from the medial origin of the labia minora (Hart line) to the hymeneal ring. The mons and labia majora cover and protect more delicate structures such as the clitoris, the clitoral hood, the labia minora, and the vestibule.

Although the modified mucous membranes of the medial labia majora, the labia minora, and periclitoral skin are generally considered to exhibit hairless mucous membrane epithelium, these areas actually are covered with partially keratinized skin that contains several structures, including subtle hair follicles, apocrine sweat glands, and ectopic sebaceous glands (Fordyce spots). These Fordyce spots are often prominent, especially on the medial aspect of these skin folds, raising a concern for genital warts in some patients. These sebaceous glands appear as small, yellow to white, lobular papules (**Fig. 1-2**).

Hart line is a variably distinct line of demarcation at the base of the medial aspect of each labium minus, separating modified mucous membrane from the mucous membrane skin of the vestibule. Nonkeratinized, non-hair-bearing squamous mucosal epithelium with mucous-secreting glands extends from Hart line to and including the vagina and the external surface of the cervix. Mucosa is defined as a membrane that lines body structures that communicate to the air, and generally produce lubricating mucus, and is nonhair bearing. Both the vagina and the vestibule are covered with mucosae, whose surfaces are variably wet (depending on estrogen status) as a result of mucus produced by associated glands and the cervix.

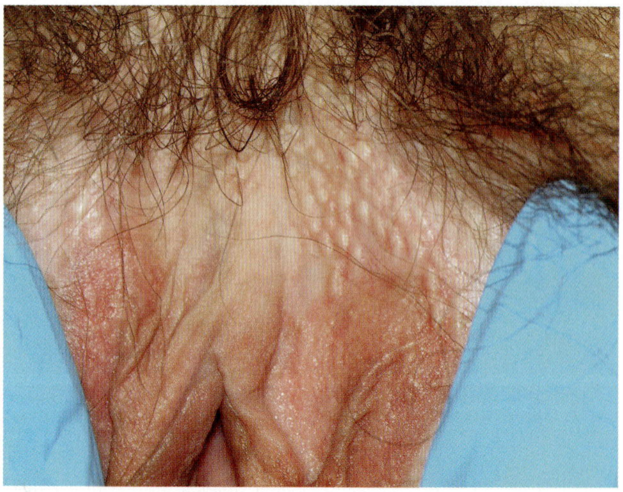

Fig. 1-2. Fordyce spots here are cream-colored papules on the medial anterior labia majora.

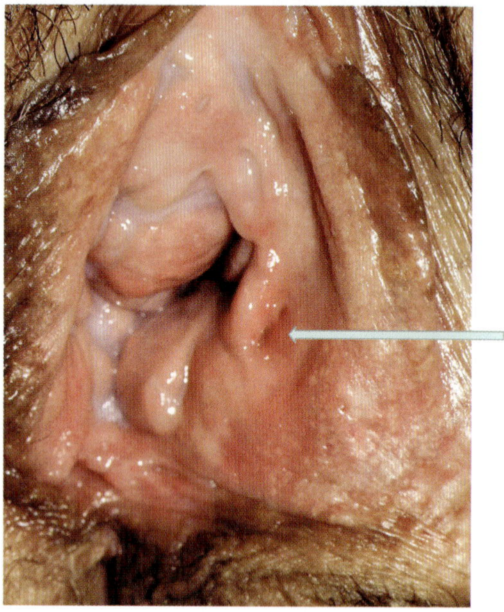

Fig. 1-3. Pits that represent the ostia of vestibular glands occur regularly abutting the lateral aspect of the hymenal caruncles (*arrow*).

The vestibule, or introitus, extends from Hart line to the hymen. Variable numbers of mucous-secreting vestibular glands open onto the mucous membrane of this area. These glands are shallow pits lined with secretory cells; these primarily open circumferentially around the external aspect of the hymeneal ring and between the hymen and urethra (**Fig. 1-3**) but are occasionally visible on other areas of the vestibule (**Fig. 1-4**). They supplement lubrication in young, well-estrogenized women. Bartholin glands are paired glands that lie under the posterior portion of the vestibule, with duct openings just outside the hymen at the 5 and 7 o'clock positions. Skene glands exit into the distal urethra.

The well-estrogenized vagina is pink with prominent rugae, although this is variable. Vaginal secretions are normally present, and these are generally white, odorless, and fairly thin, with variable volume.

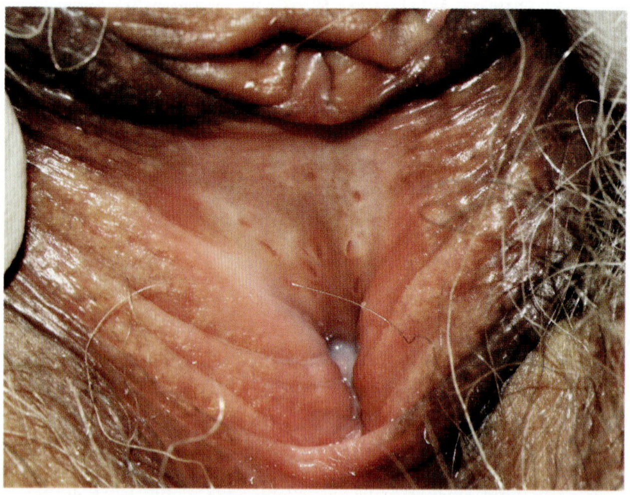

Fig. 1-4. Vestibular gland ostia also occur on other areas of the vestibule but are often very subtle. This vulva shows distinct ostia in the anterior vestibule.

The vulva undergoes marked change from birth until puberty (see Chapter 15). The skin of the mons and the lateral labia majora is characterized by fine vellus hair at birth, but with puberty, coarse terminal hair appears. In addition, the labia minora are almost absent until the onset of puberty, when estrogen appears and the labia minora elongate. The modified mucous membranes are smooth in prepubertal girls, before developing the normal sebaceous glands and redundant tissue of the estrogenized vulva. Apocrine glands become better developed with sexual maturity, and small, monomorphous papillae are common.

Likewise, after menopause and loss of estrogen, the labia minora shrink, hair diminishes, and the fat of the labia majora decreases (see Chapter 15). The normal pink color pales, sebaceous glands miniaturize, papillomatosis disappears, and the modified mucous membranes become smooth and flat. The vagina becomes pale and smooth, with minimal vaginal secretions.

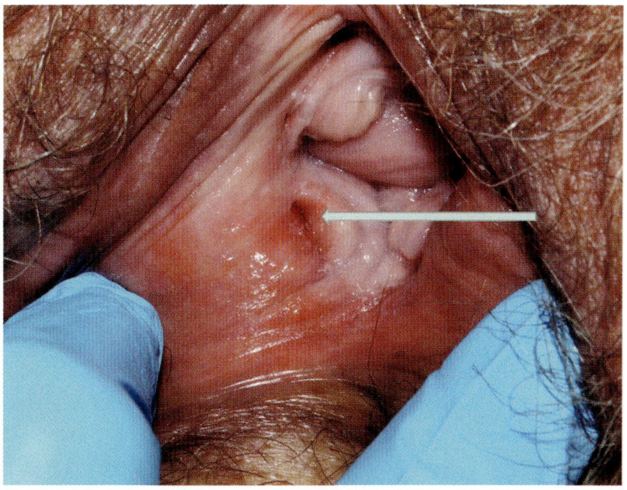

Fig. 1-6. Redness of the ostia of vestibular glands (*arrow*) is a common finding in vestibulodynia (formerly named vulvar vestibulitis). However, most often, this erythema is a normal finding, as is true in this asymptomatic woman.

## Normal Variants

A normal vulva exhibits erythema of the modified mucous membranes and vestibule, as is true of the oral mucosa, lips, and conjunctivae. Many women also show erythema of the hair-bearing labia majora normally. The degree of erythema varies widely from patient to patient, so that its significance sometimes can be difficult to ascertain. Generally, very light complected individuals and red-headed women exhibit more marked erythema than darker individuals, and the vestibule of children is sometimes remarkable normally. In one reported series of premenopausal women, 43% showed erythema (**Figs. 1-5 and 1-6**).[1] This finding is often misinterpreted by patients and their physicians as indicative of inflammation. In addition, more than half of the women with vestibular erythema report no dyspareunia, but experience pain when the area is touched with a cotton-tipped applicator (the Q-tip test). This indicates that redness and a positive Q-tip test are normal findings and do not, alone and in the absence of real-life symptoms, constitute the vestibulodynia pattern of vulvodynia, formerly called the vulvar vestibulitis syndrome.

Vulvar papillae (see Chapter 7) are also common normal variants, occurring in about one-third of premenopausal women (**Figs. 1-7 through 1-11**).[1,2] When these occur in the

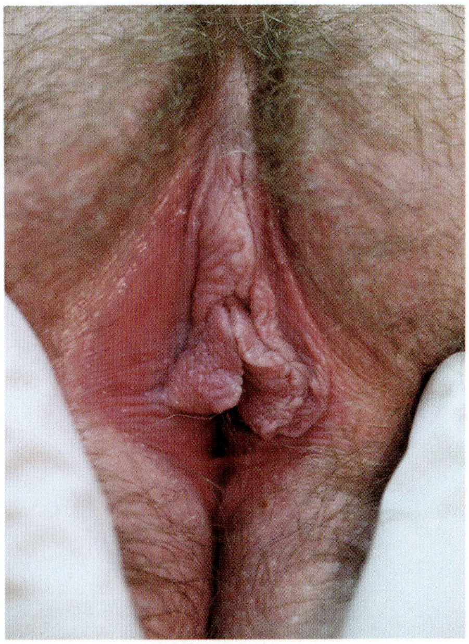

Fig. 1-5. The modified mucous membranes of the vulva normally exhibit mild erythema, as do mucous membranes of the mouth and lips. Some women, particularly those who are fair, display striking but still normal redness, so that true inflammation can be difficult to judge.

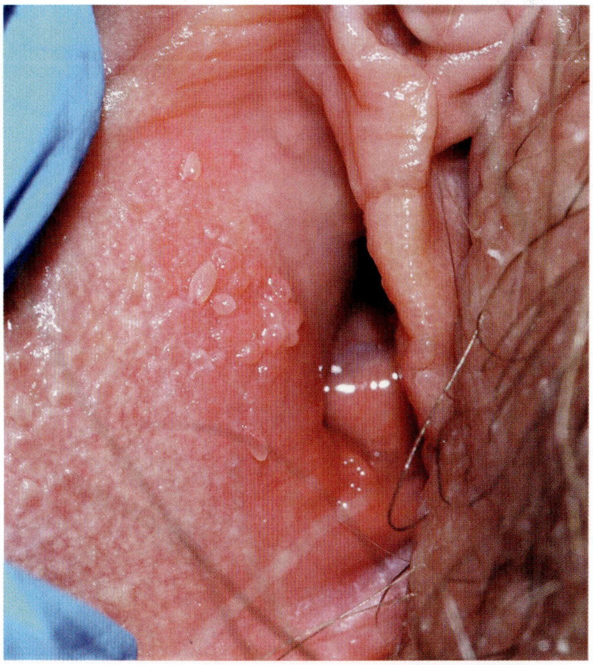

Fig. 1-7. Vulvar papillae are classically found in the vestibule and consist of symmetrical plaques of tubular papules with rounded tips, discrete to the base, unlike filiform papules of genital warts that are often fused at the base with pointed ("acuminate") tips.

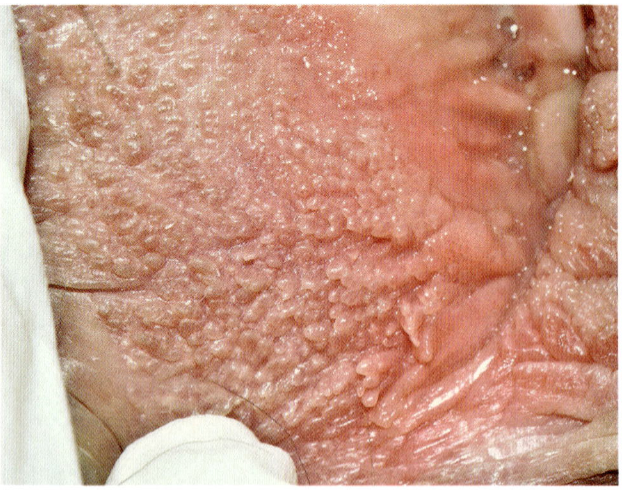

Fig. 1-8. Vulvar papillae can be short and closely set, giving a cobblestoned appearance to the skin.

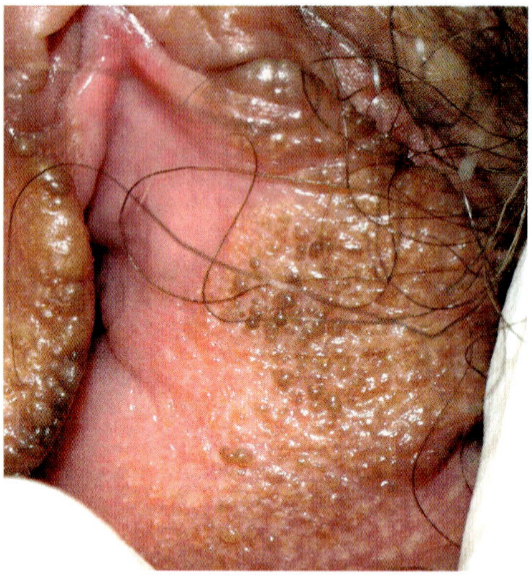

Fig. 1-10. Vulvar papillae can be more discrete and separated, and in some patients who are darkly complexioned, pigmented.

vestibule, they are called vestibular papillae, but these also occur on the medial labia minora and occasionally even on the edges of the labia minora. These variants are sometimes mistaken for signs of disease, usually condylomata acuminata. Initial descriptions of vulvar papillomatosis reported biopsies consistent with human papillomavirus (HPV) infection as the cause. However, biopsies of even normal vulvar skin often show epithelial cells that contain perinuclear vacuoles that can mimic koilocytes of HPV infection. More recent studies have evaluated for the actual presence of the virus by polymerase chain reaction. The current consensus is that vestibular papillomatosis is a variant of normal, distinct from HPV infection.[2,3] And, normal vulvar papillomatosis can be distinguished without a biopsy by the differing morphology; these small, soft, monomorphous, tubular projections of vulvar papillomatosis are distributed in a symmetrical pattern, most often long the medial aspect of the vestibule. They are also common on the bilateral medial labia minora, where they are more likely to be dome shaped and less tubular. Vulvar papillae differ from condylomata acuminata by their rounded rather than acuminate tips and symmetric pattern. Vulvar papillae are discrete to the base, whereas genital warts generally are fused at the base to adjacent lesions. Moreover, genital warts are often keratinized and appear white in this moist area.

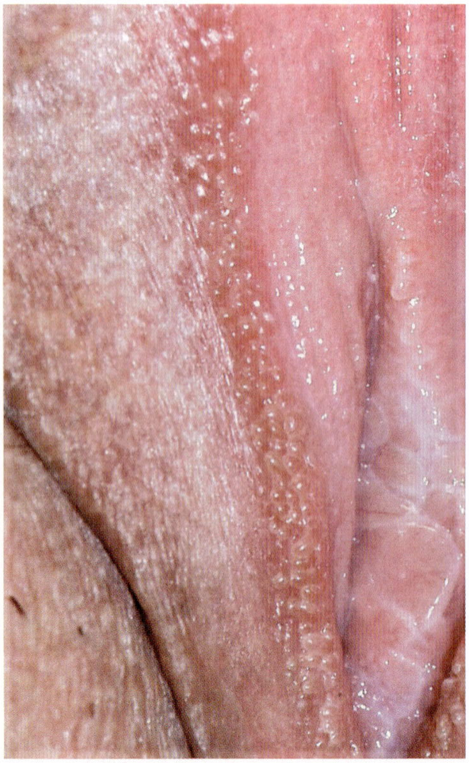

Fig. 1-9. Vulvar papillae sometimes form symmetrical lines, particularly at the edge of Hart line.

Occasionally, similar dome-shaped, smooth papules coalesce into a cobblestone texture on the inner labia minora.

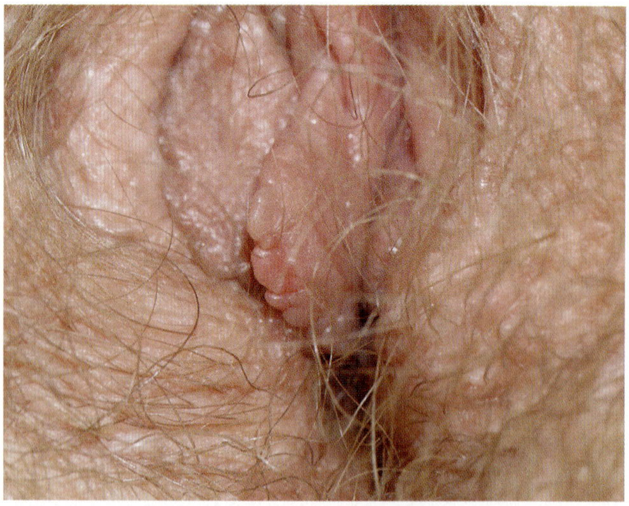

Fig. 1-11. Although vulvar papillae are found most often in the vestibule and medial labia minora, they can occur on edges of the labia minora, as seen here.

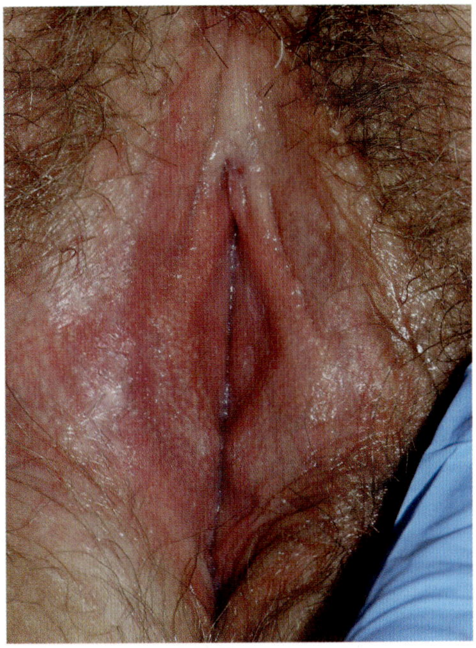

Fig. 1-12. The labia minora in this woman are very small and also display prominent Fordyce spots.

Rarely, these lesions form papules on the edge of the labia minora. These changes are also often mistaken for warts. Although vulvar papillae were once believed to produce itching or pain, they are now known to be asymptomatic.

The whitening of vulvar skin following the application of 5% acetic acid has been believed to be pathognomonic of HPV infection and intraepithelial neoplasia. Although very sensitive, this is a nonspecific finding occurring with any condition that produces hyperkeratosis or thickening of the skin.[4] Some investigators have found that 5% acetic acid predictably produces acetowhitening of all vulvar skin with prolonged contact.[1]

Labia minora exhibit wide morphologic variability. These folds of skin can be large and pendulous, so small as to be nearly absent, or very asymmetric (**Figs. 1-12 through 1-14**).

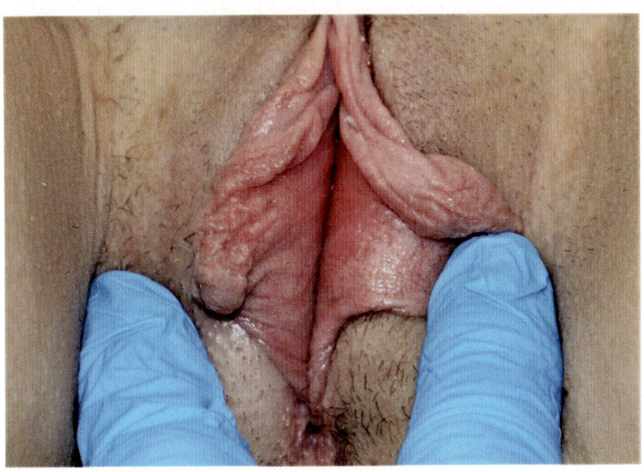

Fig. 1-13. The labia minora in this woman are large and extend far beyond the labia majora.

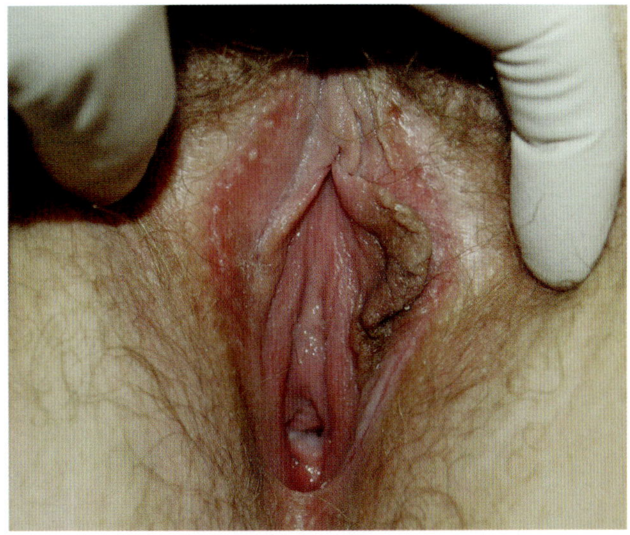

Fig. 1-14. The labia minora are often asymmetrical, with the left labium minus of this adult larger than the right.

The anterior origin of the labia minora most often is the frenulum of the clitoris, but frequently, the anterior origin is from several structures, with a contribution from the skin lateral to the clitoral hood **(Fig. 1-15)** and the posterior aspect of the labia minora can be fused **(Fig. 1-16)**.

In the past few years, labial cosmetic surgery has become fashionable for some women. Although formerly reserved for women with uncomfortable, unusually large labia minora, a labiaplasty is now being performed on women who simply do not like the appearance of the size or asymmetry of their labia minora. Studies have shown

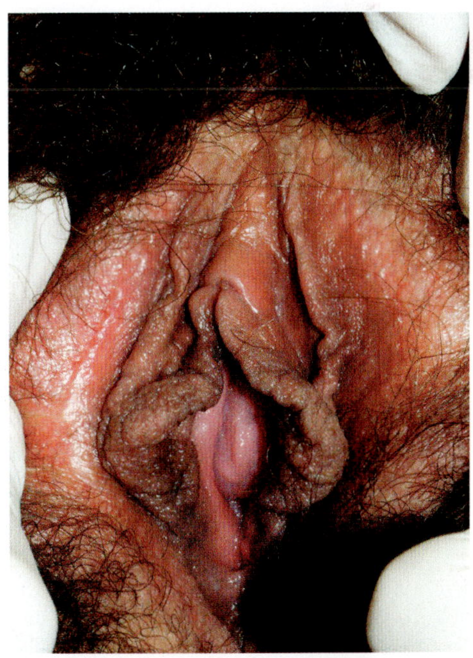

Fig. 1-15. Usually, the labia minora originate anteriorly with the clitoral frenulum, but this is variable. This patient's labia minora originate with the clitoral frenulum and the far anterior modified mucous membranes, producing redundant labia minora.

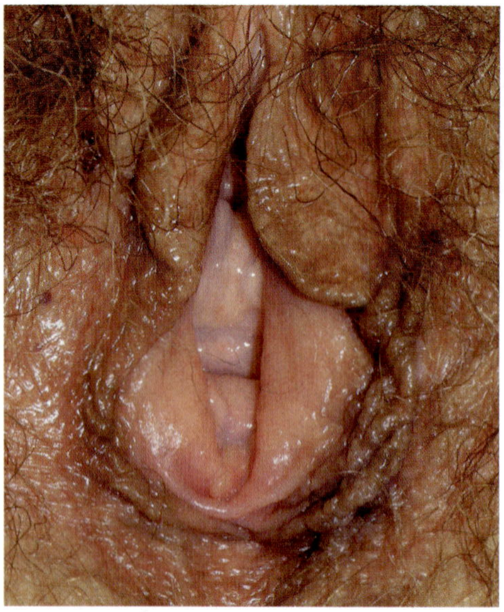

Fig. 1-16. The posterior labia minora are sometimes fused, conferring an annular appearance to the labia minora.

that most women requesting labiaplasty have labia minora within the range considered to be normal,[5] and there is no evidence that various cosmetic surgeries enhance sexual functioning.[6] Because of this, and the physical and psychological risks, guidelines for cosmetic surgery are being developed.[6]

There also is variability of the clitoral hood and the clitoris. In some, the clitoral hood is thin, with the clitoris partially exposed, and in others, the clitoral hood is thick and redundant **(Figs. 1-17 and 1-18)**. Adhesions of the clitoris to the clitoral hood are sometimes a sign of a previous scarring dermatosis; however, this is a normal finding in as many as a third of young women, with the youngest women most likely to be affected.[7]

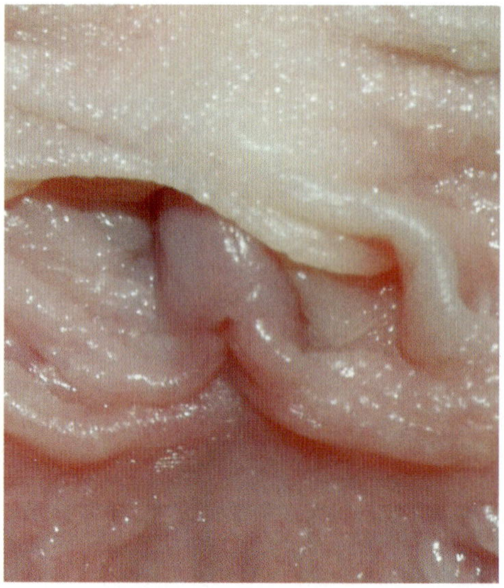

Fig. 1-17. The clitoral hood varies among normal vulvas. The clitoral hood can be thin and tight, leaving part of the clitoris exposed.

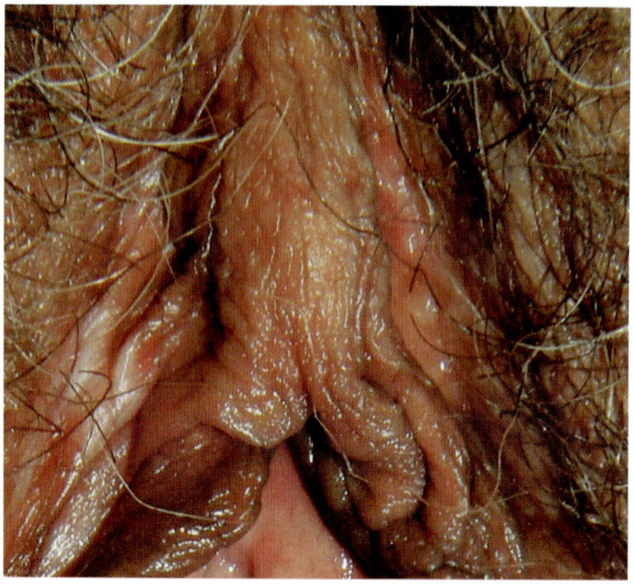

Fig. 1-18. This clitoral hood is thick and redundant.

Physiologic hyperpigmentation of the vulva is common, especially in women with a darker natural complexion, patients who are pregnant, and women with systemic hormone exposure **(Figs. 1-12 and 1-19)**. This discoloration is generally poorly demarcated and is located symmetrically on the lateral edges of the labia minora, on the perianal skin, and sometimes on the hair-bearing portion of the labia majora.

Although ectopic sebaceous glands on the modified mucous membrane skin of the vulva are regularly present in premenopausal women, some women exhibit unusually large or numerous ectopic sebaceous glands, called Fordyce spots (see Chapters 7 and 10). These structures are normal findings that are occasionally mistaken

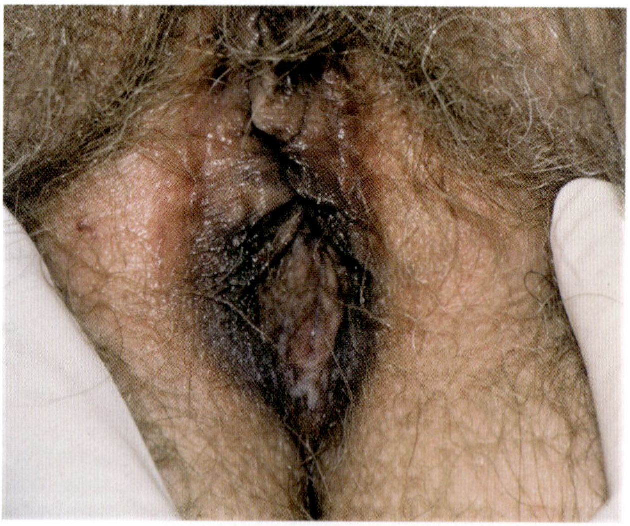

Fig. 1-19. Physiologic hyperpigmentation of anogenital skin is common, with the edges or even the entire labia minora and perianal skin most often involved; this is more marked in women who are dark complexioned, pregnant, or who have been on hormonal therapy.

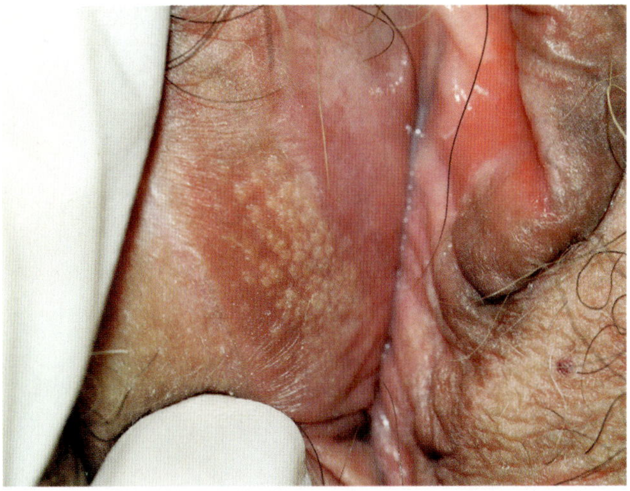

Fig. 1-20. These yellow, smooth papules are classic for Fordyce spots.

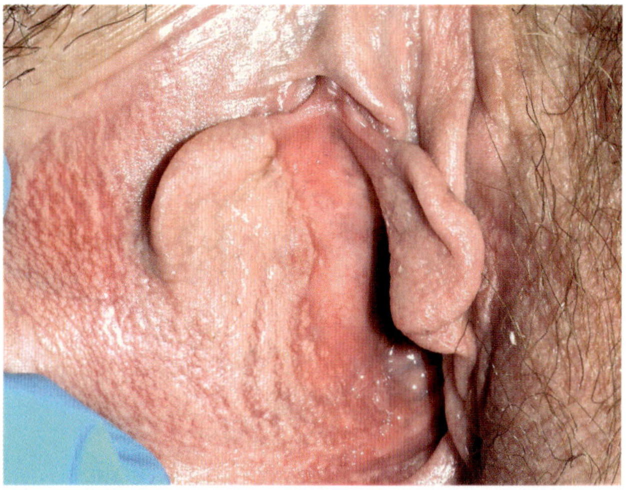

Fig. 1-22. Occasionally, the ectopic sebaceous glands coalesce into a solid plaque, as seen on the medial right labium minus, and they can form lines of sebaceous glands as displayed on the right medial labium majus.

for genital warts. However, the distribution, yellowish color, and lobular, monomorphous pattern are diagnostic for sebaceous glands. At times, these sebaceous glands combine into lines or even coalesce into plaques (**Figs. 1-20 to 1-22**).

Because very small hair follicles are present on the labia minora, firm, white, or yellowish epidermal cysts and comedones are relatively common (**Fig. 1-23**). See also Chapters 8 and 10. These are unimportant unless they become secondarily inflamed and uncomfortable.

Small, purple or red papules called angiokeratomas (see also Chapter 6) represent common, medically unimportant benign blood vessel tumors that occur on the labia majora (**Fig. 1-24**). At times, the purple lesions are so dark as to appear black and raise the incorrect specter of a tiny nodular melanoma (**Fig. 1-25**).

After menopause, the vulva changes in the absence of estrogen replacement. The labia minor regress, the mucous membranes and modified mucous membranes become pale as well as smooth, as sebaceous glands, vulvar papillae, and normal skin markings disappear (**Fig. 1-26**). The surface becomes dry. The hair on the labia majora and mons thins may nearly disappear. Although the mucous membranes are pale, the keratinized surface of the labia major is often somewhat red, possibly because of pressure from the sedentary lifestyle of many older women, overweight, and leakage (**Fig. 1-27**).

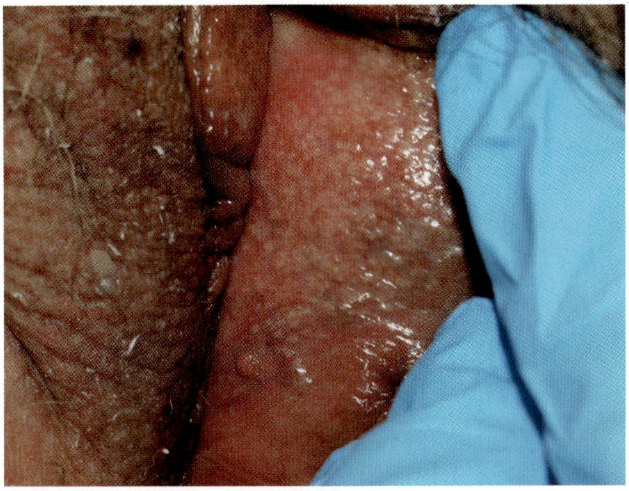

Fig. 1-21. The medial aspect of the labia minora is the most common location for Fordyce spots.

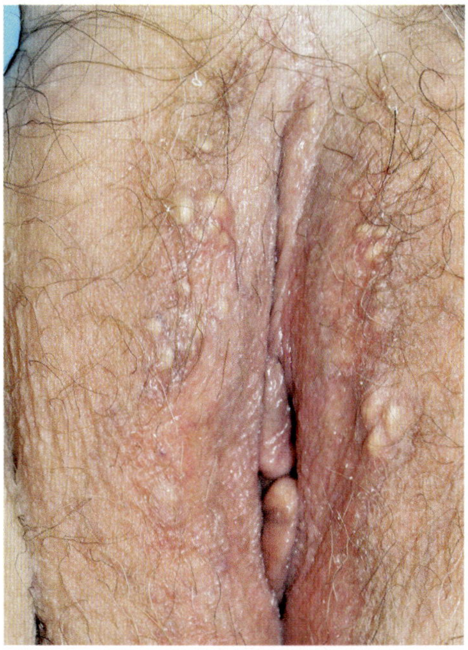

Fig. 1-23. Obstructed hair follicles fill with *white* or *yellowish* keratin debris shed from the follicular epithelium, producing epidermal cysts.

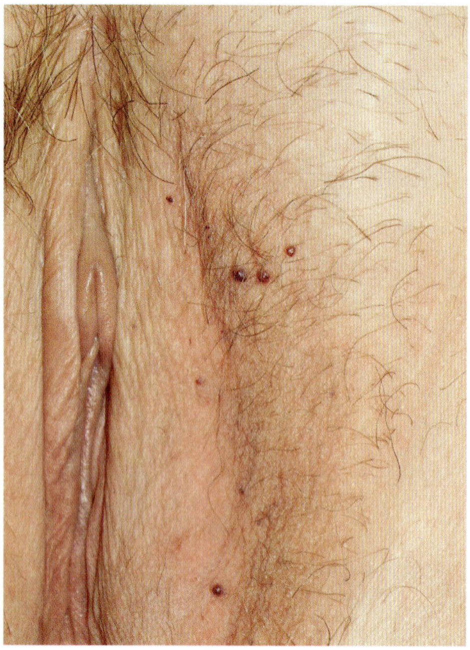

Fig. 1-24. Angiokeratomas are small blood vessel tumors that commonly show a predilection for the hair-bearing labia majora.

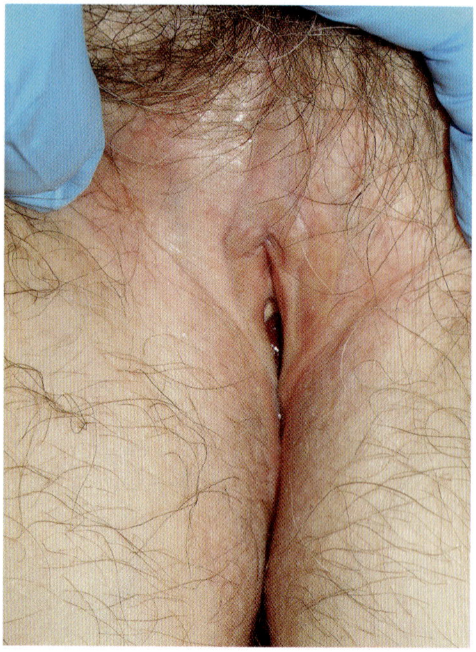

Fig. 1-26. The postmenopausal vulva differs from a well-estrogenized vulva by its pale color, by its smooth skin that lacks papillomatosis and ectopic sebaceous glands, by the partial resorption of labia minora, and by thinning hair.

## Vagina

The vagina is a tube that connects the introitus to the cervix. This structure is covered by squamous mucous membrane skin, and it is a potential space that is flattened with the anterior and posterior walls in contact. The vagina of the premenopausal woman is pink, wet, resilient vaginal skin that forms folds, or rugae. The postmenopausal, estrogen deficient generally is pale, smooth, dry, and fragile **(Fig. 1-28)**. Both obesity and frequent sexual activity can be somewhat protective in the development of an atrophic vagina. The cervix normally lies in the proximal anterior wall of the vagina, and the small pouch between the posterior cervix and the apex of the vagina is called the cul-de-sac.

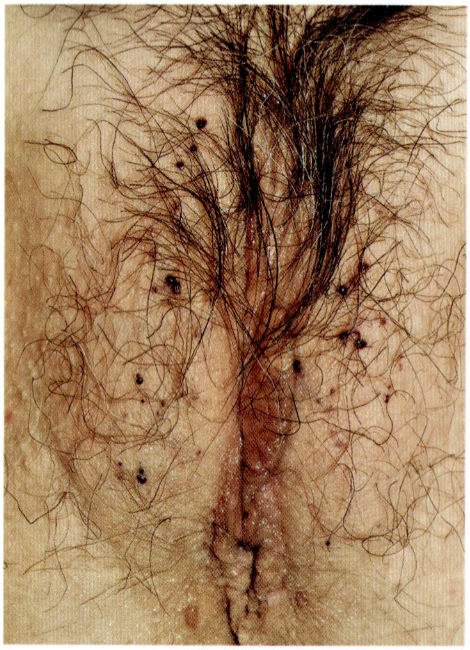

Fig. 1-25. At times, angiokeratomas can show such a *dark purple* color as to appear black, erroneously suggesting a diagnosis of nodular melanoma.

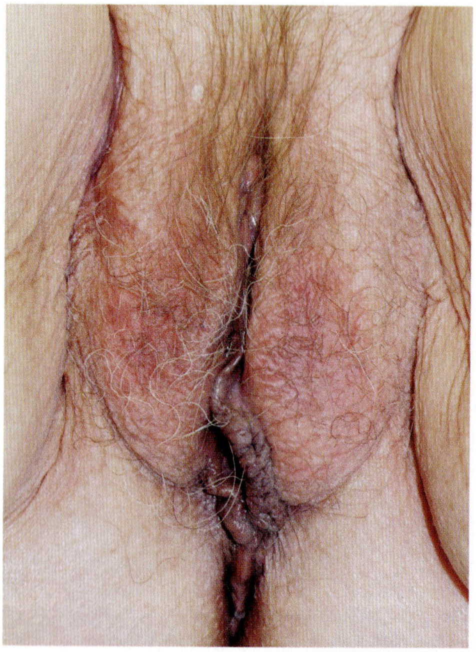

Fig. 1-27. Although the mucous membranes of the postmenopausal woman not on hormone replacement is pale, the hair-bearing labia majora is often somewhat, but asymptomatically, red, perhaps from the pressure of more time sitting and the likelihood of urinary incontinence.

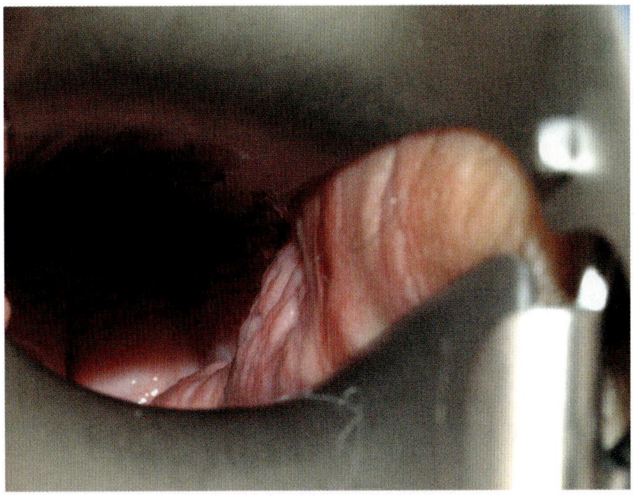

Fig. 1-28. A well-estrogenized vagina is pink, moist, with rugae of the walls.

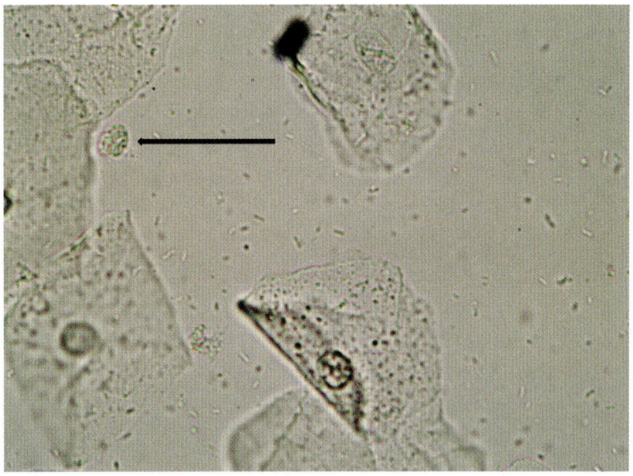

Fig. 1-29. The wet mount of a normal, premenopausal woman shows large, mature, flat, often folded epithelial cells; rods that represent lactobacilli; and fewer than one white blood cell (*arrow*) for each epithelial cell.

The vagina is rich with colonizing organisms. Lactobacilli predominate in the well-estrogenized vagina, but *Peptostreptococcus* spp, *Clostridium* spp, *Bacteroides* spp, *Fusobacterium* spp, *Prevotella* spp, *Propionibacterium* spp, *Eubacterium* spp, *Actinomyces* spp, *Veillonella* spp, *Bifidobacterium* spp, and diphtheroids spp are additional anaerobes.[8,9] Aerobes sometimes found in very small numbers include *Staphylococcus aureus, S epidermidis, Enterococcus,* faecalis, *Actinomyces, Escherichia coli,* group B *Streptococcus, Klebsiella* spp, *Proteus* spp, and *Enterobacter* spp.[10] These aerobes can act as opportunistic pathogens when found in larger numbers. Because of the lactic acid produced by lactobacilli, vaginal secretions are normally acidic, showing a pH of 3.5-5.

One study showed that as many as 16% of asymptomatic premenopausal women were found to harbor *Candida albicans* as well,[10] and after antibiotic use, this number increased to 37%.[11] A recent report found that 22% of pregnant women,[12] and diabetes is a well-known risk factor exhibit colonization.[13,14]

The microscopic evaluation of vaginal secretions is crucial in the evaluation of vaginitis. Only candidiasis and trichomonas are diagnosed with greater sensitivity by more expensive cultures or molecular studies. Secretions result from mucus, desquamated epithelial cells, and bacteria. Normal estrogenized vaginal secretions microscopically reveal large, mature, flattened, epithelial cells with small nuclei, multiple rods representing lactobacilli, and one or fewer leukocytes per epithelial cell **(Fig. 1-29)**. The borders of the epithelial cells should be crisp and sharp, without the ragged, granular appearance of a clue cell indicative of bacterial vaginosis. Fungal elements and *Trichomonas* should be absent. The pH of vaginal secretions should be lower than 5.

A nonspecific reaction to inflammation in the vagina is monomorphous red 1- to 2-mm macules, analogous to the "strawberry cervix" classic for, but not specific of, trichomonas infection.

## Normal Variants

The vaginal mucosa, like the vulva, exhibits varying degrees of normal erythema, which can be difficult to use as a measure of inflammation. One method for evaluating subtle vaginal abnormalities is by a microscopic examination of vaginal secretions (see Chapters 4 and 15). More than one white blood cell per epithelial cells suggests the presence of inflammation. However, the inflammation may be vaginal or cervical.

The vaginal walls vary from one patient to another. Rugae can be subtle or very folded. Occasionally, papillomatosis can occur in the vagina **(Fig. 1-30)**. Although vaginal HPV infection should be considered, diffuse papillae can also be a normal finding with negative HPV probes and requires no therapy.

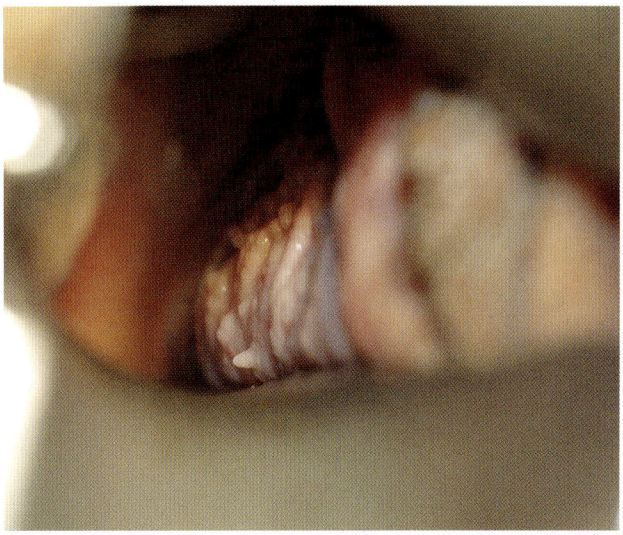

Fig. 1-30. Analogous to vulvar papillomatosis, the vagina sometimes exhibits papillae.

## Male Genitalia

The appearance of normal structures of the penis differs between circumcised males as compared to uncircumcised individuals. In addition, genital diseases of men have a different frequency of occurrence and appearance in circumcised vs uncircumcised men. Skin disease is far less common in the circumcised man, with circumcision often being curative for several diseases such as lichen sclerosus and balanitis plasmacellularis (Zoon balanitis).

The male genitalia encompass the mons pubis anteriorly, the perineum posteriorly, the scrotum posterolaterally, and the penis medially.

### Penis

The penis is composed of ectodermal, mesodermal, and endodermal structures **(Fig. 1-31)**. Three major cylindric erectile structures are enclosed by a dense white fibrous capsule, the tunica albuginea. These three structures are the paired dorsal bodies, called the corpora cavernosa, and the ventral, midline corpus spongiosum. The urethra runs through the root and body of the penis. At the distal aspect of the penis is the glans penis, and the border of the glans is called the corona, separating the glans from the shaft. The shaft of the penis is covered by keratinized epithelium, and modified mucous membrane skin is found on the glans. The slitlike opening at the distal tip of the glans is the external urethral meatus.

At the distal aspect of the penis, the overlying skin is infolded to form the prepuce (foreskin); the prepuce, in turn, covers the glans. Circumcision is the surgical removal of the prepuce. There have been heated debates for years regarding the benefits and risks of circumcision. Pain, scarring, and possible infection in newborn boys have been weighed against the increased risk of acquisition of human immunodeficiency virus and other sexually transmitted disease.[15] In addition, the risk of squamous cell carcinoma in uncircumcised men (slight, but higher than the risk in circumcised men) and the difficulty of hygiene are factors in favor of circumcision. More recently, dermatoses such as erosive lichen planus and lichen sclerosus have been shown to occur almost exclusively on the uncircumcised penis, and circumcision protects against both sexually transmitted diseases and candidiasis. However, the debate rages on, and many assert that the risks, pain, and ethics of an elective procedure on a minor who cannot give assent outweigh the small risks associated with an intact penis for the general population in an industrialized country.[16] The Canadian Paediatric Society no longer recommends routine circumcision of every boy.[17] In Germany, the circumcision of a male under the age of 14 without a medical indication is illegal and considered bodily harm.[18]

On the ventral aspect of the glans is the median fold or raphe, which extends from inferior to the opening of the urethra to the base of the glans and represents the area of fusion.

At birth, the mons pubis, the fatty pad of tissue anterior to the penis and scrotum, is characterized by fine, vellus hair. As puberty approaches, terminal hair develops. In addition, apocrine glands become better developed at this time. The penis contains both apocrine and eccrine sweat glands, and occasionally, ectopic sebaceous glands are visible.

#### Normal Variants

Ectopic sebaceous glands along the shaft of the penis are called Fordyce spots **(Fig. 1-32)**. Those ectopic sebaceous glands located on the ventral, distal shaft adjacent to the frenulum are called Tyson glands. Sebaceous glands can be mistaken for genital warts or mollusca contagiosa. In addition, pearly penile papules are found in up to 78% of

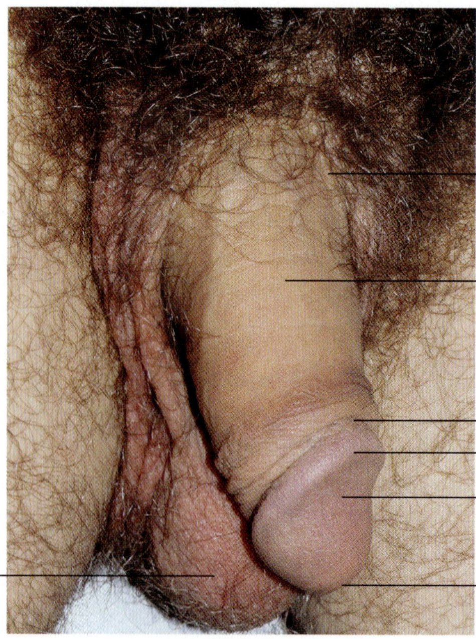


Fig. 1-31. Normal penis and scrotum.

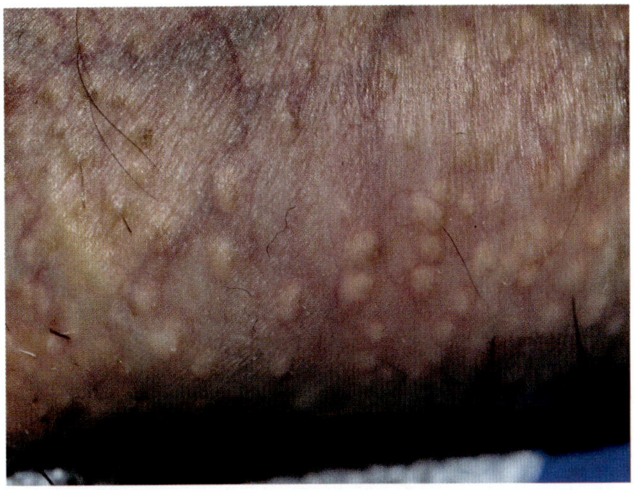

Fig. 1-32. Skin-colored to white to yellow, discrete papules on the shaft of the penis are characteristic of ectopic sebaceous glands, also called Fordyce spots.

men **(Figs. 1-33 and 1-34)** and are much more common in those who are uncircumcised and in young men.[19] These are small (1- to 2-mm) soft, monomorphous, flesh-colored papules that occur in rows around the edge of the corona (see Chapter 7). Sometimes, there are several parallel rows. These papules are sometimes elongated into papillae with rounded tips. Rarely, pearly penile papules can occur on the glans or shaft of the penis, where the diagnosis is less obvious. Like vestibular papillomatosis, pearly penile papules have been mistaken for HPV infection, but these monomorphous papules in a characteristic distribution have been found to have no association with this viral infection. For those men wanting treatment of these lesions for cosmetic reasons, $CO_2$ laser has been reported beneficial,[20] as have fractionated $CO_2$ laser,[21]

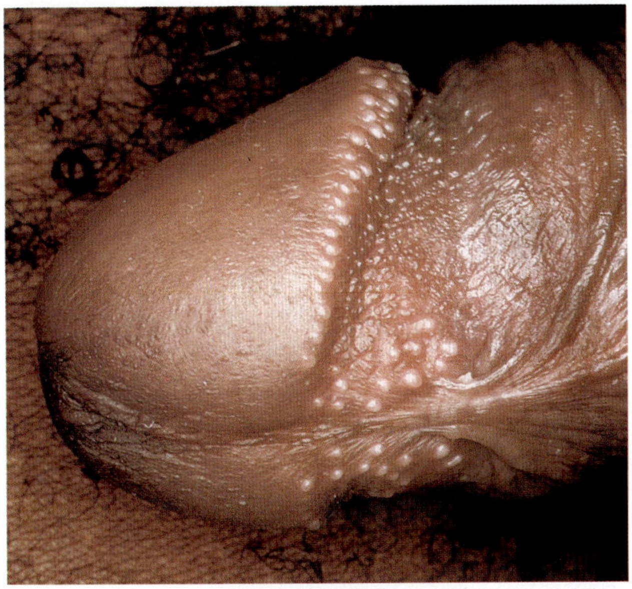

Fig. 1-33. Pearly, tiny, skin-colored to hypopigmented monomorphous papules that ring the corona of the glans in one or more rows are characteristic of pearly penile papules.

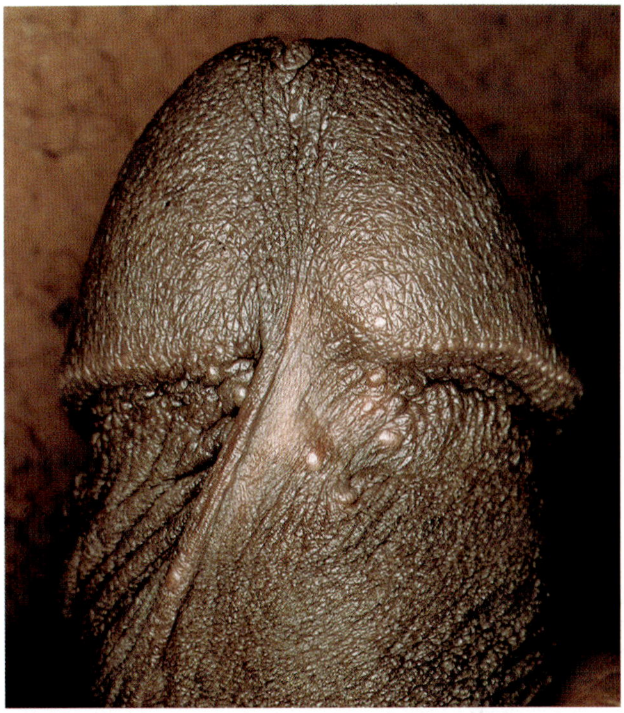

Fig. 1-34. These skin-colored papules of pearly penile papules are found primarily in uncircumcised males and can be subtle.

pulsed dye laser,[22] erbium: yttrium-aluminium-garnet laser,[23] circumcision,[24] and cryotherapy.[25]

At times, hair follicles on the shaft are prominent, making differentiation from warts, Tyson glands, and pearly penile papules of the shaft difficult.

## Scrotum

The scrotum consists of two sacs that are separated by a septum and covered with keratinized squamous epithelium. The testicles rest within the sacs, attached by the vas deferens. The scrotum, from the outside in, consists of an outer skin layer, the dartos (smooth) muscle, the external spermatic fascia with the cremasteric (skeletal) muscle, the internal spermatic fascia, and the tunica vaginalis.

### Normal Variants

Ridges or folds of skin called rugae are common on the scrotum, although some men exhibit smooth scrotal skin. The color of the scrotum ranges from moderate erythema to skin colored. Scrotum is variably red, with many showing skin-colored epithelium, others exhibiting erythema **(Fig. 1-35)**. As occurs in women, redness may not be appreciated until the patient experiences symptoms, and both the patient and health care provider misinterpret this redness as a pathologic sign of inflammation. Physiologic hyperpigmentation is common, either generalized or with accentuation of the median raphe **(Fig. 1-36)**.

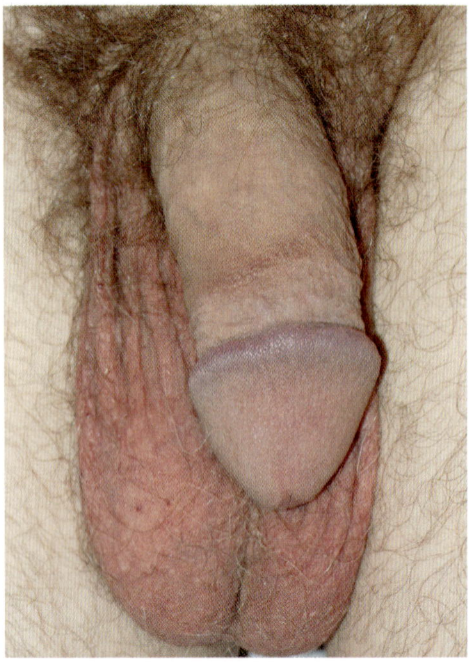

Fig. 1-35. Erythema of the scrotum is common and normal but often not noticed by the patient until symptoms occur.

Angiokeratomas are common vascular tumors of the scrotum that range from 1 to 3 mm in diameter and are most often red or purple but sometimes nearly black **(Fig. 1-37)**, and some men exhibit skin-colored or white, firm nodules that represent inconsequential scrotal epidermal cysts **(Fig. 1-38)**. Epidermal cysts occur on perianal skin of both genders **(Fig. 1-39)**.

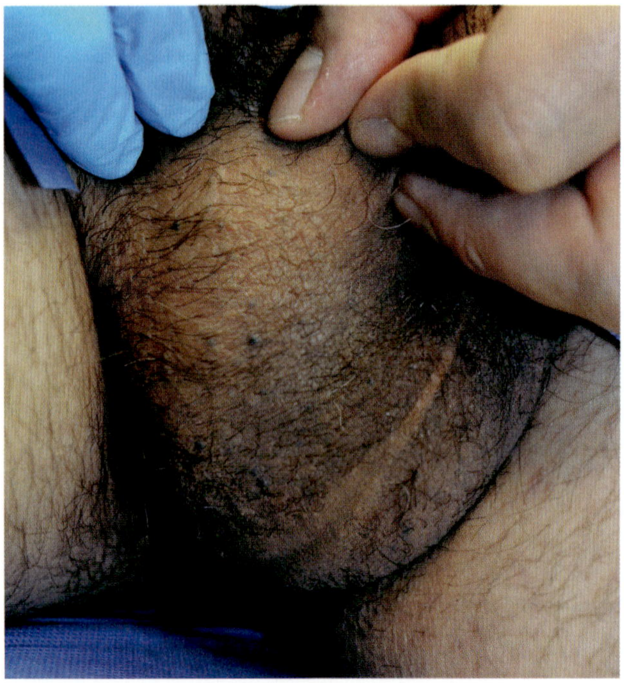

Fig. 1-36. Physiologic hyperpigmentation can occur on the scrotum of some patients, as well as near the rectal verge.

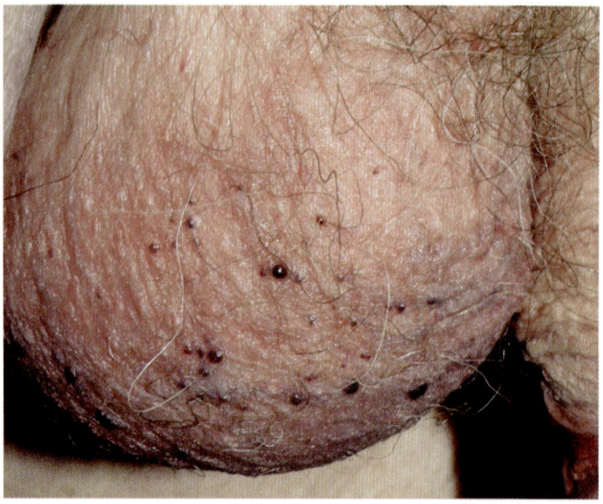

Fig. 1-37. Angiokeratomas are common, inconsequential vascular tumors on the scrotum as well as the labia majora of women.

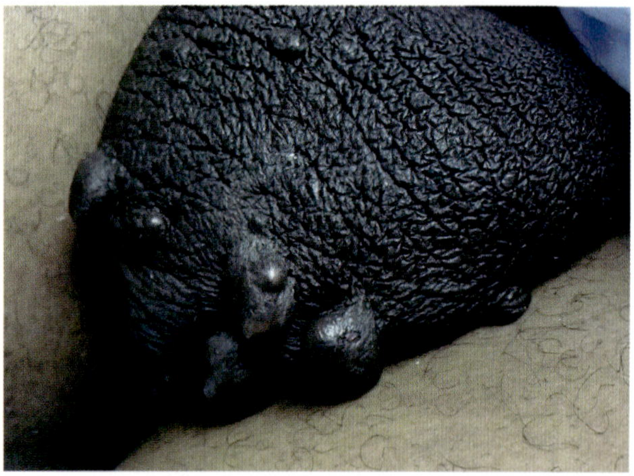

Fig. 1-38. Although epidermal scrotal cysts are common, large numbers rarely occur.

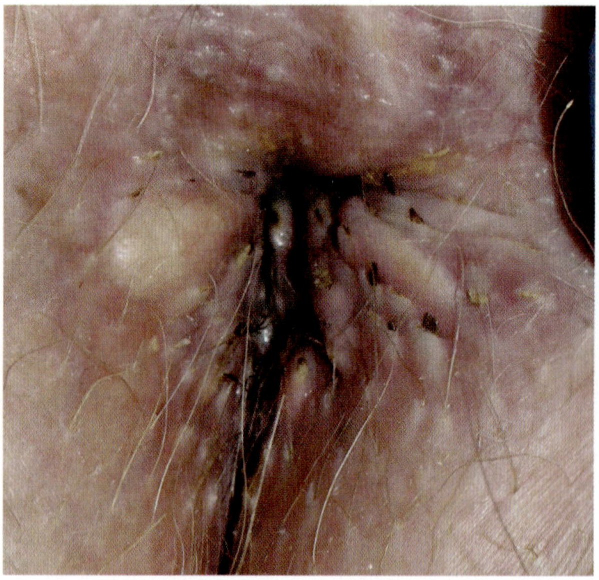

Fig. 1-39. Epidermal cysts occur in perianal skin in both men and women. The overlying comedones are seen easily in this man.

## REFERENCES


1. van Beurden M, van der Vange N, de Craen AJ, et al. Normal findings in vulvar examination and vulvoscopy. *Br J Obstet Gynaecol.* 1997;104:320-324.
2. Diaz Gonzales JM, Martinez Luna E, Pena Romero A, Molina Hernandez A, Dominguez Cherit J. Vestibular papillomatosis is a normal vulvar anatomical condition. *Dermatol Online J.* 2013;19:20032.
3. Beznos G, Coates V, Focchi J, et al. Biomolecular study of the correlation between papillomatosis of the vulvar vestibule in adolescents and human papillomavirus. *Scientific World Journal.* 2006;12(6):628-636.
4. Santoso JT, Likes W. Colposcopic acetowhitening of vulvar lesion: a validity study. *Arch Gynecol Obstet.* 2015;292:387-390.
5. Crouch NS, Deans R, Michala L, Liao LM, Creighton SM. Clinical characteristics of well women seeking labial reduction surgery: a prospective study. *BJOG.* 2011;118:1507-1510.
6. Shaw D, Lefebvre G, Bouchard C, et al. Female genital cosmetic surgery. *J Obstet Gynaecol Can.* 2013;35:1108-1114.
7. Wiesmeier E, Masongsong EV, Wiley DJ. The prevalence of examiner-diagnosed clitoral hood adhesions in a population of college-aged women. *J Low Genit Tract Dis.* 2008;12:307-310.
8. Lamont RF, Sobel JD, Akins RA, et al. The vaginal microbiome: new information about genital tract flora using molecular based techniques. *BJOG.* 2011;118:533-549.
9. Hoffman B. *Williams Gynecology.* 2nd ed. McGraw-Hill Medical; 2012:65. ISBN 978–0071716727.
10. Sharma H, Tal R, Clark NA, Segars JH. Microbiota and pelvic inflammatory disease. *Semin Reprod Med.* 2014;32(1):43-49.
11. Pirotta MV, Garland SM. Genital Candida species detected in samples from women in Melbourne, Australia, before and after treatment with antibiotics. *J Clin Microbiol.* 2006;44:3213-3217.
12. Payne MS, Cullinane M, Garland SM, et al. Detection of Candida spp. in the vagina of a cohort of nulliparous pregnant women by culture and molecular methods: is there an association between maternal vaginal and infant oral colonisation? *Aust N Z J Obstet Gynaecol.* 2016;56:179-184.
13. Gunther LSA, Martins HPR, Gimenes F, de Abreu ALP, Consolaro MEL, Svidzinski TIE. Prevalence of Candida albicans and non-albicans isolates from vaginal secretions: comparative evaluation of colonization, vaginal candidiasis and recurrent vaginal candidiasis in diabetic and non-diabetic women. *Sao Paulo Med J.* 2014;132:116-120.
14. Chatzivasileiou P, Vyzantiadis TA. Vaginal yeast colonisation: from a potential harmless condition to clinical implications and management approaches-A literature review. *Mycoses.* 2019;62:638-650.
15. Matoga M, Hosseinipour MC, Jewett S, Hoffman IF, Chasela C. Effects of HIV voluntary medical male circumcision programs on sexually transmitted infections. *Curr Opin Infect Dis.* 2021;34:50-55.
16. Earp BD. Male or female genital cutting: why 'health benefits' are morally irrelevant. *J Med Ethics.* 2021. doi:10.1136/medethics-2020-106782. Online ahead of print.
17. Sorokan ST, Finlay JC, Jefferies AL; Canadian Paediatric Society, Fetus and Newborn Committee, Infectious Diseases and Immunization Committee. Newborn male circumcision. *Paediatr Child Health.* 2015;20:311-320.
18. Rübben I, Rübben H. [Phimosis]. *Urologe A.* 2012;51:1005-1016.
19. Michajłowski I, Sobjanek M, Michajłowski J, Włodarkiewicz A, Matuszewski M. Normal variants in patients consulted in the Dermatology Clinic for lesions of the male external genitalia. *Cent European J Urol.* 2012;65:17-20.
20. Lane JE, Peterson CM, Ratz JL. Treatment of pearly penile papules with $CO_2$ laser. *Dermatol Surg.* 2002;28:617-618.
21. Gan SD, Graber EM. Treatment of pearly penile papules with fractionated $CO_2$ laser. *J Clin Aesthet Dermatol.* 2015;8:50-52.
22. Sapra P, Sapra S, Singh A. Pearly penile papules: effective therapy with pulsed dye laser. *JAMA Dermatol.* 2013;149:748-750.
23. Baumgartner J. Erbium: yttrium-aluminium-garnet (Er:YAG) laser treatment of penile pearly papules. *J Cosmet Laser Ther.* 2012;14:155-158.
24. Agha K, Alderson S, Samraj S, et al. Pearly penile papules regress in older patients and with circumcision. *Int J STD AIDS.* 2009;20:768-770.
25. Honigman AD, Dubin DP, Chu J, Lin MJ. Management of pearly penile papules: a review of the literature. *J Cutan Med Surg.* 2020;24:79-85.


## SUGGESTED READINGS


Aldahan AS, Brah TK, Nouri K. Diagnosis and management of pearly penile papules. *Am J Mens Health.* 2018;12:624-627.

Bossio JA, Pukall CF, Steele S. A review of the current state of the male circumcision literature. *J Sex Med.* 2014;11:2847-2864.

Michajłowski I, Sobjanek M, Michajłowski J, Włodarkiewicz A, Matuszewski M. Normal variants in patients consulted in the Dermatology Clinic for lesions of the male external genitalia. *Cent European J Urol.* 2012;65:17-20.

Sadowsky LM, Socik A, Burnes A, Rhodes AR. Genital angiokeratomas in adult men and women: prevalence and predisposing factors. *J Cutan Med Surg.* 2019;23:513-518.

Santoso JT, Likes W. Colposcopic acetowhitening of vulvar lesion: a validity study. *Arch Gynecol Obstet.* 2015;292:387-390.

van Beurden M, van der Vange N, de Craen AJ, et al. Normal findings in vulvar examination and vulvoscopy. *Br J Obstet Gynaecol.* 1997;104:320-324.

http://www.racgp.org.au/afp/2013/may/penile-appearance/a survey of penile lumps and bumps, normal and abnormal

# Terminology, Classification, and Diagnosis of Genital Dermatological Disorders 2

PETER J LYNCH

Diagnosis of genital dermatological disorders through the use of morphological features (see rationale for this approach below) requires that two components be understood and utilized. These are "terminology" (the definition of terms used in morphological description of mucocutaneous lesions) and "classification" (the orderly arrangement of the diseases described by this terminology into specific categories).

## Terminology

The definitions included here represent our preferences and are very similar, though not necessarily identical, to those found in standard dermatology textbooks. The minor differences, where they occur, will not interfere with the use of the diagnostic classification that follows. Note specifically that where measurements of size are given within the definitions of the lesions, these are approximate, rather than exact, measurements. For that reason, unimportant overlap may occur between smaller and larger lesions.

### Nouns (ie, Primary Lesions)

#### Macule

A macule is a small (1.5 cm or less), nonelevated, nonpalpable area of color change (**Fig. 2-1**). The surface of macules is usually smooth, though a small amount of hardly detectable powdery scale may be present.

#### Patch

A patch is a larger (>1.5 cm), nonelevated, nonpalpable area of color change (**Fig. 2-2**). It may be considered as a two-dimensional (length and width) increase in the size of a macule. Again, the surface is usually smooth but sometimes a small amount of powdery scale may be present.

#### Papule

A papule is a small (1.5 cm or less) palpable lesion (**Fig. 2-3**). Usually, but not always, a papule is visibly elevated above the surface of the surrounding tissue. A nonelevated, but palpable, lesion contained completely within the skin is still termed a papule. A papule may be considered as a one-dimensional (thickness) increase in the size of a macule. Papules may be either smooth or rough surfaced. Roughness on the surface of a papule is due to the presence of either scale or crust (see below for definitions).

#### Plaque

A plaque is a large (>1.5-cm) flat-topped, palpable lesion (**Fig. 2-4**). It may be considered as a two-dimensional (length and width) increase in the size of a papule. Plaques are usually, but not always, elevated above the surface of the surrounding tissue. As for papules, intracutaneous lesions that are palpable are termed plaques whether or not they are elevated. Likewise, plaques may be smooth or rough surfaced. Roughness on the surface of a plaque is due to the presence of either scale or crust (see below for definitions).

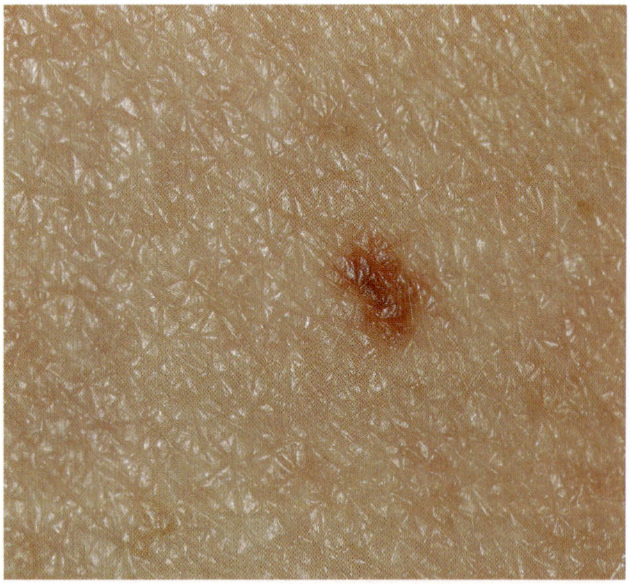

Fig. 2-1. This small nevus is a macule that shows color change only, is not palpable, and has no surface change.

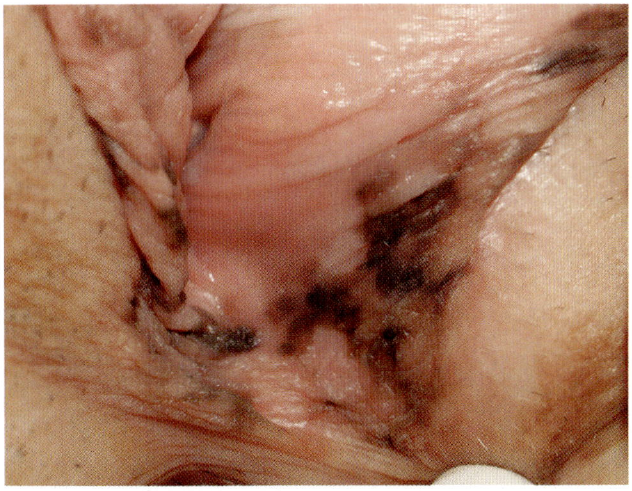

Fig. 2-2. A patch is a larger area with only color change, like this patch of irregular brown and black color of genital lentiginosis.

## Nodule

A nodule is a large (>1.5-cm) palpable lesion **(Fig. 2-5)**. It may be considered as a three-dimensional (length, width, and thickness) increase in the size of a papule. Nodules are usually smooth surfaced.

## Vesicle

A vesicle is a small (1.0-cm or less) fluid-filled blister **(Fig. 2-6)**. Conceptually, it may be considered as a fluid-filled papule. Usually, the fluid is loculated. Fluid-filled papules in which the fluid is nonloculated are known as *wheals*. Wheals only occur in urticaria (hives) and urticarial plaques. Vesicles and wheals usually can be differentiated visually. However, they can also be identified by the observation that when the surface of a blister is pierced, the fluid runs out and the blister roof collapses. When a wheal is pierced, a drop of fluid may appear on the surface, but the papule remains as it was before the piercing. When the surface of a vesicle has been removed or has disintegrated, the shallow deficit that remains is defined as an *erosion* (see below for definition). The surface of this erosion may be red and moist or may be covered with crust.

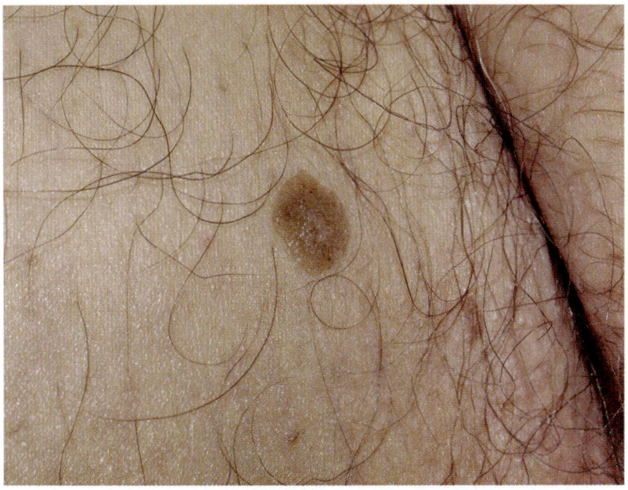

Fig. 2-3. This nevus is elevated and palpable, so it is a papule.

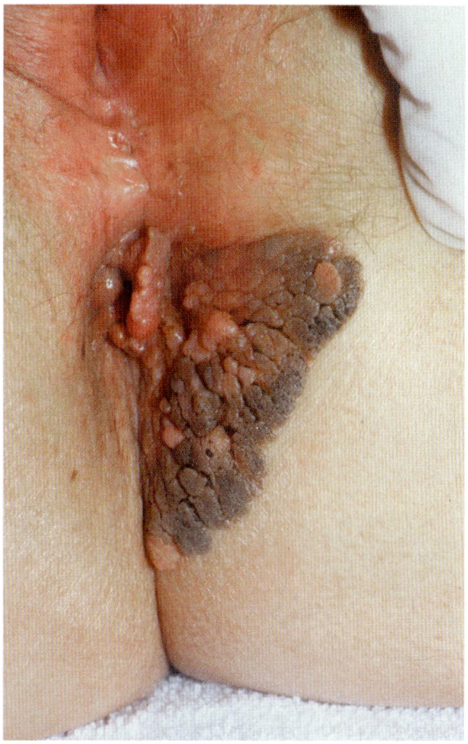

Fig. 2-4. A plaque is a large area that is palpable, such as this larger area of pigmented human papillomavirus infection.

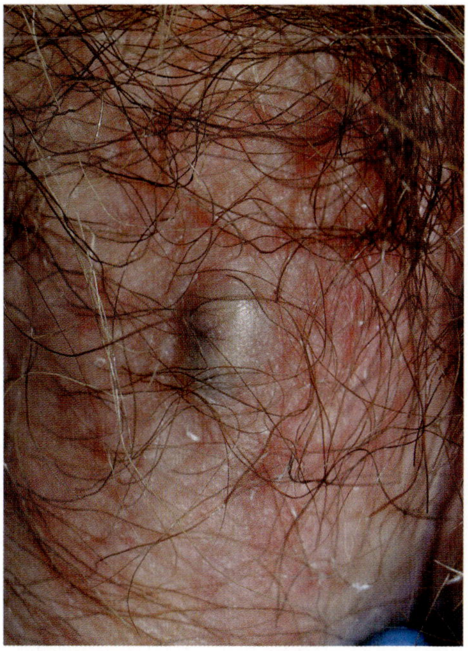

Fig. 2-5. This epidermal cyst is a typical nodule; a larger round smooth-surfaced lesion.

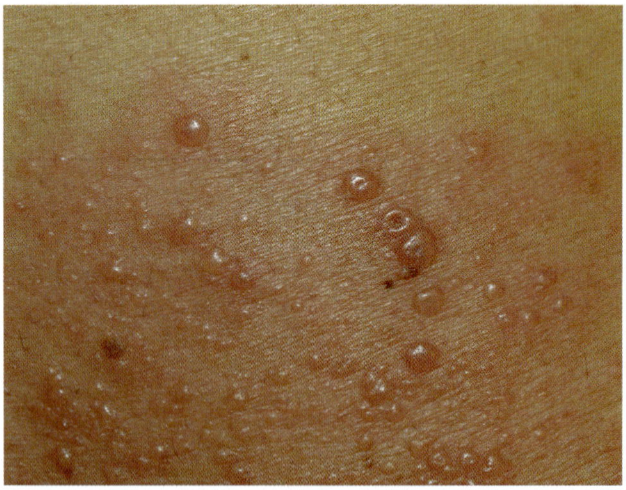

Fig. 2-6. These small fluid-filled blisters are vesicles of herpes simplex virus.

## Pustule

A pustule is a vesicle that contains visibly purulent (pus-filled) loculated fluid (**Fig. 2-7**). That is, the lesion appears opaquely white, yellow, or yellow-white. This color occurs as a result of the presence of neutrophils and other white blood cells. Note that a vesicle may turn cloudy as it ages. This change does not make it a pustule. To be a pustule, a blister must have been purulent from the time of its inception.

## Bulla (Plural: Bullae)

A bulla is a large (>1.0-cm) vesicle (**Fig. 2-8**). Here too, the fluid is loculated. Usually, the fluid is found in a single compartment occupying the whole of the lesion, but uncommonly, coalescence of closely set vesicles occurs to form a multiloculated bulla. As bullae age, they may become cloudy (see "Pustule" above). When the surface of a bulla has been removed or has disintegrated, the shallow deficit that remains is defined as *erosion*. The surface of this erosion may be red and moist or may be covered with crust.

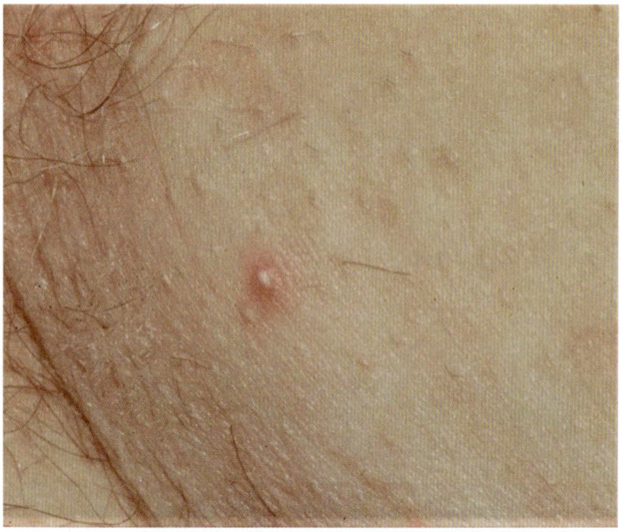

Fig. 2-7. Pustules are blisters that are filled with pus and are nearly always small, as seen in this patient with folliculitis.

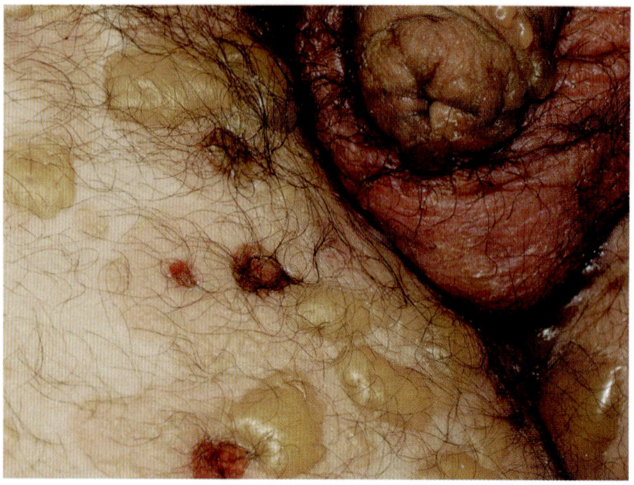

Fig. 2-8. Bullae are larger fluid-filled blisters and are characteristic of most immunobullous diseases such as bullous pemphigoid and pemphigus vulgaris.

## Erosion

An erosion is a shallow defect in the surface of the skin (**Fig. 2-9**). In this context, "shallow" means the epidermis is

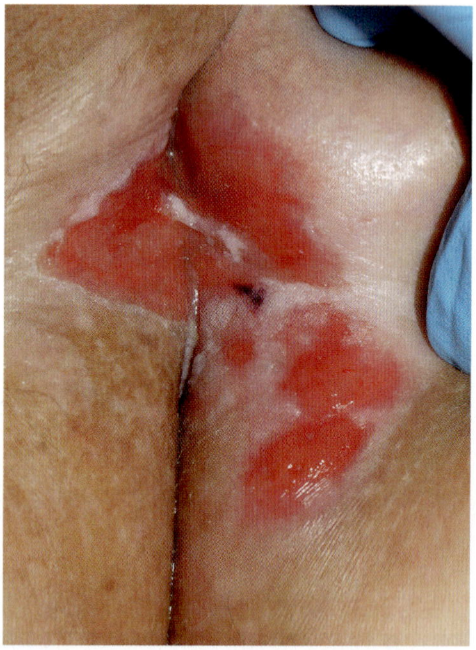

Fig. 2-9. The blister roof of benign mucous membrane pemphigoid sheared off the surface, leaving the typical superficial erosion with a red base.

missing but that the defect does not extend more deeply into the dermal component of the skin. The base of an erosion may be red and moist or the base may be covered with crust. Crust, when it is present, is yellow in color. Crust is also crumbly and fairly easily removed. If the crust is red, rather than yellow, it means that the defect is deeper (see "Ulcer" below). Erosions occur as the result of two mechanisms. They can develop as a result of trauma. Such trauma is most often due to vigorous scratching. Erosions occurring as a result of trauma are usually linear or angular in configuration. Alternatively, erosions may be nontraumatic. Nontraumatic erosions most often occur when the roof of a vesicle or bulla is removed or has disintegrated. The configuration of nontraumatic erosions is usually round and often there is a thin peripheral rim of scale. This type of scale is called "collarette" scale, and it occurs as a result of fragments of the peripheral blister roof that remain intact at the edge of a previous blister.

### Fissure

A fissure is a subtype of a nontraumatic erosion in which a thin (<1 mm in width) linear crack occurs into or through the epithelium **(Fig. 2-10)**. A fissure appears clinically as a thin red line, and due to its narrowness, it may not be recognized as a true defect in the surface of the skin unless a magnifying lens is used. Fissures generally arise in the setting of an epithelial surface that is too dry. Fissures can be viewed as analogous to the cracked surface that often occurs in the dried bed of a pond or stream.

### Ulcer

An ulcer is a deep defect in the surface of the skin **(Fig. 2-11)**. The defect is deeper than that of an erosion, and it extends into, or even through, the dermal connective tissue. These deeper defects involve significant blood vessel damage, and as a result, the base of an ulcer may contain crust that includes heme pigment as well as plasma proteins. For this reason, the crust may be red, blue, or black. When considerable fibrin is present as well, crust is usually black and is very adherent to the base of the ulcer; such crust is known as "eschar."

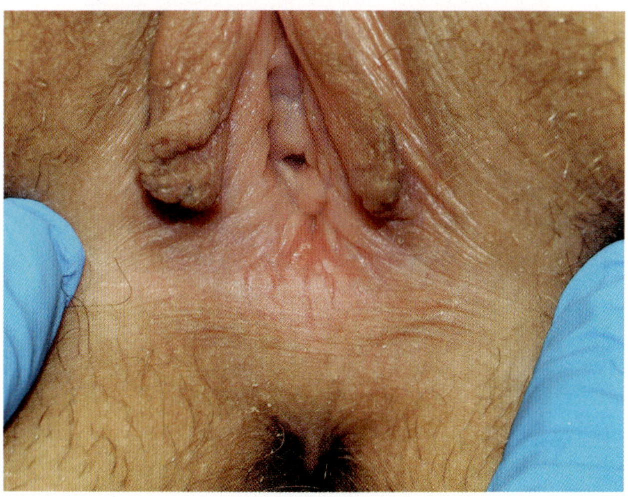

Fig. 2-10. Fine lines and cracks of fissures occur when fragile skin or skin folds are irritated or rubbed.

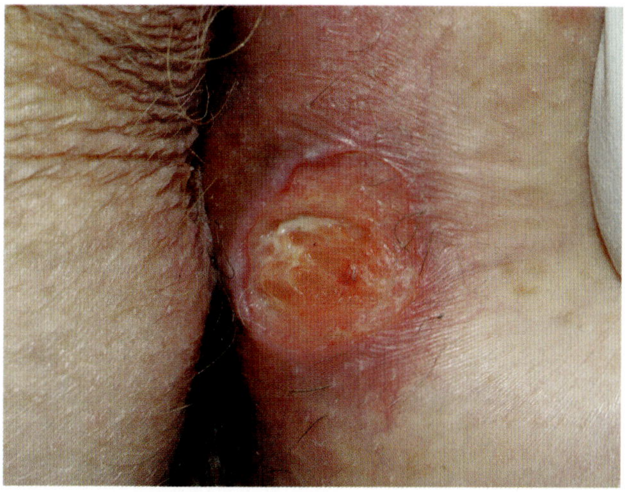

Fig. 2-11. Chronic pressure has caused an ulcer, much deeper than an erosion, and fat is visible at the base.

## Adjectives Applied to the Nouns (Primary Lesions) Listed Above

### Surface Characteristics

The surface of primary lesions may be smooth or rough. A smooth surface means that no scale or crust can be seen or palpated. A rough surface on palpation means that scale or crust is present. However, keep in mind that the roughness may be temporarily ameliorated due to patient actions such as the application of lubricants, treatment with topical creams or ointments, or toweling after bathing. A patient history regarding such activities should be obtained before deciding that a lesion's surface is smooth. A rough surface occurs as a result of scale or crust. *Scale* is due to excess keratin on the surface of a lesion. It generally occurs as a result of epithelial hyperproliferation. Scale is usually visible as gray, white, or silver "flakes" or "powder" on the surface of a lesion, but palpable roughness with no color is also due to scale. Note that thick scale when moist, as frequently occurs in the genital area, turns white. Thin scale, in the presence of moisture, may become nonapparent visually and is only recognizable by slight roughness on palpation. *Crust* is due to the presence of plasma proteins left after the water component of plasma has evaporated. It occurs as a result of an epithelial defect (erosion or ulcer). Crust is always visible and is usually yellow but, when heme pigment is present due to vascular damage, it may be red, blue, or black.

### Margination

Margination represents the zone of transition that occurs between normal and lesional tissue. This transition is best visualized as if one were looking at a vertical cross section of the skin at the transition between normal and lesional tissue. This transition can be very distinct (sharply marginated) or somewhat indistinct (poorly or diffusely marginated). Margination can be helpful in distinguishing the papulosquamous diseases (sharply marginated) from the eczematous diseases (less sharply marginated).

### Configuration

Configuration represents to the shape of the lesions when viewed from above. Most often, this shape is more-or-less round. A configuration that is gyrate (serpiginous) may occur in some lesions. This occurs most notably with urticarial lesions. Linear and angular configurations suggest a traumatic etiology, especially that due to scratching. Annular (ringlike) configurations may have a narrow peripheral border that is more elevated than is the center of the lesion. Alternatively, if the border is not elevated, the border may simply be a different color (usually red) compared to that of the center (usually tan, brown, or skin colored).

### Color

The true color of lesions can be hard to determine for several reasons. First, the color of scale or crust must be disregarded. Heavy scale obscures the true color of the underlying lesion. In this situation, the actual color has to be determined by looking at the periphery of a lesion (where there is usually less scale) or by scraping away a bit of the scale. Second, the color of crust must be ignored. Thus, an erosion with yellow crust is not a yellow lesion and an ulcer covered with eschar is not a black lesion. Actually, it is not necessary to describe the color for either an erosion or an ulcer as these lesions are classified simply as erosions or ulcers (see the "Classification" section below). Third, the term "skin colored" is used in comparison to the patient's normal skin color. A skin-colored lesion may falsely appear to be brown in a heavily pigmented person and falsely appear to be white in a very light-colored person. A lesion is skin colored only when the hue matches that of adjacent nonlesional skin. Fourth, red-colored lesions are much less apparent in those patients with racially dark skin, to the point where the redness may be almost nonapparent. This same situation occurs in heavily tanned individuals as well as in locations, such as the anogenital area, that may be hyperpigmented secondary to hormonal factors.

## Special Terminology Related to Eczematous Disease

Terminology relating to eczematous disease is often confusing and somewhat controversial. This is especially confusing for clinicians who are not dermatologists. For this reason, we are including our preferences for terminology regarding eczematous disease in this chapter. In addition, please note that some clinicians use the term "eczema" as a synonym for "atopic dermatitis." We disagree with this usage and prefer to use "eczema" for a group of disorders sharing the morphologic characteristics discussed in the three paragraphs that follow.

### Eczema

In this book, "eczema" (pronounced ECK zee ma) is used synonymously with the word "dermatitis." Eczematous (or dermatitic) lesions refer to a morphologic pattern of disease characterized by the presence of red, scaling, poorly marginated papules and plaques that display evidence of epithelial disruption or lichenification. These lesions are also usually pruritic and may be accompanied by scratching and/or erosions that occur as a result of scratching.

### Epithelial Disruption

Epithelial disruption is identified by the presence of excoriations, fissures, weeping, and/or yellow crusting (**Figs, 2-12 and 2-13**). However, if the amount of fluid from weeping onto the surface is minimal, it may only render the scale slightly yellow rather than forming as true crust.

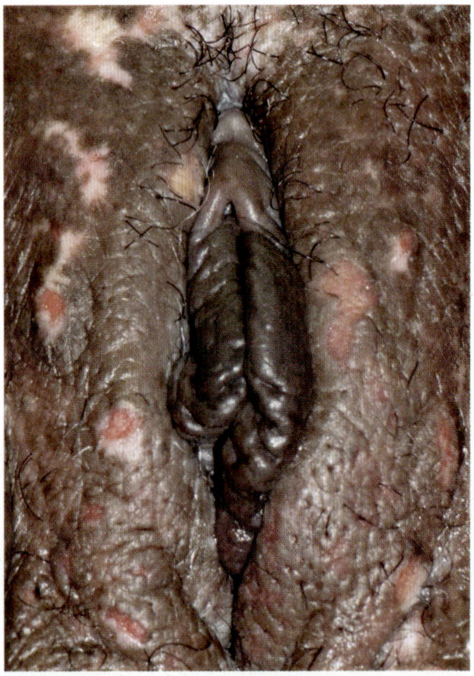

Fig. 2-12. Eczematous disease is often characterized by epithelial disruption, pictured here by scratching as seen by these excoriations, irregular erosions produced by fingernails.

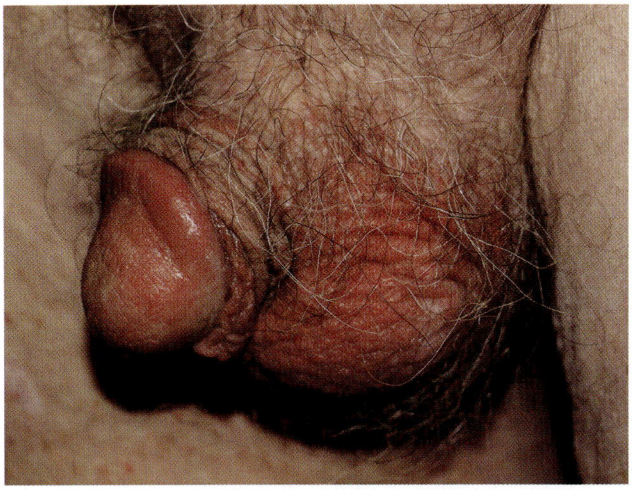

Fig. 2-13. Weeping of the skin as seen on the glans is a sign of more subtle epithelial disruption in a patient with eczematous disease.

### Lichenification

Lichenification refers to the presence of palpably thickened and rough-surfaced skin demonstrating prominent skin markings **(Fig. 2-14)**. The roughness in lichenification is due to compacted surface scale. When the scale of lichenification is dry, it partially obscures some of the redness due to underlying inflammation and usually gives the surface of the lesion a dark red, gray, or silver color. But when the compacted scale of lichenification is moist, as often occurs in the anogenital region, the color may be white. Excoriations may accompany lichenification. Lichenification occurs as a calluslike response due to chronic rubbing and scratching by way of what is known as the "itch-scratch cycle." Lichenified lesions may arise from what originally appeared to be normal skin. When the lesions are localized, this is called "lichen simplex chronicus"; when lesions are more generalized, it is called "atopic dermatitis" or "neurodermatitis." Lichenification may also be superimposed on underlying disorders such as lichen sclerosus or psoriasis.

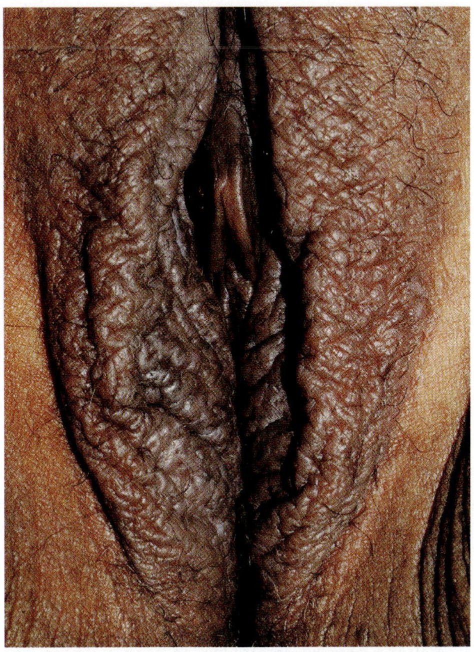

Fig. 2-14. Most often, eczematous disease of the genital skin exhibits lichenification, with accentuation of skin markings and skin that is rough and thick to palpation.

## Classification

### The Rationale for the Utilization of Classification

Classification adds order and simplicity for what otherwise would be a long list of diseases. Classifications generally contain categories into which disorders that have shared characteristics are placed. Depending on the nature of the classification utilized, a classification may or may not help a clinician identify an unrecognized disease. But note that even if disease is identified and named, an unclassified, or ungrouped, list of diseases makes it very difficult for a clinician to locate additional information about that disease. Sure, in this situation, a clinician can "look up" the disease but finding it in one's reference source is entirely dependent on the accuracy and completeness of the textbook index or the online site being used.

More importantly, what happens if you can't readily identify the disorder in question and therefore cannot put a name on it? This happens all too frequently for nondermatologists dealing with genital dermatologic disorders. When that occurs, there is no way to find, and read-up on the disorder short of having access to an atlas and then laboriously turning the pages until you happen on a photo that matches the appearance of the patient's problem. Obviously, this approach is extremely inefficient and prone to error. Simply speaking, in a clinical setting, the goal of classification should be to assist a clinician in making a diagnosis. This identification would assist one in finding additional information about the disease such as regarding therapy, pathophysiology, and needed laboratory tests.

### Approaches That Can Be Utilized for Classification

Many approaches have been used for the purpose of creating classifications. Most commonly, classifications are based either on "etiology" or "pathogenesis." However, information on either of these items is usually lacking for at least some of the diseases one is likely to place in the classification. In this situation, only some of the diseases will be classified logically; the remainder will for the most part need to be grouped randomly. Moreover, knowledge about disease etiology and pathogenesis changes rapidly as new information is discovered. This means that frequent revisions of such a classification will be necessary and makes previous editions of the classification out of date and therefore somewhat useless. Nevertheless, classification based on either etiology or pathogenesis is used in most major medical textbooks and online sources. This approach may be intellectually satisfying for the author, but it is much less satisfactory for the clinician.

A slightly better approach for the clinician might be to classify the disorders by the region of the body involved. A number of dermatology textbooks have used this approach. For example, when considering genital dermatologic problems, you might classify these disorders on the basis of specific locations within the anogenital region, such as anal, vulvar, clitoral, penile, and scrotal disorders. This approach is cumbersome, somewhat illogical, and leads to considerable redundancy simply because, as stated above, many anogenital dermatological diseases involve several, or even all, of these locations.

### The Ideal Approach for Creating a Classification of Dermatological Disorders

We believe that it makes the most sense to classify all visible anogenital dermatologic conditions on the basis of the clinical morphology. This can easily be accomplished by way of clinical examination. This approach groups the diseases on the basis of shared similarities. Thus, once you have described the disease using standard dermatologic nomenclature (see the section on "Terminology" above), one can go directly to a single group of diseases contained within the classification. Each group will have only a relatively small number of disorders. The number of diseases contained within each group will depend on the knowledge level of the audience to which the classification is addressed and would also be determined by the frequency with which members of the chosen audience might likely encounter any given disorder. In addition, the list must contain a few infrequently, or even rarely, encountered conditions (such as melanoma) that are too important for the clinician to pass over or misdiagnose. Lastly, nonvisible but symptomatic disorders (such as pruritus and pain) would of course have to be classified based solely on patient history. However, the principle of grouping those disorders having similar symptoms would remain the same as for visible disorders.

The conditions listed in a given group would essentially constitute one's list of differential diagnoses. Then, from that list, using general medical knowledge and common sense, one could quickly pick the top several candidate diagnoses. Then, to choose among these top candidates, one would turn to a textbook or online site where a few minutes of reading would usually allow one to narrow the choice to the single best diagnosis. This approach to classification even potentially allows the clinician to make a diagnosis of a disease that has never previously been encountered before. Finally, a very important benefit of such a classification is that it will only rarely require revision since it has been created using two unchanging aspects of a disorder: clinical presentation and patient history.

A classification for vulvar disorders based on this principle was developed in 2011 by the Terminology Committee of International Society for the Study of Vulvovaginal Disease (ISSVD).[1] Some of the guiding principles that were used by the committee to create this classification included (1) acceptability to ISSVD members from all specialties, (2) acceptability to ISSVD members from all countries regardless of the language used therein, and (3) sufficient simplicity and conciseness for daily clinical use. This ISSVD classification (excluding the list of diseases found within each group) is displayed in **Table 2-1**. Because this classification happens to work equally well for *male* anogenital disease, this classification, with some modification, forms the organizational basis for the disorders discussed in this book (**Table 2-2**).

The ISSVD created another quite different classification of the vulvar dermatoses in 2006.[2] Specifically, the 2006 classification was designed to be used only in those instances where making a diagnosis based on clinical

**TABLE 2-1**

**2011 ISSVD Clinical Classification of Vulvar Dermatological Disorders**

1. Skin-colored lesions
   a. Skin-colored papules and nodules
   b. Skin-colored plaques
2. Red lesions: patches and plaques
   a. Eczematous and lichenified diseases
   b. Red patches and plaques (no epithelial disruption)
3. Red lesions: papules and nodules
   a. Red papules
   b. Red nodules
4. White lesions
   a. White papules and nodules
   b. White patches and plaques
5. Dark-colored (brown, blue, gray, or black) lesions
   a. Dark-colored patches
   b. Dark-colored papules and nodules
6. Blisters
   a. Vesicles and bullae
   b. Pustules
7. Erosions and ulcers
   a. Erosions
   b. Ulcers
8. Edema
   a. Skin-colored edema
   b. Pink or red edema

Reprinted with permission from Lynch PJ, Moyal-Barraco M, Scurry J, Stockdale C. 2011 ISSVD terminology and classification of vulvar dermatological disorders: an approach to clinical diagnosis. *J Low Genit Tract Dis.* 2012;16:139-144.

**TABLE 2-2**

**Classification of Anogenital Dermatological Disorders**

1. Skin-colored lesions (Chapter 7)
   a. Skin-colored papules and nodules
   b. Skin-colored plaques
2. Red lesions: patches and plaques (Chapter 5)
   a. Eczematous and lichenified diseases
   b. Red papulosquamous patches and plaques (no epithelial disruption)
3. Red lesions: papules and nodules (Chapter 6)
   a. Red papules
   b. Red nodules
4. White lesions (Chapter 8)
   a. White papules and nodules
   b. White patches and plaques
5. Dark-colored (brown, blue, gray, or black) lesions (Chapter 9)
   a. Dark-colored patches
   b. Dark-colored papules and nodules
6. Blisters (Chapter 10)
   a. Vesicles and bullae
   b. Pustules
7. Erosions and ulcers (Chapter 11)
   a. Erosions
   b. Ulcers
8. Edema (Chapter 12)
   a. Skin-colored edema
   b. Pink or red edema
9. Nonlesional disorders (symptoms only) (Chapter 13)
   a. Pruritus (itching)
   b. Pain

appearance is not possible. In such a situation, a biopsy is necessary. In most instances, the biopsy allows the pathologist to identify a single, specific disease. However, occasionally the biopsy shows only a "histopathologic pattern" rather than a specific diagnosis. For instance, a pathologist may report an "acanthotic pattern" or a "lichenoid pattern." When this happens, the 2006 classification helps the clinician to make a clinical-pathologic correlation to arrive at a single best diagnosis. This 2006 classification is used very infrequently, and for that reason, it is not reproduced here.

## Diagnosis

### Establishing the Criteria for Diagnosis of Anogenital Dermatological Disorders

Correct diagnosis is the sine qua non for the care of any patient with any disorder. If one does not know the diagnosis, one cannot establish the cause, provide the prognosis, or institute appropriate therapy. As stated above, for patients with dermatological disorders, a working diagnosis should almost always be established on the basis of clinical morphology and/or symptoms. If necessary, this clinical diagnosis can subsequently be confirmed through procedures such as biopsy, cytology, and microbial culture (see Chapter 4).

There are two major approaches to using clinical symptoms and signs to establish a working diagnosis: the use of visual memory and the use of a morphologically determined approach. Dermatologists by virtue of repeated exposure to patients with both common and uncommon diseases almost always depend on visual memory. And, because it works for them, they consistently use that same approach when teaching medical students and other clinicians. Thus, in the classroom or at continuing medical education courses, they bombard their audience with clinical photo after clinical photo, leaving the participants with a jumbled mass of impossible to remember images of skin disease.

The use of visual memory works for the dermatologist because of sufficient, repetitive exposure to these diseases. But other clinicians, encountering fewer patients with mucocutaneous disorders, lack the opportunity for sufficient visual reinforcement to dependably recognize uncommonly and rarely encountered diseases. By analogy, these clinicians are put in the position of someone attending a large gathering where one knows very few of the guests. In spite of many introductions, the names of those they have met quickly disappear from memory. At best, on a subsequent encounter, one might remember a face as being vaguely familiar but find it impossible to identify the person by name. The same problem occurs for the nondermatologist in a clinical setting. In this situation, when faced with an unrecognized mucocutaneous disorder, one might futilely turn to a standard dermatology textbook or the internet. But the clinician quickly finds find that the diseases contained therein are almost always organized on the basis of etiology or pathophysiology. This is, of course, of no help, as one must know the diagnosis first before it is possible to make use of the material contained therein. In such a situation. one might then end up paging through the pictures hoping to stumble on a disease that matches what was just found on examination of the patient. At best, this offers a hit or miss approach, and even when it is helpful, it is an inefficient and mostly inaccurate approach to diagnosis.

A better approach, especially for anogenital dermatological disorders, is the use of an information source (such as this textbook) in which the disorders are organized on the basis of clinical morphology and/or patient history. Doing so directs the clinician to a cluster of diseases (see Table 2-2) that share similarities in appearance. This table also identifies the most appropriate chapter to turn to in this book. Then, with minimal reading about the characteristic diagnostic features for the grouped diseases together with perusal of the associated clinical photos, one can almost always arrive at a most likely diagnosis. This diagnosis can, if necessary, be confirmed by way of a biopsy or other diagnostic test (see Chapter 4). Note that this approach even allows a clinician to make a correct diagnosis of a disorder that he or she has never even previously encountered.

Of course, to use a morphologic approach such as this, one must be able to describe in dermatologic terms the features that one has seen on clinical examination. This is not very difficult because, as is true for most "foreign" languages, a relatively small number of words can serve one's basic needs. The dermatologic words that are required for this approach are listed and defined in the "Terminology" section above.

One final caveat: most mucocutaneous disorders can present with more than a single morphology. We have chosen to deal with this problem by placing the major discussion of the disease under its most prototypical presentation but mentioning the disease in other chapters should the disorder present with one of its less frequently encountered presentations. Hidradenitis suppurativa, for instance, is primarily discussed in the chapter "Red Papules and Nodules," but it is also mentioned in the chapters on ulcers and again in the chapter on edema.

## Initial Approach to the Patient History and Physical Examination

As is true in all fields of medicine, history and physical examination represent the first two steps in diagnosis. Specifically, these initial steps in the diagnosis of the vulvar component of anogenital disease have recently been reviewed.[3] The third step that of utilizing diagnostic procedures to confirm a clinical diagnosis is covered in Chapter 4.

There are at least two good approaches that can be used in obtaining the initial history. Some clinicians prefer using a questionnaire that can be completed by the patient either at home or in the office prior to first contact with the clinician. One of us (LE) utilizes this approach, and she has made her questionnaire available at her online site, www.midcharlottedermatologyresearch.com. This is quick for the clinician, allowing more time for education, but, more importantly, allows the patient to relay all information with many open-ended questions, most of which are only important to the patient's psychological comfort. This serves as therapy as well as history. This may be downloaded, modified, and subsequently used by any clinician. Alternatively, one of us (PJL) takes the initial history after the patient is placed in the examination room but, importantly, before the patient is asked to disrobe. With either alternative, a more directed history is then taken during or after the examination.

The two key points in physical examination of patients with genital problems are exposure and illumination. First, in a misguided attempt to protect patient modesty, some clinicians erroneously allow the patient to determine the extent of clothing to be removed. This leads patients to believe that they can simply pull underwear partially down or to one side whereas, in fact, all clothing covering the anogenital area must be completely removed. Second, nearly all examinations should take place with the patient lying supine on the examination table. Women can then be examined either in a "frog leg" position or with their feet in stirrups. The latter is preferred as it allows for good visualization of the anal area. Men are usually examined using the "frog leg" position as they generally resist being placed in stirrups. For men, the anal area can be examined either with the patient rolled to his side or with him standing but bending forward over the examination table. It cannot be emphasized strongly enough: the genital area in men or women cannot be adequately examined with the patient seated or standing.

Good lighting is required for all examinations. This requires use of a light separate from a fixed ceiling light. This means a light that is adequately bright and one that is flexible enough so that it can be moved to illuminate every aspect of the anogenital region. Needless to say, except in very unusual circumstances, examination of a patient of the sex opposite to that of the clinician should be carried out in the presence of a chaperone.

Once the examination is complete, the clinician should write, or enter, exactly what has been seen using the dermatological terminology described previously in this chapter. In doing so, it is helpful to first determine the noun(s), such as macule, patch, papule, plaque, that best describe the patient's problem. Once the noun (primary lesion) is determined, one can then apply the necessary adjectives such as the surface characteristics, margination, configuration, and color. If more than one lesion is present, the description should be of the most prototypical lesion.

When the description is complete, the clinician can place the patient's disease into one of the nine categories (groups) listed in **Table 2-2**. Once that is done, the clinician simply turns to the chapter related to that category. A quick perusal of the diseases discussed in that chapter allows one to put together a short list of differential diagnoses. Additional reading about each of the disorders on this short list almost always allows for identification of the single most likely diagnosis.

## REFERENCES

1. Lynch PJ, Moyal-Barraco M, Scurry J, Stockdale C. 2011 ISSVD terminology and classification of vulvar dermatological disorders: an approach to clinical diagnosis. *J Lower Genit Tract Dis.* 2012;16:139-144.
2. Lynch PJ, Moyal-Barraco M, Bogliatto F, et al. 2006 ISSVD classification of vulvar dermatoses: pathologic subsets and their clinical correlates. *J Reprod Med.* 2007;52:3-9.
3. Mauskar MM, Marathe K, Venkatesan A, Schlosser BJ, Edwards L. Vulvar diseases: approach to the patient. *J Am Acad Dermatol.* 2020;82(6):1277-1284.

# General Principles of Therapy 3

PETER J. LYNCH

This section discusses only the general principles of therapy. The specifics of individual therapeutic agents and their use for a particular disorder are contained with the discussion of the diseases as it occurs throughout this book.

## The Patient as a Person

One of the guiding principles of medical therapy is the recognition that a disorder is occurring in an individual person rather than existing as a separate, localized problem. This is particularly true for patients with genital disease where there are immense psychological, social, and sexual considerations associated with almost every problem occurring in this location. For instance, patients are highly likely to have a perception that the cause of their problem relates to improper sexual activity or to inadequate hygiene. Whether this turns out to be true, partially true, or false requires that the clinician search for the presence of anxiety, depression, guilt, or other aspects of psychological dysfunction in all patients with anogenital disorders. If one or more of these problems are identified, the clinician must offer two forms of help. First, one must offer nonjudgmental support, and second, one must either provide personal counseling or must assist the patient to obtain counseling by some other qualified professional. Failure to recognize the patient as a person, and thus overlook these responsibilities, is very likely to compromise the therapeutic outcome even when the disease itself is properly identified and treated correctly from a medical standpoint.

## Environmental Factors and Hygiene

The anogenital area represents a very hostile environment for normal function of the mucocutaneous epithelial cells that make up the barrier between us and the outside world. Some of the detrimental factors that are involved include heat, sweat, vaginal secretion, urine, feces, clothing, friction, and improper or excessive hygiene. These factors can cause disease, worsen minor problems, and/or retard normal healing.

### Sweat

Epithelial cells can generally withstand rather high temperatures but, unfortunately, with heat comes sweating. And sweat can be remarkably irritating as exemplified by the discomfort experienced when sweat gets in one's eyes during exercise on a warm day. The retention of sweat in the anogenital region leads to maceration of the mucocutaneous surface and this in turn leads to damage and possibly death of epithelial cells. This damage to the epithelial barrier allows for the exposure of cutaneous nerve endings and results in symptoms of pruritus and/or pain. The presence of this warmth and moisture also fosters the overgrowth, and often infections, due to bacteria and/or *Candida* sp. Obesity, tight clothing, and prolonged sitting (especially on vinyl or plastic seats) are often responsible for such sweat retention and maceration. It is difficult, but worth trying, to ameliorate these conditions.

### Urine, Feces, and Vaginal Discharge

In women, vaginal discharge (whether physiologic or pathologic) or urinary incontinence can cause irritation with subsequent inflammation and damage to epithelial cells. The end result is similar to that described for sweat retention. To make matters worse, women with urinary incontinence or vaginal discharge often end up using panty liners on a continual basis. The result is often even worse maceration. The cause of such vaginal secretions (see Chapter 14) should be determined and treated appropriately. Incontinence may require urologic consultation. In both sexes, fecal soiling can lead to irritation. More careful cleaning after defecation is desirable so that sweat does not liquefy and spread irritating fecal material. Usually, careful use of ordinary toilet paper is sufficient but if that causes too much irritation, Cetaphil Cleanser, Water Wipes, mineral oil, vegetable oil, or a wet soft cloth can be used for anal cleansing.

A change from tight pants (especially jeans) to looser fitting clothing can be helpful in the prevention and treatment of adverse environmental factors. The use of cotton or cotton blend underwear can also be useful. However, and in spite of the frequent admonition to use only white undergarments, the color of one's underwear has not been demonstrated to be of any particular importance. Hair dryers, even at their lowest settings, should not be used for purposes of drying. It is our opinion that changes in laundering practices, such as double rinsing and avoidance of antistatic products, are not particularly helpful.

### Excessive Hygiene

Excessive hygiene, especially in women, is frequently overlooked as an environmental irritant. Hygienic practices are rarely volunteered by patients and are, unfortunately, infrequently asked about by clinicians. A dry, chapped appearance is suggestive of too much cleansing even if a patient's history regarding washing is not helpful. More than twice daily cleansing of the anogenital area is unnecessary and is usually detrimental. Soap and water applied with the hands or with a washcloth suffices; scrubbing is never warranted. Water Wipes may also be suitable. A handheld showerhead can be used by those who are otherwise unable to reach the anogenital area.

Additional information on environmental irritation can be found under "Irritant Contact Dermatitis" in the eczematous disorders section of Chapter 5.

## The Therapeutic Use of Soaks

Soaks serve several purposes. First, they can offer symptomatic relief for both pruritus and pain. Second, they offer a gentle approach to the debridement of any crust that is present. This removal of crust decreases bacterial and yeast overgrowth and removes a mechanical impediment to wound healing. Third, soaks temporarily restore a physiologic moist environment that enhances epithelial healing. Fourth, soaks are one of the few approaches to therapy that can be safely, appropriately, and helpfully suggested by telephone before the patient can be examined.

Dermatologists historically have made somewhat of a fetish with their recommendations regarding esoteric and complicated solutions for soaks. But in reality, soaks for problems occurring in the anogenital region can be accomplished very simply by partially filling a bathtub with ordinary tap water. A sitz bath-type chair may be used for those who cannot easily get in and out of a bathtub. The water temperature should be comfortably warm rather than very hot or very cold. Nothing further needs to be added to the water and in fact many of the products sold for such purpose make the floor of a bathtub dangerously slippery. Soaking should occur for a period of 15 or 20 minutes, following which the skin should be patted, rather than rubbed, dry. The soothing effect of a soak is lost within about 30 minutes because the water quickly evaporates from the skin. This evaporative loss can be delayed by the prompt application of a lubricant (see below). Soaks may be repeated several times per day if the buildup of crust is troublesome or if the severity of pain or itching requires it.

Soaks should be considered as "first aid" and not as something to be continued indefinitely. After several days of soaks, weeping and crusting should be markedly diminished, and there will usually be no further improvement in pain or pruritus. Moreover, prolonged use of soaks may lead to detrimental excessive drying of the epithelium. A perceived need for longer use of soaks generally suggests that one's therapeutic plan requires revision.

## General Principles of Topical Therapy

Most topical products are available as creams or ointments. In the genital area, ointments are often preferred because they are less likely to cause irritation and burning as often happens with creams; the down side of ointments relates to their messiness and propensity to cause maceration if too much is applied. If this is the case, creams can be used instead. It is rarely appropriate to use gels, lotions, or solutions in the anogenital area because of their irritating properties.

Most patients have no idea how much of a topical product should be used for any one application. It is reasonable to suggest an amount about the size of a lead pencil eraser (~0.2-0.3 g). That amount, spread appropriately thinly, will usually cover the external genitalia. Note, however, that if the area to be treated is hairy, a larger amount will be required for each application. One of us (LE) instructs that far far less of a topical corticosteroid be applied, and expects a 15 g tube to last 4-5 months with daily use. Nearly all products are most appropriately applied twice a daily. Thus, if a patient is neither underusing, nor overusing, the product, a standard-sized 30-g tube, should last a month or more. Most products are also available in larger sizes (60-80 g). These larger sizes may be more economical to prescribe if the patient's disorder requires long-term therapy and if the patient is educated as to how long the larger amount should last.

Patients are often uncertain as to just where the product should be applied. Instructions in this regard should be given not only verbally but also by demonstration. For this purpose, a patient-held mirror can be used if the site is not otherwise visible to the patient.

## Lubricants

Epithelial cells are very sensitive to the amount of moisture in and around them. In the section above, we indicated that too much moisture leads to maceration and cell death. Epithelial cells are also very sensitive to too little moisture. When evaporative loss of natural moisture occurs faster than it is replaced by the underlying interstitial fluid, epithelial cells shrink in size and pull apart. In either case, disruption of the barrier layer (which is located in the outer portion of the epithelium) occurs. Such disruption allows for exposure and triggering of sensory nerve endings, resulting in pain and/or pruritus. Lubricants are used to retard evaporative loss and thus provide for a more physiologic environment and faster subsequent repair of the disrupted epithelial barrier layer.

There are two common circumstances in which the barrier layer becomes disrupted because of excessive dryness. First, and as mentioned above, this can occur as the result of excessive washing, utilization of harsh solvents, or with scrubbing rather than simple washing. The use of soap and water on the genitalia more than twice a day removes the naturally present lipids and leads to excess water loss from the epithelial cells. Second, barrier layer disruption occurs in the presence of disease-related thickening of the stratum corneum. This thickening can occur as the result of underlying inflammation or secondary to the process of lichenification (see definition in Chapter 2). In either of these two situations, interstitial moisture from the underlying dermis cannot adequately diffuse into the outermost epithelial cells. The abnormally dry epithelial cells shrink and the epithelial surface then tends to fissure, allowing even more water loss from these cells. Lubrication, by way of retarding evaporative water loss, restores a more physiologic epithelial environment and helps to alleviate the usually attendant symptoms of itching and/or pain.

Many types of lubricants are available. Those that are petrolatum based (eg, Vaseline) do not sting on application. They do a very good job of preventing evaporative water loss but are messy, sticky and, if thickly applied, may be counterproductive by way of trapping sweat. Products such as these are best used in infants and young children, though some adults find them surprisingly acceptable. Lotions, which lie at the other end of the spectrum, are liquids that can be poured or pumped out of a container. Although these are cosmetically very pleasing on intact mucocutaneous tissue, they contain very little in the way of lipids and therefore do a relatively poor job of lubricating. Moreover, most lotions contain alcohols and other chemicals that can cause stinging on application. This is particularly noticeable when applied to the tender skin of the anogenital region, especially in children. A reasonable compromise is the use of any one of the standard products ("hand creams") that are inexpensive and easily available. Though most dermatologists have a specific brand they like to recommend, we have found that allowing patients to choose the brand they prefer leads to the best compliance for use.

## Steroidal Anti-inflammatory Therapy

Anti-inflammatory therapy is the most important and most often used specific treatment in dermatology. Given the prime role for such therapy, it is dismaying to find that it is often misused. Attention must be given to the route for use (eg, topical, intralesional, or systemic), the dosage, the amount to be dispensed, and the duration of time for which the product is to be used.

### Topical Steroid Therapy

Topical steroid therapy represents the mainstay of anti-inflammatory treatment **(Figs. 3-1 and 3-2)**. The number of topical steroid products available is unmanageably large. We have found that clinicians only need to be familiar with four of these. All four are available either by brand or

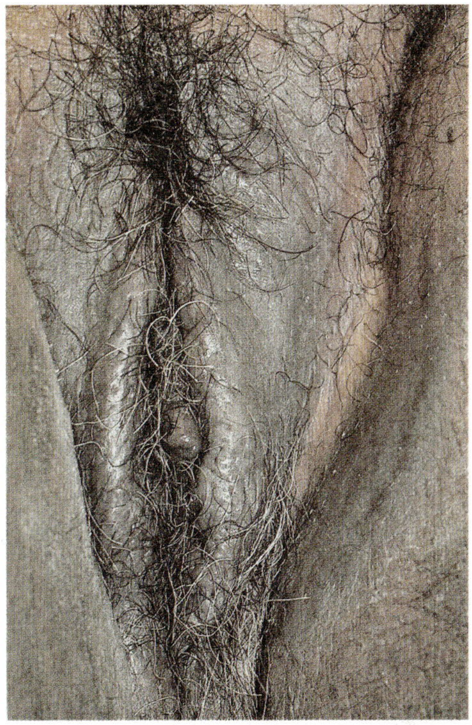

Fig. 3-1. This patient with lichen simplex chronicus reports years of excruciating pruritus, with resulting remarkable hyperpigmentation and thickening from ongoing rubbing, and even hair broken off at the surface.

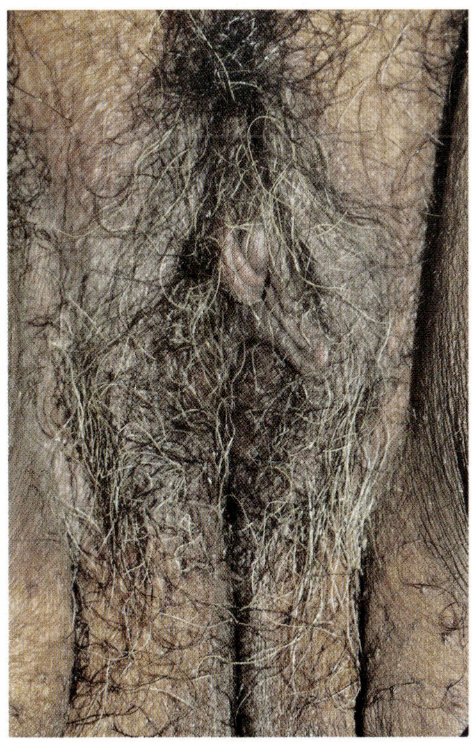

Fig. 3-2. Two months after beginning clobetasol propionate ointment daily, itching has resolved, thickness is clearing, the texture is nearly normal, and hair has regrown.

generically. The generic products can be found on most formulary lists. Advice from a dermatologist or pharmacologist might be sought in the event that one's desired topical steroid is not available and that a substitution is needed. Hydrocortisone and triamcinolone can be purchased at reasonable prices if the patient lacks insurance coverage for medications. Fluocinonide and clobetasol are appreciably more expensive but coupons (such as from GoodRx) are frequently available for somewhat more reasonable prices.

*Hydrocortisone* is a low-potency steroid. It is available as a 1.0% product (nonprescription strength) or a 2.5% product (prescription strength). Either of these is suitable as initial therapy for eczematous anogenital disorders in infants and children. Safety, even with long-term use, is excellent but their level of effectiveness is correspondingly low.

*Triamcinolone acetonide* is a mid-potency steroid. It is available in several strengths, but for the most part, only the 0.1% strength needs to be considered. Triamcinolone is appropriate for second-line therapy of eczematous disease in children and initial therapy in adults. Safety, even with long-term use, is quite good.

*Fluocinonide* is a high-potency steroid. It is available in several strengths, but only the 0.05% strength needs to be considered. It is suitable for second-line therapy of eczematous disease in adults (first line for lichen simplex chronicus) and initial therapy of papulosquamous and other noneczematous disease.

*Clobetasol propionate* is a super-potency steroid available as a 0.05% product. It is suitable for second-line therapy of lichen simplex chronicus and for first-line therapy of noneczematous disorders such as lichen sclerosus, lichen planus, and psoriasis.

From a standpoint of *systemic* adverse effects, all of the topical products described above are reasonably safe even for long-term use. When the high-potency and super-potency products are restricted to use on the modified mucous membranes of the vulvar vestibule and the glans penis, safety in terms of *cutaneous* side effects is also excellent. However, when clobetasol is used on skin (rather than on mucous membranes) or is allowed to spread onto skin due to heat and sweat, there is a fairly high risk for the development of skin atrophy, telangiectasia, and striae (**Figs. 3-3 to 3-5**). This is particularly likely to happen when used on (or is inadvertently spread onto) the upper inner thighs. It is not clear whether this can happen with the use of fluocinonide, but caution is warranted.

## Intralesional Steroid Therapy

At the practical level, triamcinolone acetonide (Kenalog) is the only steroid used for intralesional (intradermal) injection. This route of administration is used when there has been failure (due to either inadequate penetration or noncompliant use) of topically applied steroids. The commercial preparation is a 10-mg/mL multiuse vial. This product can be used at this strength or, to reduce the possibility of local atrophy, may be diluted to 5 mg/mL with equal parts of normal saline or lidocaine. An injection of 0.1 mL will spread to encompass about 1 $cm^2$; therefore, the number of injections can be planned according to the size of the involved area. As might be expected, these

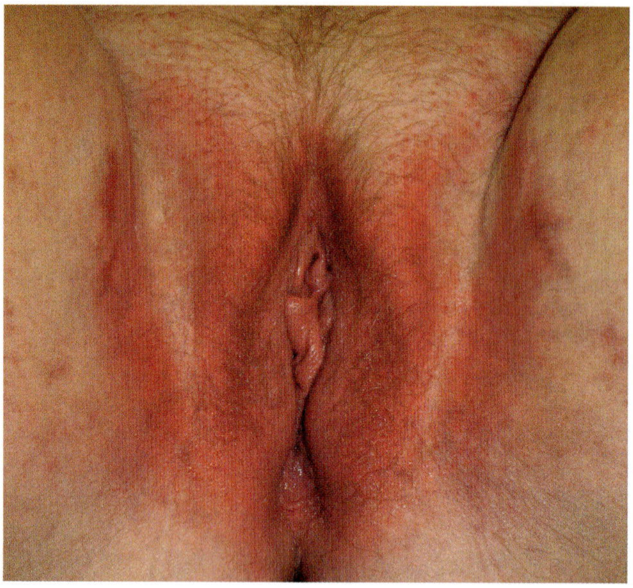

Fig. 3-3. A side effect of the chronic use of a potent topical corticosteroid that is seen almost exclusively on the nonmucous membrane skin of the vulva, and perianal area is steroid dermatitis. The skin is red, and differentiation between overuse and underuse is sometimes difficult.

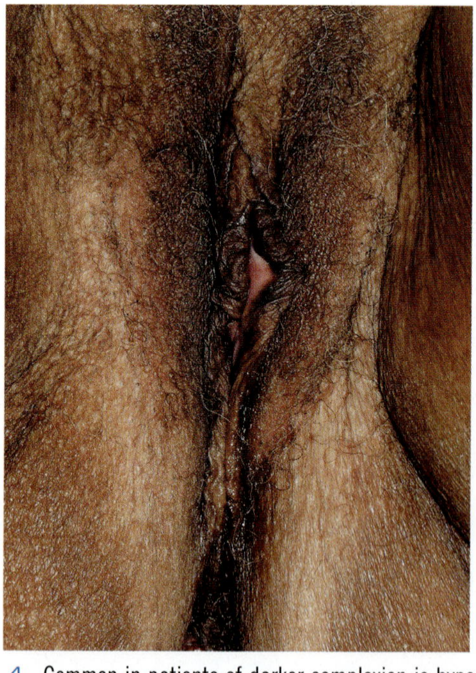

Fig. 3-4. Common in patients of darker complexion is hypopigmentation in the skin surrounding a dermatosis with use of a potent corticosteroid. Repigmentation generally occurs when the medication is discontinued or the frequency decreased.

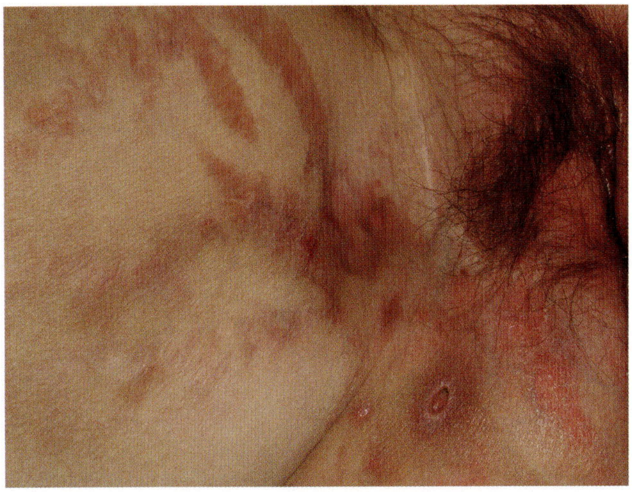

Fig. 3-5. Overuse of a potent corticosteroid can produce striae and even ulcerations. These side effects generally do not occur if a patient is counseled in the use of these medications, follow-up scheduled within 2 months, application demonstrated, and a 15-g tube dispensed without refills. The benefits greatly outweigh the risks.

injections are rather painful owing to the penetration of the needle and the tissue distension as the medication is injected. Pretreatment with topically applied 5% lidocaine or EMLA cream can help in this regard.

Several practical points should be considered in using intralesional triamcinolone. First, the stock preparation is a suspension, rather than a pure liquid, and therefore, it must be shaken before the medication is withdrawn from the vial. Likewise, the syringe in which it is contained should be shaken just prior to performing the injection. I (PJL) find that the large size of the particles in the suspension makes it difficult to withdraw and inject the product through a 30-gauge needle. Others (LE) find that a 30-guage needle is manageable. I prefer withdrawing the triamcinolone with a 27-gauge needle and usually use that size needle for injection as well. It is preferable to use a small 1-mL syringe ("tuberculin" or "diabetic" type syringe) to improve accuracy of the injected amount.

### Systemic Steroid Therapy

It is rarely necessary to use systemic steroid therapy for disorders localized to the anogenital area, though this is occasionally necessary for patients with treatment-resistant disorders such as erosive lichen planus, aphthosis major, Behçet disease, Crohn disease, hidradenitis suppurativa, chronic atopic dermatitis, and lichen simplex chronicus. Systemic steroids and/or other systemic immunomodulating agents are regularly required in immunobullous disorders, and immunomodulating agents are often used by dermatologists for psoriasis. Such systemic treatment lies outside the scope of this chapter but is discussed when each disorder is covered.

Systemic steroid therapy can be administered orally or intramuscularly. Prednisone is the oral product most often used. Generally, a daily dose of 40-60 mg is appropriate. It should be taken in the early morning so as to reduce suppression of the patient's own steroid production. In most situations, this is given, without taper, for 7-10 days. When therapy needs to be continued longer than that, the dose should be tapered both to reduce the likelihood of rebound and to allow for recovery of any hypothalamic-pituitary-adrenal suppression that has occurred.

When systemic steroids such as prednisone are used, there should be concern about blood sugar elevation, increased blood pressure, psychological problems (especially insomnia and agitation), and dangerous worsening of any underlying systemic infection. Adverse effects occurring with long-term use (osteoporosis, cataract formation, etc.) are not of concern if therapy is limited to less than a month. One of the biggest problems that occurs with use of short-term prednisone therapy is rebound of the treated disorder when the prednisone is discontinued. This is true even when the dose is tapered before it is stopped.

Systemic steroids can also be administered intramuscularly. This is the route we prefer when treating chronic eczematous disease when that condition is insufficiently responsive to topical steroid use. The product we use for intramuscular injection is triamcinolone acetonide (Kenalog). This is available in a 40 mg/mL concentration. The usual recommended dose is 40 mg (1.0 mL), but it is our opinion that this dose is too low to achieve satisfactory results. We much prefer to use 80 mg (2.0 mL). The Kenalog should be injected into the upper, outer quadrant of the buttock; we strongly advise against using the shoulder deltoid muscle to avoid the depression caused by local atrophy. A 1.5-in., 27-guage needle should be used because injection with a shorter needle leads to superficial deposition with less effectiveness and greater risk of long-lasting atrophy. As with the intralesional Kenalog product, this is a suspension, and both the vial and the syringe must be shaken before use.

There are multiple advantages related to the use of intramuscular triamcinolone. First, the clinician controls the dose. Second, there is no concern that the patient may obtain unwarranted refills. Third, there is built-in tapering of the dose (and thus less likely disease rebound) due to the depot effect and slow release of the injected medication. Fourth, fewer milligrams of steroid can be of used for a given level of anti-inflammatory effect. Fifth, there is less chance of acute adverse effect on blood pressure, blood sugar, and psyche. Sixth, the clinician determines the cost that the patient will pay, an important consideration when treating uninsured individuals.

## Nonsteroidal Anti-inflammatory Therapy

### Topical Nonsteroidal Anti-inflammatory Therapy

Long-term use of topical steroids raises concerns about systemic absorption and cutaneous side effects. To ameliorate these problems, topical calcineurin inhibitors were introduced. Two of these, pimecrolimus 1% cream (Elidel) and tacrolimus 0.03% and 0.1% ointment (Protopic), are currently being marketed. These products lessen inflammation by reducing T-cell elaboration of inflammatory cytokines. These two medications, unlike topically applied potent steroids, do not cause cutaneous telangiectasia and atrophy. For this reason, they have been widely used for facial and intertriginous eruptions. Tacrolimus 0.1% ointment appears to be slightly more effective than pimecrolimus 1% cream. Both are generally less effective than high- and super-potency topical steroids, but there have been some instances of improvement in patients where they were used following failure with topical steroids. Both products are associated with an appreciable degree of stinging and burning on application.

Controversy exists about the use of these agents for genital disease. Nearly 20 years ago, the American FDA required that a "black box" warning be included in the package information. This notice warns that the long-term safety of these agents has not been proven due to rare reports of the development of skin cancer and lymphoma following their long-term use. Most dermatologists believe that any relationship between their use and the development of malignancy is coincidental rather than causal.[1] Nevertheless, it is easy to appreciate the potential legal risk when these agents are used for the treatment of anogenital mucocutaneous disorders (such as lichen sclerosus and lichen planus) that already have an inherent risk for the development of squamous cell carcinoma.

Recently, a new *topical* antiphosphodiesterase inhibitor, crisaborole (Eucrisa) 2% ointment has been FDA approved for the treatment of mild to moderate atopic dermatitis.[2] Due to the lack of comparative studies and its high cost, we have only limited experience with it. However, to the extent that we have used it, we have not found it to be particularly effective.

### Systemic Nonsteroidal Anti-inflammatory Therapy

Multiple medications are regularly used by dermatologists as systemically administered nonsteroidal anti-inflammatory agents. These include hydroxychloroquine, cyclosporine, mycophenolate mofetil, dapsone, and a variety of other immunomodulating products to include cytotoxic agents and so-called biological medications. These are not commonly indicated for the treatment of genital disease and therefore will be discussed only where they are most likely to be used for a specific disorder rather than in this chapter.

A different approach to reduce the risk of steroid therapy has led to the introduction of anti-phosphodiesterase-4 inhibitors. The first of these was the orally administered apremilast (Otezla) that was FDA approved for the treatment of the inflammatory disorder, psoriasis.

It appears to be moderately effective for this purpose, but its high cost limits its usefulness.

## Antipruritic Therapy

Itching is an extremely distressing symptom and, for many patients, it is even more troublesome than moderate pain. It represents a major reason why patients with genital disorders seek medical help. Many agents are available for the treatment of chronic itching. The most commonly used treatments are discussed in the paragraphs that follow. The most promising new agents, most of which are either not yet FDA approved and/or are extraordinarily expensive, have been recently reviewed.[3]

### General Measures

It stands to reason that if a specific underlying disorder can be identified, treating it as effectively as possible will reduce the itching. But note that although treatment of such a disease is necessary, it often is not sufficient. This is especially true if the "itch-scratch" cycle (itching that leads to scratching that leads to more itching, more scratching, etc.) is well established. Other general approaches, as discussed previously, should include improving the local environment by way of measures to decrease sweat retention and using soaks and lubrication. These approaches can be considered as "first aid" measures and can be suggested before one even sees the patient.

### Decreasing Inflammation

Inflammation occurring as a component of any genital disorder is often associated with itching. Using any of the anti-inflammatory approaches, especially the application of topical steroids, described in the section above, almost always has a beneficial effect on pruritus when inflammation accompanies it. And, it should be noted, the use of topical steroids rarely has any adverse effect on an underlying disorder.

### Oral Antihistamines

The administration of oral antihistamines for pruritus has a time-honored place in the dermatologic armamentarium. Traditionally, the agent most often used is hydroxyzine (Atarax, Vistaril, etc.). Because of its sedative side effect, it is best administered in the evening. Note, however, that if such an antihistamine is given just before going to bed, the patient may scratch while waiting for it to take effect and also the patient may wake up in the morning feeling drowsy. Therefore, it is best to suggest taking it ~2 hours before the patient's expected bedtime. Allowing the patient to subsequently experiment with the length of the interval between dosing and bedtime increases both compliance and efficacy. The usual starting dose for hydroxyzine is 25 mg, but for a patient who is very "sensitive" to medications, it may be appropriate to start with 10 mg. This nighttime dose is then increased each week by 25 mg until there is either no more nighttime scratching, side effects prevent further increase, or a dose of 100 mg is reached. The entire evening dose is taken all at the same time. Rarely a patient may tolerate, and benefit, by taking 25 mg four times per day rather than just at night, but because of daytime drowsiness, such patients must be warned about the hazards of driving, operating machinery, and drinking alcohol.

Other antihistamines such as diphenhydramine (Benadryl) can be used instead of hydroxyzine, but most dermatologists feel that it is somewhat less effective than hydroxyzine. The dosing is the same as for hydroxyzine. Many clinicians use the "low-sedating" antihistamine cetirizine (Zyrtec) or the nonsedating antihistamines loratadine (Claritin), desloratadine (Clarinex), or fexofenadine (Allegra) for daytime treatment of itching. However, in our opinion, these agents are ineffective for the treatment of nonurticarial pruritus.

### Tricyclic Oral Medications

Use of the tricyclic agents can be remarkably effective in the treatment of both pruritus and pain. Although these drugs are approved, and marketed, primarily for the treatment of depression and anxiety, they are remarkable good antihistamines as well. As a result, these medications usually represent the second line of nighttime therapy for pruritus especially in those situations where hydroxyzine has failed. When tricyclics are used, it is not clear whether it is the psychotropic, the antihistaminic, or the sedative component that is responsible for their beneficial effect. There is, however, some consensus that those with the greatest sedative effect work better than those that are less sedating.

Doxepin (Sinequan) is the tricyclic medication most often used for the treatment of itching, though amitriptyline (Elavil) works equally well. The starting dose for either doxepin or amitriptyline is usually 25 mg taken in the evening. An initial dose of 10 mg can be used in the elderly and for those with a history of being very "sensitive" to other medications. As with hydroxyzine, it is preferable to have the patient take the medication about 2 hours before bedtime so as to increase effectiveness by the time the patient goes to bed. This also lessens "hangover" drowsiness in the morning. The nighttime dose is then increased weekly by 25 mg until either there is no more nighttime scratching, the adverse effects prevent further increase, or a dose of 100 mg is reached. The entire dose, regardless of the number of milligrams prescribed, is taken all at the same time. In addition to drowsiness, there are a number of other possible adverse effects. These include dryness of the mouth and eyes, blurred vision, arrhythmias, and many drug-drug interactions. Lest these adverse effects lead to wariness about the use of the tricyclics, it should be emphasized that they occur almost only at doses above 75 mg/day.

### Selective Serotonin Reuptake Inhibitors

Selective serotonin reuptake inhibitors (SSRIs) can be used quite effectively for daytime treatment of pruritus. These agents and their use are discussed in the section on eczematous disorders in Chapter 5.

### Topical Nonsteroidal Antipruritic Agents

Several topical products are available for topical treatment of itching. Some of the more commonly used agents include pramoxine (usually mixed with hydrocortisone), doxepin (Zonalon), benzocaine (in multiple products, notably Vagisil Cream), and lidocaine (Xylocaine). In our opinion, none of these works particularly well for itching and one of them, benzocaine, is a fairly frequent causes of allergic contact dermatitis.[4]

## Analgesic Therapy

Analgesics can be used (1) for idiopathic mucocutaneous anogenital pain (vulvodynia, penodynia, scrotodynia, and anodynia), (2) for pain associated with several dermatologic disorders (herpes zoster, erosive lichen planus, etc.), and (3) for various neuropathies. Note that opiate analgesics are essentially never indicated for use in the treatment of anogenital pain, and for that reason, they are not discussed here.

### Topical Analgesics

The most commonly recommended topical medication for genital pain is 2% or 5% lidocaine (Xylocaine). The 5% ointment is the preferred product though some patients find that "burning" on application is troublesome. If tolerated, small amount (the size of a lead pencil eraser) can be applied four or five times per day. However, note that toxic amounts of lidocaine can be absorbed from the skin and mucous membranes. For this reason, no more than 15 g should be applied in the course of a day. Many topical analgesic products, including the widely used Vagisil Cream, contain benzocaine. Benzocaine is based on the PABA molecule and is chemically unrelated to lidocaine. Unfortunately, benzocaine causes allergic contact dermatitis with considerable frequency, and for that reason, we advise against its use.[4] Other prescription-only topical analgesics, such as either generic EMLA cream or compounded tetracaine 6%/lidocaine 6%, may also be effective.

### Oral Analgesics

The tricyclic antidepressants have historically been the mainstay of therapy for genital pain of all types. These oral analgesics are used in the same doses and in the same schedules as are discussed in the section above under "Antipruritic Therapy."

Other psychotropic agents such as duloxetine (Cymbalta) and venlafaxine (Effexor and Effexor XL) are also used in the treatment of genital pain. Both of these latter agents are serotonin and norepinephrine reuptake inhibitors; venlafaxine additionally inhibits the uptake of dopamine. Neither is FDA approved for the treatment of anogenital pain. However, duloxetine, but not venlafaxine, has been approved by the FDA for the treatment of diabetic neuropathy and fibromyalgia. Both are available as generic products. Duloxetine therapy is begun in a dose of 30 mg once daily and is increased to 60 mg/day in 1 week. Venlafaxine extended release is started in a dose of 37.5 mg/day; this may be increased to 75 mg/day in a week. The total daily dose can eventually, and slowly, be increased to 225 mg/day. Both of these agents have drug-drug interactions and may have adverse central nervous system effects. Patients taking venlafaxine should have their blood pressure monitored regularly. The dose for these medications should be tapered when they are to be discontinued.

The antidepressants from the group of selective serotonin reuptake inhibitors (generally known as the SSRIs) have also been used off label in the treatment of idiopathic mucocutaneous genital pain, but most clinicians believe that they are less effective than duloxetine, venlafaxine, and the tricyclics. The use of SSRIs is further discussed in the "Eczematous Disorders" section of Chapter 5 where they are efficaciously used for daytime treatment of pruritus.

The anticonvulsants carbamazepine (Tegretol, Carbatrol), gabapentin (Neurontin), and pregabalin (Lyrica) are sometimes used in the treatment of genital pain on the basis of their approval by FDA for treatment of trigeminal neuralgia (carbamazepine), postherpetic neuralgia (gabapentin), and peripheral neuropathy and fibromyalgia (pregabalin). Carbamazepine reduces the release of the neurotransmitter, glutamate. Gabapentin and the related product, pregabalin, reduce calcium influx into nerve terminals. Gabapentin has few serious adverse effects and is the most often used of these three products. It is started in a dose of 300 mg/day and is increased weekly by 300 mg increments until relief is obtained or a total daily dose of 1800 mg (600 mg tid) is reached. Even higher dosing (up to 3600 mg/day) is possible, but little additional analgesic effect is obtained at doses above 1800 mg/day. The initial dose of pregabalin is 75 mg bid; this may be increased on a weekly basis to a total dose of no more than 300 mg bid. Carbamazepine has several potentially serious adverse effects, and we believe that it should not be used for anogenital pain.

## Antibacterial Therapy

The two most common bacterial infections of mucocutaneous genital tissue are those due to *Staphylococcus aureus* and *Streptococcus pyogenes*. For this reason, the antibacterial therapy discussed in this section will apply only to these two organisms. Therapy for other less commonly encountered infections, including those used for vaginitis and sexually transmitted disease, will be discussed as these topics are covered elsewhere in this book.

### Oral Antibiotics

The penicillin class of agents are bactericidal antibiotics that act by inhibiting the synthesis of bacterial cell walls. They are effective for streptococcal infections and non–methicillin-resistant staphylococcal infections. The most commonly used medication is dicloxacillin given in a dose of 250-500 mg qid. Other frequently used drugs in this class include penicillin V potassium in a dose of 250-500 mg qid and amoxicillin plus clavulanate (Augmentin) in a dose of 500 mg bid or tid. Allergic reactions to agents in the penicillin family are fairly common and must be inquired about before these antibiotics are prescribed.

The cephalosporins are comparable in efficacy to the penicillins for streptococcal and non–methicillin-resistant staphylococcal infections. Cephalexin (Keflex) in a dose of 250-500 mg qid is the drug most commonly used. Allergic reactions to cephalosporins do occur, but they are less common than with the penicillins. There is a 2% or 3% crossover of allergic reactions between these two groups of antibiotics.

Other antibiotics have to be considered due to the ongoing occurrence of community-associated, methicillin-resistant *S aureus* (MRSA) infections.[5] At least five generic oral antibiotics may be effective for MRSA infections. These include trimethoprim-sulfamethoxazole (1 or 2 double strength tablets bid), doxycycline (100 mg bid), minocycline (100 mg bid), rifampin (600 mg/day), and linezolid (600 mg bid). Other newer antibiotics are also available, but a discussion about them lies outside the scope of this book.[6] Vancomycin or daptomycin given intravenously are used only for the most serious, life-threatening MRSA infections. The medication used from among the oral antibiotics for MRSA infections should be based on drug sensitivity studies from patient specimen cultures and from drug resistance data for the clinician's local community.

### Topical Antibiotics

There are several nonprescription products available for the topical treatment of staphylococcal and streptococcal infections. The three most commonly used preparations are neomycin, bacitracin, and the triple antibiotic (Neosporin). The latter contains bacitracin, neomycin, and polymyxin B. All three products are applied tid or qid. These three agents have two advantages: they are inexpensive and one or another is present in almost every home. All have the drawback of causing allergic contact dermatitis with some degree of frequency.

Several other topical antibiotics are available. The following three topical antibiotics, mupirocin, retapamulin (Altabax), and ozenoxacin (Xepi) are available only by prescription. Of these, mupirocin is available as an inexpensive generic preparation. All three are as effective as neomycin, bacitracin, and triple antibiotic, and all of them have the advantage of rarely causing allergic contact dermatitis. All of these topical products currently appear to be at least moderately effective in the treatment of MRSA infections.

## Antifungal and Anticandida Therapy

The "azole" medications are very effective in the therapy of both dermatophyte fungal infections and most yeast infections due to *Candida* sp. They work by interfering with the synthesis and function of microbial cell walls. For practical purposes, the azoles have supplanted a variety of antimicrobial agents whose usefulness was restricted to either fungal infections or yeast infections.

### Topical Antifungal and Anticandida Therapy

Topically applied azoles are widely used, and effective, for both dermatophyte fungal and *Candida* yeast infection. In most instances, these agents represent the first line of treatment. Among the most frequently used products are fluconazole (Diflucan), ketoconazole (Nizoral), clotrimazole (Lotrimin), and miconazole (Micatin, Monistat). They are available either as creams or, for the latter two, as vaginal suppositories. Clotrimazole and miconazole are relatively inexpensive over-the-counter (OTC) products. All four of them are essentially equal in efficacy. Stinging with application, especially on broken skin, is troublesome for many patients. Nystatin, once the most widely used topical agent for candidiasis, is somewhat less effective than the azoles for candida infections, but its topical application causes much less burning and is therefore still a useful agent. It is not an effective anti-dermatopyte product. Therapeutic problems associated with vaginal non–*Candida albicans* yeast infections are discussed in Chapter 14. Terbinafine (Lamisil) cream and the appreciably more expensive naftifine (Naftin) cream are two OTC agents that are quite effective for dermatophyte fungal infections but are much less effective as anticandida agents.

### Oral Antifungal and Anticandida Therapy

Clinicians are gradually switching from topical to oral administration of the azoles for candidiasis in adults. This has occurred because of troublesome burning irritation from topical azoles, better patient compliance, and decreasing cost for the oral preparations. The major disadvantage is that these agents are only available with a prescription. The major products for oral use include ketoconazole, itraconazole, and fluconazole. Fluconazole is the oral product most frequently used for *Candida albicans* infections A single oral dose of 150 or 200 mg is usually sufficient to resolve the problem. For more difficult infections, fluconazole can be administered in 150 or 200 mg daily doses for as long as is necessary to clear the problem. It has a very good safety record in terms of freedom from adverse effects. However, because of its inhibition of cytochrome P-450 enzymes, there are many potential drug-drug interactions. Discussion of the medications involved in these drug-drug interactions lies outside the scope of this chapter. Because of its association with liver damage, the FDA has recommended that oral administration of ketoconazole should not be used for dermatophyte fungal infections,

Terbinafine, a member of the allylamine family, rather than the azoles, is the medication most often used when oral administration is desired for cutaneous dermatophyte fungal infections. In adults, terbinafine is administered in a dose of 250 mg/day. Numerous adverse effects, including some severe cutaneous reactions, have been reported with the use of terbinafine. It, too, inhibits cytochrome P-450 enzymes, and for that reason, it also is associated with many potential drug-drug interactions. All of the orally administered azoles mentioned above for candidiasis are also effective for dermatophyte fungal infections. All of these oral agents require a prescription, and recent data suggest increasing fungal resistance when they are used for the treatment of dermatophytosis.

## Antiviral Therapy

Several drugs are available for the treatment of infections due to herpes simplex virus (HSV) and varicella-zoster virus (VZV). Only those available for oral administration are included here as the topical agents are, in our opinion, relatively ineffective. The three products widely available for oral administration include acyclovir (Zovirax), valacyclovir (Valtrex), and famciclovir (Famvir). All of three require a prescription, and all are available as generic products. Of these, acyclovir is the least expensive, but valacyclovir is more widely prescribed because of a simpler administration schedule. All of these medications are nucleoside analogues and have a similar mechanism of action whereby they are phosphorylated by viral thymidine kinase into very potent inhibitors of viral DNA polymerase. All three are equally safe and, in appropriate dosage, are equally effective. The recommended doses vary with the use of each of them. Dosage for these agents is discussed in Chapter 10.

There are no fully effective systemic medications for other genital viral infections such as molluscum contagiosum, HPV-induced warts, and HPV-related malignancies. For the most part, these are treated with destructive methods or surgical removal, even though some topical therapies are available. These treatments are discussed in the chapters related to these disorders.

## REFERENCES

1. Hanna S, Zip C, Shear NH. What is the risk of harm associated with topical calcineurin inhibitors? *J Cutan Med Surg.* 2019;23(4_suppl):19S-26S. doi:10.1177/1203475419857688
2. Guttman-Yassky E, Hanifin JM, Boguniewicz M, et al. The role of phosphodiesterase 4 in the pathophysiology of atopic dermatitis and the perspective for its inhibition. *Exp Dermatol.* 2019;28(1):3-10. doi:10.1111/exd.13808
3. Reszke R, Krajewski P, Szepietowski JC. Emerging therapeutic options for chronic pruritus. *Am J Clin Dermatol.* 2020;21(5):601-618. doi:10.1007/s40257-020-00534-y
4. Cheng HS, Fernández-Peñas P. Allergic contact dermatitis of the anogenital region in men and women. *J Low Genit Tract Dis.* 2020;24(2):221-224. doi:10.1097/LGT.0000000000000516
5. Turner NA, Sharma-Kuinkel BK, Maskarinec SA, et al. Methicillin-resistant *Staphylococcus aureus*: an overview of basic and clinical research. *Nat Rev Microbiol.* 2019;17:203-218. doi:10.1038/s41579-018-0147-4
6. Bassetti M, Carnelutti A, Castaldo N, Peghin M. Important new therapies for methicillin-resistant *Staphylococcus aureus. Expert Opin Pharmacother.* 2019;20(18):2317-2334. doi:10.1080/14656566.2019.1675637

# Diagnostic and Therapeutic Procedures 4

LIBBY EDWARDS

Unlike many specialties, diagnostic and therapeutic procedures for outpatient anogenital diseases generally are limited. For skin disease, the area of abnormality is visible, so that the evaluation and management of this area rarely require expensive imaging or depend upon sophisticated equipment or the assistance of multiple specialties. However, complex urologic and gynecologic surgical procedures to correct structural abnormalities are beyond the scope of this book.

For the majority of patients, the relevant aspects of evaluation are a brief and directed history, careful visual examination, microscopy of vaginal fluid or the scale of some skin conditions, and, at times, a fungal culture or a skin biopsy. The careful inspection of the skin requires only a good light, stirrups for women, and, often, simple magnification of a headband magnifier that can be ordered online for under $30 **(Fig. 4-1)**. Examination with a colposcope and use of acetic acid or toluene blue are not needed.[1] In fact, a recent study of 400 women showed an overall concordance rate of only 53.9% of the vulvoscopic appearance of HSIL (high-grade squamous intraepithelial lesion), LSIL (low-grade squamous intraepithelial lesion), and carcinoma compared to the biopsy findings.[2] However, familiarity with normal structures and variants of anogenital skin is important (see Chapter 1), as is an understanding of variable presentations of classic skin diseases in damp, thin skin folds. Often, the diagnosis of skin disease on the genitalia is obvious, with classic signs such as the crinkling white skin of lichen sclerosus and further evaluation for the primary abnormality is unnecessary.

However, the typical morphology of skin disease on dry, keratinized skin often is modified in the folds of genital skin. Intertriginous areas often are somewhat pink normally, and moisture, heat, and friction obscure scale and change the appearance of dermatoses **(Fig. 4-2)**. When the morphology of skin diseases is atypical or nonspecific, there are methods for narrowing down possibilities when a firm diagnosis cannot be made and for formulating empiric therapy.

For those diseases that display objective abnormalities, the cause is nearly always infection, tumor, or noninfectious inflammation that is often immune mediated. Even when the exact diagnosis cannot be ascertained by examination or biopsy, infection and tumor can be ruled out by cultures and biopsies. Most visible skin disease that is not tumor or infection is corticosteroid responsive. Sometimes a definitive diagnosis cannot be made, and when easily diagnosed and dangerous conditions have ruled out, a trial of presumptive therapy is reasonable and often beneficial.

The management of genital skin diseases is usually inexpensive, but often time-consuming, because careful and sensitive patient education generally is required, and attention to multifactorial processes such as secondary infection, estrogen deficiency, and irritant contact dermatitis is important. Except for radiation therapy and the surgical removal of growths, the therapy of most genital disorders is medical, consisting of self-administered oral and topical medications. There are several office procedures, however, including intralesional therapy, cryotherapy, unroofing procedures for cysts and sinus tracts of hidradenitis suppurativa, and lysis of adhesions of scarring dermatoses that are simple and enhance the patients' quality of life.

## Diagnostic Procedures

The diagnostic procedures for genital skin diseases are performed in the office or at the bedside. Only careful eyes, a microscope, glass slides and cover-slips, 10%-20% potassium hydroxide (KOH), and normal saline are required for the majority of patients. Although these procedures are easy and quick to perform, the interpretation of the microscopic findings requires experience. Therefore, unexpected results or a poor response to therapy should be further evaluated by appropriate cultures, molecular studies, or biopsies to corroborate the microscopic findings.

The use of a speculum allows for visualization of the vaginal walls and sampling of vaginal fluid for microscopic examination and culture. Clinicians who care for women with vulvar dermatoses or vulvar pain should invest in a small narrow, straight Pederson speculum, which produces far less distention of the introitus and less pain on insertion than does the standard Graves speculum with its bulbous tip **(Fig. 4-3)**. Although the visualization of the cervix is more difficult with the Pederson speculum, the cervix is generally not crucial to the diagnosis

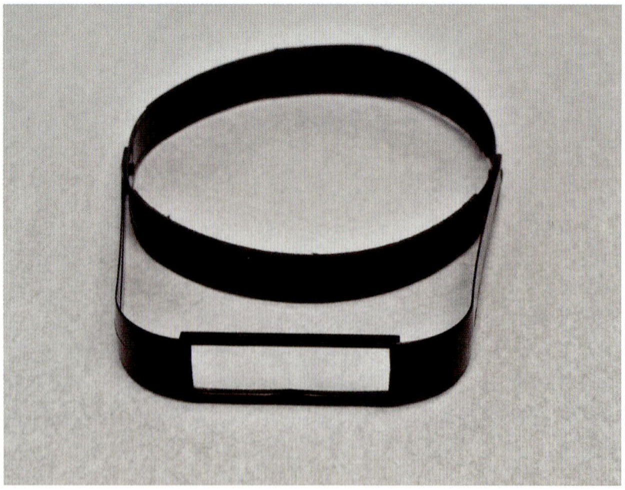

Fig. 4-1. This headband magnifier is available online in 2021 for $28 and allows for good visualization of finer skin structures.

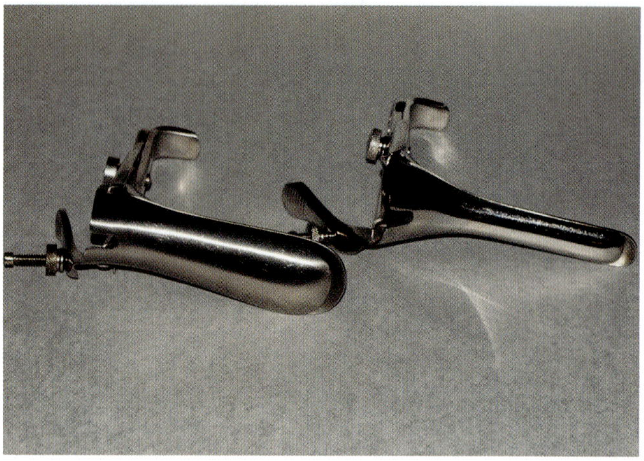

Fig. 4-3. The regular Graves speculum has a bulbous tip designed to expose the cervix for a Papanicolaou smear; this can be uncomfortable and unnecessary for women with introital pain due to skin disease or vulvodynia. A small Pederson speculum with the narrow straight blades is more comfortable and generally adequate.

and management of vulvovaginal skin diseases. A pediatric speculum is occasionally useful for those patients with severe pain with insertion of a speculum.

## Clinical Examination *(See Also Chapter 3)*

By far the most important diagnostic "procedure" is a careful examination of the skin. History is relatively unimportant, since this area is visible. For older providers, inexpensive magnification is important, and for all examiners, proper exposure of the area and a good light are necessary.

Dermatologists are familiar with the diagnosis of skin disease by morphologic appearance. However, skin disease in the genital area is modified by the location that exhibits less scale, less well-demarcated plaques, and frequent erosions rather than intact blisters. Formulation of a diagnosis is challenging at times, but an organized approach can be extremely useful (**Table 4-1**).

To help deal with this difficulty, the International Society for the Study of Vulvovaginal Disease (ISSVD) has developed a clinical diagnostic classification based on the appearance of the skin for vulvovaginal skin disease, which is also useful for male genital disease (**Table 4-2**). This classification forms the basic outline for this book. When the diagnosis is not obvious from the appearance of the skin alone, a biopsy is generally performed. Unfortunately, when the presentation of the skin disease clinically is nonspecific, the biopsies are often nonspecific as well. However, even when a biopsy is not diagnostic, the biopsy adds information. A second ISSVD classification,

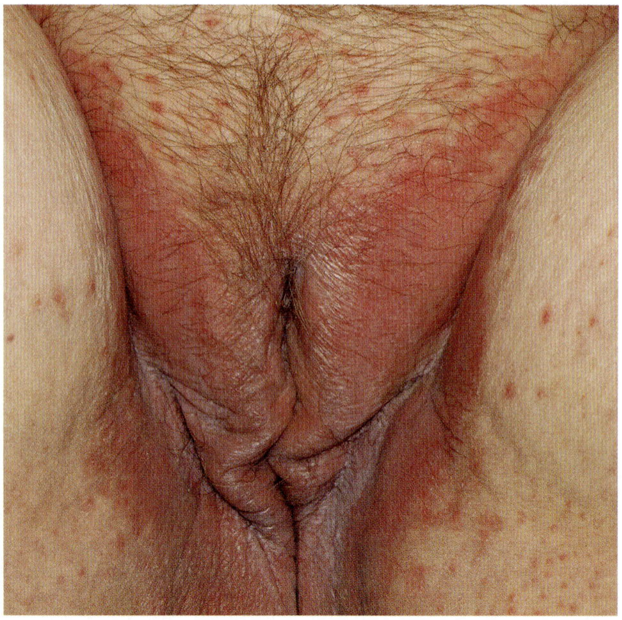

Fig. 4-2. Psoriasis is usually a skin disease characterized by heavy white scale, but on damp genital skin, the scale is inapparent.

### TABLE 4-1

### Diagnosis of Unknown Skin Disease

- Categorize by color and other visible changes (ie, red patch, white disorders, pustules), and see appropriate chapters in this book for differential diagnosis. If no diagnosis;
- Perform indicated microscopy and/or cultures. If no diagnosis;
- Biopsy. If no diagnosis;
  - Generate differential diagnosis according to clinical appearance (**Table 4-2**)
  - Correlate with histologic classification and differential diagnosis (**Table 4-3**) to narrow options and either formulate additional investigation or treat presumptively

that of the appearance on biopsy, can be used (Table 4-3). Cross-referencing the clinical diagnostic classification with the histologic classification narrows the differential diagnosis. The best dermatopathologists, when the diagnosis is not obvious, give not only a microscopic description with pertinent negatives but also suggest possible clinical diagnoses that would be consistent with the histology. For other clinicians without this benefit, the histologic classification can be used to glean this information.

For example, the differential diagnosis of a red patch can be gleaned from Table 4-2; item 2 is red patches and plaques, sending the clinician to Chapter 5. This chapter contains diseases in the differential diagnosis of red patches and plaques, including; allergic or irritant contact dermatitis, atopic dermatitis (eczema), lichen simplex chronicus, *Candida*, lichen planus, Zoon vulvitis/balanitis, Hailey-Hailey disease, extramammary Paget disease, differentiated vulvar intraepithelial neoplasia, penile intraepithelial neoplasia, high-grade squamous intraepithelial neoplasia, and eczema from rubbing and scratching superimposed on dermatitis; the differential diagnosis can be narrowed to eczema (atopic dermatitis) and contact dermatitis.

**TABLE 4-2**

**2011 ISSVD Clinical Classification of Vulvar Dermatological Disorders and Chapters That Discuss the Differential Diagnosis of Each Classification**

1. Skin-colored lesions (Chapter 7)
   a. Skin-colored papules and nodules
   b. Skin-colored plaques
2. Red lesions: patches and plaques (Chapter 5)
   a. Eczematous and lichenified diseases
   b. Red patches and plaques (no epithelial disruption)
3. Red lesions: papules and nodules (Chapter 6)
   a. Red papules
   b. Red nodules
4. White lesions (Chapter 8)
   a. White papules and nodules
   b. White patches and plaques
5. Dark-colored (brown, blue, gray, or black) lesions (Chapter 9)
   a. Dark-colored patches
   b. Dark-colored papules and nodules
6. Blisters (Chapter 10)
   a. Vesicles and bullae
   b. Pustules
7. Erosions and ulcers (Chapter 11)
   a. Erosions
   b. Ulcers
8. Edema (Chapter 12)
   a. Skin-colored edema
   b. Pink or red edema

(Reprinted with permission from Lynch PJ, Moyal-Barraco M, Scurry J, Stockdale C. 2011 ISSVD terminology and classification of vulvar dermatological disorders: an approach to clinical diagnosis. *J Low Genit Tract Dis.* 2012;16:139-144.)

**TABLE 4-3**

**2006 ISSVD Histologic Classification of Vulvar Dermatological Disorders**

- Spongiotic pattern (edema of the epidermis)
  - Atopic dermatitis
  - Allergic contact dermatitis
- Acanthotic pattern (thickened epidermis)—formerly squamous cell hyperplasia and psoriasiform dermatitis
  - Psoriasis
  - Lichen simplex chronicus
- Lichenoid pattern (lymphocytes in the upper dermis abutting the dermal-epidermal junction
  - Lichen sclerosus
  - Lichen planus
- Dermal homogenization pattern
  - Lichen sclerosus
- Vesiculobullous pattern
  - Pemphigoid
  - Linear IgA disease
- Acanthotic pattern (loss of attachment between epidermal cells)
  - Hailey-Hailey disease
  - Papular genitocrural acantholysis
- Granulomatous pattern—inflammation consisting of histiocytes and other white blood cells, especially mononuclear cells, as well as giant cells
  - Crohn disease
  - Melkersson-Rosenthal syndrome
  - Hidradenitis suppurativa
- Vasculopathic pattern
  - Aphthous ulcer
  - Behçet disease
  - Plasma cell mucositis

## Cytologic Smears

The microscopic evaluation of scale and vaginal fluid is crucial to the diagnosis of some types of vaginitis and for the diagnosis of tinea in a setting that could alternatively represent psoriasis, contact dermatitis, lichen simplex chronicus, erythrasma, etc. In the case of the evaluation of vaginal infections, even a self-collected swab can be far, far more useful than a telephone diagnosis on the basis

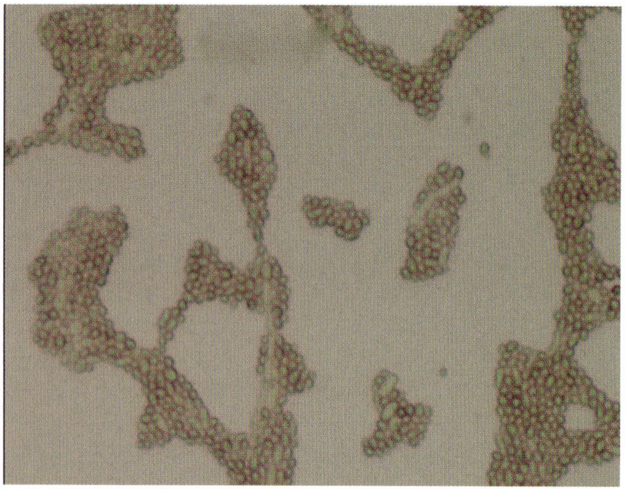

Fig. 4-4. A vaginal swab from a patient with candidiasis left in a culturette tube for 2 days shows obvious sheets of budding yeast without mycelia.

of symptoms.3 We have found that women can be given a culturette tube to capture vaginal fluid and mail to the office with excellent concordance to testing in the office for candidiasis, bacterial vaginosis, and estrogen maturation index. Most culturette brands yield obvious sheets of buds after 48 hours, but some can take as long as a week to become positive (Fig. 4-4).

Sadly, more and more gynecology offices have no microscope, severely limiting the evaluation of vaginitis.

## Fungal Preparations

Fungal preparations are essential to the diagnosis of some anogenital diseases. Men generally interpret all anogenital itching as produced by "jock itch" or tinea infection, whereas women assume that all vulvovaginal itching represents a yeast infection. The confirmation or elimination of these conditions is vital.

KOH 10%-20% solution is a basic agent that dissolves the keratin of epithelial (squamous) cells, allowing spores as well as fungal hyphae and pseudohyphae to be seen more clearly. The reliability of this test depends on the choice of the lesion to be sampled, adequate dissolution of cells so fungal elements are best visualized, and the experience of the examiner in distinguishing fungal elements from artifacts such as hair, fabric fibers, cell membranes, and fractures in crusts.

A fungal preparation of vaginal fluid is much easier than that of scale from skin, because there are fewer artifacts, and the fragile mucosal squamous epithelial cells dissolve quickly. However, some infections may produce a small number of organisms that are missed on microscopic examination. Vaginal secretions are collected with a cotton-tipped applicator from secretions remaining on the blade of the withdrawn speculum, from a pool of secretions within the vagina (avoiding the cervical os) or by gently rolling the cotton tip along the vaginal walls when there is no pool of vaginal secretions. Then, a dot of vaginal fluid is touched to the slide, rather than smeared on, which can distort the preparation. Care should be taken to avoid a too-thick preparation that prevents a careful examination. If the vagina is dry and there are no obvious secretions, then the cotton tip should be rolled onto the slide.

The best areas of skin to sample for tinea cruris (dermatophytosis) or cutaneous candidiasis include the peripheral scale from plaques of tinea, and pustule roofs, or white, cheesy material produced by suspected yeast. These elements are removed by gently scraping with the rounded surface of a number 15 scalpel blade. In the damp areas of the genitalia, the sample usually adheres to the scalpel blade and can be wiped onto the glass slide. Dry, hair-bearing skin should be moistened with water so that the scale sticks to the blade until it is smeared onto the slide.

Once the vaginal secretions or scale is applied to the glass slide, a drop of KOH is placed on the material to dissolve the keratin from cells and to enhance the visibility of fungal elements. A coverslip is applied, and firm pressure with slight agitation of the coverslip with the back of a fingernail or a pencil eraser (to avoid distracting fingerprints on the coverslip) flattens and augments the dissolution of keratin. Although the nonkeratinized epithelial (squamous) cells in vaginal smears deteriorate quickly after exposure to KOH, the scale of keratinized skin requires further attention to dissolve so that fungi and yeasts can be easily detected. The examiner can use KOH mixed with dimethyl sulfoxide or DMSO (available at medical supply facilities) to enhance dissolution. Or the examiner can simply allow 10-15 minutes for the KOH to disintegrate the cells. In addition, scale dissolves more quickly after addition of KOH if the slide is gently warmed over an alcohol flame.

Fungal elements are best visualized by lowering the condenser to increase the contrast between fungi elements and epithelial cells. Spores, buds, and hyphal elements appear refractile and sometimes very slightly green, and these are much smaller than common artifacts, such as hair and fibers. Dermatophytes appear as branching, septate hyphae that cross over cell membranes (Fig. 4-5). *Candida albicans* and *Candida tropicalis* appear as budding yeasts with hyphae or nonseptate, branching pseudohyphae (Fig. 4-6). At times, cell membranes in the process of dissolving resemble hyphae or pseudohyphae (Fig. 4-7). When this is suspected, pressure and slight agitation of the coverslip disrupts the cell membranes more efficiently and differentiates between true hyphae/pseudohyphae and this artifact. Non-*albicans/tropicalis* species of yeast are characterized by buds without mycelia (Fig. 4-8). The specific dermatophyte species of tinea cruris cannot be recognized from the smear. A culture is required to speciate a dermatophyte on the rare occasion that this is desired. Oil droplets and air bubbles can be

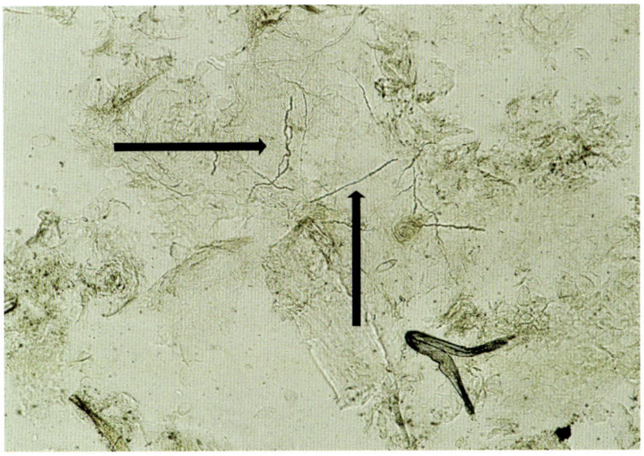

Fig. 4-5. A fungal preparation of skin cells scraped from the surface of tinea shows long dark hyphae (*arrows*) that are easily visible when the squamous cells dissolve from the KOH.

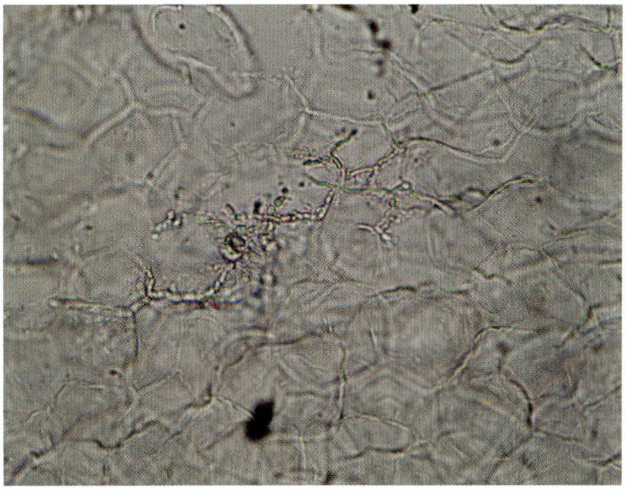

Fig. 4-7. When cell membranes are only partially dissolved, they can mimic the branching hyphae of tinea and candidiasis.

confused with yeast buds at times, but the variability in size and very round shape distinguish these from yeast buds **(Fig. 4-9)**. "Tinea" versicolor (which occurs uncommonly in the genital area) is a misnomer because it is a yeast rather than a dermatophyte or true "tinea" infection. It exhibits short, curved hyphae and spores/buds microscopically **(Fig. 4-10)**.

## Saline "Wet Mount" Preparation (See Also Chapter 14)

Information from an examination of vaginal secretions is sometimes extremely important in the evaluation of the vulva since irritating or infected vaginal secretions touch the vulva. A microscopic evaluation of vaginal secretions using normal saline under a coverslip permits an evaluation of the morphology of cells, a screen for inflammation and estrogen effect, and a crude survey of colonizing and infecting organisms. The diagnosis of bacterial vaginosis can be made only with a wet mount that shows clue cells and the absence of lactobacilli in conjunction with a positive whiff test and a pH >4.5.

A common mistake in the interpretation of a wet mount is a quick directed scan for yeast and clue cells, although even more common is submission of secretions for expensive molecular testing for infection with the incorrect assumption that this covers all causes of vaginitis. Secretions are collected as described above for evaluation for *Candida* spp. However, the secretions are transferred from the cotton-tipped applicator by touching (if abundant) or gently rolling (if scant) onto the glass slide. Care should be taken to avoid the thick application of secretions, which interferes with visualization.

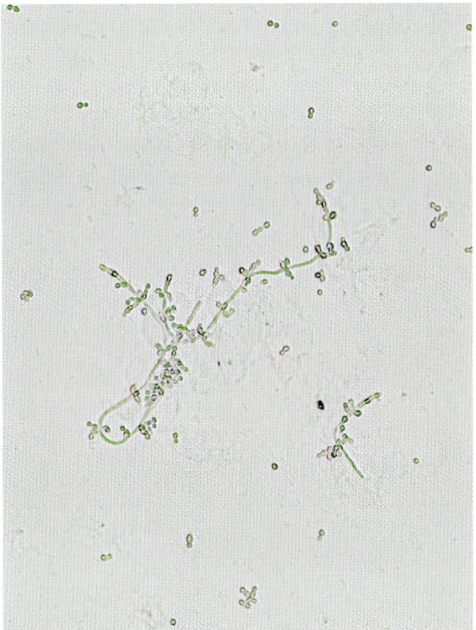

Fig. 4-6. Candidiasis shows not only branching mycelia but also budding yeast on higher power.

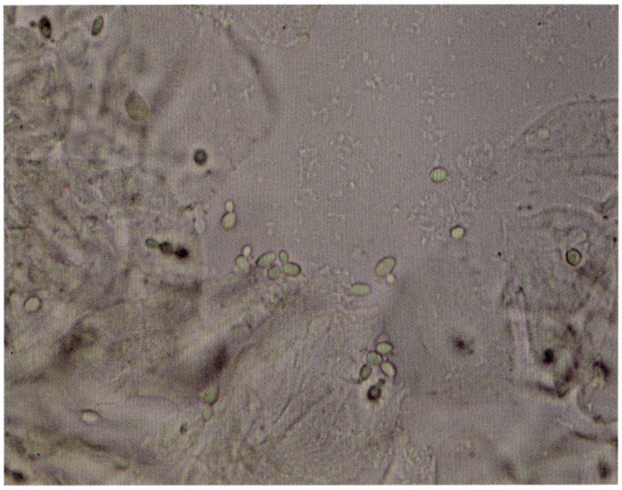

Fig. 4-8. Non-albicans *Candida* shows only buds, without mycelia, on wet mount. These elongated almost caplet-shaped buds represent *Candida krusei*.

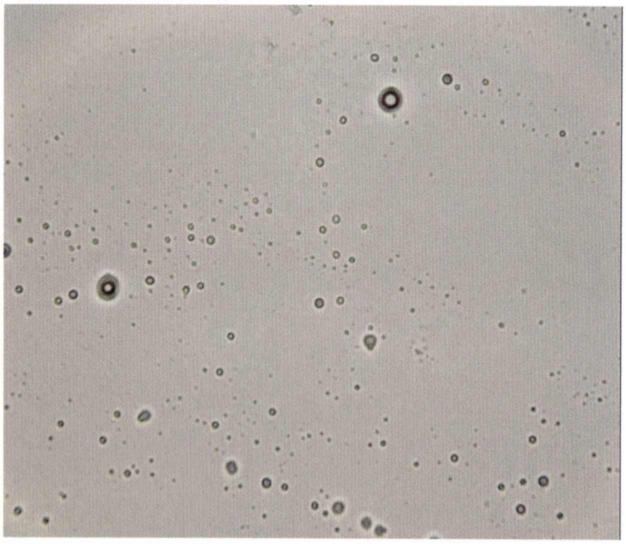

Fig. 4-9. Air bubbles or oil droplets can mimic buds of yeast. However, these do not exhibit budding, and they show marked variability in size compared to the buds of non-albicans *Candida*.

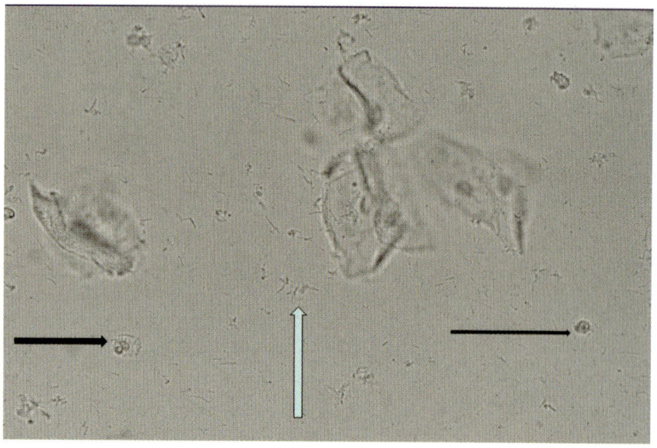

Fig. 4-11. A wet mount is crucial in the diagnosis of chronic vulvovaginal symptoms; squamous cells should be large, flat, folded, and mature, there should be only one white blood cell (*black arrows*) per squamous epithelial cell, and bacteria should be predominately the small rods of lactobacilli (*blue arrow*).

Some clinicians prefer inserting the cotton-tipped applicator into a test tube and adding a few drops of saline to dilute the secretions and separate the cells to better evaluate the morphology. This author has tried both methods but has found that the evaluation of white blood cells is problematic when the vaginal secretions are first diluted. First, inflammatory cells stick to the sides of a test tube (and the sides of a culturette tube if secretions on the cotton-tipped applicator are inserted into a culturette tube for later evaluation). Second, the sample is diluted so that detection of lactobacilli can be difficult.

A knowledge of the normal components of vaginal secretions and common artefacts is needed to evaluate vaginal secretions beyond the absence of yeast, clue cells, and trichomonads **(Fig. 4-11)**. Mature epithelial cells shed from a well-estrogenized vaginal epithelium appear as large, often folded, polygonal cells with abundant cytoplasm and a small, condensed nucleus. A crude maturation index can be performed, in which the degree of maturation of epithelial cells is estimated (and this is all that is needed for the evaluation of vulvar discomfort). Immature epithelial cells, or parabasal cells, are much smaller and rounder than mature cells, with proportionately larger nuclei **(Fig. 4-12)**. These less mature cells are seen in several settings and serve as a marker for atrophic, estrogen-deficient vaginal epithelium, erosions of the epithelium, and rapidly proliferative inflamed vaginal mucosa. Clue cells are a distinct abnormality of epithelial cells that are pathognomonic for bacterial vaginosis. These clue cells occur when bacteria adhere to epithelial cells and obscure the sharp borders of the cells so that the

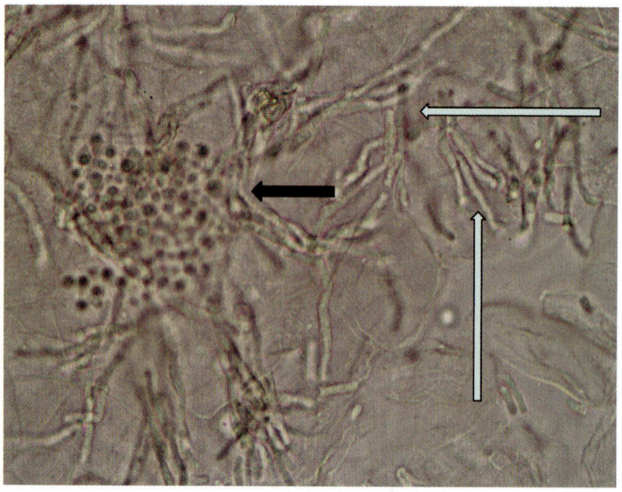

Fig. 4-10. Uncommon on anogenital skin is pityriasis ("tinea") versicolor; this fungal preparation shows clusters of buds (*black arrow*) and short hyphe (*blue arrows*) that generally do not branch.

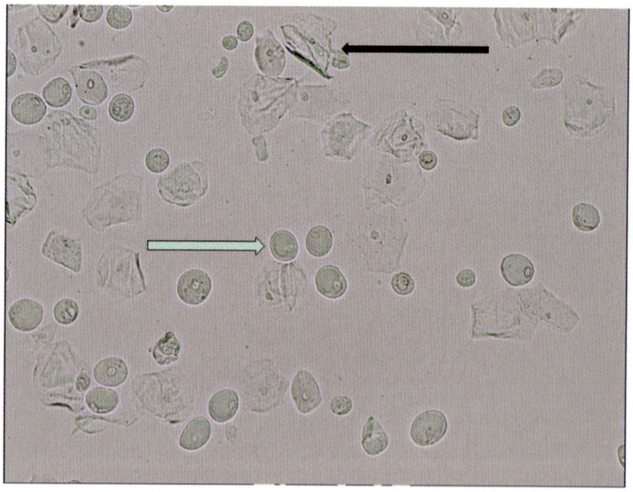

Fig. 4-12. These round cells represent parabasal cells (*blue arrow*), immature epithelial cells shed from thin estrogen-deficient vaginal walls, and normal flat, folded mature squamous epithelial cells are scant (*black arrow*).

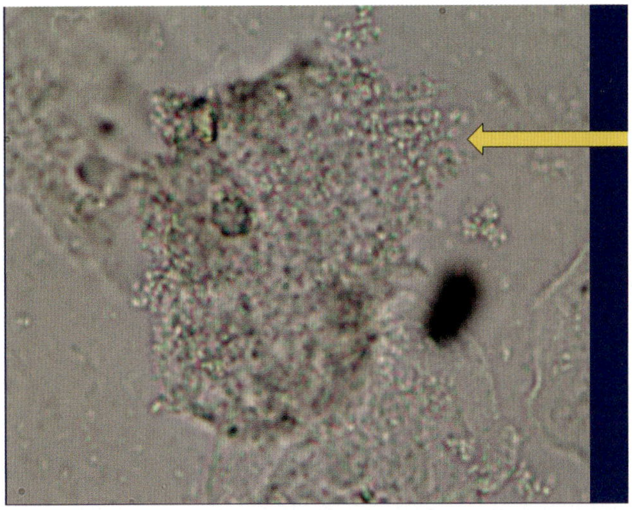

Fig. 4-13. The presence of clue cells, epithelial cells coated with bacteria so that the borders are ragged (*arrow*), is pathognomonic for bacterial vaginosis, and a more important sign than the presence of bacteria that suggests this diagnosis on molecular testing.

edge appears ragged and the cytoplasm appears granular (Fig. 4-13).

Although many different organisms are normal vaginal inhabitants, lactobacilli are the most common bacteria seen on a saline preparation of normal vaginal secretions of a well-estrogenized woman. These appear as rods of variable lengths. Occasionally, lactobacilli attach to each other from end to end, to form very long filaments, formerly believed to represent *Leptothrix* (Fig. 4-14). These strands are sometimes confused with the hyphae of *C albicans or C tropicalis*. However, the filaments of lactobacilli are smaller in caliber than yeast, and these are nonbranching, when compared to the hyphae and pseudohyphae of *C albicans*.

Other parameters evaluable from a saline preparation are the numbers and types of white blood cells. Leukocytes are regularly present, normally at a ratio of 1:1 or less with epithelial cells. Inflammation, which can be produced by *Trichomonas* infection, an irritated or superinfected atrophic vagina, erosive vaginal dermatoses, or desquamative inflammatory vaginitis, is characterized by an increase in white blood cells (Fig. 4-15). The inflammatory cells can be either lymphocytes or neutrophils, but there is no published information on the implications of this difference. Some clinicians believe that bacterial infections (excluding bacterial vaginosis) are more likely to be characterized by neutrophilic inflammation, whereas noninfectious inflamed dermatoses, such as lichen planus, are more likely to result in an influx of lymphocytes. This author has found this distinction to be unreliable.

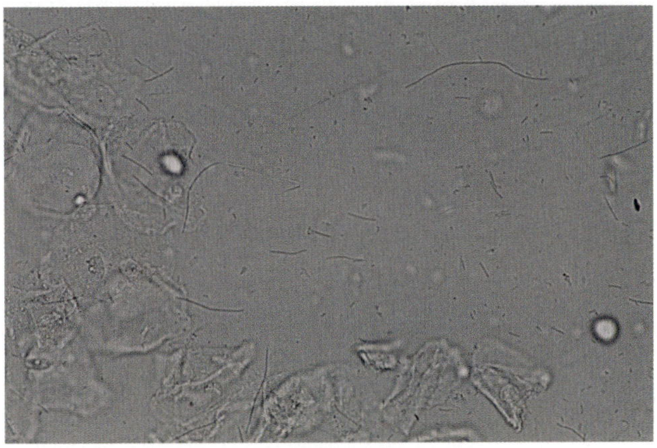

Fig. 4-14. Sometimes, lactobacilli line up end to end to form long filaments. Although some believe this occurs as a result of treatment for candidiasis and causes symptoms of itching and irritation, these authors find this to represent a normal variant.

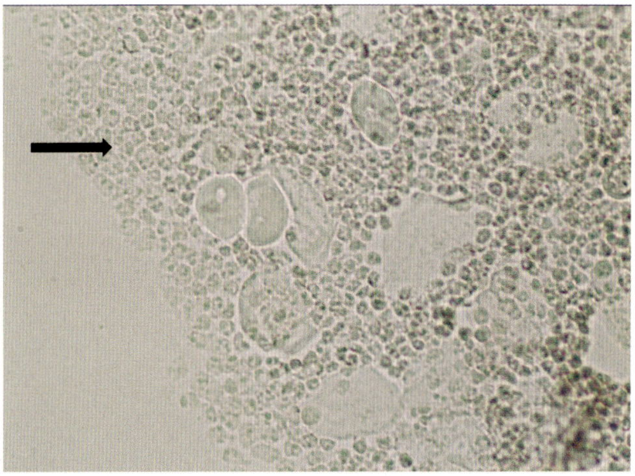

Fig. 4-15. Inflammation is characterized by increased numbers of white blood cells (*arrow*); this wet mount shows sheets of lymphocytes. Vaginal inflammation is often characterized by the presence of round parabasal cells as well.

## Microscopic Examination for Infestations

The three infestations that produce marked anogenital symptoms are scabies, pinworms, and pubic lice. Lice and their nits can be seen by the very careful naked eye or the simple magnifiers mentioned earlier, although a low-power microscopic examination of a hair with a nit is more conclusive.

The most important aspects of an evaluable scabies preparation are the correction selection of a burrow and the aggressive rather than gentle removal of the affected epidermis. The microscopic confirmation of scabies is often difficult and requires practice. The average patient with scabies has few mites despite widespread rash, most of which results from the immunologic response to the mite and the secondary eczema produced by itching and rubbing. Although one would expect a burrow to present as a linear papule, the burrow of these microscopic parasites actually appear as burrow an edematous, oval papule, with the best burrows for sampling being unscratched. Usually, even those patients with genital

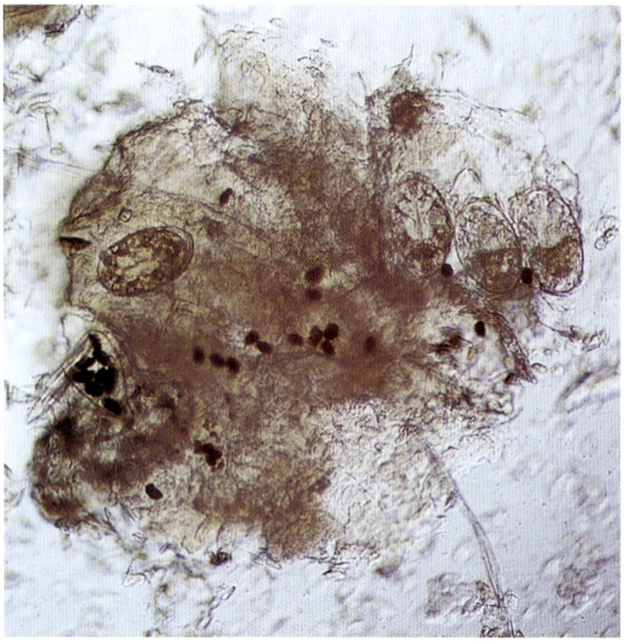

Fig. 4-16. Skin scrapings for scabies is difficult, because the identification of an appropriate site is tricky, and small numbers of mites can cause widespread itching and skin disease. However, the ova and brown feces (scybala) are more often obtained and are diagnostic as well.

scabies have more accessible and appropriate burrows between fingers or on the ventral wrists. The classic nodules of scabies most common on the penis and scrotum are not appropriate for scraping, as the mite is usually deeper in the skin. A thin layer of epidermis is shaved with a number 15 scalpel blade, and the skin specimen is laid flat on a glass slide. A drop of normal saline or immersion oil is applied to the material, and a coverslip is affixed. The presence of ova, feces (scybala), or the mite itself is definitive evidence of infestation **(Fig. 4-16)**. The mite, if present, is not subtle and is rarely missed. Eggs are regular, smooth, and fairly large, so they also are usually identified without difficulty. Scybala, however, are regular, clustered, small, golden brown globules that require some experience to identify with confidence. A negative scraping does not eliminate scabies as a diagnosis. A biopsy adds information in the absence of a positive scraping, by either identification of the mite or by the presence of eosinophils, suggests a parasite of some type. A biopsy can also be useful in the patient with genital scabietic nodules but no burrows since that biopsy specimen will be interpreted as an arthropod bite consistent with but not diagnostic of scabies, although the mite usually is not identified.

Nocturnal perianal pruritus suggests pinworm infestation, especially in children. The "Scotch-tape test" can usually diagnose this condition. Before the patient arises in the morning, the perianal skin is stretched to evert the distal mucosa slightly. The sticky side of cellophane tape is applied to the anus to affix ova deposited during the night. The tape is then stuck to a glass slide and is examined microscopically under low power. Multiple, monomorphous ova are generally easily identified when pinworms are present.

### Tzanck Preparation

When performed by experienced examiners, Tzanck smears can confirm the presence of a herpetic blister, but these cannot distinguish between herpes simplex virus and varicella-zoster virus (herpes zoster and chicken pox). Some very practiced clinicians can tentatively detect abnormalities consistent with pemphigus vulgaris with this test.

Classically, the base of an erosion left by an unroofed blister is scraped with a number 15 scalpel blade, and the material on the blade is transferred to a glass slide. However, a newer study suggests that an examination of the blister roof is twice as likely to produce visible giant cells.4 Giemsa or Papanicolaou stain is applied to reveal nuclear characteristics of cells. A Tzanck preparation a herpes (simplex or zoster) blister base shows extremely large, multinucleated epithelial cells and intracytoplasmic inclusions. However, the correct interpretation of Tzanck smears requires experience, and results from even confident dermatologists can exhibit poor intraobserver and interobserver reproducibility.2 In general, this test should be confirmed by direct viral identification (immunofluorescent antibody testing, *in situ* hybridation, or polymerase chain reaction technique), culture (although false negatives are very common in some laboratories or clinical situations), or biopsy (sensitive and quick but also does not differentiate herpes simplex from herpes zoster) if there is any question as to the correct diagnosis

### Gram Stains

When treating genital disease, most clinicians do not use Gram stains for vaginal secretions or skin afflicted by other common diseases, because a culture is required for identification and sensitivities of genital pathogens. Gram stains are now considered by some to be the gold standard for the diagnosis of bacterial vaginosis, but this is not needed as a wet mount showing the presence of clue cells, and a positive whiff test are pathognomonic for bacterial vaginosis, require less than a minute, and are nearly free.

## Cultures

Cultures for bacteria and yeast are laboratory investigations that are occasionally essential and cost-effective in the diagnosis of genital symptoms. The most common use of a culture in this area of medicine is a fungal culture for yeast. This is used for vaginitis when suspected yeast is unidentified on a KOH preparation or when candidiasis is unresponsive to therapy. This is also important when intertrigo dermatitis, redness, and maceration of skin folds, with clinical yeast, are unresponsive to antifungal therapy. In this age of methicillin-resistant *Staphylococcus aureus*, cultures of folliculitis, suspected perianal streptococcal disease, and especially furuculosis are indicated to direct appropriate antibiotic therapy.

## Molecular Studies

Nucleic acid probes are newer, accurate modalities for the diagnosis of infection. Originally used in the management of genital diseases primarily for the identification of herpes simplex virus infection, polymerase chain reaction technique sometimes requires several days for results but is far more accurate than a herpes culture. Point-of-care nucleic acid probes now are used for vaginitis panels and yield results in <1 hour. These are excellent for infections, except for bacterial vaginosis, and this does not provide information on estrogen deficiency or the noninfectious inflammation of desquamative inflammatory vaginitis or vaginal lichen planus. Although molecular testing identifies the presence of bacteria associated with bacterial vaginosis, these bacteria are sometimes present while not producing the pathognomonic signs of clue cells, lack of lactobacilli, a positive whiff test, and relatively high pH.

Molecular testing for organisms has become an extraordinarily common tool for the diagnosis of vaginitis because of their simplicity. A simple swab of the base of an erosion of possible herpes simplex virus or varicella-zoster virus infection can produce a definitive and reliable answer; cervical swabs for *Chlamydia* or gonorrhea; a swab of an ulcer for syphilis, chancroid, lymphogranuloma venereum; vaginal secretions for trichomonas; swabs of skin for human papillomavirus (HPV) detection and typing are additional tests that are available. Vaginitis panels evaluate for multiple species of *Candida* and various organisms typical for bacterial vaginosis. Although the cost of PCR has decreased remarkably over the past 15 years, these panels can be quite expensive and generally yield less useful information than a wet mount and fungal culture in the investigation of vaginitis, except for testing for trichomonas.

## Dermoscopy

Dermoscopy is a newer means of evaluating the epidermis and upper dermis with a dermatoscope, a specialized handheld magnifier that, when touched or held very closely to the skin, reveals otherwise invisible structures.5 Dermoscopy is especially useful for the evaluation of pigmented lesions, sometimes allowing avoidance of a biopsy.6 Dermoscopy also can be useful in the diagnosis of scabies, and it may aid in the identification of pediculosis pubis, although this organism also can be seen with simple magnification. Dermoscopy can also confirm a diagnosis of molluscum contagiosum in the occasional patient without pathognomonic lesions. Although this form of examination is becoming more common and there are reports of its use in genital dermatology, the examiner must put the face close to the genital skin. This tends to limit dermoscopy for most providers to the occasional worrisome pigmented lesion. There are now cameras that can be attached to the dermatoscope, minimizing the close proximity needed.

## Skin Biopsies

Because skin and mucosa are superficial, obtaining a specimen for evaluation is simple, quick, safe, and relatively painless when done properly. Be aware; charges for a skin biopsy are significantly higher than those for a vulvar or vaginal biopsy, but lower than for a penile biopsy. Fortunately, the vulva and vagina are lined with epithelium, and this author codes these as skin biopsies. The clinical hallmarks that differentiate different inflammatory, infectious, and neoplastic diseases are often less characteristic and more nonspecific when occurring in skin folds and on damp skin. Therefore, a histologic evaluation of the skin may be indicated in an attempt to render a definitive diagnosis. However, if a skin finding is not easily diagnosed on the basis of the clinical appearance, the histologic appearance is often nondiagnostic as well, particularly for inflammatory dermatoses.

A skin biopsy is not an objective laboratory test, but rather consists of another clinician who examines the skin and gives an opinion on histologic changes that may or may not provide a diagnosis. Still, a biopsy provides further information to help formulate a diagnosis and often rules out some processes, as in the case of *in situ* malignancies that mimic inflammatory skin diseases. Just as a clinical differential diagnosis of skin diseases is formulated by the appearance of the skin, the histologic differential diagnosis is formulated by the microscopic appearance of a biopsy specimen (Chapter 2: "Terminology, Classification, and Diagnosis of Genital Disorders"). These two differential diagnoses can then be cross-referenced in order to narrow down possibilities. If a diagnosis is not possible on biopsy, an experienced pathologist often lists possible diagnoses under comments with the histologic description.

The provider who performs the biopsy can maximize the chances of both obtaining useful information and the experience for the patient (**Table 4-4**). This begins by choosing the appropriate lesion and taking care not to damage the specimen. Choosing a dermatopathologist or pathologist with a special interest in skin rather than a generalist to interpret the biopsy is important, and providing that person with a thoughtful differential diagnosis also ensures that the microscopist is armed with the best information to make a realistic diagnosis.

TABLE 4-4

**Genital Biopsy Tips**

- Advise patients in advance that the biopsy may not give a definitive diagnosis, but it will give more information and rule out malignancies
- For anxious patients, offer topical anesthesia before definitive local anesthesia. Compounded tetracaine 6%/lidocaine 6%, eutectic mixture of local anesthesia, lidocaine 5% ointment
- Definitive anesthesia with lidocaine1% with epinephrine and then wait 10 minutes for epinephrine to produce vasoconstriction to minimize bleeding, especially for punch biopsies
- Only biopsy visible abnormalities
- Avoid the midline when possible
- Use a punch biopsy for tumors, pigmented lesions, or firm skin
- Consider a shave biopsy for superficial dermatoses, blisters, or erosions
- Send skin biopsy specimens to a dermatopathologist or a gynecologic pathologist with a special interest and expertise in skin disease
- List a differential diagnosis on the pathology requisition
- Use the ISSVD histologic classification to interpret nondiagnostic, descriptive biopsy results

## Where to Biopsy

The usefulness of a skin biopsy depends in part upon selection of the correct areas to sample. The choice of site depends upon the disease being biopsied.

The sample of an erosion or ulcer is best obtained from the edge so that the transition of normal epithelium to the ulcer or erosion is visible to the pathologist; the complete absence of epithelium makes a definitive diagnosis of many skin diseases impossible if the sample is from the middle of the lesion (Fig. 4-17). However, if the ulcer is firm, an additional sample of the firm area should be obtained in case the lesion represents an ulcerated or eroded tumor (Fig. 4-18). Likewise, a blistering condition should include the edge of the blister, and if a small vesicle is present, this can be removed in its entirety (Fig. 4-19). The biopsy of a blisters and erosion should be taken from the newest possible lesion, since reparative changes occur quickly, hindering the diagnosis. A tumor is biopsied from the thickest area, and sometimes several biopsies may be required (Fig. 4-20). Generally, a biopsy of a papule or plaque should include involved skin only (Fig. 4-21). In those skin diseases that show white epithelium, this white skin should be sampled (Fig. 4-22). Very old, healing lesions of any skin disease are usually poor choices of sites.

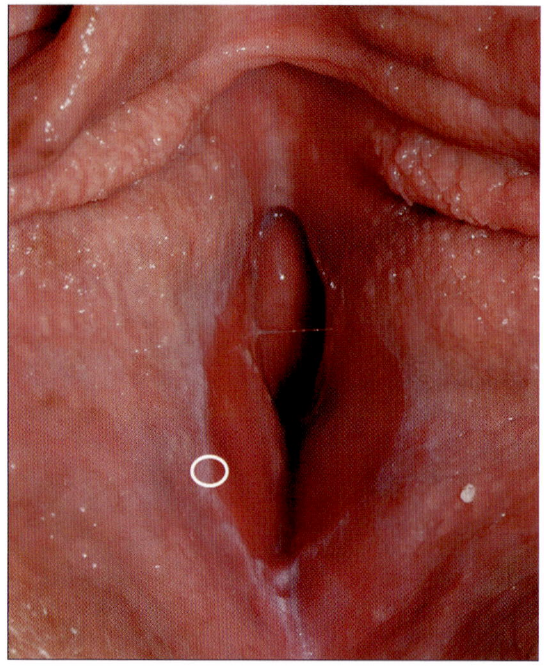

Fig. 4-17. The edge of an erosive or ulcerative disease should be sampled, since diagnostic changes on biopsy are likely to be in the epithelium.

Biopsies generally are not useful when there are no skin changes. For example, a patient with pain but no visible abnormalities does not benefit from a biopsy. This includes the modest erythema often present in the vestibule of a woman or the scrotum of some men. However, a biopsy is sometimes warranted when there is doubt as to

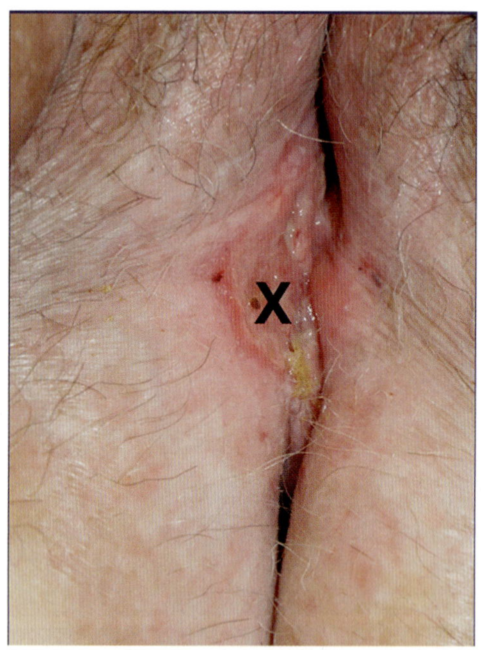


Fig. 4-18. Although the edge of an erosion is generally the best site for a biopsy, this erosion was firm to palpation, so a malignancy was considered. This indurated base was biopsied, showing a squamous cell carcinoma.

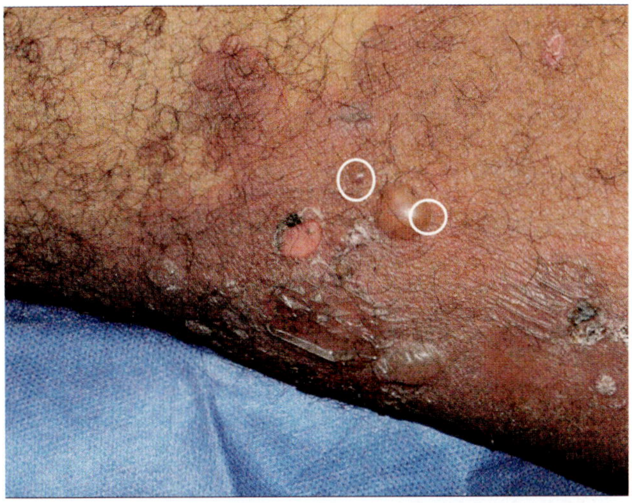

Fig. 4-19. Blistering diseases are best diagnosed when the pathologist can see the transition from normal skin to the blister; therefore, an entire small vesicle can be removed or the edge of a blister.

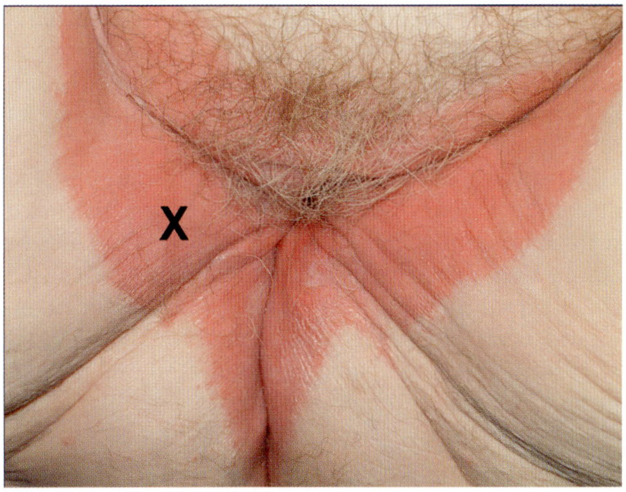


Fig. 4-21. A plaque or papule can be biopsied from fully involved skin without surrounding normal areas.

the significance of mild erythema, when a patient is adamant that their symptoms are due to inflammation rather than a condition, such as a pain syndrome, or to evaluate the activity of a known, treated disease, such as the significance of pallor in treated lichen sclerosus. The provider should be aware that a biopsy of normal genital skin often yields a histologic description of mild nonspecific chronic perivascular inflammation with acanthosis and hyperkeratosis. Therefore, mild inflammation on biopsy should not be mistaken for clinical disease.

When possible, avoid the midline and skin creases. These areas do not heal well.

Usually, multiple biopsies are only required if there are lesions with different morphologies. However, in the case of a malignancy, several biopsies may be useful in determining the best estimate of tumor thickness.

## Anesthesia

Whatever the skin biopsy technique, local anesthesia is indicated. This can be achieved quickly by infiltrating skin under the biopsy site with 0.5-1.0 mL of lidocaine 1% with epinephrine, using a 30-gauge needle. When possible, the provider should wait about 10 minutes to perform the procedure; the epinephrine produces vasoconstriction

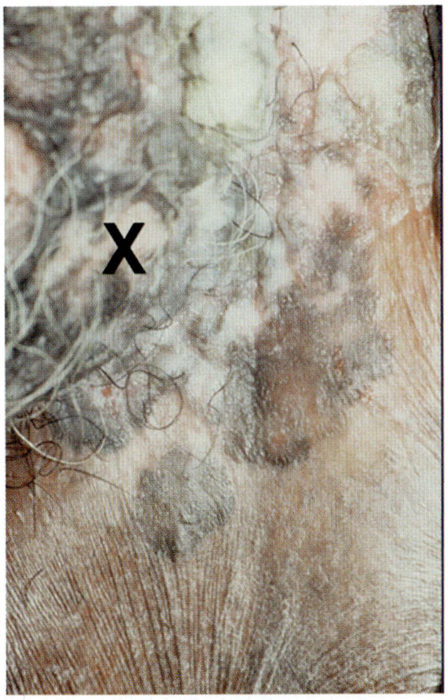


Fig. 4-20. A tumor generally should be sampled from the thickest area.

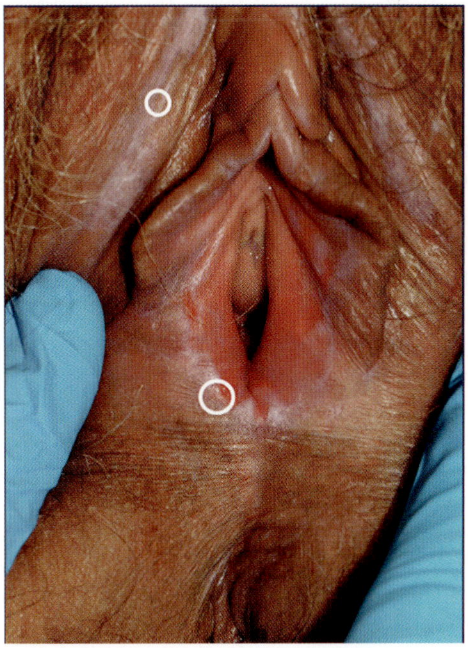

Fig. 4-22. When white areas are present, these often have high yield for a diagnosis.

and minimizes bleeding in this area of loose connective tissue. Epinephrine should be avoided in deep injections, such as blocks on the penile shaft, to prevent ischemia, but superficial anesthesia that includes epinephrine for skin biopsies is indicated and well tolerated.

Patients who are especially anxious appreciate pretreatment with a newer-generation potent topical anesthetic such as lidocaine 2.5%/prilocaine 2.5% or 4% lidocaine cream. Even more useful and well tolerated for biopsies and other uncomfortable procedures is compounded tetracaine 6%/lidocaine 6% ointment. A very thick layer of cream applied to genital skin and modified mucous membranes for 20-30 minutes partially anesthetizes the skin. If the patient is scheduled for a biopsy at a later date, patient-applied anesthetic every 15 minutes for about 2 hours before the procedure is most effective (Lynnette Margesson, MD, personal communication). These agents should not be inserted into the vagina because of the increased risk of absorption, and the vagina is less sensitive to injections than external genital skin.

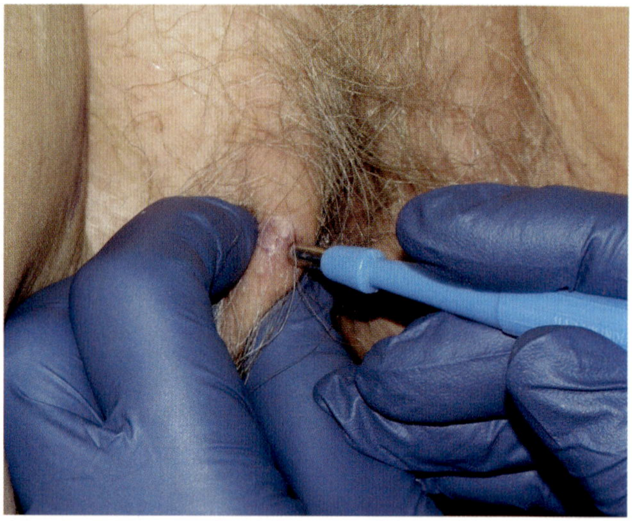

Fig. 4-23. A punch biopsy is the preferred biopsy technique when all layers of skin should be included, such as when a tumor is suspected. The punch is screwed with a back and forth rotary motion into the skin.

## Genital Skin Biopsy Techniques

The skin of the external genitalia and perianal area can be sampled by punch biopsy, shave biopsy, scissors excision, or by forceps intended to biopsy the cervix. Another useful technique is modification of the shave biopsy with use of a sharp curette.

The choice of technique depends on the possible diagnosis, the configuration of the lesion, and the location. Although some clinicians use these biopsy forceps for the vulva, this will not be discussed here because this method tends to crush the tissue, which interferes with interpretation, and the sample is often larger than required. The punch and shave biopsy techniques allow for smaller specimens and more precise sampling without the crush artifact.

A punch biopsy samples all levels of the skin; epithelium, dermis, and subcutaneous fat. Pigmented lesions, indurated lesions, and suspected neoplasms are investigated with a punch biopsy because the base of the lesion can be critical in diagnosing and assessing the prognosis of the tumor. Small lesions can be completely excised with a punch that is greater in diameter than the lesion.

A punch instrument is a cylindrical blade (generally 3-5 mm, with 3.5 commonly an adequate size that does not leave a large defect) that is applied to anesthetized tissues and, with both a rotary motion and gentle downward pressure, cuts through the epidermis and into fat, up to the hub of the punch biopsy instrument (**Figs 4-23 and 4-24**). Often, the biopsy sample remains attached at the base, and care should be taken not to crush the tissue with forceps as the plug is lifted out and the base is snipped. Rather than gripping the retained sample with forceps, the attached biopsy can be snagged and lifted with a needle, while curved iris scissors pointed toward the base of the defect detach the specimen at the base (**Fig. 4-25**). Many clinicians close punch biopsy sites with suture, whereas others leave small defects open. The suture material used is dependent on the location and the size of the lesion. Generally, keratinized, clinically hair-bearing skin is closed with fairly stiff nonabsorbable suture such as nylon. However, moist mucosa and modified mucous membrane can be closed with more comfortable, soft, absorbable sutures such as glycoprotein acid (Vicryl). Soft, nonabsorbable suture such as silk that requires removal may also be used. However, the braiding of silk somewhat predisposes to bacterial infections, and nonabsorbable sutures require a return visit for removal.

The shave biopsy is more superficial than the full-thickness punch, and this can be used with superficial dermatoses such as suspected lichen sclerosus and lichen

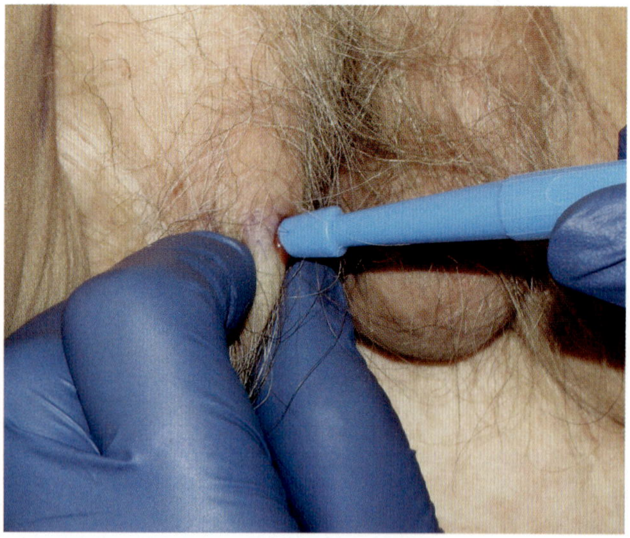

Fig. 4-24. The punch is normally driven up to the hub, so that all layers including the superficial subcutaneous tissue is sampled.

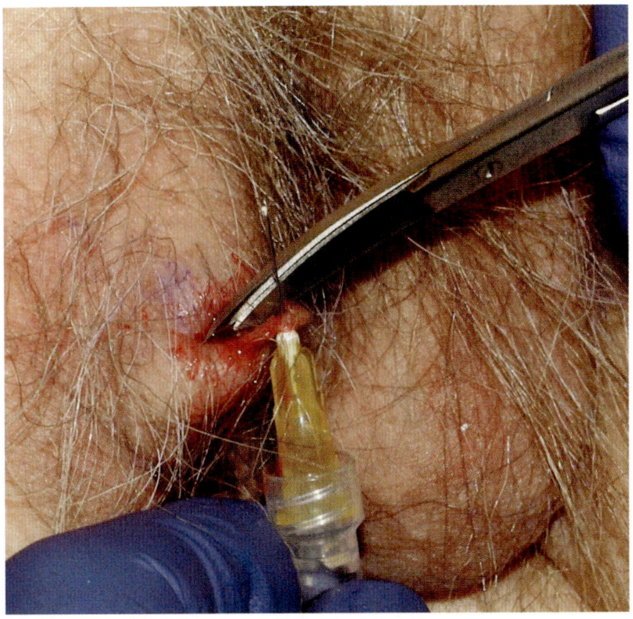

Fig. 4-25. When the skin sample remains attached at the base, care should be taken to avoid crushing it with forceps. Rather, it can be tethered with the needle that was used for anesthetizing the skin, while the tips of curved iris scissors are pointed into the biopsy hole to snip the specimen off at the base.

planus. It is also used when the roof of a fragile blister could be torn from the surface by the rotary motion of punch biopsy procedures. A shave or scissors excision is also used for the removal of a benign exophytic lesion such as a skin tag, wart, or seborrheic keratosis. The shave biopsy has the advantage of producing a more superficial biopsy site, which bleeds less, heals more quickly, and has no need for sutures. A disadvantage is that some experience is needed to ensure an adequate depth sample; if only epithelium is procured, a diagnosis usually cannot be made.

A traditional shave biopsy is performed with a number 15 scalpel blade or a double-edged razor (**Fig 4-26**). The skin is pinched into a tense mound, and then a sample is obtained well into but not through the dermis; the wound does not gape open and require suturing, and scarring is minimized.

A shave biopsy is difficult to perform on the very thin, fragile, and slippery skin of the non–hair-bearing portion of the vulva or the uncircumcised glans or inner foreskin. There are two modifications of the shave that make this more convenient. Removal of tissue with curved iris scissors is variation of a shave biopsy, which is useful on these surfaces. To avoid crush injury by forceps to this fragile skin, any 5-0 or 6-0 suture is placed through the lesional skin **(Fig. 4-27)**. The skin is then lifted by the suture, and the now exophytic skin is snipped off with curved iris scissors **(Figs. 4-28 and 4-29)**.

Hemostasis is required for these biopsies except in the case of a punch biopsy closed with a suture. Aluminum chloride, ferric chloride, or ferric subsulfate is applied to

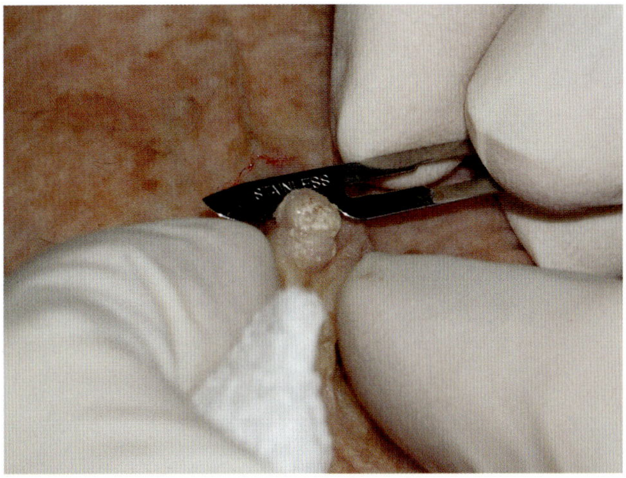

Fig. 4-26. A shave biopsy is appropriate for superficial lesions and is adequate for most inflammatory skin diseases. This has the advantage of quick healing.

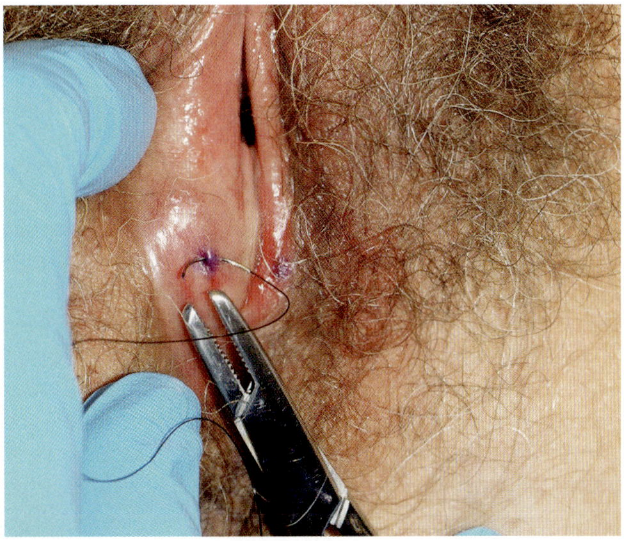

Fig. 4-27. Thin genital skin is often difficult to grasp for a shave biopsy, especially when it is wet, and forceps crush the tissue. On this skin, the lesion can be stabilized with a suture.

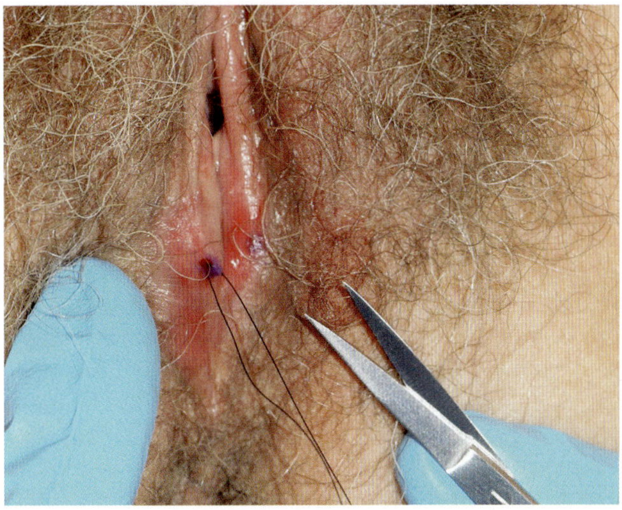

Fig. 4-28. The area to be biopsied is lifted by the suture.

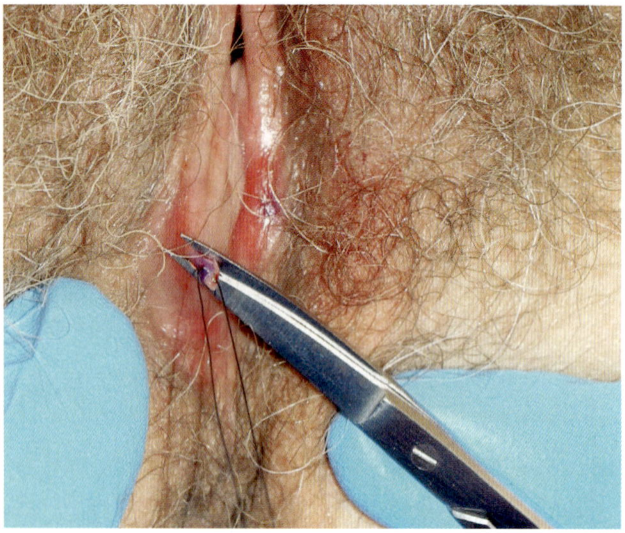

Fig. 4-29. The tips of curved iris scissors can snip the lesion with good accuracy.

the base of the biopsy site as a chemical cautery agent, to produce less tissue damage than electrocautery or silver nitrate. This author prefers aluminum chloride 20% (sold over the counter as Drysol for excessively sweaty palms and soles) because iron-containing chemical cauteries occasionally stain the skin brown/black. Sometimes hemostasis of a punch biopsy presents a challenge. Other than closing with a suture, the insertion of a small pledget of a gelatin sponge (Gelfoam) is useful when needed.

For uncommon genital processes that are likely to extend deeply into the subcutaneous tissues, such as suspected large-vessel vasculitis, necrotizing fasciitis, or panniculitis (inflammation of the fat), a deep incisional biopsy or surgical exploration is indicated.

## Vaginal Biopsy Technique

Obtaining a vaginal biopsy is more challenging. The distal vagina can sometimes be biopsied with a punch biopsy in the same manner as the external genitalia, especially when the anterior or posterior vaginal is exteriorized due to a cystocele or a rectocele. More often, the vaginal walls are not easily accessible. For most vaginal biopsies, cervical biopsy forceps are required. The vagina is anesthetized, usually requiring a syringe extender to reach the proximal vagina **(Fig. 4-30)**. Then, the biopsy forceps are used. This can be easy with a quick bite of the forceps, or the biopsy forceps may slide off the soft and slippery vaginal walls. When needed, skin hooks or a tenaculum can be used to stabilize the vaginal wall to prevent it from sliding away.

### Acetic Acid Examination

The application of 5% acetic acid (white vinegar) produces whitening of any thick or hyperkeratotic epithelium. This

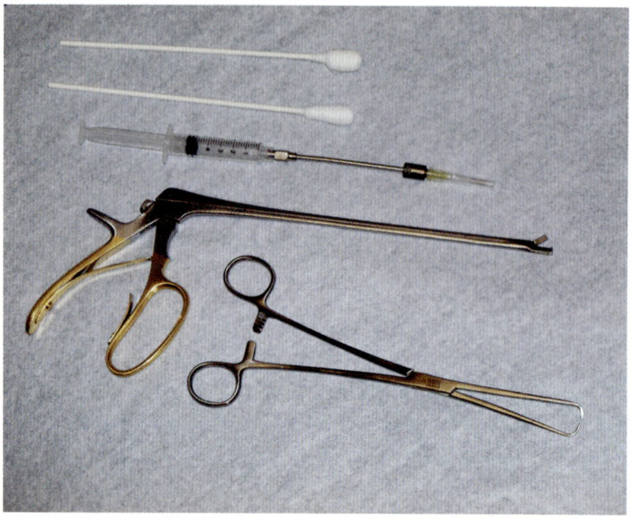

Fig. 4-30. Instruments required for a biopsy of the vaginal walls include a syringe of lidocaine 1% with epinephrine with a needle extender when more proximal vaginal lesions require anesthesia. Cervical forceps are required to remove the biopsy specimen. A cervical tenaculum can be useful to stabilize the tissue when the forceps slide off the soft and slippery vaginal epithelium.

technique originally was used to allow for identification of subtle HPV-induced lesions and to allow for early and complete treatment **(Fig. 4-31)**. However, any hyperkeratotic or inflammatory epithelial conditions whiten in response to the application of acetic acid, thus making this a sensitive but nonspecific finding.7 In addition, even normal vulvar epithelium becomes white after more extended contact with acetic acid **(Fig. 4-32)**.

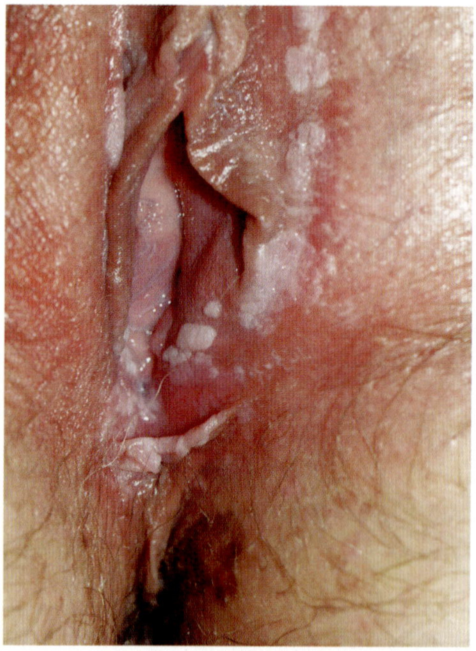

Fig. 4-31. The application of 5% acetic acid accentuates subtle hyperkeratotic lesions, such as the flat warts on the lateral inferior left labium majus, helping to guide therapy at times.

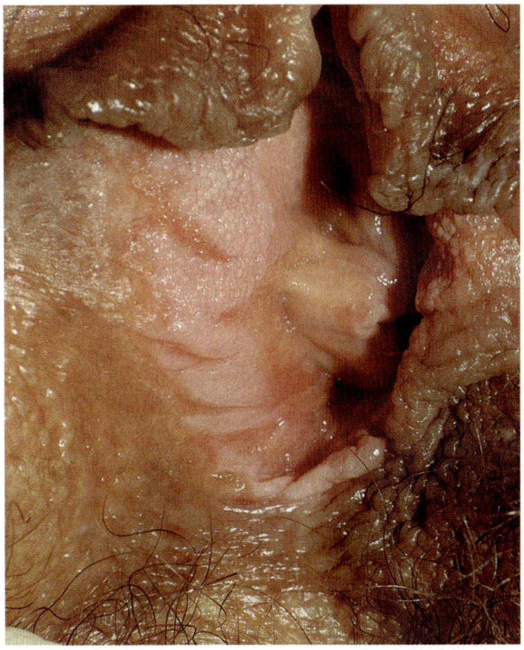

Fig. 4-32. Unfortunately, acetic acid nonspecifically produces white color of any hyperkeratotic lesion, and even turns normal mucous membrane and modified mucous membrane white with prolonged contact.

The application of acetic acid produces burning, and many clinicians believe that this acetic acid test should not be performed routinely because of this discomfort and its poor specificity. Visual inspection alone with simple magnification is accurate in evaluating the extent of clinical abnormalities, and the value of the identification and treatment of subclinical infection has not been shown. When evaluating the extent of high-grade squamous intraepithelial lesions or differentiated intraepithelial neoplasia, acetowhitening is very sensitive but with poor specificity. Clearly, acetowhite changes should be further investigated by biopsy, and many if not most vulvologists do not use acetic acid examinations.

### Wood Light Examination

The Wood light is a handheld apparatus that contains a filter that blocks all low-intensity ultraviolet light except for a band of light between 320 and 400 nm. The Wood light initially was used in detecting fungal infections of the scalp, but it is now much more useful for the identification of other conditions. This is a procedure only occasionally helpful to the genital clinician, with erythrasma being its primary use. However, a Wood light examination of tinea corporis, tinea versicolor, and epidermal disorders of pigmentation is occasionally helpful.

Erythrasma, an intertriginous infection caused by *Corynebacterium minutissimum*, produces a bright coral red fluorescence. This fluorescence is the result of a water-soluble porphyrin, and this fluorescence can be negative if the area was recently washed.

Uncommon dermatophyte fungi such as *Microsporum audouinii*, *M canis*, and *Trichophyton schoenleinii* produce a blue-green fluorescence, although most superficial fungal infections do not fluoresce, so a lack of fluorescence is usual for tinea cruris.

Pityriasis "tinea" versicolor, which characteristically presents as either hypopigmented or hyperpigmented scaly patches on the trunk, can be seen occasionally on the abdomen and thighs. A Wood light accentuates the lesions, and a dull green fluorescence is sometimes evident as well.

Localization of melanin pigment is facilitated with a Wood light examination. Melanin in the epidermis absorbs long-wave ultraviolet light, so that epidermal pigmentation is accentuated, whereas dermal pigment is relatively inapparent. In postinflammatory hyperpigmentation, the localization of melanin beneath the epidermis and in melanophages results in little color contrast with surrounding skin. However, the epidermal pigment occurring in melanoma, physiologic hyperpigmentation, and lentigines is accentuated. In addition, the depigmentation of vitiligo is accentuated by loss of melanin in the epidermis, whereas hypopigmented processes such as postinflammatory hypopigmentation show little contrast with surrounding skin.

Unfortunately, common foreign bodies such as lint and some topical medications fluoresce, so that the simple presence of fluorescence is unhelpful. Only when a characteristic pattern of fluorescence is correlated with the clinical appearance of a disease is this test useful.

## Therapeutic Procedures

The common office therapeutic procedures required for the management of benign anogenital diseases are usually simple and safe in the hands of careful generalists. Intralesional corticosteroid administration and cautious cryotherapy belong in the domain of the primary care provider.

### Cryotherapy

Cryotherapy consists of destruction of tissues by freezing. The crystallization of intracellular fluid and subsequent thaw results in cell death. Rapid freezing and slow thawing maximize destruction. Melanocytes are the most sensitive cells in the skin to low temperatures, followed by keratinocytes and, finally, fibroblasts. As a result, hypopigmentation may be a permanent consequence of vigorous cryotherapy, although posttreatment hyperpigmentation sometimes occurs but usually is transient. Cryotherapy is generally considered simple, safe, and effective even when performed by inexperienced clinicians, but the variable freezing duration required for ablation of different skin lesions depending on location, size, and cells of origin

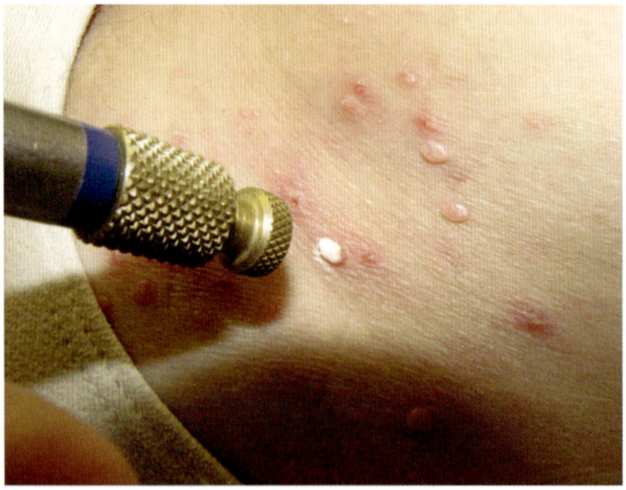

Fig. 4-33. Cryotherapy is most efficiently applied with a liquid nitrogen sprayer or cryogen gun, but this requires some practice to limit the area of freezing to the lesion without damaging surrounding tissue. Alternatively, liquid nitrogen can be applied with a cotton-tipped applicator, a slower but more precise method for many nondermatology providers.

makes this a therapy that requires some experience and care to perform well.

Liquid nitrogen, the most common cryogen used in dermatology, has a temperature of −196 °C. This agent produces marked burning with application, so patients appreciate pretreatment with a topical anesthetic such as the compounded tetracaine 6%/lidocaine 6% ointment applied generously before the appointment. Liquid nitrogen is delivered most often with either a cotton-tipped swab gently touched to the lesion or a handheld spray unit **(Fig. 4-33)**. The nozzle is directed at the center of the lesion, and short bursts of spray are applied.

Cryotherapy of the external genitalia is limited to the treatment of warts, molluscum contagiosum, seborrheic keratoses, and, by experienced clinicians and under some circumstances, high-grade squamous intraepithelial lesions. Unbiopsied pigmented lesions that are not clearly a seborrheic keratosis or a benign anogenital wart and most malignant or destructive tumors on the genitalia are usually poor candidates for cryotherapy rather than removal techniques that allow for the evaluation of surgical margins.

### Intralesional Corticosteroid Therapy

Inflammatory processes such as an inflamed epidermal cyst or an aphthous ulcer are too deep to respond to topical corticosteroids, but these often clear quickly with the injection of a corticosteroid. The medication remains in the skin for about 1 month. Also, skin diseases at times respond incompletely to topical corticosteroids, and intralesional administration can prompt improvement. This is a good management tool for the occasional patient who applies medication incorrectly or to the wrong area, producing healing that can be maintained with a lower-potency topical agent. Intralesional corticosteroids also have the advantage of avoiding systemic exposure to significant amounts of oral medication or risking the perilesional skin to the atrophy caused by a steroid cream that spreads from treated skin. In addition, thickened areas such as hypertrophic scars or prurigo nodules thin more rapidly in response to injections of a corticosteroid than the application of topical medications that cannot penetrate deeply.

Some patients appreciate the offer of topical anesthesia before injection. Because the injection of lidocaine is much more painful that the administration of intralesional corticosteroid, the skin should not be anesthetized initially with injectable lidocaine, nor should lidocaine be added to the corticosteroid solution. As before a biopsy, lidocaine 2.5%/prilocaine 2.5% cream or lidocaine 4% cream can be applied liberally every 15 minutes for about 2 hours before the procedure, or compounded tetracaine 6%/lidocaine 6% can be applied 15-30 minutes before injection.

For inflammatory conditions, triamcinolone acetonide 10 mg/mL is diluted with normal saline to a concentration of about 5 mg/mL (0.5 mL normal saline and 0.5 mL triamcinolone acetonide). Or, the provider can simply inject a smaller amount of undiluted medication. The volume injected depends upon the size of the area treated. About 0.1 mL is injected in each square centimeter, using a 30-gauge needle. A very early inflamed cyst of hidradenitis suppurativa is often improved in 1 day, whereas more recalcitrant causes of inflammation such as lichen planus may require 2 weeks **(Figs. 4-34 to 4-36)**.

Hypertrophic lesions require undiluted triamcinolone acetonide, 10 mg/mL, to decrease the thickness and produce the intended side effect of relative atrophy **(Figs. 4-37 and 4-38)**. Possible adverse reactions include atrophy

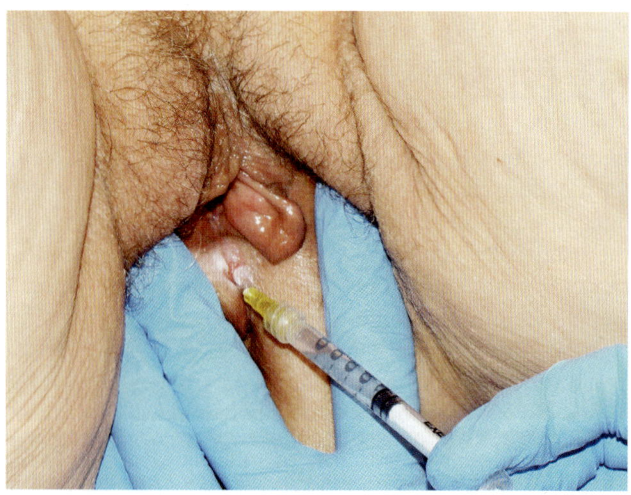

Fig. 4-34. This resistant hyperkeratotic area of lichen sclerosus was benign on biopsy and responded to 0.2 mL of triamcinolone acetonide 10 mg/mL injected into the middle of the thick lesion.

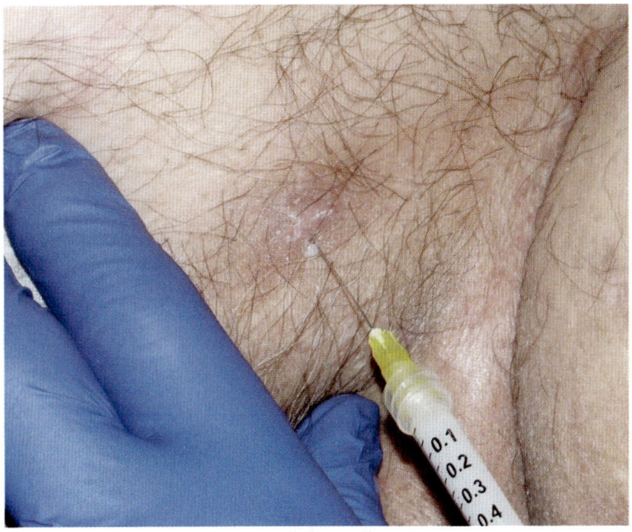


Fig. 4-35. This early but painful cyst of hidradenitis suppurativa was much improved the next morning after an injection of 0.2 mL of triamcinolone acetonide 10 mg/mL. Older, fluctuant cysts do not benefit as much because the medication is diluted within the purulent sac.

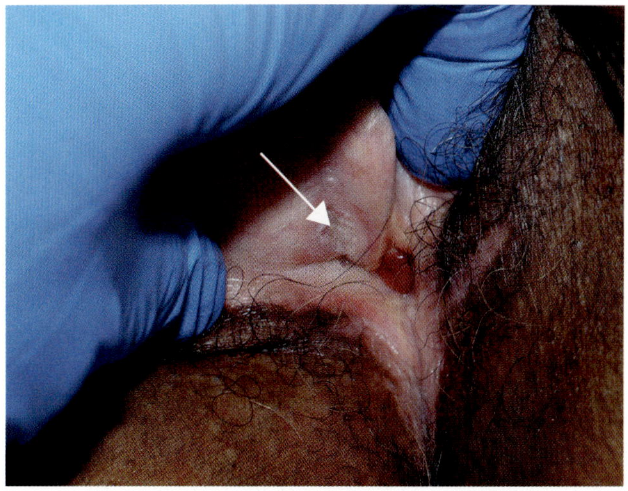

Fig. 4-37. This ulcer with a hyperkeratotic base did not respond to topical corticosteroids and had shown banal histology on biopsy in the past. It was treated with triamcinolone acetonide 10 mg/mL, 0.3 mL injected into the base of the lesion.

of adjacent skin as well as hypopigmentation if too much medication is injected or it is injected near the edges.

## Nonablative Laser

Nonablative lasers, especially fractional $CO_2$ laser (Mona Lisa Touch, FemTouch) have become popular and lucrative therapeutic tools with many gynecologists. Also used for cosmetic practices in resurfacing the skin for individuals with scarring and pigmentary changes, the fractional $CO_2$ lasers have only U.S. FDA device indication approval for vaginal estrogen deficiency in the practice of gynecologic medicine.8 Unlike traditional ablative $CO_2$ laser, nonablative lasers do not function by the destruction of skin. Very tiny superficial holes are produced in the epithelium and underlying dermis by short blasts in a grid pattern, so that each hole is surrounded by untreated tissue. This method also avoids overheating that ablates the epithelium. In addition, the nonablative photothermal erbium:yttrium aluminum garnet (erbium:YAG) crystal laser have been shown to be useful for the treatment of vaginal atrophy from estrogen deficiency. Laser waves act by heating connective tissue in the vaginal wall, thereby inducing collagen contraction, new collagen synthesis, vascularization, and growth factor infiltration. The net effect is increased thickness and restored elasticity and moisture of the vaginal mucosa.

Unfortunately, many providers use these lasers without data for other conditions, most notably lichen sclerosus,

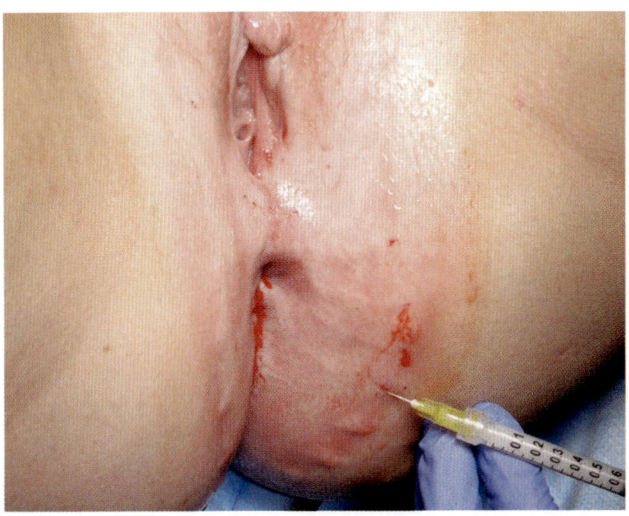

Fig. 4-36. Intralesional triamcinolone acetonide 10/mL was injected just under the surface of the skin into the dermis of the entire plaque of lichen sclerosus in this woman who was not psychologically able to apply her topical medication.

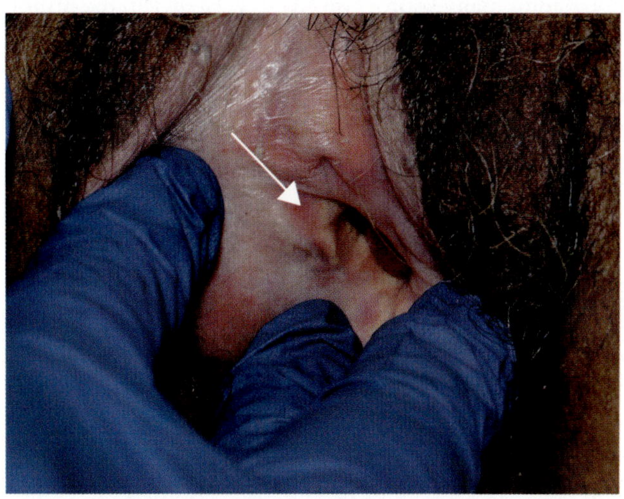

Fig. 4-38. Five weeks after the intralesional injection, the ulcer and hyperkeratosis have resolved.

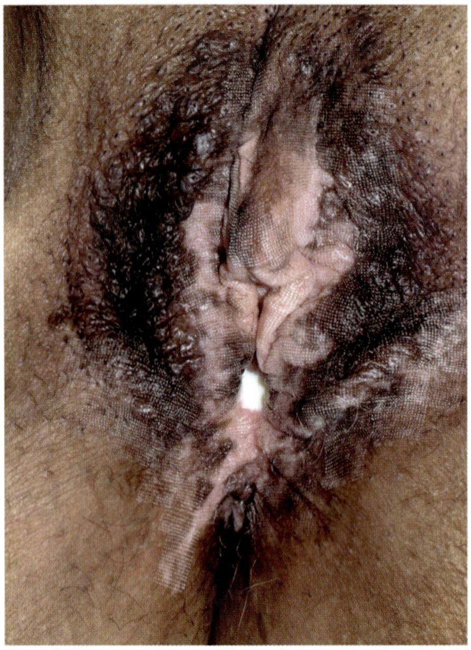

Fig. 4-39. Fractional $CO_2$ laser produces a fine grid of tiny white burns as seen here immediately following therapy for recalcitrant lichen sclerosus. Unlike traditional ablative $CO_2$ laser, damage is minimal and recovery swift.

lichen planus, and vulvodynia. Both the FDA and the ISSVD have officially condemned this practice of use in unstudied diseases.9 Although early data suggest a benefit for lichen sclerosus, there are no data for the use of these lasers in other skin conditions or pain syndromes (Fig. 4-39).

## Office Surgical Procedures

Well-known surgical procedures such as excision with suture closure or complicated procedures such as skin flaps and grafts are not discussed here, but these are detailed in many sources on surgery. However, the minor office procedures below generally have been developed informally by vulvologists and are not discussed in other venues. As such, there are no procedure codes for reimbursement. We are adding codes that we have found successful for compensation.

### Unroofing Sinus Tracts and Chronic Cysts of Hidradenitis Suppurativa

Patients with hidradenitis suppurativa (see Chapter 6, "Red Papules and Nodules") develop obstructed hair follicles and resulting epidermoid cysts. These cysts often rupture and drain to the surface, sometimes producing chronic draining sinus tracts that continually drain and heal over, just to open and again drain. Often, adjacent cysts rupture and chronic sinus tracts interconnect nearby cysts. These lesions never heal, and the treatment

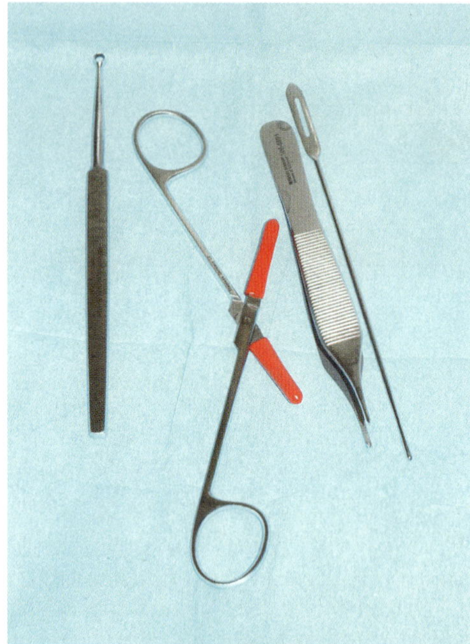

Fig. 4-40. A curette, curved iris scissors, forceps with teeth, and a lacrimal duct probe are the only necessary tools.

is surgical. Excision with suture closure can be performed, but adequate margins to remove the entire sinus tracts are required for definitive removal. A quick and tissue-sparing technique with very low recurrence involves deroofing of individual cysts and sinus tracts with curettage of the base (Fig. 4-40).

The chronically draining area is identified, and following anesthesia, a lacrimal duct probe is inserted into the surface opening and probed to the farthest extent of the sinus tract (Figs. 4-41 and 4-42). Curved iris scissors cut along the probe to open the cyst and sinus tract, and the skin edges are excised to leave a marsupialized cyst (Figs. 4-43 to 4-45). Then, the skin edges are beveled to produce sloped shoulders of the edges, which produce less scarring than would a sharp step off (Fig. 4-46). All edges of the

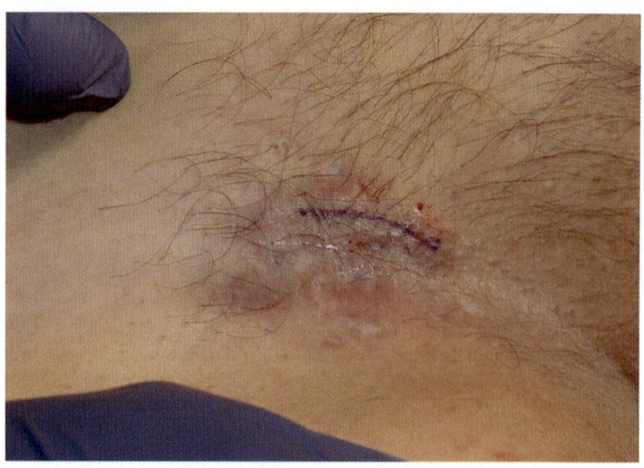

Fig. 4-41. A 3-cm linear sinus tract is identified, and the surface marked in case anesthesia makes the boundaries of the area less clear.

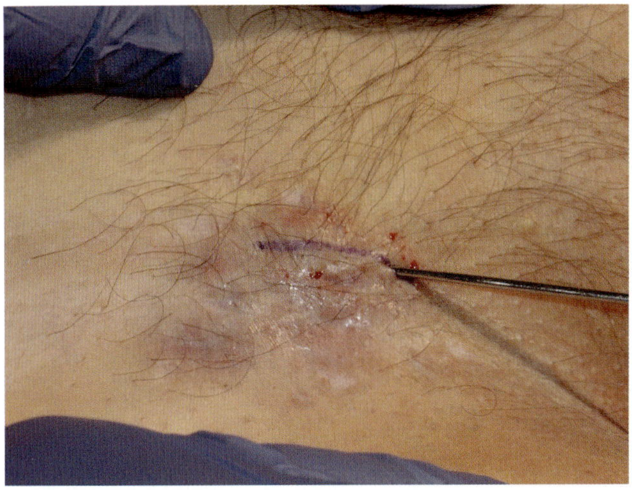

Fig. 4-42. A lacrimal duct probe is inserted at the opening of the sinus and gently advanced to the end of the sinus tract.

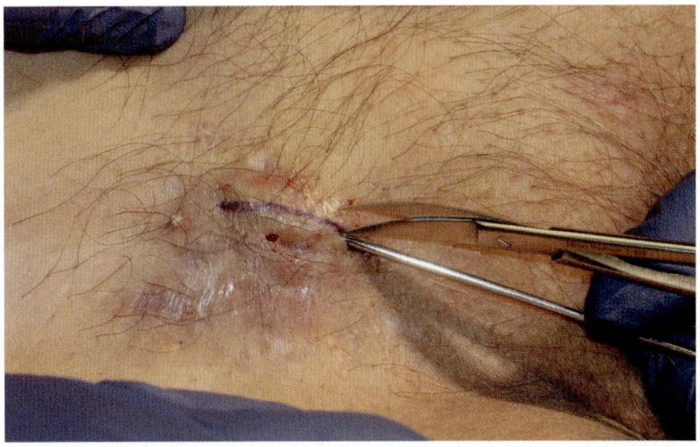

Fig. 4-43. Curved iris scissors are used to incise over the lacrimal duct probe along the top of the sinus tract.

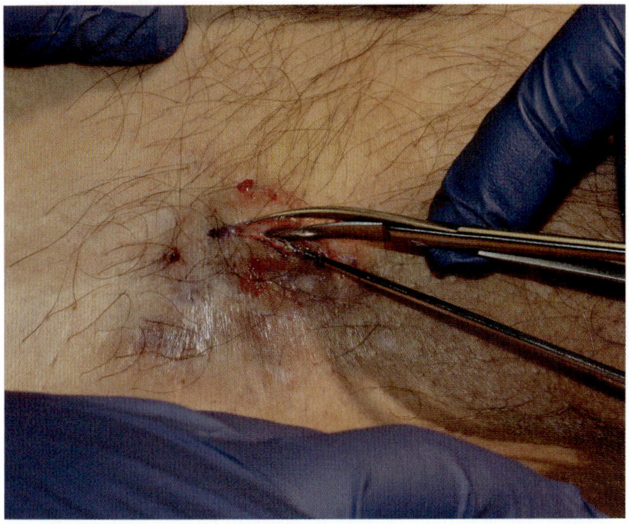

Fig. 4-44. Scissors open the roof of the sinus tract and allow better visualization.

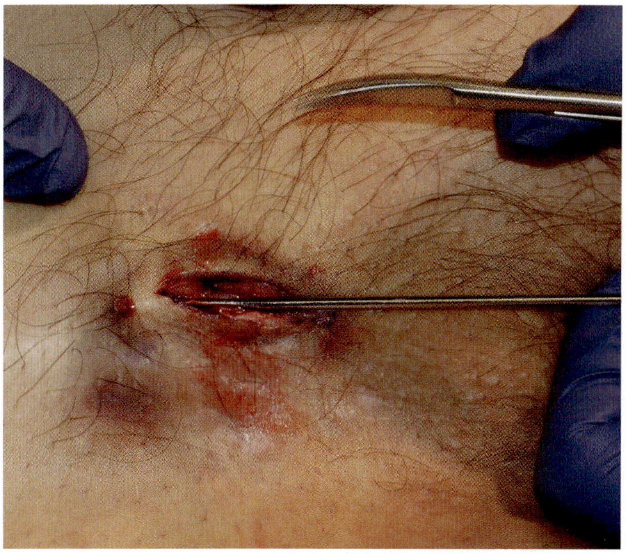

Fig. 4-45. The probe is used to ensure that the entire tract has been identified and unroofed.

cyst are probed with the lacrimal duct probe to investigate for connections to adjacent cysts, and any cords of sinus tracts are followed and opened (**Figs. 4-47 and 4-48**). The base of the cyst and sinus tracts is covered with a gelatinous material that is removed with a blunt curette or by scrubbing with dry gauze (**Figs. 4-49 and 4-50**). Hemostasis is achieved by chemical cautery with aluminum chloride or ferric chloride.

The open area is covered with petroleum jelly and gauze, and the patient soaks the area twice daily until healed, replacing the gauze dressing. The ultimate cosmetic outcome is usually quite good. Although the chronic cyst and sinus tract clear, this does not prevent the development of additional lesions (**Fig. 4-51**).

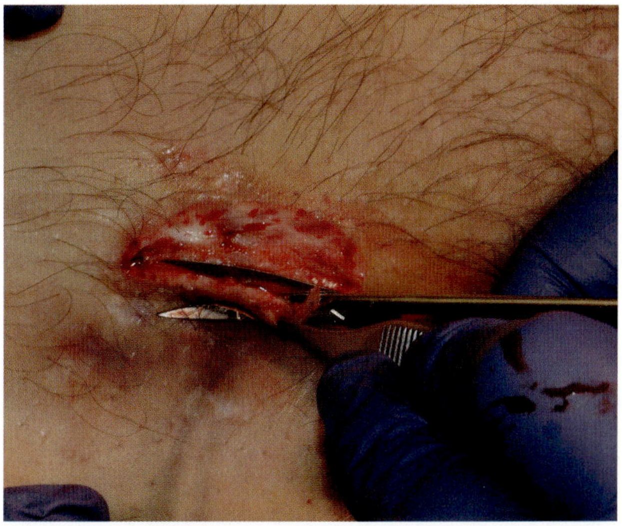

Fig. 4-46. The steep edges of the unroofed tract would not heal easily or with an acceptable scar; therefore, the edges are trimmed and beveled to make the sides sloped.

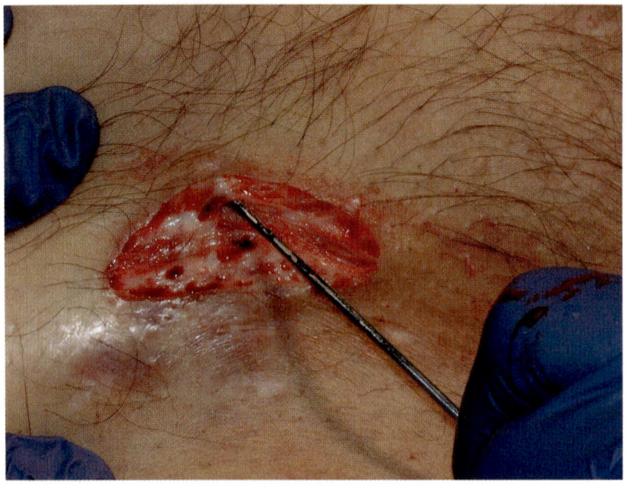

Fig. 4-47. All edges of the sinus tract are explored with the probe, and a small additional tract is identified.

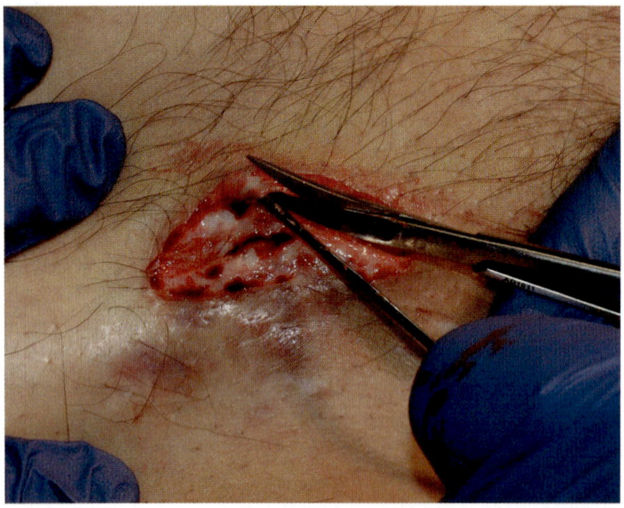

Fig. 4-48. This additional short tract is unroofed.

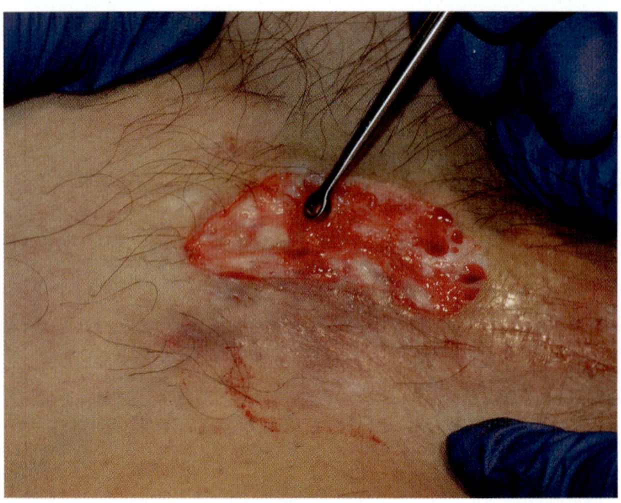

Fig. 4-49. The base of these cysts and tracts is covered with a gelatinous material that is removed with a curette.

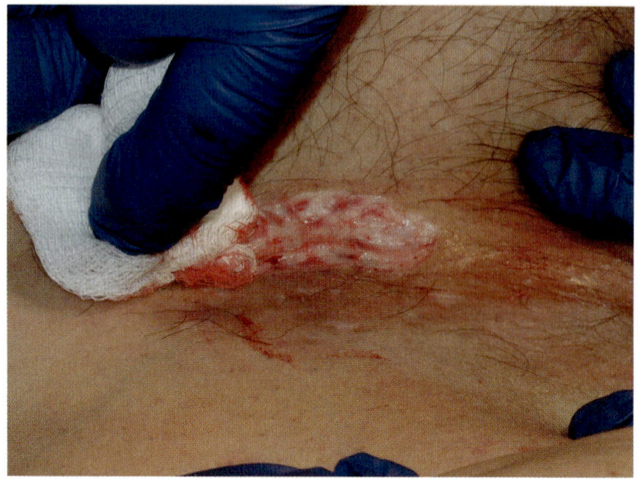

Fig. 4-50. Any additional gelatinous material and contents are scrubbed off with dry gauze, and hemostasis is achieved with aluminum chloride or other chemical cautery, or light hyfrecation/electrocautery.

This can be coded as "unroofing hidradenitis" 11462 for inguinal nodules and 11470 for perianal/perineal lesions.

Small discrete chronically draining cysts can be opened with a punch biopsy, the base curetted, and the defect closed with sutures.

## Lysis of Midline Adhesions in Scarring Vulvar Skin Diseases

Lichen sclerosus and lichen planus often result in midline adhesions of the introitus, more often anteriorly but also posteriorly at times (**Fig. 4-52**). This produces fragility in some women, with recurrent fissuring over the line of adhesion, and sufficient narrowing of the vestibule to comfortable prevent sexual activity. Rarely, and nearly always in the case of lichen planus, the scarring is so severe as to prevent urination, sometimes requiring urgent surgery.

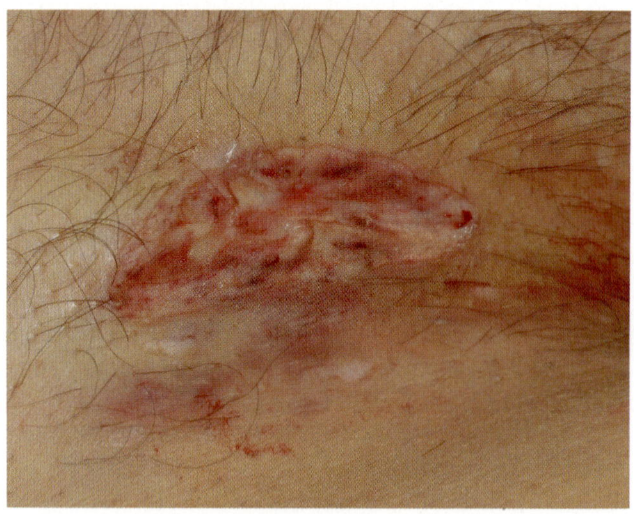

Fig. 4-51. The final defect is clean and dry, and is left to heal by secondary intention while covered with gauze covered in petroleum jelly.

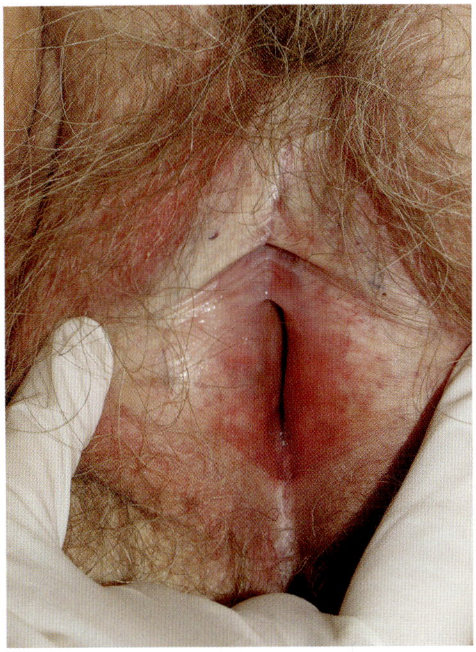

Fig. 4-52. Although these anterior midline synechiae do not significantly narrow the introitus, there is repeated painful tearing with sexual activity despite adequate control of the underlying lichen sclerosus.

These adhesions often can be lysed easily in the office, but scrupulous postoperative care is essential to prevent immediate recurrence of scarring, and good control of the underlying disease is important except in the case of urinary retention, when this luxury is not possible. Marked scarring with lichen planus can be thicker and deeper, with adherence to underlying structures, so that outpatient lysis should not be performed if the area is not well exposed in the setting of lichen planus.

Anteriorly, there is usually a vertical line of demarcation where the medial labia majora have fused (**Fig. 4-53**).

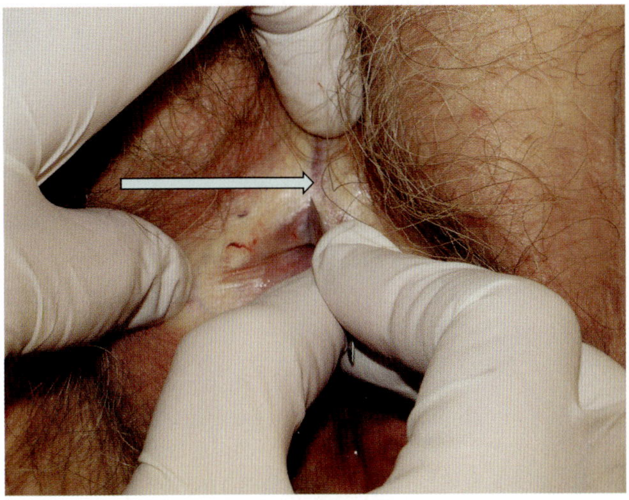

Fig. 4-53. Following topical and injected anesthesia, a nick in the midline scar of the larger scar is made; there is usually a remaining line of demarcation where the skin edges have scarred together (*arrow*).

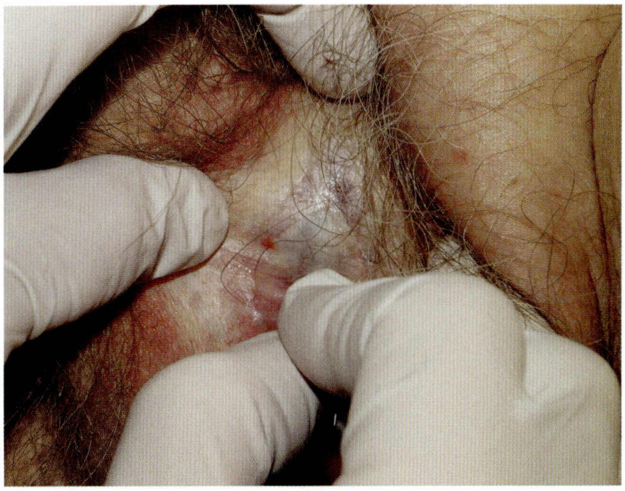

Fig. 4-54. When the edge of the adhesion is nicked, the skin edges can usually be peeled apart with gentle lateral traction.

This and surrounding skin are anesthetized with lidocaine 1% with epinephrine, having been pretreated in this author's office with topical compounded tetracaine 6%/ lidocaine 6% for 15-30 minutes.

The edge of the line of fusion is nicked with a number 15 scalpel blade (**Fig. 4-53**), and often, the skin then can be separated manually, with the skin edges peeling apart, particularly in the case of lichen sclerosus, where the scarring is often less dense (**Figs. 4-54 to 4-56**). Otherwise, the skin is separated along the original line of scarring with the scalpel blade.

On the posterior modified mucous membranes, these diseases often produce a band of tissue that may not show this line of fusion. This can be treated in the same way, or this band can be snipped, and the skin edges closed. However, this author finds that the sutures often pull though and healing then occurs by secondary intention.

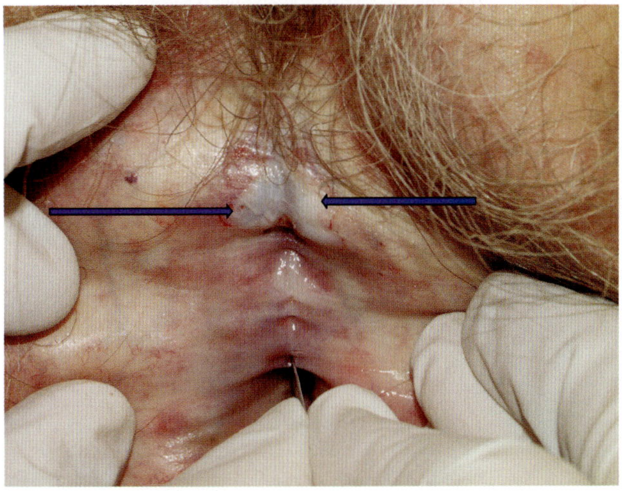

Fig. 4-55. These *arrows* show the area where the line of adhesion was, while the edge of the inferior adhesion is nicked.

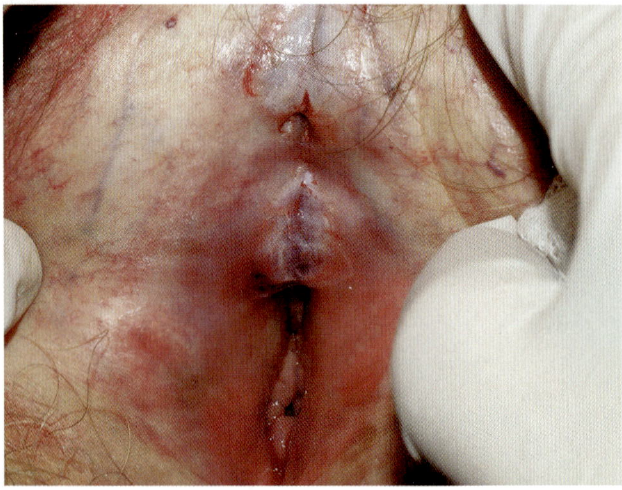

Fig. 4-56. Both adhesions have been lysed; the inferior scar was less well demarcated, and several cautious and superficial incisions were made to separate the scar, since the edges did not peel back easily.

Postoperatively, unless sutures are placed, use of dilators is crucial to maintain the caliber of the introitus, which can begin to scar shut almost immediately. The area should be soaked (in a tub or sitz bath) three times a day, and followed by insertion of a well-lubricated dilator after pretreatment with a narcotic analgesic when needed **(Fig. 4-57)**. The set of dilators must be ordered (Amazon) in advance, and the largest dilator that is easily inserted should be used. Very frequent rechecks in the office are important to ensure that these older women are able to follow through with this regimen and that scarring is not recurring.

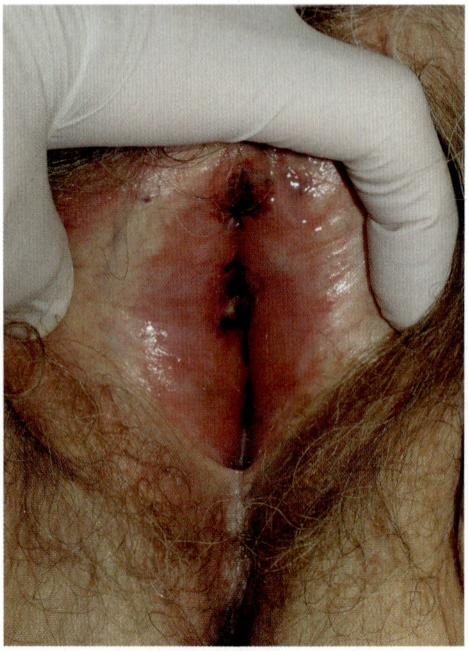

Fig. 4-57. A week later, with aggressive home care, including tub soaks, thrice daily dilators, and copious petroleum jelly, healing is progressing without recurrence of scar.

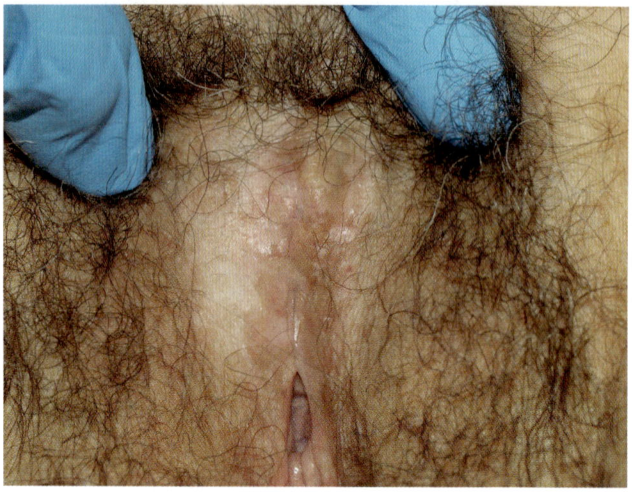

Fig. 4-58. Lichen sclerosus often produces scarring of the clitoral hood over the clitoris, decreasing sensation and producing psychological distress to the patient.

The procedure code for these procedures is 56441, "lysis of labial adhesions." When sutures are placed, a repair is added as after an excision, depending upon the length of the repair.

## Lysis of Adhesions of the Clitoral Hood

Lichen sclerosus and lichen planus often produce clitoral phimosis, where the edges of the clitoral hood to scar together, so that the clitoral hood cannot be retracted to expose the clitoris **(Fig. 4-58)**. Although many women find that, after control of their skin disease and attention to estrogen deficiency, this does not interfere with sexual functioning, other women discover that there is loss of sensation and ask that the clitoris be uncovered. When the scarring is superficial, a relatively minor office procedure can uncover the clitoris. Whereas there are several different methods, the following is quick and gives a reasonable cosmetic result. This should not be performed until there is good control of the skin disease.

Again, as above, pretreatment with 15-30 minutes of tetracaine 6%/lidocaine 6% is followed by lidocaine 1% with epinephrine instilled into the clitoral hood. A dorsal slit is performed, and the edges of the incision are closed with a soft absorbable suture such as glycoprotein acid (Vicryl) **(Fig. 4-59)**.

## Incision of Clitoral Pseudocysts

When the clitoral hood scars in some women with lichen sclerosus, much less often with lichen sclerosus, there can be entrapment of keratin debris within the closed clitoral hood **(Fig. 4-60)**. This is usually asymptomatic, requiring no therapy. When the pseudocyst is large, produces a decrease in sensation, or is recurrently inflamed from rupture, surgical management is indicated.

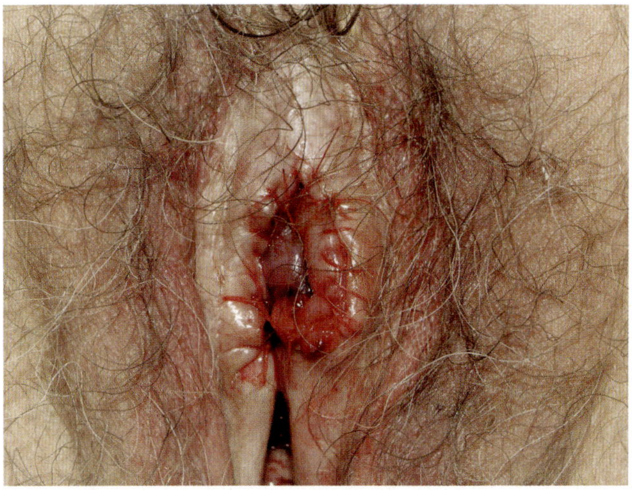

Fig. 4-59. A dorsal slit can be made over the clitoris and the edges oversewn to prevent immediate recurrent.

The area is again anesthetized as above, and a midline incision is performed, with removal of the pseudocyst contents. The edges of the incision are oversewn with a soft absorbable suture to marsupialize the cyst, producing the same result as lysing clitoral adhesions.

### Surgery for Vestibulodynia (Vulvar Vestibulitis Syndrome, Vestibulitis)

This is beyond the scope of this book, but the procedure used for this condition is describes briefly in Chapter 13, which discusses genital pain and vestibulodynia.

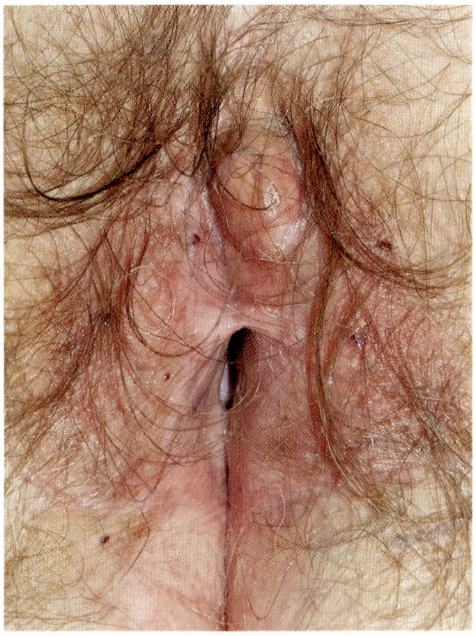

Fig. 4-60. Entrapment of keratin debris under the clitoral hood produces the clitoral pseudocyst, which can be remedied with a dorsal slit, removal of the keratin, and the edges oversewn to prevent immediate adherence of the skin edges and recurrence of the pseudocyst.

## Conclusion

The diagnostic and therapeutic procedures used in the management of benign anogenital diseases are generally straightforward and can be performed by any careful provider who pays attention. The use of these is far more beneficial to the patient than repetitive empiric treatment for *Candida*, bacterial vaginosis, and tinea.

## REFERENCES


1. Micheletti L, Bogliatto F, Lynch PJ. Vulvoscopy: review of a diagnostic approach requiring clarification. *J Reprod Med.* 2008;53:179-182.
2. Stuebs FA, Mehlhorn G, Gass P, et al. Concordance rate of vulvoscopic findings in detecting early vulvar neoplasia. *Gynecol Oncol.* 2020;157:463-468.
3. Khan Z, Bhargava A, Mittal P, et al. Evaluation of reliability of self-collected vaginal swabs over physician-collected samples for diagnosis of bacterial vaginosis, candidiasis and trichomoniasis, in a resource-limited setting: a cross-sectional study in India. *BMJ Open.* 2019;9:e025013.
4. Yamamoto T, Aoyama Y. Detection of multinucleated giant cells in differentiated keratinocytes with herpes simplex virus and varicella zoster virus infections by modified Tzanck smear method. *J Dermatol.* 2021;48:21-27.
5. Borghi A, Virgili A, Corazza M. Dermoscopy of inflammatory genital diseases: practical insights. *Dermatol Clin.* 2018;36:451-461.
6. Vaccari S, Barisani A, Salvini C, et al. Thin vulvar melanoma; a challenging diagnosis. Dermoscopic features of a case series. *Clin Exp Dermatol.* 2020;45:187-193.
7. Santoso JT, Likes W. Colposcopic acetowhitening of vulvar lesion: a validity study. *Arch Gynecol Obstet.* 2015;292:387-390.
8. D'oria O, Giannini A, Prata G, et al. Non-invasive treatment of vulvovaginal atrophy in menopause with CO2 laser. *Minerva Obstet Gynecol.* 2021;73:127-134. doi:10.23736/S0026-4784.20.04612-2
9. Preti M, Vieira-Baptista P, Digesu GA, et al. The clinical role of LASER for vulvar and vaginal treatments in gynecology and female urology: an ICS/ISSVD best practice consensus document. *J Low Genit Tract Dis.* 2019;23:151-160.


## SUGGESTED READINGS


D'oria O, Giannini A, Prata G, et al. Non-invasive treatment of vulvovaginal atrophy in menopause with CO2 laser. *Minerva Obstet Gynecol.* 2021;73:127-134. doi:10.23736/S0026-4784.20.04612-2

Errichetti E. Dermoscopy in general dermatology (non-neoplastic dermatoses): pitfalls and tips. *Int J Dermatol..* 2021;60:653-660. doi:10.1111/ijd.15427

Errichetti E, Ankad BS, Sonthalia S, et al. Dermoscopy in general dermatology (non-neoplastic dermatoses) of skin of colour: a comparative retrospective study by the International Dermoscopy Society. *Eur J Dermatol.* 2020;30:688-698. doi:10.1684/ejd.2020.3928

Mauskar MM, Marathe K, Venkatesan A, Schlosser BJ, Edwards L. Vulvar diseases: approach to the patient. *J Am Acad Dermatol.* 2020;82:1277-1284.

https://dermnetnz.org/cme/dermoscopy-course

# Red Disorders: Patches and Plaques 5

PETER J. LYNCH AND LIBBY EDWARDS

Many different "rashes" present with red patches and plaques. When these disorders occur on dry, keratinized skin, they usually exhibit distinct differentiating features that indicate a specific diagnosis. However, when these conditions occur on warm, moist skin such as the anogenital region, they more often display nonspecific erythema with no, or only barely visible, scale **(Fig. 5-1)**. Therefore, making a diagnosis on the basis of examination alone may not be possible. Other approaches, such as whole-body examination, eliciting a history of itching, listing of locally applied contactants, obtaining microbial cultures, and performing biopsies, may be necessary. In spite of all this, at times, a definitive diagnosis just cannot be made. When this occurs, and when culture and biopsy have ruled out infections and malignancy, symptomatic therapy is permissible. Such therapy usually includes the use of topical steroids to reduce itching and the redness related to underlying inflammation. Please note that, in the absence of significant infection, such topical steroid treatment will rarely, if ever, be detrimental to the underlying disorder.

## SECTION A: DERMATITIS AND LICHENIFICATION

Anogenital pruritus occurs in two settings. It may arise from visibly normal-appearing tissue ("primary" pruritus) or it may occur as part of an already visible disorder ("secondary" pruritus). The red patches and plaques that have an "eczematous" appearance are discussed here in Section A. These include both examples of primary pruritus (atopic dermatitis and lichen simplex chronicus [LSC]) and examples of secondary pruritus (contact dermatitis and seborrheic dermatitis). Primary pruritus that uncommonly presents with an eczematous appearance such as idiopathic ("essential") pruritus is discussed in Chapter 13. And, those instances of secondary pruritus that less frequently demonstrate an eczematous appearance secondary to the itching (eg, psoriasis, lichen sclerosus, and tinea cruris) are dealt with as these individual disorders are covered throughout the book.

Conceptually, it is worth trying to separate primary from secondary pruritus, but since some scratching often occurs in both settings, the clinical appearance at the time of examination may not allow one to separate the two processes. When that is the case, treatment specifically directed toward the cessation of scratching may allow for correct identification. That is, if the scratching can be stopped, the scratched tissue will either return to normal (primary pruritus) or will likely reveal the nature of the underlying disorder (secondary pruritus).

Obviously it is important, then, to understand what constitutes an "eczematous" appearance.

The following is a short review of terminology for dermatitic/eczematous disorders previously covered in Chapter 2. The two adjectives "eczematous" and "dermatitic" (which like the nouns "eczema" and "dermatitis") are synonyms, and they can be defined morphologically. The morphologic appearance of the eczematous disease is classically defined by the presence of solid plaques or plaques made up of closely set red papules. These plaques are characterized by (1) poorly marginated borders, (2) overlying scale, and (3) the presence of epithelial disruption and/or lichenification. *Epithelial*

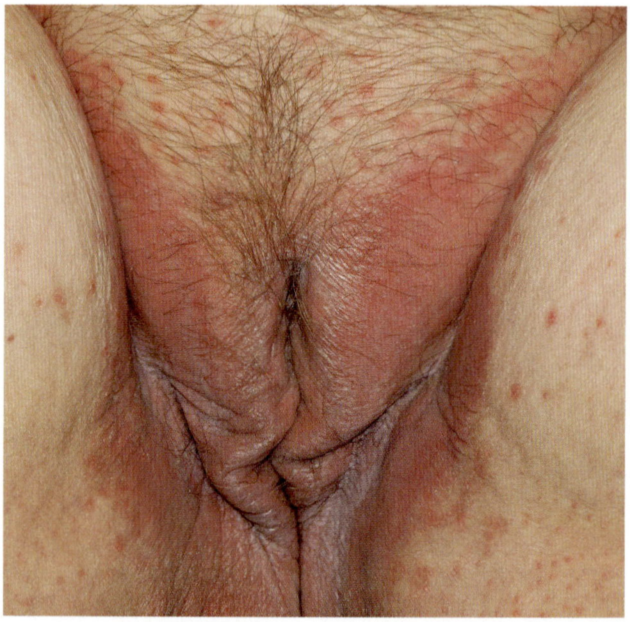

Fig. 5-1. Red, scaling diseases in damp skin folds often do not show obvious scale; this woman has psoriasis that appears shiny rather than showing the classic heavy white scale of psoriasis in other locations.

*disruption* is most often noted by the presence of excoriations, but other signs of epithelial disruption may also be present. These include weeping, crusting, fissuring, or the presence of yellow-colored scale. This yellow color is owing to the presence of small amounts of plasma that coats the otherwise gray, white, or silver color of scale. When rubbing is more prominent than scratching, the calluslike response of lichenification may supplant much of the evidence for epithelial disruption. *Lichenification* is recognized clinically by three features: (1) palpably thickened skin, (2) exaggerated skin markings, and (3) lichen-type scale. Lichen-type scale, because of its tight adherence to the underlying epithelium, is more or less colorless when dry but whitens when it absorbs moisture. This whitening often happens in the anogenital area because of retained sweat.

Lesions possessing an eczematous clinical appearance have a characteristic histological appearance as well. This microscopic appearance on biopsy demonstrates *spongiotic inflammation* (inflammatory cells accompanied by intercellular and intracellular edema within the epithelium) when the process is acute and by *acanthosis* (epithelial thickening often termed "psoriasiform dermatitis") when the process is chronic and lichenified. This is the microscopic appearance common to all of the disorders discussed in Section A of this chapter. Since all of these eczematous disorders share this common histologic appearance, pathologists are usually unable to separately identify each of the conditions that exist within the general category of eczematous disease. For this reason, when the pathologist reports either "spongiotic dermatitis" or "psoriasiform dermatitis," it is usually necessary for the clinician to make a clinical-pathologic correlation in order to arrive at a more specific diagnosis.[1]

## Atopic Dermatitis and Lichen Simplex Chronicus

Atopic dermatitis and LSC are examples of primary pruritus in which itching occurs in clinically normal-appearing tissue. This itching leads to vigorous scratching and/or rubbing. The nomenclature regarding atopic dermatitis and its variants is somewhat complex and controversial. The term "atopy" has been defined in many ways, but most often, the definition includes a genetic predisposition for the development of hypersensitivity wherein IgE-mediated reactions occur as a result of exposure to common environmental antigens. Thus, atopic individuals frequently develop allergic rhinitis (hay fever), asthma, and/or atopic dermatitis. A semantic problem arises when an eczematous eruption occurs in an individual who lacks a personal or prominent family history of hay fever or asthma. In this setting, the eczematous process has variously been termed neurodermatitis, infantile eczema, childhood eczema, or LSC. Given the lack of consensus regarding the diagnostic criteria for atopic dermatitis and in view of the fact that these eczematous eruptions share the presence of the "itch-scratch cycle" (see below and Chapter 2), I believe it is best, or at least less confusing, to use the term atopic dermatitis (for the *multifocal* form of the disorder) and LSC (for the *localized* form of the disorder) of the condition regardless of whether or not the individual has other clinical evidence of atopy. Moreover, since anogenital eczematous involvement very often occurs in the absence of eczematous disease elsewhere, we will generally refer to it as LSC.

### Clinical Presentation

#### Epidemiology

Atopic dermatitis in its multifocal form is a very common disorder with a point prevalence of about 4%-5% of adults in Western countries.[2] The localized form of atopic dermatitis, anogenital LSC, occurs in both sexes and at all ages. It is commonly encountered in those who are adults, and in this group, there is evidence that it occurs in women a little more frequently than in men.[3] It occurs a little less frequently in children, but when it does, we believe that boys are affected somewhat more often than do girls. The prevalence and incidence of localized anogenital LSC are not known with certainty, but in one of the larger studies, such patients accounted for 1.5% of all visits to a dermatology clinic.[4] Based on a few older studies, discussion at conferences, and our own experience, it is probably the single most common symptomatic condition involving the anogenital area.

#### History

Possibly because of embarrassment, patients with genital LSC rarely seek medical attention until the problem has been present for weeks or months. Often, the itching arises subtly, but in women (who do not frequently look at their vulvas), a specific event, such as vaginal discharge (perceived to be a yeast infection), will be identified by many of the patients as the initial trigger. Once itching has developed, scratching almost inevitably follows. Most patients describe the itching as severe and find that nothing in terms of home remedies or over-the-counter medications relieves it. In the most intractable cases, patients will scratch until pain caused by excoriation replaces the pruritus. However, some patients will shift from scratching to rubbing (with resulting lichenification) since they find that they can alleviate some of the itching without causing the pain and tissue damage that arises with excoriation.

In time, a vicious circle of itching followed by scratching, followed by more itching and more scratching develops. This is termed the "itch-scratch cycle." I believe that the presence of this itch-scratch cycle is the pathognomonic and defining characteristic of atopic dermatitis and LSC wherever it occurs on the body. Often, patients are conscious of the scratching and yet continue to scratch "because I can't make myself stop" or "because it feels so good to scratch." Others are unaware of their scratching and tend to think that they scratch very little. This is quite analogous to the lack of awareness that a person often develops with habit tics such fingernail biting and knuckle cracking.

Scratching during the daytime primarily occurs after using the toilet, when changing clothes after work, and in the evening when one gets undressed for bed. Scratching almost always also occurs episodically at night during the lighter stages of non-REM sleep, and it is associated with an abnormal increase in the number of partial awakenings.[5,6] I have termed this nocturnal scratching the "Penelope phenomenon" based on Homer tale of Odysseus (Ulysses) and his wife Penelope.[7] When Odysseus lingered for many years on his voyage home from the Trojan War, Penelope was urged to declare that he had died and that she should marry one of her many suitors. She agreed to do so but only after she had completed weaving a funeral shroud for her dying father-in-law. During the day, she wove the shroud, but at night, when everyone was sleeping, she would undo most of the previous daytime weaving. This "Penelope phenomenon" thus represents the nighttime scratching that undoes the benefits of what otherwise might be a good daytime therapeutic program.

## Examination

As indicated above, LSC shares the morphological characteristics of all eczematous diseases. This includes erythematous, poorly marginated, scaling papules and

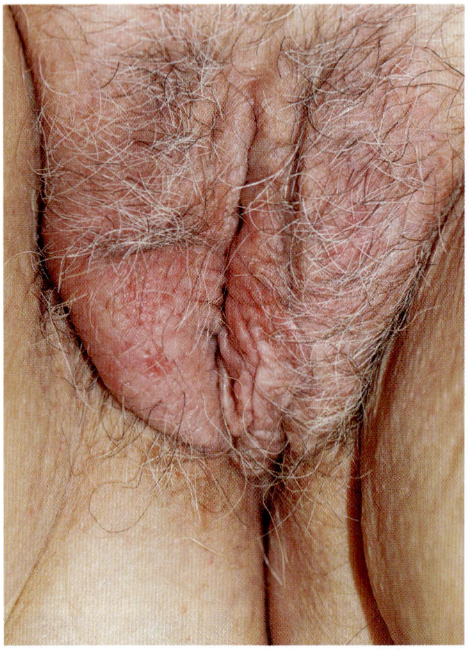

Fig. 5-2. Classic lichen simplex chronicus exhibits poorly demarcated erythematous lichenification, seen here on the hair-bearing surface of the labia majora. There is an irregular erosion from scratching as well.

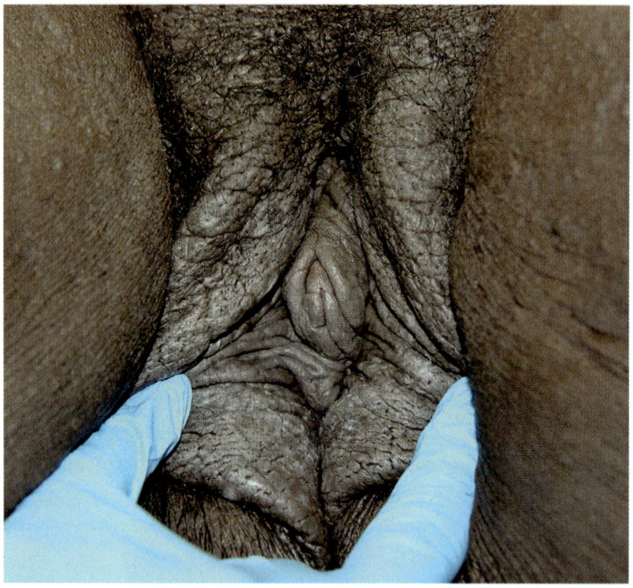

Fig. 5-3. This woman has remarkably thickened skin from rubbing and scratching, with classic deepened skin markings. Rather than erythema, this patient of color shows surface white color from hydrated epithelium.

plaques with evidence of epithelial disruption and/or lichenification **(Figs. 5-2 through 5-8)**. But in contrast to other eczematous diseases, the severity of excoriation and/or lichenification often allows for correct clinical identification. This may not be true in mild cases where the warm, moist environment of the anogenital area might obscure some of the characteristic morphological features. Thus, scale may not be as visibly apparent (though it can still be recognized by at least some roughness on palpation) as it is with LSC in other dryer regions of the body **(Figs. 5-8 and 5-9)**. This scale is hydrophilic, and when it takes up water, it whitens. The white color can be fairly prominent when a patient first undresses but decreases with time as evaporation reduces the moisture content of the surface epithelium **(Figs. 5-10 to 5-12)**. Moreover, deep scratching may destroy or remove melanocytes, leaving hypopigmented areas when the scratch marks heal **(Fig. 5-13)**. Alternatively, if rubbing supplants scratching, the involved area may become hyperpigmented due to chronic inflammatory stimulation of melanocytes. Such hyperpigmentation can decrease the apparentness of erythema, leading one to underestimate the amount of inflammation that is present **(Figs. 5-14 and 5-15)**. Hyperpigmentation is especially likely to develop in patients with naturally dark skin.

Genital LSC in women primarily occurs on the outer aspects of the labia majora though involvement of the labia minora is sometimes seen. In men, the scrotum is the predominant site of involvement, but the base, or even the entire shaft, of the penis are sometimes affected **(Fig. 5-16)**. In both sexes, there may be involvement of the anal and/or perianal area **(Fig. 5-17)**.

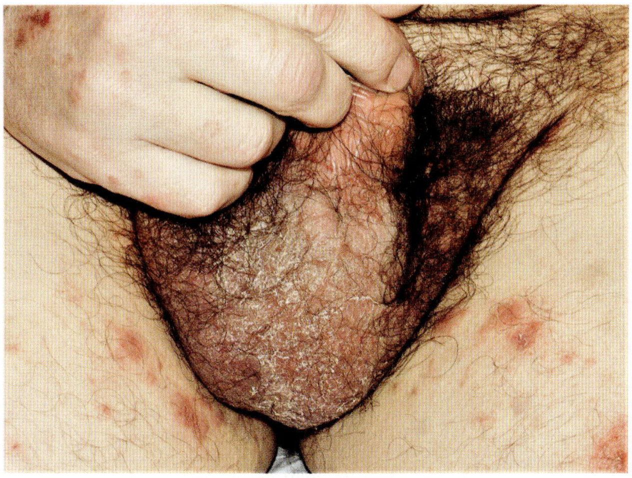

Fig. 5-4. Scale is abundant, as is redness on the scrotum of this man with severe pruritus who had recently been admitted to the hospital with an incorrect diagnosis of cellulitis.

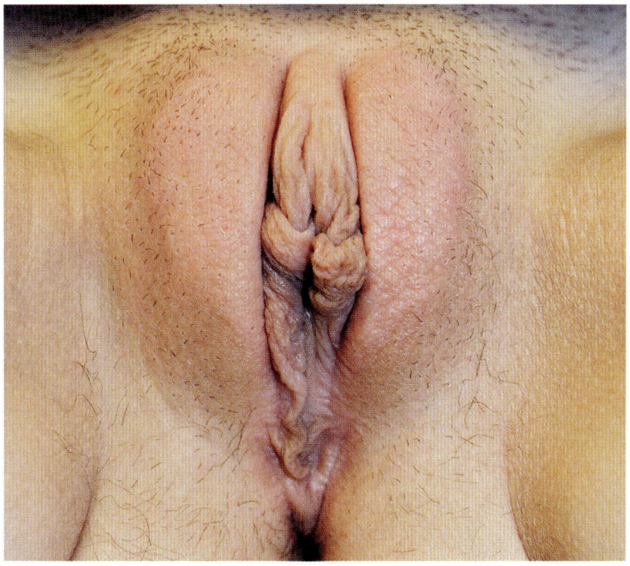

Fig. 5-5. The prominent lichenification produces thicker skin without the usual softer folds of the labia majora.

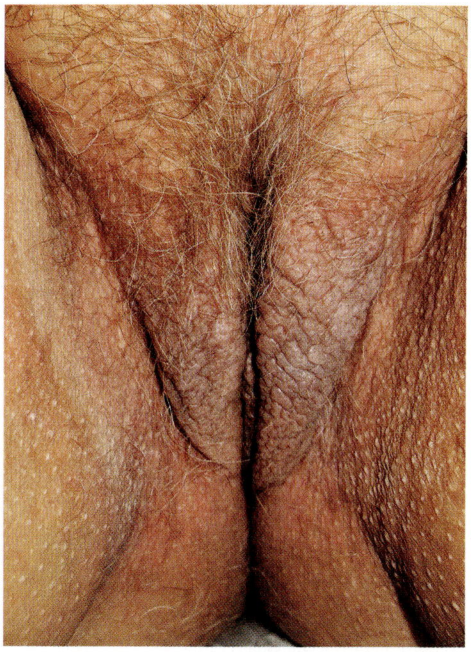

Fig. 5-6. Poorly demarcated red plaques with lichenification are classic for LSC; her lichenification is more prominent on the left labium majus than the right.

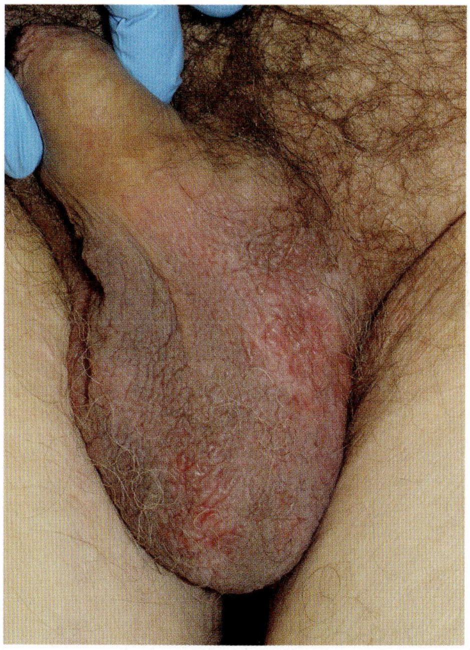

Fig. 5-7. Lichen simplex chronicus of the male genitalia is usually on the scrotum and again exhibits poorly demarcated erythema, lichenification, and superficial erosions produced by chronic rubbing and scratching.

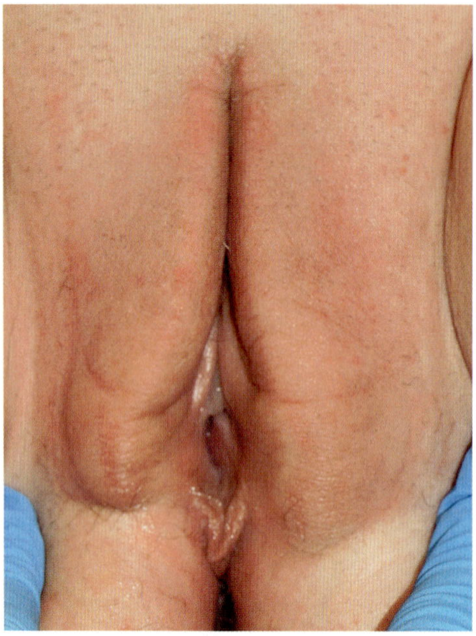

Fig. 5-8. Although the thickened labia majora in this patient do not appear to have scale because of the damp environment, the surface is rough to the touch, signifying the presence of scale.

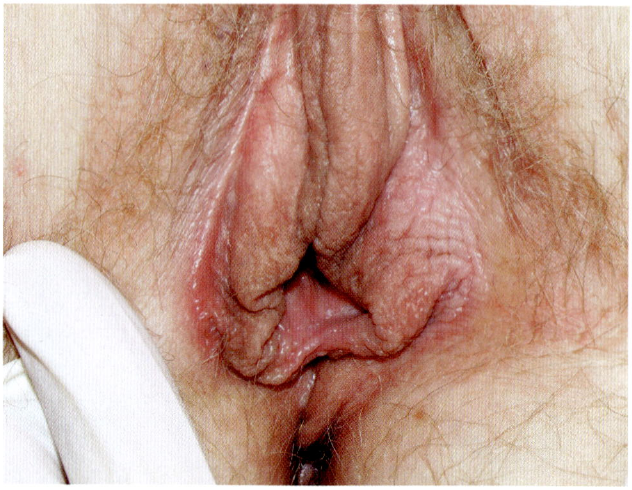

Fig. 5-10. This patient with unilateral lichenification of LSC also shows white surface discoloration from the damp environment.

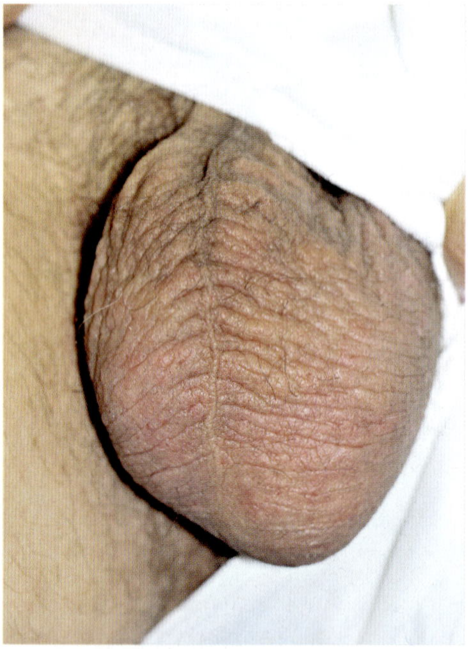

Fig. 5-9. The surface of the scrotum again is very rough in this patient with lichen simplex chronicus, in contrast to the apparent non-scaling appearance.

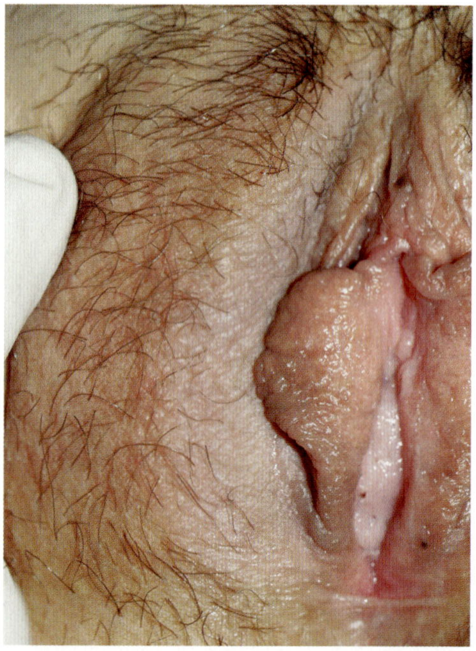

Fig. 5-11. Fairly often, LSC is unilateral, as seen here in this woman with LSC on the medial right labium majus, white from the environment.

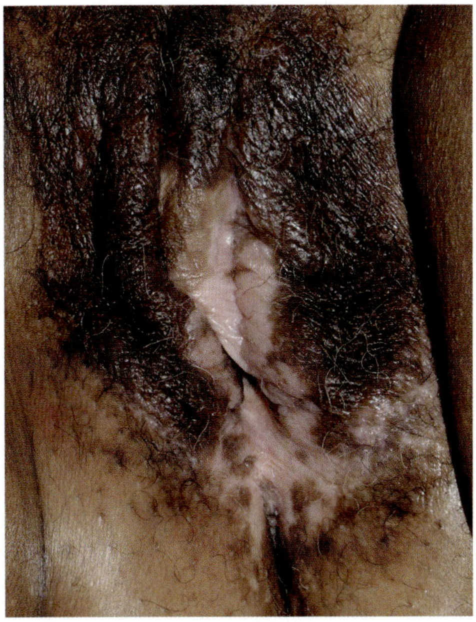

Fig. 5-12. The inflammation and damage of rubbing can precipitate vitiligo, where this disease of depigmentation occurs preferentially in areas of trauma or irritation; this is more easily seen in patients who are darkly pigmented and can be mistaken for lichen sclerosus. The hyperpigmented, thickened skin represents LSC.

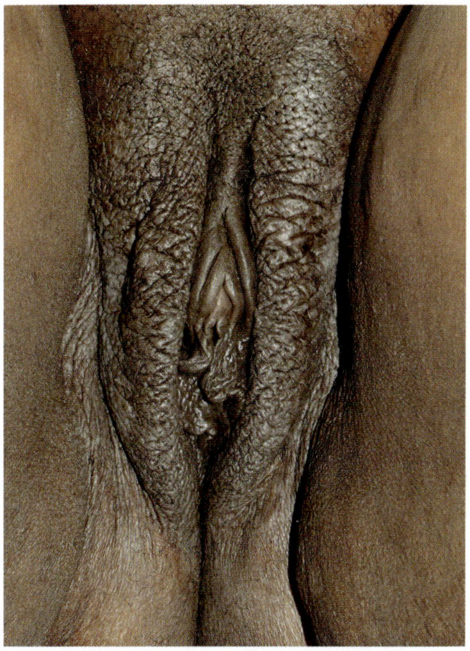

Fig. 5-14. Inflammation in dark-complexioned people appears hyperpigmented rather than red. Sometimes, lichenification and the compact, lichenoid scale appear shiny, as though the skin has been polished from the frequent rubbing.

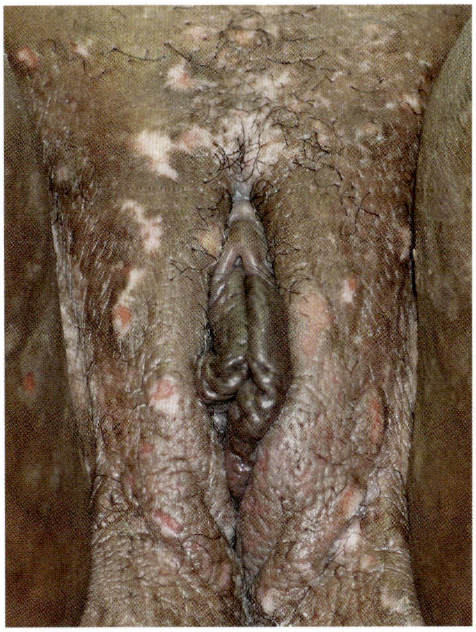

Fig. 5-13. This vulva shows white linear lesions where melanocytes were removed by forceful scratching.

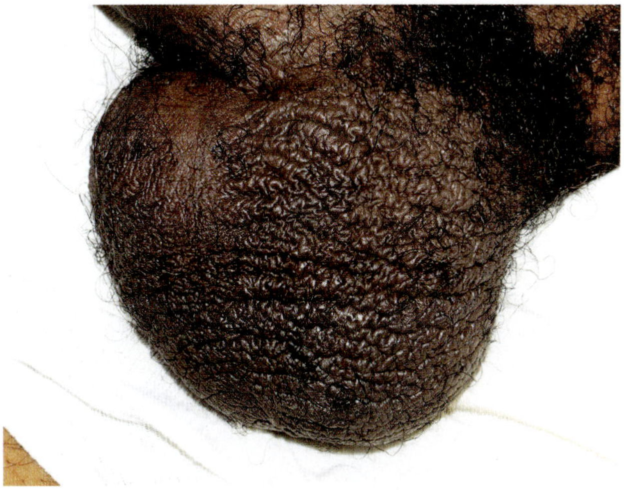

Fig. 5-15. This scrotum shows dark brown lichenification, due both erythema seen through dark skin and coexisting postinflammatory hyperpigmentation.

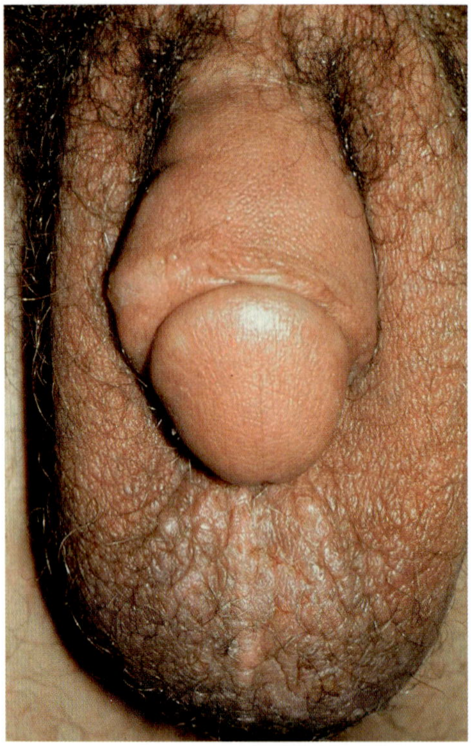

Fig. 5-16. Although male LSC is usually scrotal, sometimes the penis is involved as well; in addition to classic scrotal LSC, the penile shaft is both lichenified and thickened from underlying fibrosis from years of rubbing and scratching.

## Diagnosis

The diagnosis of LSC is usually made on the basis of the clinical findings. Dermoscopy can be a useful diagnostic tool in those providers who are skilled in this technique.

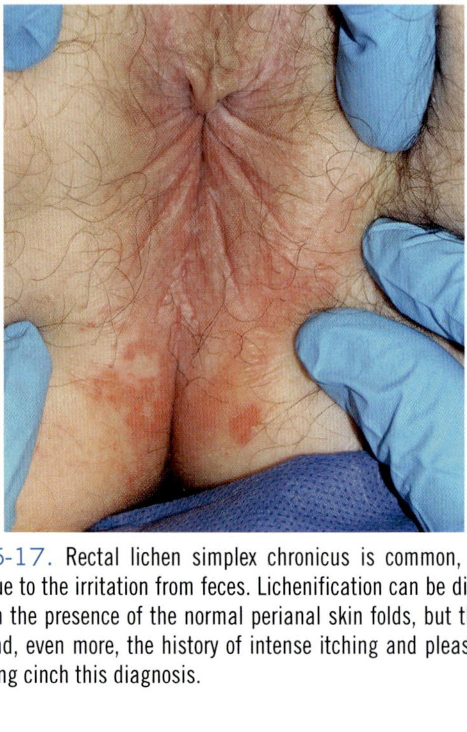

Fig. 5-17. Rectal lichen simplex chronicus is common, at least partly due to the irritation from feces. Lichenification can be difficult to gauge in the presence of the normal perianal skin folds, but these fissures and, even more, the history of intense itching and pleasure with scratching cinch this diagnosis.

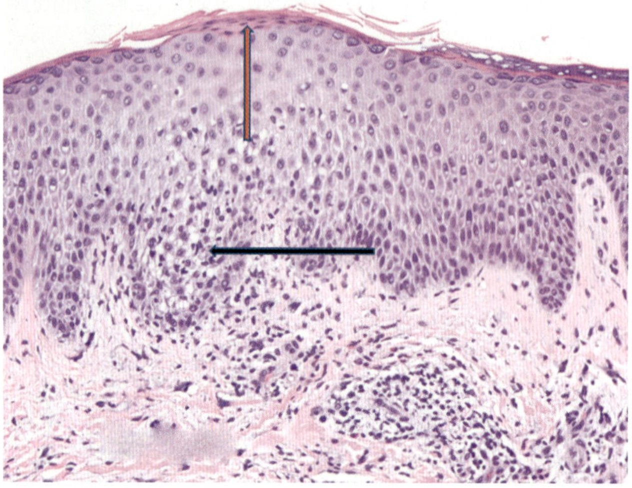

Fig. 5-18. A biopsy of scratched, red LSC/eczema shows spongiosis, which is edema of the epidermis, manifested by increased intercellular spaces (*black arrow*) and mild, focal parakeratosis, where there are nuclei seen in the stratum corneum (*red arrow*). (Courtesy of Jason Reutter, MD.)

The surface shows dotted vessels in clusters or distributed randomly as well as yellow crusts.[8]

In some instances, it is not clear whether the LSC is arising *de novo* (primary LSC) or is superimposed on another underlying dermatological problem (secondary LSC). One might think that biopsy could identify the presence of any underlying problem in the setting of secondary LSC, but this is often not true. In the acute phase of LSC, spongiotic inflammation will be prominent. Spongiosis is also present in contact dermatitis and seborrheic dermatitis.

Even more confusion can occur when chronic LSC is biopsied **(Figs. 5-18 and 5-19)**. This is particularly likely to happen when LSC overlies genital psoriasis but is also common with tinea cruris in men and lichen sclerosus in women. In this situation, the pathology report is often signed out as

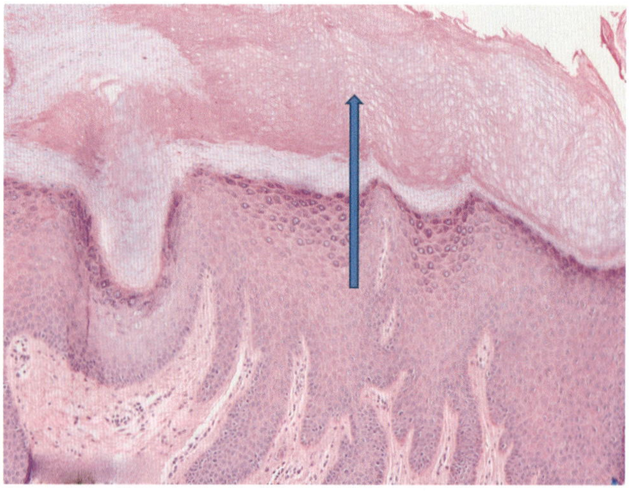

Fig. 5-19. Rubbed, lichenified lichen simplex chronicus shows remarkable thick hyperkeratosis (*arrow*) and acanthosis, thickening of the epidermis. (Courtesy of Jason Reutter, MD.)

"psoriasiform dermatitis," which will not offer the clinician much diagnostic help. If this occurs, the clinician will have to undertake clinical-pathologic correlation.[1]

Because candidiasis is the condition most commonly associated with the development of LSC in women, culture and/or KOH examination for associated candidiasis will be worthwhile. In men, if the upper inner thighs are involved, it may be useful to obtain a KOH and/or culture for dermatophyte fungi associated with tinea cruris. Psoriasis can be very similar in appearance to LSC, especially in the anogenital area where LSC may be superimposed on plaques of psoriasis. Unfortunately, as noted above, biopsy may not be helpful in separating psoriasis from LSC. In women, helpful clues to the presence of psoriasis would be the presence of more typical psoriatic plaques at characteristic sites elsewhere, the identification of typical psoriatic nail changes, and/or the presence of psoriatic arthritis. LSC frequently overlies vulvar lichen sclerosus and may obscure the typical clinical characteristics of this condition. However, architectural damage such as the presence of clitoral hooding, loss of the labia minora, or the presence of purpura would help to identify associated lichen sclerosus. At both the clinical and histological level, LSC can be confused with the often rather benign appearance of differentiated (non–human papillomavirus related) vulvar intraepithelial neoplasia (dVIN). Moreover, the frequent histological presence of epithelial acanthosis, similar to that seen in LSC, immediately adjacent to the carcinoma raises a question of what, if any, relationship might exist between LSC and the development of genital squamous cell carcinoma (see also the section on female squamous cell carcinoma in Chapter 7).

**LICHEN SIMPLEX CHRONICUS — Diagnosis**

- History of intense itching and pleasure with scratching
- Morphology of poorly demarcated lichenification, excoriation, scale, which may be subtle
- Erythema or, in darker complexioned patients, hyperpigmentation

## Pathophysiology

The cause of LSC/atopic dermatitis is multifactorial and has recently been reviewed.[8] A large proportion of the patients who develop LSC have a personal or immediate family history of hay fever, asthma, or eczematous skin disease and thus are presumably atopic. But it is still not clear just how atopy results in the development of LSC. There is increasing appreciation that many, if not most, patients with atopic dermatitis possess both genetic (notably mutations in the filaggrin gene) and nongenetic defects that interfere with the normal development of the outer ("barrier") layer of the epidermis. These barrier layer defects (microfissures) allow for greater transepidermal water loss and thus greater than normal dryness (xerosis) of the skin. These same defects also allow easier exposure and processing of both irritants and allergens. It also seems likely that these defects allow easier triggering of the terminal branches of sensory nerves that carry itch and light pain.

Even though peripheral eosinophilia and elevated serum IgE levels are frequently present, atopic dermatitis is different from other atopic disorders in that the immune dysfunction associated with the disorder is T-cell mediated rather than occurring as a type I IgE–related humoral dysfunction such as occurs in hay fever and asthma. Atopic dermatitis appears to involve the TH2 component of the cell-mediated immune system, along with related interleukins (IL-4, IL-13, IL-31), and this process likely plays an important role in the pruritus, the increased serum IgE levels, and peripheral eosinophilia.[9,10]

In addition to such peripheral abnormalities, it seems likely that there are also important central aspects such as a fairly marked adverse effect on the quality of life.[10] Possibly, there is a heightened appreciation for itching at the level of the sensory cortex and an innate tendency for the frequently present sleep disorder, attention deficit/hyperactivity disorder, and maybe even for the development of obsessive-compulsive–like scratching that characterizes the itch-scratch cycle in LSC.[10] Some clinicians also believe that patients with atopic dermatitis, and by extrapolation, some of those with LSC, have mild to moderate psychological abnormalities such as heightened anxiety levels, depression, stress vulnerability, and obsessive-compulsive traits that may play a role in causation and worsening of the disease.[10-12] Moreover, some clinicians, myself included, believe that there is a predilection for internalization of anger and hostility that is distinctive for patients with atopic dermatitis.

At the clinical level, it is apparent that irritant factors involving the local environment, such as heat and sweating, trigger both the initiation and continuation of the itching and scratching that is so characteristic in the disorder. As opposed to this important role for contact *irritants*, the role of contact *allergens* is much more controversial. A significant proportion of patients with anogenital LSC/atopic dermatitis are reported to have positive patch tests that are deemed to be clinically relevant.[3] However, data indicating that removal of the offending agents lead to amelioration of the problem are lacking. Based on our personal experience, we believe that patch testing in patients with anogenital LSC is rarely necessary or justifiable.

## Management

LSC is a chronic disease. Left untreated, the itch-scratch cycle persists indefinitely, although it can be episodic rather than consistently present. This process is extremely discomforting for the patient, and it may lead

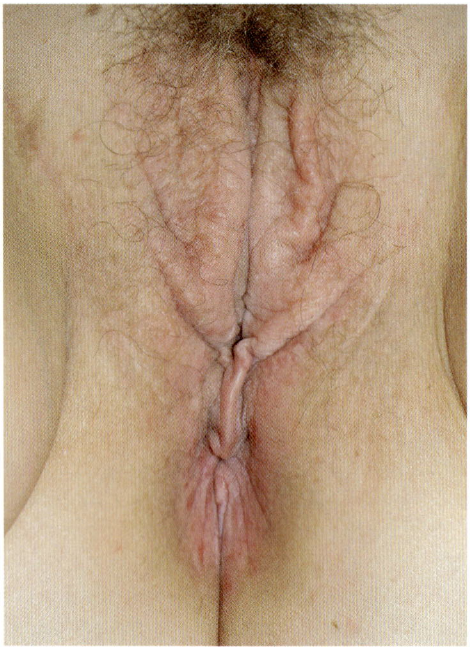

Fig. 5-20. Lichenified lichen simplex chronicus before treatment.

to a significant decrement in quality of life.[10] Other troublesome sequelae may include hyperpigmentation and hypopigmentation due to either activation or destruction of melanocytes, respectively. Treatment for LSC can be extremely effective **(Figs. 5-20 and 5-21)**. Approach to therapy includes five basic steps: (1) improvement in the local environment to reduce the triggering that leads to itching and scratching, (2) restoration of normal barrier layer function, (3) reduction in inflammation, (4) cessation of the itch-scratch cycle, and (5) identification and treatment for any detrimental psychological factors that may be present.

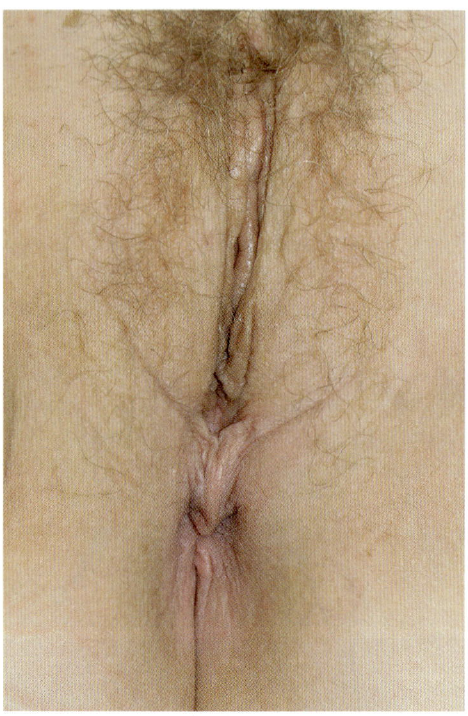

Fig. 5-21. Five weeks later, the LSC has cleared and the vulva appears normal.

**LICHEN SIMPLEX CHRONICUS — Management**

- Improvement in the local environment; attention to irritants such as overwashing, harsh soaps, panty liners, incontinence, obesity, etc.
- Reduction of inflammation; superpotent corticosteroid ointment such as daily clobetasol to gain control, then slow taper with less frequent application or lower potency until the skin appears normal
- Nighttime sedation to suppress scratching
- Attention to psychological factors; SSRI for depression/anxiety when needed

### Improvement in the Local Environment

As mentioned previously, heat and sweat act as provoking factors for the development of itching, scratching, and inflammation. Removing or reducing these factors is certainly desirable but is more difficult to do than one might expect. Immediate steps include a change to less occlusive, less tight-fitting clothing and the use of materials (such as cotton and cotton-blends) that allow for better movement of air. Other approaches we recommend include the avoidance of prolonged sitting, the use of cloth rather than vinyl for seating surfaces, and the use of cooler temperatures in the workspace or home. Weight loss can help those who are obese by way of decreasing intertriginous surface area and reducing frictional rubbing through body movement. Note that the use of a hair dryer even on its lowest temperature settings in an attempt to dry the area is not helpful, and in most instances, it is detrimental.

Other irritants such as fecal contamination, urinary incontinence, and vaginal secretions should be dealt with. Treatment of fecal and urinary incontinence lies outside the scope of this chapter; additional medical consultation will probably be necessary for amelioration of these two factors. Vaginal discharge needs to be properly diagnosed and treated (see Chapter 14), and the continual use of panty liners should be discouraged. Asking patients about the frequency and nature of their anogenital hygiene is important because many patients, particularly women, think of the anogenital area as a site "that is especially dirty." Excessive hygiene especially using water that is too hot, harsh cleaning products, and excessive scrubbing removes natural skin lubricants and thus can cause irritation. Contrary to decades of physician recommendations, such as using only white underwear, the avoidance of dyes in clothing lacks documented scientific merit. Again, contrary to popular opinion, laundering practices for underwear (number of rinses, avoidance of certain detergents, discontinuation of antistatic dryer strips, etc.) are for practical purposes never an important triggering factor.

### Restoration of Barrier Layer Function

Barrier layer dysfunction occurs in all patients with atopic dermatitis/LSC. This dysfunction can occur as a result of genetic factors that interfere with epithelial cell differentiation, irritant factors mentioned above, and physical disruption of the surface epithelium due to scratching and rubbing. The approach to all three of these factors involves the use of lubrication. Since lubricants are covered in detail in Chapter 3, this material will not be repeated here. Irritants are dealt with in the preceding two paragraphs. Reduction of itching, scratching, and rubbing is covered in the several paragraphs that follow.

### Reduction in Inflammation

Steroids, used topically or systemically, are the *sine qua non* for the treatment of inflammation. This subject is covered thoroughly in the section titled "Anti-inflammatory Therapy" of Chapter 3 and, other than mention of a few important principles, will not be repeated here. First, the strength of the topical steroid must be appropriate both for patient safety and the task at hand. Low- and mid-potency steroids such as hydrocortisone and triamcinolone are usually ineffective in anogenital LSC/atopic dermatitis. Second, an ointment vehicle, rather than a cream, will be better tolerated and adds a bit of lubrication. Third, topical steroids must be continued for a month or more after the clinical symptoms and signs have regressed. However, after clinical clearing, the frequency of application and/or the potency of the topical steroid should be tapered. A lengthy duration of therapy is necessary because microscopic evidence of inflammation remains for a considerable period of time after clinical improvement, or even resolution, is noted. Fourth, if topical steroids have not been effective after a month of treatment, consider the use of systemic steroid therapy. While a "burst" of prednisone can work, it is usually too short to be maximally effective, and in addition, rebound often occurs shortly after the last pills are administered. For this, and other, reasons, we prefer the use of intramuscularly administered triamcinolone acetonide (Kenalog) as described in Chapter 3.

Occasionally, a patient requires additional anti-inflammatory medication. There are several topical options. The use of nonsteroidal topical calcineurin inhibitors tacrolimus and pimecrolimus (see Chapter 3) in an attempt to reduce the side effects of prolonged steroid use may be considered, but the stinging on application and efficacy less than mid- and high-potency topical steroids represent significant limitations.[13] Crisaborole ointment has also been available for several years, approved in the United States as a nonsteroidal medication for atopic dermatitis. This medication has not found a useful place in the practical treatment of inflammatory dermatoses. At the time of this writing, the Food and Drug Administration has accepted ruxolitinib cream, a janus kinase inhibitor, for priority review for atopic dermatitis.

Until recently, the only systemic anti-inflammatory agents used routinely for eczematous diseases were corticosteroids. Cyclosporine is very effective but dangerous for long-term use. However, the development of biologic medications for inflammatory diseases has exploded in the last 20 years. Dupilumab (Dupixent) is the only currently available biologic medication used for eczematous diseases, and this medication has shown remarkable benefit with a good safety profile for patients with recalcitrant disease.[14,15] This medication blocks IL-4 and IL-13 signaling. There are a number of additional biologic agents in development for eczema, including lebrikizumab, tralokinumab, nemolizumab, tezepelumab, and ISB 830.[16]

### Breaking the Itch-Scratch Cycle

This is probably the single most important aspect in the treatment of LSC. Unfortunately, it is also the most often overlooked. Fortunately, the presence of clothing, a conscious attempt to control scratching, and embarrassment associated with genital scratching tend to reduce much of daytime scratching. However, these constraints are lessened when the patient is at home in the evening and are removed completely while sleeping. Thus, the nighttime scratching that characteristically is present with the itch-scratch cycle remains in place. Approaches for the treatment of nighttime rubbing and scratching are thoroughly covered in Chapter 3, but several major principles are worth reviewing here. First, nighttime scratching occurs periodically while the patient is in the lighter stages of non-REM sleep.[5,6] Nonhabituating medications with a sedative effect such as the first generation of antihistamines and certain tricyclics work well for this purpose. Second, the dose of the medication chosen should be increased weekly until nighttime scratching ceases or until the risks of side effects caution against any further increase. Third, the medication should be taken about 2 hours before going to bed to both prevent scratching before actually falling asleep and to reduce possible morning "hangover." Fourth, the medication should be taken every evening rather than on an "as necessary" basis.

In many instances, sedating therapy for nighttime scratching obviates the need to treat daytime itching with medications, such as hydroxyzine, that can cause sleepiness, inept driving, or dangerous operation of machinery. However, some patients will still experience significant daytime pruritus. Many clinicians prescribe nonsedating antihistamines for these individuals. Unfortunately, this approach does not work well probably because histamine plays only a minor role in the itching associated with atopic dermatitis and LSC. In this situation, I prefer the use of selective serotonin reuptake inhibitors (SSRIs). It is not clear whether these agents work because of their beneficial effect on anxiety and depression or whether they diminish the obsessive-compulsive component of chronic scratching. There is limited support for this approach in the medical literature.[17,18] Further information on the use of SSRIs can be found in Chapter 3.

### Identification and Treatment of Detrimental Psychological Components

Anxiety and/or depression are regularly present in patients with LSC.[12,19] Most patients will not volunteer this information unless it is directly sought by a clinician. Even then, the importance of psychological factors tends to be minimized by patients, and thus, clinician questioning in this area should occur not just initially but also periodically at the time of return visits. Some controversy exists as to whether these psychological factors play a role in the etiology of the LSC/atopic dermatitis or whether they are secondary to the presence of these disorders. It is my opinion, supported by some published data, that they frequently play a role in causation. But, either way, once identified, treatment, generally with SSRIs as described in Chapter 3, can be quite helpful.

In addition to the common problems of anxiety and depression, patients with LSC/atopic dermatitis may also experience sexual dysfunction.[20,21] Although most of us would not consider ourselves as expert in the area of sexual counseling, giving patients an opportunity to discuss this aspect of their lives, either with us or with a trained therapist, can be quite beneficial in the treatment of patients with anogenital LSC.

## Irritant Contact Dermatitis

Irritant contact dermatitis is an eczematous reaction that develops in response to an exogenous substance that can cause inflammation when applied to the skin of *any* individual. Thus, all individuals have the potential for developing *irritant* contact dermatitis, whereas only patients specifically sensitized to an allergen develop *allergic* contact dermatitis (ACD).

### Clinical Presentation

The prevalence of irritant contact dermatitis involving the anogenital area is unknown. However, a major study indicated that irritant contact dermatitis accounted for about 15% of all patients with anogenital problems referred to dermatologists for patch testing (see the supplementary online content for Ref.[3]). Irritant contact dermatitis is often divided into two categories: chronic and acute irritant contact dermatitis.

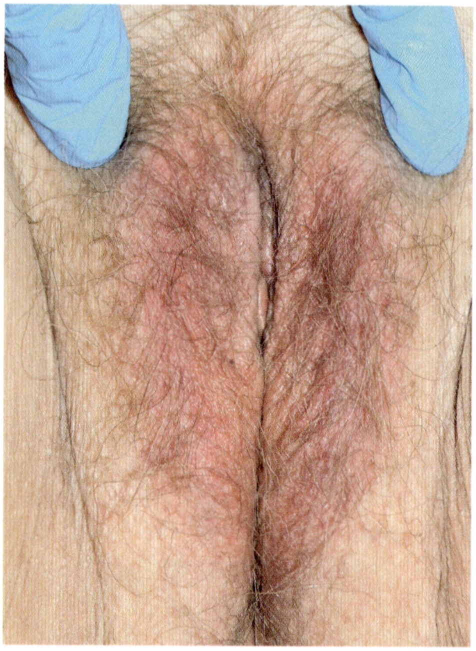

Fig. 5-22. This erythematous plaque is typical of chronic irritant dermatitis, here produced by washing with soap and water multiple times each day.

*Chronic* irritant contact dermatitis is usually manifested by symptoms of irritation, burning, pain, soreness, or rawness. Note that in some patients, especially those who are genetically atopic, the irritant can also cause itching and can initiate an itch-scratch cycle. Generally, chronic irritant contact dermatitis presents as a poorly demarcated, slightly scaly erythematous patch or slightly elevated plaque. Little or no edema is present **(Fig. 5-22)**. The red hues sometimes occur at the dusky red or brown-red end of the erythema spectrum **(Fig. 5-23)**. Often, there

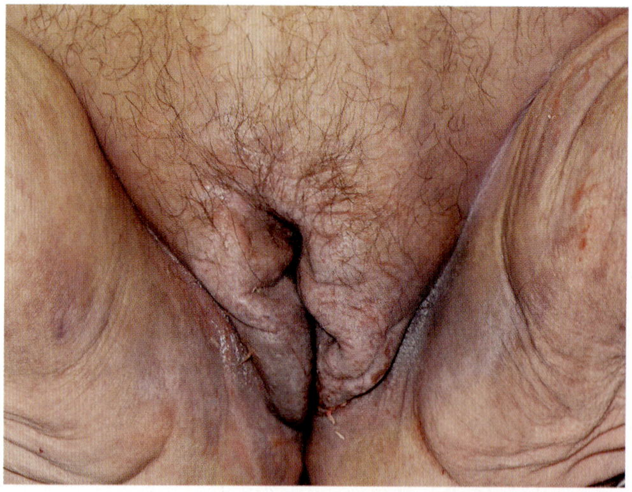

Fig. 5-23. The red-brown color of this poorly demarcated plaque of irritant contact dermatitis is characteristic and produced here by chronic incontinence.

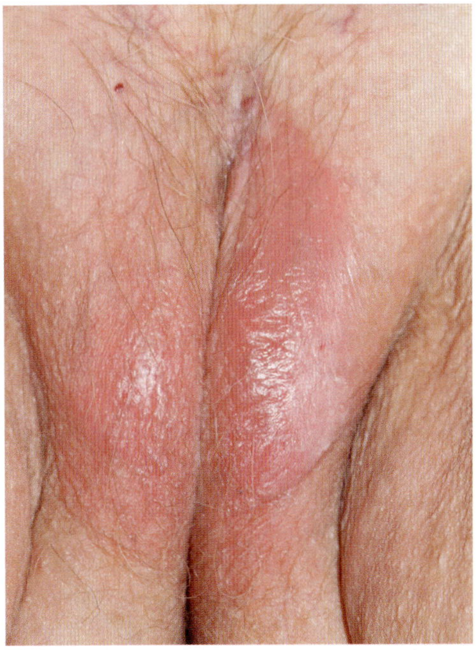

Fig. 5-24. At times, irritant dermatitis can appear red and glazed, as seen here in this patient who was using witch hazel on the vulva to stop itching.

is a dry, glazed, fissured, chapped appearance **(Figs. 5-24 and 5-25)**. If the irritant in question triggers itching and scratching, the morphology will be indistinguishable from that of LSC.

Acute irritant contact dermatitis is essentially a chemical "burn." It is characterized as a rapid development of erythema, edema, and sometimes blistering shortly after the contact occurs **(Fig. 5-26)**. Poorly keratinized skin, such as the modified mucous membranes of the vulva, the glans penis, and the inner aspect of the prepuce, is very fragile, and blister roofs are shed quickly, forming erosions or even ulcers **(Fig. 5-27)**. On the more resilient

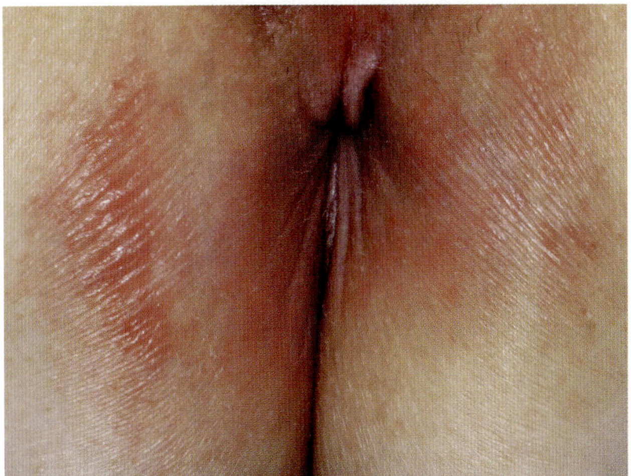

Fig. 5-25. The shiny, chapped appearance of this irritant contact dermatitis was produced by diarrhea.

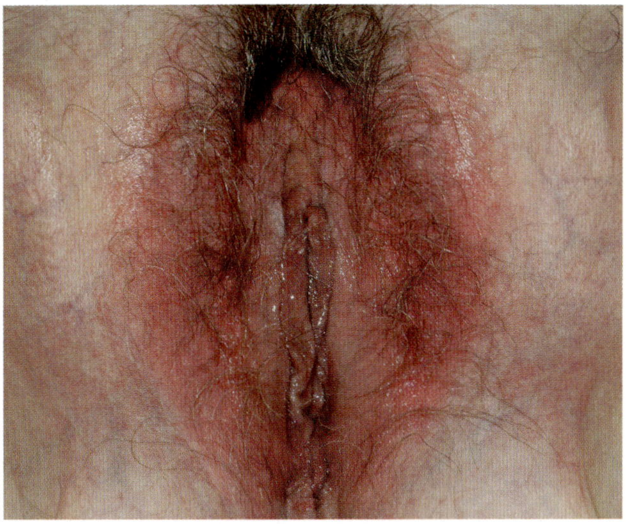

Fig. 5-26. Caustic substances, including chronic exposure to urine and feces can produce erosions and ulcerations.

keratinized skin, blisters may remain visible for a day or two before they also become unroofed, leaving erosions or ulcers **(Fig. 5-28)**.

## Diagnosis

The diagnosis of *chronic* irritant contact dermatitis is made on the appearance, as described above, together with a history that suggests undue exposure to soap, water, sweat, urine, feces, vaginal discharge, or the less

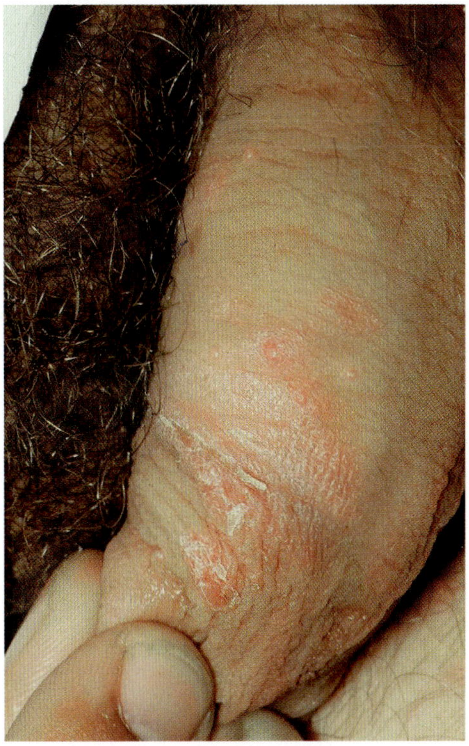

Fig. 5-27. Scale and sloughing of the skin remain after this man used an over-the-counter medication to remove a bump on the penile shaft.

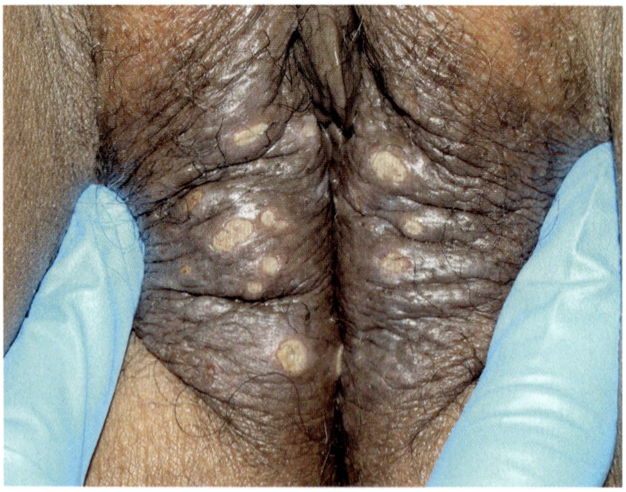

Fig. 5-28. Blisters eventuated into ulcers after application of sinecatechins for genital warts.

frequently encountered irritants listed in Table 5-1 and in the section on pathogenesis. Dermoscopy shows the changes associated with all eczematous disease as discussed in the section above on atopic dermatitis, without specific signs of irritant contact dermatitis.[8] Biopsy is rarely necessary, and if carried out, generally shows only nonspecific spongiosis and superficial perivascular lymphocytic inflammation. Sometimes epithelial acanthosis is also present. Thus, the histology only indicates that there is an eczematous process without specifically pointing toward an irritant contact etiology. In this situation, clinicopathologic correlation will be necessary.[1] The differential diagnoses for chronic irritant contact dermatitis are primarily the other eczematous diseases, especially LSC, as described above. Differentiation from allergic dermatitis can be problematic. Patch testing to identify specific allergens may be helpful in this regard. Uncommon and rare conditions that can mimic chronic irritant contact dermatitis include candidiasis, extramammary Paget disease (EMPD), Hailey-Hailey disease, and Darier disease.

The diagnosis of *acute* irritant contact dermatitis is more easily accomplished because of the very short interval between exposure and development of inflammation. Thus, patients can almost always remember and identify the contactant that caused the problem. Most often, the products responsible are medications that have been recently applied by medical personnel (Table 5-1). On the rare occasions where such a history is not forthcoming, one should consider the possibility of either obsessive-compulsive disorder or factitial disease caused by the patient or the patients' care takers. Biopsy is not useful in acute irritant contact dermatitis as the histology only shows nonspecific inflammation and disruption or destruction of the epithelium without pointing to a single, definite cause.

TABLE 5-1

**Common Causes of Irritant Contact Dermatitis**

**Weak irritants** *(chronic irritant contact dermatitis)*
- Excessive hygiene; too frequent washing
- Sweat
- Urine
- Feces
- Depilatories
- Vaginal lubricants
- Vaginal discharge
- Panty liners
- Menstrual pads
- Spermicides
- Preservatives and stabilizers
  - *Candida* sp. Proteins

**Strong irritants** *(acute irritant contact dermatitis)*
- Salicylic acid
- Podophyllin, podophyllotoxin
- Imiquimod
- Fluorouracil
- Cantharidin
- Trichloroacetic, bichloracetic acid

**IRRITANT CONTACT DERMATITIS — Diagnosis**

- Morphology of red slightly scaling plaque, sometimes dusky or chapped and fissured (chronic), or sudden onset of redness, edema, and sometimes blisters, even erosions (acute)
- History of undue exposure to soap, water, sweat, urine, feces, vaginal discharge, or less frequently encountered irritants listed in text and table

## Pathophysiology

Irritant contact dermatitis can be caused either by repeated exposure to a weak irritant (chronic irritant contact dermatitis) or by one, or only a few, exposures to a very strong irritant (acute irritant contact dermatitis) (Table 5-1). The most common causes of *chronic* irritant contact dermatitis are overexposure to soap and water and chronic exposure to urine or feces in a diapered infant or an incontinent adult (Figs. 5-29 and 5-30). Other chronic irritants include douches, feminine hygiene products, depilatories, personal lubricants, and spermicides. An often overlooked irritant is the presence of candidiasis where the candidal proteins can cause irritation quite apart from true infection. Because repeated

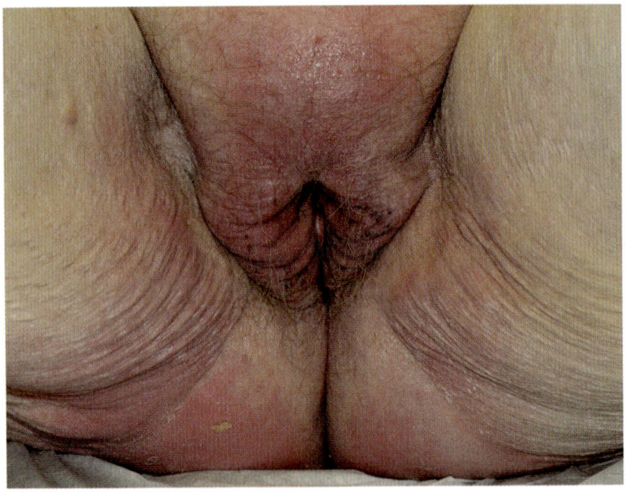

Fig. 5-29. Incontinence produced this irritant contact dermatitis, with dusky erythema and shiny, glazed skin.

exposure is necessary for the development of irritant contact dermatitis and because the symptoms and signs develop gradually, the patient is frequently unaware that the offending substance is irritating and is causing his or her problem.

*Acute* irritant contact dermatitis is produced by one or only a few exposures to a very strong irritant. This exposure is regularly accompanied by a very short duration of time between the contact and the development of pain and inflammation. For this reason, the patient usually recognizes what caused the problem, although he or she frequently misinterprets this as an allergic reaction rather than as irritation. The most common causes of acute irritant contact dermatitis include various treatments for genital warts, such as trichloroacetic and bichloracetic acids, podophyllin products, imiquimod, and cantharidin. Some patients with very sensitive skin can experience acute irritant contact dermatitis to the vehicles of the cream, gel, or solution used in topical medications and lubricants. This is most often the result of chemicals such as alcohol, propylene glycol, and polyethylene glycol. Acute irritant contact dermatitis can also be experienced with topical use of the calcineurin inhibitors and with the "azole" group of anticandidal/antifungal creams. Lastly, keep in mind that patients will sometimes apply very unorthodox products to their genitalia in misguided attempts to clean an area that is perceived to be "dirty" or "odorous." We have seen reactions to things such as lye, kerosene, and bleach.

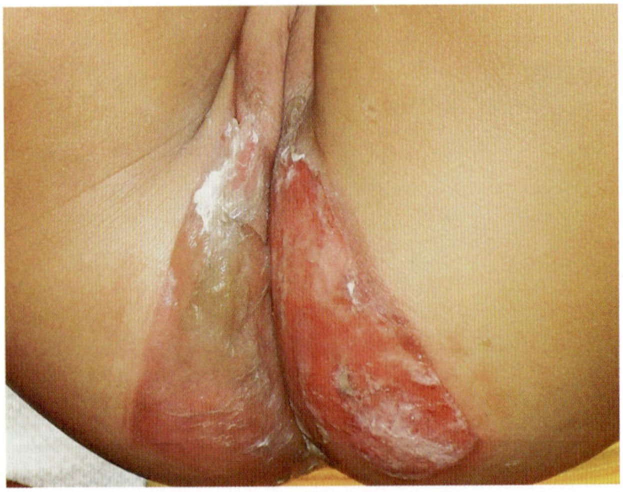

Fig. 5-30. This child was reported to child protective services for this blistering eruption, which was actually caused by diarrheal stool held against the skin overnight by an occlusive diaper.

## Management

The most important aspects of therapy are the identification and elimination of all irritants. Irritant contact dermatitis in the genital area is often multifactorial, so that anything applied to the anogenital area to include all medications, soaps, antiseptics, douches, and powders should be discontinued. Vigorous cleansing should also be stopped. Note, however, that some patients become "addicted" to certain behaviors, and as a result, there may be very poor compliance with instructions to cease these ritualistic behaviors. After the offending agent or agents are discontinued and use of a mid-potency topical corticosteroid ointment has been instituted, the dermatitis quickly improves. If the skin is dry and chapped, lubricants (see Chapter 3) may be useful. Infants and diapered adults may require the use of a simple "barrier" product such as zinc oxide ointment to keep urine and feces away from the skin. In those instances where itching or pain is really troublesome, prednisone, at a dose of 40 mg each morning for a few days, can improve this symptom until healing is well underway, at which point a topical corticosteroid can be substituted.

The pain and burning of acute irritant contact dermatitis can be minimized through the use of tepid tap water bathtub soaks several times a day for the first few days. Lubrication with a thin layer of petrolatum should be applied immediately following each soak. Nighttime sedation and oral analgesics may be necessary for several days. Topical analgesics should be avoided as they may cause additional discomfort and may even worsen the problem through the development of an allergic reaction.

**IRRITANT CONTACT DERMATITIS — Management**

- Identification and elimination of contactants
- Mid-potency topical corticosteroid such as triamcinolone 0.1% ointment
- When dry and cracked, lubrication
- If associated with incontinence/diarrhea, barrier paste such as zinc oxide

## Allergic Contact Dermatitis

As opposed to *irritant* contact dermatitis wherein all individuals are potentially capable of developing a reaction, ACD requires immunological processing. This is a more restrictive process and only a limited number of individuals exposed to a potential allergen will develop ACD at the time of their subsequent contact with the offending agent.

### Clinical Presentation

Controversy exists regarding the frequency with which ACD of the anogenital region occurs. In the past, nearly all of the published material on prevalence dealt with clinically diagnosed vulvar involvement in women. However, more recently, the publications regarding ACD come from patch test clinics. These reports contain much more information on the perianal area and the genitalia in both men and women.[3,22-24] These studies suggest that one or more clinically relevant positive patch test will be found in 40%-50% of all patients sent for patch testing.

There is, however, a problem with the data from patch test clinics. This difficulty revolves around determining which positive patch tests are actually clinically relevant. Most clinicians just assume that if the patient has applied something containing the allergen, it is relevant. This is not always true! Second, patients with "dermatitis" of all types frequently have several positive patch tests to common allergens. It is not known what role, if any, one or more of these allergens play in the pathogenesis of their dermatitis. This is particularly true for patients who actually have atopic dermatitis rather than ACD.[25]

Allergic contact dermatitis is clinically characterized by the presence of poorly marginated, bright red, edematous patches and plaques. Scale is generally less prominent than it is in both atopic dermatitis/LSC and irritant contact dermatitis. Pruritus is regularly present and, in some instances, can be quite problematic. Not surprisingly, this frequently results in superimposed development of the itch-scratch cycle and the clinical signs of LSC. Sometimes vesicles, usually minute in size (representing macroscopic evidence of histologic spongiosis), stud the surface of the erythematous plaques **(Fig. 5-31)**. Occasionally, odd shapes (linear or angular) are found **(Fig. 5-32 and 5-33)**. These generally occur by way of irregular application of medications applied with the finger tips. The labia majora are usually involved in women and both the penis and the scrotum may be affected in men **(Figs. 5-34 and 5-35)**. Anal and perianal involvement is commonly found in both sexes.[24]

Allergic contact *urticaria* is a rarely encountered, separate, and distinct disorder from ACD. The appearance can be either that of tissue swelling (angioedema) or can develop as urticarial papules (wheals, hives) and plaques that are entirely similar to those that occur with

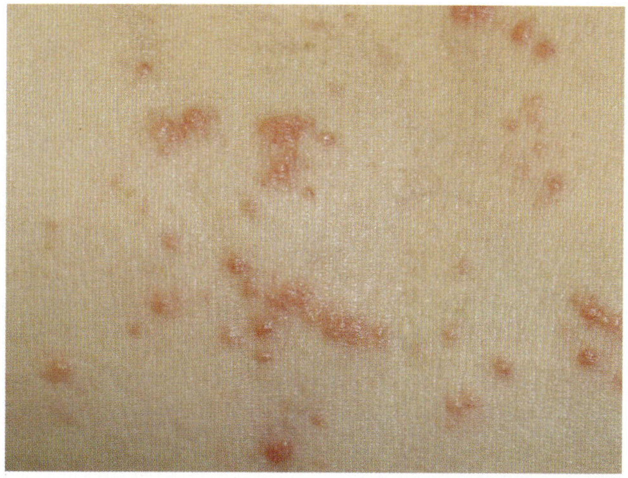

Fig. 5-31. These small, coalescing, firm vesicles are classic for allergic contact dermatitis.

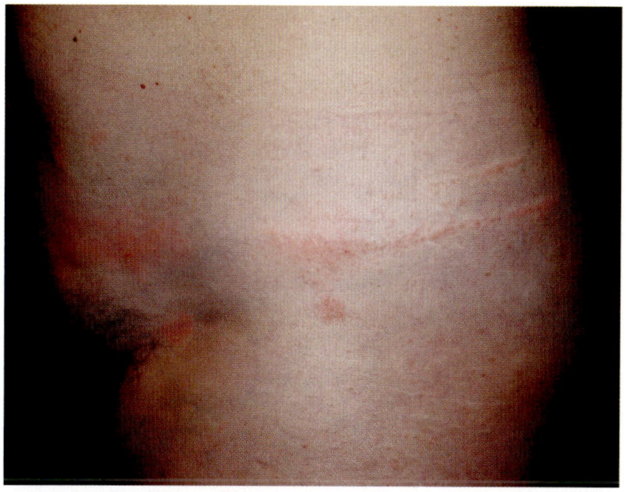

Fig. 5-32. Linear plaques of fine vesicles are pathognomonic for allergic contact dermatitis to plants such as poison ivy.

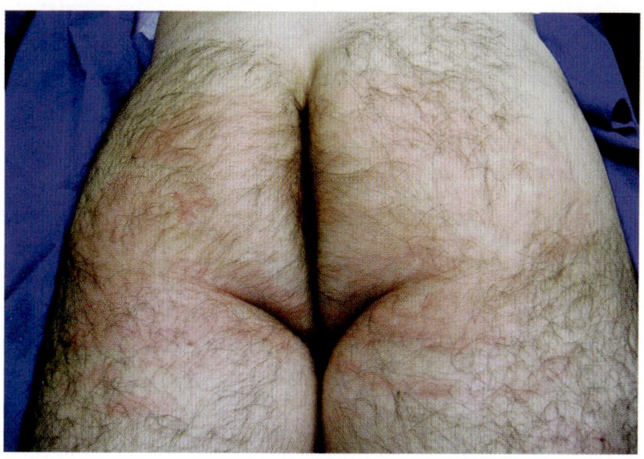

Fig. 5-33. The unusual distribution of this red, scaling plaque on the buttocks and posterior thighs is consistent with the cause of this man's allergic contact dermatitis; a teak toilet seat.

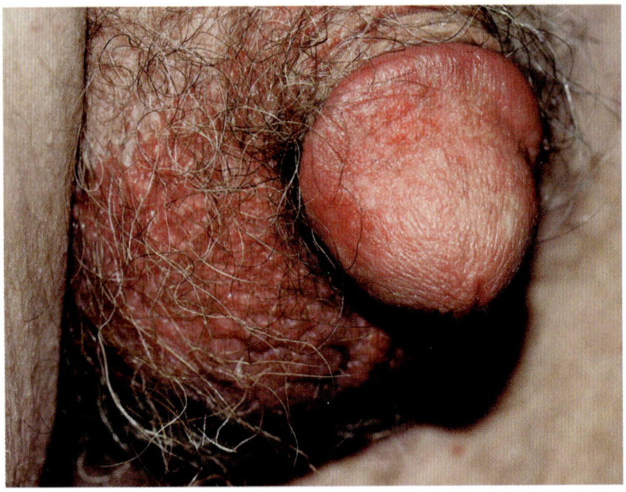

Fig. 5-34. These red, exudative lesions were produced by the application of triple antibiotic ointment, which contains the very strong antigen, neomycin.

garden-variety urticaria. Unlike the situation with allergic contact *dermatitis*, there is no clinical evidence of epithelial abnormalities. Such reactions are usually easy to recognize because of the rapid development of the urticarial reaction within minutes after contact has taken place. This allergic contact urticaria is particularly likely to occur in those who have become sensitized to latex or seminal fluid.

## Diagnosis

The diagnosis of ACD is most often made on a clinical basis. The role of patch testing for patients with eczematous disease of the genitalia is controversial. Some clinicians believe that a diagnosis of ACD is often missed unless all patients presenting with an eczematous morphology are patch tested.[26] We believe, in accordance with Bayes theorem, that patch testing is best carried out only

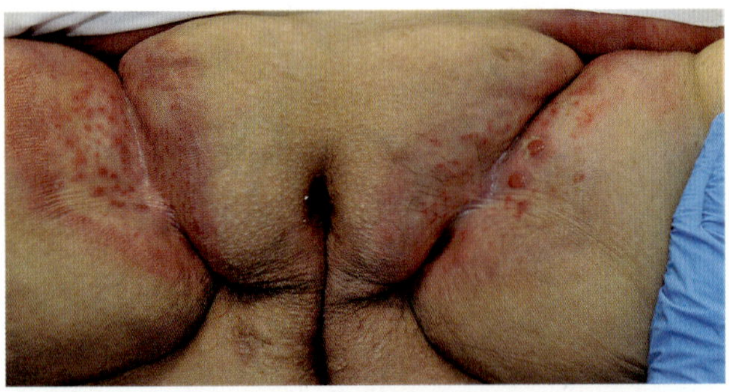

Fig. 5-35. An unusual but distinctive pattern of contact dermatitis is called granuloma gluteale infantum (in children) or adultorum (in adults), also called pseudowarts, occurs only on anogenital skin. Discrete nodules with superficial erosion, sometimes on normal skin, sometimes on red plaques, are characteristic. This woman was applying an over-the-counter anti-itch preparation that contained both the allergen benzocaine and the irritant resorcinol.

for highly suspected patients so as to reduce the large number of false-positive results that occur when testing is carried out in a relatively unselected population. Moreover, the simple presence of a positive patch test does not prove that the disease in question is due to that allergen. It is necessary first to confirm that the presence of that allergen was present in one or another of the products coming in contact with the anogenital tissue of the patient who tested positive and, second, to obtain marked clinical improvement when use of the offending product is discontinued. Absolute proof, however, would require a new contact with the suspected product to see whether the dermatitis redevelops. Not surprisingly, this latter approach is almost always rejected by the patient!

Dermoscopy shows the changes associated with all eczematous disease as discussed in the section above on atopic dermatitis, without specific signs of ACD.[8] Biopsy is not likely to be helpful because the principle findings of spongiosis and acanthosis are essentially identical to those of patients with any of the other eczematous diseases. In spite of this, some pathologists and clinicians believe that the presence of eosinophils in the inflammatory infiltrate of the biopsy suggests a high likelihood of ACD.

All of the eczematous disorders, as described in this chapter, need to be considered in one's list of differential diagnoses. In addition, one should bear in mind the possibility that preceding or concomitant candidiasis and/or dermatophyte fungal infection (tinea cruris) may also be present.

**ALLERGIC CONTACT DERMATITIS Diagnosis**

- Morphology of poorly marginated, bright red, edematous patches and plaques. Scale is often inapparent, but sometimes there are vesicles.
- Confirmed by discontinuation of any potential contactants and response to therapy; if required, patch testing and response to withdrawal of potential relevant contactant.

## Pathophysiology

Allergic contact dermatitis represents a cell-mediated, delayed-type (type IV) hypersensitivity reaction. It arises when a substance, acting as an antigen, is processed by macrophages (Langerhans cells) in the epidermis and that it is then presented to the T-cell immune system. This results in the development, activation, and proliferation of antigen-specific T cells. These cells return to the skin at the time of the next contact with the allergen, resulting in the clinical development of ACD.[24]

The agents causing ACD in the anogenital area, based on patch testing, have recently been reviewed.[3,22-24] The most commonly incriminated of these products can be placed into several groups: medications, anesthetics,

**TABLE 5-2**

**Common Causes of Allergic Contact Dermatitis**

| Common Causes of Allergic Contact Dermatitis |
|---|
| **Medications** |
| Benzocaine (Vagisil) |
| Dibucaine (Nupercainal) |
| Lidocaine |
| Neomycin |
| Bacitracin |
| Corticosteroids (hydrocortisone butyrate, budesonide, etc.) |
| Spermicides |
| Diphenhydramine |
| **Vehicles, preservatives, and stabilizers** |
| Quaternium-15 |
| Propylene glycol |
| Parabens |
| Isothiazolinones |
| Metabisulfites |
| Lubricants |
| Lanolin (wool alcohols) |
| **Fragrances** |
| Cinnamic aldehyde |
| Balsam of Peru |

fragrances, stabilizers, and preservatives. Some of most frequently identified specific agents within these groups are further detailed in Table 5-2. Note that positive patch tests occur quite often with several topically applied corticosteroids and with vehicles, preservatives, and stabilizers found in almost all personal hygiene, cosmetic, and topical medical products. Our own experience suggests that all of these latter products infrequently cause problems, but in instances of recalcitrant anogenital dermatitis, discontinuation of all topically applied agents including corticosteroids and lubricants other than petrolatum is warranted. Then, if this is followed by improvement, agents can be added back one at a time in an attempt to identify the specific culprit.

A special situation occurs in patients who are allergic to seminal fluid and latex.[27] These represent a type I, IgE-mediated, immediate reaction in which angioedema and urticarial papules and plaques arise within minutes of contact. This situation usually presents as contact urticaria and it occurs very infrequently. Nevertheless, it is mentioned here because of the very real potential for anaphylaxis to occur in such situations.

A number of commonly used products are not listed here or in tables because of controversy about their ability to cause either allergic or irritant reactions. These include soaps, laundry detergents, fabric softeners, antistatic sheets, medicated wipes, toilet paper (scented or unscented), menstrual pads, and other feminine hygiene agents. In our opinion, normal use of these products rarely leads to anogenital allergic or irritant contact dermatitis.

### Management

The first step in therapy of ACD is the identification and subsequent elimination of the most likely offending agent. If the allergen can be identified either clinically or through patch testing, the patient needs to be instructed regarding the products wherein these agents are found in order to avoid future contact. This can be difficult because some allergens can be found in multiple, often apparently innocuous, and unsuspected sources. Information regarding the potential sources of these allergens can be found in most standard dermatological textbooks. In instances of suspected ACD where a specific contactant cannot be identified, it may be necessary to counsel the patient to avoid all topical agents other than clear water and petrolatum.

After the elimination of the contactant, the symptoms of itching and discomfort that are present in ACD can be improved with tepid soaks or sitz baths used for the first few days while waiting for more specific therapy to "kick in." Oral prednisone, at a dose of 40 mg for 5 days, will bring rapid improvement in severe ACD, and if the correct allergen has been identified and removed, rebound is unlikely to occur when the steroids are stopped. If the reaction is milder, a high-potency topical corticosteroid such as fluocinonide 0.05% ointment can be applied twice daily for a week or until healing is complete. Nighttime sedation can be added if itching and scratching continue to be problematic (see "antipruritics" in Chapter 3).

Once a patient has become sensitized to an allergen, re-exposure will quickly lead to reappearance of the contact dermatitis. Patients should be made aware that this immunological memory can last for many years and that contact with even a very small quantity of the antigen can result in an allergic reaction.

**ALLERGIC CONTACT DERMATITIS Management**

- Identification and elimination of contactants
- Cool soaks or sitz baths the first few days
- If severe, prednisone 40-60 mg for about 5 days; if milder, a high-potency topical corticosteroid such as fluocinonide 0.05% ointment twice
- Nighttime sedation for itching and to prevent initiation of the itch-scratch cycle

## Seborrheic Dermatitis and Intertrigo

Seborrheic dermatitis is placed in this section rather than in the section on papulosquamous disorders because two

characteristic features of eczematous disease are generally present: epithelial disruption on clinical examination and spongiosis on biopsy. The epithelial disruption in seborrheic dermatitis is not usually visible in the form of erosions, weeping, or fissures but instead is recognized by the yellow color of the scale. This color was originally thought due to sebum coating the scale but that assumption is incorrect as sebum is actually colorless. In reality, the yellow hue occurs as the result of small amounts of serum that escape to the surface through microscopic disruption of the barrier layer, and this serum then coats the surface scale.

Seborrheic dermatitis occurs most commonly on the scalp. It develops in this location because hair and partially exfoliated epithelial cells (anchored by scalp hair) trap heat, sweat, and insensible perspiration. Scalp involvement is also frequently accompanied by development of the disorder in semi-intertriginous locations such as the nasal and retroauricular folds. It also commonly occurs in the inguinal region and gluteal cleft where it is closely linked to intertrigo occurring in these anogenital locations[28] (see the following paragraphs).

## Clinical Presentation

Seborrheic dermatitis is usually easily identified because of the presence of characteristic yellow scale when it occurs in hairy areas such as the scalp. On the other hand, it is controversial as to whether a similar eruption, but with little or no scale, occurring in nonhairy intertriginous folds should be termed intertrigo or seborrheic dermatitis. For the purposes of this chapter, intertriginous redness with no scale will be termed intertrigo. The term seborrheic dermatitis will be reserved for the occurrence of intertriginous redness accompanied by slight presence of yellow scale.

The clinical appearance of intertrigo and seborrheic dermatitis is that of poorly marginated, erythematous patches, or very slightly raised plaques, occurring in folded areas where moisture such as sweat or urine is retained. Early on, scale will not be apparent (intertrigo) but, left untreated and with the passage of time, the chronic inflammation will result in epithelial proliferation and the gradual development of scale, thus taking on the clinical appearance of seborrheic dermatitis (**Figs. 5-36 through 5-38**). Often the scale is not loose but rather more attached, resulting in a glazed, shiny, or chapped appearance. If itching is present, resultant scratching may lead to the superimposition of excoriations and/or lichenification thus presenting the appearance of LSC.

Not surprisingly, because of anatomic differences, this process is encountered more frequently in women than in men and in those who are obese rather than those who are slender. Other environmental irritation such as high ambient temperature, high relative humidity, and occlusive clothing will also increase the frequency with which this phenomenon occurs. The diagnosis of anogenital seborrheic dermatitis is infrequently made in adults but is often identified in the anogenital area of infants as well as at additional sites such as the scalp, retroauricular folds, and axillae. Cases in

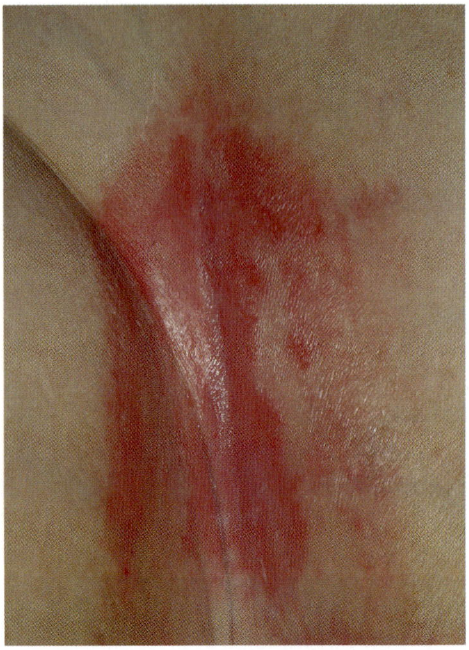

Fig. 5-36. Intertrigo dermatitis appears as poorly demarcated inflamed plaques in skin folds, often with inapparent scale.

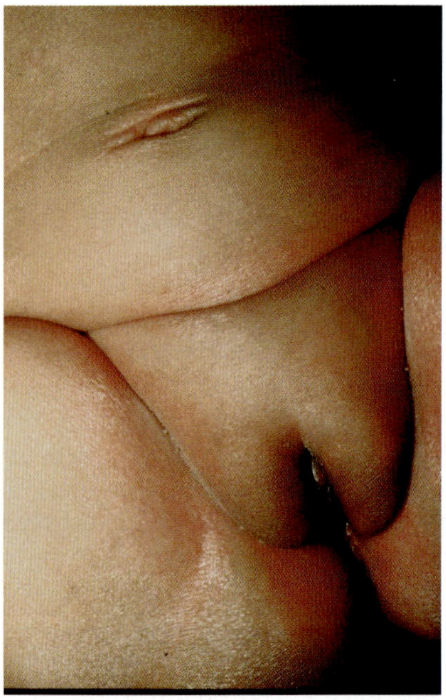

Fig. 5-37. This intertrigo dermatitis from seborrheic dermatitis shows scale and inflammation manifested by hyperpigmentation.

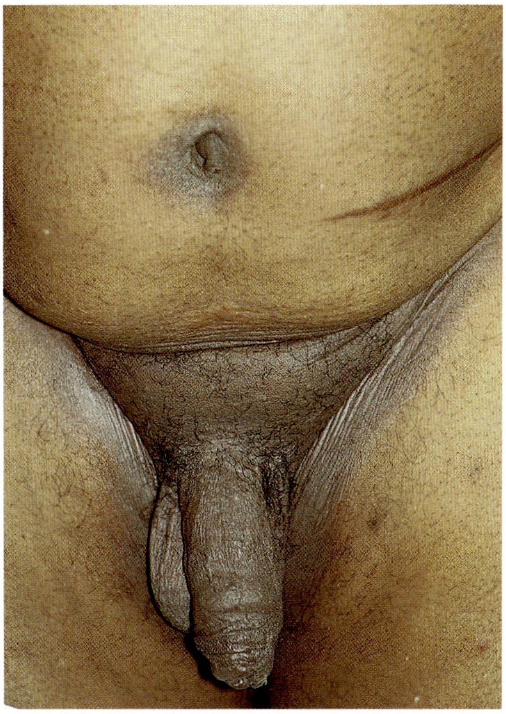

Fig. 5-38. Seborrheic dermatitis on the body, with erythema and scale in skin folds, is more common in children than in adults.

adults most often develop in incontinent patients who, analogously, remain diapered for long periods of time. It may also develop in those adults who are morbidly obese.

## Diagnosis

The diagnosis is made on a clinical basis; biopsy reveals only the generic changes found in all eczematous diseases. Dermoscopy of seborrhea on the face shows dotted vessels in a patchy distribution and fine yellowish scale with or without white scale. At times, there may be orange-yellowish areas and whitish structureless areas.[8] The major consideration in differential diagnosis is psoriasis of the inverse type. This condition is sometime called "sebopsoriasis" to indicate the possible overlap of these conditions and the difficulty in differentiating between them. In most instances, this differentiation will be based on whether or not other more classical sharply marginated plaques of psoriasis can be found at non-intertriginous sites elsewhere. Superimposition of candidiasis occurs with some frequency in intertrigo and seborrheic dermatitis occurring at intertriginous locations. The presence of minute pustules either disseminated throughout the main portion of the patches or occurring at the periphery as "satellite" lesions suggest that candidiasis is also present. Erythrasma, putatively caused by the bacterium *Corynebacterium minutissimum*, must also be included in the list of differential diagnoses (see erythrasma in the papulosquamous section of this chapter).

**SEBORRHEIC DERMATITIS/INTERTRIGO — Diagnosis**

- Morphology of red scaling plaques in the skin folds of the inguinal creases, umbilicus; erythema and scale of the scalp, ears, and central face
- Scale often yellowish
- Primarily in infants, or in adults who are unable to wash regularly—those who are debilitated, homeless, very obese, or with Parkinson disease or another neurologic disorder

## Pathophysiology

The pathogenesis of intertrigo and seborrheic dermatitis results from maceration, defined as the presence of too much moisture retained in folded areas for too long a time. The viability of epithelial cells depends on, among other constraints, an appropriate amount of water in and around them. When the immediate environment around epithelial cells is either too wet or too dry, these cells can perish. The resultant disruption of the epithelial barrier incites inflammation, and the presence of chronic inflammation creates epithelial proliferation and the consequent development of scale. This warm, moist environment, when it occurs in the anogenital area, often also leads to the development of secondary candidiasis, which in turn causes further persistent inflammation.

Dermatology textbooks and most review articles indicate that seborrheic dermatitis occurs directly as an overgrowth of the yeasts, *Malassezia* sp., that are normally resident in hair follicles. However, it seems likely to me that the overgrowth of these yeasts occurs as a result of, rather than the cause of, the inflammation found in seborrheic dermatitis. This supposition is supported by three observations: (1) steroids work just as well as the antimicrobial "azoles" (see below), (2) topical steroids do not worsen the situation even though they would be expected to lead to very favorable environment for yeast and bacterial overgrowth, and (3) the "azoles" have a fairly marked anti-inflammatory effect as well as an antimicrobial property and that could be at least part of the mechanism through which they are effective.[29]

## Management

Left untreated, intertrigo and seborrheic dermatitis becomes chronic conditions that wax and wane over time. On the other hand, there is usually an excellent and rapid response to therapy. The first step in treatment is to improve the environment as much as possible through the reduction of heat and moisture (such as in diapered infants or incontinent adults), marked improvement can be obtained with topical agents.

Topically applied "azoles," such as ketoconazole, usually represent the initial therapeutic approach by most

clinicians.[30] These products are recommended based on the belief that the process is caused by *Malassezia* sp. and by a desire to avoid the adverse effects (atrophy, striae, microbial overgrowth, etc.) of topical steroids applied on a prolonged basis at intertriginous sites. Alternatively, the use of low-potency (2.5% hydrocortisone) or mid-potency (triamcinolone acetonide 0.1%) steroid creams or ointments is equally efficacious, sting less, work faster, and equally safe when used for relatively short periods of time.

Topical calcineurin inhibitors such as tacrolimus and pimecrolimus can be used for their steroid-sparing effects, although stinging and burning limit patient acceptability (see calcineurin inhibitors in Chapter 3). Unfortunately, because of the difficulty in achieving long-term improvement in the environmental conditions that precipitated the condition in the first place, recurrences are common and retreatment is often necessary. Treatment of seborrheic dermatitis of the scalp, if such is present, seems to be helpful both in improving anogenital disease and preventing recurrences.

**SEBORRHEIC DERMATITIS/INTERTRIGO — Management**

- Minimize heat, moisture
- Mild topical corticosteroid such as hydrocortisone 2.5% cream if not too irritated, otherwise ointment, or triamcinolone ointment 0.1% or 0.025%

## SECTION B: PAPULOSQUAMOUS AND OTHER NONECZEMATOUS DISORDERS

The papulosquamous disorders are those characterized by inflamed plaques, patches, or papules that are well demarcated and, on dry, keratinized skin, show scale. This scale is often subtle or even absent on damp skin or modified mucous membranes. These disorders are often, but not always, pruritic, so there may or may not be signs of rubbing and scratching. Those patients who itch may rub and scratch so much that they produce overlying eczema/LSC, that makes a diagnosis difficult or impossible without a biopsy (which still may be confused by these changes from rubbing) or without first clearing of the eczema.

For sorting through these conditions to make a diagnosis, papulosquamous diseases are divided into those that are generally plaques (lesions that are larger than 1.5 cm) and those that are papules (smaller than 1.5 cm). There is, of course, overlap.

### Psoriasis

Psoriasis is a common skin disease that often affects genital skin in addition to the classic locations on the elbows, scalp, and knees. However, psoriasis fairly often only affects the anogenital skin, without other typical signs of psoriasis.

#### Clinical Presentation

Psoriasis is an autoimmune skin condition, occurring in 2%-3% of people. Males and females are affected equally, and in the United States, 1.3% of African Americans develop psoriasis compared to 3.5% of White individuals (National Psoriasis Foundation). This condition occurs at all ages but begins most often in young adults. There is a familial predisposition, with one in three patients reporting a family history of psoriasis.

Typical untreated psoriasis vulgaris (common psoriasis) exhibits well-demarcated, thick plaques with white scale that is so dense that the underlying red color is sometimes obscured (**Figs. 5-39 through 5-41**). Patients often report severe itching, but this is not universal. The elbows, knees, and scalp are the most common areas affected, but some patients have more severe disease with generalized involvement. Because the ultraviolet radiation of sunlight generally clears psoriasis, the face is usually spared.

The variant of psoriasis that presents with prominent genital involvement is called inverse psoriasis. Inverse psoriasis involves skin folds preferentially and often spares the classic dry, keratinized knees, elbows, and scalps. The axillae, inframammary skin, umbilicus, gluteal cleft, crural creases, and genitalia are the most common areas affected. Psoriasis in these moist skin folds, unlike psoriasis on dry, keratinized skin, generally shows erythema without visible, or at least without thickened, scale. The skin is red, often smooth, and either exhibits a glazed appearance or yellowish scale/desquamation (**Figs. 5-42 through 5-48**).

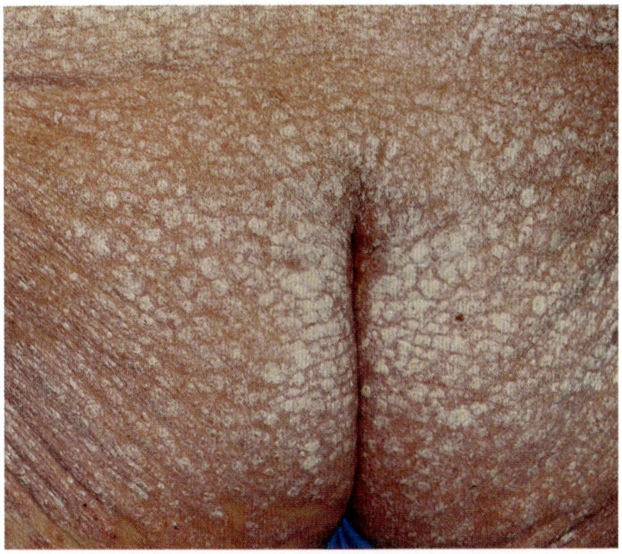

Fig. 5-39. Classic psoriasis vulgaris is manifested by heavy white scale on dry, extragenital skin.

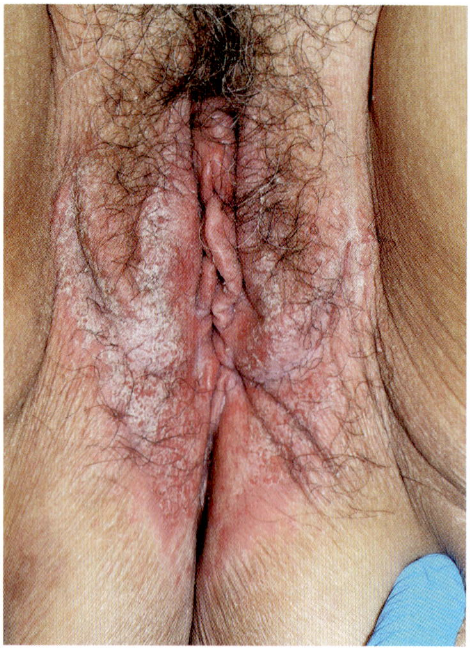

Fig. 5-40. Rarely, psoriasis presents as red plaques with coarse scale on genital skin.

Psoriasis occurring in skin folds is usually far thinner than psoriasis on other skin. Sometimes, the borders are less well demarcated, and there may be satellite lesions that mimic candidiasis **(Fig. 5-49)**. Also, yeast may coexist with intertriginous psoriasis.

Psoriasis predominantly affects the hair-bearing vulva of women, mostly sparing the modified mucous membranes and vagina. However, psoriasis often is located on the glans penis in addition to the penile shaft, scrotum, and groin.

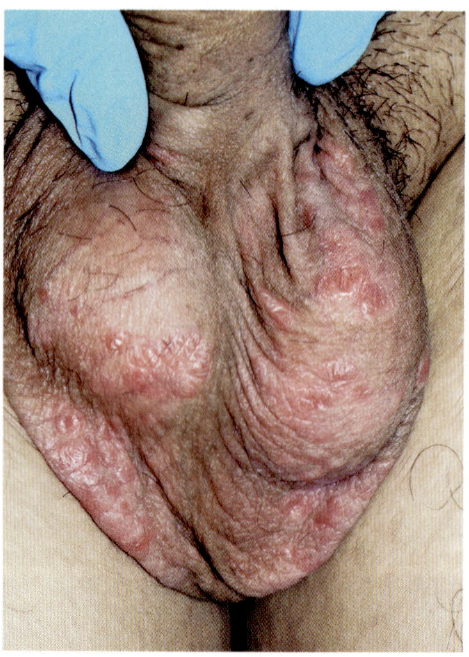

Fig. 5-41. These red, scaling, well-demarcated, coalescing plaques on the scrotum are classic for psoriasis.

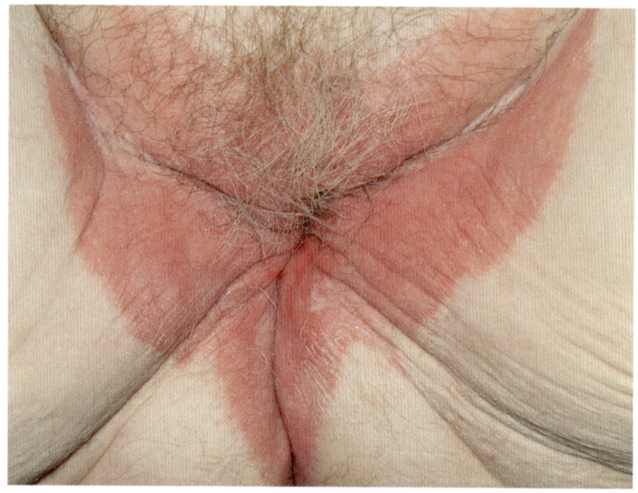

Fig. 5-42. Far more common than classic scaling plaques is the well-demarcated, red, shiny plaque of inverse psoriasis.

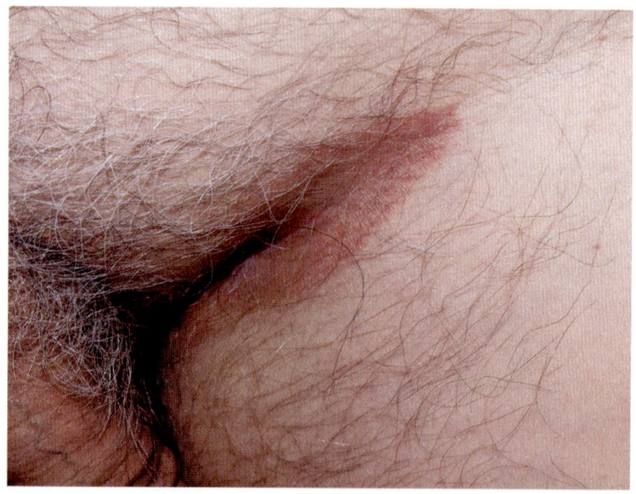

Fig. 5-43. The crural crease is a common location for inverse psoriasis in both men and women.

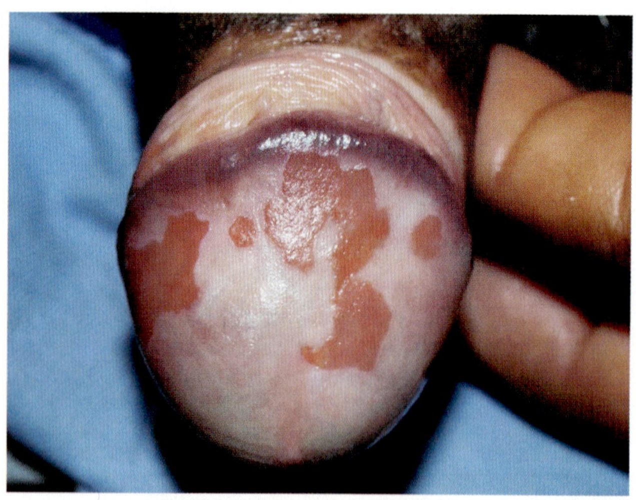

Fig. 5-44. These nonscaling papules of psoriasis are nonspecific in appearance and could also represent lichen planus, flat warts, or high-grade squamous intraepithelial lesion (dysplasia due to human papillomavirus infection).

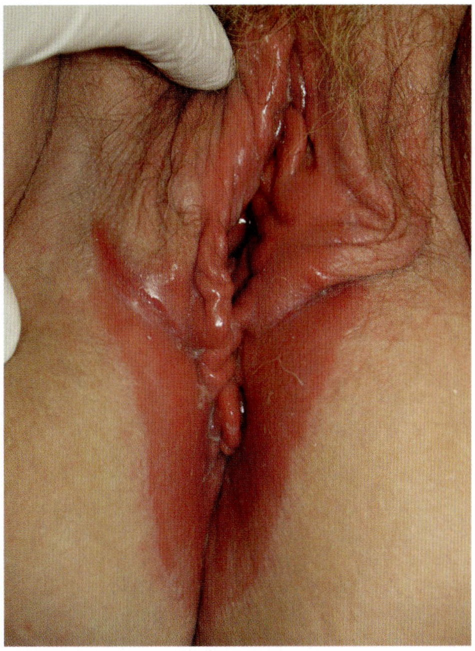

Fig. 5-45. Fissures and puffiness of the modified mucous membranes are common in patients with inverse psoriasis.

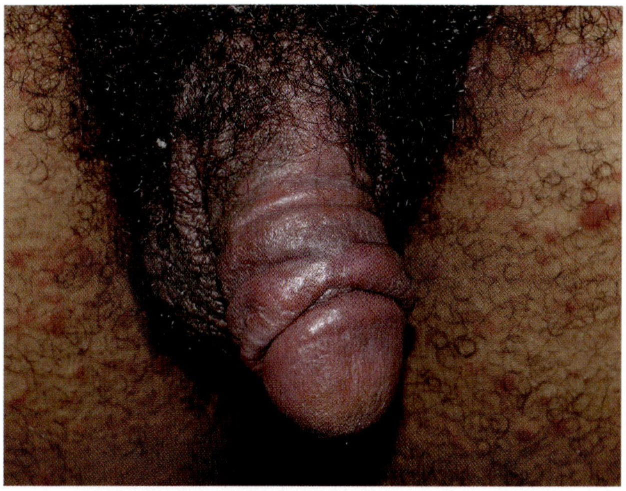

Fig. 5-47. Inverse psoriasis is manifested by nonspecific inflammation and scale of the penis in this man. The diagnosis is suspected on examination but must be confirmed by the identification of typical psoriasis in other areas or a biopsy.

About 20% of patients exhibit the isomorphic phenomenon (previously called the Koebner phenomenon), in which psoriasis occurs in areas of irritation or injury. This partially explains the distribution of lesions, including the elbows and knees, as well as the frequent involvement of the genitalia, an area subject to friction and occlusion.

An additional form of psoriasis is called guttate (which means resembling drops) psoriasis, where lesions are papules rather than plaques, primarily affecting the trunk and extremities rather than the genital area. Pustular psoriasis is characterized by plaques of pustules or crusting. This variant is discussed in Chapter 10. Psoriasis sometimes generalizes into erythrodermic psoriasis, so that generalized confluent erythema, scale, and sometimes exudation are indistinguishable from generalized eczema, seborrhea, or a medication reaction, but erythrodermic psoriasis is not the problem of the genital clinician.

Psoriasis often produces nail abnormalities in addition to inflammatory skin lesions. Most common are small nail pits **(Fig. 5-50)**, not to be confused with simple irregularity or rippling of the surface that occurs with any inflammatory process of the fingertips. Also fairly specific are "oil drop spots" **(Fig. 5-51)**. These are brownish-red discolorations of the nail plate. A third form of nail psoriasis, onycholysis, is much less specific. Onycholysis refers to lifting of the nail from the underlying surface due to any of several conditions, in this case from psoriasis of the nail bed. The scale and keratin debris under the nail can be indistinguishable from a fungal infection of the nail

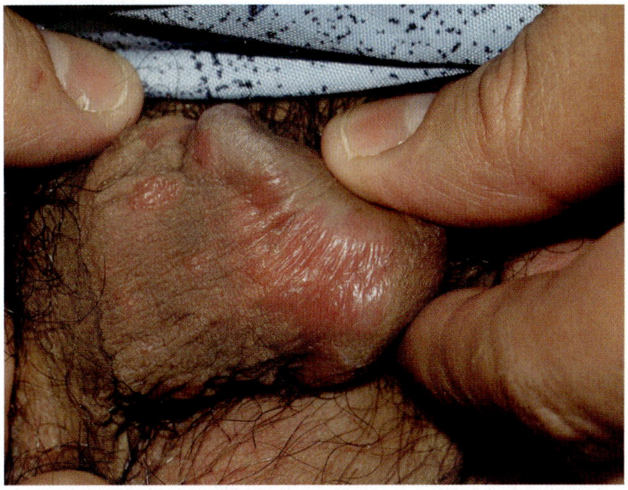

Fig. 5-46. These papules on the glans and shaft have the characteristic shiny glazed scale of genital psoriasis.

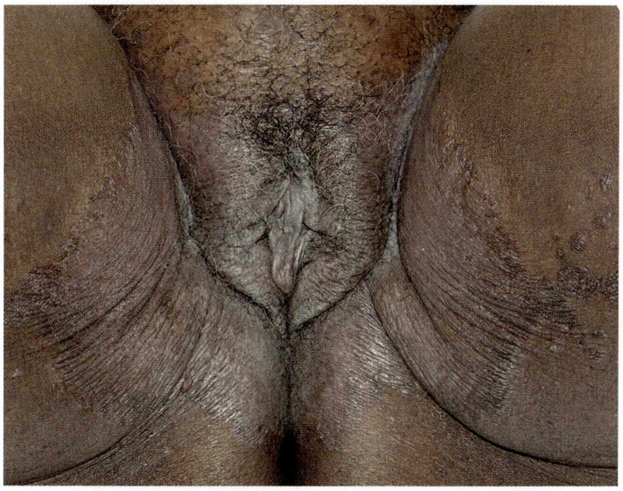

Fig. 5-48. This plaque of psoriasis, like other inflammatory diseases in patients of color, appears hyperpigmented rather than red.

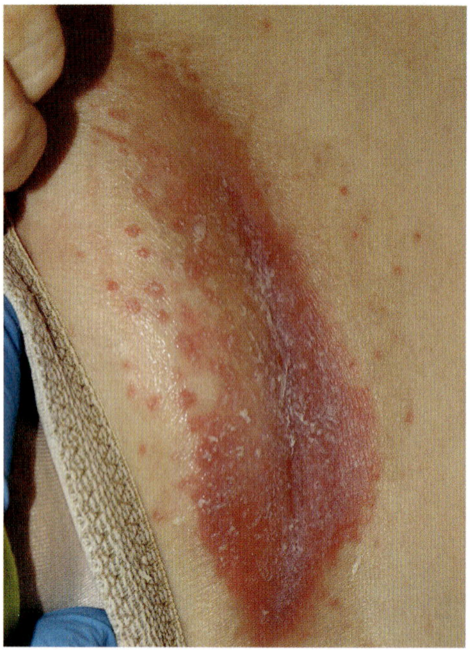

Fig. 5-49. Intertriginous psoriasis can easily be mistaken for candidiasis; this patient even shows satellite lesions and white macerated skin that would normally suggest yeast infection.

**(Fig. 5-51)**. These nail changes, when present, serve as clues to the diagnosis of psoriasis in the patient with nonspecific anogenital red plaques, although the absence of nail changes is common in patients with psoriasis.

Psoriasis is not only a cutaneous disease. The most well-known extracutaneous sign of psoriasis is arthritis, occurring in about 30% of individuals with psoriasis.[31] This ranges from pain with minimal inflammation that resembles osteoarthritis to severe, deforming, and mutilating arthritis. However, recent evidence suggests that

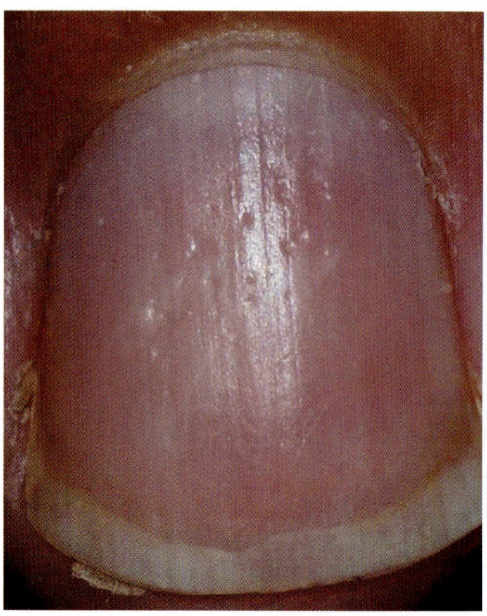

Fig. 5-50. These nail pits are nearly pathognomonic for the presence of psoriasis.

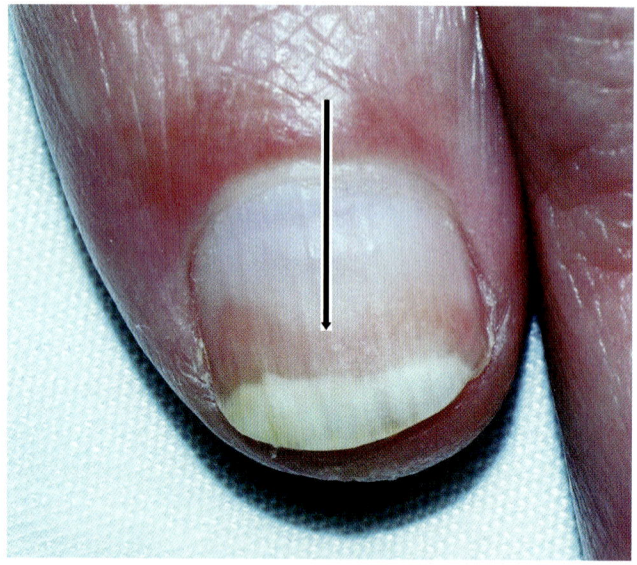

Fig. 5-51. Oil drop spots of psoriasis are spots of yellow/orange discoloration that indicate psoriasis under the nail plate (*arrow*). Then, the nail plate loses adhesion with the nail bed, and the nail lifts as is beginning here, mimicking a fungal infection.

psoriasis (not necessarily anogenital) may be associated with vulvar lichen sclerosus, with 7.5%-17% of women with lichen sclerosus reporting the presence of psoriasis.[32,33]

There is a well-known association of psoriasis with the metabolic syndrome, to include cardiovascular disease, obesity, hypertension, diabetes, and dyslipidemia.[34,35] Patients with psoriasis and diabetes are more likely to experience complications of diabetes than those without diabetes.[36] Alcoholic liver disease as well as nonalcoholic fatty liver disease, inflammatory bowel disease, and chronic kidney disease are also increased in the setting of psoriasis. The risk of dying from a malignancy is 41% higher in patients with psoriasis,[37] but this pure association with psoriasis is confounded by the increase in alcoholism and tobacco use in patients with psoriasis, the immunosuppressive therapies provided for psoriasis, and sun exposure for the management of the skin disease. However, lymphoma and especially cutaneous T-cell lymphoma appears to be a certain association.

Depression, anxiety, alcohol dependence, and nicotine dependence are known issues for patients with psoriasis, and a recent study reports these issues in about 50% of patients.[38] The psychological effects are compounded in patients with anogenital involvement.

## Diagnosis

Psoriasis of the genitalia can be diagnosed with confidence when morphologically consistent plaques in this area are associated with typical psoriasis of the elbows and knees, scalp, and nails. Not uncommonly, only the genitalia are affected. Then, the diagnosis becomes more difficult.

Dermoscopy can be useful for the diagnosis of psoriasis, particularly inverse psoriasis where heavy scale does not obscure the underlying vascular pattern. Lower magnification shows monomorphous tiny red spots on an erythematous background. Higher magnification shows these red spots to consist of small convoluted, branched capillaries, called "bushy" capillaries.[39]

More traditional is an attempt at confirmation on biopsy. However, a nondiagnostic biopsy, such as "psoriasiform dermatitis," is very common, and this does not rule out psoriasis as a cause of the eruption.

The classic but nonspecific histologic picture of psoriasis includes marked thickening of the epidermis with regular elongation of the rete pegs and suprapapillary thinning. Hyperkeratosis and parakeratosis are prominent, and there is an absence of the granular layer. More specific histologic findings are collections of neutrophils just under the stratum corneum of the thinned suprapapillary epidermis (spongiform pustules of Kogoj) and in the overlying parakeratotic layer (Munro microabscesses) **(Fig. 5-52)**. In the genital area and other skin folds, the thickening is generally less pronounced than found in biopsies of common psoriasis, but spongiosis (edema of the epidermis) is more common **(Fig. 5-53)**.

The differential diagnosis includes tinea cruris and candidiasis, which can be nearly indistinguishable. And, candidiasis especially can coexist with inverse psoriasis. However, in immunocompetent patients, tinea cruris usually spares the scrotum and penis, whereas these structures are often prominently affected with psoriasis. In addition, tinea cruris is uncommon in women. Cutaneous candidiasis frequently shows satellite pustules or erosions but can resemble and coexist with psoriasis. LSC, intraepithelial neoplasia (previously called, in this area, Bowen disease, squamous cell carcinoma *in situ*, erythroplasia of Queyrat in men, and vulvar intraepithelial neoplasia on the vulva),

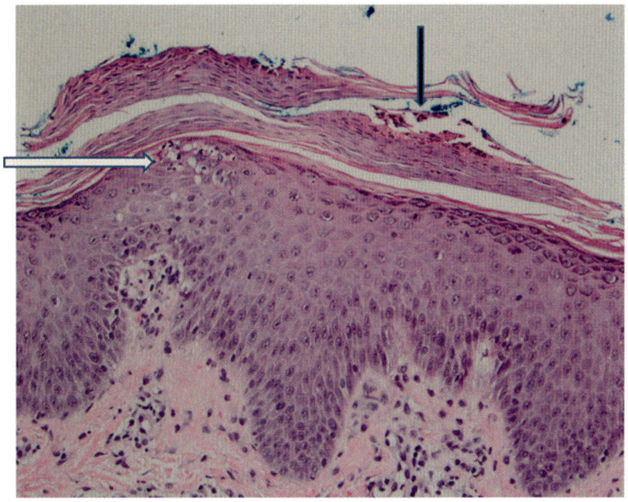

Fig. 5-52. This biopsy of classic psoriasis with heavy scale shows typical collections of neutrophils in the upper epidermis (*white arrow*) as well as in the stratum corneum (*black arrow*). The epidermis is somewhat thick, with elongated rete ridges. (Courtesy of Jason Reutter, MD.)

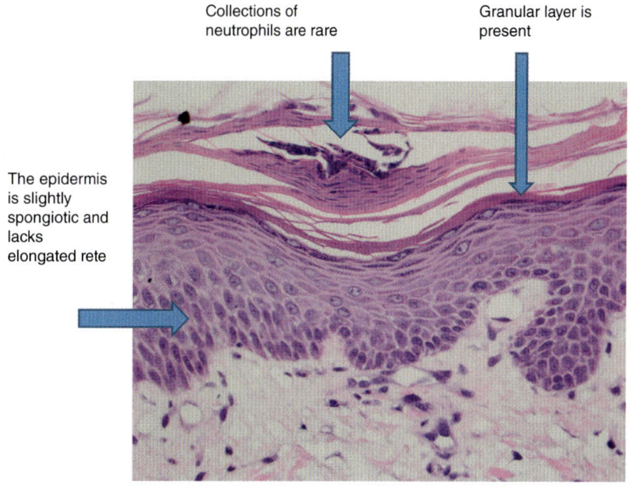


Fig. 5-53. The histologic picture of inverse psoriasis is less specific, with a thinner epidermis, loss of the rete, and with slight spongiosis, or edema of the epidermis manifested by a clear space around individual cells (*arrows*). The neutrophils in the epidermis and stratum corneum are uncommon compared to common psoriasis. (Courtesy of Jason Reutter, MD.)

and Paget disease are all red, scaling diseases that can be confused with psoriasis. Lichen planus on the glans penis is sometimes indistinguishable from smaller papules of psoriasis of this area. Seborrheic dermatitis, especially in infants, can appear very similar to psoriasis and shows the same pattern of distribution as inverse psoriasis, accentuating the scalp, axillae, umbilicus, and anogenital skin.

**PSORIASIS** — **Diagnosis**

- Morphology of well-demarcated red plaques; in dry areas with heavy white scale, in skin folds often with red glazed appearance and inapparent scale
- Accentuated in crural creases, often also in umbilicus, gluteal cleft, axillae, under breasts
- Negative testing for candidiasis
- Biopsy often shows psoriasiform dermatitis rather than psoriasis

## Pathophysiology

The thickened plaques of psoriasis result from unusually rapid proliferation of the epidermis. Replacement of the epidermis is 4-6 times faster for psoriatic epithelium than for normal skin, producing much thicker skin with more remarkable scale. The underlying etiology is multifactorial, including chronic type 1 helper ($T_H1$) T-cell– and $T_H17$-mediated inflammation, monocyte and neutrophil modulation, increased oxidative stress, endothelial cell dysfunction, and angiogenesis.[35] Other factors include a genetic predisposition and environmental issues serving as factors. Smoking, obesity, and alcohol excess worsen psoriasis as well. In addition, classic triggers for the development of psoriasis include streptococcal disease, sunburn, and human immunodeficiency virus infection. Some medications are associated with the development or worsening of psoriasis, including lithium and nonsteroidal anti-inflammatory medications.

## Management

First-line therapy for genital psoriasis is, as always, patient education and improvement of the local environment, especially since so many of these patients are obese. Control of irritants such as bacterial and fungal infection, maceration from moisture, and irritation from overwashing and topical medications can remarkably improve symptoms. Nighttime sedation for patients with significant itching also improves the quality of life. Patients should be informed of the association of psoriasis with the metabolic syndrome and the importance of weight control, and attention to blood pressure, glucose, and lipids in the avoidance of end-organ disease. They should also be advised of the chronic nature of psoriasis, which can be controlled but not cured.

Then, topical corticosteroid administration is the mainstay of treatment for anogenital psoriasis, which usually responds better to topical therapy than psoriasis of other body sites. Potent steroids such as fluocinonide 0.05% (Lidex) or ultrapotent medications such as clobetasol propionate (Temovate) and halobetasol propionate can be used initially, producing very quick improvement, with prompt tapering of potency as tolerated to preparations that can be used more safely for long periods of time, such as triamcinolone 0.1% or desonide 0.05%. Or, another means of decreasing potency is the use of the same high or ultrapotent preparation less often, such as 3 days a week.

For genital psoriasis not adequately controlled with this treatment, addition of (not substitution by) a vitamin D derivative can be useful. These include calcipotriene (Dovonex) and calcitriol (Vectical) cream and ointment, but there is a 1- to 2-month delay before maximal improvement. Alternatively, a combination of betamethasone dipropionate and calcipotriene ointment (Taclonex) can be used once daily. However, this potent corticosteroid-containing medication used chronically in skin folds can produce thinning and striae. Topical tar can be useful on some skin surfaces but are irritating and best avoided on genital skin, as are topical retinoids, salicylic acid, and anthralin.

Although not approved by the Food and Drug Administration for psoriasis, low-quality studies suggest that tacrolimus ointment, and less so, pimecrolimus cream, can be beneficial for the thinner skin of skin folds and facial psoriasis when topical corticosteroids provide suboptimal improvement.[40] These immunomodulators sometimes sting with application, and they are expensive, but they do not produce atrophy or steroid dermatitis.

Although ultraviolet light is frequently used for psoriasis, this treatment is of little use on the genitalia. First, the delivery of ultraviolet light to this area is logistically difficult. Second, an increase in penile squamous cell carcinomas is known to occur in patients treated on a long-term basis with ultraviolet light.

Severe genital psoriasis often is not adequately controlled with safe long-term local therapy. These patients frequently require systemic therapy, classically with oral methotrexate or, less often, acitretin. More recently, immunosuppressive biologic agents typically administered by self-injection at home (etanercept, adalimumab, certolizumab pegol, golimumab, secukinumab, ixekizumab, brodalumab, and guselkumab) are convenient, safe, and effective. Infliximab is given by intravenous infusion. Apremilast is an oral medication for moderate psoriasis, also an immune modifier, which requires no laboratory monitoring. All of these medications are expensive, with delayed activity requiring about a month for onset of improvement. Not only do these systemic medications manage psoriasis very well in most patients, but there is evidence that systemic therapies may improve underlying cardiovascular risk.[41] However, the metabolic syndrome and obesity can require higher doses of biologic therapies and may be associated with both decreased drug effect survival and premature discontinuation of medication.

Psoriasis is a chronic disease for which there is no cure, although control is usually achieved with topical medication. Many patients with psoriasis are psychologically incapacitated by their disease.[42] The constant production of scale, the disfigurement of their skin, and the incurable nature of the disease are hard for many patients to tolerate. People with genital psoriasis must also deal with the sexual ramifications of this chronic genital abnormality, so aggressive treatment of their psoriasis as well as counseling can be crucial.[43] Patients should be urged to join the National Psoriasis Foundation, which provides information and support to those living with psoriasis. Also, patients with significant psoriasis should be made aware of the comorbidities of the disease and referred to a primary care physician for evaluation and treatment of any obesity or alcoholism and for counseling regarding the prevention of cardiovascular disease.

**PSORIASIS** — **Management**

- As for lichen simplex chronicus when itchy. Improve local environment.
- Topical corticosteroid ointment, superpotent to midpotent, immediately taper to least frequent dosing or lower potency when controlled and follow for side effects.
- Nighttime sedation to suppress scratching when pruritic.
- Add calcipotriene or calcitriol if a topical corticosteroid not sufficient.
- Add tacrolimus 0.1% or pimecrolimus 1% twice daily if needed.
- Use systemic therapy if topical therapy is not adequate.

## Tinea Cruris (Jock Itch)

Men often blame any anogenital itching of this common disease.

### Clinical Presentation

Tinea cruris occurs far most often in men. There is no predisposition for any race, but the most common age is middle age and is extremely uncommon in children. Tinea cruris is usually associated with tinea pedis and onychomycosis, which serve as a reservoir for the organism, so that recurrence is common.

Most often, the visible lesions of tinea cruris are limited to the proximal, medial thighs. Classically, plaques are erythematous and well demarcated, with accentuation of scale peripherally **(Figs. 5-54 and 5-55)**. Many patients, particularly those with prominent hair in the area, exhibit red papules, nodules, or pustules within the plaque that represent extension of the infection to the follicular epithelium (fungal folliculitis) **(Fig. 5-56)**.

Occasionally, the plaque extends to the buttocks and scrotum, and in women, the plaque may extend to the labia majora and mons pubis. This is most likely to occur when patients are immunosuppressed or have been using a topical corticosteroid for the itching **(Fig. 5-57)**. Immunocompetent patients not using topical corticosteroids do not experience dermatophyte infections of the shaft or glans of the penis.

### Diagnosis

Most often, tinea cruris can be diagnosed by clinical morphology alone. The location of the proximal, medial thighs with sparing of the scrotum and penis, and the pattern of peripheral scale or peeling, often with central clearing that gives the classic "ringworm" appearance. When needed, the diagnosis is confirmed by the identification of hyphae on microscopic examination of scale scraped from the scaling edge of the plaque. Biopsies are only obtained if the diagnosis is unsuspected or a fungal preparation is negative and the rash is unresponsive to

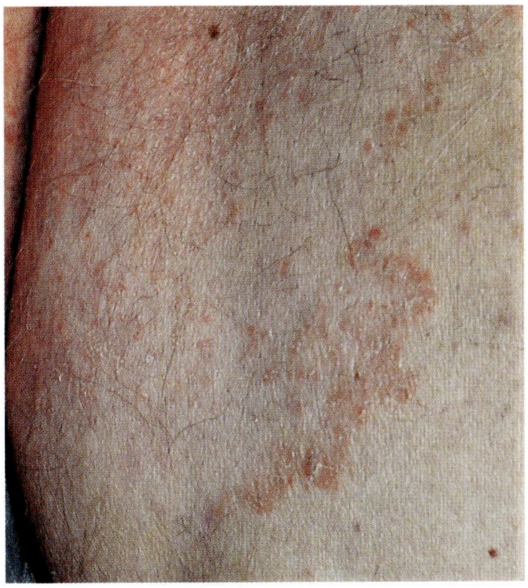

Fig. 5-54. The proximal, medial thigh of men is the most common location for tinea cruris. Accentuation of the periphery of the plaque is typical.

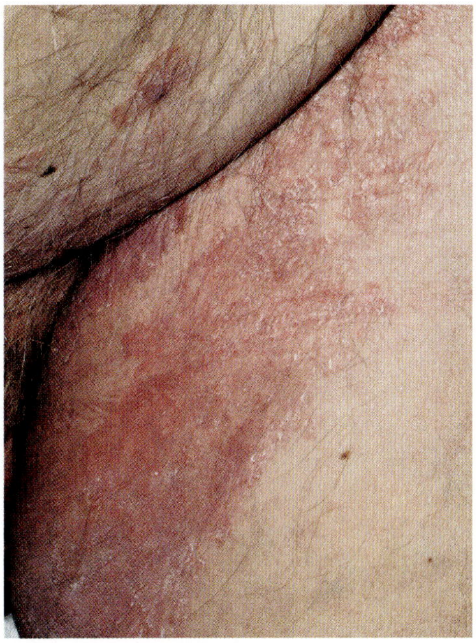

Fig. 5-55. A close examination of the edge of the plaque shows peripheral scale that, under microscopic examination, shows abundant branching hyphae.

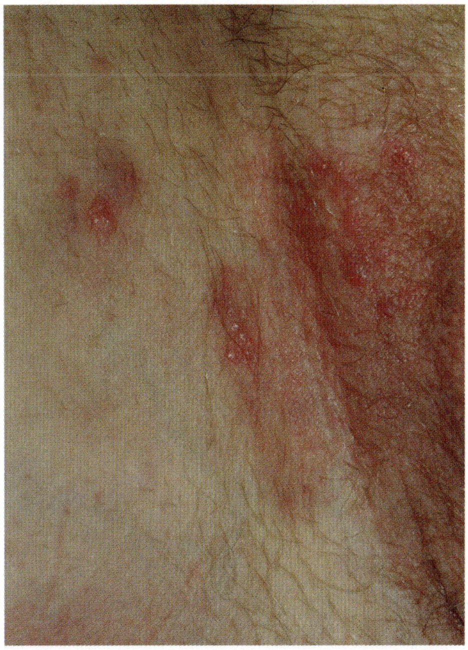

Fig. 5-56. The use of a topical antifungal and corticosteroid combination cream has cleared much of scale from these plaques of tinea cruris, but it has not penetrated into the infected peripheral hair follicles, leaving red nodules of fungal folliculitis.

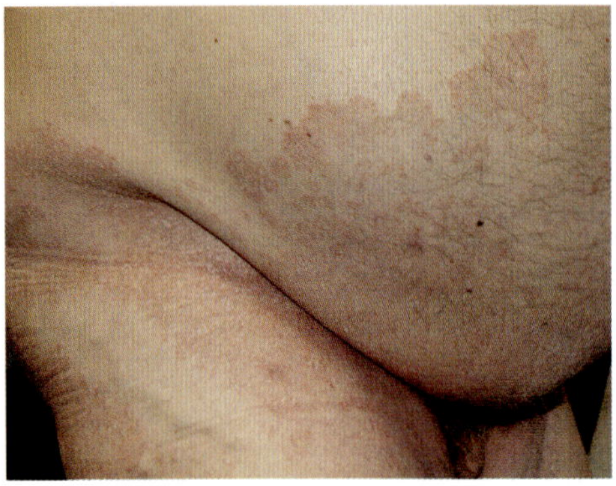

Fig. 5-57. This elderly man immunosuppressed by virtue of age has tinea not only in the genital area but also in the abdomen, legs down to his knees, buttocks, and half-way up his back.

therapy. The specific findings are those of hyphae in the stratum corneum, best visualized with special stains, usually periodic acid-Schiff reaction or the methenamine silver nitrate method. Otherwise, the findings are the same as those of eczema.

There are specific signs of dermatophytosis on dermoscopy, although these are generally not needed since a microscopic preparation confirms the diagnosis. These changes include typical hair changes such as Morse code hairs (hair with horizontal white bands), deformable (bent) hairs, translucent hairs, comma and cork screw hairs, and perifollicular scaling.[44,45]

The diseases most often confused with tinea cruris are eczema (LSC), psoriasis, and, especially in women, candidiasis. Eczema generally is less well demarcated, and it usually prominently affects the scrotum and labia majora. Psoriasis can be nearly indistinguishable, but an examination of other skin surfaces often reveals typical scalp psoriasis, involvement of elbows or knees or nail pits. Seborrheic dermatitis, irritant and ACD, Paget disease, and differentiated intraepithelial neoplasia, previously called Bowen disease or squamous cell carcinoma *in situ*, should also be considered.

**TINEA CRURIS** — **Diagnosis**

- Morphology of well-demarcated red plaques primarily on the proximal, medial thighs of men; generally sparing the scrotum and penis, sometimes extending to the buttocks. Accentuation of scale at the periphery of the plaque, usually associated with fungal toenails.
- Skin scraping for microscopic fungal preparation shows hyphae/positive dermatophyte culture.
- Response to antifungal.

## Pathophysiology

Tinea cruris is produced by dermatophyte fungi infecting the very uppermost layer of the keratinized anogenital skin, the stratum corneum. The predominant species are *Epidermophyton floccosum* and *Trichophyton rubrum*, with *T mentagrophytes* and *T verrucosum* responsible at times. These organisms are ubiquitous, and even immunocompetent patients sometimes experience recurrent infection. Usually, these patients also exhibit tinea pedis and onychomycosis, which serve as a source for autoinoculation. Fomites also contribute to the spread of this fungal infection.

## Management

Topical antifungal medications are usually the mainstay of treatment for tinea cruris. However, in the setting of skin covered with coarse hair, the fungus can tracked down the stratum corneum of hair follicles, producing papules, pustules, or nodules; these patients require an oral medication since topical therapy does not penetrate sufficiently for clearing.

Those plaques showing only erythema and scale generally can be cleared with a topical medication. The counter topical azoles clotrimazole and miconazole are inexpensive and effective, with prescription azoles also useful but often very expensive (oxiconazole, sulconazole, efinaconazole, and luliconazole), and prescription econazole and ketoconazole inexpensive and generally covered by insurance. The allylamines and related medications, over-the-counter terbinafine and prescription butenafine, and naftifine are extremely effective against dermatophytes as well, but less useful for candidiasis in the case of a mistaken or second diagnosis of yeast. In addition, there are increasing reports of dermatophyte drug resistance, particularly involving terbinafine.[46,47]

Although quite useful in the treatment of genital candidiasis, nystatin has no activity against the dermatophyte fungi of tinea cruris. Ciclopirox, haloprogin, iodoquinol, tolnaftate are older therapies that are useful as well.

At times, tinea cruris is especially inflamed and red or extremely itchy. These patients improve more quickly if a topical corticosteroid such as triamcinolone 0.1% cream is used concomitantly for the first few days. Although, theoretically, a corticosteroid should decrease the cure rate, some evidence suggests that this is not true.[48] Some clinicians use a commercial combination of clotrimazole and betamethasone dipropionate (Lotrisone). Although this combination is very convenient for the first few days, it contains a high-potency cortisone that should not be used on the proximal, medial thighs for a prolonged period because of the propensity of the medial thighs to develop striae, and the topical corticosteroid should be needed only for the first few days of therapy. An alternative rational approach to this problem is the addition of an inexpensive mid-potency corticosteroid such as triamcinolone 0.1% to the antifungal medication just for the first few days so those early anti-inflammatory actions are provided, and the topical antifungal medication is continued until the skin is clear.

Patients with follicular involvement characterized by papules or pustules within the plaque require oral therapy, because topical medication does not penetrate sufficiently to eradicate organisms within follicles. Sometimes, tinea cruris of skin containing dense, thick hair even without obvious follicular involvement is incompletely treated with a topical medication. There are several effective and safe oral medications for patients with very widespread disease, plaques within very hairy areas, and patients with pustules or nodules within plaques indicating follicular involvement.

Fluconazole at a dose of 100-200 mg/d, itraconazole at 200 mg/d, or terbinafine at 250 mg/d are very effective, and these are usually well tolerated. For the length of time (1-2 weeks) required to treat tinea cruris, laboratory testing is not required for patients without preexisting liver disease. Coadministration of itraconazole with cisapride (Propulsid), pimozide, and quinidine can precipitate cardiac arrhythmia, and this medication has multiple other interactions that require careful monitoring. Similarly, fluconazole can increase levels or actions of coumarin-type anticoagulants, phenytoin, cyclosporine, theophylline, terfenadine, and tacrolimus. There are about 400 additional potential interactions, and this list is growing, but these are not clinically relevant unless fluconazole is given daily. The Food and Drug Administration has withdrawn indication approval for oral ketoconazole for candidiasis and other fungal skin infections because of the risk of medication interactions and the occasional occurrence of liver and adrenal disease. Although time-honored and effective, griseofulvin at 500 mg administered twice daily with fatty food or whole milk for better absorption, has a disadvantage of frequent nausea as well as headache. Hepatotoxicity is a concern of many clinicians, but this is very uncommon, and laboratory testing is no longer the standard of care for the duration required to clear tinea cruris.

Often, tinea cruris is recurrent, with the reservoir being a dermatophyte infection of the toenails. Patients should be advised that recurrence is not failure of the medication, and they should either restart the antifungal cream with recurrences, or simply apply the medication daily to suppress recurrences. Some patients with recurrent tinea cruris may benefit from a longer course of an oral antifungal medication to clear the nail disease. The most common regimens for fungal nail infections consist of terbinafine at 250 mg/d for 3 months or itraconazole at 200 mg twice daily for 1 week of each month for 3 months. Fluconazole at 200 mg/wk until the nail grows out (about 1 year) is also effective. These therapies clear the nails of many but far from all patients, and recurrence of onychomycosis after treatment is usual.

**TINEA CRURIS — Management**

- If no follicular involvement, any topical antifungal therapy with miconazole or any azole, terbinafine or any allylamine, and ciclopirox, haloprogin, iodoquinol, and tolnaftate is required.
- If there is follicular involvement, systemic therapy with fluconazole, itraconazole, terbinafine, or griseofulvin is required.
- For recurrences, ongoing topical therapy may be required, or treatment of fungal toenails that serve as a reservoir.

## Erythrasma

Erythrasma is a genital skin infection that is found most often in men and mimics tinea cruris.

### Clinical Presentation

Most common in men in warm climates, and erythrasma is also found more often in those who are obese, in the presence of diabetes, patients with darker natural complexions, and in those who sweat heavily. Erythrasma affects the proximal, medial thighs and crural crease. Tan-pink, lightly scaling or finely wrinkled, well-demarcated plaques are characteristic. Patients with darker complexions often exhibit more hyperpigmentation than erythema (Figs. 5-58 and 5-59). Unlike tinea cruris, these plaques are solid, without peripheral scale or central clearing. The scrotum, penis, and vulva are generally not affected.

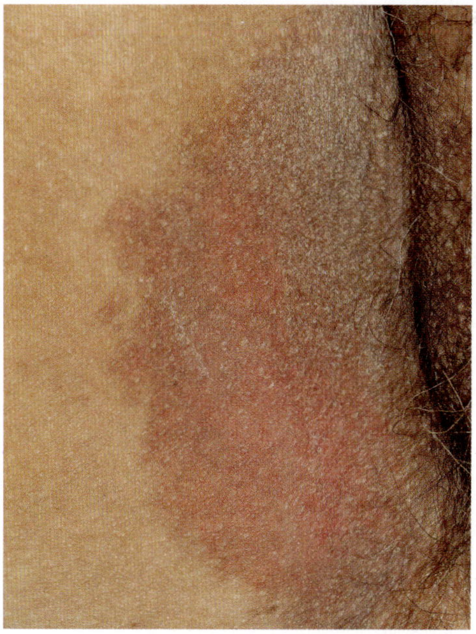

Fig. 5-58. Erythrasma superficially resembles tinea cruris due to the location of the red plaques. However, there is no peripheral accentuation of scale, and the color is often more tan/red.

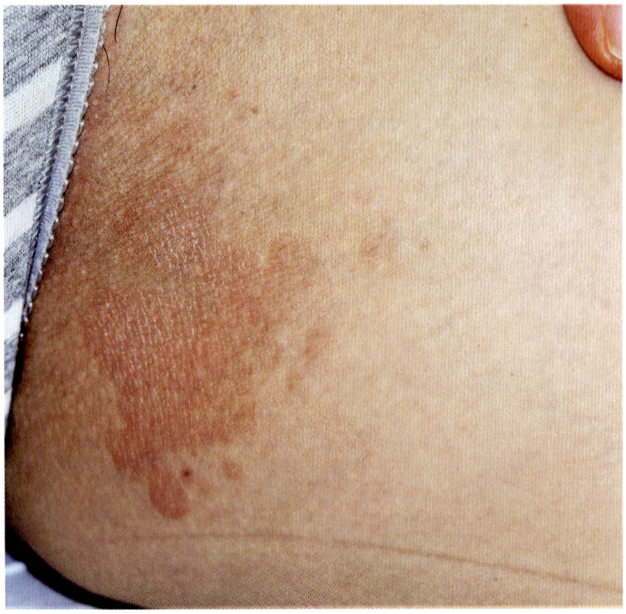

Fig. 5-59. This solid plaque shows the fine scale and wrinkling, as well as the tan color of erythrasma.

### Diagnosis

The diagnosis is made principally by the appearance of the skin, with confirmation either by characteristic coral-pink fluorescence when examined with Wood light or by response to therapy.

Tinea cruris is the disease most likely to be confused with erythrasma. Tinea cruris, also seen primarily in men, shares the same location and pattern. However, unlike erythrasma, tinea cruris usually exhibits peripheral scaling and some degree of central clearing. A fungal preparation of peripheral scale in a patient with tinea cruris shows branching long hyphae. Diseases that less often mimic erythrasma include eczema, which is characterized by prominent involvement of the scrotum or vulva with poorly demarcated plaques and is extremely pruritic. Psoriasis also frequently affects the genitalia itself but often is associated with other signs of psoriasis, such as knee, elbow, and scalp involvement and nail pits.

**ERYTHRASMA — Diagnosis**

- Morphology of pink or tan well-demarcated patches on the proximal, medial thighs with subtle scale and no peripheral accentuation of scale
- Negative skin scrapings for tinea
- Coral pink fluorescence with a Wood lamp
- Response to therapy

### Pathophysiology

Erythrasma is caused by the bacterium *C minutissimum*. Found on the feet and in skin folds such as the axillae, inframammary skin, and genital area, it is most prevalent in warmer, more humid environments.

### Management

Medications for erythrasma include erythromycin at 500 mg two times daily for 1-2 weeks, a single dose of clarithromycin,[49] topical erythromycin twice daily, and mupirocin.[50] Erythrasma is generally cleared by fusidic acid, but this is not available in the United States. Recurrence and a need for retreatment or even long-term application of medication are fairly common.

**ERYTHRASMA — Management**

- Erythromycin 500 mg bid for 1-2 weeks or topically twice daily
- Clarithromycin 1 g once
- Mupirocin applied twice daily

## Candidiasis

Candidiasis is a fungal infection most often found in the genital area and mouth. On anogenital skin, it commonly presents as a red plaque easily confused with psoriasis or tinea cruris, but sometimes with small pustules. Candidiasis is especially known for its etiology of yeast vaginitis (see also Chapters 10 and 13).

### Clinical Presentation

Cutaneous candidiasis produces red plaques that affect predominantly warm, damp areas such as the modified mucous membranes of the vulva, skin folds of the crural creases, the gluteal cleft, and under the pannus and breasts (**Figs. 5-60 to 5-62**). These plaques classically exhibit satellite pustules or collarettes that represent unroofed pustules and peripheral peeling (**Fig. 5-63**). This infection is usually accompanied by *Candida* vaginitis in premenopausal women or those on estrogen replacement. Most often seen in premenopausal women, vulvar candidiasis is manifested by edema and redness of the modified mucous membranes and often fissuring of skin folds (**Figs. 5-64 and 5-65**).

Additional risk factors for cutaneous candidiasis include obesity, incontinence, diabetes, and immunosuppression.

In addition to the crural crease, the glans penis is prominently affected in uncircumcised men (**Fig. 5-66**). Penile candidiasis is very uncommon in immunocompetent, circumcised men. However, following intercourse with women with *Candida* vaginitis, some men experience transient, irritation, itching, and poorly demarcated patchy erythema of the glans.

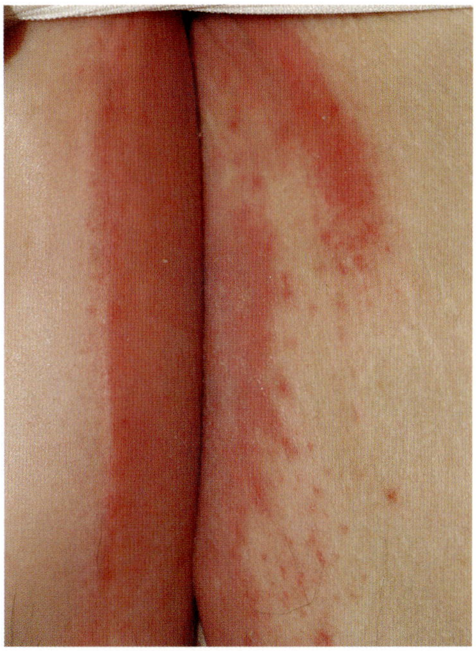

Fig. 5-60. Candida intertrigo presents as red plaques, often with satellite papules or pustules; this can be indistinguishable from inverse psoriasis.

## Diagnosis

Most often, the diagnosis is made by the appearance and confirmed by the identification of hyphae, pseudohyphae, and budding yeast on a microscopic smear of scale from the periphery of the plaques or of a pustule roof. In atypical or recalcitrant cases, a fungal culture is indicated to ensure the correct diagnosis. Dermoscopy may show a sparse white coating.[51] A biopsy is neither necessary nor desirable for the diagnosis. However, the histologic findings of cutaneous candidiasis are those of pseudohyphae and hyphae invading the stratum corneum and infiltration of the epidermis with neutrophils that form subcorneal pustules. In addition, dermoscopy is not particularly useful for this diagnosis.

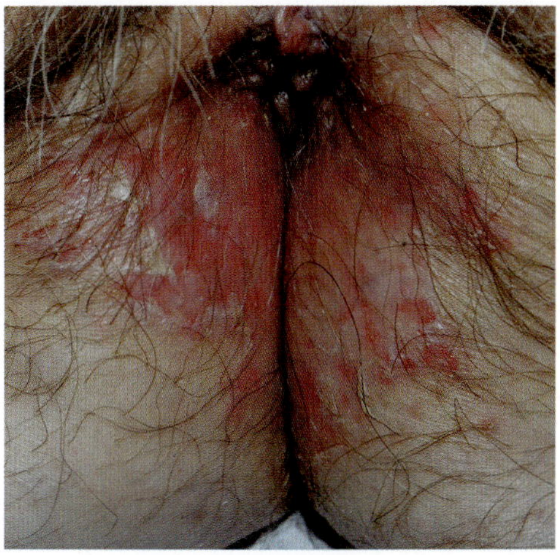

Fig. 5-61. Rectal skin is a skin fold sometimes affected by yeast, which is not surprising since yeast often colonizes the intestines.

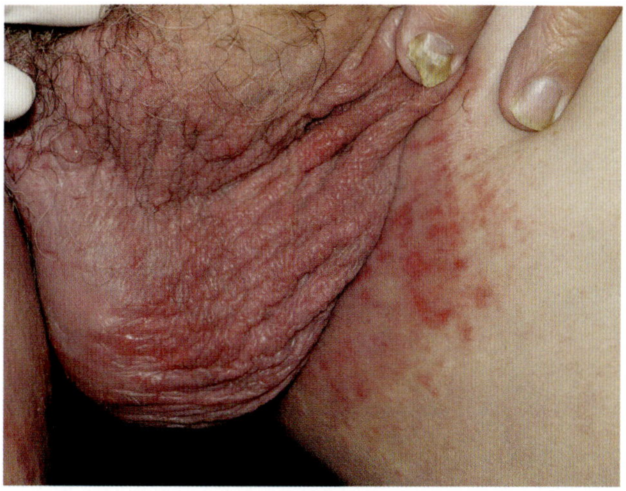

Fig. 5-62. Although generally thought of as an infection of women, intertrigo yeast occurs in men as well, especially those with incontinence or immunosuppression.

*Candida* can both be mistaken for and coexist with atopic dermatitis/eczema, LSC, irritant and ACD, psoriasis, and tinea cruris. The lack of symmetry and the pattern of Paget disease and Bowen disease make both conditions less likely to produce confusion in women, but Bowen disease of the glans penis can be indistinguishable from *Candida* balanitis.

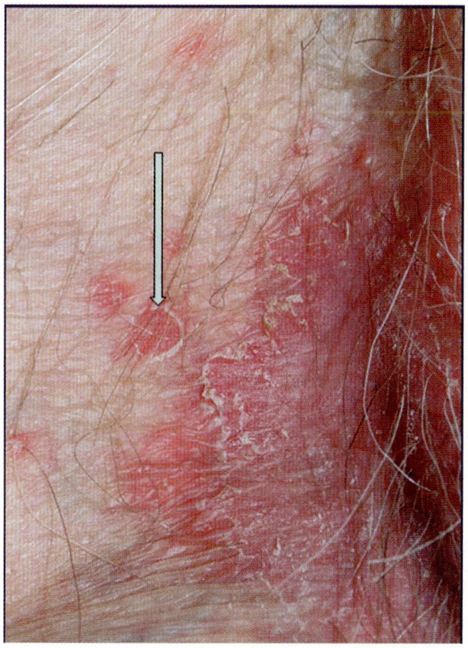

Fig. 5-63. Peripheral peeling rather than scale is classic for yeast. There is a collarette that shows the original blistering nature of the eruption, but the pustules are so superficial and fragile that they rupture early, leaving the edges of the blister (*arrow*).

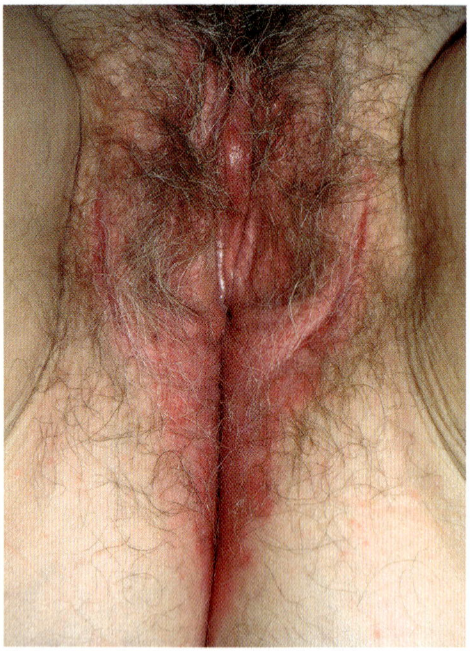

Fig. 5-64. Poorly demarcated deep erythema and fissuring are characteristic of vulvar candidiasis, as are fissures as seen in the labiocrural crease bilaterally.

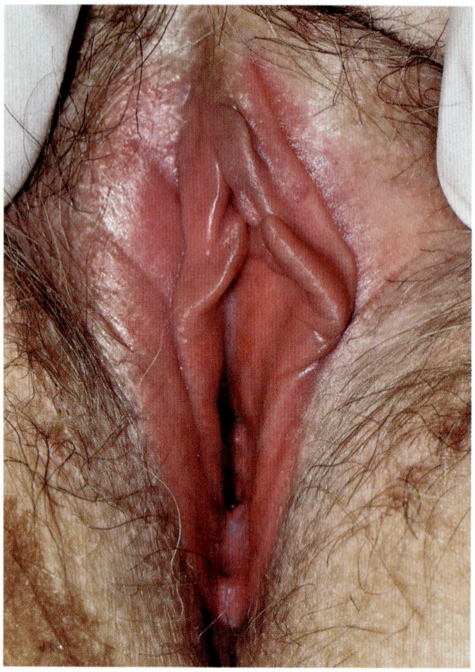

Fig. 5-65. The modified mucous membranes are edematous and red due to candidiasis, as are fine fissures in skin creases.

*CANDIDA* **Diagnosis**

- Morphology of patches, often with satellite papules, pustules, or desquamation, accentuated in skin folds most often in inguinal creases, on the vulva and scrotum of those with diabetes, obesity, incontinence
- Red puffy modified mucous membranes and mucous membranes of the vulva vagina
- Indistinguishable from inverse psoriasis
- Positive microscopic scrapings with mycelia and yeast, or, if needed, positive culture

## Pathophysiology

Cutaneous candidiasis is nearly always produced by the yeast *Candida albicans*. Although nonalbicans *Candida* species such as *Candida glabrata* now produce about 10% of vaginal yeast infection, this is not true of cutaneous yeast infections. As noted above, local factors such as incontinence, retention of sweat, and heat provide a favorable environment for this fungus. In addition, obesity, diabetes mellitus, immunosuppression by virtue of disease or medications, and the administration of systemic antibiotics also predispose to yeast infections.

## Management

Topical therapy is very effective for cutaneous candidiasis. Nystatin and all of the topical azoles (clotrimazole, miconazole, tioconazole, terconazole, ketoconazole, etc.) are beneficial for this problem. Evaluation of the vagina for candidiasis or empiric vaginal therapy is important for women, since treatment of the vulva without treatment of the vagina often results in relapse if that reservoir is not eliminated. One oral dose of fluconazole (Diflucan), 150 mg, treats both the vagina and minor skin involvement, and this is effective for *Candida* balanitis. The

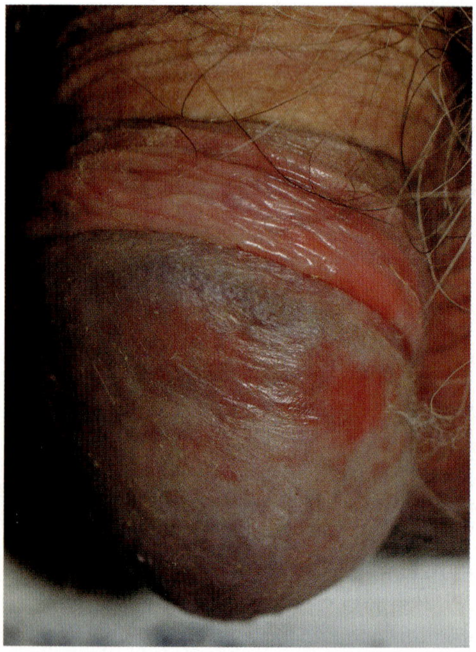

Fig. 5-66. Penile candidiasis is a condition of the uncircumcised male; the nonspecific red papules can be difficult to differentiate from lichen planus, psoriasis, and dysplasia associated with HPV.

clinical trials that evaluated the efficacy of one tablet of fluconazole for vulvovaginal candidiasis did not report the results on those patients with marked cutaneous involvement, so many clinicians administer a second tablet a few days later and/or supplement fluconazole with a topical antifungal medication. Although reasonable, there are no data to support this.

The occasional patient with very inflammatory, exudative cutaneous disease experiences burning and stinging with the use of creams, which contain irritants. Finding an azole in an ointment base can be challenging, but either nystatin ointment or daily oral therapy such as fluconazole 100 mg/d, or itraconazole 200 mg/d, for a week or until healing is underway, and a topical medication can be comfortably substituted. Although only 150 mg is approved by the Food and Drug Administration for candidiasis, this is approved as a one-dose regimen only. The 100 and 200 mg dosage sizes often are more easily approved by insurance companies for multiple tablets. Again, oral ketoconazole has lost indication approval due to safety concerns. Terbinafine is less useful for yeast than for dermatophyte forms of fungus, and griseofulvin is not effective against yeast forms. Alleviation of chronic moisture, control of diabetes, and improvement in immunosuppression help to prevent recurrent or chronic disease. An miconazole, clotrimazole, or nystatin powder can help to prevent recurrence and encourage dryness.

***CANDIDA*** **Management**

- Any topical azole cream (miconazole, clotrimazole, etc.) once or twice daily until clear, or nystatin ointment (less irritating) for external genitalia.
- Vagina can be treated with fluconazole 150-200 mg once, or any intravaginal azole (7-day formulations are least irritating).
- For those with extensive or very inflammatory disease, oral fluconazole 100 mg daily until controlled can be used.

## Perianal Bacterial Dermatitis (Also Called Perianal Infectious Dermatitis, Perianal Streptococcal Dermatitis, Perianal Streptococcal Cellulitis)

Perianal streptococcal dermatitis is a superficial infection of perianal skin that sometimes affects the penis/scrotum or vulva and vagina, where this may be called bacterial vulvitis, vaginitis, or balanitis[52] (see also Chapter 15). Although the causative organism is most often group A hemolytic *Streptococcus*, group B *Streptococcus* and *Staphylococcus aureus* have been reported as well. This is most often a pediatric disease affecting young children, but it can also affect both the genitalia and perianal skin of adults. Most information in the literature addresses the disease in childhood.

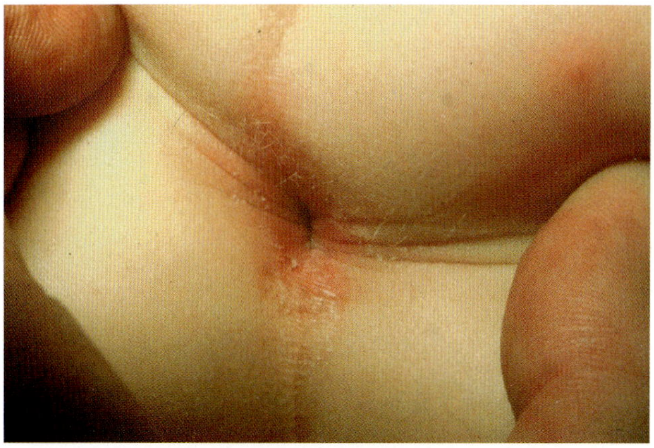

Fig. 5-67. Perianal bacterial infection is usually a disease of small children, manifested by poorly demarcated scale, and sometimes crusting and fissuring, often clinically misdiagnosed as yeast.

Patients describe persistent pain or pruritus, painful defecation, and blood-streaked stools that have been unresponsive to antifungal and corticosteroid medications. Erythema, fissuring, fragility, crusting, exudation, and/or erosion of the perianal skin (**Figs. 5-67 through 5-69**) are typical on examination. Occasionally, the scrotum and penis are involved, and the vulva may also exhibit similar abnormalities, usually associated with an erythematous vaginal mucosa and a purulent vaginal discharge. In addition, throat cultures are often positive, even in the absence of symptoms.[53]

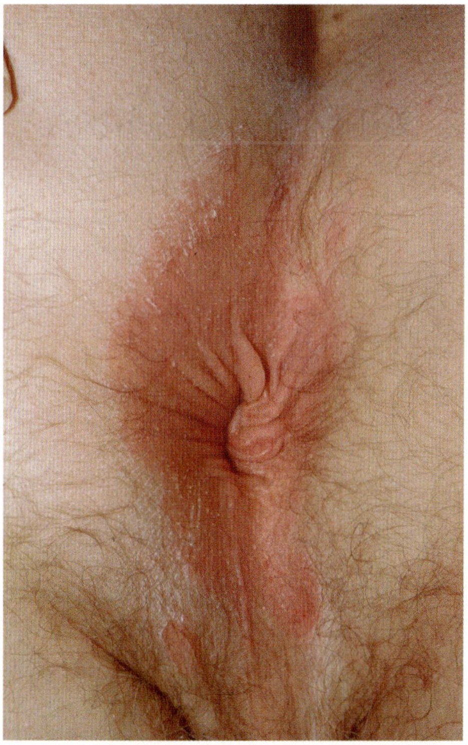

Fig. 5-68. This 56-year-old physician had empirically treated himself for fungal infection and eczema before a routine culture showed group A *Streptococcus* infection. The plaque cleared quickly with amoxicillin.

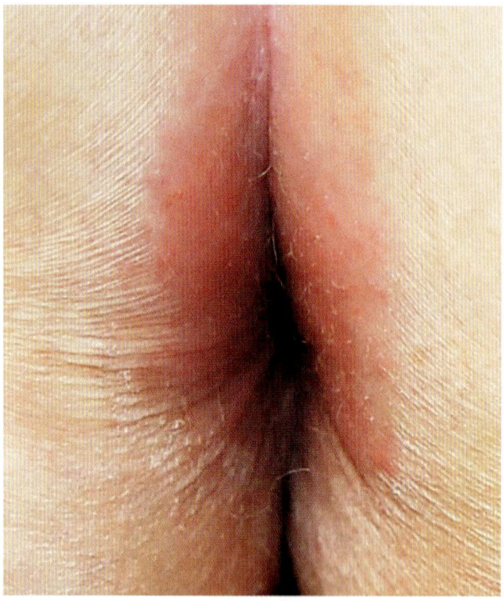

Fig. 5-69. This woman reports burning and irritation, and a culture of this red plaque with fissures showed group A *Streptococcus* and confirmed her diagnosis.

The skin should be cultured to confirm the diagnosis and to identify the causative organism and, if *S aureus*, the sensitivities. The treatment consists of oral antibiotics that cover both streptococci and *S aureus* while awaiting culture results. Even in patients with group A *Streptococcus*, cephalosporins are more effective than penicillin.[54] Because of the tendency for recurrence, some clinicians have advocated antibiotic therapy for several weeks.[55] More rapid improvement may occur with the addition of a potent topical antibiotic such as mupirocin ointment several times a day for the first week. Recurrences are common.

## Lichen Planus

Lichen planus is a relatively common dermatosis of anogenital skin, but only rarely with the morphology of red papules and plaques. Much more common is the erosive variant (see Chapter 11), and it exhibits various morphologic appearances and symptoms (see also Chapters 8, 9, and 13). This disease is discussed primarily in Chapter 11. The morphologic variant is partially dependent on the location of the disease, and many patients exhibit several different forms of lichen planus. The least common form in women and the most common form in circumcised men is that of red plaques and papules.

### Clinical Presentation

Papular lichen planus is most often pruritic, sometimes accompanied by irritation or rawness. Lichen planus of dry, keratinized skin is usually manifested by violaceous or dull red, red-brown, or pink, well-demarcated, flat-topped papules **(Fig. 5-70)**. Although the classic location of papular lichen planus is the ventral aspect of the wrist, this form of lichen planus can be found on other dry skin surfaces but almost never on the face.

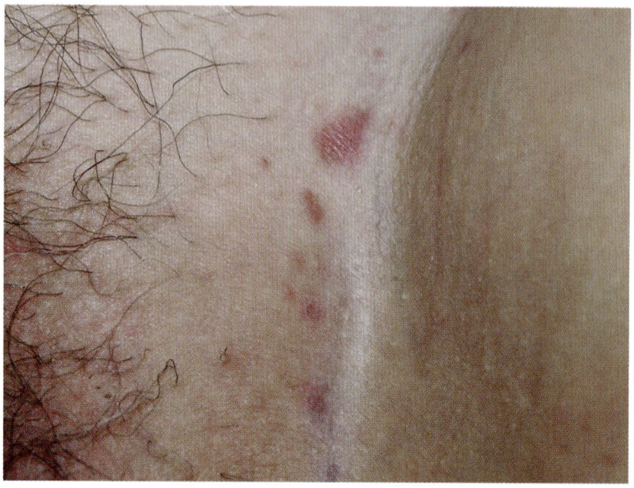

Fig. 5-70. These shiny, red flat-topped papules are typical for lichen planus.

A common location for genital papular lichen planus is the glans penis. These lesions are usually well demarcated, red, flat topped, and shiny **(Figs. 5-71 and 5-72)**. Occasionally, the lesions are annular, hypopigmented, or hyperpigmented. The crural creases and proximal, medial thighs are sometimes involved **(Fig. 5-72)**. Papular lichen planus occurring in women is found most often on the hair-bearing labia majora, crural creases, and proximal, medial thighs **(Figs. 5-73 and 5-74)**.

Papular lichen planus of the genitalia often is accompanied by erosive, atrophic red, or brown papules or plaques, or white, reticulate mucous membrane or

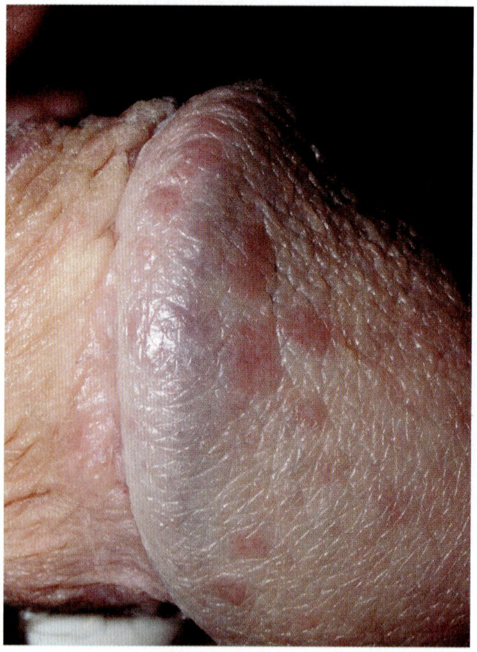

Fig. 5-71. Lichen planus on the circumcised glans is most often well demarcated, red, and flat topped.

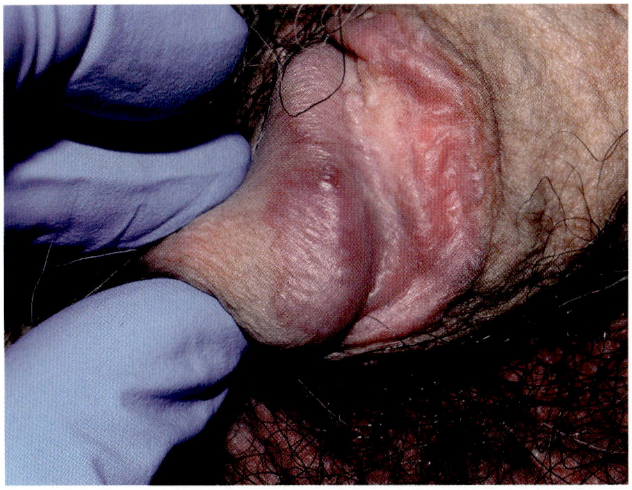

Fig. 5-72. This lichen planus of the glans and ventral prepuce shows a lavender, well-demarcated, flat-topped plaque, that is also typical for this diagnosis.

modified mucous membrane lichen planus, of the vulva, vagina, or mouth. Pathognomonic mucosal lesions are white, linear, branching papules that often form a fernlike or lacy pattern **(Fig. 5-75)**. Common but nonspecific are red, atrophic, smooth patches, or red erosions, although a careful examination often shows diagnostic white papules **(Fig. 5-76)**. Sometimes, red, atrophic patches of mucosal lichen planus can be difficult to differentiate from actual erosions of mucosal lichen planus **(Fig. 5-75)**. Even when the vaginal epithelium appears generally normal, nonspecific inflammatory vaginitis characterized by a large number of white blood cells and an increased proportion of parabasal (immature epithelial) cells is common (see Chapter 13). Since most women with vulvovaginal lichen planus are postmenopausal, a wet mount of vaginal lichen planus in this group cannot be differentiated from atrophic vaginitis in postmenopausal women who are not on estrogen replacement. Response to topical estrogen is

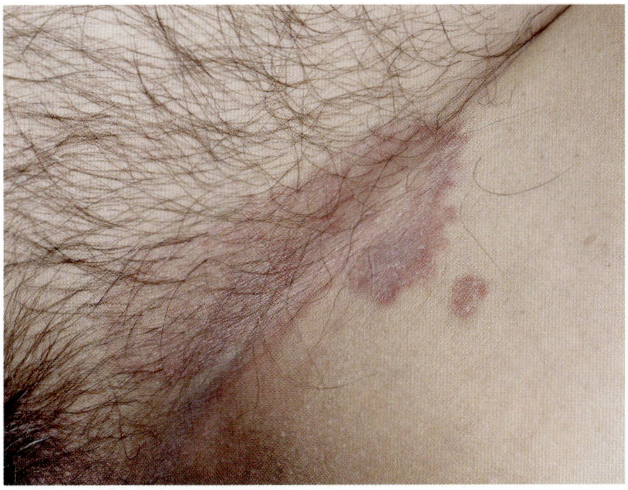

Fig. 5-73. Sometimes, lichen planus can show a brown-pink color, with more coarse scale that does not appear shiny.

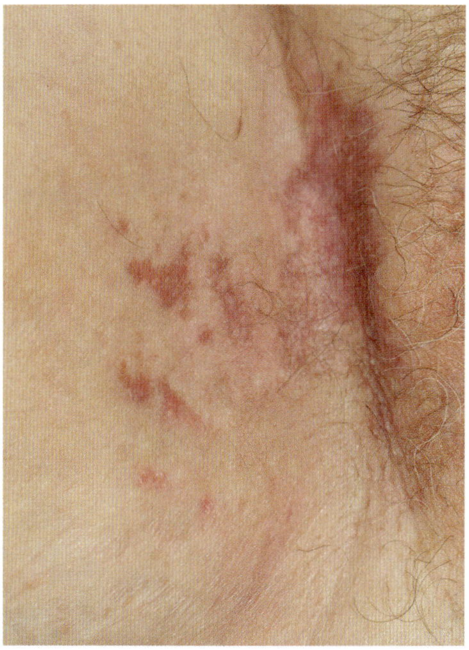

Fig. 5-74. The pink/brown coalescing flat papules are nonspecific and either a biopsy or the identification of more typical lichen planus would be required for diagnosis.

required both for separation of these two entities and for maximal patient comfort.

## Diagnosis

The diagnosis of lichen planus is made on the basis of clinical morphology and is confirmed either by finding diagnostic

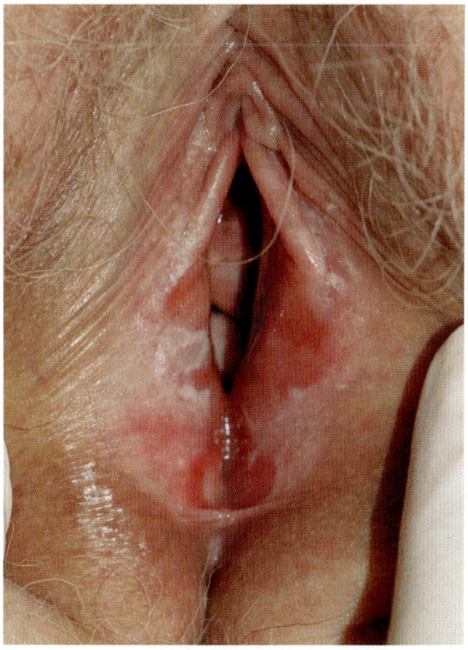

Fig. 5-75. The vulvar vestibule shows an atrophic red plaque with surrounding white linear and annular plaques that announce the diagnosis of lichen planus.

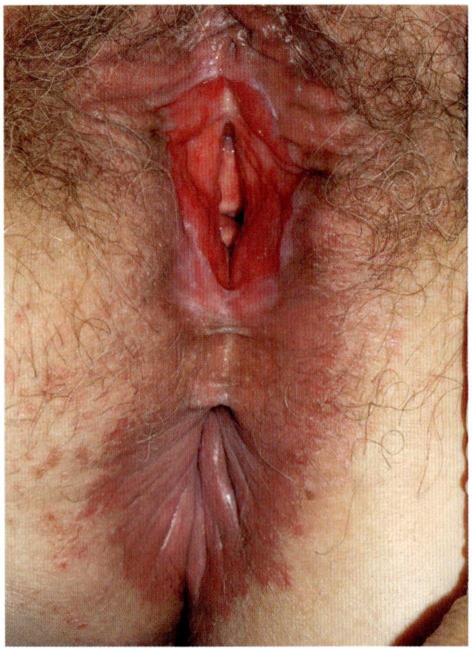

Fig. 5-76. This patient has typical erosive vulvar lichen planus, and an accompanying dusky red, edematous plaque of perianal lichen planus.

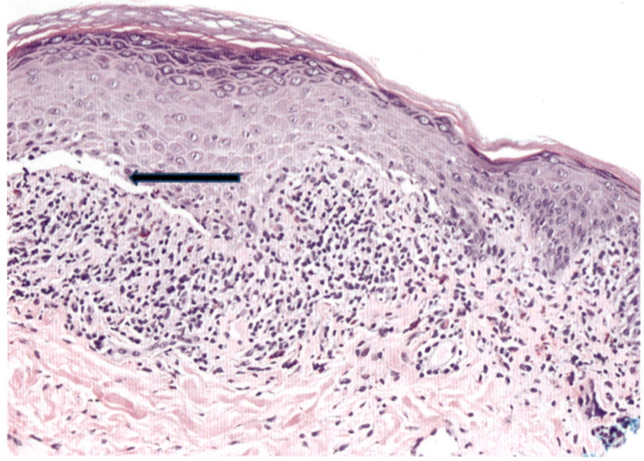

Fig. 5-77. A biopsy of red, papular lichen planus on keratinized skin is manifested by chronic inflammation hugs and disrupts the basal layer of the epidermis, here producing detachment of the epidermis from the dermis (*arrow*). (Courtesy of Jason Reutter, MD.)

white, reticular or fernlike white, or by characteristic histology on biopsy. In addition, dermoscopy highlights the classic clinical finding of Wickham striae, fine network–like white lines. Less often, linear, "radial streaming," annular, round, delicate secondary striae branching from the centered whitish venation, linked together at either end, mimicking the crystal structure of snow, and "starry sky" (clustered, follicular white dots) aspect may occur.[7] In darker skinned individuals, these striae cam appear blue. Some resolving or scarred dermatoses can exhibit similar striae.[7] A biopsy of papular lichen planus shows thickening of the epidermis in a regular, saw-toothed pattern **(Fig. 5-77)**. In addition, there is prominence of the granular cell layer and an absence of parakeratosis. A bandlike mononuclear infiltrate present in the upper epidermis tightly hugs the dermal-epidermal junction and produces some areas of vacuolar degeneration of the basal cell layer. Scattered within the epidermis are individual dyskeratotic keratinocytes.

Papular lichen planus of the glans penis and vulva can be indistinguishable high-grade squamous intraepithelial lesion (HSIL) (Bowenoid papulosis, squamous cell carcinoma *in situ* due to human papillomavirus [HPV] infection) or from differentiated intraepithelial neoplasia (Bowen disease, erythroplasia of Queyrat, squamous cell carcinoma *in situ* in the setting of chronic skin disease, primarily lichen sclerosus or lichen planus). Psoriasis, candidiasis, and plasma cell mucositis (Zoon) can also mimic popular lichen planus of the glans. The white and eroded patches and plaques on the modified mucous membranes of the vulva or the uncircumcised glans can be mistaken for pemphigus vulgaris, mucous membrane pemphigoid, herpes simplex virus infection, or candidiasis.

**PAPULAR LICHEN PLANUS — Diagnosis**

- Morphology of well-demarcated, red flat-topped papules on dry, keratinized skin, sometimes with overlying white striae, often accompanied by erosions of the uncircumcised penis or vagina or modified mucous membranes of the vulva
- Often with oral erosions or white striae of the buccal mucosae
- Biopsy showing changes of lichen planus

## Pathophysiology

Lichen planus is believed to be a disease of cell-mediated autoimmunity. In addition to data suggesting this origin, the histologic findings of lichen planus are similar to those of graft vs host disease. Also, lichen planus responds to immunosuppressant medications.

## Management

Generally, papular lichen planus is self-limited, and resolution usually occurs within several years, unlike the chronic course of erosive disease. If it is not symptomatic, treatment is not necessary. The scarring and malignancy that can occur with erosive disease do not occur with popular disease on keratinized skin. Papular lichen planus on keratinized skin is usually adequately treated with a topical corticosteroid. However, the lesions usually do not resolve but only fade somewhat and itch less. Unfortunately, a rather high-potency preparation is required, and spread of this medication to the surrounding inner thighs and crural crease is likely to produce atrophy.

Other therapies include a short burst of oral prednisone at 40-60 mg/d, oral retinoids such as tretinoin cream (starting at the lowest concentration of 0.025% as this is very irritating on genital skin), and oral hydroxychloroquine. Careful attention to the vagina is imperative, since accompanying vaginal erosive disease can occur in association with papular vulvar disease, with introital irritation due to irritant contact dermatitis from the inflammatory discharge, and narrowing or even permanent obliteration of the vaginal space. Vaginal lichen planus is discussed in Chapter 13. Management of lichen planus is discussed in detail in Chapter 11.

**PAPULAR LICHEN PLANUS — Management**

- Superpotent topical corticosteroid such as clobetasol ointment if symptomatic, with careful follow-up for side effects
- Surveillance of the vagina and mouth for accompanying erosive disease

## Pityriasis Rosea

Pityriasis rose a (PR) is a very common skin disease, which does not preferentially affect the genital skin but typically involves the trunk where it often extends to the bathing trunk area. When this occurs in the genital area, it is often misdiagnosed.

Pityriasis rosea is most common in adolescents and young adults. Sometimes pruritic, pityriasis rosea is typically characterized by 0.5- to 1.5-cm, oval, pink papules **(Figs. 5-78 and 5-79)**. These papules, which appear nearly macular, exhibit very subtle scale that is often missed on examination, and sometimes the surface must be scuffed with a fingernail to raise the fine granular scale. These papules are usually aligned with the long axis of the oval lesion lying along skin lines on the trunk. Individual lesions often demonstrate a collarette of scale. Most often, one larger (and sometimes round rather than oval) lesion, the herald patch, is noted by the patient. The diagnosis is made by the morphology and setting. Dermoscopy shows a background of erythema with dots of red vessels in a nonspecific pattern, with white or brown scale.[56] Brown dots are also common.

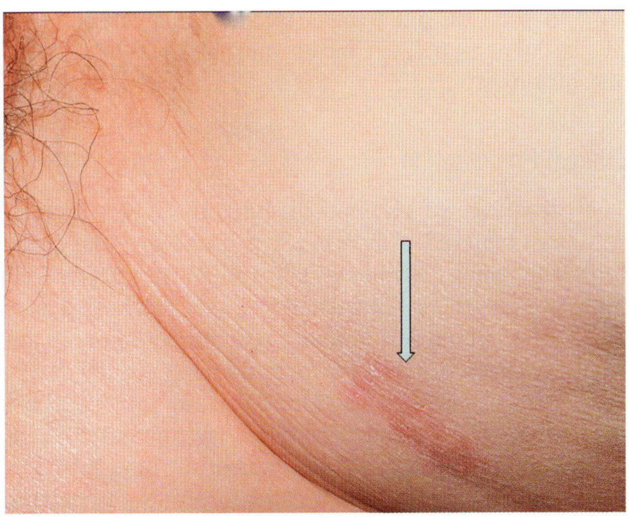

Fig. 5-78. Pityriasis rosea is manifested by pink, lightly scaling papules that are oval and lie in the natural skin lines (*arrow*); these should be accompanied by extragenital lesions as well.

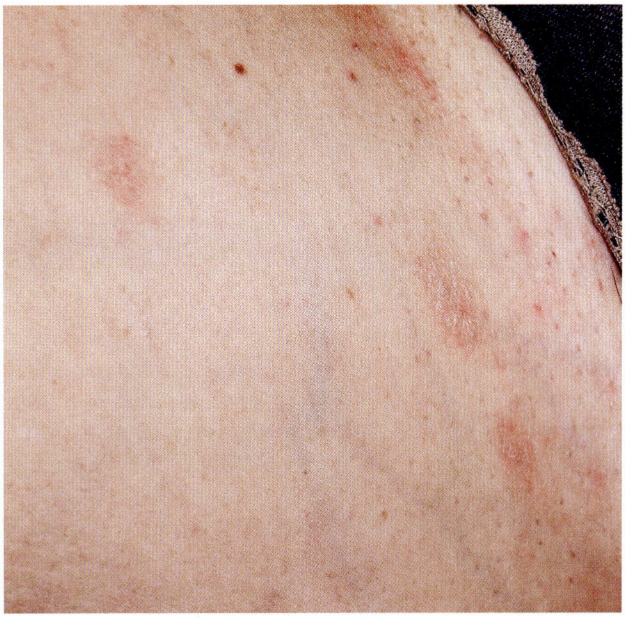

Fig. 5-79. Pityriasis rosea lesions are discrete and multiple, with the oval axis all lying parallel to each other.

The primary disease to be considered in the differential diagnosis is secondary syphilis. However, secondary syphilis exhibits generalized lymphadenopathy, and unlike pityriasis rosea, palmar lesions are common with that disease as well. Syphilis serology should be performed when there is any question of the diagnosis. Additional skin diseases that can resemble pityriasis rosea include guttate psoriasis and the red variant of papular lichen planus. Occasionally, medications can produce a pityriasis rosea like eruption; implicated agents include clozapine, lamotrigine, rituximab, nortriptyline, interferon alpha, bupropion, and HPV vaccinations. However, PR is common, so some of these occurrences could be coincidental. Guttate psoriasis usually exhibits more obvious scale but can mimic PR at times.

The cause of pityriasis rosea is unknown, but many believe that it is a reaction to a mild viral infection. Recently, herpesviruses-6 and -7 have been suggested as causes, and acyclovir has been shown to shorten the course. There have been recent reports of increased numbers of pityriasis rosea and pityriasis rosea–like rashes in association with COVID-19, likely due to reactivation of HSV-6/7.[57,58] In very symptomatic patients, a short course of oral prednisolone produced much improved and shorter course, but ultimate recurrence was higher.[59]

Exposure to ultraviolet light is useful, and topical corticosteroids reduce itching. Pityriasis rosea is self-limited, generally lasting about 2 months, but it can recur. A recent report suggests that pregnant women may be at risk for complications and fetal loss due to reactivation of HSV-6 and HSV-7.[60]

## Pityriasis (Tinea) Versicolor

Although called *tinea* versicolor in the past, this fungus infection is not produced by a dermatophyte (tinea) but rather by a yeast form. Pityriasis versicolor does not often affect the genital skin, but sometimes it extends from its usual location from the upper trunk to the lower trunk and keratinized genital skin, including the penile shaft. More common in teenagers and young adults, pityriasis versicolor is usually asymptomatic. Lesions are pink, tan, or hypopigmented, hence the name "versicolor." Individual papules are well demarcated and usually affect the upper chest and back most prominently, with coalescence of 2- to 10-mm papules into larger plaques **(Figs. 5-80 and 5-81)**. Although the surface is lightly scaling, this scaling is so subtle that the skin surface often must be scratched to raise visible scale.

The cause of pityriasis versicolor is various *Malassezia* spp, organisms that are ubiquitous. This infection is not generally spread from person to person, but rather contracted from the environment by a host whose immune system does not mount an adequate defense. These are not patients with clinically significant immune suppression, but treatment of pityriasis versicolor is regularly followed by recurrence.

Therapy consists of any topical azole, including clotrimazole, miconazole, or econazole once or twice daily. Very wide spread pityriasis versicolor is best treated orally, and options include itraconazole 200 mg/d for 5 or 7 days and fluconazole 300 mg/wk for 2 weeks, and a recent trial showed benefit with topical adapalene as well.[61,62] Either regular use of an azole cream to prevent recurrence or the prompt reinstitution of therapy with new lesions is usual therapy.

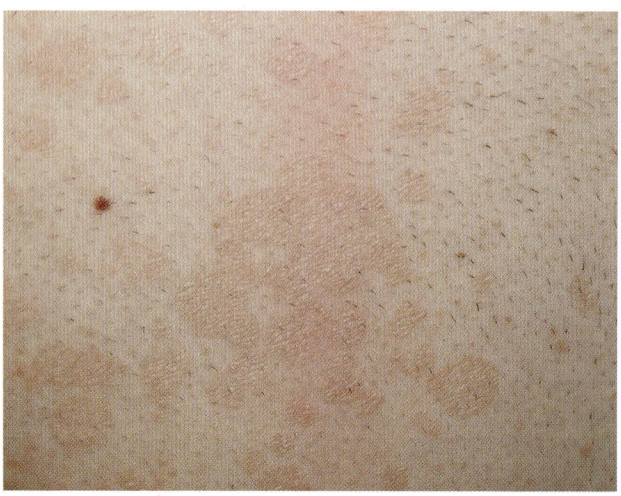

Fig. 5-80. Pityriasis (tinea) versicolor is a yeast infection that appears as small, coalescing flat papules with fine scale; the lesions can be pink, tan, or even hypopigmented; hence, the name "versicolor."

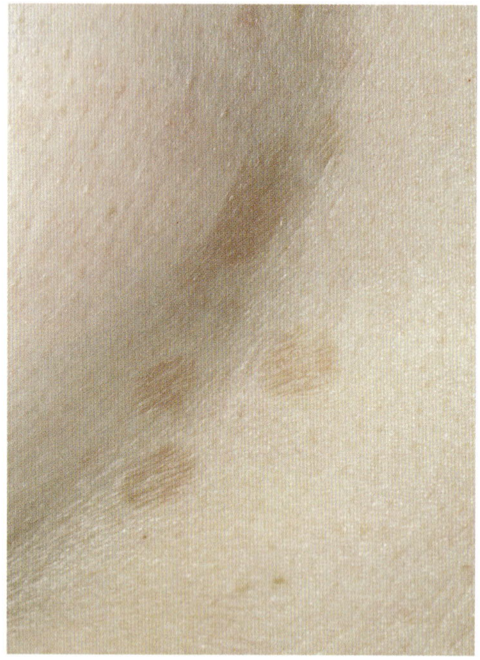

Fig. 5-81. Although pityriasis (tinea) versicolor occasionally occurs in the bathing trunk area, it is much more common on the upper trunk.

## Plasma Cell Mucositis (Plasma Cell Vulvitis and Balanitis, Zoon Mucositis, Vulvitis Plasmacellularis, and Balanitis Circumscripta Plasmacellularis)

This is an uncommon, poorly understood disease of genital skin and, less often (never seen by this author), oral mucosa that is defined by its morphologic appearance and histology.

### Clinical Presentation

The prevalence of plasma cell mucositis is not known. Although believed to be rare, it is probably more common than realized. Although few women with plasma cell mucositis have been reported, this author has treated over 27 patients (all but two women) with this condition in the past 20 years in her solo practice and observed the development of plasma cell vulvitis in existing patients. This disease is found at all postpubertal ages, although there are reports of childhood Zoon balanitis. There seems to be no racial predilection in the literature, although I have seen this exclusively in Caucasian individuals. Plasma cell mucositis has been reported more often in men than in women.

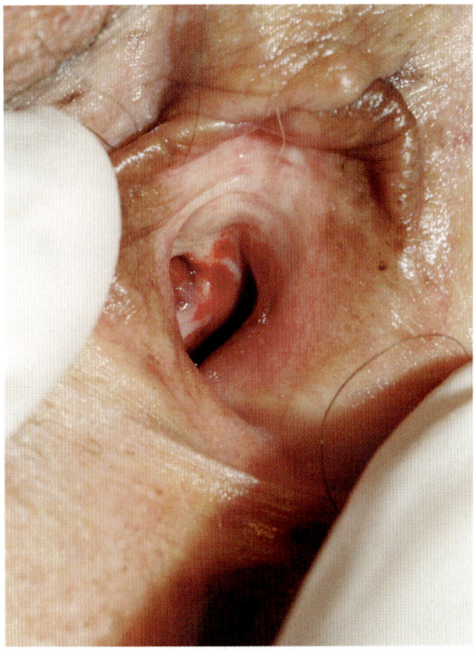

Fig. 5-82. This blood-red periurethral and vestibular patch is typical for early plasma cell vulvitis; this actually does represent purpura.

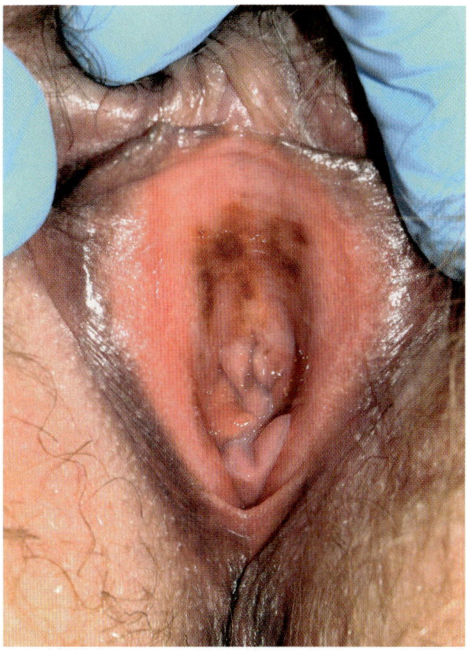

Fig. 5-84. Older lesions of plasma cell vulvitis show brown colors from the iron in the purpuric lesions.

Plasma cell mucositis presents as a glistening, nonblanching, deep red to rusty red to deep brown/black, well-demarcated, usually solitary plaque that is easily eroded and may bleed (**Figs. 5-82 through 5-88**). This is generally stable, without spontaneously waxing, waning, or migrating to other areas. When occurring on the glans, it is seen only in uncircumcised men. Lesions of plasma cell mucositis have no obvious scale, and they may be characterized by itching, soreness, or burning, but they may be asymptomatic. This condition is not related to any other skin or systemic disease. There are reports, in addition to my experience, of coexistence of plasma cell mucositis with lichen planus and lichen sclerosus.[63]

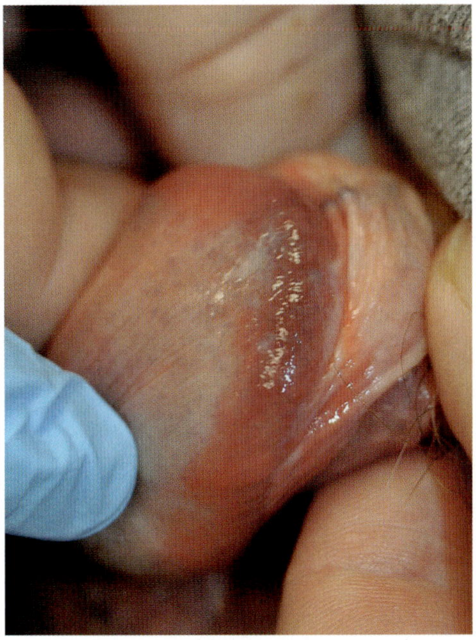

Fig. 5-83. The deep dusky patch of plasma cell mucositis on the corona is surrounded by an orange color of old purpura at the edge of the lesion.

## Diagnosis

The diagnosis of plasma cell mucositis is made by the presence of the typical deep red, well-demarcated color change, and histologic appearance. Dermoscopy of plasma cell balanitis shows focal or diffuse orange-yellowish structureless areas and fairly focused curved vessels that can be serpentine or convoluted.[64] How-

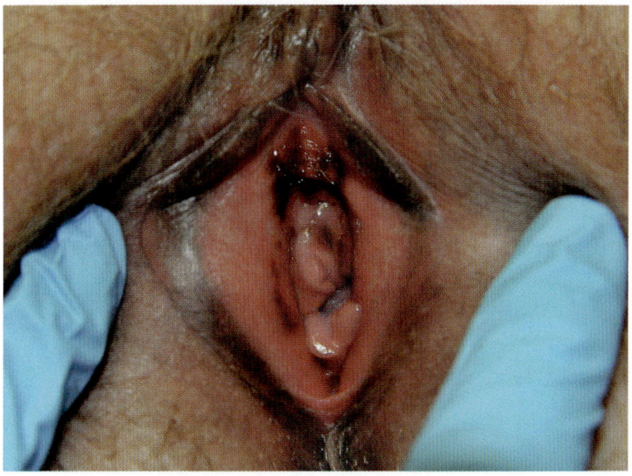

Fig. 5-85. With time, lesions of plasma cell mucositis can become even darker brown, sometimes nearly black.

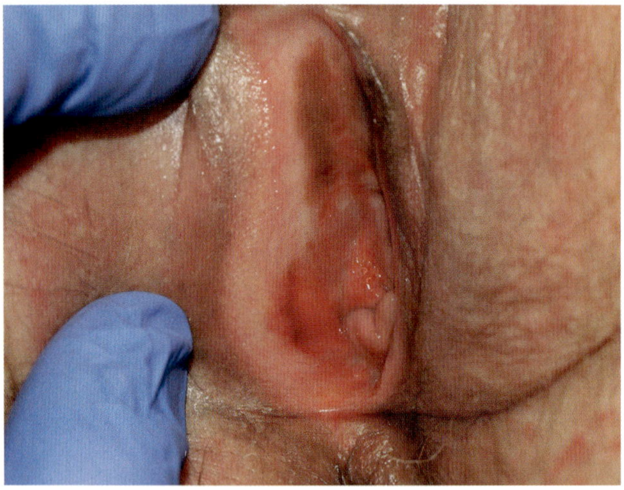

Fig. 5-86. Plasma cell mucositis is nearly always on mucous membranes. This rusty color is typical.

ever, a biopsy is required for definitive diagnosis and to rule out other red patches and erosions **(Fig. 5-89)**. A biopsy is characterized by a thinned and flattened epidermis composed of keratinocytes that are diamond shaped, sometimes necrotic, and separated by intercellular edema. There is an upper dermal infiltrate of plasma cells.

Any red well-demarcated plaque should be considered, with erosive lichen planus arguably the most difficult to differentiate at times. However, plasma cell mucositis does not scar, and also unlike erosive lichen planus, this condition does not usually eventuate into squamous cell carcinoma. Psoriasis on moist skin can mimic plasma cell mucositis, and both candidiasis and differentiated intraepithelial neoplasia (squamous cell carcinoma *in situ*) are also conditions in the differential diagnosis.

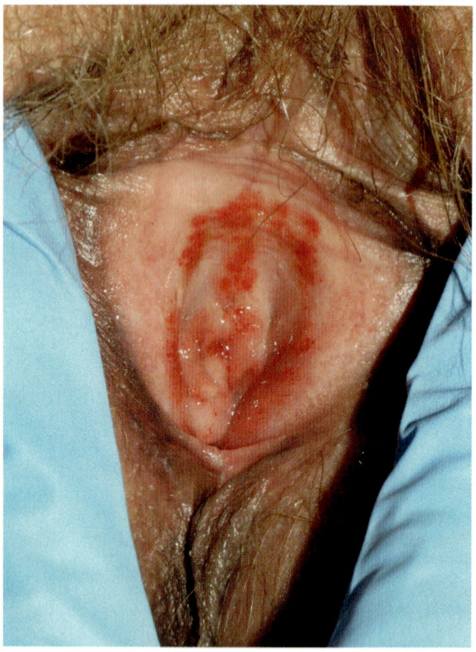

Fig. 5-88. Well-demarcated red macules in the vestibule are characteristic of plasma cell vulvitis.

**PLASMA CELL MUCOSITIS — Diagnosis**

- Distinctive morphology of well-demarcated purpuric deep red, orange-red, or brown-red patches on modified mucous membrane or mucous membranes of the vulva and glans penis or ventral prepuce
- Confirmed by a characteristic biopsy showing a dense upper dermal inflammatory infiltrate containing many plasma cells, as well as effacement of the epidermis with lozenge-shaped keratinocytes

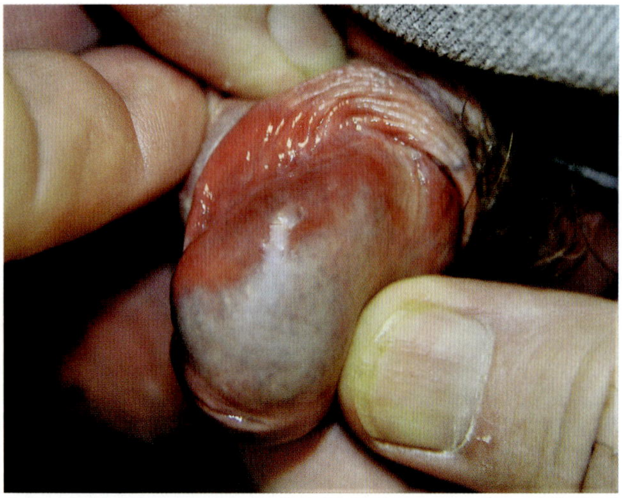

Fig. 5-87. Plasma cell mucositis presents as red, moist, usually well-demarcated papules or plaques that often mimic lichen planus.

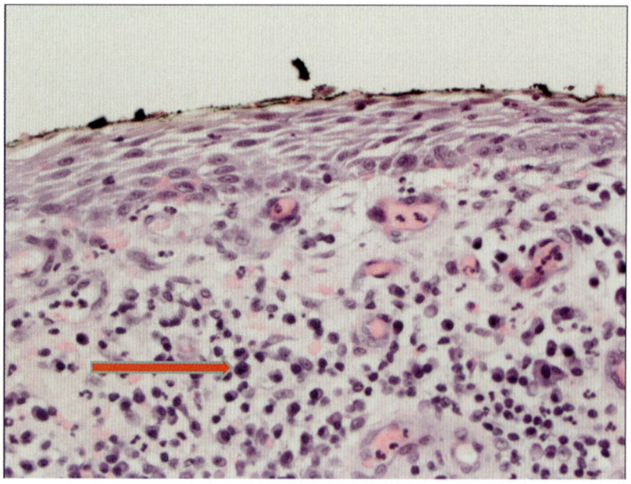

Fig. 5-89. Plasma cell mucositis is characterized histologically by an atrophic, flattened epidermis with "lozenge"-shaped epithelial cells and dermal inflammation with a large numbers of plasma cells (*arrow*). (Courtesy of Jason Reutter, MD.)

### Pathophysiology

The cause of plasma cell mucositis is unknown, and some do not believe that this represents a specific entity, but rather a nonspecific inflammatory reactive pattern. However, plasma cell mucositis is a useful term to indicate this very characteristic presentation.

Some have postulated an association with lichen planus and, anecdotally, two women with vulvar lichen planus treated successfully by this author later developed plasma cell mucositis, and one patient with lichen planus has developed plasma cell vulvitis.

### Management

There is no satisfactory therapy, and there are no studies that evaluate therapies. Circumcision is the overwhelming treatment of choice for plasma cell balanitis in uncircumcised men.[65] Anecdotal reports have shown potent topical steroids to be useful, and intralesional corticosteroids sometimes clear lesions. Imiquimod and the calcineurin inhibitors tacrolimus ointment and pimecrolimus cream have been reported to be variably useful, and a report of betamethasone valerate 0.1% mixed with fusidic acid 2% was useful in some patients.[66] One report of ablative erbium:YAG laser treatment reported success with 17 of 20 men with plasma cell balanitis.[67] Photodynamic therapy has been less successful; 1 of 6 men with plasma cell balanitis had improvement, although there is an additional favorable case report.[68,69] Carbon dioxide laser has been used.[70] A compounded topical therapy consisting of clobetasol, oxytetracycline, and nystatin has been found useful by some, but there is no supporting data (personal communication, Lynne Margesson, MD). Be aware, however, that there are rare reports of squamous cell carcinoma occurring in patients with plasma cell balanitis,[71,72] and I have one patient with clitoral phimosis and plasma cell vulvitis affecting that area, so care should be taken to follow patients for these potential issues.

**PLASMA CELL MUCOSITIS — Management**

- Superpotent topical corticosteroids such as clobetasol ointment once or twice daily, then
- Intralesional corticosteroids, such as intralesional triamcinolone 10 mg/mL, then
- Tacrolimus 0.1%/pimecrolimus 1% twice daily, then consider
- Destruction with $CO_2$ laser or photodynamic therapy

## Vestibulodynia (Vulvar Vestibulitis Syndrome, Vestibular Adenitis)

Vestibulodynia is a localized pain syndrome, especially entry dyspareunia, which is primarily discussed in Chapter 13. This condition is defined as sensations of pain, including burning, stinging, rawness, soreness, irritation, tearing, aching in the absence of objective relevant physical findings, and laboratory abnormalities. Itching is absent or a minor symptom. However, most patients describe redness and swelling. These are abnormalities that are difficult to gauge in an area that normally shows variable degrees of redness.

The classic finding in vestibulodynia is poorly demarcated erythema surrounding ostia of vestibular glands located adjacent to the external aspect of the hymenal caruncles (Fig. 5-90). On biopsy, however, the mild chronic nonspecific inflammation is the same as that found in the normal, nonpainful vestibule.

The diagnosis of this syndrome is one of exclusion, with correction of any infection, estrogen deficiency, cutaneous abnormalities, and specific neuropathic syndromes such as postherpetic neuralgia. A diagnostic workup requires only a careful normal visual examination, a normal wet mount, and, possibly, a negative fungal culture. Then, treatment consists of oral medication for neuropathic pain, pelvic floor physical therapy for the usually occurring pelvic muscle dysfunction, and attention to psychological aspects including anxiety, depression, and sexual dysfunction. The most definitive and effective therapy, but also the last resort because it is not generally needed, it is painful with a significant recovery time, and it is expensive, is a vestibulectomy. This procedure, which is most effective when performed in a setting of adequate oral medication and physical therapy, is the surgical removal of painful skin and is useful when the pain is absolutely localized to the vestibule.

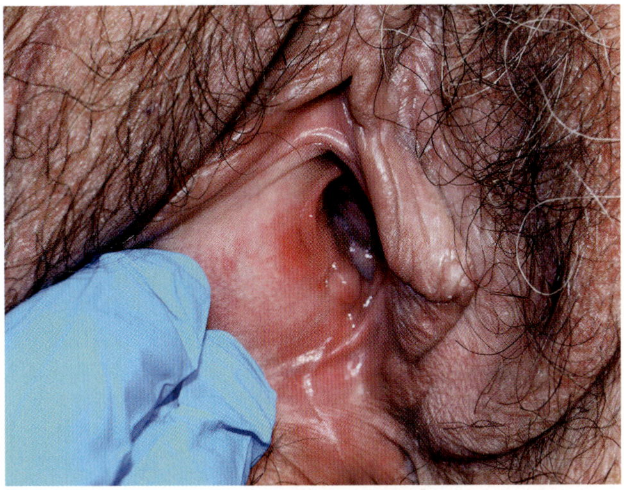

Fig. 5-90. Erythema around the ostia of vestibular glands in patients with vestibulodynia (previously called vulvar vestibulitis) suggested initially that this was an inflammatory condition. However, these red areas are also seen in asymptomatic women, and biopsies show no more inflammation in women with vestibulodynia than is seen in women without symptoms.

## Red Scrotum Syndrome

Red scrotum syndrome is one name for a sensation of scrotal burning or rawness in the absence of objective skin disease other than a variable degrees of erythema. This does not refer to one, well-accepted condition. Some clinicians consider this a synonym for corticosteroid dermatitis (also called steroid addiction),[73] whereas others feel that this is rebound erythema following the use of corticosteroids, or erythromelalgia.[74] Some use this as a designation for the pain syndrome called scrotodynia and is analogous to vulvodynia, with the degree of erythema falling into the normal range, but the patient is adamant that the redness is new. Some feel that this represents neuropathic discomfort.[75] Finally, some journal articles report red scrotum syndrome as an inflammatory dermatitis produced by corticosteroid use, sometimes persisting for years after cessation, and responding to doxycycline.[76] Therefore, various reports are likely referring to different conditions. And, because nearly all chronic inflammatory genital skin diseases receive empiric antifungal medications and corticosteroid therapy, implicating the corticosteroid as the etiology may be tenuous, especially when the time course is distant.

The unifying concept is that the patient describes burning and macular redness (Fig. 5-91). Therefore, the patient with the complaint of scrotal discomfort and redness should be evaluated for skin disease and fungal infection ruled out, although fungal infection is generally on the proximal, medial thighs rather than the scrotum. Generally, only itching, not burning, irritation, or pain, responds to corticosteroids, and a 1-week trial is a sufficient diagnostic trial to ascertain the presence of a steroid-responsive dermatosis. A 1-week course is insufficient to cause corticosteroid side effects. Therapies that have been tried include avoidance of topical corticosteroids, a trial of doxycycline for its anti-inflammatory effects, and medications such as pregabalin for neuropathic pain.[75,77] Patients who seem especially anxious, especially those worried about undiagnosed infection and sexually transmitted disease, need further time and evaluation (see Chapter 13).

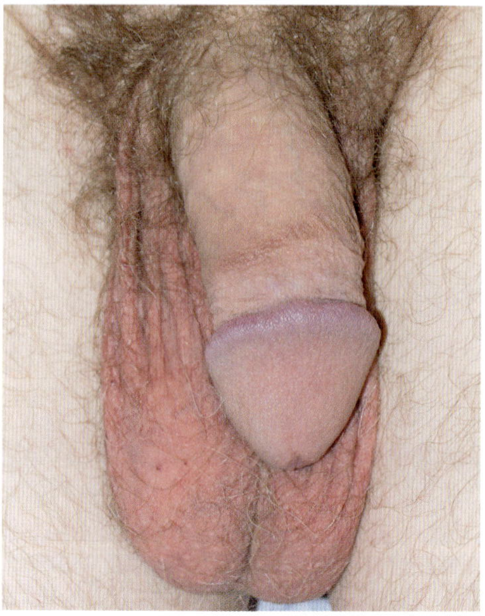

Fig. 5-91. The redness of the scrotum reported by men with red scrotum syndrome/scrotodynia is generally within the normal range of erythema.

These authors believe that red scrotum syndrome often is a condition analogous to vestibulodynia/vulvodynia in women, but often associated in men with even more remarkable anxiety and sexual dysfunction. This author believes that there is an enormous range of dysfunction in these men, with some responding promptly to oral therapy for neuropathy and others either unwilling to accept this diagnosis and therapy or unresponsive to treatment.

## Steroid Dermatitis (Steroid Addiction)

This characteristic response to topical corticosteroids occurs only on genital and facial skin, and only in response to rather potent formulations used chronically. This is a condition recognized by dermatologists and vulvologists but not one easily found in the literature.

### Clinical Presentation

Steroid dermatitis, sometimes referred to as steroid addiction syndrome, consists of redness with, usually, stinging and burning occurring primarily on the genital or facial skin of women in response to chronic potent corticosteroid use.[78] There are two primary forms, papulopustular (steroid rosacea) and erythematoedematous subtypes, and this author most often sees the erythematoedematous type.

This reversible but uncomfortable condition occurs on the dry, keratinized skin, primarily on the labia majora, and mons and results in poorly demarcated, dusky red, and generally nonscaling patches (Figs. 5-92 and 5-93).

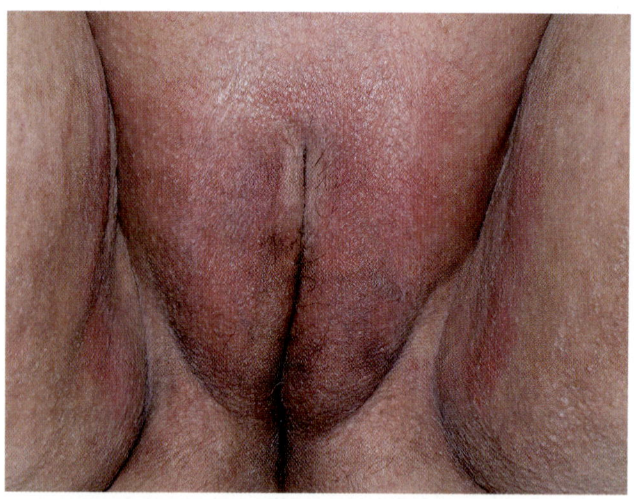

Fig. 5-92. Steroid dermatitis is dusky redness from overuse of topical steroids on the dry, hair-bearing skin, generally of the vulva.

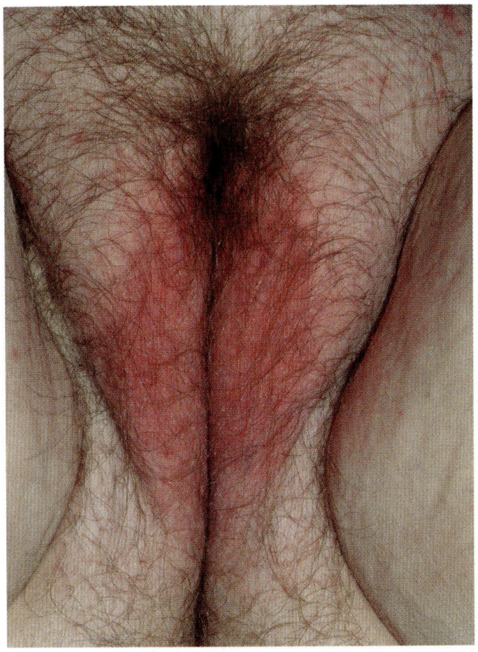

Fig. 5-93. Unintentional spread of a potent topical corticosteroid is often the cause of steroid dermatitis; this underscores the importance of showing the patient what a tiny amount of medication is used and showing the patient exactly where it is to be applied.

Dermoscopy or even a careful examination with a hand lens yields telangiectasias.

### Diagnosis

The diagnosis of corticosteroid dermatitis is made by the presence of poorly demarcated redness and burning, most often of the labia majora or scrotum, in a setting of chronic corticosteroid use. The conundrum for the clinician sometimes is the question of whether redness and symptoms are the result of the undertreatment of an underlying primary red skin disease, or the development steroid dermatitis from overuse of the steroid. However, primary skin diseases such as eczema, LSC, lichen sclerosus, contact dermatitis, and psoriasis, the most common diseases treated with topical corticosteroids, produce itching, whereas steroid dermatitis produces burning. Because patients with steroid dermatitis experience rebound worsening of redness and burning discontinuation of the corticosteroid, improvement with discontinuation of medication cannot be used as a diagnostic criterion.

In addition to undertreated red dermatoses, candidiasis should be considered in the differential diagnosis, and steroid dermatitis can be confused with or coexist with scrotodynia or vulvodynia that exhibit erythema and have been treated with topical corticosteroids.

### Pathophysiology

The cause of corticosteroid dermatitis is not known, and why this is generally limited to facial and genital skin is a mystery.

### Management

The management of steroid dermatitis consists of withdrawal of the corticosteroid. Classic is a flare of symptoms when medication is discontinued, with improvement requiring a month or longer, although most patients do well. Supportive care such as cool tap water soaks, topical lidocaine, and reassurance is usually useful, and low-potency corticosteroids such as hydrocortisone 1-2.5% ointment can serve as a bridge if needed. Flares generally consist of slight worsening of redness and edema, but papules and pustules have been described.

If patients are adequately warned that flares are expected and will remit, most tolerate the increased discomfort. At 1-month follow-up, the skin generally has improved, although erythema often persists, since redness due to telangiectasias does not resolve, but becomes asymptomatic.

## Extramammary Paget Disease

Paget disease is an uncommon adenocarcinoma occurring primarily on anogenital or breast skin. When occurring on skin over the breast, Paget disease is always indicative of underlying breast carcinoma. EMPD is heterogeneous, occurring either as a primary malignancy, arising within the epidermis, or as a secondary process, arising from underlying malignancy. The underlying tumor is most often genitourinary or gastrointestinal in origin.

### Clinical Presentation

Extramammary Paget disease presents most often in people over 50 years of age and much more often in women than in men. However, in the past 40 years, the incidence has increased in men by 3.2% per year, with men of African genetic background having four times less Paget disease and Asian/Pacific Islander men having four times more compared to White men.[79] Invasive extramammary Paget's has more than doubled in the United States in the past 30 years.[80] Chronic pruritus is the most common initial symptom, occurring in most patients, with pain and exudation less common complaints. As expected, there is a poor response to topical corticosteroids and other anti-inflammatory medications.

The most common location for EMPD is on the vulva, both the keratinized skin and modified mucous membrane surfaces, as well as the perianal skin. Less common are the perineum, scrotum, mons, and penis. EMPD presents as a well-demarcated red plaque with a scaling or moist surface, often with islands of white epithelium (**Figs. 5-94 through 5-97**). Erosions are common as well. Pigmented EMPD is a well-recognized variant.

The proportion of patients with EMPD who have associated underlying malignancy is arguable. Often quoted is 15% to 30% of patients with an associated malignancy, although one of the largest series reports only 4%,[81] and a

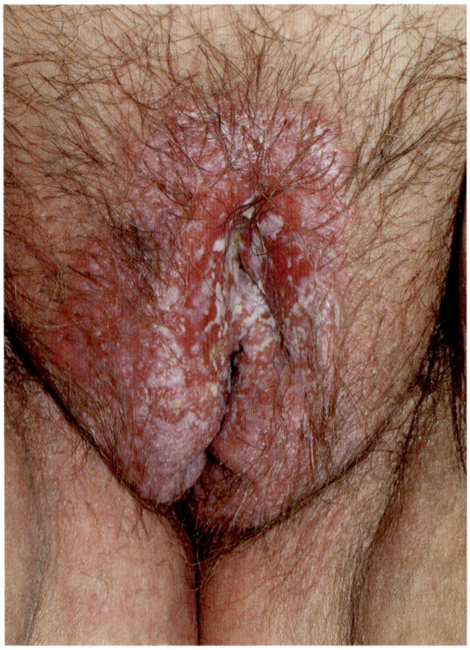

Fig. 5-94. A red plaque with white islands of hyperkeratosis is classic for extramammary Paget disease.

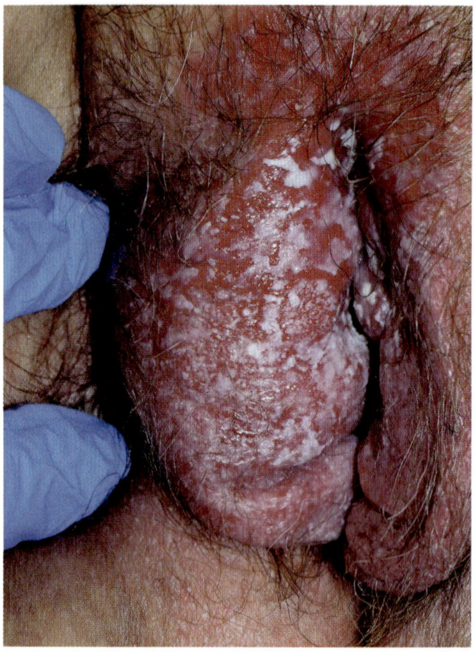

Fig. 5-96. Women are more affected by EMPD than men, especially in Western countries.

large series of Asian men with EMPD showed 8% of men with accompanying malignancies.[82] Even primary EMPD can invade and metastasize, although this is usually an indolent disease. Invasion, nodules within the plaque, and lymph node involvement are, not surprisingly, poor prognostic signs. Patients with underlying carcinomas have a much poorer prognosis.

## Diagnosis

The diagnosis of Paget disease is made by clinical suspicion and confirmed by biopsy. The dermoscopic appearance of EMPD is not well characterized due to its uncommon occurrence, but most lesion show milky-red areas.[83] Most patients experience delayed diagnosis because the appearance mimics several benign skin diseases. A skin biopsy of Paget disease shows an epidermis with scattered large clear cells that exhibit nuclear atypia **(Fig. 5-98)**. These cells are often seen in hair follicles and sweat gland ducts. Often, there is an underlying chronic inflammatory infiltrate.

Paget disease closely resembles eczema, LSC, eczematized tinea, contact dermatitis, and rubbed or scratched psoriasis. It can also resemble lesions of squamous atypia such as HSIL and differentiated intraepithelial neoplasia, formerly called squamous cell carcinoma *in situ*, Bowen

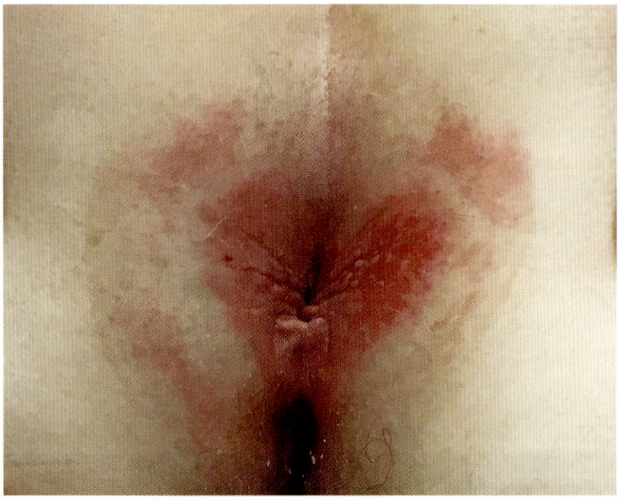

Fig. 5-95. Extramammary Paget disease can be confused with eczema, but the white islands of hyperkeratosis is a strong indication of this condition.

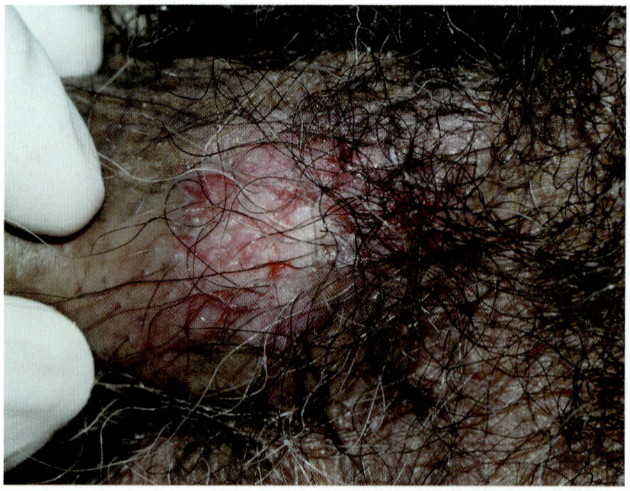

Fig. 5-97. This small plaque of EMPD on the proximal shaft of the penis is somewhat less characteristic, with more impressive diffuse hyperkeratosis suggestive of squamous cell carcinoma.

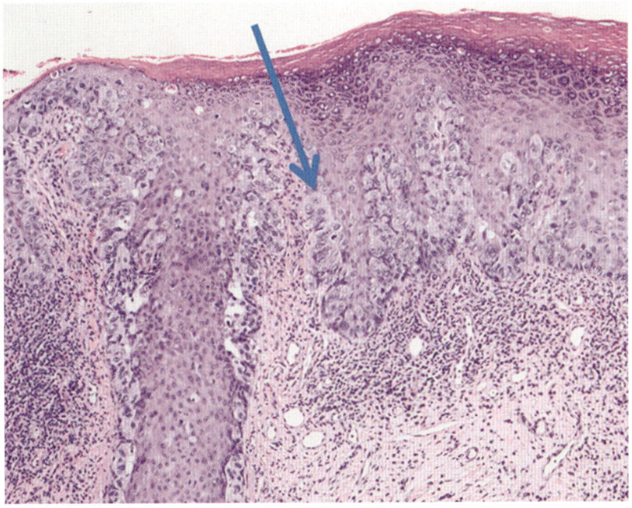

Fig. 5-98. The histology of EMPD is characteristic; large atypical cells with light pink cytoplasm and large nuclei contrast with normal cells (*arrow*). (Courtesy of Jason Reutter, MD.)

disease, Bowenoid papulosis, erythroplasia of Queyrat, vulvar intraepithelial neoplasia, etc. Pigmented Paget disease can mimic superficial spreading melanoma.

**EXTRAMAMMARY PAGET DISEASE Diagnosis**

- Morphology of red plaque with scale, erosion, or exudation and islands of white epithelium can occur on the dry, keratinized skin or modified mucous membranes.
- Confirmed on biopsy.

### Pathophysiology

Extramammary Paget disease is a malignancy whose cause is controversial. Primary disease appears to arise from the epidermis; this may be from cells of apocrine gland origin in the epidermis, from keratinocytes, or from Toker cells of mammarylike glands of the vulva. Secondary EMPD arises from cells that migrate from the underlying adenocarcinoma. There are no known precipitating causes for Paget disease other than the underlying adenocarcinoma of secondary Paget disease.

### Management

By default, as there are no large well-designed studies, surgery is the most widely accepted treatment of choice.[84,85] This allows not only for removal of the tumor but for evaluation of the entire lesion for dermal invasion; those patients with <1 mm of invasion rarely die of their disease or experience metastasis. Local recurrences are usual and expected for both invasive and *in situ* EMPD and require management with excision or topical therapy.

More recently, reports of Mohs micrographic surgery (MMS) suggest that this technique to be superior, with wide local excision showing a 2.5 times higher recurrence compared to MMS.[86] A recent case report has proposed that a removal technique evaluating both the peripheral and the mucosal borders by MMS may lower the recurrence rate further.[87]

For patients who are not surgical candidates or who refuse surgery, there is increasing evidence that topical imiquimod is useful,[84] and both imiquimod and radiation therapy are leading nonsurgical therapies.[88] Less useful options include photodynamic therapy, which showed a response rate of almost 60% in a recent review of the literature. This modality was most useful in combination with other therapies and for recurrent lesions, previously treated lesions, and selected invasive lesions.[89]

Extramammary Paget disease extending more than 1 mm into the dermis can rapidly progress and metastasize. The prognosis of disease associated with underlying adenocarcinomas is also dependent upon the state of this related malignancy. Patients should undergo screening evaluation for genitourinary carcinoma or a gastrointestinal malignancy because these can certainly cause death if they are not detected and treated adequately. Immunohistochemical investigations can help to differentiate between primary and secondary Paget disease.

**EXTRAMAMMARY PAGET DISEASE Management**

- Excision
- For those who are not surgical candidates or in combination with surgery
- Imiquimod topically
- Radiation therapy

## Squamous Cell Carcinoma *In Situ*/Squamous Intraepithelial Neoplasia/Squamous Intraepithelial Lesion (Primarily Discussed in Chapter 7)

There are two forms of anogenital squamous intraepithelial neoplasia, that occurring as a result of HPV infection and that occurring in association with lichen sclerosus or lichen planus. In the past, these were grouped together as intraepithelial neoplasia (vulvar intraepithelial neoplasia I, II, III; penile intraepithelial neoplasia I, II, III, etc., depending upon the severity of dysplasia). This terminology led to confusion regarding the malignant potential—or lack thereof.

The more common form of squamous intraepithelial lesion is that produced by oncogenic forms of HPV infection, and the new designation for this is HSIL. The more aggressive but less common form is now termed differentiated intraepithelial neoplasia, the proper name for full-thickness dysplasia of the epidermis generally related to lichen sclerosus or lichen planus and unassociated with HPV infection.

A third form of *in situ* squamous cell carcinoma that affects keratinized skin, not necessarily of the anogenital area and unassociated with either HPV or chronic lichen sclerosus or lichen planus, is Bowen disease. The cause is often unclear.

## High-Grade Squamous Intraepithelial Lesion

Although often asymptomatic, these HPV-induced skin lesions of HSIL can be pruritic or patients may describe irritation. Lesions are most often multiple small, skin-colored, brown, red, or white papules in younger patients at higher risk for this sexually transmitted disease. These sometimes coalesce into plaques, especially in immunosuppressed individuals who are at higher risk for an aggressive course (**Figs. 5-99 to 5-102**). "Warts" that are flat-topped and, in light-complexioned patients, hyperpigmented are especially suspicious for HSIL. Treatment is by excision or destruction, with careful evaluation of the cervix and rectal areas, which have a greater risk of rapid invasion and metastasis. Imiquimod is sometimes used.

Differentiated Vulvar, Penile, and Anal Intraepithelial Neoplasia III, VIN III, PIN III, AIN III (Squamous Cell Carcinoma *In Situ*, Erythroplasia of Queyrat).

Differentiated intraepithelial neoplasia has many different morphologic appearances, and one is red patches or plaques.

### Clinical Presentation

Differentiated vulvar intraepithelial neoplasia (dVIN), differentiated penile intraepithelial neoplasia (dPIN), and differentiated anal intraepithelial neoplasia (dAIN) are seen at an older age, following years of poorly controlled lichen sclerosus or, less often, lichen planus. This lesion is more often solitary. The morphology discussed in this chapter is red, usually well demarcated, and generally smooth surfaced (**Fig. 5-103**). Other appearances discussed in other chapters include hyperkeratotic, firm white papules and plaques, erosions, or even hyperpigmented lesions. The perianal area, perineum, glans penis (where this condition is called erythroplasia of Queyrat), and vulva are common areas.

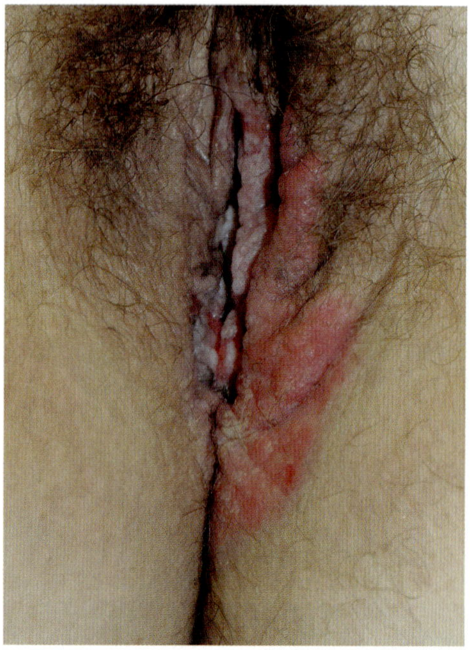

Fig. 5-99. This red, verrucous plaque of the left labium majus and surrounding skin is HPV-induced high-grade squamous intraepithelial lesion or squamous cell carcinoma.

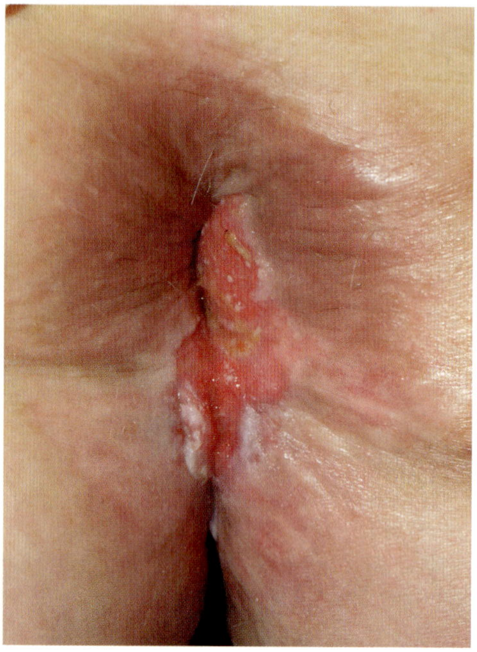

Fig. 5-100. HSIL is common on perianal skin of both men and women.

### Diagnosis

Differentiated intraepithelial neoplasia is diagnosed on clinical suspicion and is confirmed by skin biopsy. A skin

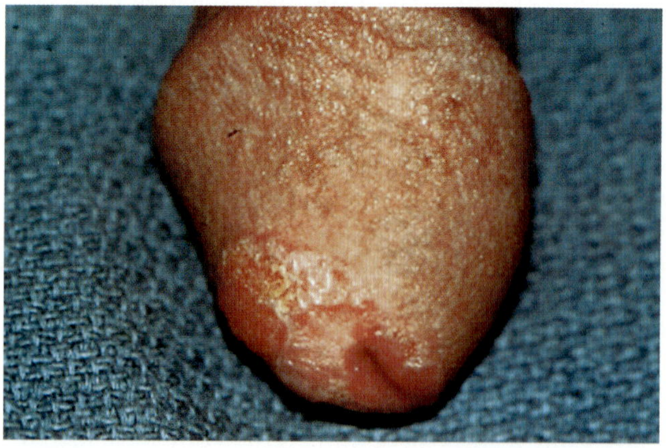

Fig. 5-101. This red plaque on the glans represents HSIL or HPV-induced squamous cell carcinoma *in situ*. (Courtesy of Dr. Chris Tiegland.)

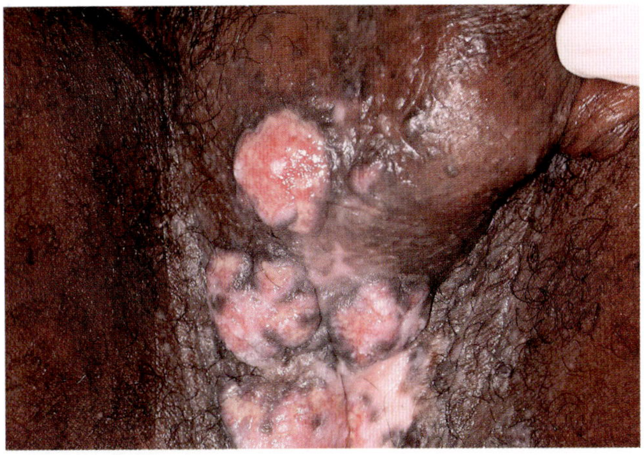

Fig. 5-102. This immunosuppressed patient with genital warts experienced progression to red verrucous areas of HSIL, now with areas of squamous cell carcinoma.

biopsy shows full-thickness dysplasia of the epithelium, but there is no invasion of these cells through the basement membrane into the dermis, as occurs in invasive squamous cell carcinoma.

This condition can be difficult to distinguish from psoriasis, lichen planus, candidiasis, especially on the glans penis.

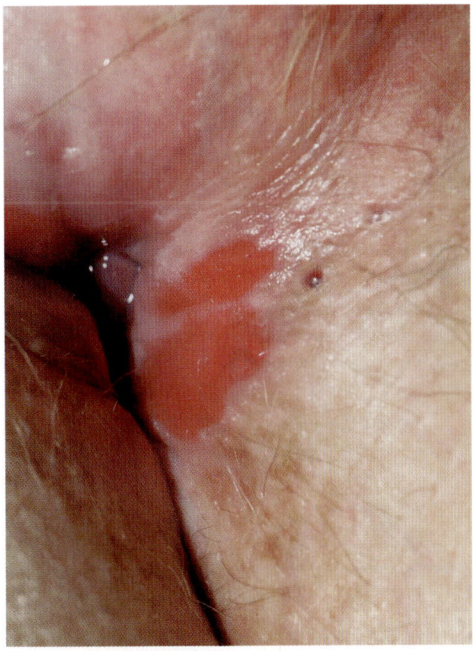

Fig. 5-103. Differentiated intraepithelial neoplasia is much more common in women, because this is related to lichen sclerosus as in this patient, or lichen planus, both diseases that occur more often in women, and primarily only in uncircumcised men. This red patch of dVIN could be plasma cell vulvitis or lichen planus, but its association with the obvious lichen sclerosus, and her history of a vulvectomy for past squamous cell carcinoma strongly suggests the correct diagnosis.

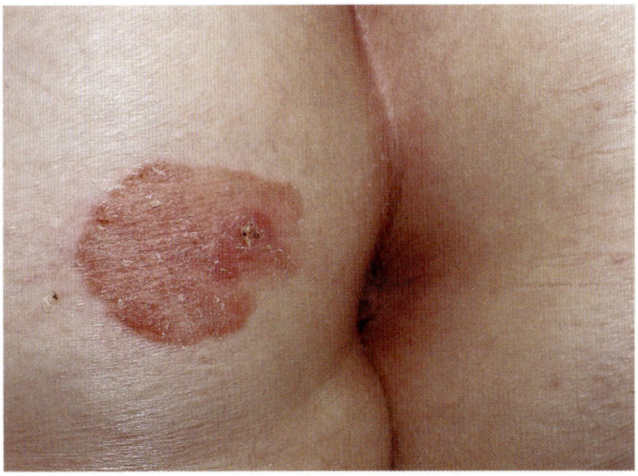

Fig. 5-104. This well-demarcated, red scaling plaque of Bowen disease (SCC *in situ* of unknown cause) on keratinized skin can resemble a solitary plaque of psoriasis or lichen planus and appears more like an inflammatory condition than tumor.

### Pathophysiology

Differentiated intraepithelial neoplasia occur as a result of some chronic dermatoses, most notably lichen sclerosus and lichen planus, following years of poor control.

### Management

Differentiated intraepithelial neoplasia is treated by surgical excision, which confers the advantage of a histologic evaluation for invasion of the entire area, or ablation. More recently, topical imiquimod cream has shown in small series to sometimes clear this condition and is reasonable in poor surgical candidates.

### Bowen Disease

Patients with squamous cell carcinoma *in situ* of keratinized skin unassociated with HPV infection or underlying lichen sclerosus or lichen planus have the morphologic type called Bowen disease. Very uncommon on anogenital skin, these lesions are nearly always produced not only by chronic sun exposure but also by arsenic exposure, such as found in some well water. Often, the cause is not known. These lesions are generally asymptomatic and indolent. Clinically, Bowen disease exhibits a well-demarcated, usually solitary red, and scaling plaque on the keratinized skin surface **(Fig. 5-104)**. Treatment is by excision or destruction.

## REFERENCES

1. Lynch PJ, Moyal-Barracco M, Bogliatto F, et al. 2006 ISSVD classification of vulvar dermatoses: pathologic subsets and their clinical correlates. *J Reprod Med.* 2007;52:3-9.
2. Barbarot S, Auziere S, Gadkari A, et al. Epidemiology of atopic dermatitis in adults: results from an international survey. *Allergy.* 2018;73(6):1284-1293. doi:10.1111/all.13401

3. Warshaw EM, Kimyon RS, Silverberg JI, et al. Evaluation of patch test findings in patients with anogenital dermatitis. *JAMA Dermatol.* 2020;156(1):85-91. doi:10.1001/jamadermatol.2019.3844
4. Rajalakshmi R, Devinder MT, Telanseri JJ, Amiya KN. Lichen simplex chronicus of anogenital region: a clinico-etiological study. *Indian J Dermatol Venereol Leprol.* 2011;77:28-36.
5. Kaaz K, Szepietowski JC, Matusiak Ł. Influence of itch and pain on sleep quality in atopic dermatitis and psoriasis. *Acta Derm Venereol.* 2019;99(2):175-180. doi:10.2340/00015555-3065
6. Treister AD, Stefek H, Grimaldi D, et al. Sleep and limb movement characteristics of children with atopic dermatitis coincidentally undergoing clinical polysomnography. *J Clin Sleep Med.* 2019;15(8):1107-1113. doi:10.5664/jcsm.7800
7. Lynch PJ. Lichen simplex chronicus (atopic/neurodermatitis) of the anogenital region. *Dermatol Ther.* 2004;17:8-19.
8. Errichetti E. Dermoscopy of inflammatory dermatoses (inflammoscopy): an up-to-date overview. *Dermatol Pract Concept.* 2019;9:169-180. doi:10.5826/dpc.0903a01
9. Grobe W, Bieber T, Novak N. Pathophysiology of atopic dermatitis. *J Dtsch Dermatol Ges.* 2019;17(4):433-440. doi:10.1111/ddg.13819
10. McKenzie AN. Type-2 innate lymphoid cells in asthma and allergy. *Ann Am Thorac Soc.* 2014;11(Suppl 5):S263-S270.
11. Kouris A, Christodoulou C, Efstathiou V, et al. Comparative study of quality of life and obsessive-compulsive tendencies in patients with chronic hand eczema and lichen simplex chronicus. *Dermatitis.* 2016;27(3):127-130. doi:10.1097/DER.0000000000000180
12. Cheng BT, Silverberg JI. Depression and psychological distress in US adults with atopic dermatitis. *Ann Allergy Asthma Immunol.* 2019;123(2):179-185. doi:10.1016/j.anai.2019.06.002
13. Fiorillo L, Marcoux D, Ramien M. Contemporary role of topical calcineurin inhibitors: a pediatric dermatology perspective. *J Cutan Med Surg.* 2019;23(4_suppl):11S-18S. doi:10.1177/1203475419857975
14. Deleuran M, Thaçi D, Beck LA, de Bruin-Weller M, et al. Dupilumab shows long-term safety and efficacy in patients with moderate to severe atopic dermatitis enrolled in a phase 3 open-label extension study. *J Am Acad Dermatol.* 2020;82(2):377-388. doi:10.1016/j.jaad.2019.07.074
15. Seegräber M, Srour J, Walter A, Knop M, Wollenberg A. Dupilumab for treatment of atopic dermatitis. *Expert Rev Clin Pharmacol.* 2018;11(5):467-474. doi:10.1080/17512433.2018.1449642
16. Ratchataswan T, Banzon TM, Thyssen JP, Weidinger S, Guttman-Yassky E, Phipatanakul W. Biologics for treatment of atopic dermatitis: current status and future prospect. *J Allergy Clin Immunol Pract.* 2021;9:1053-1065.
17. Kouwenhoven TA, van de Kerkhof PCM, Kamsteeg M. Use of oral antidepressants in patients with chronic pruritus: a systematic review. *J Am Acad Dermatol.* 2017;77(6):1068-1073.e7. doi:10.1016/j.jaad.2017.08.025
18. Farmer WS, Marathe KS. Atopic dermatitis: managing the itch. *Adv Exp Med Biol.* 2017;1027:161-177. doi:10.1007/978-3-319-64804-0_13
19. Cheng BT, Fishbein AB, Silverberg JI. Mental health symptoms and functional impairment in children with atopic dermatitis. *Dermatitis.* 2021;32(5):353-361.
20. Corazza M, Virgili A, Toni G, et al. Pictorial representation of illness and self-measure to assess the perceived burden in patients with chronic inflammatory vulvar diseases: an observational study. *J Eur Acad Dermatol Venereol.* 2020;34(11):2645-2651. doi:10.1111/jdv.16637
21. Misery L, Taïeb C, Schollhammer M, Bertolus S, et al. Psychological consequences of the most common dermatoses: data from the Objectifs Peau study. *Acta Derm Venereol.* 2020;100(13):adv00175. doi:10.2340/00015555-3531
22. Foley CC, White S, Merry S, Nolan U, et al. Understanding the role of cutaneous allergy testing in anogenital dermatoses: a retrospective evaluation of contact sensitization in anogenital dermatoses. *Int J Dermatol.* 2019;58(7):806-810. doi:10.1111/ijd.14360
23. Cheng HS, Fernández-Peñas P. Allergic contact dermatitis of the anogenital region in men and women. *J Low Genit Tract Dis.* 2020;24(2):221-224. doi:10.1097/LGT.0000000000000516
24. Gilissen L, Schollaert I, Huygens S, Goossens A. Iatrogenic allergic contact dermatitis in the (peri)anal and genital area. *Contact Dermatitis.* 2021;84(6):431-438. doi:10.1111/cod.13764
25. Owen JL, Vakharia PP, Silverberg JI. The role and diagnosis of allergic contact dermatitis in patients with atopic dermatitis. *Am J Clin Dermatol.* 2018;19(3):293-302. doi:10.1007/s40257-017-0340-7
26. Brites GS, Ferreira I, Sebastião AI, et al. Allergic contact dermatitis: from pathophysiology to development of new preventive strategies. *Pharmacol Res.* 2020;162:105282. doi:10.1016/j.phrs.2020.105282
27. Caminati M, Giorgis V, Palterer B, Racca F, Salvottini C, Rossi O. Allergy and sexual behaviours: an update. *Clin Rev Allergy Immunol.* 2019;56(3):269-277. doi:10.1007/s12016-017-8618-3
28. Everink IHJ, Kottner J, van Haastregt JCM, Halfens R, Schols JMGA. Skin areas, clinical severity, duration and risk factors of intertrigo: a secondary data analysis. *J Tissue Viability.* 2021;30(1):102-107. doi:10.1016/j.jtv.2020.12.005
29. Beck KR, Telisman L, van Koppen CJ, Thompson GR III, Odermatt A. Molecular mechanisms of posaconazole- and itraconazole-induced pseudohyperaldosteronism and assessment of other systemically used azole antifungals. *J Steroid Biochem Mol Biol.* 2020;199:105605. doi:10.1016/j.jsbmb.2020.105605
30. Borda LJ, Perper M, Keri JE. Treatment of seborrheic dermatitis: a comprehensive review. *J Dermatolog Treat.* 2019;30(2):158-169. doi:10.1080/09546634.2018.1473554
31. Mease PJ, Gladman DD, Papp KA, et al. Prevalence of rheumatologist-diagnosed psoriatic arthritis in patients with psoriasis in European/North American dermatology clinics. *J Am Acad Dermatol.* 2013;69(5):729-735.
32. Eberz B, Berghold A, Regauer S. High prevalence of concomitant anogenital lichen sclerosus and extragenital psoriasis in adult women. *Obstet Gynecol.* 2008;111(5):1143-1147. doi:10.1097/AOG.0b013e31816fdcdf
33. Susan Simpkin S, Oakley A. Clinical review of 202 patients with vulval lichen sclerosus: a possible association with psoriasis. *Australas J Dermatol.* 2007;48(1):28-31. doi:10.1111/j.1440-0960.2007.00322.x
34. Lin I-C, Heck JE, Chen L, Feldman SR. Psoriasis severity and cardiometabolic risk factors in a representative US National Study. *Am J Clin Dermatol.* 2021;22(5):719-730. doi:10.1007/s40257-021-00600-z
35. Takeshita J, Grewal S, Langan SM, et al. Psoriasis and comorbid diseases Part I. Epidemiology. *J Am Acad Dermatol.* 2017;76:377-390. doi:10.1016/j.jaad.2016.07.064
36. Armstrong AW, Guerin A, Sundaram M, et al. Psoriasis and risk of diabetes-associated microvascular and macrovascular complications. *J Am Acad Dermatol.* 2015;72:968-977.e2.
37. Abuabara K, Azfar RS, Shin DB, et al. Cause-specific mortality in patients with severe psoriasis: a population-based cohort study in the U.K. *Br J Dermatol.* 2010;163:586-592.

38. Sondermann W, Fiege O, Körber A, Scherbaum N. Psychological burden of psoriatic patients in a German university hospital dermatology department. *J Dermatol.* 2021;48(6):794-806. doi:10.1111/1346-8138.15721
39. Micali G, Verzì AE, Giuffrida G, et al. Inverse psoriasis: from diagnosis to current treatment options. *Clin Cosmet Investig Dermatol.* 2019;12:953-959.
40. Reynolds KA, Pithadia DJ, Lee EB, Wu JJ. Treatments for inverse psoriasis: a systematic review. *J Dermatolog Treat.* 2020;31(8):786-793. doi:10.1080/09546634.2019.1620912
41. Egeberg A, Skov L, Joshi AA, et al. The relationship between duration of psoriasis, vascular inflammation, and cardiovascular events. *J Am Acad Dermatol.* 2017;77:650-656.
42. da Silva N, Augustin M, Langenbruch A, et al. Disease burden and treatment needs of patients with psoriasis in sexually-sensitive and visible body areas: results from a large-scale survey in routine care. *Eur J Dermatol.* 2020;30:267-278.
43. Lukmanji A, Basmadjian RB, Vallerand IA, Patten SB, Tang KL. Risk of depression in patients with psoriatic disease: a systematic review and meta-analysis. *J Cutan Med Surg.* 2021;25(3):257-270. doi:10.1177/1203475420977477
44. Bhat YJ, Keen A, Hassan I, Latif I, Bashir S. Can dermoscopy serve as a diagnostic tool in dermatophytosis? A pilot study. *Indian Dermatol Online J.* 2019;10(5):530-535. doi:10.4103/idoj.IDOJ_423_18
45. Sonthalia S, Ankad BS, Goldust M, Jha AK. Dermoscopy—a simple and rapid in vivo diagnostic technique for tinea incognito. *An Bras Dermatol.* 2019;94:612-614. doi:10.1016/j.abd.2019.09.017
46. Gupta AK, Renaud HJ, Quinlan EM, Shear NH, Piguet V. The growing problem of antifungal resistance in onychomycosis and other superficial mycoses. *Am J Clin Dermatol.* 2021;22(2):149-157. doi:10.1007/s40257-020-00580-6
47. Gaurav V, Bhattacharya SN, Sharma N, et al. Terbinafine resistance in dermatophytes: time to revisit alternate antifungal therapy. *Mycol Med.* 2020;31(1):101087. doi:10.1016/j.mycmed.2020.101087
48. van Zuuren EJ, Fedorowicz Z, El-Gohary M. Evidence-based topical treatments for tinea cruris and tinea corporis: a summary of a Cochrane systematic review. *Br J Dermatol.* 2015;172:616-641.
49. Avci O, Tanyildizi T, Kusku E. A comparison between the effectiveness of erythromycin, single-dose clarithromycin and topical fusidic acid in the treatment of erythrasma. *J Dermatolog Treat.* 2013;24:70-74.
50. Greywal T, Cohen PR. Erythrasma: a report of nine men successfully managed with mupirocin 2% ointment monotherapy. *Dermatol Online J.* 2017;23:13030. https://www.ncbi.nlm.nih.gov/pubmed/28537862
51. Errichetti E, Lallas A, Di Stefani A, et al. Accuracy of dermoscopy in distinguishing erythroplasia of Queyrat from common forms of chronic balanitis: results from a multicentric observational study. *J Eur Acad Dermatol Venereol.* 2019;33(5):966-972.
52. Liegeon AL, Berville S, Wendling-Héraud J, Micheline Moyal-Barracco M. Group A streptococcal vulvitis in adult women: clinical features and association with psoriasis. *J Low Genit Tract Dis.* 2019;23(4):287-289. doi:10.1097/LGT.0000000000000492
53. Serban ED. Perianal infectious dermatitis: an underdiagnosed, unremitting and stubborn condition. *World J Clin Pediatr.* 2018;7:89-104. doi:10.5409/wjcp.v7.i4.89
54. Heath C, Desai N, Silverberg NB. Recent microbiological shifts in perianal bacterial dermatitis: *Staphylococcus aureus* predominance. *Pediatr Dermatol.* 2009;26:696-700.
55. Olson D, Edmonson MB. Outcomes in children treated for perineal group A beta-hemolytic streptococcal dermatitis. *Pediatr Infect Dis J.* 2011;30:933-936.
56. Makhecha M, Singh T, Khatib Y. Dermoscopy differentiates guttate psoriasis from a mimicker—pityriasis rosea. *Dermatol Pract Concept.* 2021;11:e2021138. doi:10.5826/dpc.1101a138
57. Drago F, Ciccarese G, Rebora A, Parodi A. Human herpesvirus-6, -7, and Epstein-Barr virus reactivation in pityriasis rosea during COVID-19. *J Med Virol.* 2021;93:1850-1851. doi:10.1002/jmv.26549
58. Wang CJ, Worswick S. Cutaneous manifestations of COVID-19. *Dermatol Online J.* 2021;27:13030/qt2m54r7nv.
59. Sonthalia S, Kumar A, Zawar V. Double-blind randomized placebo-controlled trial to evaluate the efficacy and safety of short-course low-dose oral prednisolone in pityriasis rosea. *J Dermatolog Treat.* 2018;29:617-622. doi:10.1080/09546634.2018.1430302
60. Rebora A, Ciccarese G, Herzum A, Parodi A, Drago F. Pityriasis rosea and other infectious eruptions during pregnancy: possible life-threatening health conditions for the fetus. *Clin Dermatol.* 2020;38:105-112. doi:10.1016/j.clindermatol.2019.10.020
61. Gupta AK, Lane D, Paquet M. Systematic review of systemic treatments for tinea versicolor and evidence-based dosing regimen recommendations. *J Cutan Med Surg.* 2014;18:79-90.
62. Shi TW, Ren XK, Yu HX, Tang YB. Roles of adapalene in the treatment of pityriasis versicolor. *Dermatology.* 2012;224(2):184-188.
63. Delaleu J, Cavelier-Balloy B, Bagot M, Fouéré S, Dauendorffer JN. Zoon's plasma cell balanitis associated with male genital lichen sclerosus. *JAAD Case Rep.* 2020;6:670-672. doi:10.1016/j.jdcr.2020.05.018
64. Errichetti E, Stinco G. Dermoscopy in general dermatology: a practical overview. *Dermatol Ther (Heidelb).* 2016;6:471-507. doi:10.1007/s13555-016-0141-6
65. Kumar B, Narang T, Dass Radotra B, Gupta S. Plasma cell balanitis: clinicopathologic study of 112 cases and treatment modalities. *J Cutan Med Surg.* 2006;10(1):11-15.
66. Virgili A, Borghi A, Minghetti S, Corazza M. Comparative study on topical immunomodulatory and anti-inflammatory treatments for plasma cellvulvitis: long-term efficacy and safety. *J Eur Acad Dermatol Venereol.* 2015;29(3):507-514.
67. Wollina U. Ablative erbium:YAG laser treatment of idiopathic chronic inflammatory non-cicatricial balanoposthitis (Zoon's disease)—a series of 20 patients with long-term outcome. *J Cosmet Laser Ther.* 2010;12(3):120-123.
68. Calzavara-Pinton PG, Rossi MT, Aronson E, Sala R; Italian Group For Photodynamic Therapy. A retrospective analysis of real-life practice of off-label photodynamic therapy using methyl aminolevulinate (MAL-PDT) in 20 Italian dermatology departments. Part 1: inflammatory and aesthetic indications. *Photochem Photobiol Sci.* 2013;12(1):148-157.
69. Pinto-Almeida T, Vilaça S, Amorim I, Costa V, Alves R, Selores M. Complete resolution of Zoon balanitis with photodynamic therapy—a new therapeutic option? *Eur J Dermatol.* 2012;22(4):540-541.
70. Retamar RA, Kien MC, Chouela EN. Zoon's balanitis: presentation of 15 patients, five treated with a carbon dioxide laser. *Int J Dermatol.* 2003;42:305-307.

71. Balato N, Scalvenzi M, La Bella S, Di Costanzo L. Zoon's balanitis: benign or premalignant lesion? *Case Rep Dermatol.* 2009;1:7-10. doi:10.1159/000210440
72. Starritt E, Lee S. Erythroplasia of Queyrat of the glans penis on a background of Zoon's plasma cell balanitis. *Australas J Dermatol.* 2008;49(2):103-105.
73. Verma SB, Wollina U, Das A. A curious observation of passive transfer of steroid antifungal combination creams to the scrotum in patients of tinea cruris—is this forme fruste of red scrotum syndrome? *Dermatol Ther.* 2020;33:e14212. doi:10.1111/dth.14212
74. Khalil S, Kurban M, Abbas O. Red scrotum syndrome: an update on clinicopathologic features, pathogenesis, diagnosis, and management. *J Am Acad Dermatol.* 2020;S0190-9622(20)30988-9. doi:10.1016/j.jaad.2020.05.113
75. Miller J, Leicht S. Pregabalin in the treatment of red scrotum syndrome: a report of two cases. *Dermatol Ther.* 2016;29:244-248. doi: 10.1111/dth.12354
76. Abbas O, Kibbi AG, Chedraoui A, Ghosn S. Red scrotum syndrome: successful treatment with oral doxycycline. *J Dermatolog Treat.* 2008;19:1-2. doi:10.1080/09546630802033858
77. Cardenas-de la Garza JA, Villarreal-Villarreal CD, Cuellar-Barboza A, et al. Red scrotum syndrome treatment with pregabalin: a case series. *Ann Dermatol.* 2019;31(3):320-324. doi:10.5021/ad.2019.31.3.320
78. Hajar T, Leshem YA, Hanifin JM, et al.; the National Eczema Association Task Force. A systematic review of topical corticosteroid withdrawal ("steroid addiction") in patients with atopic dermatitis and other dermatoses. *J Am Acad Dermatol.* 2015;72(3):541-549.e2.
79. Herrel LA, Weiss AD, Goodman M, et al. Extramammary Paget's disease in males: survival outcomes in 495 patients. *Ann Surg Oncol.* 2015;22(5):1625-1630.
80. Kilts TP, Long B, Glasgow AE, et al. Invasive vulvar extramammary Paget's disease in the United States. *Gynecol Oncol.* 2020;157(3):649-655. doi:10.1016/j.ygyno.2020.03.018
81. Fanning J, Lambert HC, Hale TM, et al. Paget's disease of the vulva: prevalence of associated vulvar adenocarcinoma, invasive Paget's disease, and recurrence after surgical excision. *Am J Obstet Gynecol.* 1999;180(1 Pt 1):24-27.
82. Kang Z, Zhang Q, Zhang Q, et al. Clinical and pathological characteristics of extramammary Paget's disease: report of 246 Chinese male patients. *Int J Clin Exp Pathol.* 2015;8(10):13233-13240.
83. Mun JH, Park SM, Kim GW, et al. Clinical and dermoscopic characteristics of extramammary Paget's disease: a study of 35 cases. *Br J Dermatol.* 2016;174:1104-1107. 10.1111/bjd.14300
84. Edey KA, Allan E, Murdoch JB, Cooper S, Bryant A. Interventions for the treatment of Paget's disease of the vulva. *Cochrane Database Syst Rev.* 2019;6(6):CD009245. doi:10.1002/14651858.CD009245.pub3
85. Edey KA, Allan E, Murdoch JB, Cooper S, Bryant A. Interventions for the treatment of Paget's disease of the vulva. *Cochrane Database Syst Rev.* 2013;(10):CD009245. doi:10.1002/14651858.CD009245.pub2
86. Long B, Schmitt AR, Weaver AL. A matter of margins: surgical and pathologic risk factors for recurrence in extramammary Paget's disease. *Gynecol Oncol.* 2017;147(2):358-363.
87. Chang MS, Mulvaney PM, Danesh MJ, Feltmate CM, Schmults CD. Modified peripheral and central Mohs micrographic surgery for improved margin control in extramammary Paget disease. *JAAD Case Rep.* 2020;7:71-73. doi:10.1016/j.jdcr.2020.11.002
88. Snast N, Sharon E, Ran Kaftory R, et al. Nonsurgical treatments for extramammary Paget disease: a systematic review and meta-analysis. *Dermatology.* 2020;236(6):493-499. doi:10.1159/000506832
89. Shim PJ, Zeitouni NC. Photodynamic therapy for extramammary Paget's disease: a systematic review of the literature. *Photodiagnosis Photodyn Ther.* 2020;31:101911. doi:10.1016/j.pdpdt.2020.101911

## SUGGESTED READINGS

Atzmony L, Reiter O, Hodak E, Gdalevich M, Mimouni D. Treatments for cutaneous lichen planus: a systematic review and meta-analysis. *Am J Clin Dermatol.* 2016;17(1):11-22. doi:10.1007/s40257-015-0160-6

Cartron AM, Nguyen TH, Roh YS, Kwatra MM, Kwatra SG. Janus kinase inhibitors for atopic dermatitis: a promising treatment modality. *Clin Exp Dermatol.* 2021;46(5):820-824. doi:10.1111/ced.14567

Forouzan P, Cohen PR. Erythrasma revisited: diagnosis, differential diagnoses, and comprehensive review of treatment. *Cureus.* 2020;12(9):e10733. doi:10.7759/cureus.10733

Morris CR, Hurst EA. Extramammary Paget disease: a review of the literature—Part I: History, epidemiology, pathogenesis, presentation, histopathology, and diagnostic work-up. *Dermatol Surg.* 2020;46:151-158. doi:10.1097/DSS.0000000000002064

Morris CR, Hurst EA. Extramammary Paget's disease: a review of the literature Part II: treatment and prognosis. *Dermatol Surg.* 2020;46:305-311. doi:10.1097/DSS.0000000000002240

Sahi FM, Masood A, Danawar NA, Mekaiel A, Malik BH. Association between psoriasis and depression: a traditional review. *Cureus.* 2020;12(8):e9708. doi:10.7759/cureus.9708

Sbidian E, Chaimani A, Garcia-Doval I, et al. Systemic pharmacological treatments for chronic plaque psoriasis: a network meta-analysis. *Cochrane Database Syst Rev.* 2017;12(12):CD011535. doi:10.1002/14651858.CD011535.pub2

Tier HL, Balogh EA, Bashyam AM, et al. Tolerability of and adherence to topical treatments in atopic dermatitis: a narrative review. *Dermatol Ther (Heidelb).* 2021;11(2):415-431. doi:10.1007/s13555-021-00500-4

Zhou S, Qi F, Gong Y, Zhang J, Zhu B. Biological therapies for atopic dermatitis: a systematic review. *Dermatology.* 2021;237(4):542-552. doi:10.1159/000514535

# Red Disorders: Red Papules and Nodules

# 6

PETER J. LYNCH

Anogenital disorders that present as red papules or nodules are most often either neoplasms or inflammatory lesions. *Vascular* neoplasms tend to present as bright red, dusky red, or violaceous papules and nodules with sharply demarcated borders. Red, *nonvascular* neoplasms are also sharply marginated but tend to be lighter red in color. Inflammatory papules and nodules are most often medium to dark red toward the center and tend to fade to light red or pink peripherally. They usually are less sharply marginated than red neoplasms. Most of the lesions considered in this chapter lack scale and therefore are smooth surfaced both visually and palpably. Many skin-colored papules and nodules may appear pink or red at times because of secondary inflammation or increased vascularity. This is particularly notable in patients who have a light complexion. Therefore, when encountering pink or red papules or nodules, the clinician may also need to consider the skin-colored disorders from Section A, Chapter 7. Note that some red disorders may present with a mixture of papules and nodules. In such instances, try to determine whether either papules (Section A) or nodules (Section B) represent the dominant lesions. However, at times, a mix of papules and nodules is present, and for this reason, disorders in both sections may have to be considered.

## SECTION A: RED PAPULES

### Folliculitis

Bacterial, candidal, and dermatophyte folliculitis can present as small red papules **(Figs. 6-1 and 6-2)**. The lesions are generally multiple and are often clustered. Many times a few of these lesions will have a white or yellow-white pustule at the summit. This distinguishing feature, followed by appropriate KOH preparation and/or culture from the pustule, allows for establishment of the correct diagnosis. The primary discussion of folliculitis can be found in Chapter 10.

### Keratosis Pilaris

#### Clinical Presentation

Keratosis pilaris (KP) is a noninfectious form of folliculitis. It has been extensively reviewed recently, and much of the information that follows is based on that review.[1] KP is a very common condition often occurring in an autosomal dominant pattern. There is a slight male predominance. It is more common in children and adolescents where the prevalence may be as high as 30%. KP spontaneously resolves through the teen years, and with one exception, it is not often encountered after the fourth or fifth decade. The exception revolves around what we believe is its common presence on the buttocks in adult women where it is all too often misdiagnosed as bacterial folliculitis.

The clinical appearance of KP is that of minute (1-2 mm) closely set, clustered papules. Some, but not all, of the papules will have a small hair emerging from the summit of the papule, and it not uncommon to find a few white-summited papules intermingled with the more typical completely red papules (see the following paragraph). All of the lesions are approximately the same size, and they are spaced equidistant from one another **(Figs. 6-3 and 6-4)**. This lends a monomorphic appearance to the process and is a helpful diagnostic clue.

In those individuals with the least severe involvement, the papules may be skin-colored or pink, but in most patients, both the papules and a narrow halo around them are distinctly red. A few of the larger lesions may be capped by a firm, solid, white summit (pseudopustule) consisting of compacted keratin retained in the follicular orifice. If this solid white "ball" of keratin is scraped away, it sometimes contains a fine, rolled-up hair within it. The most commonly involved sites for KP are the upper, outer arms and thighs. The buttocks are also frequently involved, and in this location, it is often misdiagnosed as bacterial folliculitis. There is a sandpaperlike, slightly rough, feel when the fingertips are lightly passed over clustered lesions. KP is usually asymptomatic though, especially in atopic individuals, pruritus can be present.

#### Diagnosis

Keratosis pilaris is diagnosed on a clinical basis. The key features include (1) a large number of closely set homogeneous papules, (2) location on lateral, upper arms, thighs, and buttocks, (3) long duration with little or no change in clinical appearance, and (4) failure to respond to antibiotic therapy.

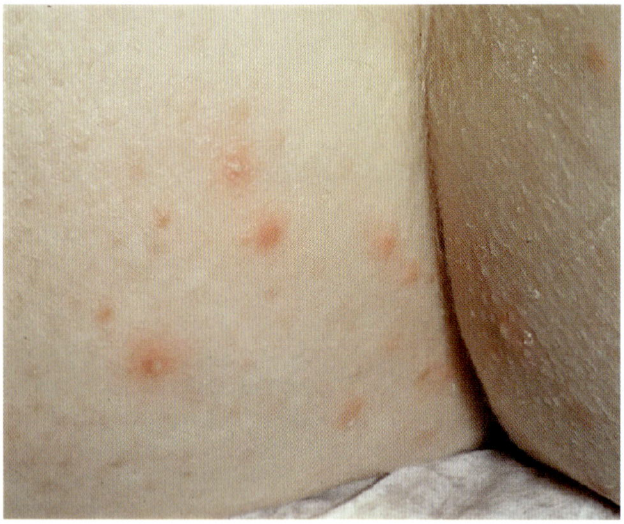

Fig. 6-1. These red papules represent a *Staphylococcal aureus* infection of the hair follicles, although the buttocks are a common location for irritant folliculitis as well. Although folliculitis is considered a pustular condition, most lesions are papules, since the pustule is often subtle and ruptures early.

**KERATOSIS PILARIS** — **Diagnosis**

- Clustered, small (1- to 2-mm) red papules
- White-capped, solid keratotic summit on a few scattered papules
- Hairs emerging from the summit of some papules
- Equidistant spacing of all the papules
- Location on the lateral arms and thighs and/or on the buttocks
- Rough, sandpaperlike feel on palpation
- Failure to respond to antibiotics

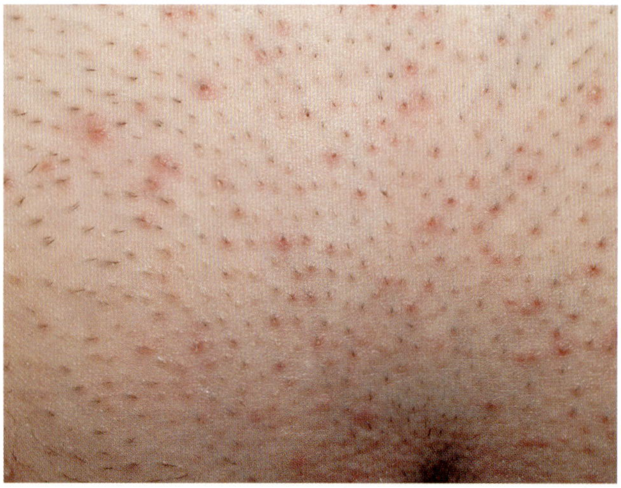

Fig. 6-2. Shaving is a common cause of irritant folliculitis, with erythema at the base of each shaved hair.

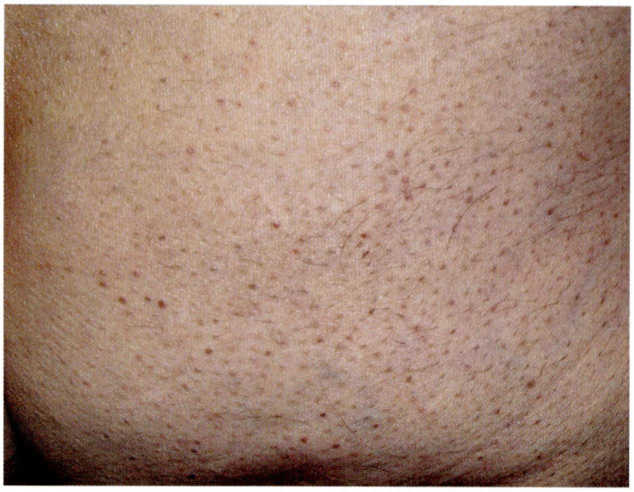

Fig. 6-3. Keratosis pilaris exhibits monomorphous, follicular papules with a keratotic plug that gives the skin a sandpapery texture; although sometimes skin-colored, many patients exhibit erythema as seen on the buttocks of this patient. This patient also had typical keratosis pilaris on the lateral, upper arms.

### Pathophysiology

Keratosis pilaris is caused by excess keratinization (keratin plugging) of the outermost portion of hair follicles. The cause of this accumulation of keratin is unknown, but it is likely related to an abnormality of keratinocyte differentiation since KP occurs primarily in those who have ichthyosis vulgaris or atopic background. These two conditions are almost always associated with keratinocyte differentiation abnormalities and are especially likely to possess mutations in the filaggrin gene. Histologically, perifollicular lymphohistiocytic inflammation surrounds these keratin plugged follicles.

### Management

No therapy is medically necessary. This happenstance is fortunate as no treatment is completely effective. Patients

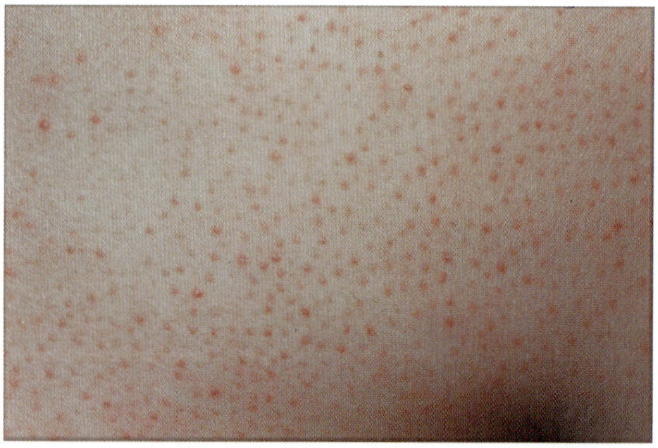

Fig. 6-4. Although keratosis pilaris sometimes appears inflamed, it is generally asymptomatic.

who are bothered by the appearance or by pruritus may periodically undertake a prolonged bathtub soak followed by the use of light abrasion with a loofah sponge or soft brush. Lubrication, especially with products containing humectants such as urea, lactic acid, or salicylic acid, improves the textural feel of the skin. Topical retinoids, while theoretically attractive as therapeutic agents, tend to increase the inflammation and thus are not routinely useful. In particularly symptomatic or severe cases, laser therapy may be considered.[2]

**KERATOSIS PILARIS** — **Management**

- 20-minute bathtub soak
- Light scrubbing with a soft brush or loofah
- Application of a moisturizer after the soak and scrub
- Cautious trial of topical retinoids

## Scabies

The primary discussion of scabies can be found in the section on Pediatric Issues in Chapter 15. Only a few summarizing points will be made here. Scabies generally occurs as a pink or red papular eruption. Characteristically a few linear vesicles or elongated edematous papules (mite burrows) will be present (**Fig. 6-5**). Dermoscopy can show these burrows with more clarity, and even occasionally show the mite itself. Typically, lesions develop in the digital web spaces, on the volar wrists, and on the elbows. However, the genitalia in males and the mammary area in adult females may be involved. It is an extremely common disorder in poor, underdeveloped countries where its prevalence is estimated at 150-200 million persons. Children are affected most often, but it certainly also occurs in infants and in sexually active adults. In Western countries today, it is most often encountered in the elderly who are housed in congregate living facilities. The most common treatment is with either topical permethrin 5% cream or oral ivermectin in a dose of 200 μg/kg. The nodular form of scabies is discussed with the nodular lesions in Section B of this chapter.

## Miscellaneous Bites and Infestations

The most common bites that occur in the anogenital area are due to chiggers. These "bites" are especially likely to occur at the waistband, in the inguinal folds, and/or on the shaft of the penis. An extensive review has recently been published.[3] Chiggers, also called harvest mites, are active during the warmer months when they colonize tall grasses and brush. The larval form of these mites latch onto exposed, nonclothing covered skin of those who contact this greenery. These mite larvae are extremely small, generally requiring magnification to be visualized. Dermoscopy can be useful for this. They then find and settle in folded areas or in spots where clothing tends to bind to the skin. They do not bite in the true sense of the word. Instead, they attach to the skin using their mouth parts, and their saliva liquefies the stratum corneum epidermal cells thus forming a "tube" through which they suck the nourishing fluid, which bathes the lower epidermal cells of the skin. This results in the development extremely pruritic, red, nonscaling, dome-shaped 0.5- to 1.0-cm papules (**Figs. 6-6 and 6-7**). Often a darker red dot, representing the feeding "tube," can be seen at the center of the papule. Clustering of multiple papules is usually present and is a distinguishing diagnostic feature for chigger bites.

The mites fall off of the host in 2-4 days, and the papules slowly resolve spontaneously. Oral antihistamines and topical steroids provide some symptomatic improvement of the itching. Prevention of chigger "bites" is the

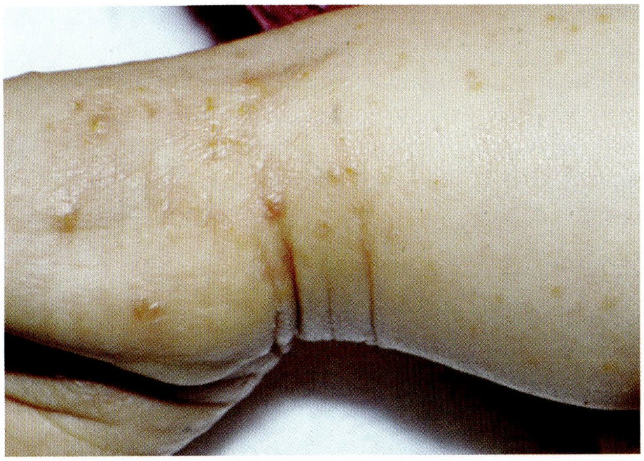

Fig. 6-5. Scabies most often occurs in skin folds as small oval papules, but sometimes red, excruciatingly pruritic red papules can occur. (Courtesy of Lynette J. Margesson.)

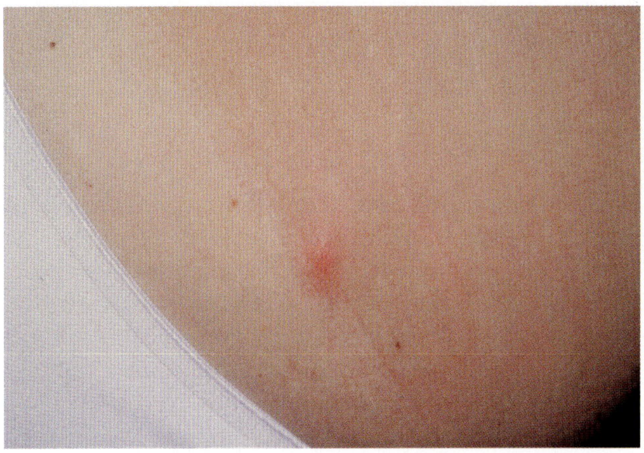

Fig. 6-6. This patient developed red, dome-shaped, nonscaling, pruritic papules around her panty line produced by chiggers after a hike. In general, these are concentrated at the panty line.

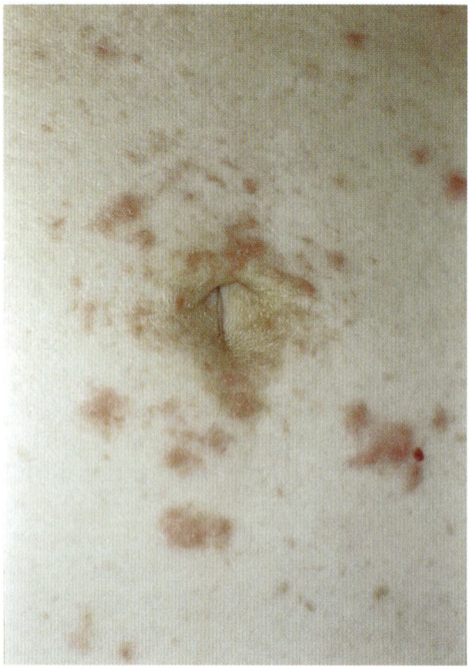

Fig. 6-7. This woman exhibits poorly demarcated pink, dome-shaped papules of insect bites on the mons and lower abdomen.

better part of therapy. This can be achieved through the use of standard insect repellents and the wearing of long sleeves and long pants.

Insect bites in the genital area, other than those due to chiggers, are otherwise uncommon because this area is usually protected by clothing. However, such bites do occur in campers and hikers who expose the genital area when urinating, defecating, or having intercourse alfresco. When these lesions do occur, they also appear as pruritic red papules. Usually only a few papules are present, and when multiple, there is much less likelihood of clustering than with chigger bites. While there is nothing that clinically identifies which insect is responsible for these bites, the likelihood that a given red papule is due to one or another type of insect can be strongly suggested by the presence of numerous eosinophils within the inflammatory infiltrate of a biopsy specimen.

## Cherry Angioma

Cherry angiomas (Campbell de Morgan spots) represent a benign neoplasm of clustered capillary blood vessels. They first appear in young adult life and thereafter slowly increase in number with age. These angiomas may be small macules at their inception but fairly quickly develop into sharply marginated dome-shaped papules that are bright red, dusky red, or even violaceous in color[4] **(Fig. 6-8)**. They vary in size from nearly flat, pinpoint lesions to 3- or 4-mm papules. The majority of light-skinned persons will have developed at least one by age 40, and the average adult may have 30 or more lesions. It is not that dark-skinned persons have fewer angiomas but rather that they are less easily visible against a darker background. A rare variant, eruptive cherry angiomas, involves the explosive development of 50 or more lesions over a very short period of time. Cherry angiomas are most commonly found on the trunk and proximal extremities but occasionally are also noted on the thighs, buttocks, pubis, and genitalia.[4]

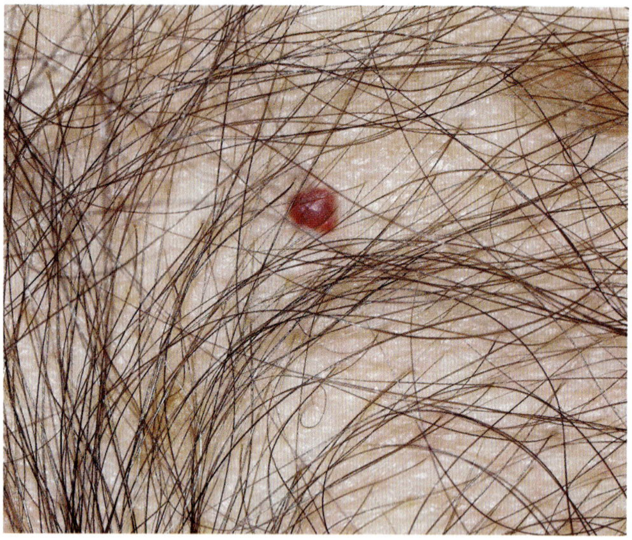

Fig. 6-8. Cherry angiomas are bright-red, well demarcated, and best seen in light complexioned individuals.

The cause of cherry angiomas is not known though the frequency of familial development suggests a genetic predisposition as does the high frequency of GNA, especially GNA14, gene mutations that occur.[5] A risk factor for the development of these angiomas is use of the alpha-adrenergic receptor blocker, tamsulosin.[4] Other possible risk factors include the presence of dyslipidemia, chronic immunosuppression, benign prostatic hypertrophy, and various malignancies. Use of the medication, clopidogrel, may reduce the likelihood of developing these angiomas.[4]

The diagnosis is made on a clinical basis. The differential diagnosis is that of angiokeratomas. Since both disorders are asymptomatic and benign, it is not always necessary to differentiate between these lesions. No treatment is necessary. Lesions that are troublesome to patients or those that bleed frequently with trauma may be excised or may be destroyed with electrosurgery, cryotherapy, or laser ablation.[6]

## Angiokeratoma

Angiokeratomas commonly occur on the genitalia and consist of clusters of ectatic, superficial cutaneous blood vessels. A recent major review has recently been published.[7] These benign papules are sometimes given the eponymous epithet of Fordyce but that name should not be confused with Fordyce spots referring to prominent sebaceous glands on the lips or genitalia. Angiokeratomas are sufficiently common to be considered as a normal variant rather than a disease. The prevalence is not known, but based on our experience, they develop in early adulthood in about 10% of men but considerably less frequently than that in women. In males, they appear as multiple 1- to 2-mm red, smooth-surfaced, dome-shaped papules occurring primarily on the scrotum and, rarely, on the penile shaft[7] (Fig. 6-9). Sometimes they are lined up as tiny ("beads on a string") outpouchings along a linear telangiectatic vessel (Fig. 6-10). Generally, 10-30 scrotal papules are present. In females, the lesions are found on the vulva, especially the labia majora, where they are fewer in number (often solitary), larger in size (3-8 mm), and darker in color (dusky red, violaceous, or blue) (Figs. 6-11 and 6-12). In both sexes, bleeding with minor trauma sometimes happens, but angiokeratomas are otherwise asymptomatic.

The diagnosis is made on a clinical basis. In men, the main differential diagnosis is cherry angiomas (Campbell de Morgan spots). Angiokeratomas found in the extremely rare, X-linked condition, angiokeratoma corporis diffusum (Anderson-Fabry disease), are individually similar in appearance, but in this life-threatening systemic disorder, they are much more numerous and occur in wider distribution pattern to include the lower trunk and upper thighs. In women, solitary, darker lesions may be confused with nevi or even melanoma, and for that reason, biopsy is usually necessary. Dermoscopy shows the vascular nature of these lesions when there is any question. Biopsy in men is not usually needed. Histologically, angiokeratomas reveal characteristic, clustered, dilated vessels in the upper dermis. The overlying epidermis is slightly

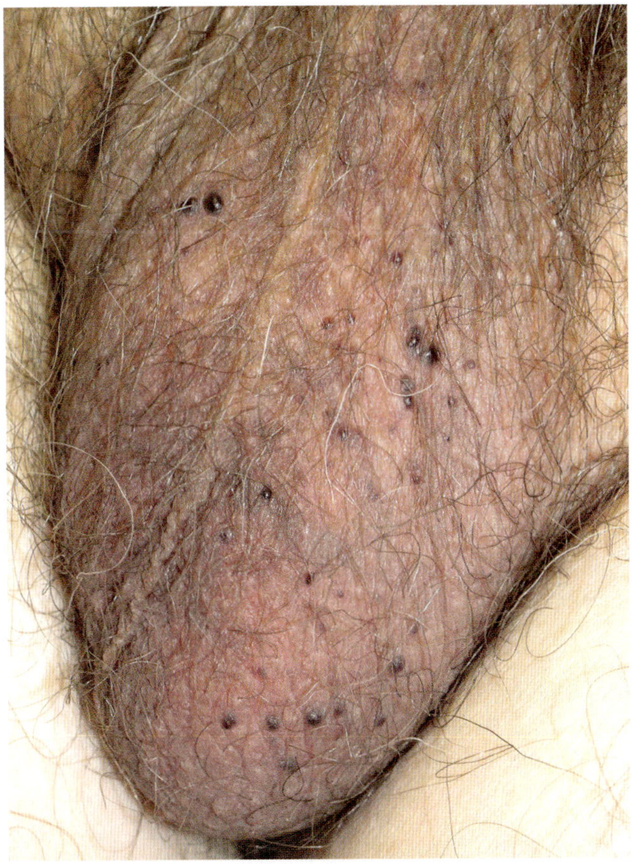

Fig. 6-9. Angiokeratomas of the scrotum are typically large in number, and generally dark purple.

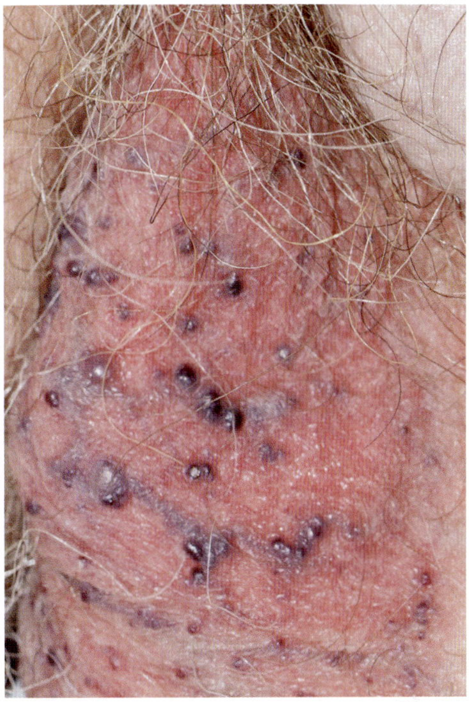

Fig. 6-10. On the scrotum, angiokeratomas sometimes align along veins resulting in this peculiar beaded pattern.

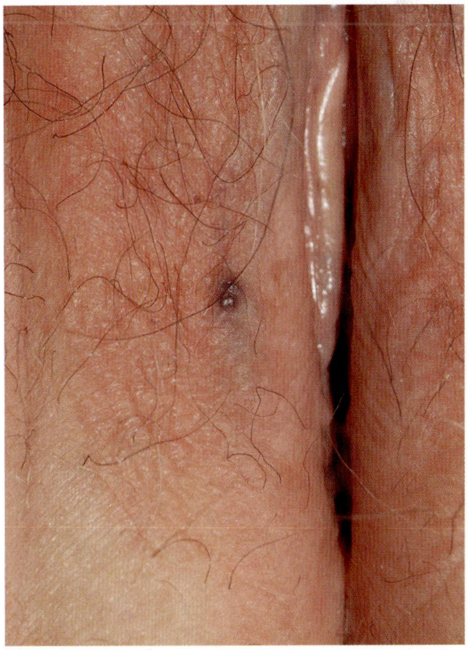

Fig. 6-11. Angiokeratomas of the vulva are more often fewer or even single in number.

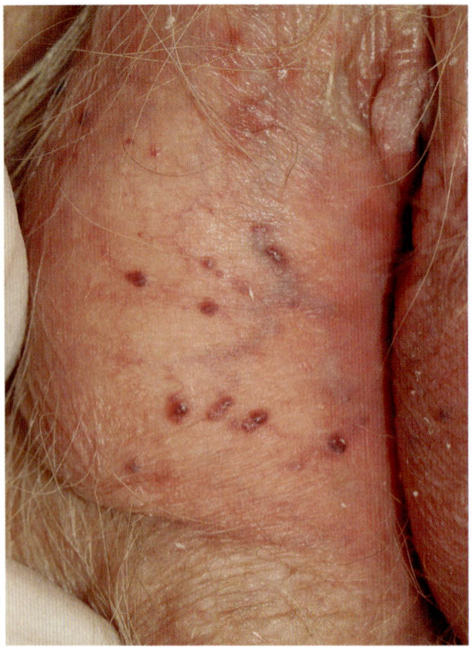

Fig. 6-12. Sometimes the vulva also displays large numbers of angiokeratomas; these range from very tiny to several millimeters and from bright red to dark purple, almost black.

thickened and elongated rete ridges usually extend into the dermis around the vessels, sometimes entirely encircling them. The cause of these lesions is unknown. However, based on their frequent occurrence along a dilated vessels on the scrotum, it is possible that they develop as saccular varices in aging, weak-walled capillaries.

## SECTION B: RED NODULES

The discussion in this section covers disorders that are primarily nodular. That is, it centers around those disorders wherein the majority of the lesions are 1.5 cm in diameter or even quite a bit larger. However, in some instances, smaller lesions (papules) may be intermingled among the larger nodules.

### Hidradenitis Suppurativa (Acne Inversa)

Hidradenitis suppurativa (HS) is a chronic disfiguring disease that is difficult to treat successfully. It is often accompanied by pain, drainage, and odor. As such, it has the potential to materially reduce the quality of life for patients affected by it. Several extensive reviews of this disease have recently been published. These include two-part articles in 2019 and 2020[8-11] and another lengthy single article in 2020.[12] These publications support nearly all of what is written below, and thus, I will not reference them for each point made.

#### Clinical Presentation

Hidradenitis suppurativa is a relatively common problem with an estimated prevalence of about 1%-2% in Western countries with a slightly higher rate elsewhere. Similarly, it affects women more often than men in the west, but men develop HS more often, and more severely, elsewhere. With the exception of familial cases, it rarely develops before age 20 and is most commonly encountered during the third and fourth decades of life. New onset after menopause is unusual, and disease activity, whenever it starts, tends to decrease slowly over time. Most clinicians believe that HS is more common in Africans and African Americans, but data to support this supposition are not very persuasive. A positive family history for HS is found in about one-third of the patients. Smoking (current and former), obesity, and a positive family history for HS are notable predisposing factors associated with its development. (See also the section on "Pathophysiology" below.) In a "chicken and egg" sort of way, it is not clear whether the association with "metabolic syndrome" (large waist circumference, abnormally high blood sugar, increased blood pressure, and elevated lipid levels) is a predisposing factor or occurs as a result of having HS. In addition, there are associations with many other medical disorders. These include inflammatory bowel disease, pyoderma gangrenosum, polycystic ovarian syndrome, arteriosclerosis, thyroid dysfunction, and arthropathic disorders. HS can also be encountered in association with severe cystic acne and dissecting cellulitis (noninfectious inflammatory cysts) of the scalp (the follicular retention triad).

The quality of life for patients with HS is very seriously impaired, perhaps more so than for patients with any other common dermatologic disease. Patients are hindered both socially and at work because of odor and drainage. Sexual intimacy becomes impossible for many of those with HS. Some patients are even rejected by the clinicians from whom they seek therapy. Severe psychological disability often occurs, and most patients with moderate to severe disease develop significant anxiety and/or depression. Not surprisingly, there is an increased risk for suicide.

Hidradenitis suppurativa begins with painful, red nodules, many of which eventually rupture and form chronic, draining sinus tracts (**Figs. 6-13 through 6-21**). The inflammatory nodules greatly resemble furuncles and are often initially misdiagnosed as such. Chronic ulcers can also develop. Both the sinus tracts and the ulcers tend to heal with thick ropelike scars (**Fig. 6-22**). In the worst instances, these scars result in contracture formation. Comedones, with black follicular plugs, are regularly found in the areas around the inflammatory lesions (**Figs. 6-23 and 6-24**). These comedones are larger than normal. The presence of two comedones separated by only 1-2 mm of normal skin ("twin" comedones) is sufficiently distinctive to represent a helpful diagnostic sign of the disorder. The older literature suggested that these "twin" black heads occurred as a result of a bifurcated follicular outlet. More recently, it has been

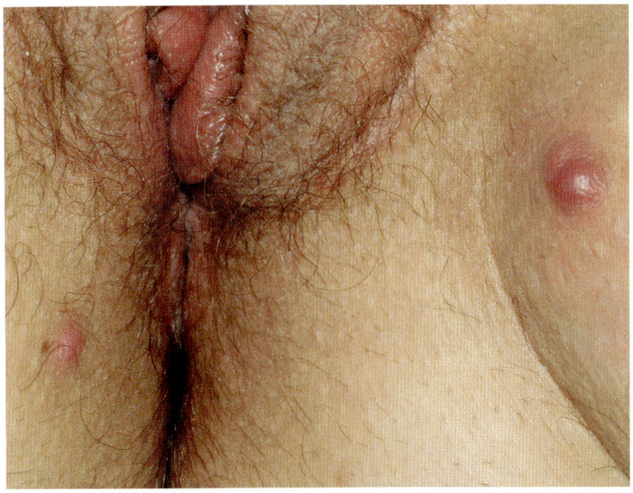

Fig. 6-13. Hidradenitis suppurativa ranges from an occasional inflamed cyst, as in this patient, to large numbers of coalescing nodules.

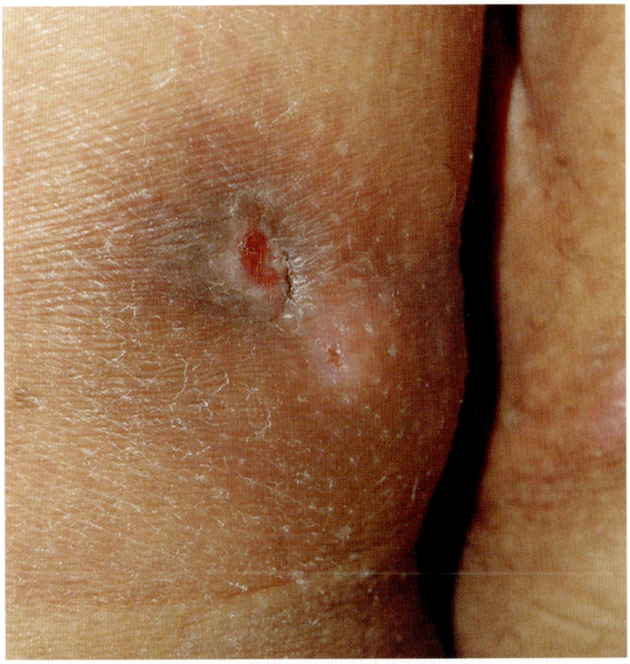

Fig. 6-14. As inflamed cysts rupture, they sometimes eventuate into chronic draining sinus tracts, surface erosions, and depressed scarring.

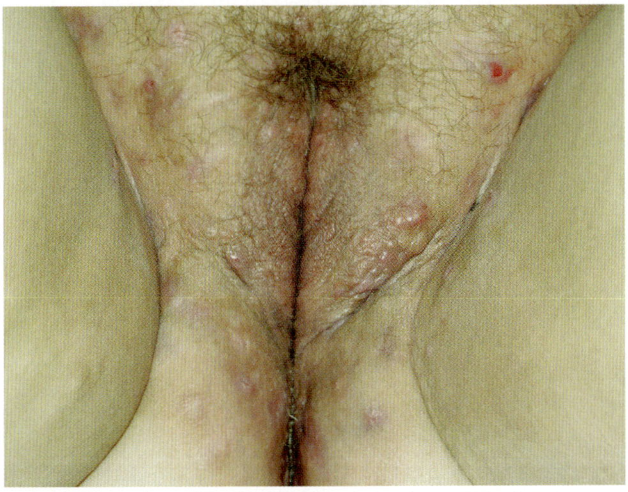

Fig. 6-15. Some people experience multiple, mostly discrete, waxing, and waning inflammatory lesions.

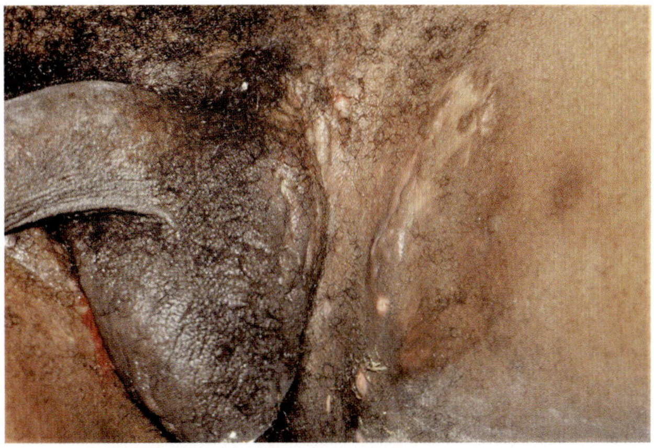

Fig. 6-16. Other individuals experience coalescing nodules that connect in the subcutaneous tissue, producing deep fibrotic scarring and induration.

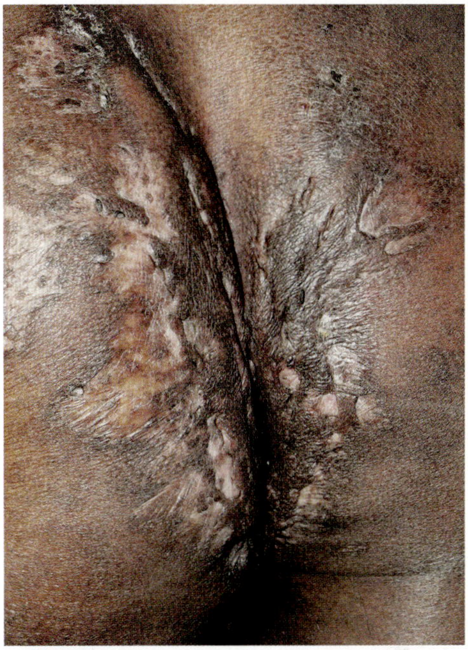

Fig. 6-17. Hidradenitis suppurativa also can affect the perianal skin and buttocks, so that even sitting is painful.

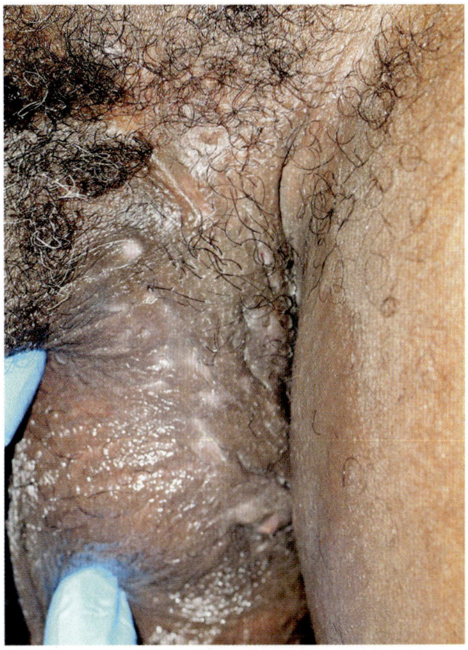

Fig. 6-18. The constant drainage from sinus tracts produces irritant contact dermatitis, odor, and rawness, as occurs in the inguinal fold of this man.

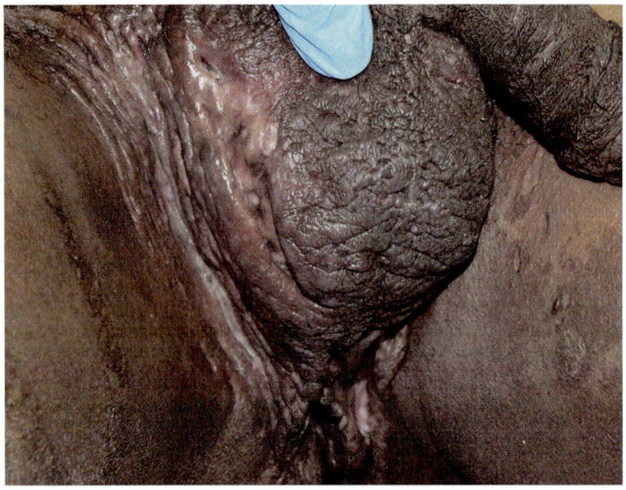

Fig. 6-19. The scarring from HS has resulted in hard, nonpitting edema of the scrotum.

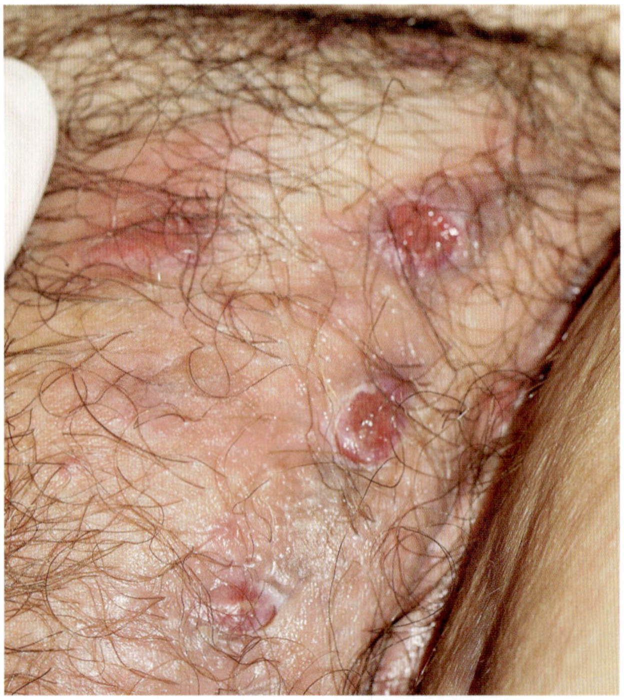

Fig. 6-20. Red, eroded, exophytic nodules sometimes form at the exit of draining sinus tracts.

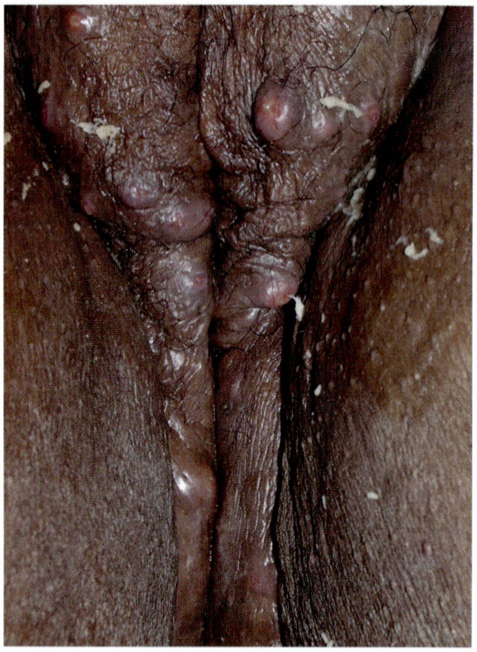

Fig. 6-21. This woman has constant wetness from her constantly draining HS cysts.

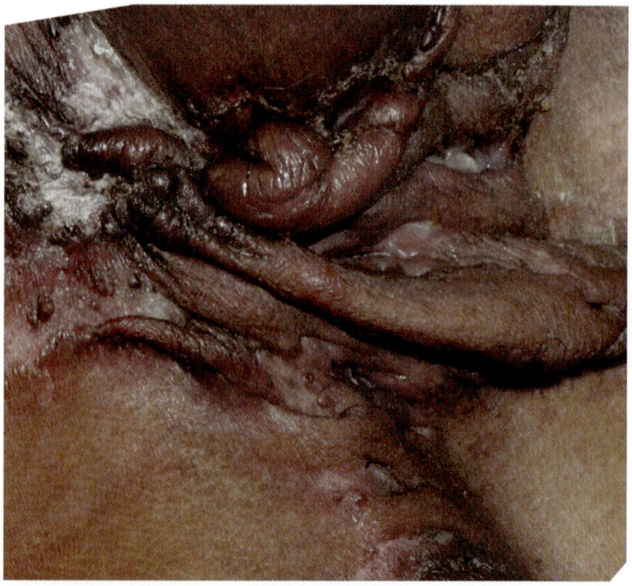

Fig. 6-22. HS occurs often in the axillae; this man has severe scarring and constant drainage from one axilla and his buttocks only.

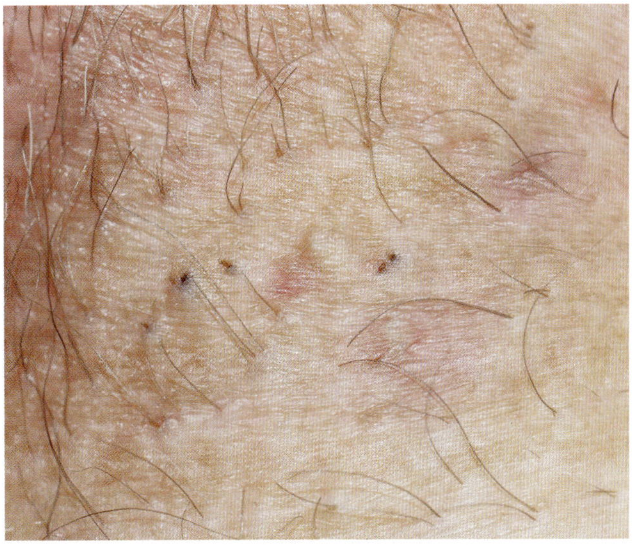

Fig. 6-23. Fairly subtle comedones, some "twin comedones," are characteristic of HS, with careful inspection.

found that at least in many instances they are pseudocomedones without attached complete hair follicles and that they form as part of the postinflammatory scarring process.[13]

The inflammatory lesions of HS occur almost solely at sites possessing hair follicles with associated apocrine glands, even though the apocrine glands themselves do not seem to be involved in the direct pathogenesis of the lesions. Because of the relationship between mammary glands and apocrine glands, it is not surprising that nearly all of the lesions of HS occur along the "milk line" that runs from the axillae through the mammary area and extends into the pubic, inguinal, genital, perineal, and perianal area. Scattered lesions (presumably related to ectopically located apocrine gland–related follicles) may be found on the buttocks and thighs. The axillae and buttocks are the locations most often affected in men; the anogenital area and the upper inner thighs are the location most commonly involved in women. Several systems for documenting the severity of HS have been proposed.

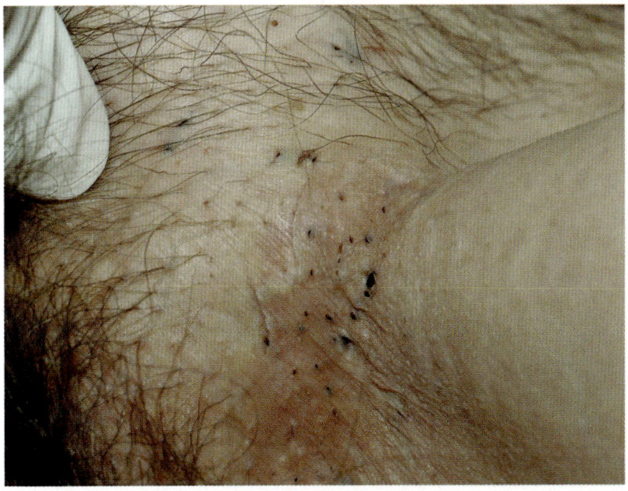

Fig. 6-24. Occasionally, comedones are quite prominent.

Of these, the Hurley staging and the Sartorius score are the two most commonly used in clinical studies; neither is often used in clinical day-to-day practice.[14]

## Diagnosis

A diagnosis of HS is made on a clinical basis.[15] The clinical features that lead to the diagnosis include (1) the presence of multiple lesions bilaterally, (2) the location of lesions within the milk line, (3) recurrence of lesions at the same site, (4) long-lasting duration (weeks to months) of individual lesions, (5) bacterial cultures that are either negative or demonstrate a multiplicity of bacterial species, and (6) failure to respond quickly (7-10 days) and completely to antibiotic therapy. Diagnostic algorithms that include many of these features have been proposed. Biopsy is rarely indicated, and because of the nonspecific inflammation that is found, it is usually not helpful if it is carried out. However, when Crohn disease is a consideration, and there is no history of bowel disease, a biopsy may be helpful to separate it from HS.

Two common diseases should be considered in the list of differential diagnoses. First, furunculosis is the condition with which HS is most often confused. Several clinical features are useful in identifying furunculosis: (1) only one or two, rather than multiple, inflammatory nodules are usually present at any one time; (2) lesions are found at random sites rather than mostly within the milk line; (3) culture reveals only a single bacterial species (almost always *Staphylococcus aureus*); and (4) there is a complete response to appropriate antibiotic therapy within 7-10 days. Second, anogenital cutaneous Crohn disease can look very much like HS. A history of bowel symptoms and signs, the lack of "twin" comedones, absence of lesions outside the anogenital region, the presence of anal fistulae, and the somewhat more distinctive histological findings on biopsy would point toward a diagnosis of Crohn disease. Note, however, that even though they appear to be entirely separate entities, there are several reports indicating that the two diseases coexist with a greater frequency than would be expected by chance. Other disorders that may present with lesions that mimic the inflammatory nodules of HS include deep fungal infections (especially in the immunosuppressed), mycobacterial infections, granuloma inguinale, and inflamed cysts of various types.[12]

**HIDRADENITIS SUPPURATIVA — Diagnosis**

- Multiple lesions are present.
- Lesions located within the milk line.
- Recurrence of lesions at the same site.
- Long duration of individual lesions.
- Little or no spontaneous regression of the overall disease.
- Cultures sterile or contain multiple species of bacteria.
- Slow and incomplete resolution with oral antibiotics.

## Pathophysiology

Multiple elements are associated with the development of HS. Some of these include *lifestyle factors.* A past or currant history of smoking is present in an astoundingly high proportion of patients. Interestingly, cessation of smoking leads to little or no improvement in the patient's HS. Obesity, with or without features of the complete metabolic syndrome (see above), is also frequently found. This obesity contributes to sweat retention and friction both of which contribute to the development of inflammation. *Genetic factors* are also important. As indicated above, nearly a third of HS patients have a positive family history of the disorder. It is worth noting that at the molecular level, some Asian patients with familial HS have gamma secretase gene mutations leading to Notch receptor deficiency. These mutations, at least in mice, lead to follicular hyperkeratosis and the development of hair follicle cysts.[12,16] *Immune factors* play a role as well. There is upregulation of interleukin-1β and tumor necrosis factor alpha both of which increase the presence of neutrophils. These neutrophils result in abscess formation with eventual rupture of involved hair follicles and purulent drainage. If this abscess-related necrosis breaks through the skin, secondary bacterial colonization and/or infection may occur. These and other similar abnormalities suggest that HS is part of the autoinflammatory spectrum of disorders and helps to explain its reported association with Crohn disease and pyoderma gangrenosum.[12,16]

## Prognosis

Hidradenitis suppurativa is an extraordinarily chronic disease extending over many years or even decades. When HS is untreated or is treated inadequately, *nondraining* abscesses eventually resolve spontaneously over the course of several months. Unfortunately, recrudescence at the same sites occurs frequently. *Draining* sinuses and fistulae remain in place even longer, sometimes for years. And, of course, scars evolving from such lesions last for a lifetime. Overall, in the untreated state, there is a tendency for the process to extend locally within the field of apocrine gland–related follicles. This extension probably occurs because of inflammatory cytokine release with resultant inflammation-related destruction of adjacent follicles. Eventually, after years of activity, scarring causes the process to gradually results in spontaneous resolution.

The clinical sequelae of longstanding disease includes hypertrophic, ropelike scarring, architectural distortion of involved tissue (especially of the genitalia), and moderate to severe limitation in limb mobility. Massive, persistent vulvar or scrotal edema may develop. Moreover, cutaneous squamous cell carcinoma has been reported as occurring in chronic HS ulcers in nearly 100 patients.[17] These carcinomas have been noted more often in men and have developed primarily in the anogenital area. The pathogenesis of such malignancy is unknown, but it seems to be related to persistent inflammation and scarring in a manner analogous to the development of squamous cell carcinoma (Marjolin ulcers) in longstanding stasis ulcers. The prognosis for such patients is very poor.

## Management

The first step in treatment is an attempt to improve the local environment through reduction in sweat retention and body-fold friction. Weight loss is quite helpful in this regard even though it is difficult to achieve.[12] Less helpful but still worth pursuing is cessation of smoking. Medical therapy, despite its limitations, is necessary for nearly all patients but especially for patients with disseminated and/or severe disease. Discussion of such treatment can be found in several review articles.[9,11,12,14] Basically, patients with nondraining abscesses can be treated topically with long-term application of 1% clindamycin or 2% erythromycin antibiotic lotions or creams. Individual abscesses, especially if they are limited in number, can be injected intralesionally with triamcinolone acetonide (Kenalog) in a concentration of 5-10 mg/mL. Small nodules will require 0.1-0.5 mL; larger ones may need 0.5-1.0 mL.

Patients with numerous lesions should be placed on long-term oral antibiotic therapy. This treatment requires the use of those specific antibiotics possessing anti-inflammatory properties.[18] Note that these anti-inflammatory effects greatly outweigh the importance of their antimicrobial effect. The products most often used include tetracycline 250 mg qid, doxycycline 100 mg bid, and minocycline 100 mg bid. These three products appear to be equally effective. A somewhat more aggressive approach involves the simultaneous administration of clindamycin (300 mg bid) and rifampin (300 mg bid). There is, however, some concern about long-term safety when this combination therapy is used, and the increasing incidence of *Clostridium difficile* can be a concern with clindamycin. Antibiotic therapy usually results in only moderate improvement, and relapse generally occurs when such treatment is discontinued.

Hormonal therapy may be considered for women even though only meager data have been published regarding efficacy.[19] This approach is initiated with oral contraceptives (especially with those products incorporating drospirenone or cyproterone as the progestational agent) and is followed, if necessary, by spironolactone or finasteride. Patients with HS have an increased likelihood of having type 2 diabetes and, in women, polycystic ovarian syndrome. For this reason, metformin, in escalating doses to 1.5 mg daily, can be surprisingly effective for women and may even be helpful for those who do not have either of these two disorders.[20]

Systemic steroids can be used effectively for short-term amelioration of acute flares in HS. Generally, prednisone in an oral dose of 40 mg/day is administered, but relapse usually quickly follows cessation of this agent. We have had equally good results, with much less risk relapse, when 80 mg of the depot steroid triamcinolone acetonide (Kenalog-40) is injected intramuscularly into the buttock.

In spite of high cost, potential serious adverse effects, and, like all therapies for HS, the requirement for ongoing injections, there is currently considerable enthusiasm for the use of anti-inflammatory biologics.[19,21] The most widely studied of these, and the only one currently approved for HS by the U.S. FDA, is adalimumab (Humira). It is a tumor necrosis factor antagonist and has proven to be moderately effective for moderate to severe HS. This medication in no way clears all patients with HS, but it our hands has been by far the most effective therapy available other than, perhaps, dramatic weight loss in very obese patients. This medication can be life changing. There is evidence that those who do not respond well may benefit from therapeutic drug monitoring, as patients with poorer response have lower serum trough levels of medication.[22] Aggressive staff can nearly always procure adalimumab for insured patients, and patient assistance is available for those without insurance or with a large co-pay. Many other biologics are being used in clinical studies but discussion regarding the effectiveness of these agents is at this time premature. Nevertheless, I think it is worth mentioning apremilast (Otezla) because it is an oral (rather than injectable) agent, has been reasonably efficacious for HS in studies, and has an excellent safety profile requiring no follow-up laboratory testing.[23] However, because it is expensive and not FDA approved for HS, this can be more difficult to obtain for patients.

Several other systemic medications can be mentioned; none of these will be discussed in detail as their use generally falls outside the scope of nondermatologists. Oral retinoids have been tried because of their effectiveness in acne but are of very limited value in the treatment of HS. Other therapies include the administration of dapsone, cyclosporine, zinc gluconate, and metronidazole.

Given the significant limitations of medical therapy, many clinicians consider HS to be a disease for which surgery represents the best approach. Multiple surgical procedures have been used.[24] The simplest approach, incision and drainage of individual lesions, offers little long-term value and is no longer generally recommended. Marsupialization ("un-roofing"), though fairly effective, is a procedure with prolonged healing and is less often used that it was years ago (see Chapter 4). However, this is very effective for those individual chronic/recurrent draining cysts and sinus tracts, and it is an easy and quick office procedure. Surgical excision with primary closure is extremely effective for limited areas of disease. When excisional surgery for extensive disease is carried out, controversy exists as to which is the best technique. Some favor surgery with grafting, others allow for healing by secondary intention, and still others prefer staged removal with primary closures for each stage.

Unfortunately, many clinicians are hesitant to perform surgery for HS because of two concerns. First, they fear that wound infection will develop owing to the draining pus in and around the surgical field. In answer to this concern, it must be noted that the pus present in HS is usually sterile and there has been no reported increase in wound infections beyond that which might occur in the absence of this purulent drainage. Second, they view the development of new lesions at the surgical margin, which frequently occurs, as surgical failure. However, the lesions that occur at the surgical margin usually represent "new" lesions rather than "recurrences," and these may be excised effectively at a later date on an "as necessary" basis. Importantly, patient satisfaction with surgical procedures for HS is really quite high and is almost always higher than the satisfaction expressed by the surgeons who performed it.

Various forms of light-based therapy and laser therapy have some enthusiastic backers,[25] but they are not currently "mainstream" approaches. The same is true for radiotherapy (X-ray therapy).[26] For that reason, discussion of these latter three treatments will not be further pursued in this chapter.

**HIDRADENITIS SUPPURATIVA** — **Management**

- Prolonged antibiotic therapy for its anti-inflammatory effect
- Hormonal therapy for women
- Adalimumab and other "biologics" for moderate to severe disease
- Surgical excision of involved areas

## Furunculosis ("Boils")

Furuncles develop as a deep form of bacterial folliculitis and usually present as a solitary, red, dome-shaped nodule **(Figs. 6-25 and 6-26)**. Most are 2-4 cm in diameter. They are painful, warm, and tender to touch. On palpation, they may be firm or have a central soft area of fluctuance. The surface may be either intact or broken down, in which case there is usually purulent ("pus") drainage. The term "abscess" is used for similar infections, presenting with a similar appearance, occurring at a nonfollicular site. Closely clustered furuncles are called carbuncles.

Furuncles and abscesses are almost always caused by *S aureus* infection, and in about half of the cases, these bacteria are methicillin-resistant *Staphylococcal aureus* (MRSA). Moreover, these staphylococcal organisms frequently carry the Panton-Valentine leukocidin virulence factor. This factor causes neutrophil lysis and lysosomal enzyme release that consequently favors development of tissue necrosis and purulence.[27] The warm, moist environment of the anogenital area facilitates the development of these lesions as does skin-to-skin friction such as occurs with obesity, sexual intercourse, and some forms of exercise. Debility,

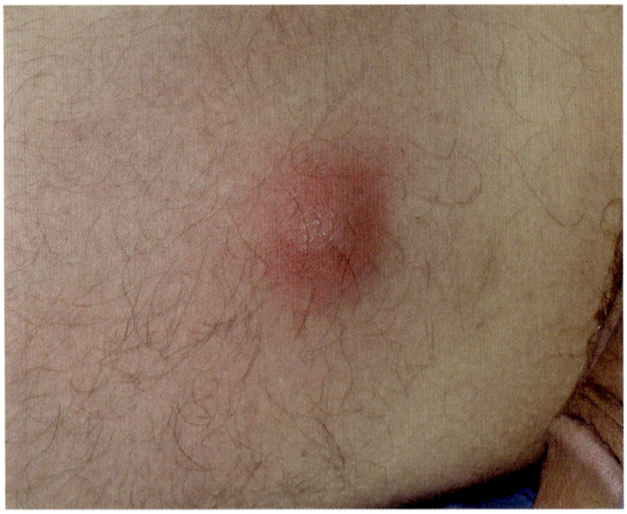

Fig. 6-25. This painful, red nodule could represent a furuncle, a bacterial infection, or an inflamed cyst. Only a culture can tell for sure, and this is indicated to ascertain sensitivities.

immunocompromised, corticosteroid therapy, atopic dermatitis, diabetes, alcoholism, poor personal hygiene, and nasal colonization with *S aureus* may act as cofactors in causation. Notably individuals who are chronic nasal carriers of *S aureus* tend to have frequently recurring lesions.[28]

The inflammatory nodules of HS are regularly confused with furuncles. However, the presence of multiple nodules, their location at characteristic sites, the culture of multiple species of bacteria rather than only *S aureus*, and the failure to quickly and fully respond to antibiotic therapy usually allow for correct identification of HS.

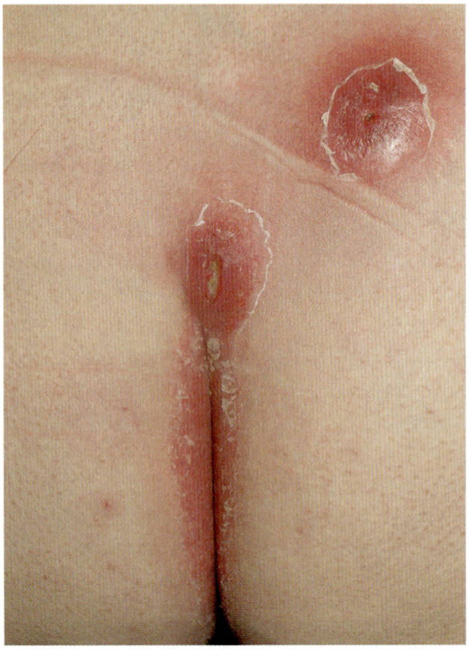

Fig. 6-26. This patient has poorly controlled inverse psoriasis, with scaling skin, which is often colonized with *Staphylococcus aureus*. There were no noted preceding cysts, and a culture yielded methicillin-resistant *S aureus*.

Inflamed cysts are also similar in appearance to furuncles. For such cysts, there is generally a history of a previous noninflamed nodule (preexisting noninflamed cyst) at that same site. This history together with a poor response to antibiotic therapy allows for correct identification. Other conditions to consider in the list of differential diagnoses for disorders occurring in the anogenital region include pilonidal cysts and Crohn disease. If the lesion is very large and nonpurulent, cellulitis and the early stage of necrotizing fasciitis should also be considered.

The diagnosis is generally made on a clinical basis; confirmation by bacterial culture is possible only if the lesion is fluctuant and pus can be sampled; needle aspiration of solid lesions rarely provides enough fluid for culture. Small, relatively asymptomatic lesions may clear spontaneously. For all other furuncles, whether or not culture is possible, those oral antibiotics that are generally effective against MRSA, such as doxycycline or trimethoprim-sulfamethoxazole, should be considered as first-line therapy.[27] Then, for those lesions that have been cultured, appropriate changes in antibiotics can be made after sensitivity results have been returned. Use of parenteral antibiotics for seriously ill, hospitalized patients lies outside the scope of discussion in this chapter. Finally, although warm, wet compresses are often recommended, there is little factual published evidence to support their use.

## Inflamed Cysts

Most cysts occurring in the anogenital region are not inflamed and therefore are skin-colored and asymptomatic. As such, the primary discussion of these lesions can be found in Chapter 7. However, sometimes these cysts become inflamed. In this situation, a patient may present with a red, tender nodule. Inflammation occurring in or around a cyst develops as the result of cyst wall leakage, or rupture, with release of cyst contents into the surrounding connective tissue. These cyst contents subsequently induce a foreign body-type inflammatory reaction. It should be noted that many clinicians speak of these inflamed cysts as being infected but, in fact, infection is a very unlikely event. Infection can occur, however, if an inflamed cyst has undergone necrosis and drains to the skin surface.

Noninflamed cysts are usually asymptomatic, but inflamed cysts are generally tender and painful. When a patient initially presents with an inflamed cyst, the first (mistaken) consideration often is that of a furuncle. Correct diagnosis of an inflamed cyst is usually possible based on the history of a preexisting, nontender, skin-colored lesion. This observation together with an unchanging size for a week or more and a failure to respond quickly and completely with antibiotic therapy allows for correct clinical identification. The type of cysts most like to become inflamed include epidermoid ("sebaceous") cysts (**Fig. 6-27**), pilonidal cysts (**Fig. 6-28**), and Bartholin duct cysts (**Fig. 6-29**). Other conditions to be considered in

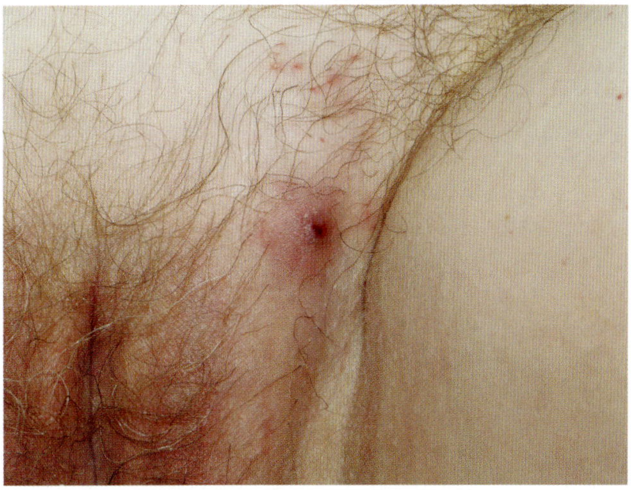

Fig. 6-27. This nodule was as red and painful as a furuncle produced by infection, but a culture was negative, showing a diagnosis of an inflamed cyst.

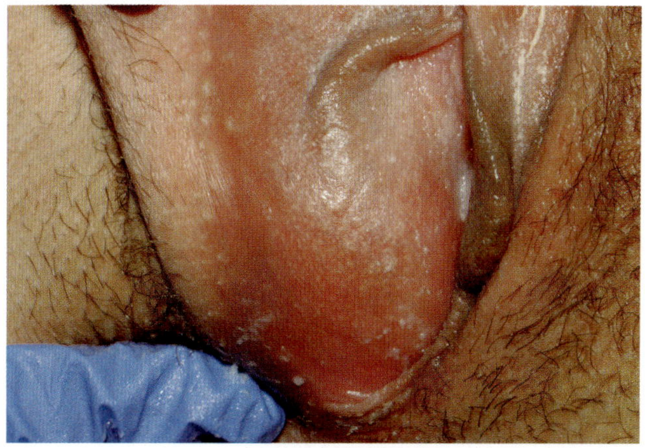

Fig. 6-29. An abscess of Bartholin gland duct cyst presents as a diffuse, painful, red swelling of the vulva underlying the posterior vestibule and labium majus, and transected by the interlabial fold. (From transparency.)

the list of differential diagnoses include cutaneous Crohn disease and HS.

The treatment of inflamed cysts depends partly on the type of cyst involved. But in most instances, incision and drainage with bacterial culture of the contents is a desirable first step. If the cyst cavity is quite large, packing it with sterile iodoform gauze may be warranted. Antibiotics are often administered, even though infection is rarely present in intact cysts. Often, there is some improvement with antibiotics, but this presumably is more related to the anti-inflammatory property of most antibiotics rather than to any direct antimicrobial effect.[18] Soaks and sitz baths with warm tap water are often recommended, but there are few data to support their use.

Not all cysts need to be completely excised though the recurrence rate is fairly high if this is not carried out. In any event, definitive, complete excision of the cyst is best delayed until the initial inflammation has resolved as this leads to better recognition of the actual size of the lesion to be removed. The excision of pilonidal and Bartholin cysts requires special expertise, and discussion of this topic lies beyond the scope of this chapter.

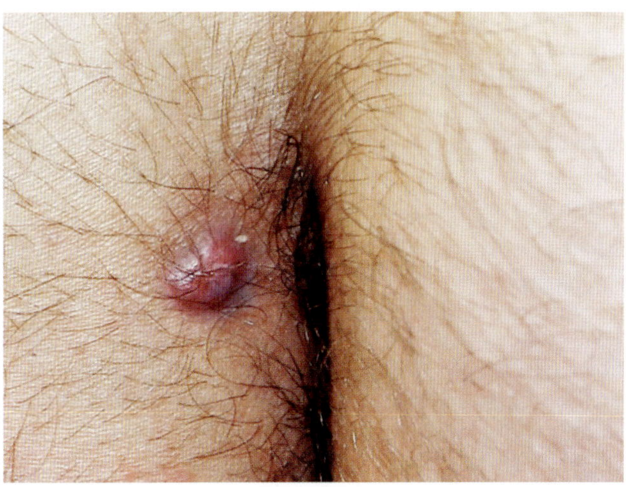

Fig. 6-28. This nodule of a pilonidal cyst has been annoying for this man for years; although it would appear to be an easy office removal, it may be very deep and should only be removed in an operating room where the depth of the lesion can be explored.

## Inflamed Bartholin Gland Cysts

See Skin-Colored Nodules in Chapter 7.

# SECTION C: MISCELLANEOUS, UNCOMMON RED PAPULES AND NODULES

## Prurigo Nodularis (Picker Nodule)

### Clinical Presentation

Prurigo nodularis (PN) occurs in patients who chronically scratch, pick, or gouge at a small area of skin.[29-31] Prolonged scratching produces a calluslike reaction as epithelial cells proliferate and produce increased amounts of keratin in response to chronic trauma. Individual lesions are 0.5- to 2.0-cm pink, red, or brown-red papules and nodules usually with overlying excoriation or ulceration (**Figs. 6-30 and 6-31**). The surface is palpably rough due to the presence of the compacted scale and crust. Erosion and bleeding are sometimes also present. Generally, no primary lesions are seen, but occasionally, a coexisting underlying problem, such as folliculitis, is found having served as a focus for the initial scratching.

Prurigo nodules may occur anywhere on the body especially on the extensor surface of the extremities. When lesions develop in the anogenital area, they are

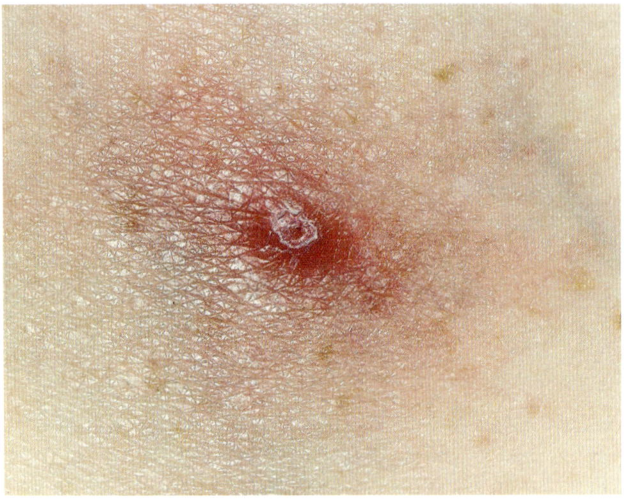

Fig. 6-30. These prurigo nodules are typical in their dusky erythema and superficial erosion from picking.

likely to be found on the labia majora in women, on the scrotum in men, and in the pubic area in both sexes. Picking may start as a result of pruritus, but habitual picking, often at the completely subconscious level, plays the major role in the perpetuation of these lesions. PN occurs more often in women than in men and more frequently develops in African Americans than in Caucasians, when they appear more brown than red. A history of atopy and/or atopic dermatitis is frequently present. Other underlying pruritic disorders that may provoke PN include HIV infection, hematological malignancies, chronic renal disease, and various autoimmune disorders. Notably, a few patients (falsely) express the belief that "bugs" or "fibers" are present in the skin and that their picking only occurs in an attempt to remove them (see "delusions of parasitosis" in the section on psychosexual issues in Chapter 15).

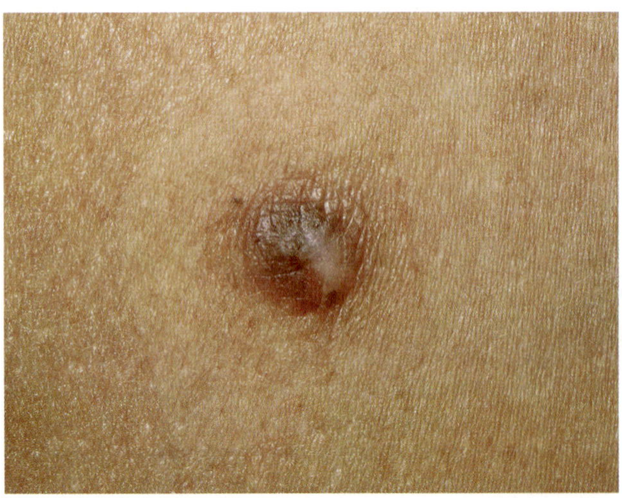

Fig. 6-31. Prurigo nodules are most common in people of African genetic background, and in that skin color, inflammatory conditions such as prurigo nodules tend to be brown rather than red.

## Diagnosis

The diagnosis is made by the clinical appearance and a history of scratching or picking. Occasionally, the scratching occurs at the subconscious level in which case the history of picking may be denied. Biopsy is not usually necessary, but if carried out, demonstrates the presence of lichenification with the histological features of epidermal hyperkeratosis, acanthosis, and irregular downward proliferation of the rete ridges. Inflammatory cells (eosinophils, T lymphocytes, and mast cells) are present in the dermis, and there is proliferation of dermal nerve fibers. Elevated levels of interleukin-31 (IL-31), substance P, and calcitonin gene–related peptide can be demonstrated. The differential diagnoses for PN occurring in the anogenital area includes Fox-Fordyce disease (especially in women), nodular scabies (particularly in males), and pseudowarts (usually in infants and diapered adults). Fox-Fordyce disease is discussed in Chapter 7, and the latter two disorders are covered further on in this chapter.

**PRURIGO NODULARIS — Diagnosis**

- Excoriated, rough-surfaced papules or nodules
- History of habitual scratching or picking
- Occasional belief that "something is in the skin and must be removed"
- Confirmation by biopsy, if necessary

## Pathophysiology

The pathophysiology of these nodules is not well understood but is probably related to neuroimmune dysregulation, which then causes a protective calluslike response of epithelial cells to the chronic trauma of picking, scratching, and rubbing.[29] The process is analogous to that occurring with the itch-scratch cycle that results in lichenification (see Chapter 2), but, because the scratching is so localized, papules and nodules are formed rather than plaques. Some degree of psychological dysfunction (especially anxiety and depression) is regularly present. The intensity and repetitiveness of the picking has many features of an obsessive-compulsive disorder.

## Management

Treatment consists of the identification and, where possible, elimination of any underlying pruritic condition, such as folliculitis that initiates the picking. Patients with anxiety or depression (a common occurrence) should have these psychological issues addressed. Individual lesions can be treated fairly effectively by intralesional injections of 0.2-0.5 mL of triamcinolone acetonide (Kenalog) 10 mg/mL. A light freeze with liquid nitrogen may help temporarily because such very cold temperatures selectively destroy the nerve endings that convey the pruritus before causing other types of tissue damage. High-potency topical steroid therapy is usually prescribed but, used alone, this approach is rarely of much help. Nighttime sedation with hydroxyzine or a tricyclic medication such as doxepin can minimize scratching during sleep. An orally administered selective serotonin reuptake inhibitor (SSRI), used in doses recommended for the treatment of obsessive-compulsive disease, can be very beneficial. In the most severe cases, administration of one of the atypical antipsychotic agents may be worth trying. The use of these latter medications is further discussed in Chapter 3.

Phototherapy (narrow band UVB and PUVA) is generally helpful if it is available. Immunosuppressive therapy with methotrexate or cyclosporine represents "third-line" treatment. Not surprisingly, several "biologicals" have been reported as useful. Dupilumab (Dupixent), already FDA approved for atopic dermatitis, has been used successfully[32] and nemolizumab (Galderma), an IL-31 receptor antagonist, granted modified U.S. FDA approval, has also been demonstrated as helpful.[33]

**PRURIGO NODULARIS** **Management**

- Intralesional steroid injection, triamcinolone 10 mg/mL, 0.2-0.5 mL each lesion
- Trial of brief, light liquid nitrogen therapy
- Hydroxyzine or doxepin, 25 mg 2 hours before bedtime. Increase to 75 mg, if necessary
- SSRI, such as citalopram, if daytime therapy is necessary

## Pyogenic Granuloma

This reactive neoplasm is most commonly encountered on the oral mucosa and on the fingers in children and pregnant women. The genitalia are not a usual site of predilection, but there have been a few reported cases involving these areas **(Figs. 6-32 and 6-33)**. Moreover, we believe that they occur more commonly at anogenital sites than these infrequent reports suggest. Clinically, pyogenic granuloma presents as one or more, red or violaceous small nodules, about 1.5-2.0 cm in diameter. When multiple lesions are present, they usually occur in a cluster. Individual pyogenic granulomas may be slightly pedunculated (ie, "pinched in" at the base). Because the surface epithelium of these lesions is markedly thinned, they tend to have a glistening surface that bleeds easily following minimal trauma. The diagnosis is generally apparent on clinical examination, but many of the lesions discussed in this chapter should be considered in the list of differential diagnoses. Importantly, amelanotic melanoma can closely mimic the appearance of pyogenic granuloma.[34] For this reason, biopsy confirmation of a clinical diagnosis is usually warranted.

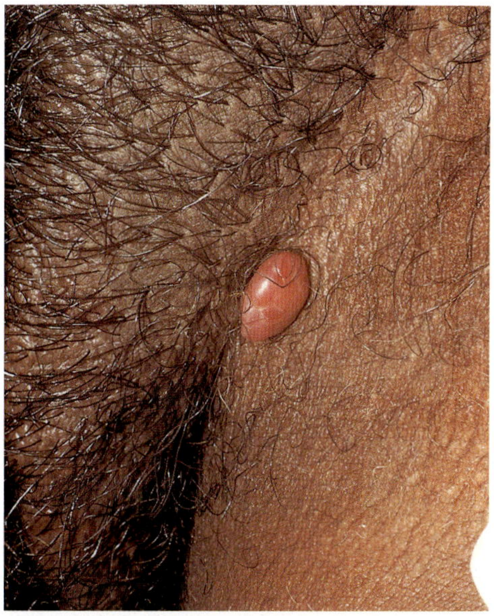

Fig. 6-32. A pyogenic granuloma is recognizable by its pedunculated morphology and red surface.

Pyogenic granuloma is a benign reactive neoplasm. Bleeding represents the only important complication of these lesions. The cause of pyogenic granuloma is not known, but in many cases, they arise after trauma, perhaps developing as a result of disturbed normal reparative angiogenesis. Since these lesions occur with much increased frequency during pregnancy and in the prepubertal years of childhood, it is possible that hormonal factors play a role in their pathogenesis.

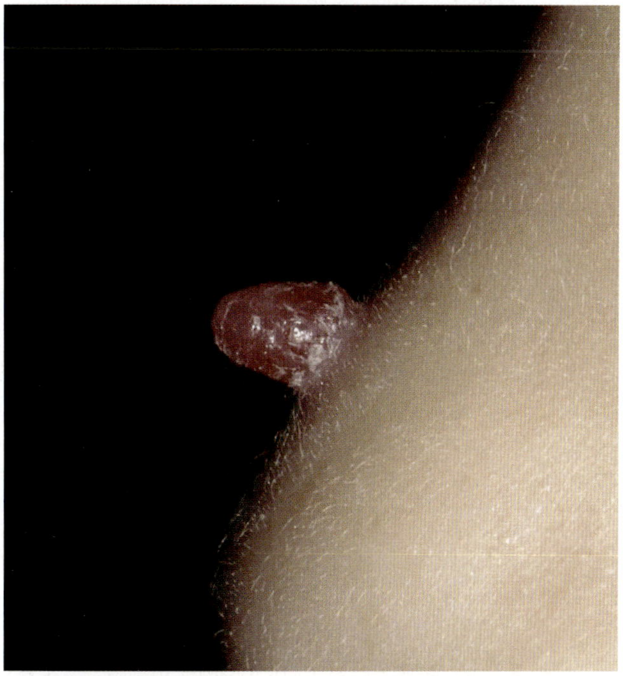

Fig. 6-33. This pyogenic granuloma is a classic nodule with a red, glistening surface.

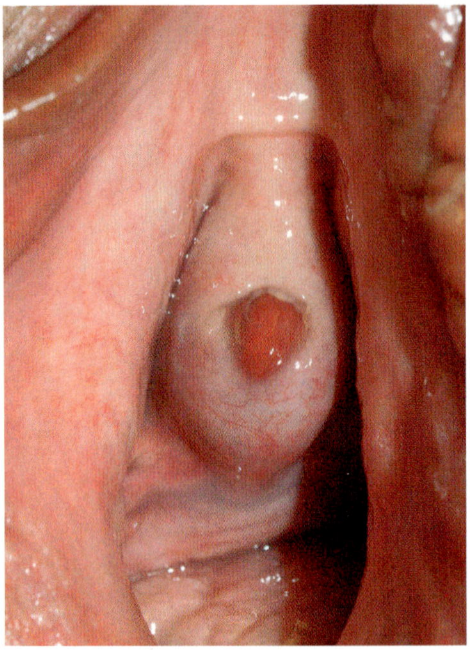

Fig. 6-34. Urethral caruncles are regular occurrences in postmenopausal women and appear inflamed and uncomfortable, but generally are asymptomatic.

The treatment of choice is shave excision at the level of the surrounding skin. This provides a good specimen for histological examination. The base of the excision should be treated with electrosurgery as otherwise bleeding may ensue and the recurrence rate is unacceptably high.

## Urethral Caruncle

Urethral caruncle occurs in middle-aged and elderly women though a very few instances have been reported in female children.[35] It appears as a solitary red papule at the urethral meatus **(Figs. 6-34 and 6-35)**. Such caruncles are 1 cm or less in diameter and are usually either pedunculated (pinched in at the base) or dome- shaped. Most are located at the posterior lip of the urethra. They are asymptomatic, but the surface is friable, and for this reason, they are often discovered by the patient because of mild hematuria or the presence of blood on the toilet tissue after wiping. Others are only found at the time of a routine gynecological examination. Urethral caruncles differ from urethral prolapse in that caruncles are focal and prolapse is circumferential. Microscopic features include vascular dilatation and an infiltration of neutrophils in a loose connective tissue stroma.

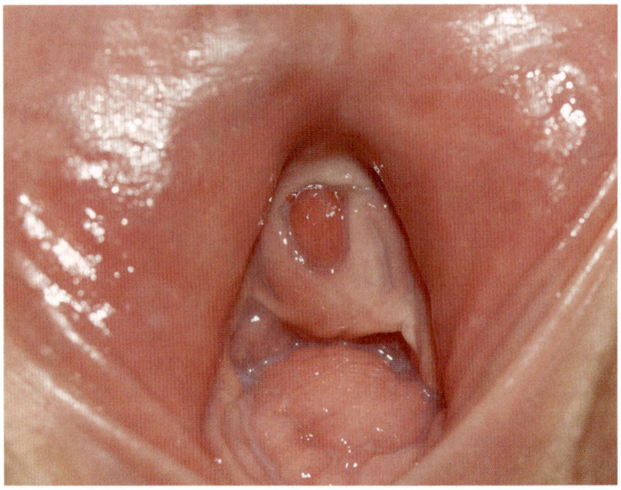

Fig. 6-35. Urethral caruncles are sometimes large, but at other times are small and subtle.

The cause is unknown, but because they occur almost entirely in postmenopausal women, estrogen deficiency is suspected. Asymptomatic small lesions may be left untreated. If treatment is desirable, several options are available.[35] Topical estrogen therapy is worth trying, though even when it is successful, recurrences are common when applications are discontinued. If topical therapy does not result in regression, the lesion can be removed by shave excision at the base of the lesion. Light electrosurgery after removal is desirable to achieve hemostasis and prevent recurrence. The removed specimen should be submitted for histological examination to rule out other types of urethral tumors.

## Urethral Prolapse

Prolapse of the urethra is seen only in females, and it occurs primarily in African and African American Black premenarchal girls and in White postmenopausal women.[36] It presents as a red, edematous circumferential cuff consisting of prolapsed urethral mucous membrane. The cuff almost always completely surrounds the urethral meatus **(Fig. 6-36)**. This disorder may be asymptomatic, but

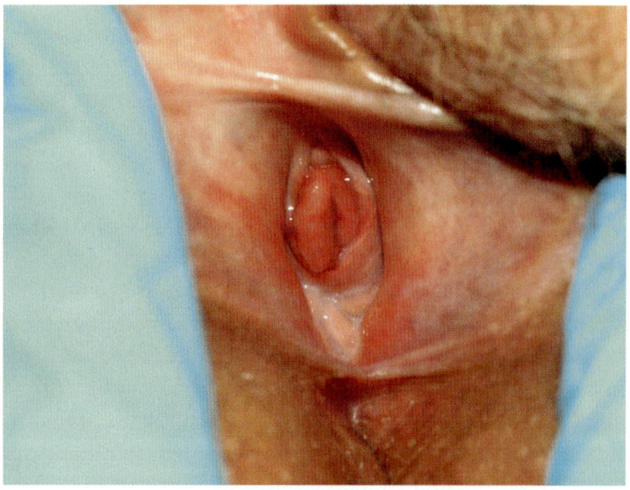

Fig. 6-36. Although urethral prolapse resembles a urethral caruncle, the erythematous nodule is circumferential around the meatus, thus making a doughnut shape with the urethral opening in the center.

both in children and adult women, bleeding, dysuria, and palpable presence of a mass with or without symptoms of local discomfort may be present. The diagnosis is usually made on visual examination and can be confirmed, if necessary, by insertion of a urinary catheter in the center of the lesion and noting the presence of urine. Biopsy is rarely necessary, but if carried out, the histological features are those of normal urethral epithelium with a variable amount of nonspecific underlying inflammation.

The cause of urethral prolapse is unknown. Because it mostly occurs in prepubertal girls and postmenopausal women, estrogen deficiency is likely to play a significant role. Rarely, it occurs as a congenital abnormality, but most often, the prolapse seems to be precipitated by trauma or pelvic straining, especially in those who are overweight. Topical estrogen therapy and manual reduction of the prolapse are often successful, but relapse is common. Surgical excision, ligation, or electrosurgical destruction is sometimes necessary.

## Vulvar and Perineal Endometriosis

### Clinical Presentation

The presence of endometrial tissue in ectopic cutaneous and mucosal sites is a relatively uncommon condition that presents as a papule, nodule, or plaque of highly variable size and color. Endometriosis of the vulva and perineum can be *primary* (arising in unscarred tissue) or, much more commonly, *secondary* (occurring at a previous surgical site). Usually only a solitary lesion is present, but rarely, there can be several clustered lesions. Endometriosis can be located in the vulvar vestibule (where they are likely to be mistaken for a Bartholin duct cyst), on the keratinizing epithelium of the labia majora and, most often, on the perineum in women who have had an episiotomy.[37,38] Small superficial lesions occur as a pink, red, violaceous, brown, or skin-colored, smooth-surfaced papule or nodule. Larger and deeper lesions are usually skin-colored, red-brown, blue, or violaceous **(Fig. 6-37)**. The average size is about 2 cm.

### Diagnosis

Recognition can usually be made on a clinical basis because characteristically these nodules enlarge and become painful at the same time as uterine menstruation. Regression to original size occurs after menstruation. Biopsy, revealing endometrial tissue, will confirm a clinically suspected diagnosis. Conditions included in the differential diagnosis include hidradenoma papilliferum, pyogenic granuloma, vascular tumors, and inflamed cysts. Other secondarily inflamed tumors may also mimic vulvar endometriosis.

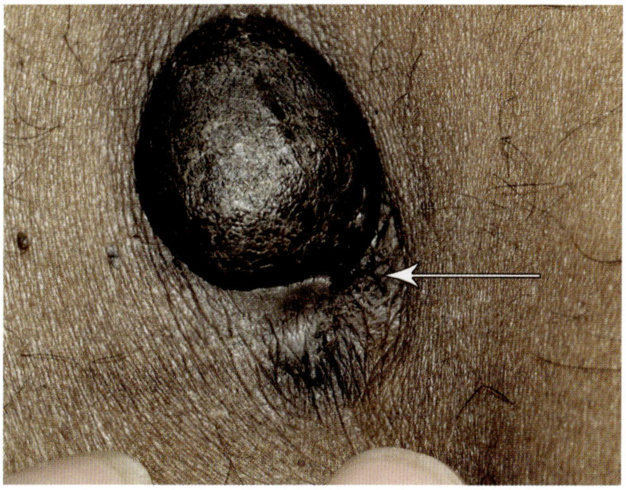

Fig. 6-37. Nodules of cutaneous endometriosis are dome-shaped and nondescript, but this lesion enlarged during menses, and bleeding occurred from one edge (*arrow*).

**ENDOMETRIOSIS — Diagnosis**

- Usually, a solitary lesion located on or within the vulva
- Color variable
- Surface smooth and intact
- Enlargement and discomfort during menses; regression afterward

### Pathophysiology

Cutaneous endometriosis develops when endometrial tissue arises spontaneously (rare) ectopically or is accidentally implanted (relatively common), at an extrapelvic location. The latter occurs most often at an episiotomy site but can also occur as a result of menstrual flow containing microscopic bits of endometrial tissue. Development of visible vulvar endometriosis lesions may lag behind actual endometrial implantation by months to years.

### Management and Prognosis

Encroachment into the anal sphincter may occur, and there have been reports of carcinoma developing in longstanding lesions. Wide surgical excision is usually adequate for small lesions. However, recurrence happens fairly often, especially with larger lesions. These larger lesions may require hormonal menstrual suppression with gonadotropin-releasing hormone agonists following surgical resection.[38]

**ENDOMETRIOSIS — Management**

- Surgical excision
- Laser ablation is possible after biopsy
- Expect a high rate of recurrence
- Postsurgical hormonal suppression of ovulation

## Hematoma

Hematomas represent a loculated collection of blood secondary to trauma. They occur rather easily within the vulva and scrotum because of the loose, distensible connective tissue at these sites and the postural dependent location of the genitalia. Usually in men, and sometimes in women, they occur following accidental or sexual trauma (Fig. 6-38). In women, vulvar hematomas occur most often at the time of vaginal delivery or after episiotomy.[39] The clinical appearance is that of acute or subacute nodular swelling accompanied by poorly demarcated, nonblanching purple discoloration. After the first few days, the original violaceous color is replaced by hues of yellow, green, and brown. Nontraumatic loculation of blood (strictly speaking not hematomas) can also occur, and because of the red-purple color, these can mimic the appearance of hematomas. In women, for instance, this type of loculation could develop as hematocolpos wherein menstrual blood is trapped inside the vagina by an imperforate hymen. In boys and men, such an example may occur as varicoceles.

Depending on the nature of the trauma resulting in a hematoma, the possibility of urethral rupture, testicular damage, and/or intrapelvic tissue damage should be considered. Imaging can be quite helpful in evaluation of this possibility.[39] Treatment of genital hematoma is usually expectant and conservative. Soaks and pain control can be useful. Surgical incision and evacuation of a clot may be necessary in instances of larger or expanding hematomas.[40]

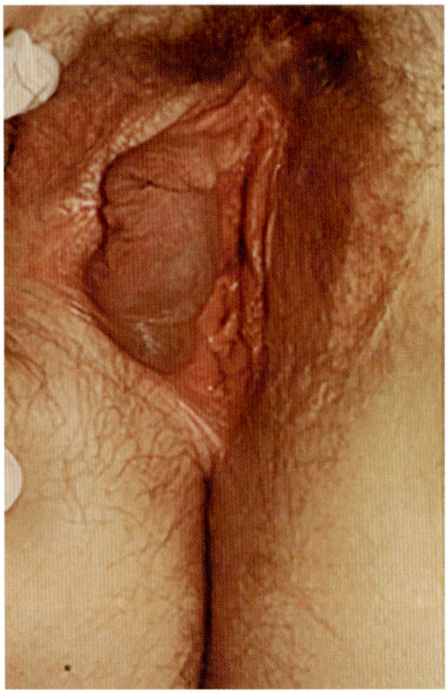

Fig. 6-38. The loose connective tissue of the vulva results in a space occupying hematoma fairly easily.

## Hidradenoma Papilliferum (Mammarylike Gland Adenoma)

Hidradenoma papilliferum (HP) is an uncommon neoplasm of the female anogenital area.[41,42] It develops primarily in middle-aged and older women. In nearly all instances, the nodules are solitary and most are papules or small nodules (1.5-3 cm). They are usually skin-colored but often have a faintly pink hue. Some appear cystic and others appear solid. The skin surface may be smooth in which case the lesions are asymptomatic but about one-third are ulcerated with attendant bleeding and discomfort (Fig. 6-39). Characteristically, HP are located in the interlabial sulcus (in the grove between the labium majus and labium minus) of the vulva, but occasionally, it develops on the labia majora, the labia minora, the perineum, or in the perianal region. The most common entities in the differential diagnosis are epidermoid cysts and fibromas. The diagnosis may be suggested clinically, especially for nodules located in the interlabial sulcus, but biopsy should be carried out for confirmation.

Hidradenoma papilliferum was originally thought to be an apocrine gland tumor, but it is now known that it is an adenoma derived from anogenital mammarylike glands. As such, HP can be viewed as analogous to intraductal papilloma of the breast. For this reason, it should not be surprising that a high frequency of activating mutations in *PIC3CA* gene, known to occur frequently in mammary intraductal papillomas, are also commonly found in HP.[43] In spite of these mutations, it is essentially a benign neoplasm with only very rare cases of ductal carcinoma found at the time of biopsy. The treatment is surgical excision, and recurrence is infrequent.

## Nodular Scabies

Scabies is primarily covered in the pediatric section of Chapter 15; only the nodular form of the infestation

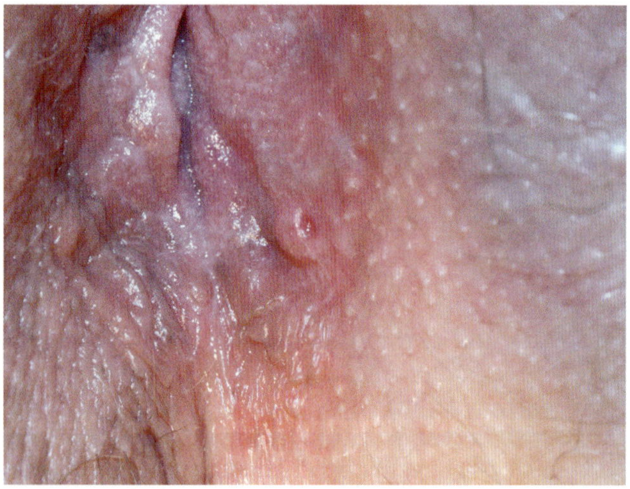

Fig. 6-39. This hidradenoma papilliferum shows the typical location near the interlabial sulcus and the typical morphology of a red papule with a central dell.

will be considered here. Scabies, including nodular scabies, has been recently well reviewed.[44] Nodular scabies occurs as a type 4 delayed hypersensitivity reaction to mite parts, eggs, and feces (scybala). It occurs weeks or months after the initial lesions of scabies are first noted and mostly develops after successful treatment of active disease. Assuming adequate treatment has previously been carried out, these nodules contain no live organisms and thus are not a cause of transmission to others.

The distribution of lesions, however, does not correspond to that of classical scabies as there is a special predilection for lesions to be located on the glans penis, penile shaft, and scrotum of boys and men. The reason for this site and gender predilection is unknown. Nevertheless, nodular lesions can also sometimes develop elsewhere in both sexes. When this happens, the pubic region, groin, buttocks, and axillae are most frequently involved. The lesions of nodular scabies may be papules or nodules or a mixture of both. They are dome-shaped, red to brown-red in color, and are usually 5-20 mm in diameter **(Figs. 6-40 and 6-41)**. Itching is notably intense. As a result, the surface of some of the lesions may demonstrate either scaling, due to long-term rubbing, or erosion because of vigorous scratching.

The clinical features of nodular scabies overlap appreciably with the lesions of PN, and for this reason, these two entities may be clinically indistinguishable. However, a diagnosis of nodular scabies is often suggested on the basis of lesion location, history of previously treated scabies, and urtication (Darier sign) when lightly scratched by the clinician. When the clinical diagnosis is uncertain, biopsy should be performed. Microscopically, mite parts, ova, or feces are usually found in the stratum corneum, and this observation is accompanied by a notable inflammatory infiltrate of eosinophils located in the dermis.

Left untreated, the lesions of nodular scabies may persist for months but do eventually resolve spontaneously.

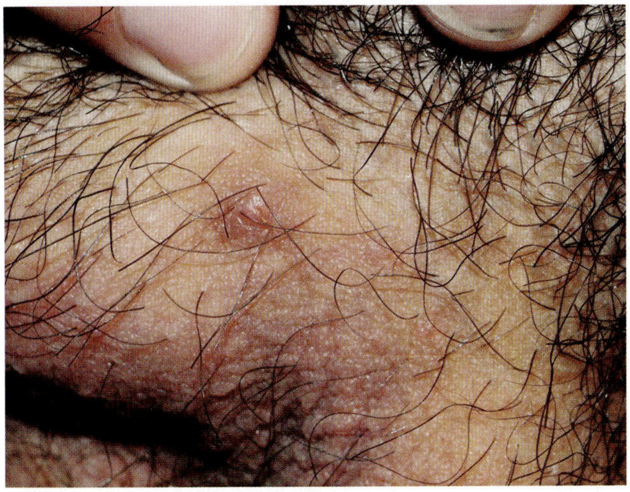

Fig. 6-40. Nodular scabies shows a predilection for the penis, scrotum, and axillae.

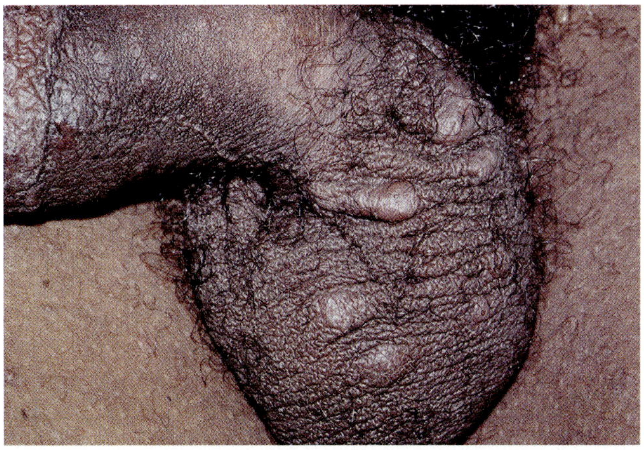

Fig. 6-41. Nodular scabies in patients with dark skin, like other inflammatory conditions in dark skin, often does not show the red color.

Assuming that the patient has been successfully treated for more generalized infestation, repeated application of scabicides or oral therapy with ivermectin is not helpful. The use of high-potency topical steroids or light liquid nitrogen therapy may ameliorate, but seldom abolishes, the pruritus. Improvement in both the pruritus and a reduction in size of the lesions can more reliably be obtained with intralesional injections of 0.2-0.4 mL of triamcinolone acetonide (Kenalog), at a concentration of 10 mg/mL, into each lesion.

## Kaposi Sarcoma

Kaposi sarcoma (KS) is a low-grade malignancy of endothelial cell origin. The lesions of Kaposi sarcoma are dome-shaped, dusky red-brown, or violaceous papules or nodules **(Fig. 6-42)**. Similarly colored, flat-topped patches and plaques may also occur. Nearly all types of cutaneous

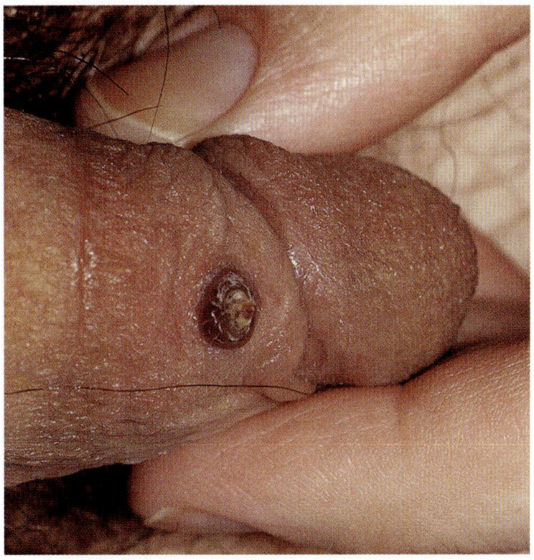

Fig. 6-42. Purple or purple/brown is the most common color of Kaposi sarcoma in a White patient. The setting of HIV makes the diagnosis much easier.

Kaposi sarcoma are asymptomatic. There are four forms of Kaposi sarcoma: (1) HIV/AIDS-related type; (2) "classical" leg involvement in older, mostly Jewish, men; (3) African endemic type; and (4) transplant-related type, all of which appear to be caused by Kaposi sarcoma–associated herpes virus, also known as human herpes virus type-8.[45] Interestingly, and for reasons not well understood, men predominate with all four variations of KS. The most common types of Kaposi sarcoma found in Western countries are those associated with significant immune suppression such as occurs in patients with HIV/AIDS and in those individuals who have undergone organ transplantation. Not surprisingly, the prevalence of Kaposi sarcoma has decreased appreciably in the last decade since the institution of highly effective antiretroviral therapy for individuals with HIV infection.

In Kaposi sarcoma of the immunosuppressed, lesions are most commonly found on the trunk and on mucosal surfaces of the mouth. There is no particular predilection for the anogenital area, but lesions occasionally do occur at this location. Presumably because Kaposi sarcoma occurs more frequently in men, penile involvement is the most commonly reported genital lesion. There are only a very few case reports involving the vulva. Treatment is usually unnecessary for limited numbers of asymptomatic small tumors, but if therapy is desired, individual lesions can be treated with cryotherapy, radiation, surgical excision, or intralesional vinblastine or vincristine.[46] Chemotherapy is desirable and effective for widespread, disfiguring lesions or for systemic Kaposi sarcoma, but use of this treatment falls outside the scope of this book.

## Diaper Granulomas (Diaper Dermatitis of Jacquet, Granuloma Gluteale Infantum)

Many clinicians, including ourselves, believe that the entities listed in the title, together with those known as erosive diaper dermatitis and perianal pseudoverrucous papules and nodules (PPPN), are variants of a single disorder. Regardless of which name is used, lesions occur in the chronically diapered area as discreet flat-topped or dome-shaped papules and nodules. Less often closely set papules may appear as a plaque. Lesion color is quite variable and may be pink, red, brown-red, or violaceous **(Figs. 6-43 and 6-44)**. Because the surface is made up of a hydrophilic thickened stratum corneum, lesions may appear white when they are wet and macerated. The surface of lesions may be intact, eroded, or ulcerated. Most of the papules and nodules are about 1 cm in diameter, but larger lesions are also fairly common. Sparing of the inguinal folds is a characteristic feature. Secondary colonization or infection with *Candida* species happens frequently. This disorder is not commonly encountered in Western countries but is seen with considerable frequency in those areas where chronic diarrhea is rampant.[47]

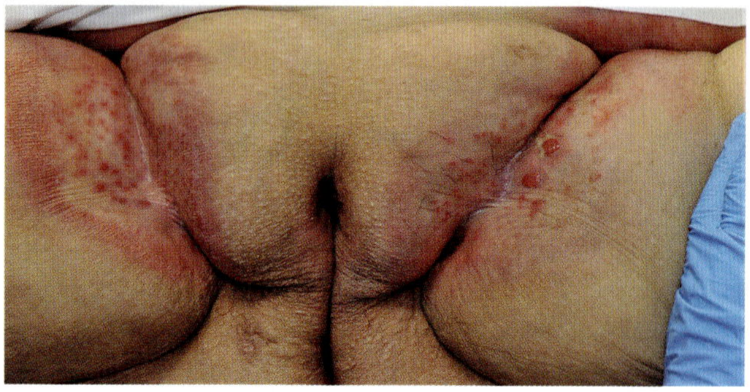

Fig. 6-43. Benzocaine applied to irritant contact dermatitis associated with incontinence has produced these eroded papules in the groin. Although the most common cause of pseudowarts in an adult is the use of benzocaine, this woman has experienced this unusual form of contact dermatitis from constant incontinence.

This condition presumably arises as a calluslike, protective reaction to chronic irritation of skin exposed to a continually wet environment. For that reason, the lesions occur in both diapered infants and in incontinent bedridden and diapered adults. The chronic irritation can be due to urine and/or feces. Rarely, similar problems occur where appliances are attached to the skin at peristomal sites. Conditions such as HPV infection (warts), condyloma lata, nodular scabies, PN, mastocytomas, and Langerhans cell histiocytosis should be considered on one's list of differential diagnoses.[48] The diagnosis is usually made on a clinical basis though biopsy can be considered when it seems prudent to rule out these other disorders.

Treatment requires improvement in the local environment notably obtaining a reduction in the amount and duration of retained urine, sweat, or feces. Skin protective products such as zinc oxide ointment, petrolatum-based products, or topically applied liquid sucralfate are modestly helpful. Controversy exists regarding the usefulness of topical steroids as some clinicians believe that these agents actually worsen the problem and may even play a role in its etiology. This

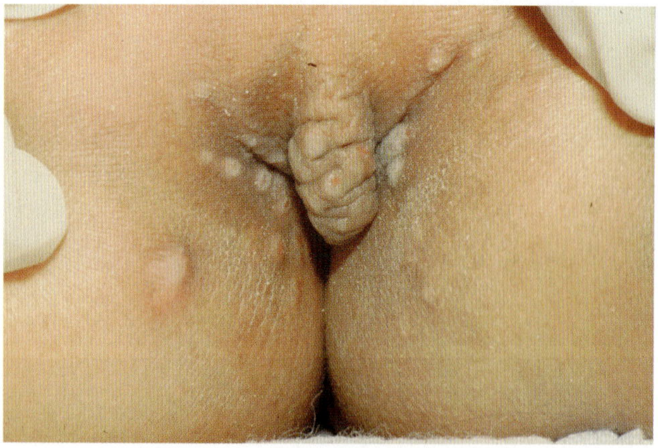

Fig. 6-44. This child with ambiguous genitalia has chronic incontinence, resulting in these eroded nodules of pseudowarts.

author (PJL), however, has found time-limited use of high-potency topical steroids to be helpful. Concomitant anticandidal therapy is usually warranted. Rarely, systemic steroids, administered either orally or intramuscularly, are necessary.

## Langerhans Cell Histiocytosis

Langerhans cells are dendritic antigen-presenting cells that are resident in the skin, mucous membranes, and other organs. Histologically, they are characterized by CD1a, CD207 (Langerin), and S100 positivity. Proliferation of these cells, usually clonal in type, occurs in a variety of conditions varying from single lesions involving only one organ, such as the skin, to widely disseminated systemic disease. These disparate disorders were historically grouped as "histiocytosis X" but are now preferentially categorized as "Langerhans cell histiocytosis." The most common entity of this group (Letterer-Siwe disease) occurs as a disseminated condition in infants and children with skin lesions that commonly involve the anogenital area **(Fig. 6-45)**. It is discussed in the Pediatric section of Chapter 15.

In the less often encountered adult variation of Langerhans cell histiocytosis, skin lesions may develop in the anogenital area.[49] Fewer than 50 vulvar cases have been reported; penile and scrotal cases are even less common. Anogenital skin lesions are quite pleomorphic in appearance. Those developing on or near the genitalia may occur as skin-colored, pink, or red papules, nodules, or plaques. The surface of these lesions may be intact, eroded, or ulcerated. Separately ulcers, often linear ("knife cut") in type, may also be present.

It is important to appreciate that genital lesions may occur as part of already present systemic disease or may be primary in the skin. And it should be understood that some of the patients thought to have lesions that appeared to be primary in the skin subsequently developed systemic disease.[50] For this reason, all patients should be evaluated for potential systemic involvement not only at the time of diagnosis but periodically thereafter. A few instances of malignant transformation have been reported as occurring in residual or recurrent cutaneous disease. Evaluation and treatment of Langerhans cell histiocytosis will not be discussed as this lies outside the scope of this chapter.

## Sarcoidosis

About 25%-35% of patients with systemic sarcoidosis have, or will develop, skin lesions. However, fewer than 20 cases have been recorded in men and women as being present in the anogenital region.[51,52] The cutaneous lesions of sarcoid can occur as papules, nodules, and plaques; the surface may be intact or ulcerated. Cutaneous lesions may be skin-colored, red, brown-red, or even darkly pigmented **(Fig. 6-46)**. They are usually asymptomatic and have a predilection for developing in scar tissue. Biopsy reveals noncaseating (ie, nonnecrotic) granulomas that are typically present in sarcoidal tissue. Sarcoidosis occurring as primary (with no recognized systemic involvement) has been recorded for cutaneous lesions found at extragenital sites, but the patients who have had anogenital lesions (probably because of delay in detection and diagnosis in this location) were found to have systemic disease at the time their mucocutaneous lesions were identified.

## Crohn Disease

Crohn disease in the anogenital area generally presents with ulcers (often of "knife cut" linear morphology), fis-

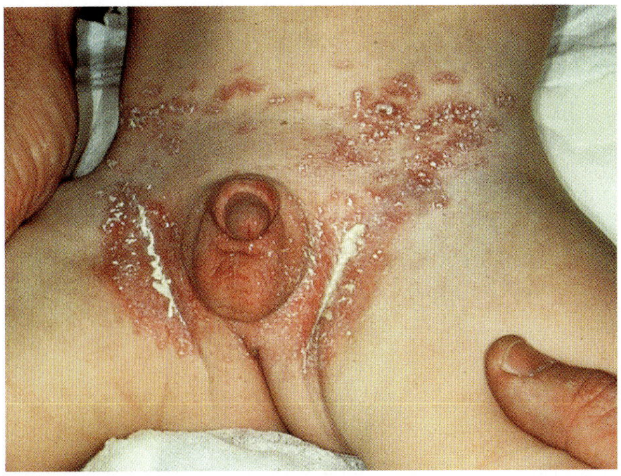

Fig. 6-45. Langerhans histiocytosis is sometimes likened morphologically to seborrheic dermatitis in children; however, the closely set red papules that often have yellowish scale are more indurated.

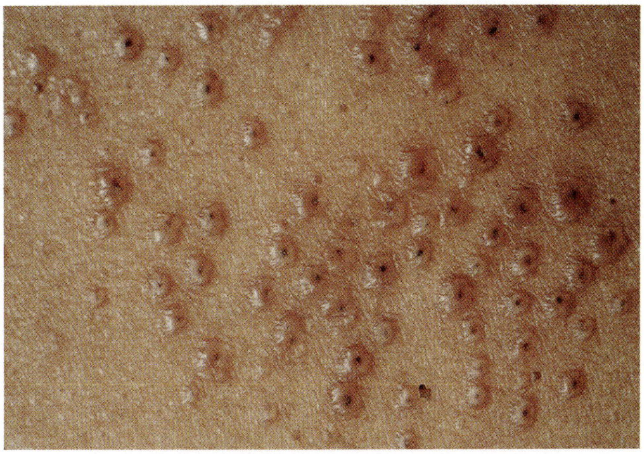

Fig. 6-46. These shiny translucent papules are classic for sarcoidosis, although this condition is famous for its ability to mimic many different appearances and colors.

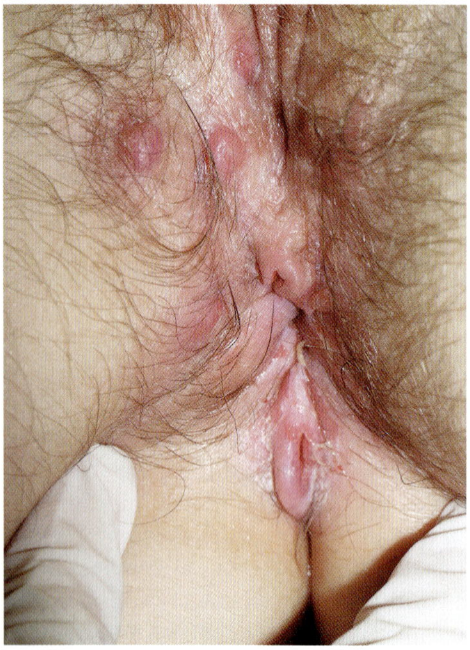

Fig. 6-47. Crohn disease here shows several red nodules, and there is a red nodule around the draining perianal sinus tract or fistula.

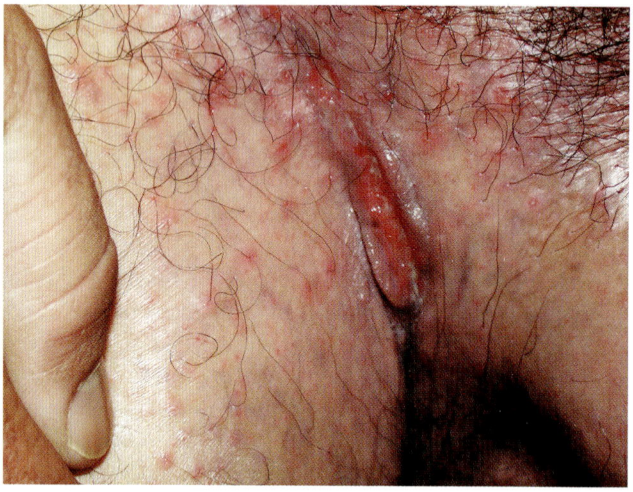

Fig. 6-49. The inguinal crease in this man shows the linear red nodules of Crohn disease surrounding the ulcers.

tulae, and genital edema (**Figs. 6-47 through 6-49**). The primary coverage for Crohn disease is in the Ulcer section of Chapter 11. However, along with these ulcers, there may also be erythematous perianal skin tags as well as dome-shaped red papules and nodules. All of these lesions are quite similar in appearance to those that occur in HS, thus sometimes making it difficult to clinically separate these two disorders.

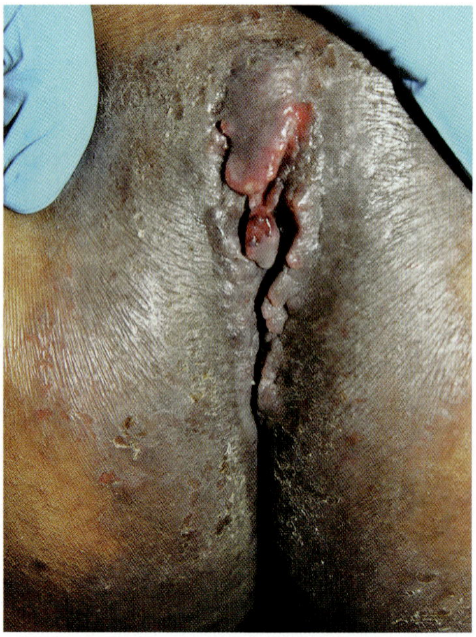

Fig. 6-48. The classic knifelike ulceration of cutaneous Crohn disease shows heaped red borders of Crohn disease.

## Vulvar Sebaceous Adenitis

Sebaceous adenitis (vulvar Fordyce adenitis) is a more recently recognized cause of chronic painful red papules and nodules found primarily on the labia minora or medial labia majora in the area of Fordyce spots (**Fig. 6-50**). Characterized recently in a review of the literature, these papules were found between the ages of 16 and 60, with a median age at diagnosis of 36 years.[53] Occasionally associated with vulvar acne or hidradenitis, this condition is generally treated with a tetracycline such as doxycycline or minocycline, or an antiandrogen such as spironolactone or (not available in the United States) cyproterone acetate. Recalcitrant cases respond to isotretinoin.

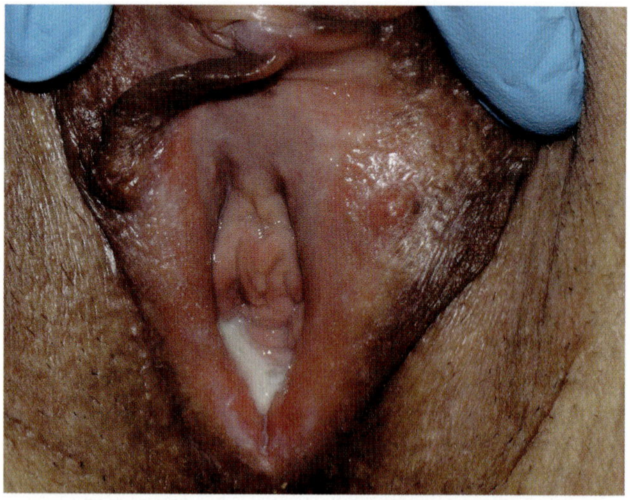

Fig. 6-50. The tender, red nodule on the medial left labium minus is typical of vulvar sebaceous adenitis.

## REFERENCES


1. Wang JF, Orlow SJ. Keratosis pilaris and its subtypes: associations, new molecular and pharmacologic etiologies, and therapeutic options. *Am J Clin Dermatol.* 2018;19(5):733-757. doi:10.1007/s40257-018-0368-3
2. Maghfour J, Ly S, Haidari W, Taylor SL, Feldman SR. Treatment of keratosis pilaris and its variants: a systematic review. *J Dermatolog Treat.* 2022;33:1231–1242. doi:10.1080/09546634.2020.1818678
3. Alexander L, Buckley CJ. Chigger bites. In: *StatPearls* [Internet]. StatPearls Publishing; 2020.
4. Nazer RI, Bashihab RH, Al-Madani WH, Omair AA, AlJasser MI. Cherry angioma: a case–control study. *J Family Community Med.* 2020;27(2):109-113. doi:10.4103/jfcm.JFCM_293_19
5. Liau JY, Lee JC, Tsai JH, Chen CC, et al. High frequency of GNA14, GNAQ, and GNA11 mutations in cherry hemangioma: a histopathological and molecular study of 85 cases indicating GNA14 as the most commonly mutated gene in vascular neoplasms. *Mod Pathol.* 2019;32(11):1657-1665. doi:10.1038/s41379-019-0284-y
6. Buslach N, Foulad DP, Saedi N, Mesinkovska NA. Treatment modalities for cherry angiomas: a systematic review. *Dermatol Surg.* 2020;46(12):1691-1697. doi:10.1097/DSS.0000000000002791
7. Cohen PR, Celano NJ. Penile Angiokeratomas (PEAKERs) revisited: a comprehensive review. *Dermatol Ther (Heidelb).* 2020;10(4):551-567. doi:10.1007/s13555-020-00399-3
8. Alikhan A, Sayed C, Alavi A, Alhusayen R, et al. North American clinical management guidelines for hidradenitis suppurativa: a publication from the United States and Canadian Hidradenitis Suppurativa Foundations: part I: diagnosis, evaluation, and the use of complementary and procedural management. *J Am Acad Dermatol.* 2019;81(1):76-90. doi:10.1016/j.jaad.2019.02.067
9. Alikhan A, Sayed C, Alavi A, Alhusayen R, et al. North American clinical management guidelines for hidradenitis suppurativa: a publication from the United States and Canadian Hidradenitis Suppurativa Foundations: part II: topical, intralesional, and systemic medical management. *J Am Acad Dermatol.* 2019;81(1):91-101. doi:10.1016/j.jaad.2019.02.068
10. Goldburg SR, Strober BE, Payette MJ. Hidradenitis suppurativa: epidemiology, clinical presentation, and pathogenesis. *J Am Acad Dermatol.* 2020;82(5):1045-1058. doi:10.1016/j.jaad.2019.08.090
11. Goldburg SR, Strober BE, Payette MJ. Hidradenitis suppurativa: current and emerging treatments. *J Am Acad Dermatol.* 2020;82(5):1061-1082. doi:10.1016/j.jaad.2019.08.089
12. Sabat R, Jemec GBE, Matusiak Ł, Kimball AB, et al. Hidradenitis suppurativa. *Nat Rev Dis Primers.* 2020;6(1):18. doi:10.1038/s41572-020-0149-1
13. Lacarrubba F, Musumeci ML, Nasca MR, Verzì AE, et al. Double-ended pseudocomedones in hidradenitis suppurativa: clinical, dermoscopic, and histopatho-logical correlation. *Acta Derm Venereol.* 2017;97(6):763-764. doi:10.2340/00015555-2601
14. Patel K, Liu L, Ahn B, Silfvast-Kaiser AS, Paek SY. Hidradenitis suppurativa for the nondermatology clinician. *Proc (Bayl Univ Med Cent).* 2020;33(4):586-591. doi:10.1080/08998280.2020.1793643
15. Revuz JE, Jemec GB. Diagnosing hidradenitis suppurativa. *Dermatol Clin.* 2016;34(1):1-5. doi:10.1016/j.det.2015.08.009
16. Nomura T. Hidradenitis suppurativa as a potential subtype of autoinflammatory keratinization disease. *Front Immunol.* 2020;11:847. doi:10.3389/fimmu.2020.00847
17. Kohorst JJ, Shah KK, Hallemeier CL, Baum CL, Davis MDP. Squamous cell carcinoma in perineal, perianal, and gluteal hidradenitis suppurativa: experience in 12 patients. *Dermatol Surg.* 2019;45(4):519-526. doi:10.1097/DSS.0000000000001713
18. Huckle AW, Fairclough LC, Todd I. Prophylactic antibiotic use in COPD and the potential anti-inflammatory activities of antibiotics. *Respir Care.* 2018;63(5):609-619. doi:10.4187/respcare.05943
19. Folkes AS, Hawatmeh FZ, Wong A, Kerdel FA. Emerging drugs for the treatment of hidradenitis suppurativa. *Expert Opin Emerg Drugs.* 2020;25(3):201-211. doi:10.1080/14728214.2020.1787984
20. Jennings L, Hambly R, Hughes R, Moriarty B, Kirby B. Metformin use in hidradenitis suppurativa. *J Dermatolog Treat.* 2020;31:261-263. doi:10.1080/09546634.2019.1592100
21. Abdalla T, Lowes MA, Kaur N, Micheletti RG, Steinhart AH, Alavi A. Is there a role for therapeutic drug monitoring in patients with hidradenitis suppurativa on tumor necrosis factor-alpha inhibitors? *Am J Clin Dermatol.* 2021;22(2):139-147. doi:10.1007/s40257-020-00579-z
22. Flood KS, Porter ML, Kimball AB. Biologic treatment for hidradenitis suppurativa. *Am J Clin Dermatol.* 2019;20(5):625-638. doi:10.1007/s40257-019-00439-5
23. Maloney NJ, Zhao J, Tegtmeyer K, Lee EY, Cheng K. Off-label studies on apremilast in dermatology: a review. *J Dermatolog Treat.* 2020;31(2):131-140. doi:10.1080/09546634.2019.1589641
24. Vellaichamy G, Braunberger TL, Nahhas AF, Hamzavi IH. Surgical procedures for hidradenitis suppurativa. *Cutis.* 2018;102(1):13-16.
25. Lyons AB, Townsend SM, Turk D, et al. Laser and light-based treatment modalities for the management of hidradenitis suppurativa. *Am J Clin Dermatol.* 2020;21(2):237-243. doi:10.1007/s40257-019-00491-1
26. Thompson AM, Seivright J, Atluri S, et al. Radiotherapy for hidradenitis suppurativa: a systematic review. *Dermatology.* 2021;237:357–364. doi:10.1159/000514027
27. Hatlen TJ, Miller LG. Staphylococcal skin and soft tissue infections. *Infect Dis Clin North Am.* 2021;35(1):81-105. doi:10.1016/j.idc.2020.10.003
28. Nowicka D, Grywalska E. *Staphylococcus aureus* and host immunity in recurrent furunculosis. *Dermatology.* 2019;235(4):295-305. doi:10.1159/000499184
29. Williams KA, Roh YS, Brown I, et al. Pathophysiology, diagnosis, and pharmacological treatment of prurigo nodularis. *Expert Rev Clin Pharmacol.* 2021;14(1):67-77. doi:10.1080/17512433.2021.1852080
30. Huang AH, Williams KA, Kwatra SG. Prurigo nodularis: epidemiology and clinical features. *J Am Acad Dermatol.* 2020;83(6):1559-1565. doi:10.1016/j.jaad.2020.04.183
31. Williams KA, Huang AH, Belzberg M, Kwatra SG. Prurigo nodularis: pathogenesis and management. *J Am Acad Dermatol.* 2020;83(6):1567-1575. doi:10.1016/j.jaad.2020.04.182
32. Holm JG, Agner T, Sand C, Thomsen SF. Dupilumab for prurigo nodularis: case series and review of the literature. *Dermatol Ther.* 2020;33(2):e13222. doi:10.1111/dth.13222

33. Ständer S, Yosipovitch G, Legat FJ, et al. Trial of nemolizumab in moderate-to-severe prurigo nodularis. *N Engl J Med.* 2020;382(8):706-716. doi:10.1056/NEJMoa1908316
34. Moshe M, Levi A, Ad-El D, et al. Malignant melanoma clinically mimicking pyogenic granuloma: comparison of clinical evaluation and histopathology. *Melanoma Res.* 2018;28(4):363-367. doi:10.1097/CMR.0000000000000451
35. Verma V, Pradhan A. Management of urethral caruncle: a systematic review of the current literature. *Eur J Obstet Gynecol Reprod Biol.* 2020;248:5-8. doi:10.1016/j.ejogrb.2020.03.001
36. Fornari A, Gressler M, Murari JCL. Urethral prolapse: a case series and literature review. *J Obstet Gynaecol India.* 2020;70(2):158-162. doi:10.1007/s13224-019-01288-2
37. Corazza M, Schettini N, Pedriali M, Toni G, Borghi A. Vulvar endometriosis. A clinical, histological and dermoscopic riddle. *J Eur Acad Dermatol Venereol.* 2020;34(7):e321-e322. doi:10.1111/jdv.16257
38. Liu Y, Pi R, Luo H, et al. Characteristics and long-term outcomes of perineal endometriosis: a retrospective study. *Medicine (Baltimore).* 2020;99(23):e20638. doi:10.1097/MD.0000000000020638
39. Bellussi F, Cataneo I, Dodaro MG, et al. The use of ultrasound in the evaluation of postpartum paravaginal hematomas. *Am J Obstet Gynecol MFM.* 2019;1(1):82-88. doi:10.1016/j.ajogmf.2019.03.002
40. Lapresa Alcalde MV, Hernández Hernández E, Bustillo Alfonso S, Doyague Sánchez MJ. Non-obstetric traumatic vulvar hematoma: conservative or surgical approach? A case report. *Case Rep Womens Health.* 2019;22:e00109. doi:10.1016/j.crwh.2019.e00109
41. El-Khoury J, Renald MH, Plantier F, Avril MF, Moyal-Barracco M. Vulvar hidradenoma papilliferum (HP) is located on the sites of mammary-like anogenital glands (MLAGs): analysis of the photographs of 52 tumors. *J Am Acad Dermatol.* 2016;75(2):380-384. doi:10.1016/j.jaad.2016.01.034
42. Konstantinova AM, Michal M, Kacerovska D, et al. Hidradenoma papilliferum: a clinicopathologic study of 264 tumors from 261 patients, with emphasis on mammary-type alterations. *Am J Dermatopathol.* 2016;38(8):598-607. doi:10.1097/DAD.0000000000000495
43. Liau JY, Lan J, Hong JB, et al. Frequent PIK3CA-activating mutations in hidradenoma papilliferums. *Hum Pathol.* 2016;55:57-62. doi:10.1016/j.humpath.2016.04.014
44. Leung AKC, Lam JM, Leong KF. Scabies: a neglected global disease. *Curr Pediatr Rev.* 2020;16(1):33-42. doi:10.2174/1573396315666190717114131
45. Cesarman E, Damania B, Krown SE, et al. Kaposi sarcoma. *Nat Rev Dis Primers.* 2019;5(1):9. doi:10.1038/s41572-019-0060-9
46. Etemad SA, Dewan AK. Kaposi sarcoma updates. *Dermatol Clin.* 2019;37(4):505-517. doi:10.1016/j.det.2019.05.008
47. Abu-Alhaija H, Zayed E, Abu-Alhaija B. Anogenital papular lesions in children five year old and younger: gender differences. *Med Arch.* 2020;74(1):28-33. doi:10.5455/medarh.2020.74.28-33
48. Ramos Pinheiro R, Matos-Pires E, Baptista J, Lencastre A. Granuloma gluteale infantum: a re-emerging complication of diaper dermatitis. *Pediatrics.* 2018;141(2):e20162064. doi:10.1542/peds.2016-2064
49. Sirka CS, Sethy M, Rout AN, Sahu K. Langerhans cell histiocytosis of vulva and perineum. *Indian J Dermatol Venereol Leprol.* 2021;87(1):75-77. doi:10.25259/IJDVL_399_20
50. Wieland R, Flanagan J, Everett E, Mount S. Langerhans cell histiocytosis limited to the female genital tract: a review of literature with three additional cases. *Gynecol Oncol Rep.* 2017;22:4-8. doi:10.1016/j.gore.2017.08.005
51. Pereira IB, Khan A. Sarcoidosis rare cutaneous manifestations: vulval and perianal involvement. *J Obstet Gynaecol.* 2017;37(4):539-540. doi:10.1080/01443615.2016.1256964
52. Al-Riyami HA, Al-Kiyumi MH, Al-Harthi RR, Al-Mahrezi AM. Sarcoidosis presenting as a penile lesion: a case report. *Oman Med J.* 2020;35(1):e94. doi:10.5001/omj.2020.12
53. Poizeau F, Plantier F, Bell H, Moyal-Barracco M. Vulvar Fordyce adenitis: a cohort of 45 women. *Ann Dermatol Venereol.* 2021;148:221-227.

## SUGGESTED READINGS

Alexander L, Buckley CJ. Chigger bites. In: *StatPearls* [Internet]. StatPearls Publishing; 2020.

Alikhan A, Sayed C, Alavi A, et al. North American clinical management guidelines for hidradenitis suppurativa: a publication from the United States and Canadian Hidradenitis Suppurativa Foundations: part I: diagnosis, evaluation, and the use of complementary and procedural management. *J Am Acad Dermatol.* 2019;81(1):76-90. doi:10.1016/j.jaad.2019.02.067

Alikhan A, Sayed C, Alavi A, et al. North American clinical management guidelines for hidradenitis suppurativa: a publication from the United States and Canadian Hidradenitis Suppurativa Foundations: part II: topical, intralesional, and systemic medical management. *J Am Acad Dermatol.* 2019;81(1):91-101. doi:10.1016/j.jaad.2019.02.068

Goldburg SR, Strober BE, Payette MJ. Hidradenitis suppurativa: epidemiology, clinical presentation, and pathogenesis. *J Am Acad Dermatol.* 2020;82(5):1045-1058. doi:10.1016/j.jaad.2019.08.090

Goldburg SR, Strober BE, Payette MJ. Hidradenitis suppurativa: current and emerging treatments. *J Am Acad Dermatol.* 2020;82(5):1061-1082. doi:10.1016/j.jaad.2019.08.089

Maghfour J, Ly S, Haidari W, Taylor SL, Feldman SR. Treatment of keratosis pilaris and its variants: a systematic review. *J Dermatolog Treat.* 2022;33:1231-1242. doi:10.1080/09546634.2020.1818678

# Skin-Colored Disorders 7

PETER J. LYNCH

## SECTION A: SKIN-COLORED PAPULES

"Skin colored" refers to those disorders whose color is of the same hue as the patient's surrounding normal tissue. Thus, in a darkly pigmented person, skin-colored lesions would be tan or brown, whereas in a lighter pigmented person, skin-colored lesions would be almost totally nonpigmented or white. Likewise, skin-colored lesions on a pink or red mucosal surface will be pink or red. Skin-colored lesions may be benign or malignant.

### Genital Warts

Genital warts are caused by infection with human papillomavirus (HPV). These viruses cause common benign neoplasms and are significant because of (1) their transmissibility, (2) the association of some HPV types with the development of malignancy, and (3) our current inability to eradicate latent HPV from infected tissue. In contrast with herpes simplex virus (HSV) where there are just two viral types, HSV 1 and HSV 2, there are over 200 HPV types; about one-quarter of which can infect the anogenital region.[1]

### Clinical Presentation

Most anogenital HPV infections occur at a subclinical and asymptomatic level, and only a small percentage (about 10%) of those infected will develop clinical lesions in the form of genital warts and precancerous lesions. *Asymptomatic* anogenital infection due to HPV is extremely common. Most (75%-90%) sexually active individuals will become infected in their lifetime making HPV the most commonly transmitted sexually transmitted disease (STD) agent in the world.[1] Moreover, about 10%-20% of men and women in their 20s and 30s have evidence of HPV infection. This rate decreases with age, declining to about 5% in older persons. Not surprisingly, the rates are even higher in special groups such as prisoners, patients who attend an STD clinic, and men who have sex with men (MSM). On the other hand, the prevalence of *symptomatic* anogenital infection (anogenital warts and precancerous lesions) based on genital examination varies from country to country and is ~0.1%-5% in men and women worldwide. Importantly, there is evidence that HPV vaccination is reducing these prevalence figures.[2]

Human papillomavirus infection is quite transmissible and the major risk factor for acquisition of the virus relates to sexual activity. Specifically, the risk of infection correlates best with age at first intercourse and the number of past sexual partners. Another important risk factor is that of immunosuppression due to HIV/AIDS and organ transplantation.[1] Most HPV transmission occurs by way of vaginal and anal intercourse, but other forms of sexual activity with skin-to-skin contact also result in high transmission rates. In contrast, among children with anogenital warts, probably most transmission occurs through self-inoculation and innocent nonsexual contact. Though the evidence is not conclusive, condom use and male circumcision appear to decrease the risk of transmission.

There are four major morphologic variants of genital warts. Those found in persistently moist areas tend to be skin colored, filiform (eg, tall and narrow) with or without a brushlike tip (Fig. 7-1). This variant is appropriately

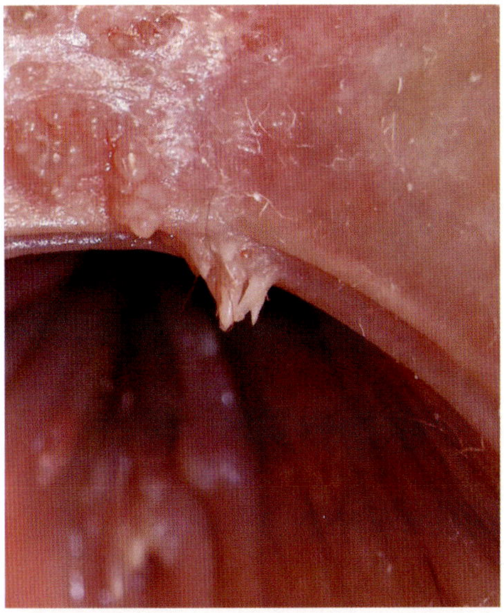

Fig. 7-1. The acuminate, or spiky, shape of this genital wart give the name to the condyloma acuminatum morphology of external genital warts.

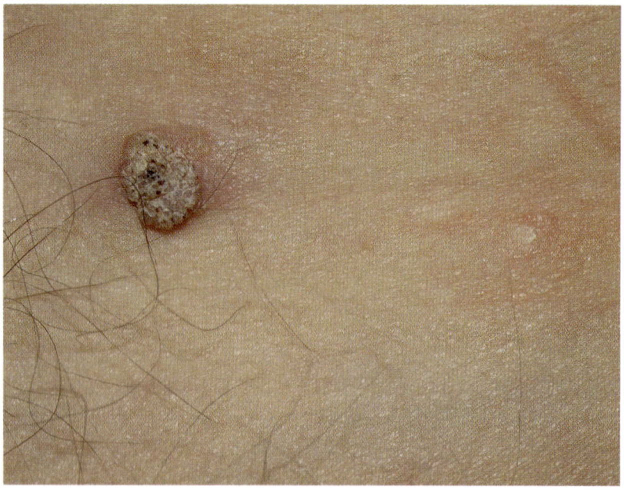

Fig. 7-2. This wart shows the morphology of a common wart; these are found on the dry, more keratinized skin and shows a very rough, keratotic surface.

termed "condyloma acuminatum" (pl: condylomata acuminata) and, strictly speaking, is the only form of warts for which this term should be used. The second variant occurring in the anogenital area is verruca vulgaris (common warts) **(Figs. 7-2 and 7-3)**. These are skin colored and similar in appearance to hand warts. They are about as wide (5-10 mm) as they are tall and typically have palpable, if not visible, surface roughness due to the presence of scale; there may also be a visible brushlike surface on the top of these lesions. They are located on the drier aspects of the anogenital tissue. The third variant is represented as smooth-surfaced, flat-topped, or dome-shaped papules that are wider than they are tall **(Figs. 7-4 and 7-5)**. These are usually 3-15 mm in diameter and can occur on either moist or dry surfaces. While often skin colored, these flat-topped warts may be pink, red, brown, or black. Finally, large globular warts, 2-4 cm in diameter, correspond to the fourth variant **(Fig. 7-6)**. They have a smooth but often cauliflowerlike surface and are skin colored, pink, or red in hue. This type of lesion is often termed a giant condyloma or Buschke-Lowenstein tumor.

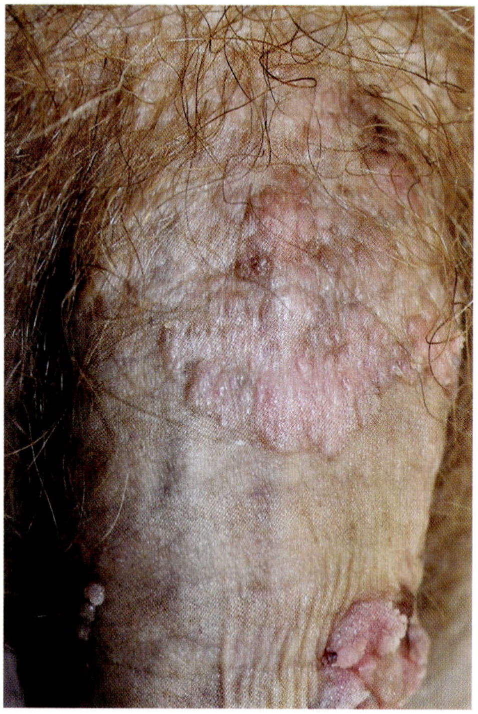

Fig. 7-4. The proximal shaft shows an extensive shaft flat wart.

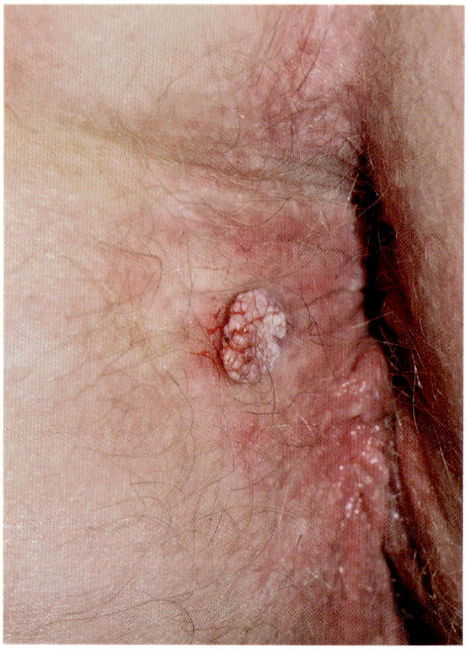

Fig. 7-3. This wart is as tall as it is wide, as is typical of the morphology of a common wart.

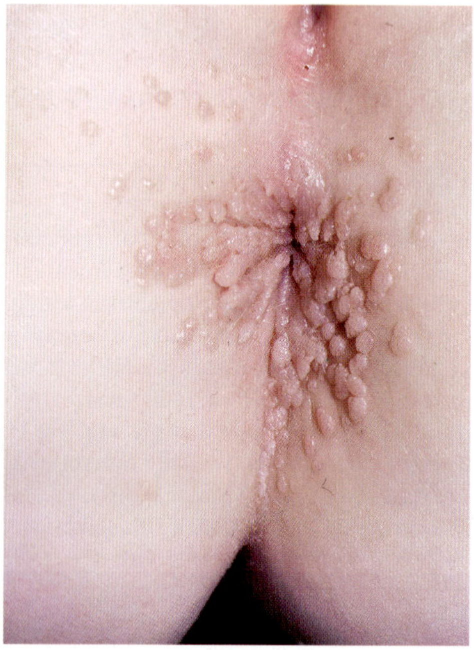

Fig. 7-5. These perianal warts are mostly wider than they are tall, with a smooth surface.

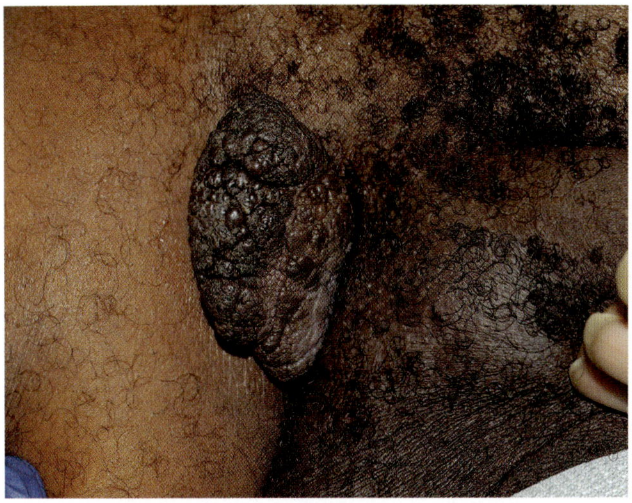

Fig. 7-6. Unusually large, globular warts are called giant condylomata or Buschke-Lowenstein tumors.

Genital warts occur most often in individuals between the ages of 16 and 25 years. Although genital warts are usually asymptomatic, they occasionally produce itching and/or irritation. The number and size of lesions in an infected individual presumably depend on the immunologic resistance that the host can mount against the infecting virus. Thus, some individuals with very good immune response may have only a few small lesions that disappear spontaneously or respond readily to treatment. Other patients with lesser immune response exhibit numerous small and large lesions that can be resistant to most attempts at therapy.

In men, most genital warts occur on the shaft of the penis and, less frequently, the glans, foreskin, scrotum, groin, and periurethral or intraurethral area. Perianal and anal warts occur most commonly in men who have anal coitus with men but also can develop in heterosexual men who do not have anal intercourse. In women, genital warts occur most commonly around the vaginal introitus, the vulvar vestibule, and the surrounding anogenital skin. Approximately half of women with vulvar warts have evidence of cervical HPV infection. Women may develop perianal warts, and, not surprisingly, their presence at this site is especially likely in those who participate in receptive anal intercourse.

## Diagnosis

A diagnosis of anogenital warts is generally made on a clinical basis. However, biopsy is required for two types of warts, described as the third and fourth variants above. These are the flat-topped, smooth-surfaced lesions and the giant condylomata. Histological examination is necessary in these two variants because *in situ* or invasive squamous cell carcinoma (SCC) may be present in these otherwise clinically normal-appearing HPV infections. In an attempt to better identify genital warts, some clinicians apply 5% acetic acid (common vinegar) to the anogenital area for several minutes prior to visual examination. Whitening suggests where warts are present, but we believe that neither the specificity nor sensitivity of this procedure is high enough for this technique to be recommended. Low-power magnification, usually with a lamp containing a centrally mounted magnifying glass surrounded by a circular fluorescent bulb, can be helpful in detecting small lesions. Gynecologists and dermatologists sometimes examine the anogenital area with high magnification using a colposcope or a dermatoscope. Dermoscopic findings have been described as showing a fingerlike appearance with highly vascular-patterned features surrounded by whitish halos.[3] Colposcopy, along with scraping for a cytological specimen, as is true for cervical HPV infection, is especially useful for identifying anal HPV infection. This is particularly true for HIV-positive women who participate in anal intercourse and MSM.[4] I believe, that with this one exception, such highly magnified approach has little usefulness and greatly increases the duration and cost of the examination.

Biopsy can confirm a clinical diagnosis of genital warts, and it is highly recommended under certain circumstances such as for individuals with the third or fourth variants of genital warts. The histologic hallmarks include variable acanthosis often with elongation of the rete ridges. The presence of koilocytosis (vacuolated cells with dark pyknotic nuclei) is particularly helpful. True koilocytosis occurs throughout most layers of the epidermis. Pathologists who are not expert in cutaneous pathology often overcall this feature, failing to realize that scattered vacuolated cells (usually without nuclear change) are normally present in anogenital tissue. About 250 molecular tests for determining the specific HPV type or types are commercially available.[5] Because of the identification of low-risk and high-risk HPV types, there has been slowly increasing enthusiasm over the use of HPV typing. However, at the current time, we believe that treatment and follow-up of patients can largely still be based on the degree of dysplasia, if any, identified on biopsy. Viral cultures cannot be carried out as HPV does not grow in artificial media.

Many conditions must be considered in the list of differential diagnoses for genital warts. In women, vestibular papillomatosis can easily be confused with genital warts. Patients with this condition have closely set, minute, hemispherical papules, arranged in a cobblestone-like pattern, within the vulvar vestibule **(Fig. 7-7)**. This is a normal physiologic variant that needs no therapy. The equivalent disorder in men, pearly penile papules (PPP), consists of one or two rows of minute papules encircling the corona of the glans penis **(Fig. 7-8)**. Other conditions to be considered include molluscum contagiosum, common

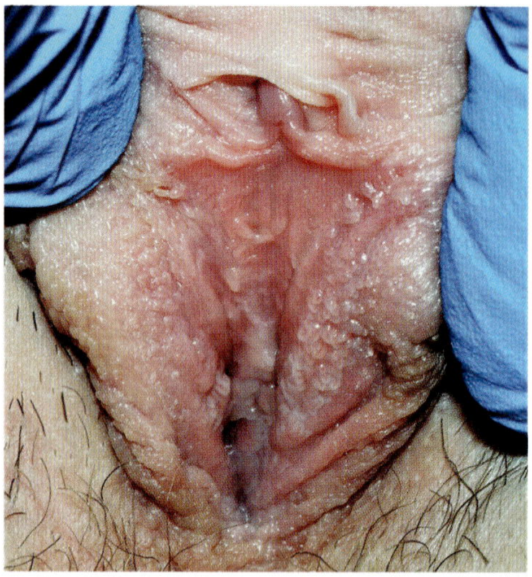

Fig. 7-7. Vulvar papillae resemble genital warts but are differentiated by their rounded rather than spiky tips, and the fact that each papilla is discrete to the base rather than fused as is common with warts.

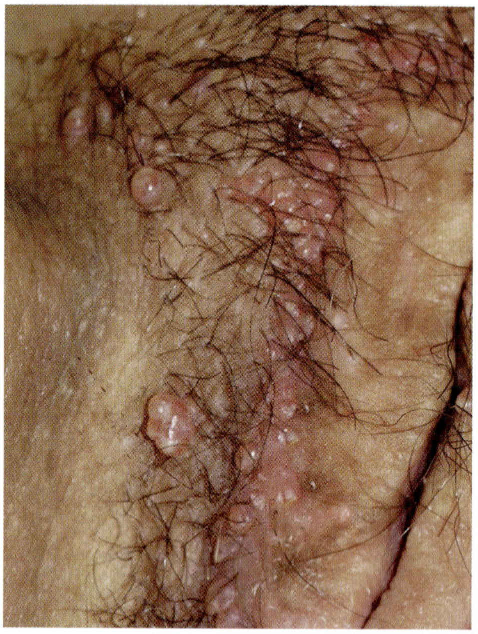

Fig. 7-9. This patient has lymphangiectasias (also called secondary lymphangioma circumscriptum) extruding through the surface of the skin due to chronic edema resulting from pelvic surgery.

skin tags, lymphangiectasia, elephantiasis from chronic edema, and enlarged sebaceous glands (Fordyce spots) (**Figs. 7-9 to 7-12**). As indicated above, both *in situ* and invasive HPV-related SCC may have an identical appearance in the third and fourth variants of warts, flat-topped papules, and plaques or large globular lesions.

## Pathophysiology

Human papillomaviruses are grouped into five genera of which only the alpha and beta genera are important to clinicians. Viruses of both the alpha and beta genera can cause latent (asymptomatic) infections. On the other hand, it is primarily viruses from the alpha genus that are responsible for the vast majority of benign and malignant mucosal and cutaneous lesions (symptomatic infections) in the anogenital region.[1] These alpha papilloma viruses are further divided into "high-risk," "uncertain risk," and "low-risk" categories. Anogenital infection may occur with viruses from any one of these three categories. The average incubation period is about 3 months. Approximately 90% of clinically recognizable infections are due to four HPV types. The vast majority of these are caused by low-risk types HPV 6 and 11, and the remainder are mostly due to high-risk types HPV 16 and 18. It is not possible clinically to determine which of these HPV types represents the cause of genital lesions. Coinfection with multiple HPV types happens fairly often.

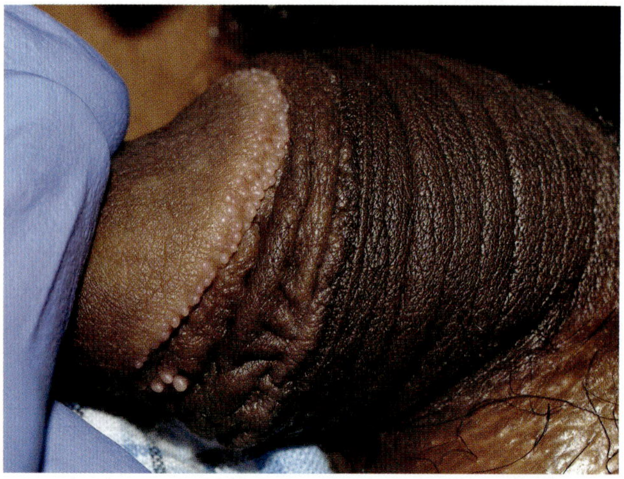

Fig. 7-8. Pearly penile papules are monomorphous skin-colored or white papules arranged in one or more rows around the corona, and seen almost exclusively in uncircumcised men.

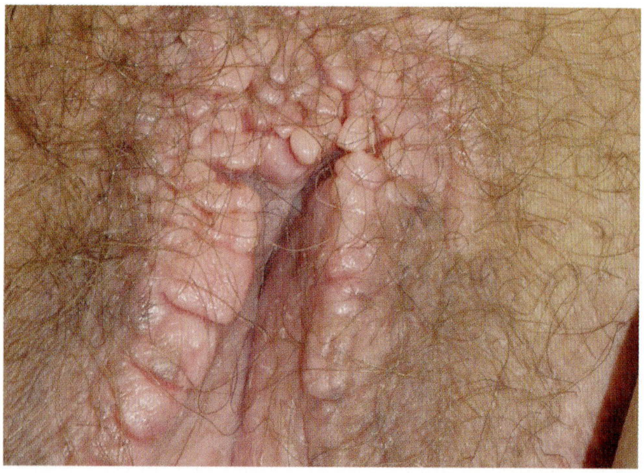

Fig. 7-10. Elephantiasis is a peculiar skin reaction to chronic edema, consisting of firm nodules that can mimic genital warts; this patient had only modest edema on the basis of erosive lichen planus.

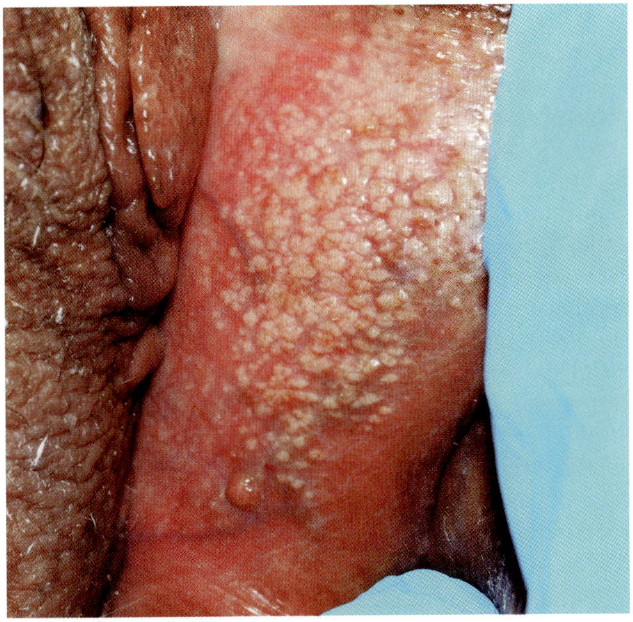

Fig. 7-11. Fordyce spots are ectopic sebaceous glands that are found on the modified mucous membranes of the vulva, here on the medial left labium minus. Although these are regularly found in premenopausal women, this patient has unusually prominent lesions that can be confused with flat warts.

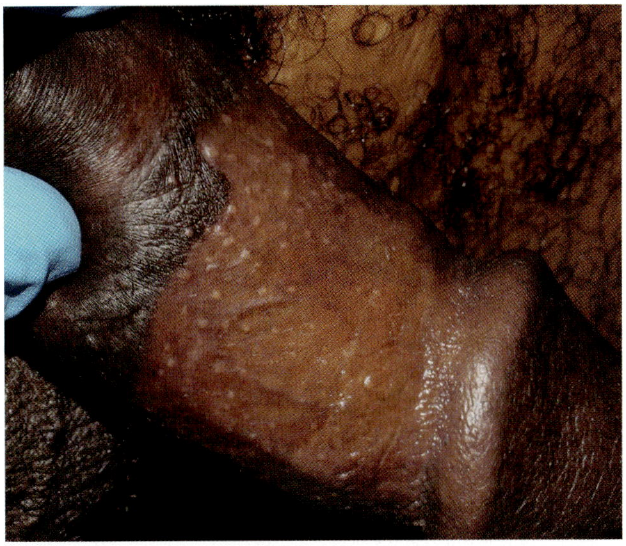

Fig. 7-12. Ectopic sebaceous glands occur on the shaft of the penis as well, seen here as discrete small light papules; he also has hyperpigmented flat warts on the proximal shaft.

**GENITAL WARTS** — **Diagnosis**

- Most commonly occur in sexually active individuals 15-30 years of age.
- Four clinical variants: (1) filiform warts, (2) verruca vulgaris, (3) flat-topped papules/plaques, and (4) large globular nodules.
- Lesions may be skin colored, pink, red, brown, or black.
- Biopsy, especially for the third and fourth variants, is necessary to confirm diagnosis and to rule out malignancy.
- Consider the possibility of cervical involvement in women and anal involvement in both sexes.

## Prognosis

Information on the duration of asymptomatic HPV infections in which no visible lesions are present (by far the most common type of infection) is based mostly on older serological data that involve the detection of antibodies to the HPV L1 protein. Unfortunately, since the virus exists only in epidermal cells above the basement membrane (where only limited antigen processing can occur), these data are highly suspect. However, they do suggest that immune clearance occurs in a matter of a few months for most infections with low-risk virus types and a little longer (about a year) for most high-risk types. But it is also recognized that latency, with a persistent very low viral load, occurs in an unknown percentage of cases. Presumably the likelihood of latency is higher with high-risk virus types and is also higher in those who have some degree of immunosuppression. Clearance also occurs more rapidly in younger individuals than in those who are older, probably based on more robust immune response in young people.

Spontaneous resolution of visible warts occurs when an HPV-specific cell-mediated immune (CMI) response develops. Resolution without treatment, if it is to occur, takes on average several months. Unfortunately, those warts containing high-risk HPV types and those occurring in immunosuppressed patients are likely to remain in place longer or even indefinitely. This CMI response, rather than humoral immunity, appears to be much more important for lesion resolution. This belief is based on four observations. First, the titer and timing of antibody response do not correlate well with resolution of warts; second, many patients with visible lesions are not seropositive; third, many patients who are seropositive do not currently have clinically detectable infection; and fourth, individuals with significantly depressed CMI, notably those with HIV-AIDS, are more easily infected, have larger numbers of lesions, and rarely clear their lesions spontaneously.

## Management

In spite of the potential for resolution, most anogenital warts should be treated to reduce contagion occurring through sexual activity and other skin-to-skin contact. This is particularly important because it is not possible to determine clinically which warts contain foci of dysplastic change. However, it is extremely important to note that treatment only eradicates visible lesions; latent virus can remain in place indefinitely. This leads to high recurrences rates regardless of the type of treatment used.

Before considering treatment options, clinicians should consider whether or not biopsy of one or more lesions should be undertaken. As indicated above, flat-topped warts (regardless of color) and large globular warts should be biopsied because of the possibility that *in situ* or invasive SCC may be present. Shave biopsy is acceptable for flat-topped warts. On the other hand, local excision is preferred for large globular warts for three reasons: deeper penetration (even when there is no dermal invasion); risk of missing true dermal invasion; risk of sampling error in these large lesions. Filiform lesions and those mimicking hand warts (see above) may be treated without biopsy due to the very low likelihood that dysplasia will be present.

Multiple approaches to treatment are available.[6-8] Treatment needs to be individualized for each patient as no single therapy is universally preferable. One of the first priorities in the treatment process is the education of patients regarding the contagious aspects of the viral infection, the likelihood of recurrence after therapy, and, in some instances, the potential for malignant transformation. After this has been accomplished, input from the patient should be sought as to whether the treatment is to be undertaken by the patient (patient-based therapy) or by the clinician (clinician-based therapy). Cost and, in the United States, insurance coverage also should be taken into consideration. Lastly, for clinician-based therapy, availability of equipment and the provider experience will influence the choice of therapy.

*Patient-based therapy.* There are four medications, all requiring a prescription, available for patient-based therapy: 0.5% podophyllotoxin (Condylox), 3.75% imiquimod (Zyclara) or 5% imiquimod (Aldara), and 15% sinecatechins (Veregen). Podophyllotoxin solution or cream is applied to the warts twice daily for 3 days followed by 4 days without treatment. This is usually carried out for 4 or 5 weeks, and note that podophyllotoxin is contraindicated for use during pregnancy. Imiquimod 3.75% or 5% cream is applied once daily two or three times per week (on alternate days) for up to 16 weeks. Sinecatechins 15% ointment (Veregen) is applied three times per day for up to 16 weeks. Adverse effects of redness, burning, pain, and erosion occur with all four of these products. Clearance rates (about 50%-75%) are slightly better with podophyllotoxin; recurrence rates (about 25%-35%) are approximately similar for all four medications.[6,8]

*Clinician-based therapy* can be either medical or procedural. The *medical* approach consists of the application of trichloroacetic acid (80%-90%) carried out very carefully in the office at 2- or 3-week intervals. Clearance rates of 70%-80% have been reported, but recurrence rates are similar to those with patient-based therapy as described above.[7] Burning on application is troublesome for patients, and ulcer formation is possible if too much is applied. Nevertheless, it is a reasonable approach when the warts are relatively nonkeratotic and the number and size of the lesions are small. It has the advantage of not requiring specialized equipment. Another medical approach, the application of 25% podophyllin, is no longer recommended.

Clinician-based *procedural* therapy includes cryotherapy, electrosurgical destruction, laser destruction, and surgical excision.[6] With *cryotherapy*, liquid nitrogen is sprayed (or is applied by probe or with cotton-tipped applicators) at 2- to 3-week intervals. *Electrosurgical destruction* (electrofulguration, electrodessication) is carried out under local anesthesia. Other electrosurgical approaches using loop excision or a bipolar Bovie-type apparatus can also be used. *Laser therapy*, generally with a $CO_2$ laser, can also be considered, but the cost of this equipment, and thus the cost of treatment, is quite high. *Surgical excision* is most often accomplished with a tangential shave or scissors-snip technique; rarely elliptical excision might be considered. All three of these ablative approaches result in clearance rates of close to 90%, but recurrence rates remain high. Drawbacks to procedural therapy include the possibility of secondary infection, potentially long healing time, scarring, and, with all but cryotherapy, the necessity for local anesthesia.

The choice of which medical or procedural approach is taken depends on patient preference and on the experience level of the clinician. For most patients, I (PJL) prefer either electrosurgical destruction or removal with scissors "snip" or tangential shave excision. If bleeding persists, it can be stopped with very light electrosurgery to the base. These two approaches are time honored, inexpensive, and do not depend on patient compliance. Moreover, only a single clinic visit is generally necessary, and the patient leaves the clinic with the knowledge that he or she is free of most or even all of the visible lesions. Of course, if the number and size of the warts are large, staged eradication at monthly intervals may be necessary.

Anogenital warts in children present a special problem because of the concern that sexual abuse may have taken place. However, for children under the age of 2, it is not likely that the transmission occurred through sexual contact.[1] Anogenital warts in these very young children may have arisen through normal parental contact, autoinoculation, or by way of contagion from an infected birth canal. A greater level of concern about sexual abuse exists for those over the age of 4, and in any case, inquiry by an experienced clinician or by other skilled interviewers must be carried for all children with anogenital warts.

## Vaccination

The best approach for HPV infection (and lesions associated with this infection) is to prevent it from occurring in the first place. During the last two decades, three HPV vaccines have been approved in most countries.[9] These include Cervarix, Gardasil, and Gardasil 9. All three vaccines are directed against the HPV L1 structural protein and do not contain any part of the HPV that would allow for viral replication following vaccination.[9]

*Cervarix* is a bivalent vaccine that is directed toward HPV 16 and 18, the two HPV types that are associated with the development of about 70% of anogenital malignancies. *Gardasil* is a quadrivalent vaccine that offers the same protection against HPV 16 and 18 as well as against HPV 6 and 11, the two low-risk types that cause about 90% of benign anogenital warts. *Gardasil 9* is a nonavalent vaccine that is designed to prevent infection from HPV types 6, 11, 16, 18, 31, 33, 45, 53, and 58 thus covering the risk of ~90% of cervical and other anogenital malignancies. Interestingly, though all three of these vaccines were originally approved by the U.S. FDA, Gardasil 9 is the only one currently available in the United States.

All three vaccines are administered by way of three intramuscular injections administered over a 6-month period of time with the second injection given 1-2 months after the first. The third injection is administered at about the 6th month. Although three doses are recommended for adults, there is evidence that for children two doses are sufficient. All three vaccines are preferably given before sexual debut (usually at age 9-11) because the vaccines have no efficacy against their HPV types once infection with them has occurred. Catch-up vaccination (to offer protection against those HPV types that have not as yet been acquired) is recommended for those teenagers and adults who have not been vaccinated earlier.

Safety of these vaccines is excellent with no serious safety concerns having so far been detected.[9] Vaccination is not specifically recommended for pregnant women but appears to be safe when it is administered. The efficacy of HPV vaccination is also excellent. When vaccines are given to those with no evidence of previous HPV infection (HPV-naive group), there is at least 90% prevention of HPV-related anogenital malignancy.[9] And when the quadrivalent vaccine is administered to the HPV-naive group, there is almost complete protection against the development of anogenital warts.[9] Studies have shown that this protection lasts for at least 6-10 years. Unfortunately, in the real world, the prevalence of vaccination, and the lateness in life with which vaccines are often administered, limits the efficacy to appreciably lower protection rates. Female vaccination rates are higher than for men, but fortunately, there is some evidence of "herd immunity" for heterosexual men as the rate of vaccination for women rises.

**GENITAL WARTS — Management**

- Home therapy with imiquimod or podophyllotoxin
- Office therapy with liquid nitrogen or trichloroacetic acid
- Office therapy with electrosurgery, excision, or laser ablation
- Follow-up for recurrences and development of new warts
- Check for sexual abuse in children with anogenital warts
- Prevent infection with vaccination before sexual debut

## Molluscum Contagiosum

Infection with molluscum contagiosum virus (MCV) is common, benign and self-limited. It can be viewed as more of a nuisance than a threat to health or well-being. A review of the subject was published in 2019 and many of the points that follow are related to that review.[10]

### Clinical Presentation

Molluscum contagiosum (MC) is a common infection that occurs primarily in children, and less often, in sexually active older individuals and in those who are immunologically compromised. In children ages 1-4 years, the incidence rates in the United Kingdom and North America appear to be about 0.1%-1.5% per year. The point prevalence rate for children worldwide averages <3% or 4%. Though controversial today, historically, it has been believed that children with atopic dermatitis ("eczema") and those who are frequent swimmers may be predisposed to acquire the infection.[10] Sexual abuse as a cause of MC essentially does not occur. Spread (hetero-inoculation) among children in families is possible but occurs infrequently. Auto-inoculation is also possible. Adults account for only a small portion of all MC infections. The majority of such infections occur in those sexually active young adults and in those who compete in close skin-to-skin contact sports such as wrestling. In addition, individuals who are immunosuppressed either by illness or through immunosuppressive therapy are predisposed to infection together with more numerous and somewhat larger lesions. Infection rates are similar between males and females. Transmission occurs primarily by skin-to-skin contact and is facilitated by damage to the epidermal barrier layer.

The lesions of molluscum contagiosum are skin colored, pink, white, or, occasionally, translucent ("water warts") hemispherical papules 3-8 mm in diameter **(Figs. 7-13 and 7-14)**. Uncommonly, a light red halo forms

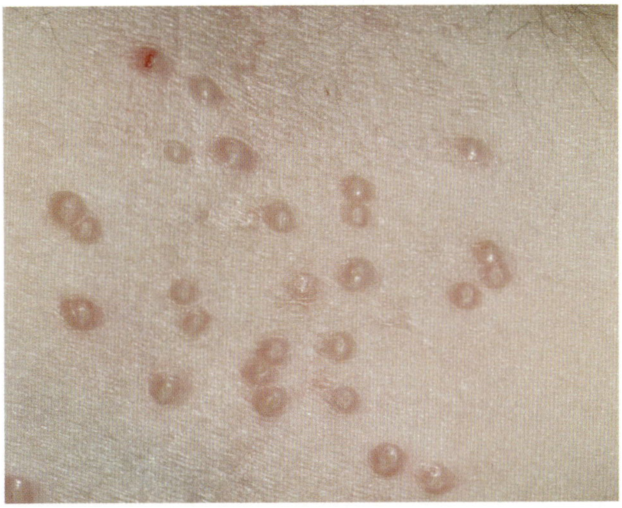

Fig. 7-13. These dome-shaped shiny discrete papules are typical for mollusca contagiosa.

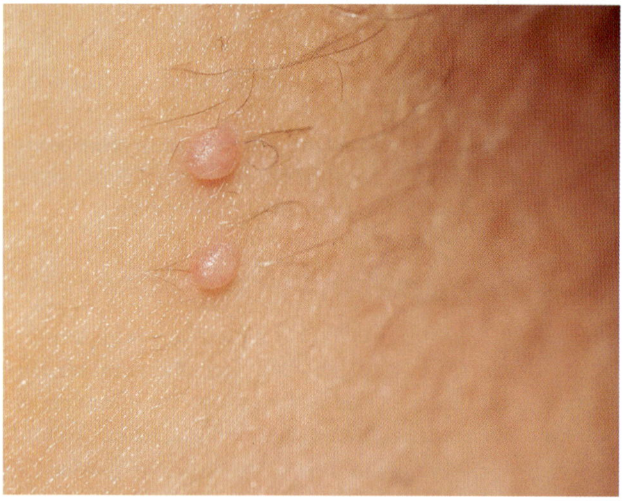

Fig. 7-14. Although providers look for a central dell as a diagnostic sign on lesions of mollusca contagiosa, most lesions do not show this useful hint.

around the molluscum papule.[10] Rarely, and mostly in immunocompromised patients, giant lesions are encountered. Patients with intact immunity generally have 15-50 lesions at any one time; some of these may appear in a clustered group. Most of the lesions develop on keratinizing epithelial skin, but they rarely also occur on mucous membranes. The skin surrounding lesions is usually normal in appearance, but redness and eczematous changes may occur circumferentially.[10] Sometimes early during the resolution stage ("the beginning of the end"), individual MC develop brisk, red inflammation **(Fig. 7-15)**.

The fully developed papules of molluscum contagiosum characteristically have a central depression or umbilication. However, many lesions, especially early and small lesions, lack this feature **(Fig. 7-16)**. Although this umbilication may not be seen in every lesion, a careful examination, especially with magnification, usually allows one to find at least a few of these characteristic umbilicated lesions. Molluscum contagiosum is typically asymptomatic, but some patients may experience low-grade pruritus. Lesions in children may be found anywhere on the skin but occur most often on the trunk. In sexually active women, MC are commonly located on the mons, the medial thighs, and the buttocks. In both genders, they may develop on the genitalia.

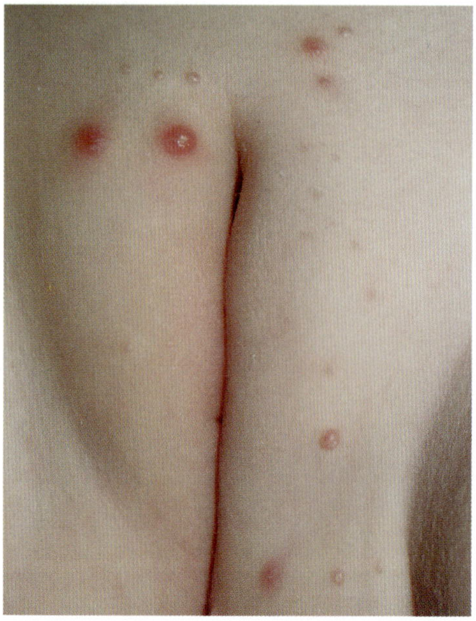

Fig. 7-15. Mollusca contagiosa are not a sign of sexual abuse in children, and the inflamed lesions here suggest that her lesions are entering a resolution phase.

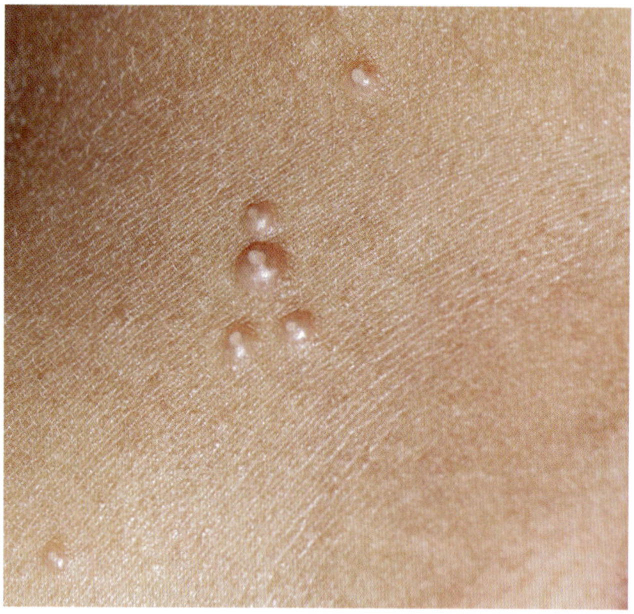

Fig. 7-16. These mollusca contagiosa all show the central umbilication, cinching the diagnosis.

## Diagnosis

The diagnosis, especially when umbilicated lesions are present, is usually made on a clinical basis. Sometimes, the diagnosis can be confusing, and dermoscopy is useful. Magnification enhances the central umbilication and shows polylobular white-to-yellow amorphous structures and peripheral crown vessels.[10] Otherwise, confirmation of a clinical diagnosis is possible through removal of a lesion by curettage with subsequently "mashing" and spreading it out on a microscope slide; this reveals a typical small white "molluscum body." A shave biopsy submitted for microscopic observation may be appropriate if the clinical appearance is atypical. The histologic findings include pathognomonic features of intracytoplasmic inclusion bodies ("Henderson-Patterson" bodies) made up of globular viral proteins.

The list of differential diagnoses includes HPV infection (genital warts), scabies, hidradenoma papilliferum, lymphangiectasia, and, in men, PPP and lichen nitidus. Genital warts are not usually hemispherical and often have a rough, rather than smooth, surface. The lesions of scabies occur in a characteristic distribution pattern (web spaces, axillary folds, areolae, and penis), and small linear burrows can usually be found. The small papules and vesicles of lymphangiectasia contain fluid when pierced with a needle. The lesions in lichen nitidus are more numerous, mostly flat-topped, and more morphologically homogenous. PPP occur only on the corona and sometimes coronal sulcus of the glans penis.

**MOLLUSCUM CONTAGIOSUM — Diagnosis**

- Small, smooth, dome-shaped papules.
- White, pink, translucent, or skin colored.
- Umbilication at the summit is characteristic.
- Bright red color may occur when lesions undergo resolution.
- Confirm by curettage and microscopic examination for a molluscum body.

### Pathophysiology

Molluscum contagiosum is caused by the MCV, which is a very large DNA poxvirus. There are four MCV virus types (c.f. two for HSV and 200 plus for HPV).[10] Most infections are caused by MCV 1; some by MCV 2. Infection due to MCV 3 and 4 is quite rare. There are no significant differences in appearance or distribution for infections caused by the four MCV types. MC infection only involves epidermal cells. As indicated above, transmission is primarily by skin-to-skin contact, but a lesser role for fomites may also be possible. The incubation period after inoculation of the virus averages about 4-8 weeks, but much longer intervals have been reported. Virus latency in epidermal cells does not seem to occur. MCV cannot be cultured using artificial media.

Resolution of the infection is associated with the development of both a humoral and a CMI response. Antibodies to MCV are found in most patients with molluscum contagiosum. However, the timing of antibody appearance and the titer levels do not closely parallel the severity or duration of the infection. One's CMI response is much more important than antibodies in resolving the infection. The onset of the CMI is sometimes clinically apparent by the development of inflammation with accompanying redness in and around individual lesions. Once such inflamed lesions are present, total resolution of all lesions usually follows within about a month.

## Management

In *immunocompetent* patients, untreated individual lesions of molluscum contagiosum resolve spontaneously over a matter of several months. But, "seeding" of virus into surrounding skin or at distant sites frequently occurs such that new lesions develop while old ones are resolving. The total duration of the entire infection averages about 2 years; however, considerably shorter and longer time frames (such as 12-36 months) have been reported. On the other hand, in *immunocompromised* persons, the number of lesions is larger, the variability in size is greater and spontaneous resolution takes much longer or may not occur at all. Secondary bacterial infection is possible, but it is often "overcalled" because of the CMI-related reddening before spontaneous resolution or because of induced inflammation following treatment.

All of the treatments currently available are controversial or problematic in one way or another. Specifically, there is no evidence-based consensus as to what constitutes the best treatment.[10,11] For this reason, most clinicians advise "watchful waiting" rather than active therapy, especially for pediatric patients. For adults and for patients who insist on treatment, both medical and procedural approaches are possible.

### Office Medical Management

Cantharidin 0.9% solution is applied very carefully to individual papules in order to prevent contact with the normal surrounding skin. Special care must be taken if cantharidin is used in intertriginous areas so as to prevent unwanted secondary bacterial infection or spread of the applied solution. For lesions in the anogenital area, it is useful to apply a loose bandage (such as a Band-Aid) over treated lesions to prevent spread of the cantharidin due to friction and retained sweat. Many clinicians advise that the cantharidin be washed off 6-8 hours after application, but I (PJL) have not found it necessary to do so. In any event, a blister develops within 24 hours at the cantharidin application site and the lesion is eventually sloughed off about a week later when the blister roof peels away. Because new lesions will likely continue to appear, several office visits for repeated applications are usually necessary. Cantharidin is painlessness when initially applied, and for this reason, it is most often the treatment of choice for children. Mild pain and irritation may occur later. The clearance rate for individually treated lesions approaches 100%, and patient (or parent) satisfaction is quite high.

Trichloroacetic acid 85% solution can be applied, but even more carefully, so that the solution does not run off of the papule onto normal skin, causing necrosis and possible scaring. This approach is quite effective, but it is somewhat painful within moments of application. All treated lesions are likely to be destroyed with a single application, but several treatments will be required for new lesions as they appear.

### Home Medical Management

Five percent imiquimod cream may be used at home, and the method in which it is used is identical to that described in the section above on genital warts. Home application decreases patient embarrassment for MC occurring in the anogenital area and also reduces the number and expense of multiple office visits. However, this therapeutic approach is accompanied by considerable discomfort due to inflammation at the application site. Moreover, the duration of treatment required is long enough to hamper patient compliance. Finally, there is even some controversy as to whether or not imiquimod therapy actually out-performs its vehicle and thus may be just a placebo.

Potassium hydroxide (KOH), usually in a concentration of 10%, can also be applied to individual MC papules at home. The recommended frequency of application varies from once every other day to twice a day. In any event, it is applied until inflammation occurs. It appears that 10% KOH solution and imiquimod are about equally effective and are about equally irritating. Perhaps, the effectiveness of both depends on the inflammation they cause, which might in turn initiate the cell-mediated immunity that results in clearing the infection.

Many other medical approaches are possible, but limited experience with them and a lack of studies regarding their effectiveness restrict our recommendation for their use. Some of these, which will not be further discussed, include podophyllotoxin, glycolic acid, lactic acid, salicylic acid, retinoids, benzoyl peroxide, tea tree oil, injected interferon alpha, and oral cimetidine.

### Procedural Management

The most commonly used procedural approaches are cryotherapy and curettage. Liquid nitrogen cryotherapy is used in the same manner as is used for warts (q.v. "Genital Warts" in this chapter). It can be applied using a spray technique or with a probe and is available in most gynecology and almost all dermatology offices. A total freeze time of about 10-15 seconds is recommended, and this can be obtained either in a single freeze or in a freeze-thaw-freeze cycle. It is moderately painful and moderately effective, but as for all therapy, several visits are necessary to treat new MC as they develop.

Curettage, in which the lesion is scraped away with the edge of a skin curette, is also moderately painful, but the fact that all visible lesions are completely removed after the first treatment session leads to high patient satisfaction. Because of discomfort, both cryotherapy and curettage are best used for adults, especially when the number of lesions is small. In the hands of a skilled operator, the likeliness of adverse effects such as scaring is quite small.

Several other procedural approaches are available. Electrosurgery is very effective, but use of this approach is limited because MC are very superficial and, unfortunately, destruction depth with electrosurgery is somewhat difficult to control. Thus, this procedure is associated with some potential for secondary infection and scaring. Laser therapy is likewise quite effective, but its use is also restricted due to high cost and limited availability.

**MOLLUSCUM CONTAGIOSUM — Management**

- Consider observation without specific therapy in children.
- Office application of cantharidin is painless and effective.
- Liquid nitrogen cryotherapy if lesion number is large.
- Curettage for removal if lesion number is small.
- Imiquimod cream or potassium hydroxide can be considered for home therapy.

## Skin Tag (Acrochordon, Fibroepithelial Polyp)

Skin tags are common benign skin growths that affect at least half of the adult population. They begin to develop in midlife or earlier in those who are overweight. They then slowly increase in number until about age 70.[12] Small lesions are usually referred to as skin tags, whereas large lesions may be termed fibroepithelial polyps (**Figs. 7-17 and 7-18**). People with obesity, lipid disorders, acanthosis nigricans, darker skin pigmentation, and diabetes mellitus appear to be predisposed to develop skin tags.[13]

Skin tags (acrochordons) are soft, asymptomatic, skin-colored to tan papules. They are most commonly stalk-like lesions averaging 2 mm in diameter and 3-8 mm in length; they have a predilection to occur in the axillae, around the neck, and on the trunk. Small skin tags are usually numerous and somewhat clustered. Longer, larger skin tags (fibroepithelial polyps) are pedunculated with a thin (1-3 mm) base and larger (5-15 mm) body. These larger, often solitary fibroepithelial polyps are more likely to be found on the upper inner thighs, inguinal creases,

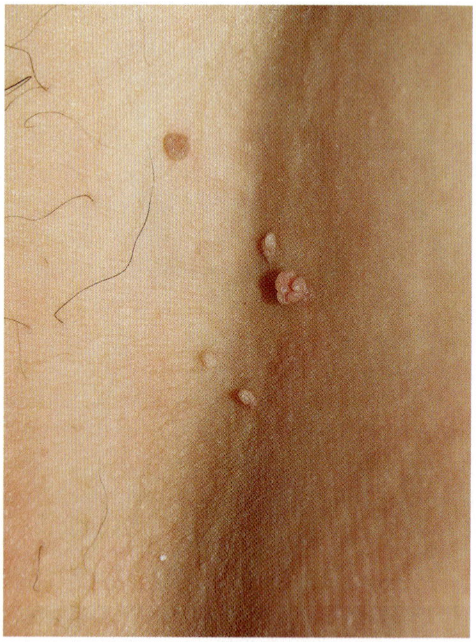

Fig. 7-17. Skin tags are small, fleshy, pedunculated papules that occur primarily in skin folds and are especially common in patients who are overweight.

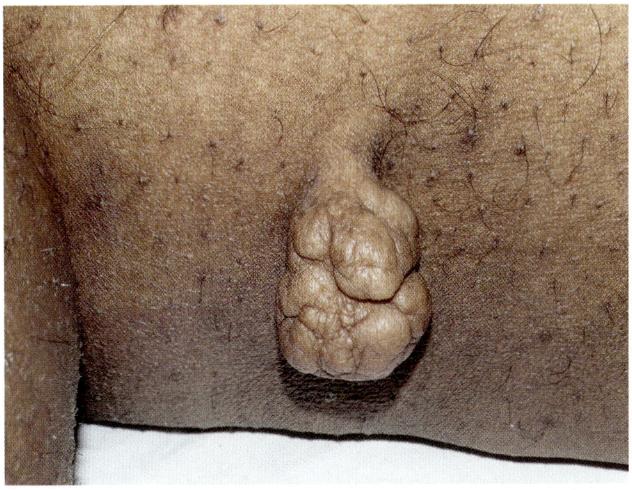

Fig. 7-18. A fibroepithelial polyp is a large, usually solitary skin tag.

and the buttocks. Skin tags are only rarely encountered on the penis and vulvar vestibule. Note, however, that skin tags (especially larger and edematous ones) are found more often than would be expected in patients with inflammatory bowel disease, especially those with Crohn disease.[14]

The diagnosis of skin tags is made on a clinical basis. Rarely, they may be confused with genital warts, intradermal nevi, and isolated neurofibromas. Skin tags are always benign, and no treatment is necessary unless they become inflamed because of skin friction, spontaneous torsion, or having been caught in clothing. In this situation, the lesions can be snipped with fine scissors. The slight bleeding that occurs can be stopped by the application of Monsel (ferric subsulfate) solution, aluminum chloride, or light electrosurgery. Silver nitrate is not a good choice for hemostasis because of the potential for skin staining. Very small skin tags can be obliterated by liquid nitrogen cryotherapy, cautery, or light electrodessication. There is an effective, but seldom recommended, home remedy in which a thread is tied tightly around the base of a lesion. A week or so later, the skin tag undergoes necrosis and both it and the ligature fall off.

## Intradermal Nevi (Dermal Nevi)

Intradermal nevi are benign neoplasms. They differ from junctional and compound nevi clinically by their lighter color and histologically by the location of the nevus cells (melanocytes) only within the dermal connective tissue. They present as soft, usually hemispherical, papules 5-15 mm in diameter **(Fig. 7-19)**. Color is variable, and they can be skin-colored, pink, or light tan. Intradermal nevi rarely occur on the penis, scrotum, or within the vulva but are encountered fairly commonly on the thighs, buttocks, and in the pubic area. These lesions need to be differentiated from basal cell carcinomas (BCCs), genital warts, molluscum contagiosum, and isolated neurofibromas.

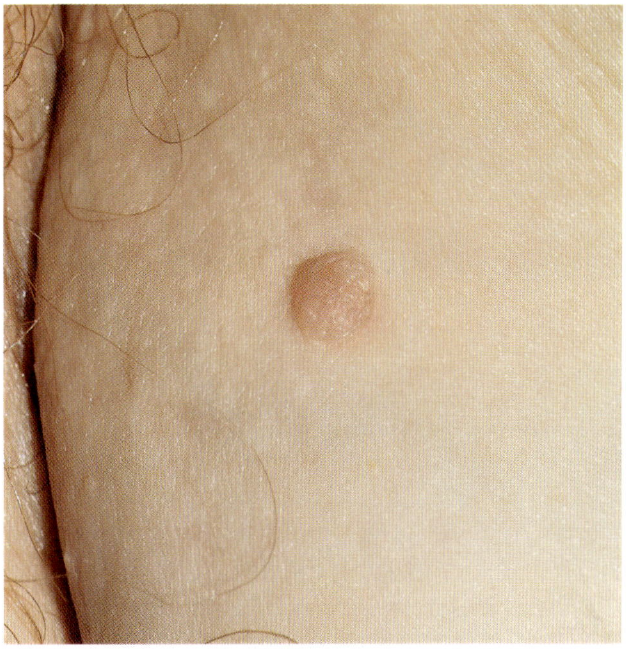

Fig. 7-19. Intradermal nevi are benign tumors of melanocytes, but these generally are skin colored, well demarcated, and soft to the touch.

In some instances, they are pedunculated enough to be confused with skin tags. They are always benign and are never precursors of melanoma. No treatment is necessary unless they are inflamed as a result of trauma. If removal is necessary, they can be shaved tangentially or excised.

## Pearly Penile Papules

Pearly penile papules are so common as to be considered a normal variant rather than as a disease (see also Chapter 1).[15] They are estimated to be present in about 25% of men, but their prevalence is higher in both uncircumcised and African American men. These papules may appear as early as at puberty, and their prevalence generally increases until the third decade of life. Although they are asymptomatic and completely benign, their presence may cause anxiety because of concern on the part of the patient, or the sexual partner, that they represent a STD. PPP are small, skin-colored, whitish, or pink papules that can be either elongated (filiform) or dome shaped (**Figs. 7-8 and 7-20 to 7-22**). The smallest lesions are only about 1 mm in diameter and height, while larger filiform lesions can be 2 mm wide and up to 4-5 mm in length. They are most commonly located on the dorsal corona of the penis, but they often entirely encircle the glans. A single row of lesions may be present, but it is not uncommon to encounter double or triple rows. Less often, they occur in the coronal sulcus or even on the distal shaft of the penis.

The diagnosis is made on the basis of the characteristic morphology and location. Dermoscopy shows a whitish pink cobblestoned or grapelike appearance with

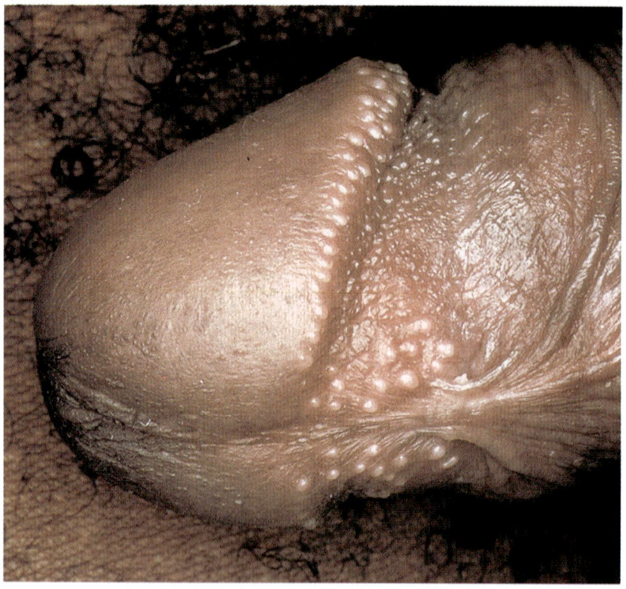

Fig. 7-20. The patient with pearly penile papules has papules clustered around the frenulum as well as around the corona.

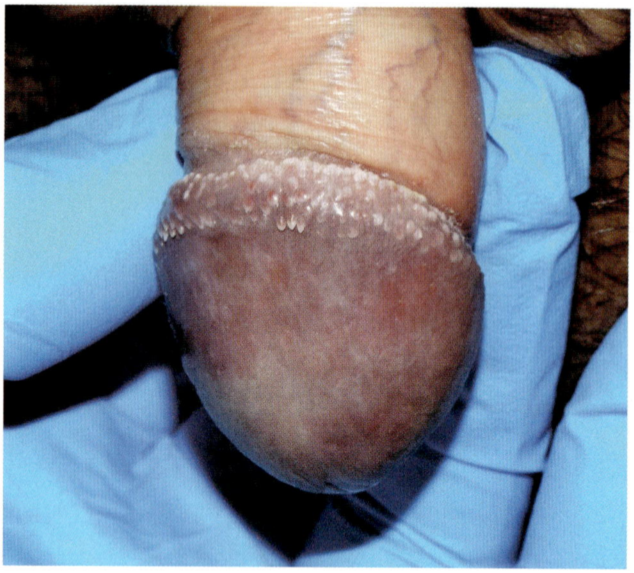

Fig. 7-22. Both dome-shaped papules and filiform lesions are evident in this man with pearly penile papules.

central dotted or commalike vessels in each papule.[16] They should be differentiated from enlarged sebaceous glands that occur on both the inner prepuce (Tyson glands) and on the distal shaft of the penis (Fordyce spots). Occasionally biopsy, demonstrating angiofibromatous histology, is needed to differentiate PPP from filiform genital warts. Treatment is unnecessary, but if the patient or the sexual partner is troubled by their presence, they can be destroyed with electrosurgery, cryotherapy, or laser ablation.[15]

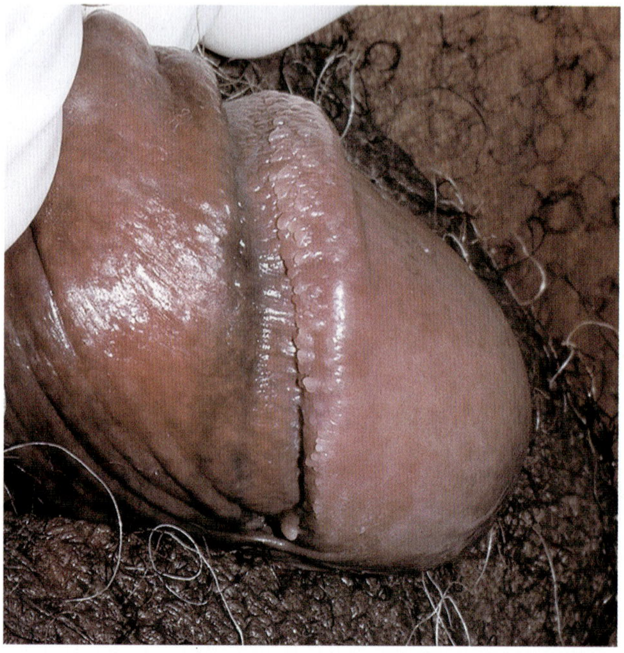

Fig. 7-21. These skin-colored, small pearly penile papules are found in a significant minority of uncircumcised men but are often subtle and overlooked.

## Vulvar Vestibular Papillomatosis

Vulvar vestibular papillomatosis (VVP) is a normal anatomic variant and can be considered as the analogue of PPP in the male.[17] Early publications described a prevalence of only 1%, but later reports, and our own clinical experience, indicate that VVP occurs in about one-third of premenopausal women (see also Chapter 1). The papillae are asymptomatic, soft, hemispherical, or slightly elongated papules with a diameter and height of about 1-2 mm. However, some filiform lesions may be as tall as 5 mm. The papules are pink or red and, as such, similar to the color of the vestibular tissue from which they arise. Sometimes only a few papules are present, but it is not uncommon to see 50-100 clustered such that the entire vestibule is carpeted with them (**Figs. 7-7, 7-23 and 7-24**).

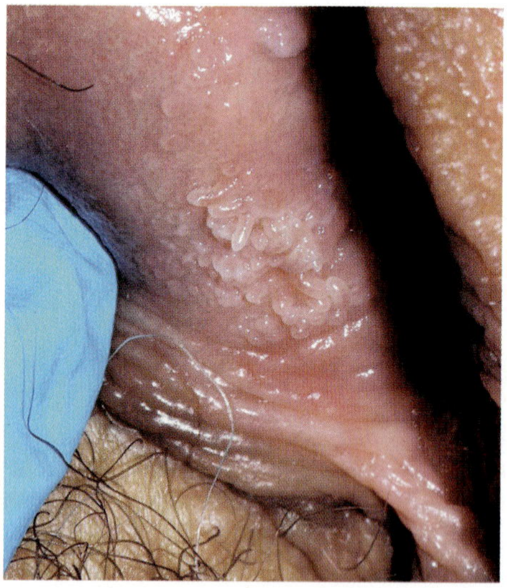

Fig. 7-23. These vestibular papillae have the typical dome-shaped tips and lesions that are discrete to the base.

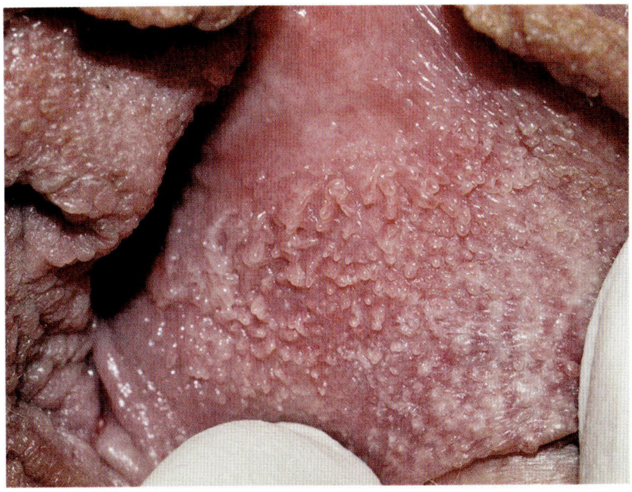

Fig. 7-24. Although these papillae are called vulvar vestibular papillae, they occur on other areas of the modified mucous membranes as well; these cover the medial labia minora.

The papules may be arranged in a cobblestone pattern, but often, on close inspection, they can be observed as occurring in linear rows **(Fig. 7-25)**.

The papules in vestibular papillomatosis must not be confused with vestibular genital warts, as indeed they were until about 30 years ago. Clinical differentiation from genital warts is based on the following characteristics of VVP: (1) the overall appearance is very homogenous with each papule being very similar in morphology to its neighbors; (2) the papules remain separate and discrete down to their base; (3) the papules are soft to touch; and (4) a linear pattern of arrangement can often be discerned. Early on, the confusion with genital warts was engendered by reports that HPV DNA was sometimes present within the papules. Today, however, there is consensus, based on special histological staining and molecular studies, that HPV DNA is present no more often than it is found in vestibules of women with no VVP.

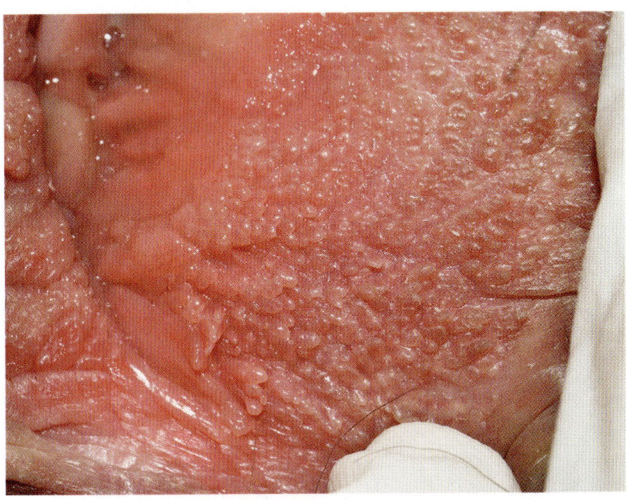

Fig. 7-25. Vulvar papillomatosis sometimes consists of smaller, dome-shaped, nearly confluent papules that confer a cobblestoned appearance to the skin.

The diagnosis is made clinically and is assisted, if necessary, by magnification via dermoscopy, colposcopy, or reflectance confocal microscopy. Dermoscopy shows profuse and irregular vascular channels in multiple cylindrical filiform projections.[17] But if biopsy is performed, the clinician (and the pathologist) should be aware that large cells, somewhat resembling the koilocytes found in genital warts, are present in normal mucosal epithelium. This sometimes results in an incorrect diagnosis of HPV infection. The papules of VVP should also be differentiated from ectopic sebaceous glands (Fordyce spots), which are fewer in number, less elevated, and more yellow in color. Because the lesions are asymptomatic, no treatment needs to be undertaken.

## Fordyce Spots, Fordyce Granules, Tyson Glands, and Sebaceous Gland Hyperplasia

All four of these entities consist of sebaceous glands. Ectopic sebaceous glands are found primarily on mucosal surfaces where pilosebaceous units do not ordinarily exist. They were originally termed Fordyce spots, Fordyce granules, and, on the modified preputial mucosa of the penis, Tyson glands.[18] Sebaceous gland hyperplasia, on the other hand, occurs as either ectopically or nonectopically placed large glands.[19] In any event, all four of these entities consist histologically of sebaceous lobules that are not attached to fully formed hair follicles as occurs with usual normal sebaceous glands. In our opinion, all of these occur on the genitalia much more commonly than suggested by the scarcity of published reports.

Fordyce spots and Fordyce granules are synonyms for small (1-3 mm), often clustered, dome-shaped papules that develop on the mucosal surfaces of the lips, the vulvar vestibule, and the non–hair-bearing portion of the penis (**Figs. 7-11, 7-12, and 7-26 to 7-29**). Tyson glands are similarly sized and shaped, clustered papules on the modified mucosal, inner surface of the prepuce. They all at first appear to have the same color as the surrounding tissue, but if the tissue surrounding them is stretched, they become more apparent and take on a more yellow-white hue.

The papules of sebaceous gland hyperplasia are larger, solitary papules that occur on the face (forehead, cheeks, and nose), areolae of the breasts (Montgomery tubercles), labia minora, labia majora, and the shaft of the penis. They average 5-10 mm in diameter and often appear umbilicated (dimpled) owing to the infundibulum (pore) into which the enlarged sebaceous lobules empty. They are usually skin colored but sometimes display a yellow-white color.

All of these sebaceous gland entities are completely benign, and they are for the most part asymptomatic. However, pruritus or pain may develop when patients are overly concerned about contagion or malignancy. Diagnosis is almost always possible on a clinical basis; biopsy will provide a conclusive answer if doubt occurs. Reassurance is usually all that is needed, but destruction or excision can be performed if necessary.

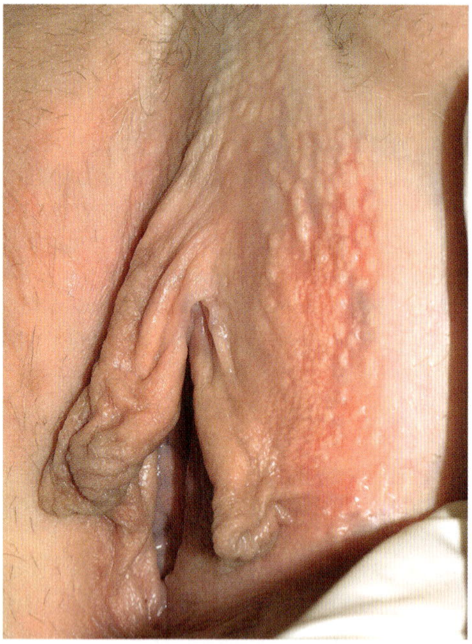

Fig. 7-26. Most prominent on the medial labia minora, Fordyce spots appear as skin-colored or yellowish flat papules.

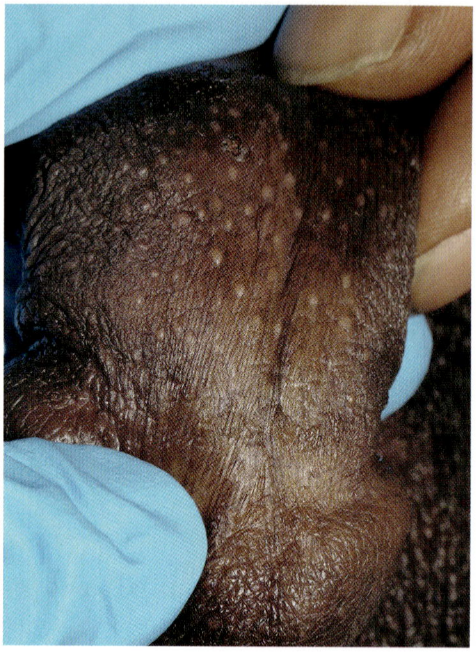

Fig. 7-28. The Fordyce spots are more obvious when the skin is stretched.

## Fox-Fordyce Disease (Apocrine Miliaria)

Fox-Fordyce disease (FFD) is an uncommon, usually pruritic, chronic inflammatory condition of apocrine gland–bearing hair follicles. FFD should not be confused with the similarly, eponymously termed sebaceous gland entities described in the section above. A thorough review has recently been published.[20] More than 90% of the reported cases have occurred in women. Interestingly, in nearly all of these women, onset developed at puberty with marked improvement or resolution at menopause. Moreover, most patients experienced perimenstrual flares and improved with pregnancy. A few familial cases have been reported.

Individual lesions are somewhat monotonous-appearing, dome-shaped follicular papules. In most affected

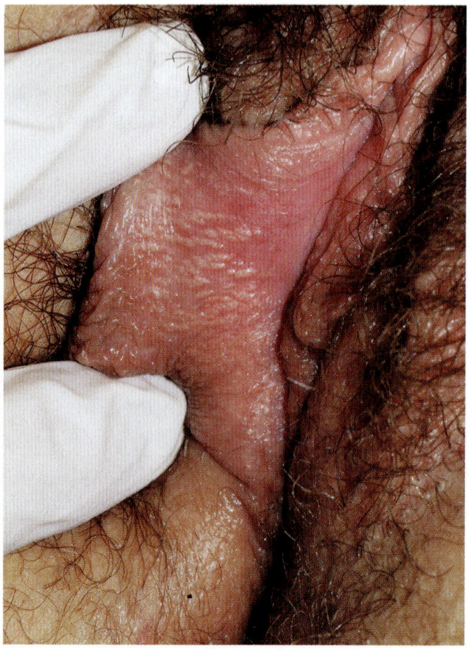

Fig. 7-27. Fordyce spots disappear at menopause unless estrogen is replaced; sometimes these lesions can be linear.

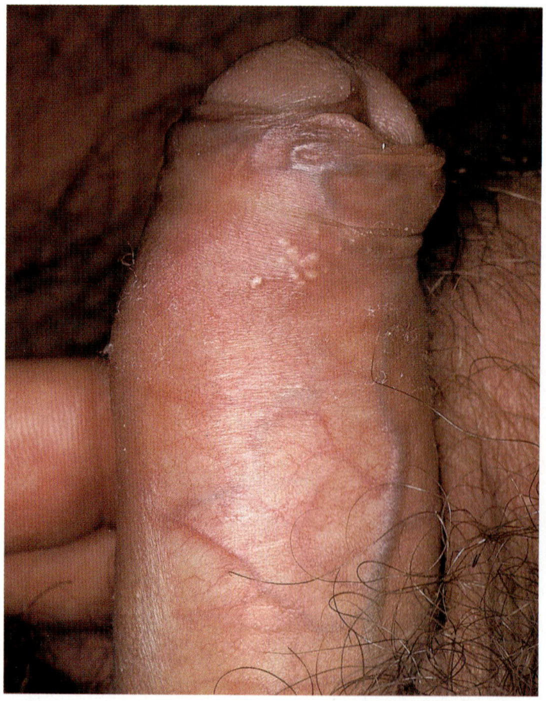

Fig. 7-29. Fordyce spots can be more subtle on more light-complexioned skin.

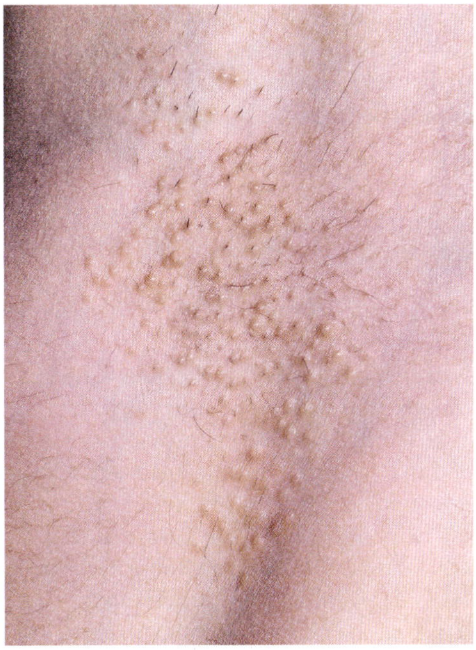

Fig. 7-30. Fox Fordyce disease exhibits dome-shaped, monomorphous, pruritic skin-colored papules in the axillae and genital area.

individuals, the papules are skin colored, but occasionally, yellow or brown hues are present. These papules are distinctive in that they are discrete and are clustered equidistantly apart and in what has been termed a cobblestone pattern. They are almost always located at sites where apocrine glands naturally occur thus, in decreasing frequency, are located in the axillae, pubic region, around the mammary areolae, and over the sternum **(Fig. 7-30)**. Somewhat surprisingly, Fox-Fordyce disease does not commonly occur on the genitalia.[21]

The diagnosis is generally possible on a clinical basis because of the characteristic distribution pattern and by the distinctive morphology of the lesions. A suspected diagnosis can be confirmed by biopsy in which transverse sectioning demonstrates infundibular dilatation and hyperkeratotic plugging of the apocrine gland duct. Spongiosis of the follicular epidermal cells is commonly present as is a perifollicular and perivascular lymphocytic inflammatory infiltrate. The presence of perifollicular foam cells is a helpful, semicharacteristic finding.

The pathogenesis of this condition is unknown. One hypothesis suggests that outlet obstruction of apocrine gland–related follicles leads to retention and dilatation of the apocrine duct and/or gland. Following this, extravasation of apocrine sweat into the surrounding dermis could then lead to inflammation and itching. The cause of the putative initiating follicular obstruction is unknown. Notably, at least 10 cases of FFD have occurred following laser therapy for hair removal, a process that leads to heat damage of the hair follicle infundibulum suggesting that trauma to apocrine gland–related follicles could play a prominent role.[22] The menstrual flares along with the timing of onset at puberty and resolution at menopause suggest that hormonal factors may be important in the pathophysiology of the disorder. Finally, a few familial cases have been published indicating that genetic aspects may also play an etiologic role.

As can be gathered from the long list of treatments that have been tried, there is no fully established therapy for FFD.[20,22] Topical steroids, topical calcineurin inhibitors, topical tretinoin cream (which is often too irritating to use effectively), and oral isotretinoin may improve symptoms in some patients. The severity of the itching improves somewhat with pregnancy and while taking oral contraceptives.

## Lichen Nitidus

Lichen nitidus (LN) is an uncommon disorder that occurs primarily in children and young adults.[23] Most reviews indicate that there is no gender preference, but in some case series and in our own experience, males seem to predominate. LN is characterized by multiple, tiny (1-2 mm), shiny, flat-topped papules that are usually skin colored but can be white or pink **(Figs. 7-31 and 7-32)**. The lesions are most often asymptomatic though some patients report mild to moderate pruritus. This eruption usually involves the trunk and upper extremities. A few reports of generalized eruptions mention involvement of the thighs and pubis. Notably, in males, the shaft of the penis is frequently and characteristically involved. No cases specifically involving the vulva appear to have been reported. In

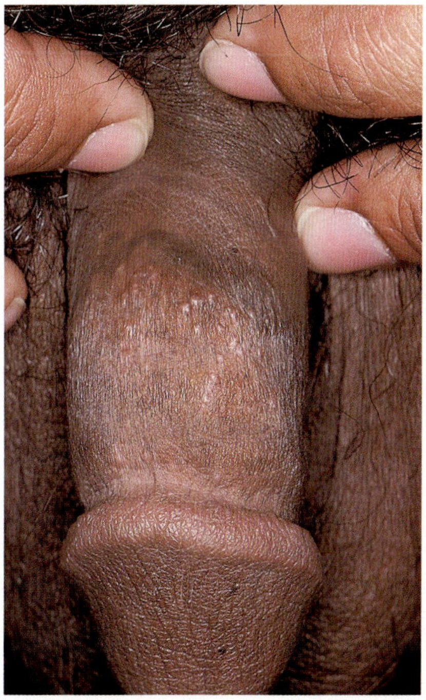

Fig. 7-31. The shaft of the penis is an area of predilection for lichen nitidus, consisting of tiny, closely set, dome-shaped papules.

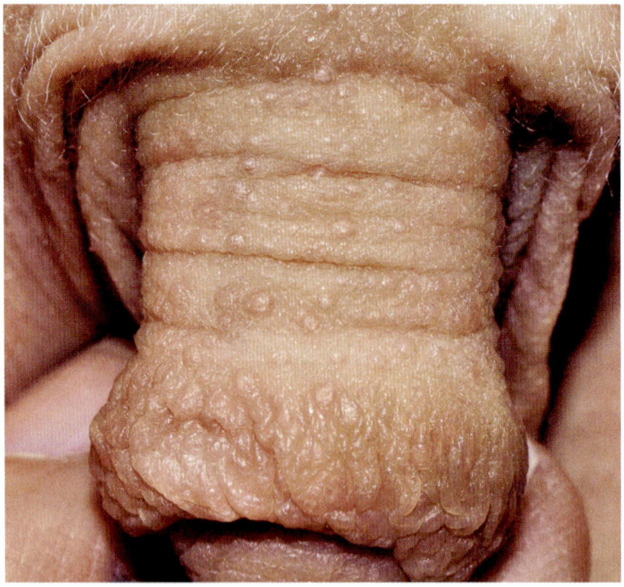

Fig. 7-32. Lichen nitidus is fairly common in children, and the penis is often affected.

most instances, the condition remits spontaneously after 6-12 months; rarely, cases have persisted for years.

The diagnosis is suspected clinically, and dermoscopy is useful. This shows small white round areas without skin markings.[24] The diagnosis may be confirmed by biopsy. Histologically, there is a unique picture of a lichenoid reaction with the presence of small, focal, lymphohistiocytic granulomas located in the papillary dermis. These granulomas are partially or completely surrounded by tongues of downward proliferating epidermis ("ball in a claw" formation). Multinucleated giant cells are generally present. Basal layer vacuolization of the epidermis occurs above the clumps of inflammatory cells.

The etiology of lichen nitidus is unknown. Originally some thought that it was a variant of lichen planus. In fact, lichen planus and lichen nitidus can rarely develop concomitantly. Today, however, it is considered to be a separate, unique disorder of unknown pathogenesis. No treatment is completely satisfactory though the application of mid- to super-potent topical steroids may hasten its resolution. But, since it is usually asymptomatic and tends to remit with time, it seems reasonable in most instances to leave it untreated.

## SECTION B: SKIN-COLORED NODULES

The same caveat applies here as is indicated for skin-colored papules: "skin colored" means that the lesion color is similar to that of the surrounding tissue whether it is skin or mucous membrane. Thus, the lesion color in a dark-skinned individual may be tan or brown, or in a light-skinned individual, the lesion color may be almost white. Lesions occurring on mucous membranes are usually pink or red. Note also that although the following disorders are listed as "nodular," there may be an admixture with some smaller papules being present as well.

### Hidradenoma Papilliferum (Mammarylike Gland Adenoma)

Hidradenoma papilliferum (HP) is a fairly common benign vulvar adnexal neoplasm. The primary discussion of this disorder can be found in Chapter 6, but a few additional comments are added here. It is a lesion that develops only in women, and it mainly occurs in the vulvar tissue of those who are middle-aged and of Caucasian decent. Most often, the lesion is solitary and is found on the vulvar labia minora and/or labia majora. It has specific predilection to develop in the interlabial sulcus.[25] Rarely, HP occurs at the anus or perianally.[26] It usually is found as a 1- to 2-cm, medium-soft to firm, asymptomatic nodule that is skin colored or red **(Figs. 7-33 and 7-34)**. The surface of the nodule may be smooth or ulcerated. Sometimes HP has a somewhat translucent, cystic-type appearance. Most lesions are asymptomatic, but pruritus, bleeding, and mild pain occur in a minority of instances. The lesions can be morphologically and dermoscopically very variable, so that diagnosis is by biopsy.

These neoplasms were originally thought to be apocrine gland–derived tumors, but they are now known to develop from apocrine-related, but separately identified, mammarylike glands that are known to be located in the anogenital area of women.[27] This new category of mammarylike gland adenomas may subsume other rare anogenital adenomas such as tubular adenomas and syringocystadenoma papilliferum. Almost all of the tumors are benign though at least a few patients have demonstrated

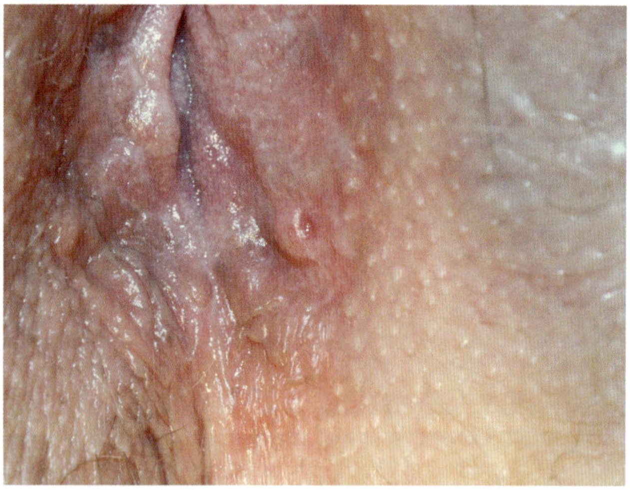

Fig. 7-33. A hidradenoma papilliferum is an uncommon tumor more often found on the vulva than male genital; it is a skin-colored, dome-shaped papule that often appears cystic, sometimes with a central dell.

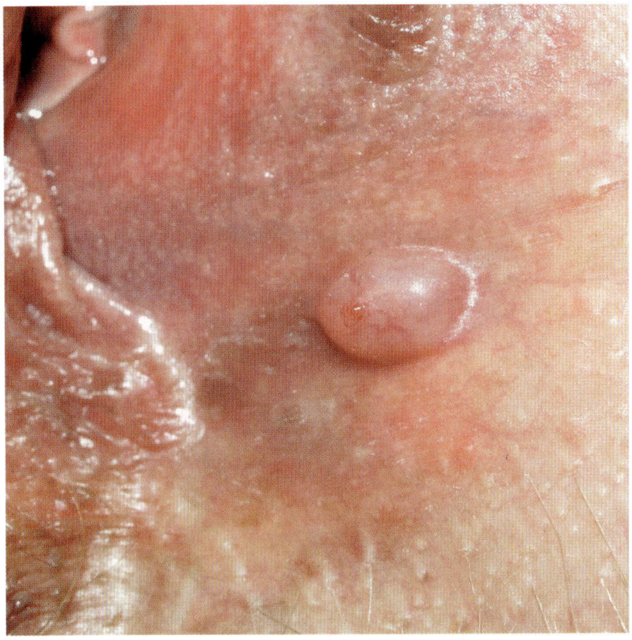

Fig. 7-34. This hidradenoma papilliferum shows a drop of mucoid material at the surface pit.

ductal carcinoma *in situ*. Interestingly, however, about 75% of biopsy specimens harbor mutations in cancer-related genes.[28] The meaning of this finding is unknown. Treatment by way of local excision is curative.

## Neurofibroma

Neurofibromas are asymptomatic, soft, skin-colored, or light tan nodules. Dermatologists generally divide them into two groups: small, solitary, superficial neurofibromas (that are not part of type 1 generalized neurofibromatosis) and larger, deeper neurofibromas (that are part of either type 5 segmental or type 1 generalized neurofibromatosis).

Small, solitary neurofibromas clinically mimic fibroepithelial polyps in that they are soft, pedunculated, and skin colored. They are, however, easily invaginated ("buttonhole sign"). One or several lesions may be present and most often occur on the lower trunk and thighs but only rarely directly involve the genitalia **(Figs. 7-35 and 7-36)**. They have no medical meaning, but if they cause irritation by catching on clothing, they can easily be "clipped" off.

Larger nodules are slightly less soft, skin colored to slightly tan, and are easily recognized as part of type 1 generalized neurofibromatosis (von Recklinghausen disease).[29] These develop along with numerous other similar nodules and scattered café au lait patches. Such lesions do not evolve into sarcomas. Even larger, nonpedunculated, slightly elongated nodules attached to underlying nerves may occur as plexiform neurofibromas.[30,31] These may occur on the genitalia (especially in a periclitoral location) as part of type 1 (generalized neurofibromatosis) or type 5 (segmental neurofibromatosis). These latter lesions do have the potential to undergo sarcomatous change and therefore should be removed by neurosurgical dissection.

## Condyloma Latum

Condylomata lata (plural) is the name used for the flat-topped papules and nodules that develop in the anogenital area during the secondary stage of syphilis.[32] These lesions are uncommonly seen in conventional office practice but are encountered with some frequency in STD clinics and occasionally in referral centers. The primary

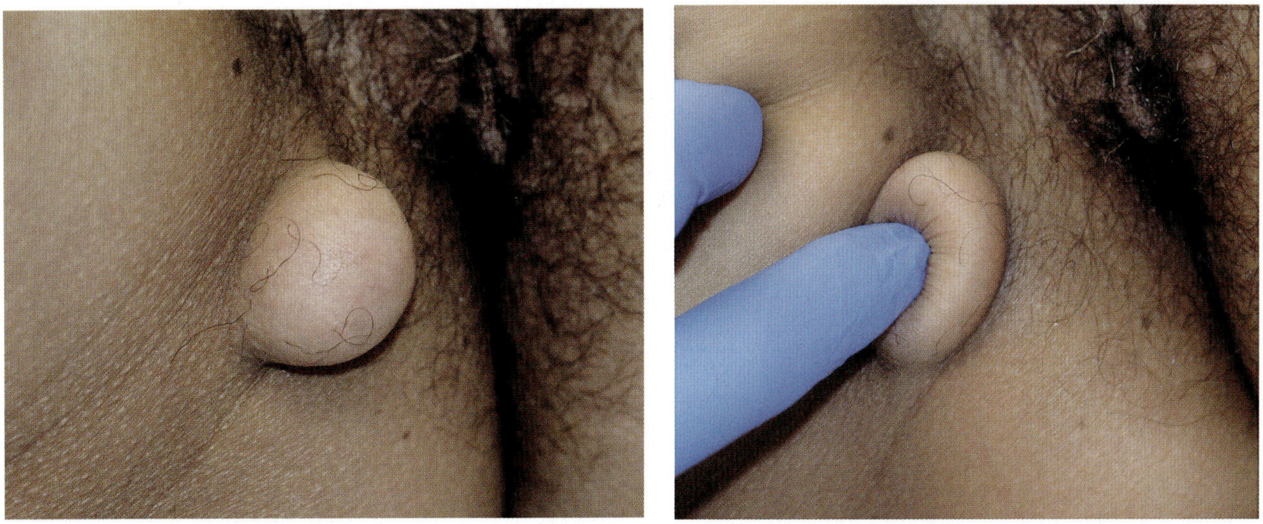

A B

Fig. 7-35. **A, B.** Although the term fibroma implies fibrotic and firm, a neurofibroma is notoriously soft and squishy, often described as feeling like a "bag of worms" on palpation. The superficial nature as well as the extraordinary softness helps to distinguish a neurofibroma from a lipoma and epidermoid cyst.

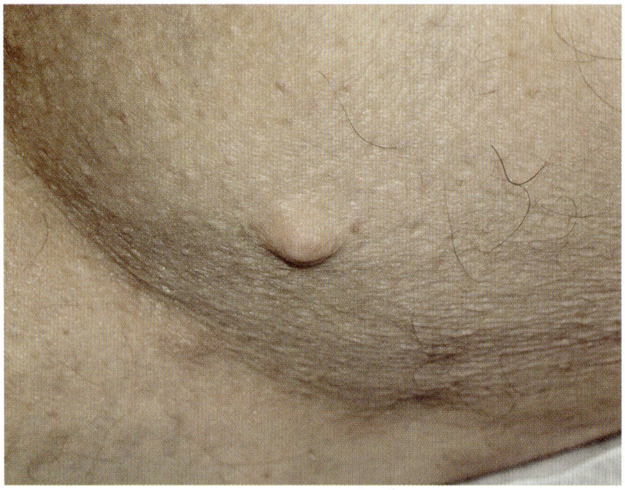

Fig. 7-36. Small neurofibromas are common, medically insignificant tumors, and often overlooked.

coverage of syphilis is located in the section on chancres in Chapter 11. Only the clinical presentation and therapy of condylomata lata will be covered here.

Condylomata lata are sharply demarcated, large (1- to 2-cm), flat-topped, skin-colored or pink nodules (Fig. 7-37). When the lesions are located on mucosae or intertriginous areas, they may exhibit a white surface because of retained moisture in the outer layers of their thickened, hyperkeratotic epidermis (Fig. 7-38). They are most commonly found on the vulva and the perianal area but can occur elsewhere on the genitalia and perigenital skin.

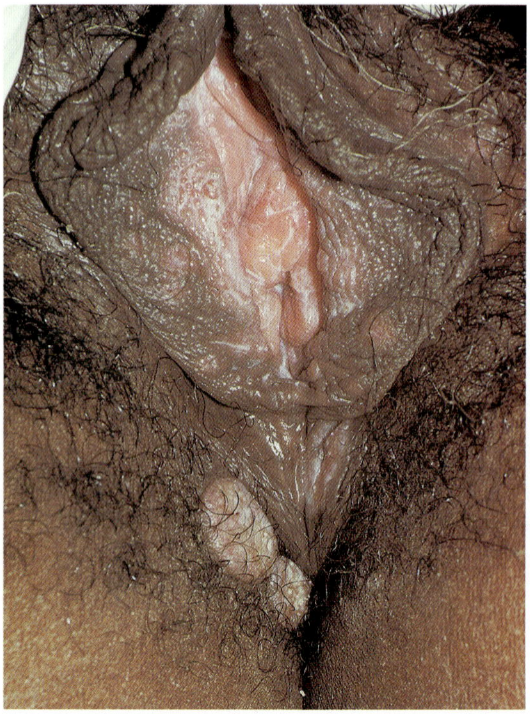

Fig. 7-37. The very flat-topped morphology of these papules is the reason for the term condyloma latum, for flat, in contradistinction to condyloma acuminata produced by HPV.

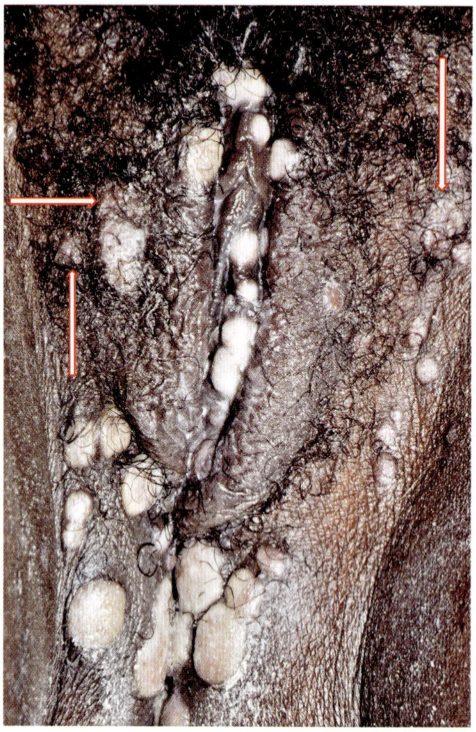

Fig. 7-38. The underlying skin-colored nature of these condylomata lata is appreciated on the more peripheral dry skin, compared to the areas that stay wet in skin folds, producing a white fibrin exudate on the surface.

Rarely, they develop at nonanogenital intertriginous sites. As opposed to the other cutaneous lesions of secondary syphilis the lesions, the surfaces of condylomata lata are teeming with spirochetes and pose a high risk for transmission to others. Condylomata lata are usually associated with other signs and symptoms of secondary syphilis such as fever, malaise, and generalized lymphadenopathy. Other skin findings of secondary syphilis such as slightly scaly red papules on the trunk, brown-red palmar and plantar papules, white patches on the oral mucous membranes, and patchy hair loss may also be present.

The clinical presentation may suggest the correct diagnosis of syphilis but confirmation is obligatory. Patients with condylomata lata almost always exhibit a positive *nontreponemal* serology such as a rapid plasma regain (RPR) or Venereal Disease Research Laboratory (VDRL) test for syphilis.[33] The only exceptions are those who are severely immunocompromised (eg, by HIV/AIDS) and those with such a high antibody titer that they exhibit the so-called prozone phenomenon. However, patients with clinically suspicious lesions, whether or not their nontreponemal test is positive, should receive a *treponemal* test such as the fluorescent treponemal antibody absorbed (FTA-ABS) test. The combination of these two kinds of test will essentially always indicate the correct diagnosis.

The lesions of condylomata lata can be confused with HPV-induced warts (condyloma acuminata) and intraepithelial neoplasia of the vulva, penis, and scrotum. If there is any question about the correct identity, a biopsy should be obtained as well as the serological tests mentioned in the paragraph above. The generally recommended treatment for secondary syphilis, including condylomata lata, is a single 2.4 million unit IM injection of benzathine penicillin G (Bicillin L-A).[33]

## Lymphogranuloma Venereum

Until recently, lymphogranuloma venereum (LGV) was rarely encountered in Western countries. However, during the last 20 years, there has been a significant rise in the number of cases reported from the United Kingdom and Europe together with a smaller increase in the United States.[34] Nearly all of this increase is accounted for by rectal infections occurring in MSM and is particularly likely to be found in those men who are HIV positive. LGV is rarely diagnosed in women probably because, in this population, the infection is often asymptomatic. The increase has been facilitated by more worldwide travel and easier social connectivity by way of online networking.

Classically, when infection occurred through heterosexual sex, the initial clinical lesion of LGV was a nonpainful, papule, pustule, or superficial ulcer. Such lesions were quite transient and, because of their asymptomatic nature, they were usually not noted or, if noted, were ignored by the patient. By and large, such patients did not seek medical attention until the onset of lymphadenopathy. Today, nearly all (90%-95%) of the patients with LGV present with proctitis; they may or may not have mild lymphadenopathy. A discussion of LGV proctitis falls outside the scope of this textbook.

The most striking feature from a standpoint of this book is the impressive lymphadenopathy (buboes) that occurs when the genitalia, rather than the rectum, are infected. Inguinal lymph nodes are most commonly affected though in some cases femoral nodes are also involved. When both sets of nodes are involved, Poupart ligament (ligamentum inguinale) creates a characteristic groove (the "groove sign") between the two groups of nodes (**Fig. 7-39**). The enlarged nodes are usually bilateral, and they are exquisitely tender. In untreated patients, nodes that have been present for some time undergo liquefaction with attendant fluctuance. Eventually, breakdown of the overlying skin occurs, resulting in the development of chronic purulent draining sinuses. Massive genital edema (elephantiasis) frequently develops. Patients with untreated proctitis develop rectal stenosis, strictures, and perianal abscess formation. Such patients may be mistaken as having Crohn disease.

Lymphogranuloma venereum is caused by the L1, L2, or L3 serovars of the bacterium, *Chlamydia trachomatis*. Nearly all of the newly reported cases in MSM have been with the L2 or L2b subvariant serovar.[34] A diagnosis of LGV is usually suspected on a clinical basis, but similar

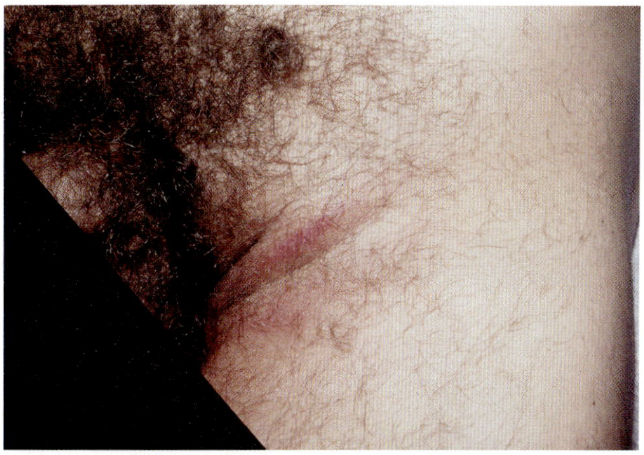

Fig. 7-39. The lymphadenopathy of LGV is exquisitely painful, becomes red, and, without treatment, can break down and form chronic draining sinuses. The groove sign is easily seen here.

adenopathy can occur in chancroid. Confirmation of the diagnosis requires identification of an LGV-type serovar from the site of infection. Previously, this had primarily been accomplished with bacterial cultures, but today, molecular techniques found only in specialized laboratories are more widely used. In situations where these tests are not available, serologic techniques can be used, but there are many problems with sensitivity and specificity.[34]

The current recommended treatment is with oral doxycycline 100 mg twice daily for 3 weeks.[34] In an attempt to obtain better compliance, single dose or short course azithromycin has also been used, but cure rates appear to be lower with this medication. Fluctuant lymph nodes should be aspirated.

## Syringomas

Syringomas are benign adnexal lesions of sweat gland or sweat duct origin. They are most often found on the face especially on and around the eyelids. They occur appreciably more frequently in women than in men. A few familial cases have been reported. Generally, they appear insidiously around the time of puberty or in young adult life; however, when asymptomatic, they may not be recognized until much later in life. Published reports of genital lesions are uncommon but both of the authors of this textbook, and others, have encountered vulvar syringomas often enough to believe that they frequently go unrecognized or at least unreported.[35] Vulvar lesions are much more common than are penile or scrotal lesions.

The clinical appearance is usually that of multiple smooth surfaced, flat-topped, or slope shouldered papules or nodules (**Figs. 7-40 and 7-41**). Ten to twenty closely set lesions, 5-20 mm in diameter, are usually present bilaterally. Less often solitary papules or nodules have been described. Most are skin colored, but white, yellow, or tan color may be present. On the vulva, they are almost

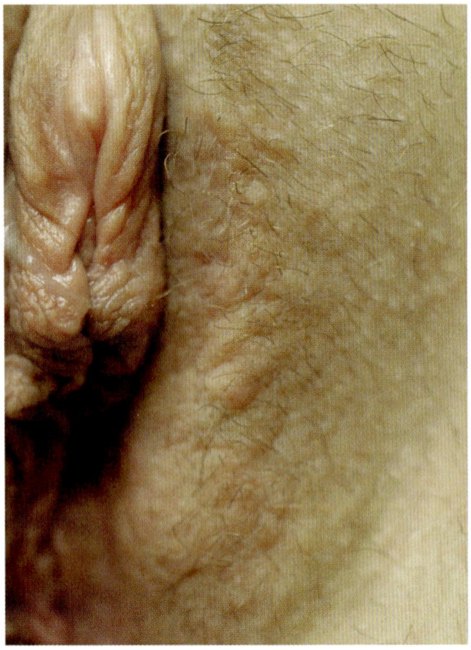

Fig. 7-40. Syringomas are skin-colored, dome-shaped papules that are sometimes subtle lesions that can mimic lichenification in itchy patients.

always located on the labia majora. In most instances, the lesions are asymptomatic.[35] However, pruritus occurs in some of the patients, and at times, it can be quite troublesome. Once present, they remain static in size and persist indefinitely.

Usually, a clinical diagnosis is possible, but dermoscopy can be useful as well. This shows glittering yellow-whitish structures, round-shaped or oval, over a fading pink background, with patchy and clustered dotted and

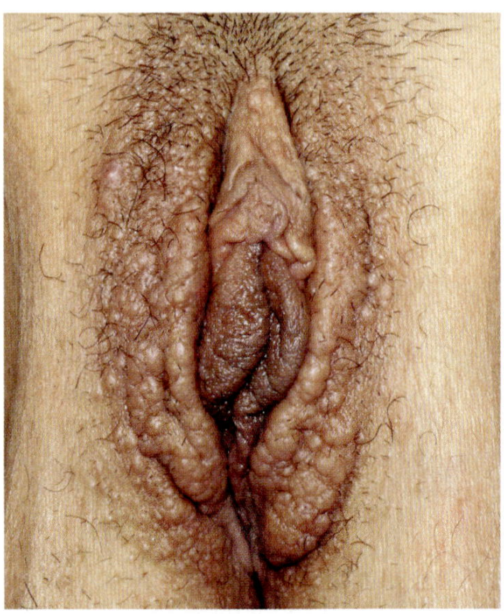

Fig. 7-41. At times, syringomas are large and mimic epidermal cysts.

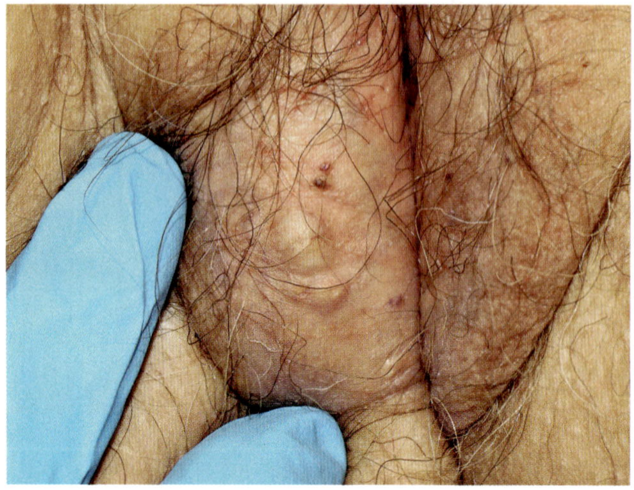

Fig. 7-42. An epidermal cyst is a white, yellow, pink, or skin-colored, dome-shaped, firm nodule; sometimes these are even bluish due to melanin in the keratin contained in the cyst.

short linear vessels.[36] However, a suspected diagnosis should be confirmed by biopsy as both their clinical and histological appearance can be confused with microcystic adnexal carcinoma.[35] The histology is that of closely set tubular structures resembling that seen in normal eccrine sweat ducts. Syringomas can be left untreated, but when severe pruritus occurs, the itching can be ameliorated by way of excision or destruction with electrosurgery, laser ablation, or cryotherapy.[35]

## Epidermal Cysts (Epidermoid Cysts)

Epidermal cysts (EC) are commonly, but erroneously, termed sebaceous cysts; they contain keratin not sebum! EC are the most common type of cysts found in the anogenital area where they occur as firm, slope-shouldered, smooth-surfaced, white, yellow-white, slightly pink or skin-colored papules or nodules **(Figs. 7-42 and 7-43)**. Very small cysts (1-2 mm) are called milia, but these are not commonly encountered in the anogenital area. The average diameter for genital EC is 0.5-2.0 cm. Noninflamed cysts are usually asymptomatic. Epidermal cysts primarily develop on the hair-bearing aspects of the genitalia. They are most commonly located on the scrotum in men and the labia majora in women. EC also occur in the periclitoral area in women[37] and as a small proportion of median raphe cysts in men **(Fig. 7-44)**.[38] One or several may be present; occasionally, there are 10-20 clustered lesions **(Fig. 7-45)**. The diagnosis is usually made on the basis of clinical appearance. Dermoscopy can be useful in atypical cases; there is ivory white background found in most, with a punctum or pore sign found in about half of cases.[39] Even more certain confirmation can be obtained when white cyst contents are visualized after

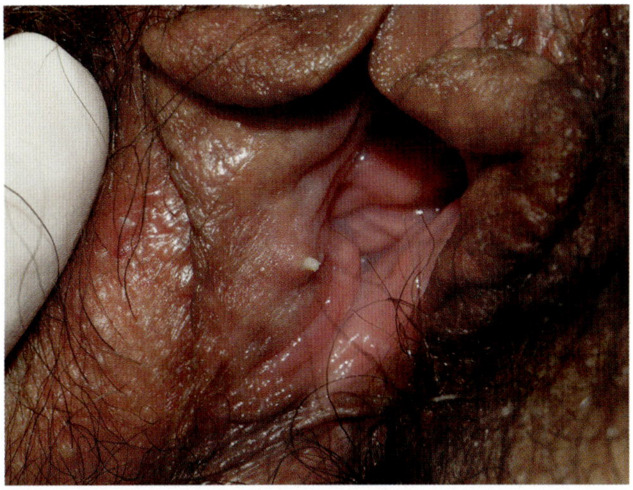

Fig. 7-43. The diagnosis of this small cyst is easily made, since the keratin from within the cyst is being extruded.

incising and gently squeezing the lesion. The differential diagnoses include the following entities. Syringomas arising on the labia majora may be confused with epidermal cysts. The lesions of molluscum contagiosum may mimic epidermal cysts, but MC lesions are more superficial and appear to sit on the surface, rather than lie within the skin. Ectopic sebaceous glands (Fordyce spots) on mucosal aspects of the genitalia may resemble milia.

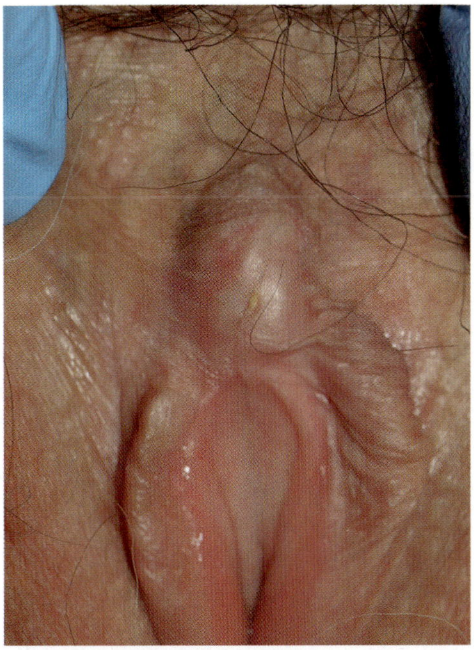

Fig. 7-44. Although these nodules found in women with scarring dermatoses are sometimes called clitoral pseudocysts, they are actually true epidermoid cysts. Desquamated keratin that is trapped under a scarred clitoral hood distends the surrounding skin, and here, a bit of white keratin can be seen peaking between the sealed tips of the clitoral hood.

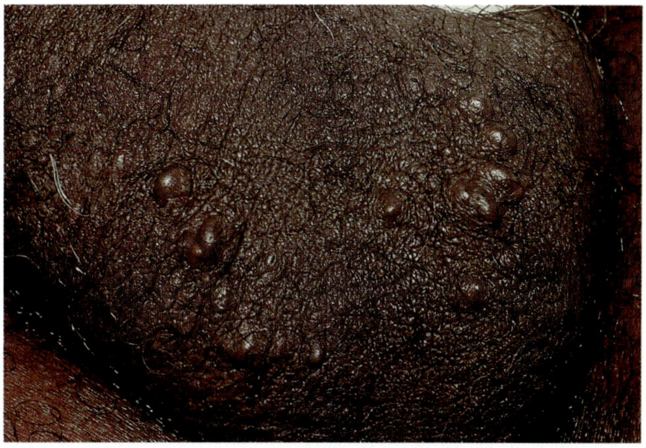

Fig. 7-45. The most common locations for larger cysts are the scrotum and labia majora.

So-called inclusion cysts arise when bits of epithelium are implanted in the skin during the course of a surgical procedure or as a result of trauma sufficient to break the surface of the skin. The term "inclusion cyst" should not otherwise be used as a general synonym for "epidermal cyst." The much more common, typical epidermal cyst found on the genitalia develops from the remnant of an anatomically malformed pilosebaceous unit that lacks a fully adequate outlet to the surface of the skin. The white material located within an epidermal cyst is keratin that is produced by keratinocytes located in the lining of the cyst wall. In men, the contents of scrotal epidermoid cysts sometimes undergo calcification. However, in some cases of calcification, the epidermal cell wall has disappeared, and in such instances, the term "idiopathic calcinosis cutis" is used instead.[40]

Epidermal cysts are medically unimportant and cause no problems unless the cyst wall leaks or ruptures. If this occurs, keratin cyst contents come into contact with the connective tissue surrounding the cyst. This keratin acts as a "foreign body" and engenders a brisk inflammatory reaction. This inflammation causes the cyst contents to liquefy into puslike material. In spite of the appearance and smell, this mixture of liquefied keratin and inflammatory cells almost always lacks pathogenic bacteria and thus does not represent true infection. Nevertheless, such lesions may clinically resemble a furuncle or an inflammatory pseudocyst such as is seen in hidradenitis suppurativa. No treatment is needed for noninflamed cysts. Inflamed cysts may be incised and drained. Most clinicians prescribe antibiotics for inflamed cysts but any beneficial effect that occurs is likely due to the anti-inflammatory, rather than the antimicrobial, properties of these antibiotics. Rarely, symptoms or patient insistence will result in a need for laser ablation or excisional removal of noninflamed cysts. Simple incision together with removal of the cyst contents is almost invariably followed by recurrence.

## Cysts of the Median Raphe

A "median raphe" represents the midline embryonic joining point of two symmetrical tissues. In the anogenital area of men, a median raphe extends from the anus forward through the perineum, along the scrotum extending onto the underside of the penis and ending at the urethral meatus on the tip of the glans. The raphe is visible and palpable as a slight ridge that is skin colored or light brown. Cyst or canals can develop anywhere along this raphe but occur most commonly on the underside of the penis. Usually, only a solitary papule or nodule, representing a single cyst, is present, but in some cases, multiple cysts are found along the raphe. The lesions appear as dome-shaped skin-colored, translucent, yellow, or tan hemispherical papules or nodules that are 2-15 mm in diameter **(Fig. 7-46)**. Most are present from birth, but slow growth and lack of symptoms generally mean they are not brought to anyone's attention until later in life. Less often they develop in adult life as "inclusion" cysts arising because of implantation of tissue that occurs as a result of skin-breaking trauma. Rarely, inflammation occurs as a result of trauma or infection. Histologically, they may be lined with either columnar or stratified squamous epithelium. No treatment is necessary for asymptomatic lesions; symptomatic or inflamed lesions (usually occurring as the result of irritation or trauma during sexual activity) can be excised. The subject has been recently reviewed.[38]

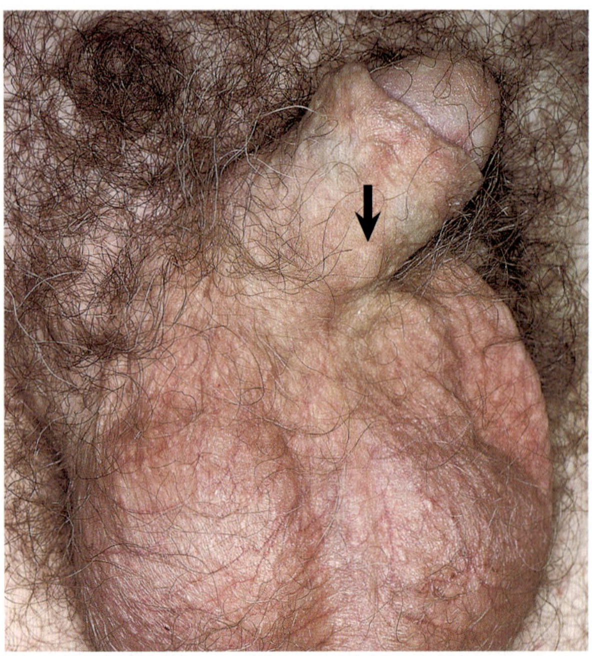

Fig. 7-46. A median raphe cyst occurs along the midline of the ventral aspect of the penis.

## Mucinous Vestibular Cysts

Mucinous vestibular cysts are located within the vulvar vestibule. These cysts develop fairly frequently though there is a surprising lack of published reports about them. Mucinous cysts presumably develop from either anatomic abnormalities or obstruction of the minor vestibular glands. A buildup of gland secretion forms these 0.5- to 2-cm soft nodules **(Figs. 7-47 and 7-48)**. They can be translucent, skin colored, yellow, or blue. Although vestibular cysts can be excised surgically, they are almost always asymptomatic and ordinarily require no treatment.

## Pilonidal Sinus (Pilonidal Cyst)

Though often termed "pilonidal cysts," these lesions lack an epithelial cyst wall and therefore are more appropriately identified as pilonidal sinuses. They arise as an acquired lesion wherein hairs, trapped in folded areas of tissue, forcibly penetrate the skin and create a foreign body inflammatory reaction.[41] Pilonidal sinus occurs more often in men than in women and is most commonly located in the sacrococcygeal area **(Fig. 7-49)**. Risk factors include obesity, sedentary lifestyle, excess body hair, and lack of good hygiene. However, locations in other sites such as the axillae, web spaces of the hands, and genitalia have been reported. Relatively few cases have been reported to have involved the vulva or penis. But most of the vulvar cases have occurred

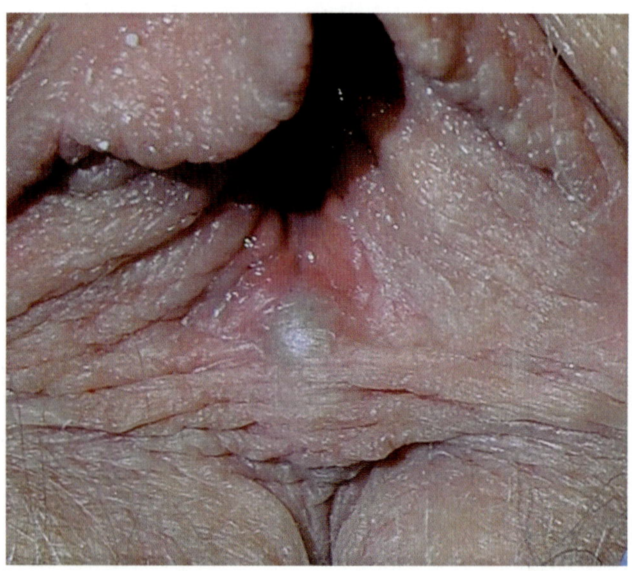

Fig. 7-47. Mucinous vestibular cysts can be skin colored, bluish, or white.

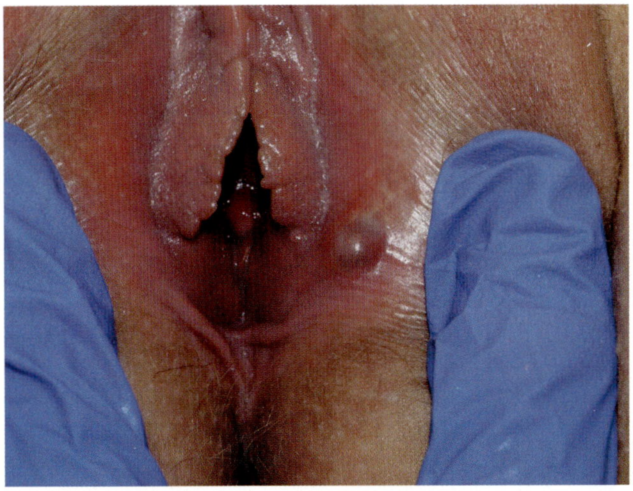

Fig. 7-48. Not all vulvar mucinous cysts are in the vestibule, but all are on some part of the mucous membranes or modified mucous membranes.

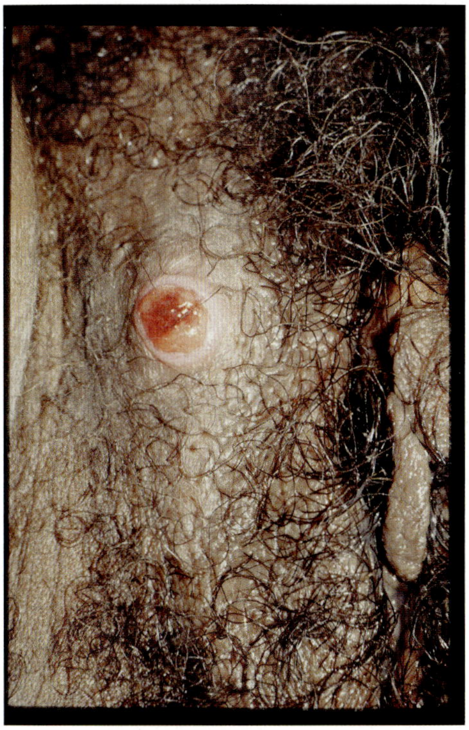

Fig. 7-50. When pilonidal cysts occur on the vulva, they are usually periclitoral.

at a periclitoral site where they develop into a clitoral or periclitoral abscess **(Fig. 7-50)**.[42] In uncircumcised men, penile lesions have been found in the coronal sulcus.[43]

Pilonidal sinus first develops as an asymptomatic, soft, skin-colored nodule that becomes red and very painful as foreign body inflammation ensues. Hairs can sometimes be seen extruding from the surface of the lesion when the folds of skin around the lesion are separated. Accumulated pus within the lesion may drain from the sinus tract. Treatment is more difficult than might be expected.[41] All of the inflamed tissue and the entire sinus tract must be completely excised preferably following laser hair ablation. Even with careful, extensive surgery, the recurrence rate is fairly high.

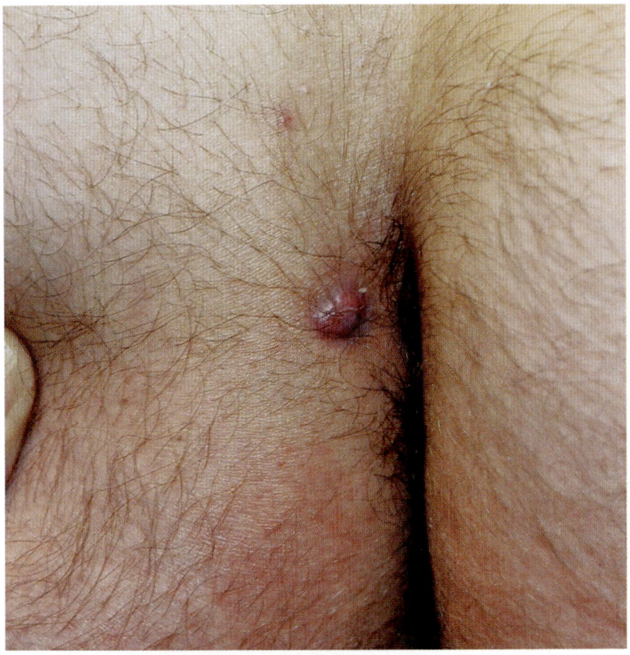

Fig. 7-49. This pilonidal cyst is in a classic location near the superior portion of the gluteal cleft; although it appears superficial and easily removable, these often are only the superior portion of a sinus tract that may require fairly extensive surgery.

## Bartholin Cysts and Abscesses

Bartholin glands (the major vestibular glands) open into the vulvar vestibule at about the 5 and 7 o'clock position, just distal to the hymeneal ring. They lie at the base of the labia minora and empty through ducts that are about 2 cm long. These glands provide a small amount of mucinous, lubricating fluid during sexual activity. A fairly recent review of the cysts and abscesses that can develop in these structures has recently been published.[44]

Bartholin duct cysts and abscesses are fairly common with a lifetime risk that is estimated at about 2%. They are most likely to occur during the third decade with the risk declining slowly after that as the glands begin to involute. Dilation of the ducts to form a cyst occurs if the outlet of the duct becomes obstructed. Such blockage results in a unilateral, tissue-colored, smooth-surfaced, slope-shouldered nodule that ranges from about 1-5 cm in diameter. Small noninflamed cysts are usually asymptomatic. They arise at the lateral aspect of the vestibule within the labium minus **(Fig. 7-51)**. The positioning of the medial wall of the labium minus directly over the approximate center of the cyst is a highly characteristic feature.

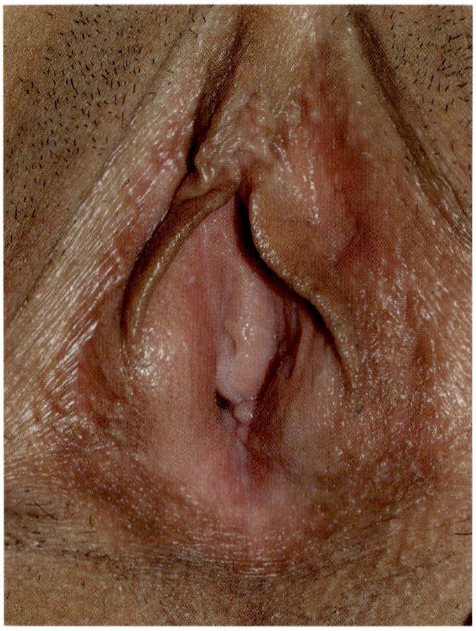

Fig. 7-51. This woman has bilateral Bartholin gland duct cysts; typically, the labium minus transects the cyst.

Bartholin cysts may become inflamed as a result of either infection or cyst rupture. The previous presence of a noninflamed cyst is not necessary for a Bartholin gland abscess to develop. The inflammation and swelling in these abscesses cause considerable pain and may be accompanied by fever. For infected cysts, it was originally believed that *Neisseria gonorrhoeae* was the most common bacterium causing the abscess formation, but today, many different bacteria, especially *Staphylococcal aureus and Escherichia coli*, are more often identified.

The diagnosis is made on a clinical basis. Noninflamed cysts contain sterile, clear mucinous fluid. Asymptomatic small cysts may be left untreated in younger women. Pus is present within an abscessed cyst or gland. Often sufficient purulent material for culture may be expressed from the ostium of the duct with gentle massage. If the lesion is too tender for such manipulation, pus for culture can be obtained by needle aspiration or by incision and drainage. Noninflamed cysts do not require treatment unless they are large enough to cause discomfort. However, because the possibility of squamous cell or adenocarcinoma increases after age 40, most clinicians recommend biopsy for cysts developing in postmenopausal women. Inflamed cysts are generally treated with oral antibiotics, and a fair number of these will then resolve. Larger or inflamed cysts can be aspirated or incised and drained to relieve discomfort. Unfortunately, cysts treated in this manner frequently recur. Appreciable controversy exists regarding what represents the most definitive management of these lesions.[45] Most gynecologists favor the placement of a Word catheter because this can be done as a fairly simple office procedure.[46] Other possibilities include marsupialization, sclerotherapy, and placement of a Jacobi ring. Detailed discussion of such therapies lies outside the scope of this book.

## Lipoma

Lipomas are common hamartomas of fat. They can develop anywhere on the body as asymptomatic, lobular, soft, skin-colored, smooth nodules. Their size is variable, but generally, it ranges from 2 to 5 cm. Genital lipomas are encountered only rarely.[46] In the vulva, lipomas are most often located in within the labia majora **(Fig. 7-52)**. Perineal lipomas, mostly occurring congenitally or in infants, are slightly more common **(Fig. 7-53)**.[47] Surgical excision is often requested by the patient because of distortion of the genitalia. The histology shows mature fat cells. Excision should also be considered because a few cases of mesenchymal malignancy have presented clinically as lipomas.

## Sclerosing Lymphangitis and Mondor Thrombophlebitis of the Penis

Nonvenereal sclerosing lymphangitis is an uncommon condition usually presenting as a very firm, linear, smooth-surfaced, ropelike, asymptomatic nodule that is located at, or just proximal to, the coronal sulcus **(Fig. 7-54)**.[48] At this site, it partially encircles or, less often, completely encircles the penis. Occasionally, the nodule branches such that there is a small perpendicular exten-

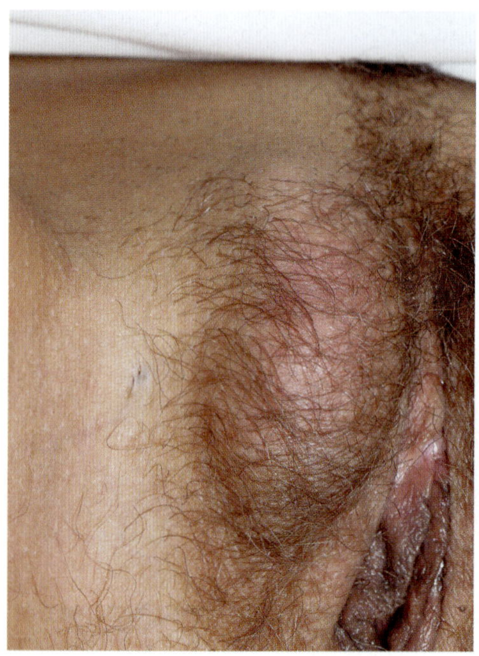

Fig. 7-52. Lipomas on the vulva are most common on the labia majora.

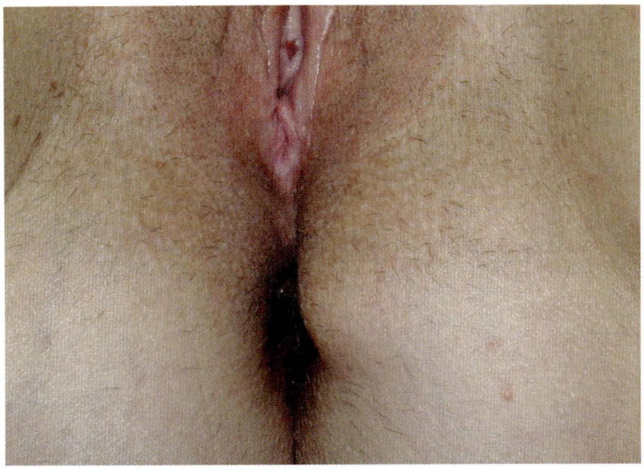

Fig. 7-53. The perineum is a fairly common location for anogenital lipomas; often the extent of these benign tumors is more easily palpated than seen.

sion a short way proximally along the shaft of the penis. The overlying skin is freely moveable over it.

The condition almost always develops within days after a prolonged period of vigorous sexual intercourse or frequent masturbation. Because of its fairly common occurrence after coitus, testing for STD should be performed even though there is no evidence that the condition itself is caused by sexually transmitted infection. Considerable controversy exists as to whether sclerosing lymphangitis represents a thrombosis of lymphatic vessels or venous vessels. In any event, sclerosing lymphangitis can be viewed as an analog of Mondor thrombophlebitis of the superficial dorsal vein of the penis and, in fact, when Mondor disease of the penis occurs distally, at or near the coronal sulcus, the two conditions may be hard to distinguish clinically.[49] First-line treatment of both of these benign conditions is avoidance of sexual activity including masturbation. If this is achieved, spontaneous resolution of both disorders can be expected within 4-6 weeks.

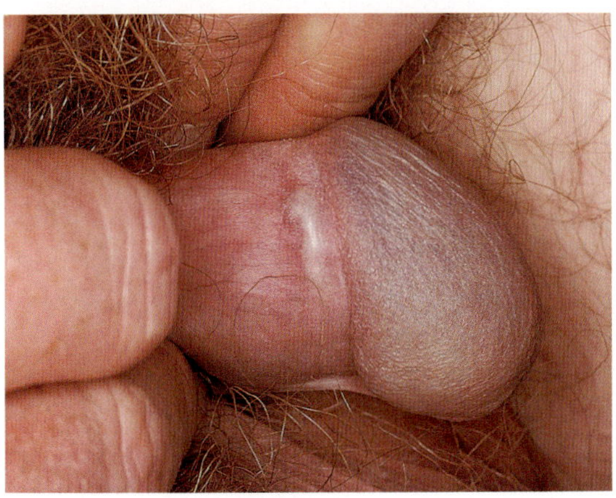

Fig. 7-54. Sclerosing lymphangitis has the characteristic appearance of a firm cord parallel to the corona.

## Squamous Cell Carcinoma of the Genitalia

In both men and women, there are two distinct pathways through which genital SCC can develop: an HPV-related pathway and HPV nonrelated pathway. The lesions that develop through each of these routes have a quite different appearance and prognosis. Lesions developing through the HPV-related pathway tend to have a more variegated appearance (pink, red, brown, black, or skin-colored papules and plaques) and a more prolonged duration between the *in situ* and the invasive stage. On the other hand, those lesions that are non–HPV-related are usually less variegated (red, white, and skin-colored nodules) with a more rapid progression between the *in situ* and invasive stages. Obviously, with all of this variability, these malignancies could have been considered in any one of several chapters, and our placement of the major discussion in this particular chapter is quite arbitrary.

## Squamous Cell Carcinoma of the Male Genitalia

### Clinical Presentation

Squamous cell carcinoma represents the vast majority of malignant tumors involving the penis and scrotum. SCC has historically been classified based on histological morphology as *in situ* tumors and *invasive* tumors. In more recent years, there has been a preference to classify them based on pathogenesis into *HPV-related* and *HPV nonrelated* tumors. We prefer the former because of simplicity and low cost. Basically, in many countries, definitive testing (determination by polymerase chain reaction) for the presence of HPV is either not available or when available is too expensive for routine use. In addition, there are quite a few false-positive and false-negative tests for HPV utilizing the least costly and most widely available technique (p16 immunostaining) for determining the presence of causative HPV. Finally, while p16 staining can identify the most common high-risk type of HPV, HPV 16, there are other high-risk HPV types that have been associated with the development of SCC.

*Noninvasive* penile SCC (penile *in situ* carcinoma—PeIN) is fairly common and can occur either on the prepuce or glans (historically termed erythroplasia of Queyrat) or on the shaft (historically called Bowen disease or Bowenoid papulosis). PeIN (except for the histologically differentiated HPV nonrelated type) tends to be multicentric wherein several lesions are often present. It occurs as flat-topped papules or plaques (**Fig. 7-55**). The latter may be as large as 2 or 3 cm in diameter. The papules and plaques of PIN on the shaft

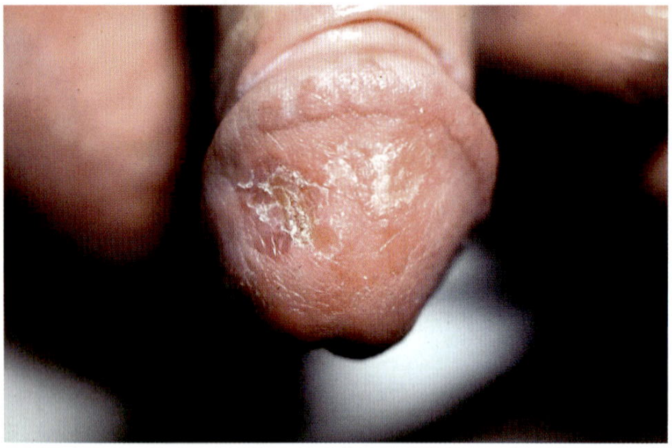

Fig. 7-55. This penile intraepithelial neoplasia (erythroplasia of Queyrat, squamous cell carcinoma *in situ*) of the glans is scaling and could be confused with psoriasis.

may be pink, red, brown, or skin colored. Those on the glans and prepuce are usually white, pink, or red. The surface of PeIN is not ulcerated and may either be smooth or, especially on the penile shaft, slightly scaly **(Fig. 7-56)**. An uncommon variant of PeIN is pseudoepitheliomatous keratotic and micaceous balanitis in which the lesion appears as thick, heaped-up scale and crust **(Fig. 7-57)**.

*Invasive* penile and scrotal SCC is an uncommon disorder in Western countries. Overall, *invasive penile* SCC accounts for only about 1% of all malignancies that occur at all locations in men.[50] Rates are somewhat higher than that in among Hispanics and African Americans in the United States, and the rates are appreciably higher for these individuals in lesser developed countries. The annual incidence of invasive penile SCC in all groups increases with age and primarily occurs after age 50. Invasive *scrotal* SCC is even less common than penile SCC and has markedly decreased in frequency as occupational exposure to causative toxins has decreased and scrotal shielding during PUVA therapy (psoralens plus ultraviolet A light) has increased.[51]

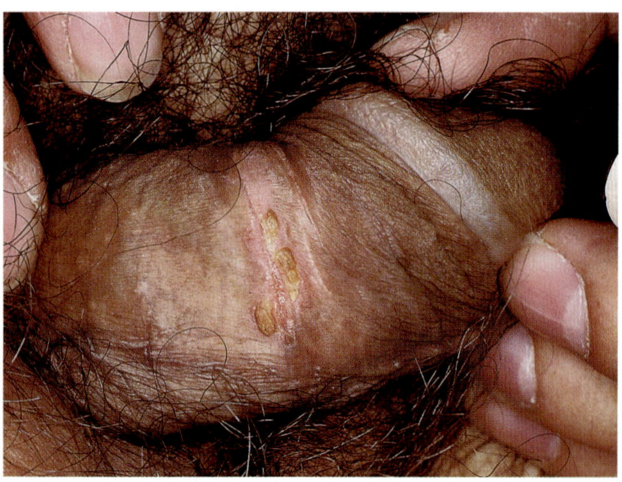

Fig. 7-56. PeIN of the shaft (Bowenoid papulosis, squamous cell carcinoma *in situ*) is generally scaling and can be skin colored, pink, or brown.

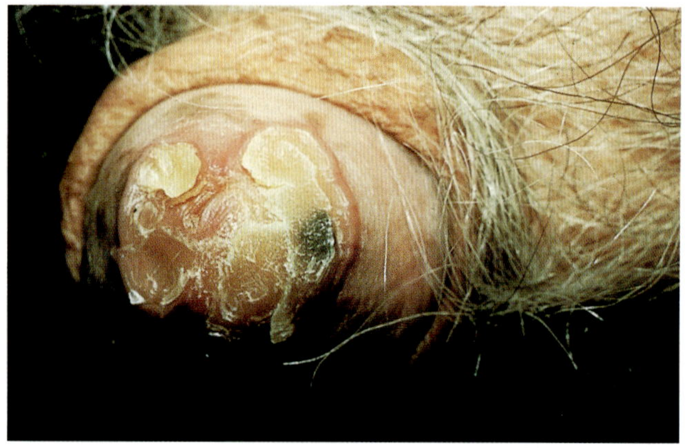

Fig. 7-57. Pseudoepitheliomatous, keratotic, and micaceous balanitis has been found to be associated with squamous cell carcinoma, lichen sclerosus, and, recently, with low-risk HPV infection in some instances; this has been treated surgically, with fluorouracil, cryotherapy, acitretin, and photodynamic therapy.

Almost all invasive SCC of the penis occurs on the glans, prepuce, and coronal sulcus. It usually presents as a 1- to 3-cm solitary nodule that is most often red or white in color **(Fig. 7-58)**. The surface in advanced lesions is often ulcerated in which case friable tissue with bleeding may be present at the base of the ulcer. Verrucous carcinoma, which accounts for only about 1% of penile

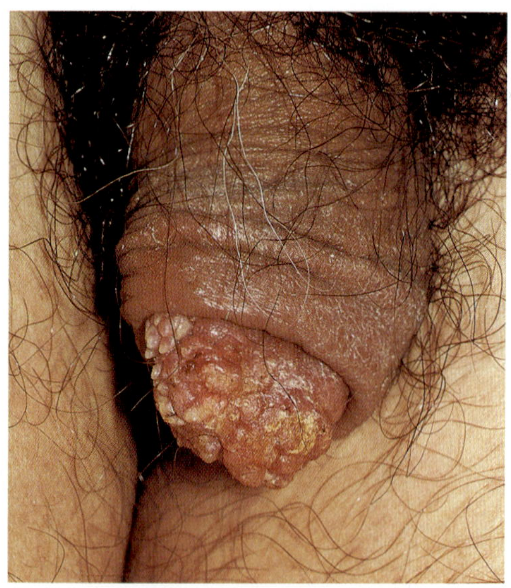

Fig. 7-58. This invasive squamous cell carcinoma shows a verrucous skin-colored mass in a typical location protruding from the glans of an uncircumcised man.

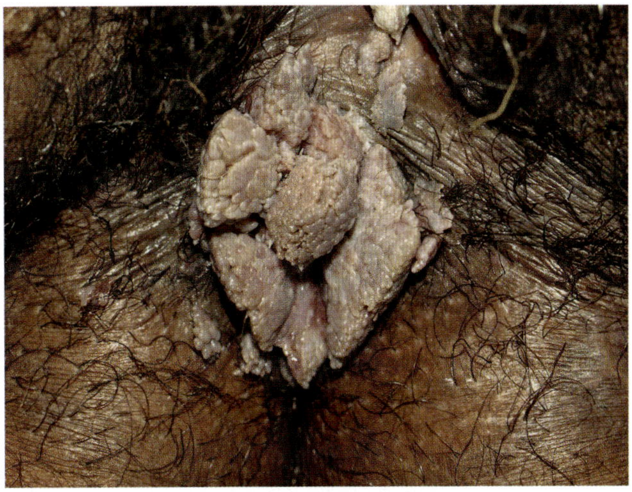

Fig. 7-59. This perianal Buschke-Lowenstein tumor is a very large wart that is clinically indistinguishable from a verrucous carcinoma.

SCC, presents as a nonscaling, cauliflowerlike, globular mass that is clinically indistinguishable from the nonmalignant, giant condyloma (Buschke-Lowenstein tumor) (**Fig. 7-59**). Regional lymphadenopathy, which is sometimes due to inflammation in the carcinoma rather than metastases, is present in about half of patients with invasive carcinoma. Note that nodal metastases can be present in nonpalpable nodes.

## Diagnosis

Though a diagnosis of penile SCC is frequently apparent on clinical findings, biopsy is always required for confirmation of the diagnosis. Histologically, penile SCC, as stated above, is divided into *in situ* (PeIN) cancer and *invasive* cancer. Of the *in situ* lesions, about 80% are positive for HPV DNA, and of the *invasive* lesions, ~50% are positive for HPV DNA.[45,47] Histologically, depending on various authors and their institutions, there are multiple subtypes of penile SCC. Suffice it to say that those placed within the "basaloid" and "warty" category are highly likely to contain high-risk HPV DNA, whereas those in the keratinizing (differentiated) and verrucous carcinoma subtypes are much less likely to contain HPV DNA.

In terms of differential diagnoses, PeIN on the shaft cannot clinically be differentiated from HPV-related warts. Likewise, verrucous carcinoma at any anogenital site cannot clinically be differentiated from the benign HPV-related giant condyloma (Buschke-Lowenstein tumor). Seborrheic keratoses on the shaft can mimic PeIN in that location. Psoriasis and lichen planus can appear very similar to PeIN on the shaft, glans, and prepuce. Extramammary Paget disease (EPD) also appears similar to PeIN, though the diameter of the plaques in EPD is usually much greater.

**SQUAMOUS CELL CARCINOMA IN MEN — Diagnosis**

- *HPV-related*: flat-topped red, brown, or skin-colored papules and plaques
  - Occur in younger men (<50).
  - Multiple lesions are usually present.
  - Most frequently located on the penile shaft, pubis, and perianal tissue.
  - Biopsy usually shows *in situ* dysplasia (PIN); much less often invasive cancer.
- *Non–HPV-related*: pink, red, white, or skin-colored papules, plaque, ulcers, or nodules
  - Occur in older men (>50).
  - Solitary lesion is usually present.
  - Most located on the glans, coronal sulcus, and inner aspect of prepuce.
  - Association with lichen sclerosus or, less often, erosive lichen planus.
  - Biopsy shows either *in situ* dysplasia or invasive cancer.

## Pathogenesis

As noted above, there appear to be two major pathways through which penile SCC develops: HPV-related and HPV nonrelated. The HPV-related pathway is more often associated with development of *in situ* dysplasia than with invasive SCC. And in this pathway, the same high-risk HPV types that are responsible for cervical carcinoma (notably HPV 16, 18, 31, 33, etc.) appear to be responsible for most of PeIN and about 50% of the invasive penile SCC.[50,52] Of these, HPV 16 is by far the most common type identified. But often multiple HPV types are found in a single tumor in which case there may be an admixture with low-risk HPV types, especially HPV 6 and 11. The situation for benign giant condyloma and verrucous carcinoma is more ambiguous. These two lesions are indistinguishable clinically and histologically, also, have many overlapping features. However, low-risk HPV types (HPV 6 or 11) are almost always found in the giant condylomas, whereas most of the verrucous carcinomas lack any HPV DNA. Risk factors for *in situ* carcinoma primarily relate to the acquisition of HPV and include early and numerous sex partners, penile-oral sex, sex with women who have cervical neoplasia and/or a history of anogenital warts.

The non-HPV pathway is less well understood but probably involves the presence of toxins (eg, tobacco smoke, retained smegma) or underlying chronic inflammatory disease such as is found in lichen planus and lichen sclerosus (aka, balanitis xerotica obliterans). There are multiple risk factors associated with the development of *invasive* penile SCC. The four most important as identified in published studies have been lack of circumcision at birth, smoking, phimosis, and lichen sclerosus (LS) of the glans. Though a relationship with lichen sclerosus seems noncontrovertible, most published series of patients suggest that only a small proportion of these with LS go on to develop malignancy. Nevertheless, in some instances of penile and vulvar SCC, histologic evidence of lichen sclerosus was sometimes found in peritumoral tissue, even though clinically LS was not visible.

### Management

Staging is appropriate for patients with penile SCC. This is usually carried out using the TNM staging system as is found in the American Joint Committee on Cancer (AJCC) 8th edition.[53] "Tis" is the TNM term used for PeIN. "T1" applies to carcinomas that invade only into the lamina propria (mucous membrane) or the most superficial connective tissue (skin). "T1" is further divided into "T1a" (no lymphovascular or perineural invasion and with favorable histologic features) and "T1b" (with lymphovascular and/or perineural invasion or with less favorable histologic features).[53]

Discussion of therapy in this chapter is restricted to *in situ* and minimally invasive carcinoma since the deeper forms require the involvement of gynecological oncologists or urologists. Historically, local excision or partial penectomy (usually with frozen section control of margins) represents the treatments of choice for Tis and T1a malignancies. Published information regarding the use of Mohs micrographic surgery is very limited. However, destructive methods (laser ablation, radiotherapy, or electrosurgery) and topical therapies (fluorouracil or imiquimod) are widely used for those instances of PeIN that are demonstrably HPV related. One problem, of course, with destructive and topical therapy is the dependence on limited biopsy sampling to assume that deeper invasion is not occurring elsewhere in the lesion.

Nevertheless, patients with Tis and T1a SCC are expected to essentially have a 100% 5-year survival. Node dissections are not carried out for Tis malignancy. Node sampling is recommended for T1a and other categories of more advanced disease since node metastases are found in about 25% of patients with no palpable nodes. Please note that, since at least 50% of penile SCC appears to be HPV-related, it is tempting to believe that HPV vaccination might prevent a significant portion of these penile SCCs; unfortunately at this time, the published data remain controversial.[54]

**SQUAMOUS CELL CARCINOMA IN MEN — Management**

*In situ* carcinoma (PeIN)
- *HPV-related:* excision or destruction with electrosurgery, laser, or topical therapy
- *Non–HPV-related*: excision or partial penectomy
- No sentinel node biopsy or node dissection

Invasive carcinoma
- Use TNM staging
- Excision for all
- If perineural or lymphovascular invasion, sentinel node biopsy
- Node dissection if more than two sentinel nodes are positive

## Squamous Cell Carcinoma of the Genitalia in Women

The spectrum of vulvar SCC includes both *in situ* vulvar intraepithelial neoplasia (VIN) and invasive SCC. VIN and invasive SCC of the vulva account for about 80%-90% of all vulvar malignancies; both are slowly increasing in frequency (see the discussion below regarding nomenclature and classification).

There are many similarities between squamous cell cancer of the genitalia in men and women. First, both develop through the same two pathways: an HPV-related one and a non–HPV-related one.[55,56] Second, squamous intraepithelial neoplasia associated with HPV infection tends to be multifocal, occurs in younger women, progresses somewhat more slowly from *in situ* disease, and when SCC does develop, it has a little better prognosis. On the other hand, intraepithelial neoplasia not associated with HPV tends to be unifocal, occurs in older women, progresses more quickly to invasion from the *in situ* stage, and when SCC does develop, it has a somewhat poorer prognosis.[55]

Third, as mentioned above in the section on SCC in men, SCC in women has historically been classified based on histological morphology as *in situ* malignancy (VIN) and *invasive* malignancy. In more recent years, there has been considerable movement toward classification of SCC based on pathogenesis into *HPV-related* and *HPV nonrelated* tumors. Many groups including the ISSVD and WHO are now specifically recommending classification and terminology for VIN that is similar to that used for cervical intraepithelial neoplasia: (1) low-grade squamous intraepithelial lesions (L-SIL) for benign warts containing low-risk HPV types, (2) high-grade squamous intraepithelial lesions (H-SIL) for what previously was termed usual VIN containing high-risk HPV types, and (3) differentiated VIN (dVIN) for intraepithelial lesions that are not HPV related.[55]

While this type of classification is logical and intellectually satisfying, we still prefer using VIN and invasive SCC at this time. Our preference is based on histological simplicity (routine histology is not 100% accurate in separating the HPV-related and the HPV nonrelated pathways) and because of the high cost or unavailability in many laboratories of definitive techniques (polymerase chain reaction, *in situ* hybridization) for detecting the presence of high-risk HPV types.

### Clinical Presentation of Vulvar Intraepithelial Neoplasia

Vulvar intraepithelial neoplasia appears to be increasing in frequency, whereas the age at which it occurs is decreasing. On the other hand, the incidence of invasive SCC is nearly stable or is barely rising. These changes are probably due to the increase in sexually transmitted papillomavirus infections some of which will be high-risk HPV types. For the same reason, the age at which invasive vulvar carcinoma occurs is falling. Unlike the situation for anogenital SCC in men, VIN and invasive SCC seem to be more common in White women than in African Americans or Hispanics. Of course, all of this is likely to change in the future based on the impressive efficacy of HPV vaccination and rising rate at which it is being administered. The clinical manifestations of VIN vary depending on whether or not the VIN is HPV related.

### HPV-Associated VIN (Also Called HSIL)

Vulvar intraepithelial neoplasia associated with HPV infection occurs almost entirely in young women, 15-50 years of age. It accounts for about 90%-95% of all VIN cases. It is most often a multifocal process in which multiple lesions are present concomitantly **(Figs. 7-60 and 7-61)**. The lesions are flat-topped papules and plaques that vary in diameter from 0.5 to 3 cm. The tissue around the lesions appears clinically normal. At times, these lesions grow into confluence resulting in the presence of even larger plaques that can occupy a large portion of the vulvar vestibule and on the keratinizing skin over the rest of the anogenital area. The color of HPV-related VIN is remarkably variable; it may be skin colored, pink, red, white, brown, or black. The surface is usually smooth or slightly scaly but, rarely, can be slightly eroded. The lesions are mostly asymptomatic, though mild itching may be present. On biopsy, a "basaloid" or "warty" pattern is usually found; p16 immunostaining is densely positive.

### HPV Nonrelated VIN

HPV nonrelated VIN (differentiated VIN, dVIN) presents quite differently. These lesions are much less common, are more frequently solitary, and occur mostly in older postmenopausal women. They occur as plaques or nodules that are usually 2-5 cm in diameter. Palpable scale, erosion, and/or ulceration are frequently present especially when VIN is superimposed on lesions of lichen sclerosus or erosive lichen planus. The lesions are red, white, or brown in color, and they develop mostly within the vestibule when the VIN is associated with lichen sclerosus or lichen planus **(Fig. 7-62)**. Uncommonly,

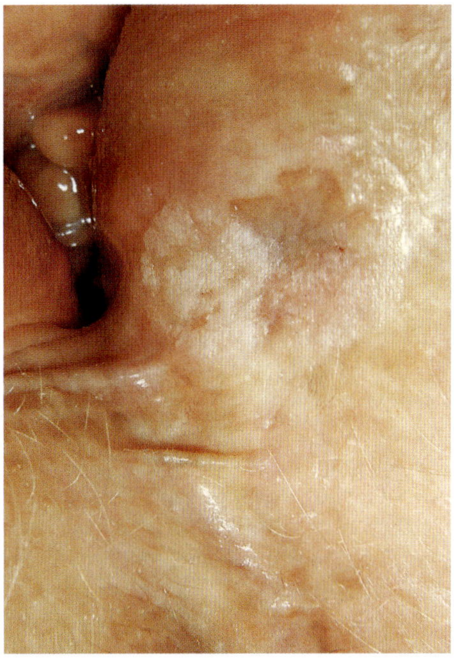

Fig. 7-61. HPV is the underlying cause of this intraepithelial neoplasia, or HSIL of the flat-topped, skin-colored to tan to white plaque on the perineum.

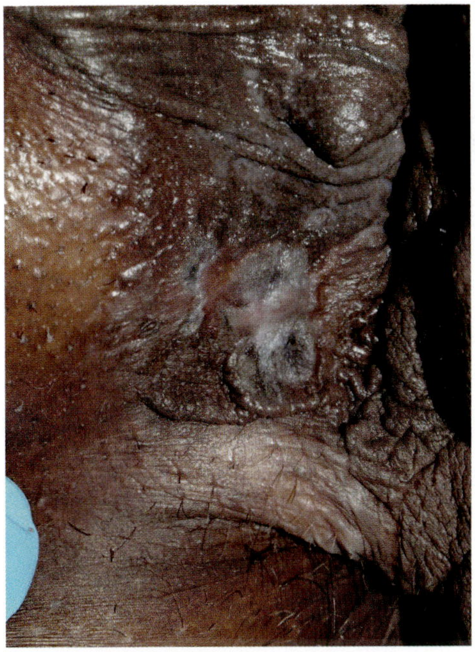

Fig. 7-60. The flattopped morphology with coalescence into a large plaque is suggestive of the correct diagnosis of HSIL.

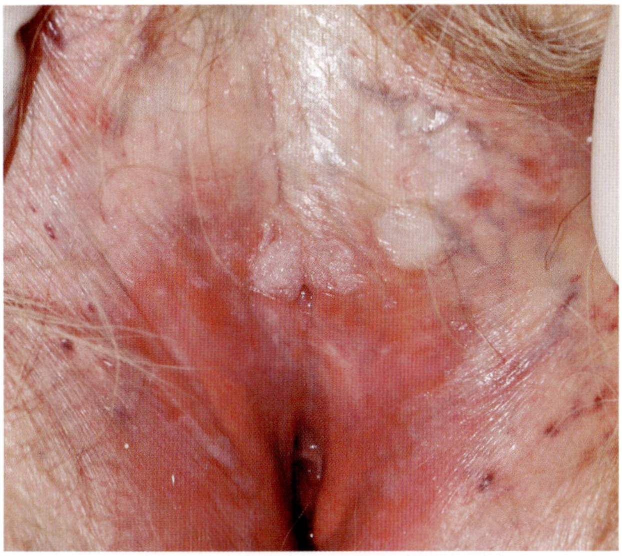

Fig. 7-62. Nearly all *in situ* squamous cell carcinoma on the basis of lichen sclerosus or lichen planus (dVIN) is red or white rather than skin colored. Although the rather rough surface suggests HPV as an etiology, the setting of lichen sclerosus and a biopsy that shows no evidence of HPV, and differentiated histology gives the correct diagnosis of dVIN, a much more aggressive form of *in situ* carcinoma.

HPV nonrelated VIN can be found on keratinizing skin anywhere in the anogenital area. Lesions overlying concomitant lichen sclerosus and erosive lichen planus are usually associated with itching, burning, or pain. Lesions arising on normal-appearing skin are more often asymptomatic, though pruritus and pain sometimes is present. Biopsy reveals a differentiated pattern, often superimposed on histologic changes compatible with lichen sclerosus. Recently two other precursor histologic patterns have been recognized, that of "differentiated exophytic vulvar intraepithelial lesion" (DEVIL) and "vulvar acanthosis with altered differentiation" (VAAD).[56] Mutation in tumor suppressor genes are found in 80%-90% of these HPV-independent VIN lesions.

In terms of differential diagnosis, VIN arising from normal skin must be differentiated from anogenital warts, psoriasis, lichen planus, and seborrheic keratoses. It may be quite difficult to separately identify VIN overlying lichen sclerosus and lichen planus from those disorders themselves. In all of these situations, biopsy is required.

*Verrucous carcinoma* is essentially identical in clinical appearance to that of benign giant condylomata (Buschke-Lowenstein tumors). It presents as a slow growing, large warty, or cauliflowerlike nodule **(Fig. 7-63)**. I have chosen to place verrucous carcinoma in this section on intraepithelial squamous neoplasms because in the majority of cases, the histologically impressive downgrowth of the rete ridges pushing deeply into the dermis, along with noncontiguous nests of epithelial cells, makes it difficult to determine whether or not the basement membrane has actually been breached.[57] At one time, it was thought that verrucous carcinoma represented malignant transformation of the HPV-related giant condylomata, but this hypothesis has fallen into disfavor for two reasons: (1) benign giant condylomata are associated only with low-risk HPV types (mostly HPV 6 and 11) and thus should not progress to cancer and (2) polymerase chain reaction (PCR) studies of verrucous carcinoma rarely reveal the presence of any HPV DNA. Today, it seems more likely that verrucous carcinoma is related to differentiated exophytic vulvar intraepithelial lesion (DEVIL) or vulvar acanthosis with altered differentiation (VAAD).[56] Notably, these conditions share somewhat similar histological morphology and have a high frequency of *PIK3CA* and *HRAS* gene mutations.[57]

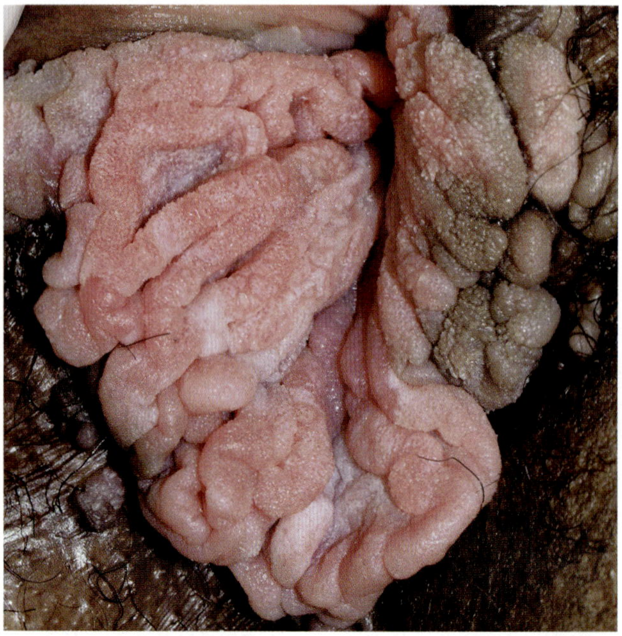

Fig. 7-63. This enormous wart showed malignant changes on pathology when it was removed.

**VULVAR INTRAEPITHELIAL NEOPLASIA (VIN) IN WOMEN — Diagnosis**

*HPV-related*: flat-topped red, brown, or skin-colored papules and plaques; younger women; multiple lesions are generally present; accounts for 85%-90% of VIN

- Location on vestibule, labia majora, perivulvar, and perianal sites.
- Biopsy shows only *in situ* carcinoma (VIN); invasion is present in only 5% of cases.

*Non–HPV-related:* pink, red, or white papule and nodule, surface rough or ulcerated; older women; usually only a solitary lesion is present; accounts for 10%-15% of VIN

- Location within vestibule and labia minora; occasionally elsewhere.
- Frequent occurrence with lichen sclerosus or, less often, lichen planus, DEVIL, VAAD.
- Biopsy often shows one or more areas of invasion.

## Clinical Presentation of Invasive Squamous Cell Carcinoma

Invasive SCC is not a common cancer, but it does have an incidence rate of about 2 or 3 per 100,000 women per year. Short of biopsy, it is not possible to determine whether one or more lesions having the appearance of HPV-related VIN (see above) harbors evidence of invasion. In fact, multiple biopsies generally are necessary just to be sure that a small area of invasion is not missed. It is true that HPV nonrelated VIN arising in lichen sclerosus or lichen planus undergoes invasion much more often than, and much more quickly than, HPV-related VIN. As a consequence, only a small minority of invasive SCC is multifocal. It is also true that most invasive SCC occurs in women over the age of 50, but it is worth noting that about 15% of such cancers develop in women under the age of 40.

Early in its evolution, minimally invasive SCC cannot be distinguished clinically from VIN. More advanced lesions occur as white, red, or skin-colored plaques or nodules. The surface is often ulcerated with the ulcer cavity containing friable tissue that bleeds easily. Itching and/or pain occur commonly.

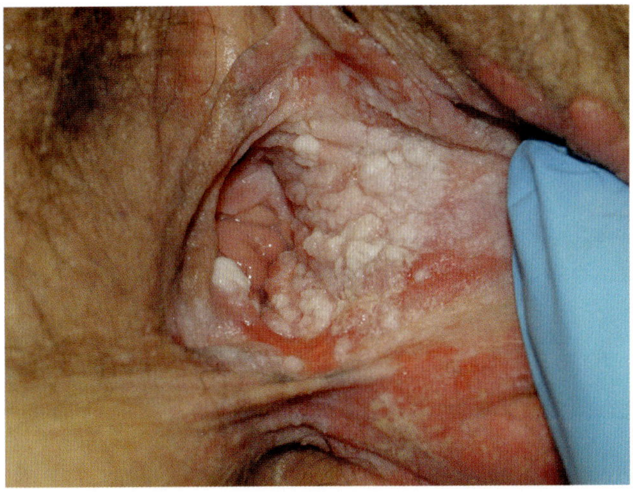

Fig. 7-64. The verrucous plaque of genital wart has enlarged and transformed into high-grade squamous intraepithelial lesion (VIN) and then invasive squamous cell carcinoma involving much of the left vulva.

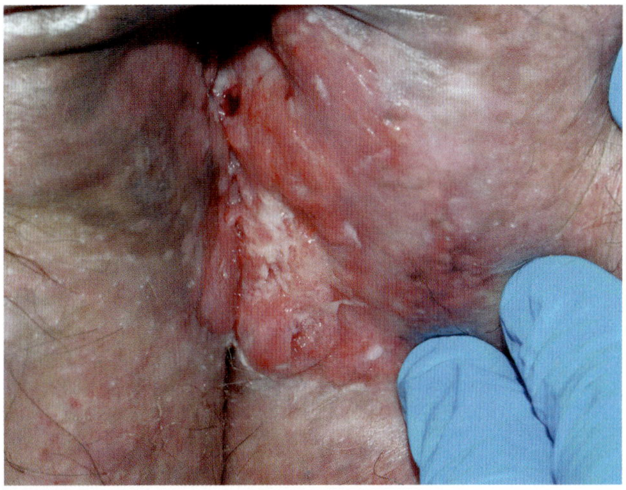

Fig. 7-65. Lichen sclerosus is well known to be associated with squamous cell carcinoma, as has occurred here, where a large skin-colored eroded tumor covers the left perineum.

In the short run, invasive SCC develops in about 10% of untreated HPV-related VIN and possibly would occur in nearly all such patients in the long run. This progression from *in situ* HPV-related disease is appreciably more common in women than it is in men **(Fig. 7-64)**. Early invasive SCC can develop with an appearance similar or identical to VIN and is especially likely to be present in patients with eroded, ulcerated, or hyperkeratotic lichen sclerosus **(Fig. 7-65)**. We believe that it can also develop in eroded plaques of lichen planus, though this view is somewhat debatable. Rarely, invasive SCC arises on completely normal tissue.

More advanced SCC appears as a bulky exophytic mass, often with ulceration and bleeding. Invasive SCC, especially with early lesions, may be asymptomatic, but in most instances, itching, pain, or bleeding alerts the patient or the clinician to its presence. When pruritus is severe, as it often is in patients with lichen sclerosus, the thickened epidermal response of lichenification occurs because of prolonged rubbing and scratching. It is controversial whether or not the epithelial cell proliferation that occurs during lichenification plays any role in the development or progress of malignancy.[56] However, it could be that lichenification was misdiagnosed when, in fact, it was part of the DEVIL or VAAD spectrum and was a true precursor of SCC (see above).[57]

## Diagnosis of VIN and Invasive Squamous Cell Carcinoma

A diagnosis of VIN or invasive SCC may be suspected clinically but must be confirmed by histopathological examination. If multiple lesions are present, or if the lesion is large, it is advisable to take several biopsies. It is especially important to biopsy (and even re-biopsy) any persistently elevated or eroded area in lichen sclerosus and lichen planus that has not completely responded to appropriate therapy.

## Pathophysiology

As indicated above, there are two pathways relating to the development of vulvar SCC: an HPV-related pathway and a non–HPV-related pathway.[55] These two pathways correlate well, but not perfectly, with separate histologic patterns: a warty or basaloid pattern in HPV-related disease and a differentiated (keratinizing) pattern for HPV nonrelated disease. The HPV-related pathway involves infection with the same high-risk HPV types (notably HPV 16 and much less often HPV 18, 31, 33, 45, 52, and 58) responsible for cervical carcinoma. This type of infection leads first to the development of warty and/or basaloid VIN (H-SIL) followed in many cases by the development of invasive carcinoma with those same histologic features. PCR studies reveal HPV DNA to be resent in the vast majority of warty and basaloid VIN and also in a similarly high percentage of invasive carcinomas with warty or basaloid histology. At the molecular level, and in the simplest terms, the HPV viral proteins E6 an E7 bind to and interfere with the effect of the p53 and retinoblastoma tumor suppressor proteins.[58]

The non–HPV-related pathway is less clear. However, recently, the importance of chronic inflammation in the development of many cancers has become more apparent. Most, but not all, differentiated VIN (dVIN) arises in the setting of the inflammatory diseases lichen sclerosus or, less often, erosive lichen planus. Approximately 70%-90% of these patients have mutations in the tumor suppressor genes that might explain the predilection to develop SCC.[56] But what of the 10% or 30% who do not harbor these mutations? Two possibilities seem to exist. First, there is a high frequency of squamous cell hyperplasia (the acanthotic changes found in lichenification) in the peritumoral tissue in some HPV nonrelated malignancies, thus raising the possibility that the chronic inflammation, induced by constant rubbing and scratching, might be involved. Second, is that the acanthosis and absence of cellular atypicality is in reality that of DEVIL or VAAD (see above). These two entities commonly contain *PIK3CA* and *HRAS* mutations that could identify them as true precursor lesions.[56,57] Finally, it should also be noted that DNA for various low-risk and high-risk HPV types is found in a small percentage of cases of differentiated VIN and associated invasive SCC. It seems most likely that such HPV DNA is there simply as an "innocent bystander," but an etiologic role cannot be completely excluded at this time.

There are multiple clinical risk factors associated with the development of VIN and invasive SCC. Smoking is the most important of these for both HPV-related and HPV nonrelated malignancy. In addition, there are several risk factors that apply only for HPV-related VIN. These are associated with acquisition of HPV at a young sexual debut, multiple sex partners, history of abnormal Pap smears, and history of anogenital warts. Immunosuppression and the use of various hormones may also play a role as risk factors.

## Management

### Staging

Both VIN and invasive SCC are staged using the tumor, nodes, metastases (TNM) approach. Both the 2016 American Joint Committee on Cancer (AJCC) classification and the 2009 Federation of Gynecology and Obstetrics (FIGO) classification are in widespread use.[59,60] Little detail will be given here since, as was true for penile cancer, management of patients with positive nodes and/or metastases goes beyond the scope of this book. The AJCC term for carcinoma *in situ* is "Tis," while there is no term for *in situ* malignancy in the FIGO system. The AJCC and the FIGO terms for early carcinoma are essentially identical (T1a and 1A) for those lesions of 2 cm or less in diameter and with stromal invasion of 1.0 mm or less. The AJCC and the FIGO terms are also similar (T1b and 1B) for those lesions >2 cm in size or with stromal invasion more than 1.0 mm.

### Management of VIN

Spontaneous regression of HPV-related VIN (H-SIL) has been reported in some young women (under age 35) and in a few patients following parturition. This possibility along with a low likelihood of malignant progression in these young women suggests that it would be reasonable to simply follow young patients without treatment for about 1 year in the hope that their strong immune responsiveness will allow for clearing of the problem. For those over 35 years with H-SIL and for all patients with differentiated type VIN (dVIN), wide local excision shortly after diagnosis is the treatment of choice.[55] There is some controversy regarding the appropriate width of margins for these excisions. Most gynecologists believe that 5 mm is sufficient for H-SIL, but some believe that differentiated VIN (dVIN) should be treated with wider margins (10 mm) because of its higher risk for recurrence and generally poorer outcome. These wider margins might be theoretically desirable, but they must be balanced with greater architectural damage, possible sexual dysfunction, and poorer quality of life. Mohs micrographic surgery should offer excellent results for VIN of all types, but unfortunately, there are too few published studies for this approach to be strongly recommended at this time.

Laser ablation or photodynamic therapy may be considered for HPV-related VIN (H-SIL), but longer postoperative pain and prolonged healing generally make these destructive techniques second-line therapy.[55] Medical therapy for H-SIL with imiquimod or cidofovir also provides quite good results and preserves normal architecture leading to some patient preference.[55] However, the biggest drawback for both ablative and medical therapy is the resultant lack of tissue for histological examination leading to the very real possibility that foci of stromal invasion might be missed.

The prognosis for VIN depends on patient age, immunocompetence, and whether the VIN is HPV related or is of the differentiated type. Patients who are immunocompromised and those with differentiated VIN appear to have an appreciably poorer prognosis. The overall prognosis of patients following excisional surgery for VIN is quite good. Nevertheless, recurrence rates are fairly high even with histologically clear margins, and ~5% of patients with treated H-SIL and 35% of those with dVIN do go on to develop invasive SCC.[55]

Recommendations for the staging of vulvar carcinoma are given in the first paragraph in this section on management. The preferred treatment for the first stage (lesions <2 cm) with invasion of no more 1.0 mm (T1a, IA) is wide local excision with margins of about 1 cm.[59] This limited form of surgery is just as effective as the historically recommended, but devastating, radical vulvectomy. Since there is very little likelihood of node involvement, patients with T1a and no palpable nodes can be spared node dissection and can be treated with observation instead. The preferred treatment for the second stage (T1b, 1B) that is, lesions >2 cm or invasion deeper than 1.0 mm and no palpable nodes is also wide local excision with margins of about 1 cm.[59] However, in this stage, while the likelihood of node involvement is still low, ipsilateral node dissection or sentinel node biopsy is recommended. The prognosis for these two stages treated as indicated above is quite good with 2-year overall survival of about 90% and 5-year survival of about 80%. Finally, as noted above, prophylactic HPV vaccination with any of the currently available vaccines has the potential to eliminate those forms of vulvar cancer that are HPV related.

**SQUAMOUS CELL CARCINOMA IN WOMEN** — **Management**

*In situ carcinoma (VIN)*

- HPV-related (usual VIN, HSIL): excision; but consider electrosurgery, laser ablation, or topical imiquimod.
- After biopsy; 1-year observation OK for women under age 35.
- Non–HPV-related (differentiated VIN, dVIN): wide local excision is mandatory.

*Invasive carcinoma*

- Use FIGO or AJCC staging.
- Excision with 1-cm margin for all.
- If >1 mm invasion, sentinel node biopsy or node dissection.

## Basal Cell Carcinoma

Basal cell carcinoma, the most frequently diagnosed of all skin malignancies on sun-exposed skin, is uncommonly encountered at clothed sites such as on the genitalia. In fact, these genital BCCs represent only about 1% of all BCCs and account for only about 5%-8% of all genital malignancies. Recently, Chinese investigators, using data gathered from 18 registries of the U.S. Surveillance, Epidemiology and End Results (SEER) database, published a review of BCCs involving the male and female genitalia.[61] This review included 1607 cases reported from 2000 to 2017, making it the largest ever such review. Much of the material presented in the next several paragraphs is based on their results.

Multiple types of BCC have been described as occurring on sun-exposed skin. Nodular BCCs are by far the most common and probably account for 90%-95% of these tumors. The second most common type is the plaquelike superficial BCC, which can simplistically be viewed as an analog of *in situ* SCC. Almost none of the reported cases of anogenital BCC indicate which type was encountered. In fact, I was able to find less than a half dozen published cases that specifically identify superficial BCCs though I suspect that there were many more. With this in mind, only the nodular form of BCC is described in this section.

### Clinical Presentation

The median age at presentation in both men and women was in the eighth decade. The range of age is, however, pretty large with half of the tumors having developed between the ages of 60 and 85 years. Almost 100% of the anogenital BCCs occur on tissues where hair follicles can be found. BCC of the genitalia predominated in women and accounted for about 85% of all the cases reported. Most occurred on the labium majus of the vulva with only a few found on the labium minus and around the clitoris. Men accounted for only 15% of the cases, and the scrotum was involved twice as often as the penis. Rarely, BCCs have been found in the perianal area. Lesions tend to have been present for a long period of time prior to diagnosis probably because they are usually asymptomatic and because many of them, especially in women, are not easily observable by the patients.

Probably for the same reasons, these neoplasms are larger than BCCs that develop at other sites. They average about 1.0-3.0 cm in diameter. Almost all lesions are solitary and they usually appear as skin-colored or pink 1.0- to 3.0-cm papules or nodules. Occasionally, tan or even brown hues are noted, especially in people of color, due to increased melanin pigmentation (**Fig. 7-66**). Early, small lesions are smooth surfaced, but about 30% of the tumors are ulcerated. Large lesions may have rolled borders.

### Diagnosis

Occasionally, the correct diagnosis is suspected clinically, but all lesions require biopsy for confirmation. Dermoscopy of the nodular BCC is characterize by arborizing vessels, large bright red branching vessels, among many other possible findings.[62] The histologic appearance is usually quite characteristic, but sometimes the pathologist has trouble distinguishing nodular BCC from other hair follicle–derived tumors and from basaloid SCCs. Disorders commonly considered in differential diagnosis include SCC and intradermal nevi. Less often, other skin-colored lesions described in this chapter will need to be considered.

**BASAL CELL CARCINOMA OF THE ANOGENITAL REGION** — **Diagnosis**

- Older men and women.
- Skin colored, pink, or, in patients of color, tan.
- Usually appear as a solitary papule or nodule.
- Lesion may be ulcerated.
- Occur only on hair-bearing, keratinizing (nonmucosal) skin.
- Location: labia majora in women; penis and scrotum in men; perianal area for both sexes.
- Biopsy for diagnosis and/or confirmation.

### Pathophysiology

Chronic ultraviolet light exposure plays a very important role for those BCC that occur on sun-exposed skin. Obviously, this is not the situation for genital lesions. All patients with Gorlin syndrome (nevoid BCC syndrome, basal cell nevus syndrome) and most with sporadic BCC have mutations in genes (especially the patched and smoothened genes) that are part of the sonic hedgehog signaling pathway. Mutations in *TP53* and polymorphisms in *MC1R* also occur. Although not documented, it seems likely that patients with anogenital BCC also have these genetic defects. It is likely that such mutations act in concert with other environmental factors such as chronic irritation and inflammation to induce the development of this malignancy in the anogenital region.[63]

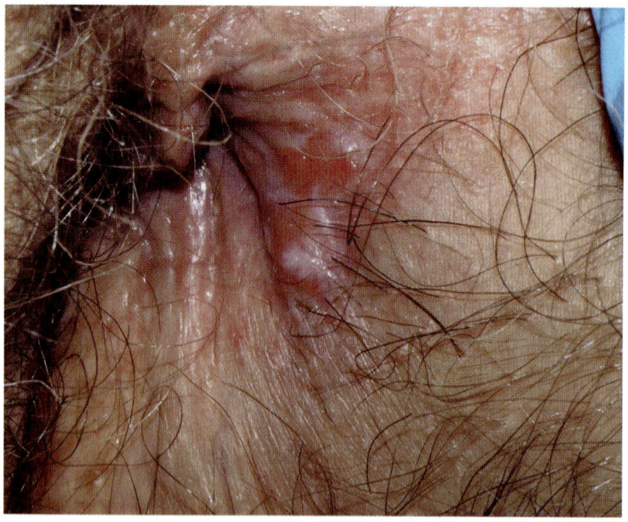

Fig. 7-66. The basal cell carcinoma is a perianal, skin-colored plaque at 3-5 o'clock with a shiny translucent surface; the lower area shows a superficial white discoloration due to hydration of a thickened surface.

## Management

Excision has historically represented the treatment of choice. But, because of their large size together with an attempt to preserve normal architecture, histological margins observed after excision may not be clear. For this reason, recurrence rates as high as 20% have been reported. Mohs micrographic surgery should be strongly considered as it combines maximum tissue sparing with the ability to obtain microscopically documented tumor-free margins at the time of the initial procedure.[64] Topical application of imiquimod cream is theoretically attractive on the basis of the excellent cosmetic outcome associated with its use. However, it is not FDA approved for nodular BCC, and experience with its use for genital BCC is limited.

The overall prognosis for BCC occurring at nongenital sites is excellent as it rarely results in metastasis. However, regional spread and metastases have been reported in 2% or 3% of anogenital BCCs. This number seems to be excessively high, but this apparent excess may be explained by the observation that patients with genital BCCs seem to have had their tumors longer, present with larger lesions, and are appreciably older (thus with a less robust immune response) than patients with lesions on other parts of the body.

**BASAL CELL CARCINOMA — Management**

- Excision for all though recurrence rates are fairly high.
- Consider Mohs micrographic surgery as recurrences are much less frequent.
- Risk of metastasis is small.
- No sentinel node biopsy.
- No node dissection unless nodes are palpable.

## REFERENCES


1. Magalhães GM, Vieira ÉC, Garcia LC, De Carvalho-Leite MLR, Guedes ACM, Araújo MG. Update on human papilloma virus—part I: epidemiology, pathogenesis, and clinical spectrum. *An Bras Dermatol.* 2021;96(1):1-16. doi:10.1016/j.abd.2020.11.003
2. Hirth J. Disparities in HPV vaccination rates and HPV prevalence in the United States: a review of the literature. *Hum Vaccin Immunother.* 2019;15(1):146-155. doi:10.1080/21645515.2018.1512453
3. Seong SH, et al. Dermoscopic findings of genital keratotic lesions: Bowenoid papulosis, seborrheic keratosis, and condyloma acuminatum. *Photodiagnosis Photodyn Ther.* 2021;36:102448. doi:10.1016/j.pdpdt.2021.102448
4. Tosato Boldrini NA, Bondi Volpini LP, de Freitas LB, et al. Anal HPV infection and correlates in HIV-infected patients attending a Sexually Transmitted Infection clinic in Brazil. *PLoS One.* 2018;13(7):e0199058. doi:10.1371/journal.pone.0199058
5. Poljak M, Oštrbenk Valenčak A, Gimpelj Domjanič G, Xu L, Arbyn M. Commercially available molecular tests for human papillomaviruses: a global overview. *Clin Microbiol Infect.* 2020;26(9):1144-1150. doi:10.1016/j.cmi.2020.03.033
6. Bertolotti A, Ferdynus C, Milpied B, Dupin N, Huiart L, Derancourt C. Local management of anogenital warts in non-immunocompromised adults: a network meta-analysis of randomized controlled trials. *Dermatol Ther (Heidelb).* 2020;10(2):249-262. doi:10.1007/s13555-020-00357-z
7. Gilson R, Nugent D, Werner RN, Ballesteros J, Ross J. 2019 IUSTI-Europe guideline for the management of anogenital warts. *J Eur Acad Dermatol Venereol.* 2020;34(8):1644-1653. doi:10.1111/jdv.16522
8. Jung JM, Jung CJ, Lee WJ, et al. Topically applied treatments for external genital warts in nonimmunocompromised patients: a systematic review and network meta-analysis. *Br J Dermatol.* 2020;183(1):24-36. doi:10.1111/bjd.18638
9. Cheng L, Wang Y, Du J. Human papillomavirus vaccines: an updated review. *Vaccines (Basel).* 2020;8(3):391. doi:10.3390/vaccines8030391
10. Meza-Romero R, Navarrete-Dechent C, Downey C. Molluscum contagiosum: an update and review of new perspectives in etiology, diagnosis, and treatment. *Clin Cosmet Investig Dermatol.* 2019;12:373-381. doi:10.2147/CCID.S187224
11. van der Wouden JC, van der Sande R, Kruithof EJ, Sollie A, van Suijlekom-Smit LW, Koning S. Interventions for cutaneous molluscum contagiosum. *Cochrane Database Syst Rev.* 2017;5(5):CD004767. doi:10.1002/14651858.CD004767.pub4
12. Pandey A, Sonthalia S. Skin tags. In: *StatPearls* [Internet]. StatPearls Publishing; 2021.
13. Platsidaki E, Vasalou V, Gerodimou M, et al. The association of various metabolic parameters with multiple skin tags. *J Clin Aesthet Dermatol.* 2018;11(10):40-43.
14. Pogacnik JS, Salgado G. Perianal Crohn's disease. *Clin Colon Rectal Surg.* 2019;32(5):377-385. doi:10.1055/s-0039-1687834
15. Honigman AD, Dubin DP, Chu J, Lin MJ. Management of pearly penile papules: a review of the literature. *J Cutan Med Surg.* 2020;24(1):79-85. doi:10.1177/1203475419887730
16. Ozeki M, Saito R, Tanaka M. Dermoscopic features of pearly penile papules. *Dermatology.* 2008;217:21-22. doi:10.1159/000118509
17. Thakare SA, Udare S. Importance of dermoscopy to diagnose vulvar vestibular papillomatosis vs. warts. *Indian Dermatol Online J.* 2020;11(4):680-681. doi:10.4103/idoj.IDOJ_463_18

18. Paolino G, Muscardin LM, Panetta C, Donati M, Donati P. Linear ectopic sebaceous hyperplasia of the penis: the last memory of Tyson's glands. *G Ital Dermatol Venereol.* 2018;153(3):429-431. doi:10.23736/S0392-0488.16.05129-4
19. Roma AA, Barry J, Pai RK, Billings SD. Sebaceous hyperplasia of the vulva: a series of cases reporting no association with the Muir-Torre syndrome. *Int J Gynecol Pathol.* 2014;33(4):437-442. doi:10.1097/PGP.0b013e31829ff21e
20. Salloum A, Bouferraa Y, Bazzi N, et al. Pathophysiology, clinical findings, and management of Fox-Fordyce disease: a systematic review. *J Cosmet Dermatol.* 2022;21:482-500. doi:10.1111/jocd.14135
21. Gurusamy L, Jegadeesan M, Jayakumar S. Fox-Fordyce disease of the vulva. *Indian J Sex Transm Dis AIDS.* 2016;37(1):65-67. doi:10.4103/0253-7184.180293
22. Byth LA, Byth J. Fox-Fordyce disease: insights from cases induced by laser hair removal. *Australas J Dermatol.* 2020;61(2):188-189. doi:10.1111/ajd.13194
23. Kundak S, Çakır Y. Pediatric lichen nitidus: a single-center experience. *Pediatr Dermatol.* 2019;36(2):189-192. doi:10.1111/pde.13749
24. Errichetti E. Dermoscopy of Inflammatory Dermatoses (Inflammoscopy): an up-to-date overview. *Dermatol Pract Concept.* 2019;9:169-180. doi:10.5826/dpc.0903a01
25. Tosti G, Salvini C, Barisani A, et al. Vulval hidradenoma papilliferum: a clinical and dermoscopic study. *Clin Exp Dermatol.* 2020;45(8):1035-1039. doi:10.1111/ced.14254
26. Seo GJ, Seo JH, Cho KJ, Cho HS. Hidradenoma papilliferum of the anus: a report of 2 cases and review of the literature. *Ann Coloproctol.* 2019;35(6):361-363. doi:10.3393/ac.2018.08.03
27. El-Khoury J, Renald MH, Plantier F, Avril MF, Moyal-Barracco M. Vulvar hidradenoma papilliferum (HP) is located on the sites of mammary-like anogenital glands (MLAGs): analysis of the photographs of 52 tumors. *J Am Acad Dermatol.* 2016;75(2):380-384. doi:10.1016/j.jaad.2016.01.034
28. Pfarr N, Allgäuer M, Steiger K, et al. Several genotypes, one phenotype: PIK3CA/AKT1 mutation-negative hidradenoma papilliferum show genetic lesions in other components of the signalling network. *Pathology.* 2019;51(4):362-368. doi:10.1016/j.pathol.2019.01.010
29. Ku S, Balasubramanian A, Kao CS, Eisenberg ML, Skinner EC. Co-manifestations of genital neurofibromatosis in a patient with neurofibromatosis type 1. *Urology.* 2020;141:e49-e50. doi:10.1016/j.urology.2020.03.030
30. Rabley A, Bayne CE, Shenoy A, DeMarco RT. Genital neurofibromatosis presenting as painful clitoromegaly. *Urology.* 2019;133:219-221. doi:10.1016/j.urology.2019.07.016
31. Banthia R, Yadav P, Agarwal R, Lal H. Plexiform neurofibromatosis of penis: a rare presentation of type 1 neurofibromatosis. *BMJ Case Rep.* 2020;13(11):e236542. doi:10.1136/bcr-2020-236542
32. Forrestel AK, Kovarik CL, Katz KA. Sexually acquired syphilis: Historical aspects, microbiology, epidemiology, and clinical manifestations. *J Am Acad Dermatol.* 2020;82(1):1-14. doi:10.1016/j.jaad.2019.02.073
33. Forrestel AK, Kovarik CL, Katz KA. Sexually acquired syphilis: laboratory diagnosis, management, and prevention. *J Am Acad Dermatol.* 2020;82(1):17-28. doi:10.1016/j.jaad.2019.02.074
34. de Vries HJC, de Barbeyrac B, de Vrieze NHN, et al. 2019 European guideline on the management of lymphogranuloma venereum. *J Eur Acad Dermatol Venereol.* 2019;33(10):1821-1828. doi:10.1111/jdv.15729
35. Garib G, Lullo JJ, Andea AA. Vulvar syringoma. *Cutis.* 2020;105(5):E7-E10.
36. Corazza C, Borghi C, Minghetti S, Ferron P, Virgili A. Dermoscopy of isolated syringoma of the vulva. *J Am Acad Dermatol.* 2017;76:S37-S39. doi:10.1016/j.jaad.2016.06.009
37. DiCarlo-Meacham AM, Dengler KL, Snitchler AN, Gruber DD. Clitoral epidermal inclusion cyst leading to anorgasmia: a case report and literature review. *J Pediatr Adolesc Gynecol.* 2020;33(3):321-323. doi:10.1016/j.jpag.2020.01.150
38. Syed MMA, Amatya B, Sitaula S. Median raphe cyst of the penis: a case report and review of the literature. *J Med Case Rep.* 2019;13(1):214. doi:10.1186/s13256-019-2133-5
39. Suh KS, et al. Usefulness of dermoscopy in the differential diagnosis of ruptured and unruptured epidermal cysts. *Ann Dermatol.* 2017;29:33-38.doi:10.5021/ad.2017.29.1.33
40. Syed MMA, Rajbhandari A, Paudel U. Idiopathic calcinosis cutis of the scrotum: a case report and review of the literature. *J Med Case Rep.* 2018;12(1):366. doi:10.1186/s13256-018-1922-6
41. Nixon AT, Garza RF. Pilonidal cyst and sinus. In: *StatPearls* [Internet]. StatPearls Publishing; 2021.
42. Kanis MJ, Momeni M, Zakashansky K. Pilonidal cyst of the clitoris. *Female Pelvic Med Reconstr Surg.* 2014;20(5):297-298. doi:10.1097/SPV.0000000000000065
43. Shanmugathas N, Yassin M, Ross C, Minhas S. Pilonidal sinus disease of the penis: a case report and review of the literature. *Andrologia.* 2021;53(1):e13837. doi:10.1111/and.13837
44. Omole F, Kelsey RC, Phillips K, Cunningham K. Bartholin duct cyst and gland abscess: office management. *Am Fam Physician.* 2019;99(12):760-766.
45. Illingworth B, Stocking K, Showell M, Kirk E, Duffy J. Evaluation of treatments for Bartholin's cyst or abscess: a systematic review. *BJOG.* 2020;127(6):671-678. doi:10.1111/1471-0528.16079
46. Reda A, Gomaa I. Vulvar lipoma: a case report. *Rev Bras Ginecol Obstet.* 2018;40(10):647-649. doi:10.1055/s-0038-1670642
47. Goto Y, Takiguchi K, Shimizu H, Go H, Tanaka H. Congenital perianal lipoma: a case report and review of the literature. *Surg Case Rep.* 2019;5(1):199. doi:10.1186/s40792-019-0753-z
48. Bhanja DB, Chakraborty S, Sil A, Panigrahi A. Non-venereal sclerosing lymphangitis of the penis. *Int J Dermatol.* 2020;59(11):e395-e396. doi:10.1111/ijd.15007
49. Foresti M, Parmiggiani A. Penile Mondor's disease: imaging in two cases. *J Radiol Case Rep.* 2020;14(12):24-30. doi:10.3941/jrcr.v14i12.3926
50. Eich ML, Del Carmen Rodriguez Pena M, Schwartz L, et al. Morphology, p16, HPV, and outcomes in squamous cell carcinoma of the penis: a multi-institutional study. *Hum Pathol.* 2020;96:79-86. doi:10.1016/j.humpath.2019.09.013
51. Zhu Y, Ye DW. Preneoplastic and primary scrotal cancer: updates on pathogenesis and diagnostic evaluation. *Urol Clin North Am.* 2016;43(4):523-530. doi:10.1016/j.ucl.2016.06.013
52. Olesen TB, Sand FL, Rasmussen CL, et al. Prevalence of human papillomavirus DNA and p16$^{INK4a}$ in penile cancer and penile intraepithelial neoplasia: a systematic review and meta-analysis. *Lancet Oncol.* 2019;20(1):145-158. doi:10.1016/S1470-2045(18)30682-X
53. Khalil MI, Kamel MH, Dhillon J, et al. What you need to know: updates in penile cancer staging. *World J Urol.* 2021;39:1413-1419. doi:10.1007/s00345-020-03302-z
54. da Costa Nunes JF, Pires S, Chade DC. Human papillomavirus vaccination and prevention of intraepithelial neoplasia and penile cancer: review article. *Curr Opin Urol.* 2020;30(2):208-212. doi:10.1097/MOU.0000000000000730

55. Lebreton M, Carton I, Brousse S, et al. Vulvar intraepithelial neoplasia: classification, epidemiology, diagnosis, and management. *J Gynecol Obstet Hum Reprod.* 2020;49(9):101801. doi:10.1016/j.jogoh.2020.101801
56. Jenkins TM, Mills AM. Putative precancerous lesions of vulvar squamous cell carcinoma. *Semin Diagn Pathol.* 2021;38(1):27-36. doi:10.1053/j.semdp.2020.09.006
57. Akbari A, Pinto A, Amemiya Y, Seth A, Mirkovic J, Parra-Herran C. Differentiated exophytic vulvar intraepithelial lesion: clinicopathologic and molecular analysis documenting its relationship with verrucous carcinoma of the vulva. *Mod Pathol.* 2020;33(10):2011-2018. doi:10.1038/s41379-020-0573-5
58. Szymonowicz KA, Chen J. Biological and clinical aspects of HPV-related cancers. *Cancer Biol Med.* 2020;17(4):864-878. doi:10.20892/j.issn.2095-3941.2020.0370
59. Rogers LJ, Cuello MA. Cancer of the vulva. *Int J Gynaecol Obstet.* 2018;143(Suppl 2):4-13. doi:10.1002/ijgo.12609
60. Le ST, Karia PS, Vollenhoven BJ, Besaw RJ, Feltmate CM, Schmults CD. Evaluation of AJCC and an alternative tumor classification system for primary vulvar squamous cell carcinoma. *J Natl Compr Canc Netw.* 2018;16(1):42-49. doi:10.6004/jnccn.2017.7022
61. Chen X, Hou Y, Chen C, Jiang G. Basal cell carcinoma of the external genitalia: a population-based analysis. *Front Oncol.* 2021;10:613533. doi:10.3389/fonc.2020.613533
62. Cameron MC, et al. Basal cell carcinoma: contemporary approaches to diagnosis, treatment, and prevention. *J Am Acad Dermatol.* 2019;80321-80339.doi:10.1016/j.jaad.2018.02.083
63. Dika E, Scarfi F, Ferracin M, et al. Basal cell carcinoma: a comprehensive review. *Int J Mol Sci.* 2020;21(15):5572. doi:10.3390/ijms21155572
64. Sinha K, Abdul-Wahab A, Calonje E, Craythorne E, Lewis FM. Basal cell carcinoma of the vulva: treatment with Mohs micrographic surgery. *Clin Exp Dermatol.* 2019;44(6):651-653. doi:10.1111/ced.13881

## SUGGESTED READINGS

Bhanja DB, Chakraborty S, Sil A, Panigrahi A. Non-venereal sclerosing lymphangitis of the penis. *Int J Dermatol.* 2020;59:e395-e396. doi:10.1111/ijd.15007

Dehlendorff C, Baandrup L, Kjaer SK. Real-world effectiveness of human papillomavirus vaccination against vulvovaginal high-grade precancerous lesions and cancers. *J Natl Cancer Inst.* 2021;113:869-874.

Iorga L, et al. Penile carcinoma and HPV infection (Review). *Exp Ther Med.* 2020;20:91-96. doi:10.3892/etm.2019.8181

Irshad U, Puckett Y. Giant condylomata acuminata of Buschke and Lowenstein. In: *StatPearls* [Internet]. StatPearls Publishing; 2021.

Leslie SW, Sajjad H, Kumar S. Genital warts. In: *StatPearls* [Internet]. StatPearls Publishing; 2021.

Salloum A, Bazzi N, Saad W, Bachour J, Mégarbané H. Pseudo-epitheliomatous keratotic and micaceous balanitis: a literature review. *Australas J Dermatol.* 2021;62:421-426.

Salloum A, Bouferraa Y, Bazzi N, et al. Pathophysiology, clinical findings, and management of Fox-Fordyce disease: a systematic review. *J Cosmet Dermatol.* 2022;21:482-500. doi:10.1111/jocd.14135

Singh N, Gilks CB. Vulval squamous cell carcinoma and its precursors. *Histopathology.* 2020;76:128-138. doi:10.1111/his.13989

Sivaraj V, Ahamed A, Gurung M, Menon-Johansso AS. Anogenital molluscum contagiosum: treatment choices. *Sex Transm Infect.* 2022;98:230. doi:10.1136/sextrans-2021-055108

Sugai S, Nishijima K, Enomoto T. Management of condyloma acuminata in pregnancy: a review. *Sex Transm Dis.* 2021;48:403-409. doi:10.1097/OLQ.0000000000001322

# White Disorders 8

LIBBY EDWARDS

White skin lesions can occur from a lack of pigment, from thick skin that is wet and hydrated, from fibrin debris at the base of an ulcer, and from substance on the skin such as cream or yeast. In the past, all white discoloration of a mucous membrane was called "leukoplakia," and this white change was believed to be a precancerous condition. Although squamous cell carcinoma and squamous dysplasia are often white, clearly not all white diseases confer an increased risk of malignant transformation.

## White Patches and Plaques

### Vitiligo

Vitiligo is almost the only acquired condition that consists of the complete loss of pigment, or depigmentation, of the skin, rather than hypopigmentation, the partial loss of color. This is a common condition, occurring in 1%-2% of the population worldwide, although it is much more easily recognized in individuals of natural darker complexions. In addition to the cosmetic concerns of this condition, there is enormous stigma associated with white patches in some cultures,[1] partly because Hansen disease (leprosy) can present with white areas.

#### Clinical Presentation

Vitiligo is characterized by asymptomatic milk-white patches with no evidence of texture change. At times, the distinction between the depigmentation of vitiligo and the hypopigmentation of other white patches can be difficult to confirm, particularly in light-complexioned individuals. A Wood light differentiates these two states, with depigmentation appearing bright white and verifying the diagnosis of vitiligo, whereas hypopigmentation shows little difference compared to surrounding unaffected. Also, vitiligo shows no crinkling, roughness, scale, lichenification, smoothness, or shininess (**Figs. 8-1 through 8-3**). The pigment loss can be patchy or extensive and confluent. Patients often present with extragenital lesions that are more distinct when surrounding skin darkens from tan.

There is a predilection for body sites that are often irritated or injured (called the isomorphic response, previously called Koebner phenomenon). This helps to explain the typical locations such as the external genitalia, skin over the metacarpal joints, and around the mouth. This also helps to explain why vitiligo sometimes occurs in the setting of an underlying skin disease such as lichen simplex chronicus (LSC) or lichen sclerosus. Although vitiligo produces no pruritus or pain, the scratching of conditions such as LSC can precipitate vitiligo. Lichen sclerosus especially is known to occur in association with vitiligo, even in association with extragenital vitiligo (**Fig. 8-4**). Then, the lichenification, excoriations, and texture change of LSC in a setting of vitiligo can confuse the examiner who is expecting no texture change or symptoms with vitiligo.

The hair within depigmented patches sometimes loses their pigment (poliosis) (**Fig. 8-5**). The last melanocytes to be disappear and the first to reappear are at the base of hair follicles; vitiligo often exhibits skin-colored follicular macules within a patch of depigmentation (**Fig. 8-6**). The border of the depigmented skin is sometimes hyperpigmented, and sometimes there are hypopigmented

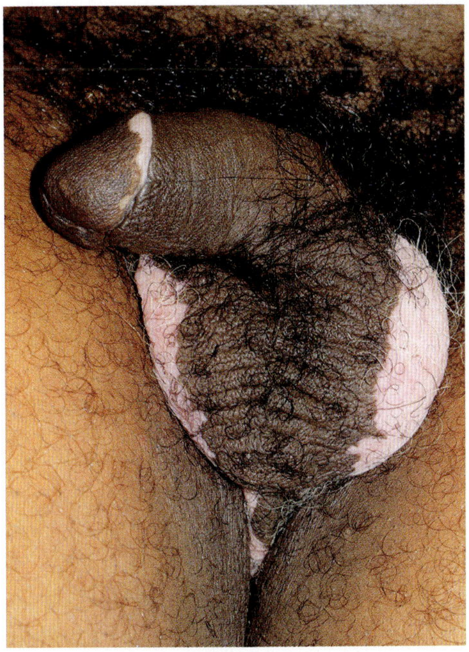

Fig. 8-1. This man has scrotal vitiligo and involvement of the corona and perineum. The patches are well demarcated and consist of color change only.

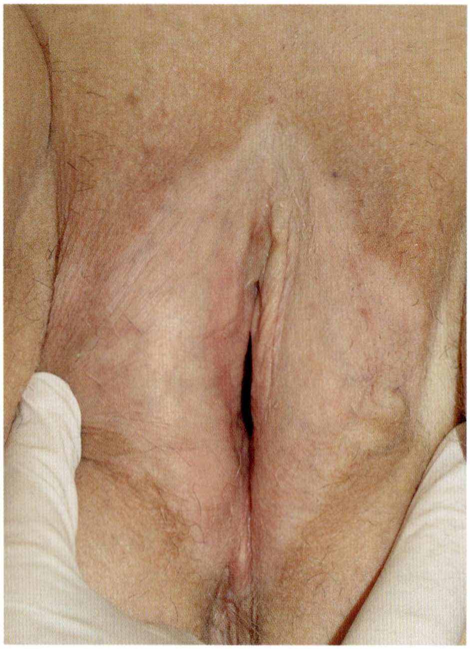

Fig. 8-2. This patch of vitiligo is easily mistaken for lichen sclerosus due to the color and distribution; however, there is no texture change, loss of architecture, or symptoms of itching or pain.

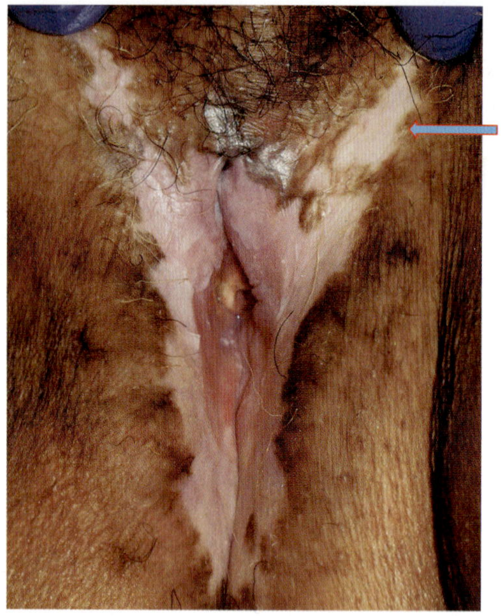

Fig. 8-4. Vitiligo is prone to occur in areas of irritation or injury; this patient has both lichen sclerosus and vitiligo. The loss of architecture and texture change shows the diagnosis of lichen sclerosus, but the white macular white patch without surface abnormality (*arrow*) is typical of vitiligo. The unusually white color of her lichen sclerosus and peripheral hyperpigmentation suggest that vitiligo is superimposed upon her plaques of lichen sclerosus as well.

macules in addition to hyperpigmentation and depigmentation **(Fig. 8-7)**. Widespread vitiligo occasionally can be difficult to differentiate from a hyperpigmented condition **(Fig. 8-8)**, where the normal skin color can be misinterpreted as hyperpigmentation in light-complexioned patients. At times, even the patient believes he or she has brown patches instead of normal skin color in a background of depigmentation.

Patients with generalized vitiligo exhibit an increase in other autoimmune diseases, especially thyroid disease, and have more circulating autoantibodies in general.

## Pathophysiology

Although there are various theories for the origin of vitiligo, an autoimmune etiology is the most prominent, with genetic factors. Vitiligo is associated with autoimmune hypothyroidism, alopecia areata, lichen sclerosus, and halo nevi, all autoimmune conditions, as well as increased autoantibodies compared unaffected individuals. Cytotoxicity from neurotransmitters has been suggested and even vitamin D deficiency.

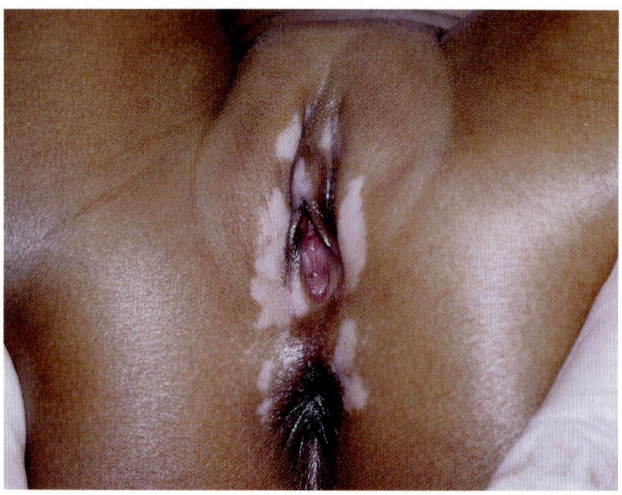

Fig. 8-3. Vitiligo is common in children, as seen in the child with coalescing macules and patches of the vulva and perianal skin.

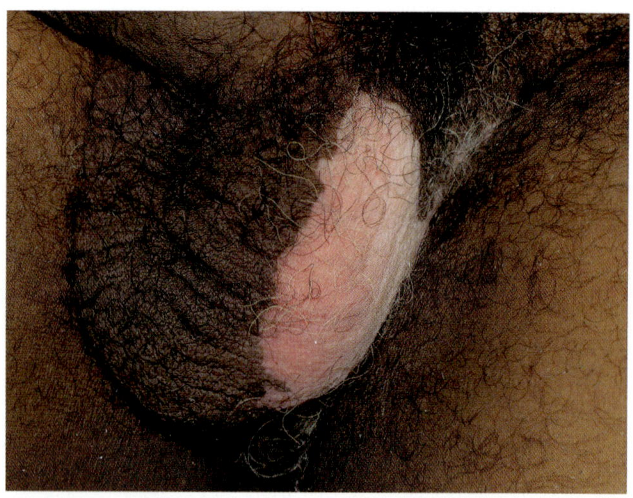

Fig. 8-5. Hair within a patch of vitiligo is often white also, an occurrence named poliosis.

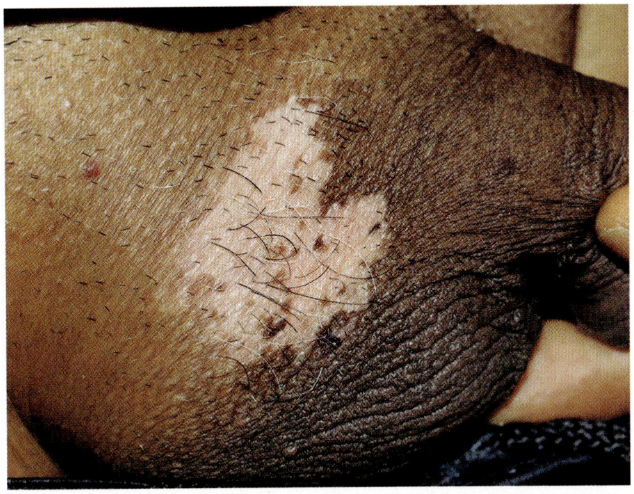

Fig. 8-6. This milk white patch exhibits the skin-colored macules of brown color from the base of follicles, the last melanocytes to be affected and the first to recover.

Occupational vitiligo can occur in the genital area in men as a result of destruction of melanocytes by exposure to *para*-tertiary-butylphenol, a substance found in resins for adhesives in the car industry. In addition, new medications such as the immune checkpoint inhibitors used in the management of malignancies and biologics used for rheumatoid arthritis, psoriasis, and inflammatory bowel disease, especially the tumor necrosis factor alpha blocker, have been shown to precipitate vitiligo.[2,3] Topical imiquimod used for anogenital warts has been associated

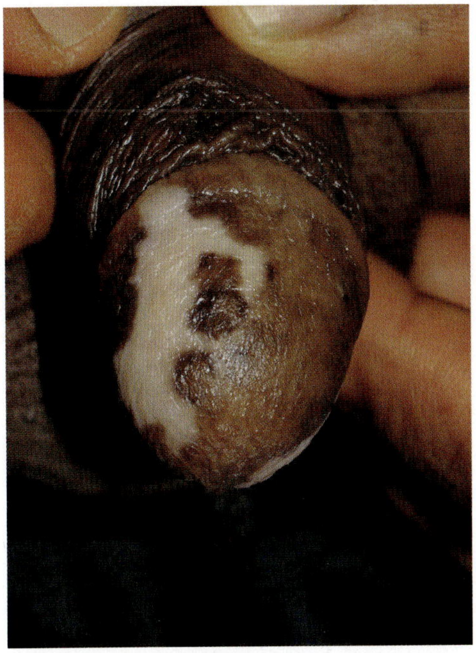

Fig. 8-7. In addition to normal skin color and white depigmentation, vitiligo sometimes exhibits hyperpigmentation, most often at the periphery of the depigmented patch as seen here. Or, there can be tan patches intermediate between depigmentation and normal skin color at times, called trichrome vitiligo.

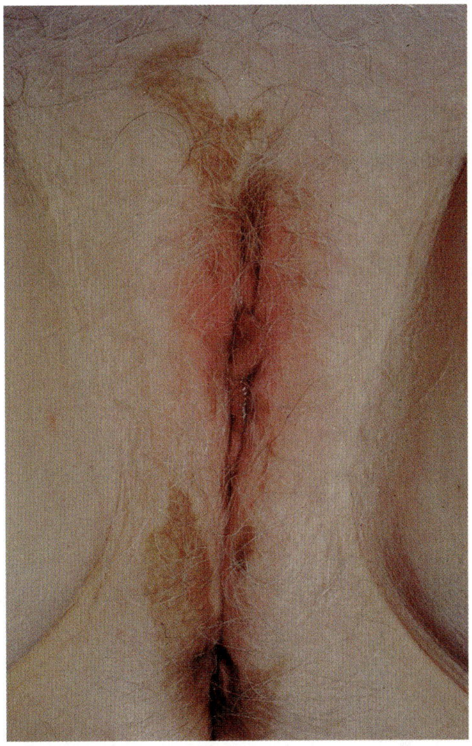

Fig. 8-8. Occasionally, the depigmentation of vitiligo is so extensive that the remaining normal skin color can be mistaken for hyperpigmentation, sometimes confusing even the patient.

with the development of vitiligo,[4-6] which may well have occurred from the cutaneous inflammation regularly produced by imiquimod. Theoretically, any destructive or inflammogenic therapy could precipitate vitiligo.

## Diagnosis

Vitiligo is diagnosed clinically by the presence of depigmentation and the absence of textural change. The diagnosis is more difficult when vitiligo occurs in a setting of underlying skin disease such as lichen sclerosus or LSC. The most specific findings on dermoscopy are well-demarcated, dense/glowing, white areas. Sometime, white hairs and perifollicular pigmentation are considered specific features of vitiligo as well.[7] A biopsy may be necessary in some cases.

Histopathologically, there is an absence of melanocytes and melanin in the epidermis. This can be difficult to discern on routine hematoxylin and eosin stains, but incubation with 0.01% 3,4-dihydroxyphenylalanine (also called dopa) stains enzymatically active melanocytes black in the basal layer, and electron microscopy can demonstrate the loss of the melanocytes. There is also a mild to moderate dermal lymphocytic infiltrate at the borders of some lesions, and melanocytes in this area often appear large with long dendrites containing melanin.

The differential diagnosis of vitiligo includes any white patch or white plaque with subtle scale or texture change.

Confusion of vitiligo with postinflammatory hypopigmentation can arise, particularly in the early lesions of vitiligo. This can be an especially difficult differentiation in black patients with hypopigmentation as a postinflammatory sequelae of an inflammatory condition such as LSC. The main differential diagnosis in the anogenital area is lichen sclerosus. This has a similar marble white color, but the textural changes in the skin of lichen sclerosus help to differentiate these conditions. The anesthetic, hypopigmented patches of Hanson disease may also mimic vitiligo, but testing for sensation within the white skin is normal in vitiligo. This condition is vanishingly rare in the United States, but immigration can widen the usual differential diagnoses. Topical corticosteroids can produce hypopigmentation, but not depigmentation, and the borders are usually poorly demarcated.

**VITILIGO — Diagnosis**

- White, well-demarcated depigmented patches
- No scale, surface change, or texture change of any kind
- Biopsy generally not necessary, and routine histology is often normal; may require dopa stains to confirm the absence of melanocytes

### Management

Vitiligo is a cosmetic issue only. However, this condition can be very upsetting to some patients, especially those in Eastern countries.[1] And, any disfigurement of the genitalia can be upsetting to many patients, resulting in sexual dysfunction and other stresses.[8,9] Because our options for successful repigmentation of vitiligo are limited at this time, the provider should be very aware of the psychological ramifications for some patients, and address or refer those individuals.

Some patients are not especially bothered by their genital vitiligo, and no therapy is required for those people. For those who wish to pursue treatment, there are medical and surgical options, although in practice, finding providers who offer the surgical options in the United States is extremely difficult. Ultraviolet light in combination with topical agents have been reported useful, but this increases the risk of squamous cell carcinoma, especially on anogenital skin. Most clinicians begin with topical therapies, especially superpotent corticosteroids, taking care to follow carefully for atrophy and other side effects.[10] One method is a trial of a potent topical corticosteroid (ie, clobetasol propionate or halobetasol propionate for no longer than 8 weeks in a cycle). When there is some repigmentation with this therapy, cycles of a corticosteroid can be used, such as 6 weeks on and 6 weeks off. Care must be taken, particularly in the genitocrural folds, inner upper thighs, and scrotum, as these areas are susceptible to steroid atrophy. Many providers also use a topical calcineurin inhibitor, tacrolimus (Protopic) or pimecrolimus (Elidel) twice a day, often in combination with the topical corticosteroid.[11] These expensive medications are often not covered by insurance for this purpose but have no side effects of atrophy or steroid dermatitis.[5] They may sting with application, and they are black-boxed by the U.S. Food and Drug Administration for the unlikely events of squamous cell carcinoma and lymphoma. Topical calcipotriol, a vitamin D analog, is sometimes used as well.[12,13]

Intravenous (not oral) corticosteroid pulses have been reported useful.[14] The biologic therapies with Janus kinase inhibitors have shown promise as well.[15] More aggressive therapies that are not routinely used include epidermal grafts and melanocyte-keratinocyte transplantation.[16,17] Although dermabrasion is usually used only to prepare recipient skin for grafts, use of dermabrasion alone with adjuvant topical 5-fluorouracil[18] and tacrolimus[19] have been shown useful. Anything that damages the skin runs the risk of worsening of the vitiligo due to the isomorphic response.

Phototherapy has been used for years for vitiligo, but it is a poor choice in the anogenital area due to the increased risk of squamous cell carcinomas that occur with chronic ultraviolet therapy. The 308-nm excimer laser has been used but appears to be less effective than calcineurin inhibitors.[20] There are early trials using fractional $CO_2$ laser alone and in combination with other therapies. A summary of a systematic Cochrane review of management for vitiligo shows that data are derived from poorly designed trials and concluded that only corticosteroids and phototherapy can be shown from data to show benefit.[21]

People with vitiligo that is widespread or cosmetically disfiguring can be treated by depigmentation therapy, where 20% monobenzylether of hydroquinone is used to depigment normal skin so that the skin does not show patches of discoloration. This medication must be compounded and has a fairly high risk of contact dermatitis. Support and reassurance are generally the most effective course for genital vitiligo.

**VITILIGO — Management**

- No satisfactory therapy for repigmenting the genital area, but the following are occasionally useful, alone or in combination:
  - Topical ultrapotent corticosteroid ointment applied bid in 6- to 8-week pulses
  - Tacrolimus or pimecrolimus applied bid ongoing
  - Calcipotriol (calcipotriene) cream applied bid
  - Ultraviolet light not practical or safe for genitalia, and confers risk of malignancy
- When large areas of the body are affected, remaining normal skin can be depigmented permanently with 20% monobenzylether of hydroquinone applied twice a day to even the skin color.

## Postinflammatory Hypopigmentation

### Clinical Presentation

Injury or inflammation of the skin can produce either hyperpigmentation or hypopigmentation. Hypopigmentation can be mild or marked, and usually, but not always, there is a history of a preceding event. The color changes are more marked in people with a natural darker complexion. Poorly demarcated hypopigmentation occurs in the distribution of the preceding inflammation or injury **(Fig. 8-9)**. The loss of pigment is often very subtle, and unless the cause of the inflammation is ongoing, the skin should show only hypopigmentation, without texture changes or scale. When the injury is severe, such as a chemical burn, the borders may be well demarcated.

### Diagnosis

The diagnosis can usually be determined by the pattern of hypopigmentation in association with the past or present existence of skin disease or injury. However, patients often either forget previous events or were unaware of them, so the lack of a consistent history is common. Dermoscopy is likely to show features of the preexisting skin condition causing the inflammation. A biopsy is only occasionally required and shows a decreased amount of melanin in the basal keratinocytes, but melanocytes are present. Pigment-ladened macrophages may be present in the underlying dermis.

The pallor of lichen sclerosus, lichen planus, and lichen simplex may be similar to and coexist with postinflammatory hypopigmentation, but the textural changes and scarring help to distinguish these disorders. Vitiligo due to depigmentation can mimic postinflammatory hypopigmentation, and Wood lamp examination can usually differentiate between the two.

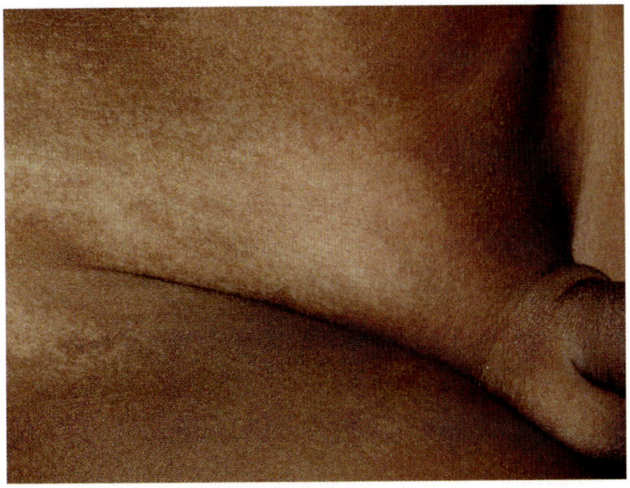

Fig. 8-9. Postinflammatory hypopigmentation shows lighter color but not the absence of color seen with vitiligo. This child has postinflammatory hypopigmentation remaining from a recent diaper dermatitis.

**POSTINFLAMMATORY HYPOPIGMENTATION — Diagnosis**

- Pattern of hypopigmentation that correlates with past known or common inflammation or injury; diaper dermatitis, lichen simplex chronicus, trauma of wart therapy, etc.
- Pale, hypopigmented patches.
- No scale or surface change, except for that associated with any ongoing underlying etiologic inflammatory process.
- Biopsy generally not necessary for diagnosis; stains show presence of melanocytes.

### Pathophysiology

Any inflammatory dermatosis or injury can leave residual hypopigmentation or hyperpigmentation in the affected areas. The underlying cause of postinflammatory hypopigmentation is injury or destruction of the melanocytes. Generally, this is short-lived and the melanocytes recover. Occasionally, scarring occurs, and the color change is permanent. Permanent hypopigmentation also is a sequelae of destructive treatments in which the melanocytes may be more susceptible to damage, as seen after cryotherapy or radiotherapy.

### Management

There is no treatment for postinflammatory hypopigmentation other than treatment of or prevention of further dermatosis or injury. The normal skin pigmentation returns spontaneously to most with time.

**POSTINFLAMMATORY HYPOPIGMENTATION — Management**

- Control of any ongoing underlying inflammatory process
- Otherwise, self-resolving; no therapies hasten repigmentation

## Lichen Sclerosus

Lichen sclerosus (LS) is a relatively common disease with a strong predilection for the anogenital skin, especially that of postmenopausal women. A recent study suggests that 0.05% of women develop anogenital lichen sclerosus,[22] which is less than that previously reported and less than the 1.6% likelihood of acquiring LS by age 80 years reported in the national Finnish registry in 2020.[23] The incidence of lichen sclerosus in men is dependent on whether or not circumcision is prevalent, since lichen sclerosus occurs almost entirely in uncircumcised males. The incidence ranges from 0.07% to 0.3%, and these are likely underestimates due to lack of familiarity of providers with

LS, embarrassment of patients, and the failure of providers to examine the penis and retract the foreskin.[24-26] In both genders, this is generally bimodal, occurring mostly in childhood and older adults; postmenopausal women and men aged 61 years and older.

The terms kraurosis vulvae and balanitis xerotica obliterans were used in the past, usually to describe advanced lichen sclerosus in women and men, respectively.

## Clinical Presentation

The most common presentation of LS is in the postmenopausal woman. However, this condition can occur at any time, including childhood. The classic presenting symptom is that of pruritus that can be excruciating, often associated with pain from erosions in the fragile skin due to rubbing and scratching or minor, otherwise inconsequential, trauma, including sexual activity. Often, lichen sclerosus is asymptomatic until an event such as a yeast infection produces symptoms that initiate irritation with resulting rubbing and scratching that perpetuates the inflammation and injury.

Constipation is a common presenting complaint in prepubertal girls, because lichen sclerosus around the rectal canal causes fissuring and painful defecation with consequent anal retention. Perianal involvement almost never occurs in boys and men.

The classic findings of lichen sclerosus consist of white papules and plaques that are usually fairly well demarcated **(Fig. 8-10)**. The clitoris is often puffy, white, and smooth,

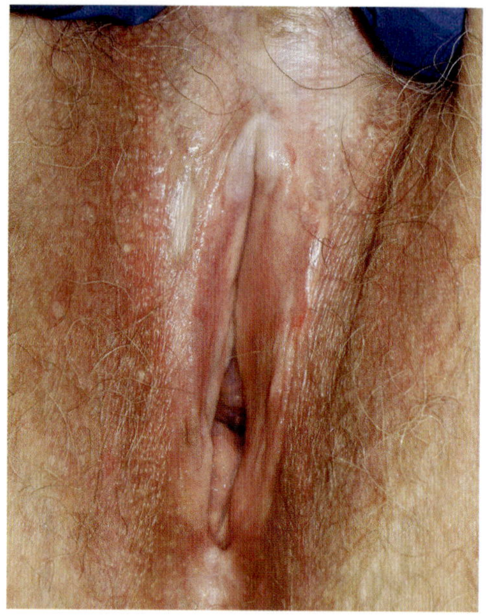

Fig. 8-11. Lichen sclerosus favors the perineum and periclitoral area; these are often the first areas affected, and the most difficult to clear.

whereas the surrounding skin characteristically is white and crinkled. In women, lichen sclerosus often first and most prominently affects the clitoral area and the perineal body **(Fig. 8-11)**. The entire modified mucous membranes and perianal skin become involved in some women, which many clinicians visualize as a figure-of-8 pattern **(Fig. 8-12)**. In the male, LS occurs on the glans and prepuce

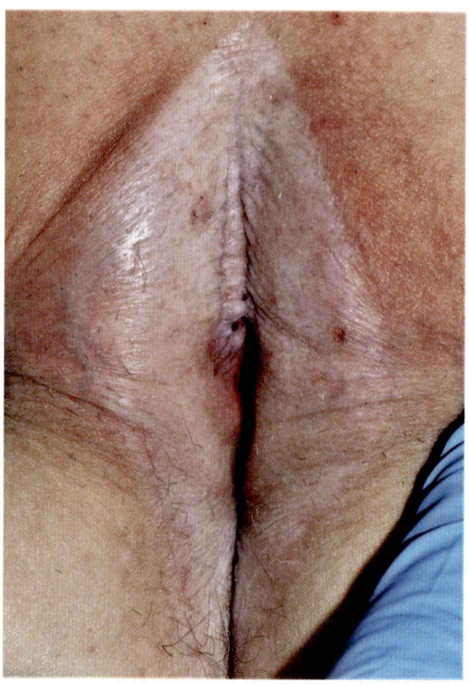

Fig. 8-10. This well-demarcated plaque of lichen sclerosus shows characteristic white color and loss of labia minora, with shiny, crinkled skin and scarring of the clitoral hood.

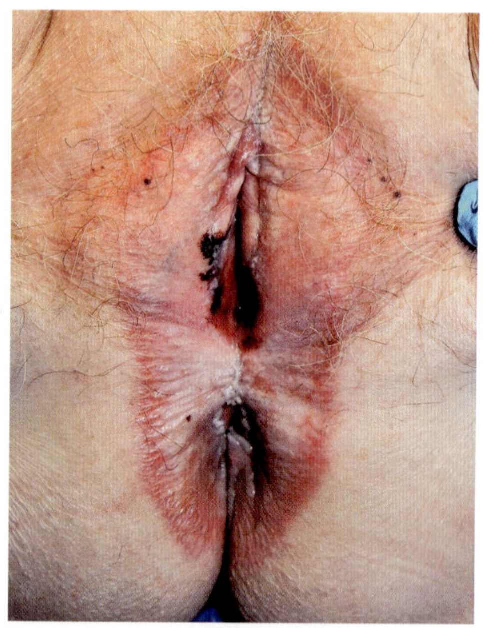

Fig. 8-12. Vulvar lichen sclerosus is often described as a figure-of-8 plaque, and this patient also exhibits purpura, puffiness of the clitoral hood and labia minora, as well as fissuring and erosion within areas of hyperkeratosis.

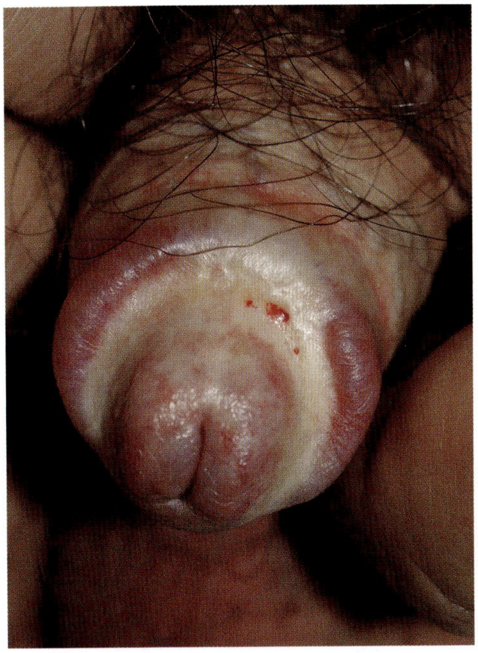

Fig. 8-13. Hypopigmentation and scarring occur in men as well, with the glans the most often affected. Vascular ectasias and angiomas occur sometimes in both men and women in areas of lichen sclerosus.

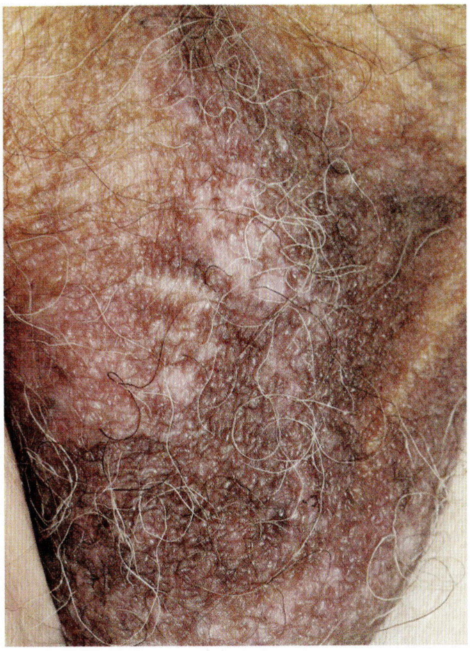

Fig. 8-15. The scrotum is not a common location for lichen sclerosus, and the linear, almost fernlike striae required a biopsy to diagnose. Even though the patient has classic penile lichen sclerosus, lichen planus and lichen sclerosus sometimes occur in the same patients.

of the penis and less commonly the shaft **(Figs. 8-13 and 8-14)**. Occasionally, the scrotum is affected **(Fig. 8-15)**.

Although hypopigmentation occurs in many skin diseases, the texture of lichen sclerosus is a strong diagnostic clue. The skin surface classically shows fine crinkling, a reliable sign of lichen sclerosus **(Fig. 8-16)**. At times, the skin can be shiny and smooth, waxy, or hyperkeratotic

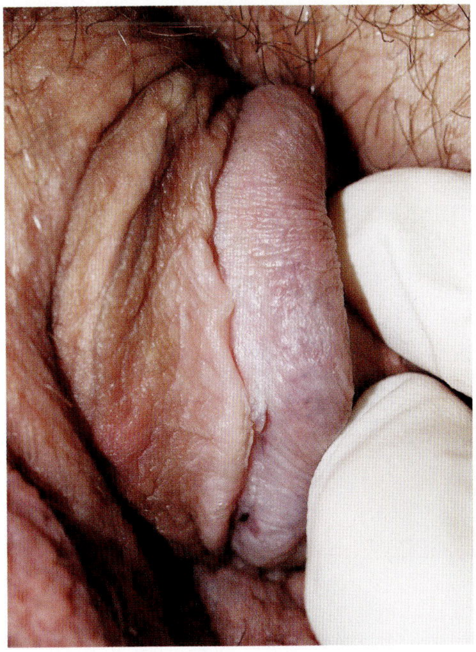

Fig. 8-14. Early agglutination of the glans to the prepuce is obvious here.

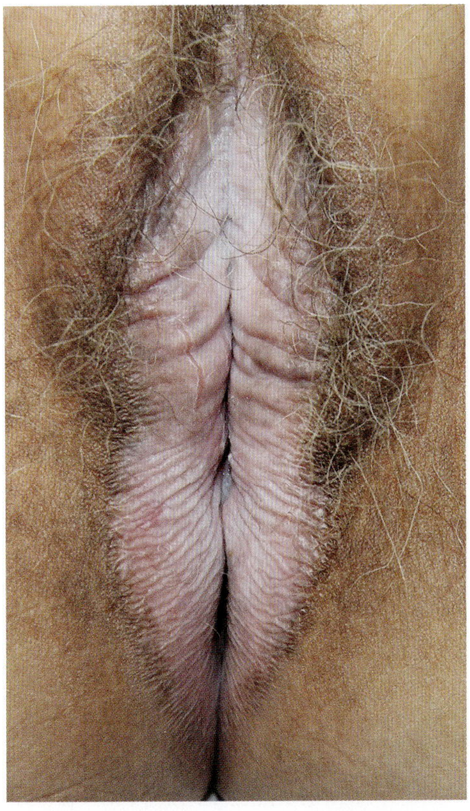

Fig. 8-16. Lichen sclerosus is typically a well-demarcated plaque of white, crinkled skin; this plaque is thick from rubbing and scratching. Occasionally, lichen sclerosus is bordered by hyperpigmentation.

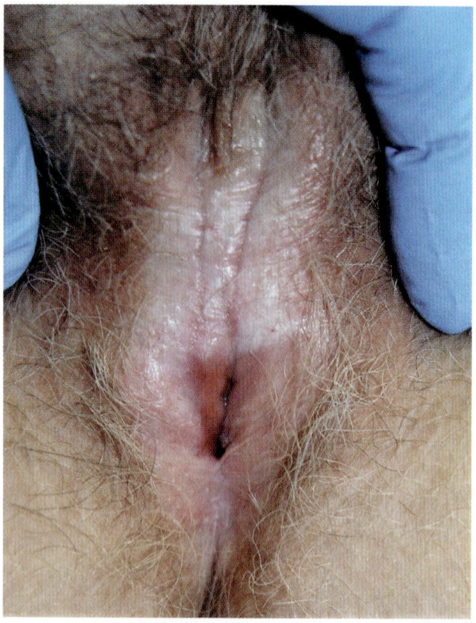

Fig. 8-17. Although crinkling is classic, sometimes lichen sclerosus is manifested by shiny epithelium; the loss of architecture is an additional feature of advanced disease.

and rough, but there are always texture changes (**Figs. 8-17 to 8-20**). Sometimes, rather than plaques, small discrete papules occur, often coalescing into plaques (**Fig. 8-21**). Ecchymosis is extremely suggestive of lichen sclerosus (**Figs. 8-12, 8-22, 8-23**). These ecchymoses can be mistaken for evidence of abuse in young girls. Additional signs include erosions or ulceration due to the fragility of lichen

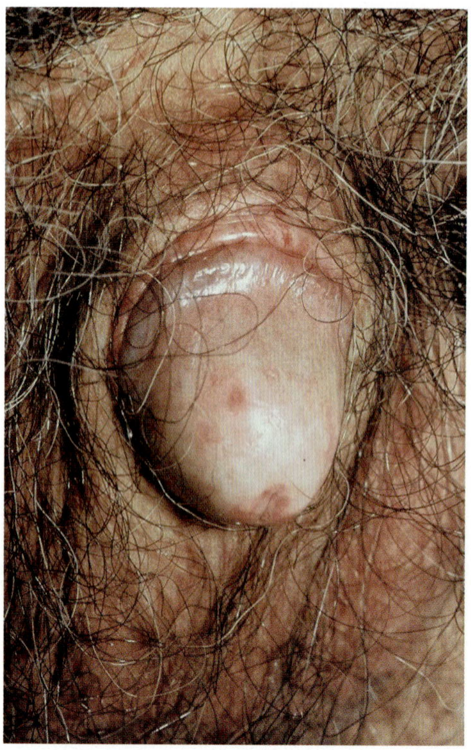

Fig. 8-18. The texture on the glans is also occasionally thin and smooth, with hypopigmentation more subtle, making the diagnosis more challenging.

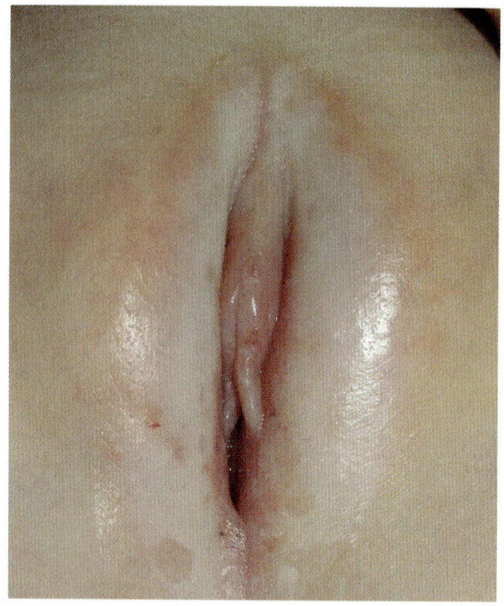

Fig. 8-19. Less often, the skin is waxy, but there is always texture change compared to normal skin in the setting of lichen sclerosus.

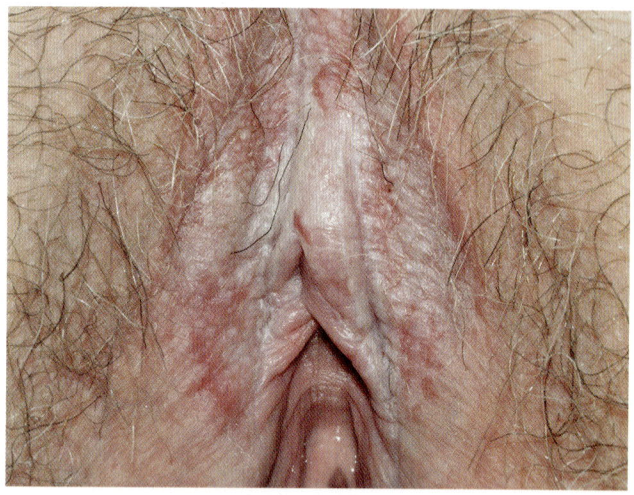

Fig. 8-20. A more thickened, hyperkeratotic texture change is often a late development, and this progression can herald a higher risk for malignant transformation.

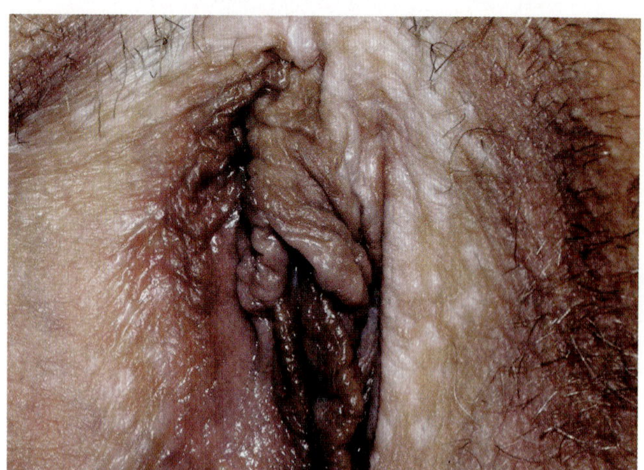

Fig. 8-21. Sometimes, lichen sclerosus can occur as small white discrete, flat-topped papules, often coalescing into plaques.

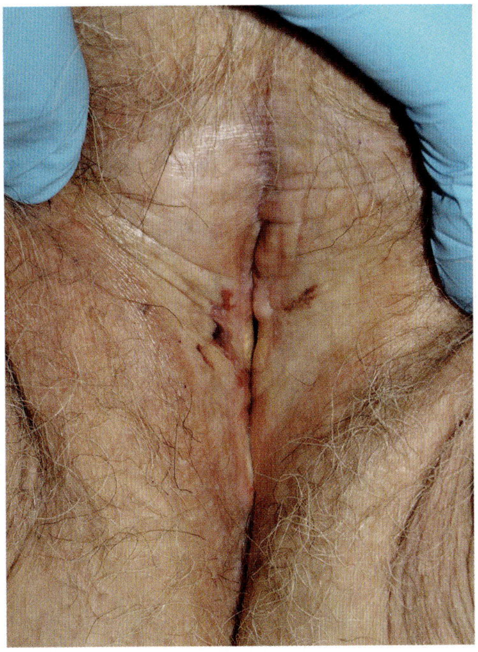

Fig. 8-22. This partially treated patient with LS could be thought to be nearly clear, were it not for the prominent purpura.

sclerosus. Hyperkeratotic plaques occur at times; sometimes as a result of rubbing and scratching, and sometimes spontaneously, which is worrisome for incipient differentiated vulvar intraepithelial neoplasia (dVIN or squamous cell carcinoma *in situ*) (**Fig. 8-23**).

In young boys, lichen sclerosus often presents with phimosis, and LS is a major cause of medical circumcisions. The lichen sclerosus is often unrecognized until the excised prepuce is examined histologically. White papules occur on the glans and ventral foreskin, producing the same white, fragile plaques that may exhibit purpura. The shaft can be involved as well.

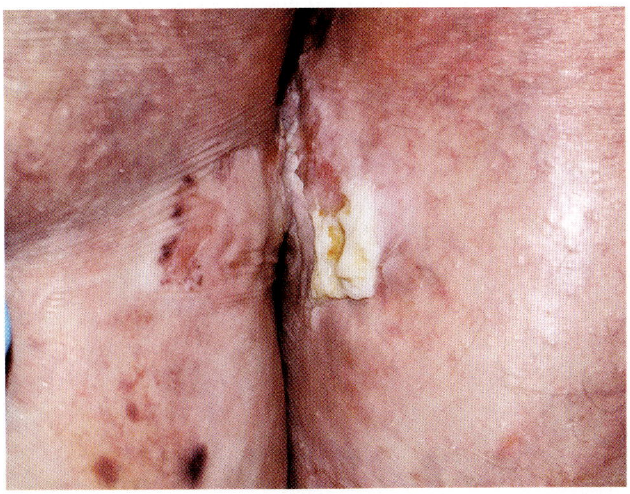

Fig. 8-23. Malignant change is most common in hyperkeratotic lesions of postmenopausal women who have had lichen sclerosus for years; lesions such as this should be immediately biopsied. This fortunately was benign, although she developed a nearby squamous cell carcinoma several years later.

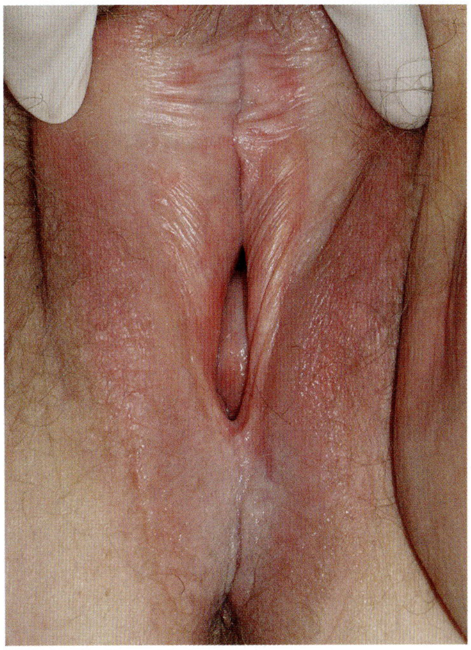

Fig. 8-24. This patient shows the resorption of labia minora and midline scarring that covers the clitoris of so many women with lichen sclerosus.

Scarring is usual in more advanced disease; in women, this is manifested by resorption of the labia minora and scarring of the clitoral hood to the clitoris, with eventual sealing of the clitoral hood, or prepuce, concealing the glans clitoris underneath (**Fig. 8-24**). At times, the pocket formed under the clitoral hood becomes impacted with keratin debris of trapped keratinocytes shed from the surface of the epithelium, forming a pseudocyst (**Fig. 8-25**).

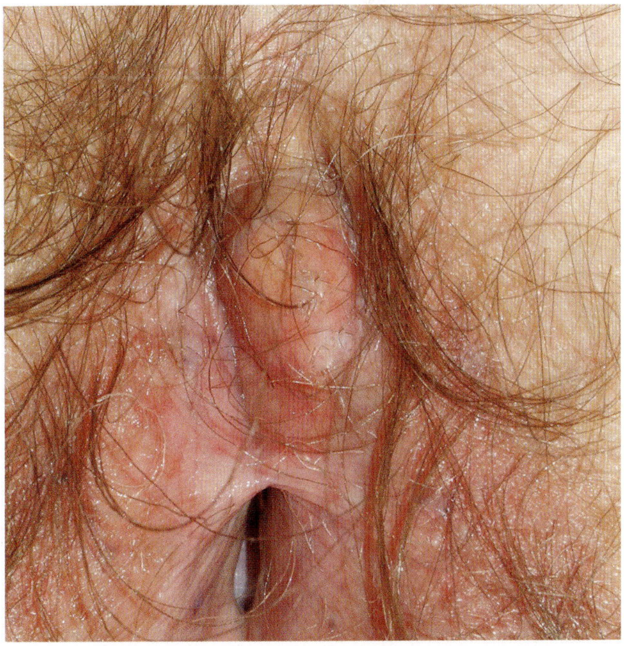

Fig. 8-25. When the tip of the clitoral hood seals together, a pseudocyst sometimes forms; desquamated keratin and epithelium are trapped in this pocket and enlarge, usually causing no significant issues. When this is uncomfortable or interferes with function, it can be opened and marsupialized or otherwise reconstructed.

Although usually asymptomatic, these pseudocysts occasionally produce discomfort from distention and decrease sensitivity of the clitoris because of the accumulated keratin between the clitoris and the skin surface. Rupture of the pseudocyst produces a brisk foreign body response, resulting in a painful, red nodule that may drain keratin and purulent material.

Midline adhesions result in introital narrowing. Lichen sclerosus usually spares the mucosal surface of the vagina, and this is sometimes discussed as a differentiating feature from lichen planus, with only four reported cases in the literature. However, this author (LE) has six patients with biopsy-proven vaginal lichen sclerosus, so vaginal LS clearly occurs more often than realized.[8-26] This usually, but not always, occurs overlying an exposed, prominent cystocele or rectocele in an area of squamous metaplasia. But, unlike occurring with lichen planus, there are no reported cases of narrowing of the vagina itself occurring with lichen sclerosus **(Fig. 8-26)**.

Since lichen sclerosus is more likely to affect uncircumcised men, the scarring leads to a gradual tightening of the prepuce and eventually phimosis. The coronal sulcus can also become obliterated with adhesions **(Fig. 8-27)**. Lichen sclerosus sometimes involves the cornified epithelium surrounding the urethral meatus and lower part of the urethra **(Fig. 8-28)**, with resulting strictures that can result in major management issues.

Occasionally, lichen sclerosus is associated with hyperpigmentation. This can be postinflammatory hyperpigmentation, a nonspecific reaction to injury **(Fig. 8-29)** or, more interestingly, lentiginosis. This condition is manifested by brown, often very dark, or variegate macules and patches that can mimic melanoma **(Fig. 8-30)**. This is discussed in more detail in Chapter 9, which addresses dark lesions. Although lentiginosis does not transform into melanoma, these changes should be taken seriously and biopsied, because there may be an increased risk of melanoma in areas of lichen sclerosus. Melanocytic nevi within plaques of LS are more atypical histologically than nevi on the unaffected vulva, and there are a number of reports of melanoma occurring within areas of LS.

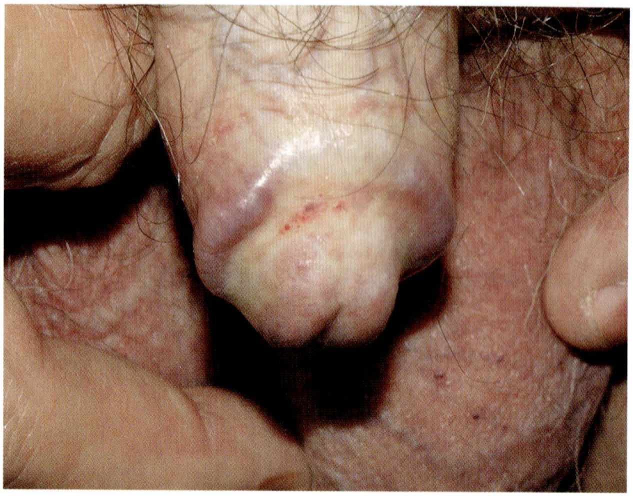

Fig. 8-27. Loss of the corona has occurred as a result of scarring from lichen sclerosus.

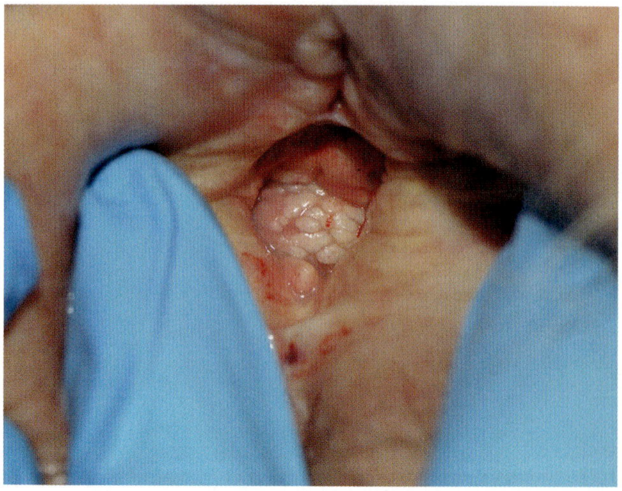

Fig. 8-26. Vaginal lichen sclerosus is believed to be very uncommon but occurs at times and primarily on the surface of an exposed rectocele or cystocele. Because most providers do not examine the vagina carefully, cases may be more common than reported.

Extragenital lichen sclerosus has been reported in 15%-20% of patients[27] **(Fig. 8-31)**. However, a review of 250 charts of this author's (LE) women with lichen sclerosus, all of whom received an initial general skin examination, showed only 6% of patients with extragenital lichen sclerosus. This correlates with my clinical impression in general. Extragenital sites occur most often on the upper back, axillae, volar aspects of the wrists, and in areas exposed to friction such as the shoulders and inframammary areas. The distribution of lesions in the friction zones can be partly explained by the isomorphic (previously called Koebner) phenomenon, in which some diseases tend to occur in areas of injury or irritation. Very rare instances of lichen sclerosus of the face, scalp nails,

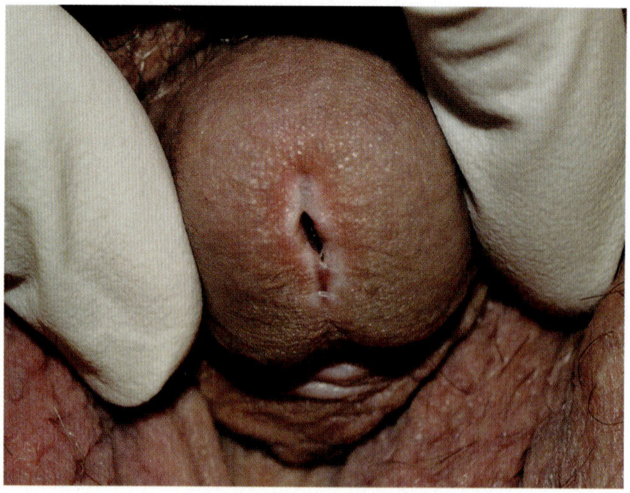

Fig. 8-28. Lichen sclerosus often affects the urethral meatus and can produce stenosis that interferes with function.

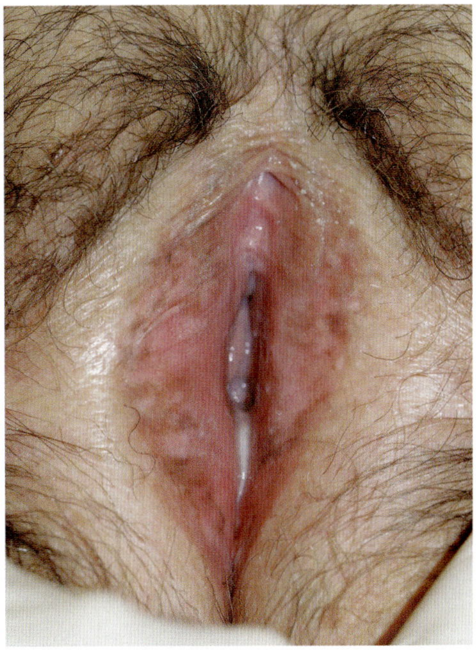

Fig. 8-29. Lichen sclerosus produces postinflammatory hyperpigmentation more often than do most other genital dermatoses, characterized by poorly demarcated patchy brown discoloration.

and mouth have all been reported. Oral lesions of lichen sclerosus are extremely uncommon, and this author, who examines the mouth of all genital patients, has never seen oral lichen sclerosus.

There is an association with the other lymphocyte-mediated disorders such as lichen planus and morphea, and some patients can develop all three conditions.

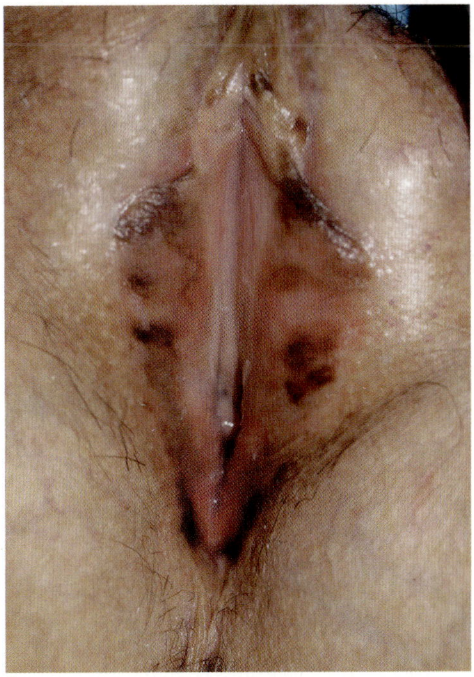

Fig. 8-30. Lentiginosis is another form of hyperpigmentation associated with lichen sclerosus, manifested by one or more patches of irregular hyperpigmentation that often exhibit multiple shades of brown, some with very dark discoloration.

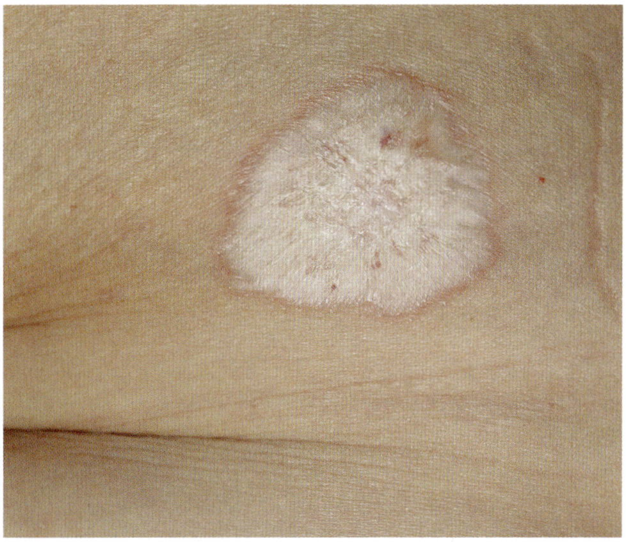

Fig. 8-31. Extragenital lichen sclerosus is most often found on the trunk and exhibits the same white discoloration with a crinkled surface; extragenital LS, however, is much less responsive to therapy, although it is generally asymptomatic and does not scar or eventuate into squamous cell carcinoma.

Vitiligo may also accompany lichen sclerosus. Psoriasis has also been found to occur more often than expected by chance **(Fig. 8-32)**,[28] and most postmenopausal women with lichen sclerosus are hypothyroid.

## Diagnosis

Although a diagnosis of lichen sclerosus can be made clinically in classic cases, lichen planus or other erosive, scarring dermatoses, or LSC sometimes mimic lichen sclerosus.

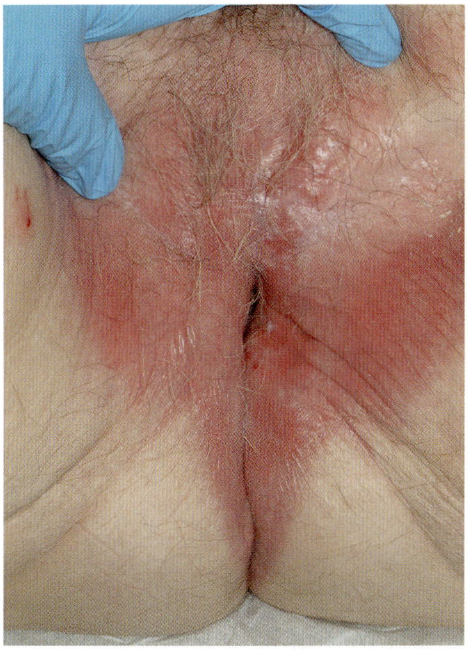

Fig. 8-32. This patient with lichen sclerosus developed superimposed psoriasis that was initially mistaken for candidiasis and contact dermatitis.

These patients should be biopsied to confirm the diagnosis. Dermoscopy shows keratotic follicular plugs, corresponding to follicular hyperkeratosis, and well-defined, bright white patches, resulting from superficial fibrosis.[29] In addition, scaling and hemorrhagic spots are specific.[29]

When there is any question, a biopsy should be performed, preferably before treatment is begun. Skin that exhibits fine crinkling or ecchymosis is the ideal site for biopsy; if there is no crinkling, then any other texture change is acceptable. Those patients without classic skin lesions often show inconclusive biopsy results.

In uncomplicated lichen sclerosus, a biopsy shows an epidermis that is hyperkeratotic, thinned, and effaced (**Fig. 8-33**). The epidermis overlies a band of hyalinization in the upper dermis with a mixed lymphocytic infiltrate immediately below it. In some areas, small foci of lichenoid change are found where the infiltrate abuts the dermoepidermal junction. At times, the epidermis exhibits the histologic features of squamous cell hyperplasia, that is, it is thickened (acanthotic). This is important as there seems to be an association with this kind of change and development of squamous cell carcinoma.

Although patients with a classic appearance do not require biopsy, photo-documentation, or at least very careful description of the clinical findings, is recommended to prevent future providers from disbelieving the diagnosis and discontinuing therapy.

The pallor, atrophy, and loss of the normal anatomic features associated with well-established lichen sclerosus raises a differential diagnosis of other diseases that produce a common end-stage picture, most notably lichen planus, mucous membrane (cicatricial) pemphigoid, and morphea. LSC can appear white and both resemble lichen sclerosus and coexist with LS. Vitiligo can mimic LS but normally has no texture change. However, because vitiligo exhibits the isomorphic phenomenon, the damage from rubbing and scratching LSC can precipitate vitiligo and mimic lichen sclerosus.

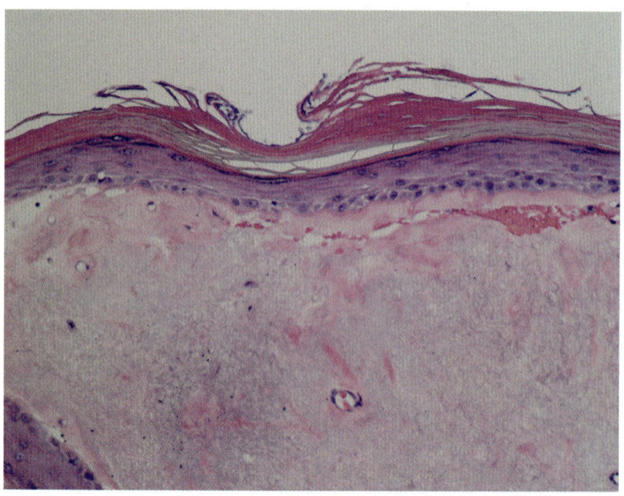

Fig. 8-33. This photomicrograph shows typical hyperkeratosis on the surface, thinning of the epithelium, and smudging of the upper dermis. This upper dermis is fragile, has separated, and produced a cleft filled with blood that is clinically manifested as purpura.

**LICHEN SCLEROSUS** — **Diagnosis**

- White, crinkled, or shiny plaques
- Involvement of the labia minora, periclitoral skin, medial labia majora, perineal body and perianal skin of women, glans penis and ventral prepuce of men.
- Scarring often prominent
- When not classic, confirmed by biopsy that shows upper dermal chronic inflammatory infiltrate, hyalinization of the upper dermis, and disruption of basement membrane

## Pathophysiology

It is a chronic lymphocyte-mediated inflammatory dermatosis with increasing evidence that it is an autoimmune-mediated disorder. There is a strong association with other autoimmune diseases particularly thyroid disease in women autoantibodies. An occasional family exhibits a strong genetic predisposition, but the majority of patients have no known affected family members. Location on the skin is important; excision of anogenital lichen sclerosus with grafting from an extragenital sight is associated with recurrence in grafted skin. However, vulvar lichen sclerosus that was grafted to the back showed regression of lichen sclerosus. Some hypothesize that there are hormonal aspects, because onset is most common in women before puberty and after menopause, possibly associated with estrogen deficiency. In men, there is increasing evidence that the retention of urine under the foreskin, or in skin folds, in obese men is a factor.[30,31]

## Management

Although the undisputed first-line therapy for lichen sclerosus is a superpotent topical corticosteroid, simply handing a patient a tube of medication is a mistake. Patient education regarding the disease, prognosis, expectations, and the chronic nature of lichen sclerosus is a central initial intervention. Avoidance of irritants such as soap or irritating panty liners is important for many. Those who have miserable pruritus should receive sedation during sleeping hours to minimize rubbing and scratching during sleep. Women with dyspareunia and estrogen deficiency should receive estrogen replacement of some type, such as estradiol cream at a dose of 1/2 g two or three times a week (see management of the atrophic vagina, Chapter 13). For men, avoidance of contact with soap and urine are important, as is the use of a barrier ointment. Some feel that pubic hair should be trimmed to avoid the irritation of trapped hair under the foreskin.[32]

Historically, the specific treatment of choice for males with lichen sclerosus has been circumcision, believed to be curative. More recently, superpotent topical corticosteroid ointments have become the treatment of choice for men as well, so that circumcision is recommended only for those who have failed medical therapy.[32] Early treatment with urethral clobetasol ointment for men with urethral involvement has been shown to help prevent and manage urethral strictures, previously treated surgically, with a high rate of recurrence.[33]

Clear first-line treatment of lichen sclerosus in women is an ultrapotent topical corticosteroid ointment (ie, clobetasol propionate 0.05%, halobetasol propionate 0.05%, betamethasone dipropionate in augmented vehicle 0.05%, or diflorasone diacetate 0.05%) (**Fig. 8-34A and B**). Randomized controlled trials, performed solely on women, have examined the effect of clobetasol only, although anecdotal experience and common sense suggest, but surely do not prove, that any ultrapotent topical corticosteroid should be beneficial. Therefore, there also are no data to support one ultrapotent steroid over another. Frequently, this is a decision made on the basis of insurance coverage and local pricing.

As for other genital dermatoses, an ointment is preferred because it is less irritating, especially in the face of painful fissures and erosions. Initially, a very small amount of this medication, far less than pea sized, is applied once or twice daily. Patients respond at varying rates, and different areas of the vulva and perianal skin also improve at different rates, with the perineum and periclitoral area often especially difficult. Therefore, therapy should be individualized, by reevaluating every 4-8 weeks for improvements and side effects, and decreasing either the potency or frequency of application as areas clear. Patients should not be treated according to symptoms, but rather according to clinical evidence of disease. Discomfort resolves long before the skin changes of lichen sclerosus clear, and symptom-guided therapy results in increased scarring and a greater risk of squamous cell carcinoma transformation. Generally, daily application can be reduced to long-term maintenance therapy after 3 or 4 months. Fifteen grams of the ointment should last at least 6 months for initial treatment.

Discontinuation of therapy regularly results in recurrence. Without treatment, there is up to a 5% risk for the development of a squamous cell carcinoma (SCC) in long-standing, vulvar lichen sclerosus (**Figs. 8-35 and 8-36**). The risk for penile SCC is less well known, but is likely less, with 1% reported in a series of 771 men.[34] There is now evidence that ongoing therapy minimizes scarring and the development of SCC in anogenital LS in women.[35]

There are no data regarding the type and frequency of maintenance therapy. Most vulvologists in the United States suppress recurrence either with a mid-potency corticosteroid ointment such as triamcinolone 0.1% daily or an ultrapotent corticosteroid ointment such as clobetasol 0.05 or halobetasol 0.05 once, three times a week (such as Monday, Wednesday, and Friday morning or night).

Penile LS that does not improve sufficiently with a topical superpotent corticosteroid should undergo circumcision.

The vast majority of women who fail to improve sufficiently usually have other issues playing a role; adherence, estrogen deficiency, contact dermatitis, infection, etc.

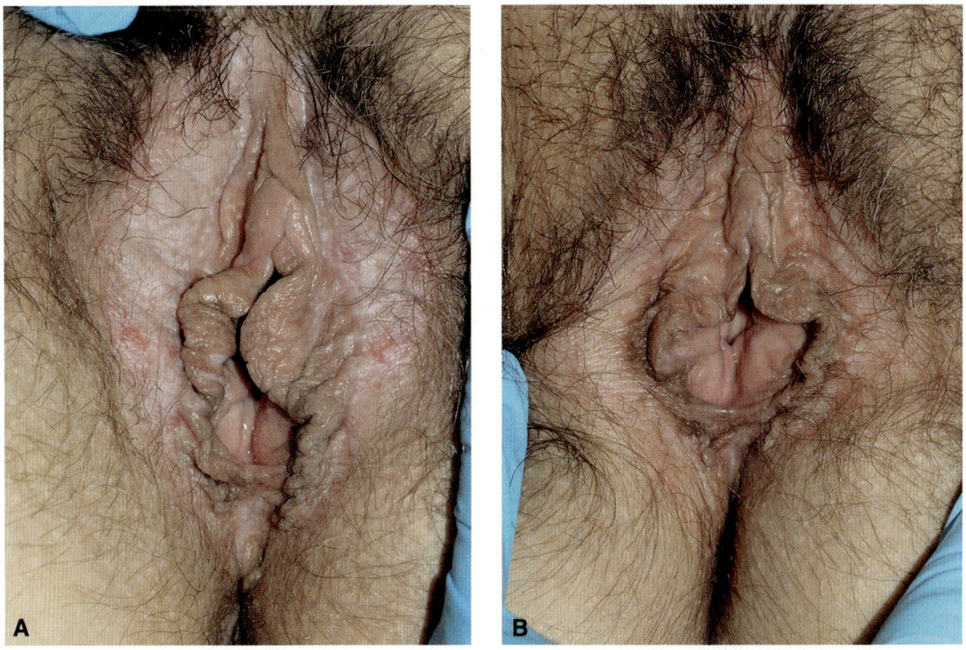


Fig. 8-34. **A.** This vulva before therapy shows a white plaque with erosions and hyperkeratosis. **B.** Five weeks after therapy with halobetasol ointment twice a day, the skin has nearly normalized; a faster response than usually occurs.

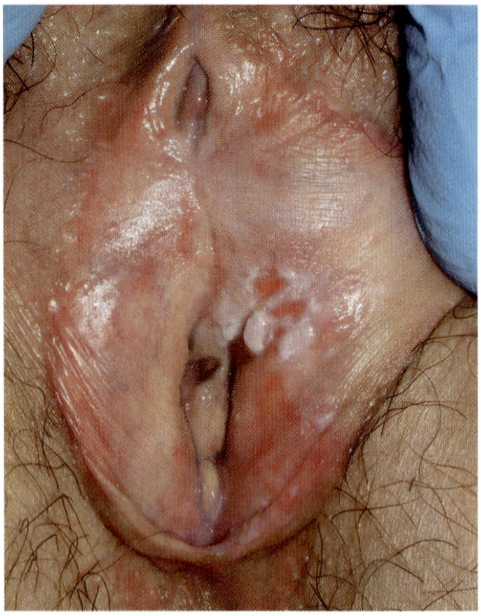

Fig. 8-35. The erosions with thick hyperkeratosis proved to represent differentiated vulvar intraepithelial neoplasia on biopsy (dVIN). Following a partial vulvectomy, dVIN has recurred.

These women should be evaluated to ensure that they are using the medication correctly and to the correct areas. Many obese or elderly patients cannot see well or reach the affected areas and do not apply medication to correct areas. Those who have developed associated differentiated intraepithelial neoplasia (histological squamous cell carcinoma *in situ*) experience nonresponse of those areas. An atrophic vagina sometimes produces symptoms of irritation or pain, and contact dermatitis, usually from an irritant, can cause symptoms similar to lichen sclerosus.

The following should only be contemplated when patients are not sufficiently improved with topical corticosteroids, when visible signs of lichen sclerosus persist, and when other causes of symptoms have been ruled out.

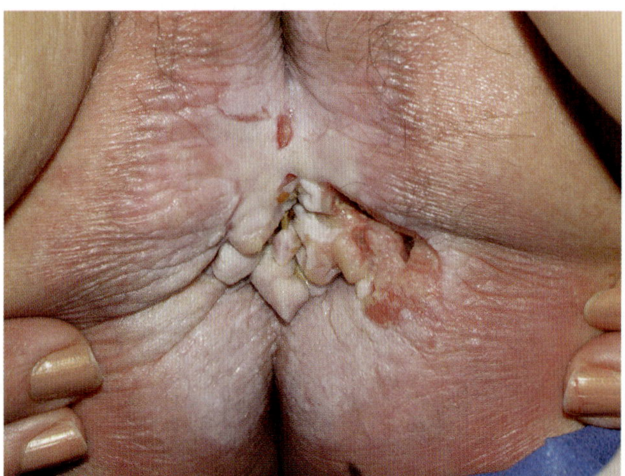

Fig. 8-36. This patient with long-standing lichen sclerosus treated according to symptoms rather than with ongoing therapy has developed invasive squamous cell carcinoma.

Then, these modalities should be added to topical corticosteroids, not replace them.

**LICHEN SCLEROSUS — Management**

- Correction of infection, local estrogen deficiency, irritant contact dermatitis, etc.
- Topical ultrapotent corticosteroid ointment (clobetasol propionate 0.05%, etc.)
  - Once or twice a day until normal texture (usually about 4 months)
  - Then once three times a week ongoing or mid-potency corticosteroid (triamcinolone 0.1%, etc.) daily to maintain control
- Tacrolimus or pimecrolimus added bid is second-line therapy
- Careful follow-up, 6-8 weeks until disease is controlled, then twice yearly, to evaluate for side effects of medication, for control of disease, for changes of malignancy

### *Other Medications*

Topical testosterone propionate is no longer used for the treatment of lichen sclerosus, and controlled studies show no advantage over vehicle. The topical calcineurin inhibitors tacrolimus and pimecrolimus have been used for lichen sclerosus that have not improved sufficiently with topical corticosteroids or in cases where there have been steroid side effects. However, these produce burning with application in most, are more expensive and often not covered by insurance, and are black-boxed by the U.S. Food and Drug Administration for the dubious events of squamous cell carcinoma and lymphoma. The improvement in lichen sclerosus is slower and the benefit less than occurs with corticosteroids.[36] When used for recalcitrant disease, calcineurin inhibitors should be added to the corticosteroid, not replace it. However, for patients who cannot apply medication in the correct amounts to the correct places, a calcineurin inhibitor may be useful, and the patient can apply any amount to the entire area.

Retinoids may be useful, but there are almost no data on this class of medications. Usually used for hyperkeratotic disease, topical retinoids generally are not tolerated due to irritation. This most recent trial evaluating the use of tretinoin cream 0.025% applied every other day showed only 18% showing objective response; presumably, resistant LS would show less benefit.[37] Oral acitretin for severe LS in men produced clearing in 12 of 33 patients receiving active medication and partial clearing of 12 of 33 patients.[38]

Vitamin D analogs are sometimes used, but there are no data. Phototherapy has also been tried[19] but is not indicated in genital lichen sclerosus because of the risk of squamous cell carcinoma.

Oral methotrexate has been used for recalcitrant lichen sclerosus with essentially no data. This has been reported useful combination with high-dose pulse intravenous corticosteroids in seven patients' extragenital lichen sclerosus,[39] which is much harder to control than genital involvement, and a recent letter reported "improvement" in half of 21 women with recalcitrant vulvar lichen sclerosus treated with 2.5-17.5 mg of methotrexate weekly from 1 to 17 months.[40] I have found methotresxate very useful in a minority of women with disease recalcitrant to topical and intralesional corticosteroids and topical calcineurin inhibitors.

## Procedures

Most often used is intralesional corticosteroids (see Chapter 4 for specifics). There are no data for this procedure, but it is regularly used by dermatologists for any steroid-responsive dermatosis that does not respond to topical therapy. It is especially useful for thickened and hyperkeratotic skin that is resistant to topical medications and for those patients who demonstrate poor adherence. This is repeated monthly until the disease is controlled.

Some providers find that intramuscular corticosteroids are useful, again with no data. Doses of 40 mg (small patients) to 80 mg (large patients) can be used. Normally, this is performed about every 3 months as needed.

Destruction of lichen sclerosus has been shown to clear lichen sclerosus; photodynamic therapy, cryotherapy, focused ultrasound (generally used for tumors), and ablative $CO_2$ laser are all often useful, although generally followed by recurrence.[41-44] In addition, I have seen lichen sclerosus (temporarily) completely clear following a blistering irritant contact reaction to a topical anesthetic applied in the office. These are counterintuitive, since lichen sclerosus is triggered by injury and irritation.

The use of fat grafting to attenuate local vessel depletion and promote healing of radiation-induced skin damage has been well documented in murine models.[45] Autologous fat grafting has been tried recently for lichen sclerosus, and the most recent prospective open study of 33 women showed improvement in symptoms and mood, and the physician-based score showed an overall improvement "to lesser or greater extent."[46] The conclusion was that further trials were needed to rule out a placebo effect.

Over the past 5 years, platelet-rich plasma therapy has received publicity, particularly among women with lichen sclerosus, as potential therapy. Case reports and open trials have been promising, but a recent double-blind, placebo-controlled trial with before and after histology showed little difference between treated and untreated women.[47] A prospective study of five men with resistant lichen sclerosus treated with platelet-rich plasma showed improvement in symptoms at 10 months, but little change visually in the skin.[48] And, a review of studies in 2019 showed weak evidence for benefit,[49] so this treatment cannot be recommended at this time.

Nonablative laser for lichen sclerosus has become popular with providers recently, and multiple reports generally showing benefit have appeared in the literature in the past 2 years, mostly case reports and small series. Although primarily used for dermatologic cosmetic procedures, and unapproved by the U.S. Food and Drug Administration for all vulvovaginal indications, the fractional CO2 laser (Mona Lisa Touch®, FemTouch®) has been used for the treatment of lichen sclerosus over the past few years. One open study of 40 women with lichen sclerosus symptomatic despite topical clobetasol found that 72.5% of women reported overall improvement of at least 66%, but white color only decreased by a disappointing 20%.[50] As of this writing, there are two controlled studies comparing topical corticosteroids to a nonablative laser, both concluding that laser was superior to topical corticosteroids. Both had flaws in methodology; among them was marked underuse of the topical corticosteroid compared to standard for the treatment of lichen sclerosus.[51,52] Still another 2021 controlled study showed no significant benefit of fractional $CO_2$ laser as monotherapy for vulvar lichen sclerosus.[53] One of very few reports of nonablative laser for lichen sclerosus in men showed a positive impact on their sexual function and quality of life, but there was no mention of objective changes.[54] Studies at this time do not give us an answer and, in fact, show us that some researchers do not understand the correct use of current first-line therapy for lichen sclerosus. A position statement by the International Society for the Study of Vulvovaginal Disease stated in 2019 that "The use of LASER in women with vulvodynia or lichen sclerosus should not be recommended in routine clinical practice."[55] With great skepticism, I treated 11 women with very recalcitrant lichen sclerosus with fractional $CO_2$ laser with concomitant superpotent topical corticosteroid. Ten did extremely well, but ongoing topical therapy was required. I suspect nonablative lasers may find a place in the management of recalcitrant lichen sclerosus when added to a topical corticosteroid.

Usually, surgery is only indicated for correction of scarring and, unless urgent, only after the skin disease is controlled. Surgery in the face of active skin disease generally results in immediate recurrence. Lysis of side-to-side adhesions that produce introital narrowing with fissuring, correction of clitoral phimosis, and unroofing clitoral pseudocysts should be delayed until the lichen sclerosus is controlled. However, men sometimes experience urethral strictures that may require urgent correction. Recurrences are common with active disease in this instance as well, so proactive therapy with clobetasol is preferred. Obviously, prompt surgery is required for squamous cell carcinoma or intraepithelial neoplasia. Rarely, for very severe disease, excision of recalcitrant disease followed by the immediate institution of maintenance topical corticosteroid ointments has been found anecdotally to prevent recurrence, as a last resort.

#### Special Issues

Most often used is intralesional experience regression of lichen sclerosus at puberty. We now know that, although the symptoms of lichen sclerosus usually improve, probably due to the appearance of estrogen, the disease only sometimes resolves. A prospective study showed that 25% of girls experienced remission.[56] A more recent study reported that 80% of postpubertal girls were asymptomatic after puberty, 70% off therapy, but these children were not examined, and postpubertal girls with active LS are well known to often be asymptomatic while experiencing ongoing silent scarring.[57] This author offers cessation of therapy at puberty with quarterly follow-up for 2 years to those girls with absolution no signs of lichen sclerosus. There is no information regarding recurrence of lichen sclerosus at menopause in these girls who appear to clear at puberty.

Hyperkeratotic lesions are often resistant to treatment, sometimes because topical medication does not penetrate easily, sometimes because the disease is more severe, and sometimes because the neoplastic process has begun. If those areas do not respond fairly promptly to topical or intralesional therapy, a biopsy is indicated to rule out differentiated vulvar intraepithelial neoplasia or squamous cell carcinoma. If the area is small, excision may be a good option, since even hyperkeratotic lesions that are banal on biopsy are sometimes observed over time to transform into squamous cell carcinoma. Retinoids are reported to be useful for hyperkeratotic lesions as well, particularly if lesions are not easily excised.

#### Follow-up

Long-term follow-up twice a year is indicated for most patients with well-controlled lichen sclerosus to evaluate for ongoing control, side effects, and any signs of early malignant transformation. The longer a patient has lichen sclerosus, the higher the risk for secondary squamous cell carcinoma. One large study showed an increase from 1.4% of women with lichen sclerosus for 24 months developing squamous cell carcinoma to 36.8% of women with disease duration at 300 months.[59] However, this study did not report treatment and control of the lichen sclerosus. Therefore, the provider should not develop a false sense of security in women who do well for years.

## Lichen Planus

Lichen planus exhibits multiple morphologies and is discussed in several chapters: 5, 9, 11, and 13, in addition to this one. On genital skin, lichen planus is most often erosive, so the primary discussion is in Chapter 11.

### Clinical Presentation

Lichen planus is an inflammatory, autoimmune lymphocyte-mediated disease that sometimes presents as white papules or plaques. Patient usually report pruritus, often associated with burning, pain, and dyspareunia, since erosive disease is often present as well.

Overlying the typical dusky red, flat-topped papules on keratinized, dry skin are the classic white striae, called Wickham striae, generally not visible without magnification. Also, pathognomonic are the lacy white striae on mucous membranes, and sometimes these appear as discrete or coalescing annular papules (Figs. 8-37 to 8-39). This appearance is most common in the mouth but occasionally occurs on the anogenital skin (Fig. 8-40). A confluent uniform, whitened epithelium that mimics lichen sclerosus is infrequently present, although crinkling and ecchymosis are absent (Figs. 8-41 and 8-42). Although the red papules and white striae of lichen sclerosus are generally unassociated with scarring, any morphology is likely to accompany erosive lichen planus, which is well known to scar.

The erosive form, discussed in Chapter 11, affects predominantly the mucosal surfaces and is often associated with adjacent white lesions (Fig. 8-43). In the syndrome of Hewitt and Pelisse, also known as the vulvovaginal-gingival syndrome, the affected areas are the gingivae, the vagina, and the vulvar vestibule. Less common is the association of erosions of the glans penis and gingivae. The areas involved have a characteristic glazed erythema or are frankly eroded and bordered by an edge of whitened hyperkeratotic epithelium. This edge is the best site for biopsy, as often the areas of glazed erythema, particularly in the vestibule, do not show the characteristic features of lichen planus, and many are reported as a plasma cell mucositis.

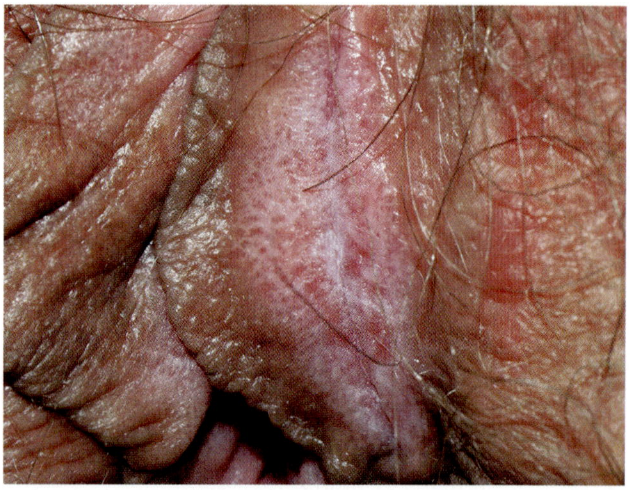

Fig. 8-37. The interlacing white papules on the lateral aspect of the labium minus is pathognomonic for lichen planus; no biopsy is needed for that diagnosis.

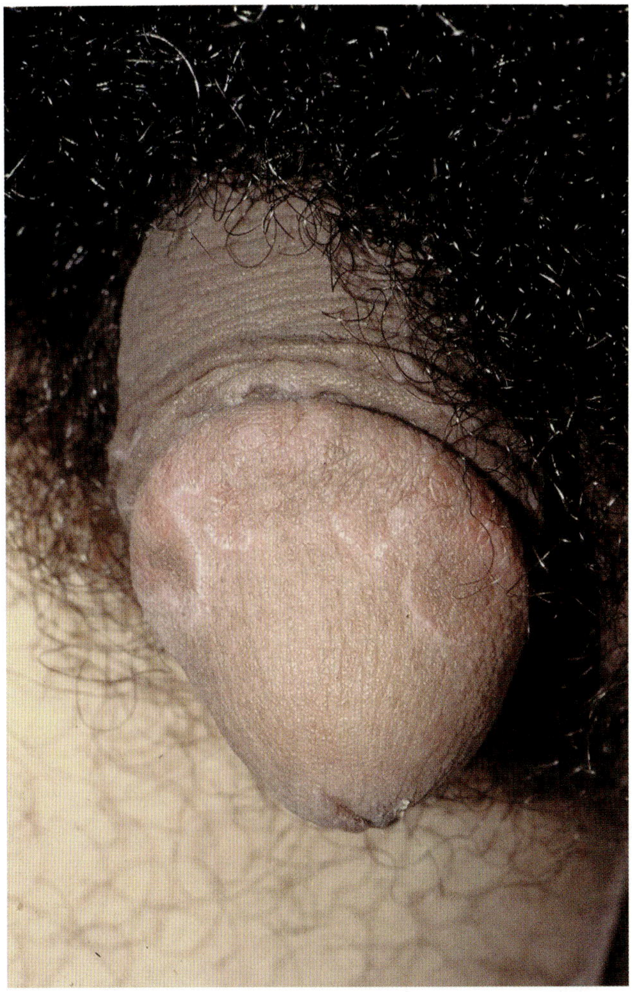

Fig. 8-38. White lesions of lichen planus are sometimes annular.

## Diagnosis

When reticulate or fernlike striae are present, the diagnosis is clinical and no biopsy is required. Dermoscopy of these lesions primarily shows magnification of the white network, lacy, or annular white pattern, which may be somewhat blue in patients with darker natural skin tones, brownish dots surrounding the striae.[58] However, "pseudo-Wickham striae" occur in skin lesions with some scarring or resolving skin lesions, especially prurigo nodules, discoid lupus erythematosus, and nodular scabies, but these have more dilated vessels.

Patients with solid white epithelium usually require a biopsy to differentiate from lichen sclerosus and, sometimes, LSC. In long-standing disease, in which there is complete loss of the vulvar architecture, lichen planus is indistinguishable from end-stage lichen sclerosus, morphea, or mucous membrane pemphigoid. White papules of lichen planus sometimes raise the possibility of candidiasis or the white papules seen on modified mucous membranes in Reiter disease. Lupus erythematosus is rare on the anogenital skins, but the lesions are very similar to lichen planus. Immunofluorescent studies should help in the differentiation. When lichen planus presents as papules or plaques of uniform, white

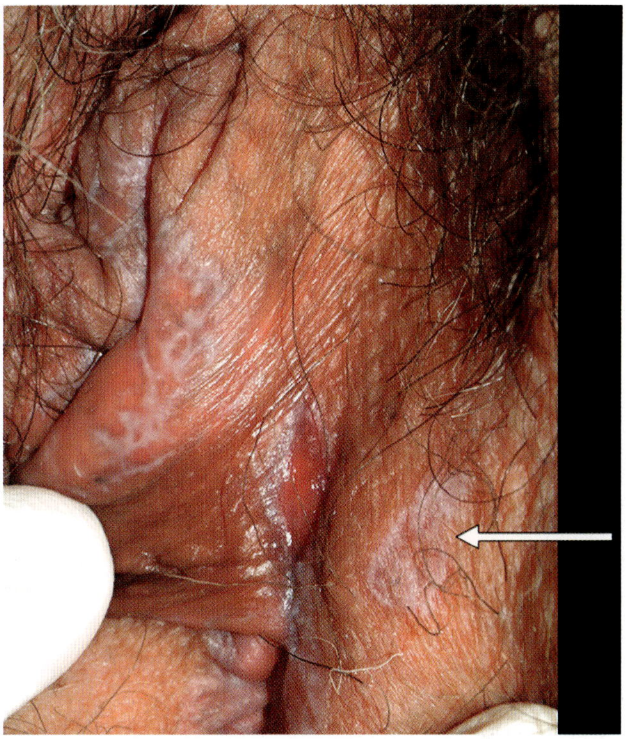

Fig. 8-39. These white interlacing and annular striae are classic for lichen planus, but sometimes lichen planus also appears as solid white epithelium (*arrow*).

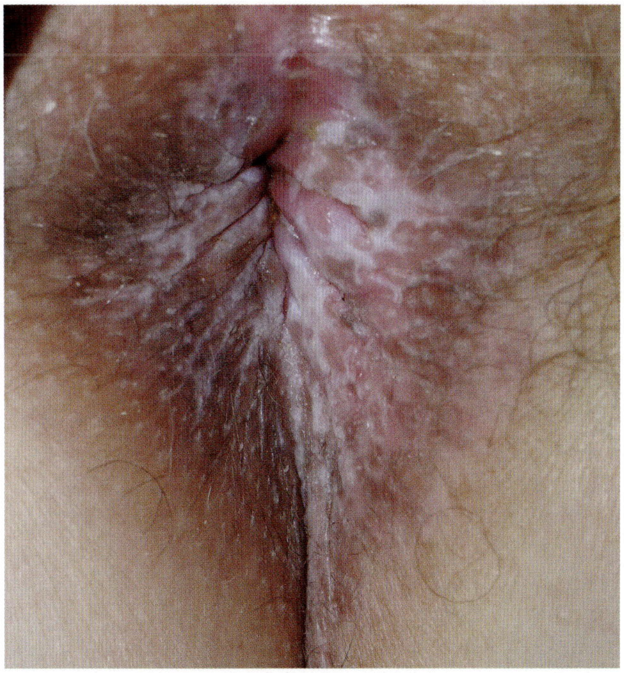

Fig. 8-40. These white lesions of lichen planus were accompanied by erosive disease just inside the rectal verge.

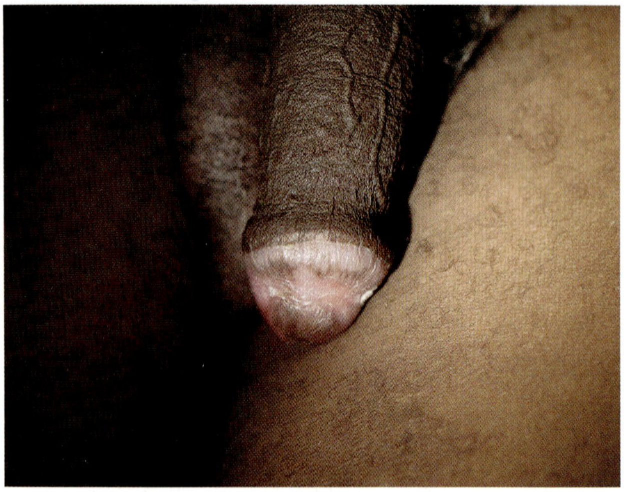

Fig. 8-41. Anogenital lichen sclerosus is sometimes solid white epithelium that can mimic lichen sclerosus.

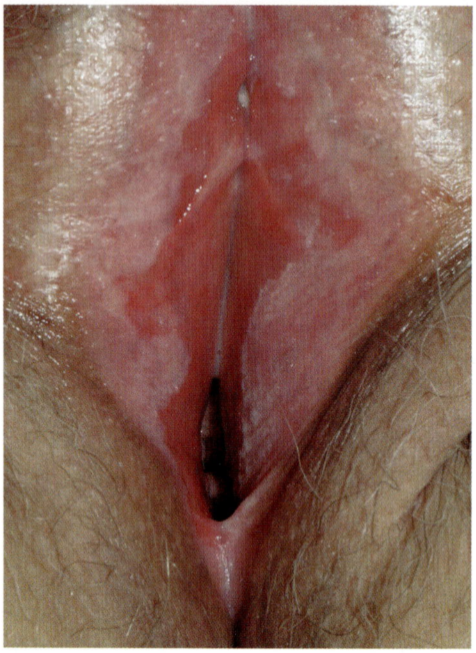

Fig. 8-42. Lichen planus is sometimes manifested by white plaques but without the crinkling that is characteristic of lichen sclerosus. The atrophic red patch or superficial erosion of the vestibule and adjacent modified mucous membrane is characteristic of LP rather than LS as well.

epithelium, a differentiation of lichen planus from lichen simplex, lichen sclerosus, macerated, psoriasis or eczema, Hailey-Hailey disease, fungal infection, and vitiligo must be made.

**LICHEN PLANUS (WHITE MORPHOLOGY) — Diagnosis**

- Women: white reticulate striae, or white epithelium, often surrounding erosions; vaginal erosions and inflammatory vaginal secretions common.
- Men: white reticulate or annular striae, flat-topped white papules most common on glans. Less often erosions with surrounding white epithelium.
- Both women and men, oral lichen planus with white striae common, +/– buccal mucosal or gingival erosions.
- Confirmed by biopsy that shows upper dermal chronic inflammatory infiltrate abutting and disrupting the basement membrane, dyskeratotic cells. Often, biopsy is interpreted as nonspecific "lichenoid dermatitis" so that diagnosis is made by clinical correlation.

### Management

First-line treatment of lichen planus consists of topical corticosteroids, usually a daily superpotent ointment such as clobetasol or halobetasol propionate, medications that usually produce sufficient response, then tapered to thrice weekly at most. Topical calcineurin inhibitors tacrolimus or pimecrolimus can be added for inadequate improvement, with the same caveats as noted above for lichen sclerosus and vitiligo. Generally, the white forms of lichen planus respond well to topical therapy.

**LICHEN PLANUS (WHITE MORPHOLOGY) — Management**

- Correction of infection, estrogen deficiency
- Women: topical ultrapotent corticosteroid ointment (clobetasol propionate 0.05%, etc.) once or twice a day until normal texture, then decrease frequency as possible to maintain control
- Tacrolimus or pimecrolimus added bid is second-line therapy; may be used with a corticosteroid for added benefit when required
- Men: circumcision if sufficiently severe, otherwise as for women
- Careful follow-up, monthly at first to evaluate for side effects of medication, for control of disease, for changes of malignancy

## Lichen Simplex Chronicus

Lichen simplex chronicus (LSC) most often presents as red (or hyperpigmented, in patients of color), lichenified plaques, and this is discussed primarily with other red plaques in Chapter 5. However, skin of LSC that is thickened by rubbing and scratching can be white when it is hydrated, as occurs in this occluded area, just as palms and soles turn white when soaked in water (**Figs. 8-44 to 8-46**). In addition, the injury of rubbing and scratching sometimes produces postinflammatory hypopigmentation. Finally, the injury of rubbing and scratching can trigger vitiligo in the predisposed patient.

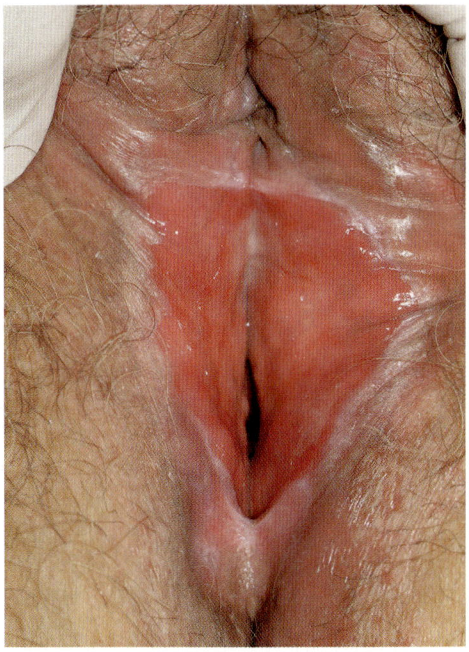

Fig. 8-43. Many erosions exhibit a rim of hypopigmentation, as does this erosion of lichen planus; however, this rim is also a nonspecific finding for many chronic erosions.

The diagnosis can usually be made on the basis of a history of intense itching and pleasure with scratching, the presence of lichenification, and a lack of genital scarring. Nevertheless, severe superimposed LSC can obscure underlying lichen sclerosus and, less often, psoriasis or contact dermatitis. If this is suspected, a biopsy should be performed. Although the presence of lichen sclerosus can generally be detected underlying LSC, the superimposed changes of LSC that confuse the morphologic diagnosis can confuse the histologic picture as well. Microscopically, a biopsy of LSC shows marked

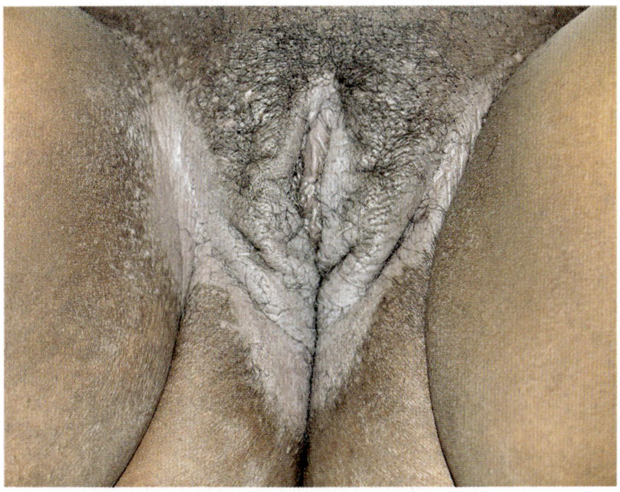

Fig. 8-44. The remarkable lichenification seen in this patient with lichen simplex chronicus is white from moisture, extending beyond the usual areas of genital wetness due to her excess weight, sweating, and occlusion.

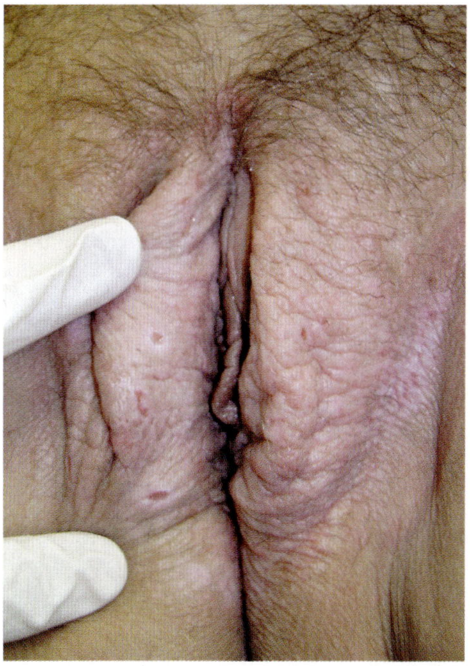

Fig. 8-45. Hydrated thickened skin from rubbing and scratching again is white; if she stays in stirrups for 15 minutes, the white color will fade. The linear and irregular erosions of excoriation are characteristic of LSC as well.

hyperkeratosis overlying an irregular psoriasiform, hyperplastic epithelium with a prominent granular cell layer. There may be a perivascular infiltrate of lymphocytes and eosinophils, and lamellar fibrosis of the papillary dermis is often seen.

Hailey-Hailey disease (benign familial pemphigus), psoriasis, extramammary Paget disease, and the

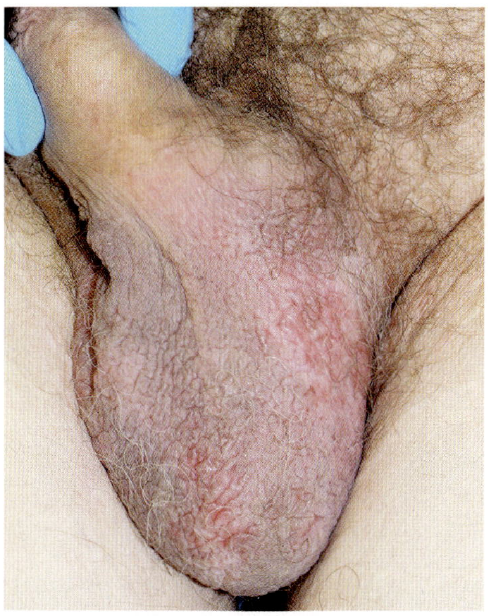

Fig. 8-46. The lichenified scrotum is white, again due to the occluded, relatively humid environment; this white color is less common on the penis and scrotum, which are dryer than the vulva and perianal skin.

hypertrophic forms of lichen planus and lichen sclerosus can all resemble LSC.

Management consists of ultrapotent topical corticosteroids, avoidance of irritants, and sedation during sleeping hours to prevent rubbing and scratching at night to help break the itch-scratch cycle (see Chapter 5). A lower-potency topical corticosteroid or less frequent dosing of the ultrapotent preparation can be substituted as the patient improves.

## Candidiasis

Although the primary lesions of candidiasis are red plaques and erosions, mucous membrane or intertriginous candidiasis, especially when severe, can exhibit white epithelium or a surface covered in a white adherent exudate, which can be removed by scraping the area **(Figs. 8-47 and 8-48)**. Other patients exhibit coalescing white papules that represent fragile pustules with macerated blister roofs **(Fig. 8-49)**. This condition is discussed in more detail in Chapter 5 (Red Plaques) and Chapter 13 (Vaginitis and Balanitis). The causative organism of candidiasis characterized by white lesions is usually *Candida albicans* or, less often, *Candida tropicalis*. Although other strains such as *Candida (Torulopsis) glabrata* and *Candida parapsilosis* rarely cause vulvovaginal symptoms, these forms of *Candida* generally produce only irritation of the mucous membrane skin of the vagina and introitus, rather than white lesions of keratinized, exterior skin.

The white lesions of vulvar or penile candidiasis are seen most often in patients who are obese, diabetic, or immunosuppressed.

Most candidal vulvitis is found in conjunction with vaginal candidiasis and the term vulvovaginitis would be a more accurate description of the problem.

Men who are not circumcised can acquire genital candidiasis through contact with affected sexual partners or, from *Candida* colonizing the bowel, especially when there is an underlying dermatosis, obesity, or incontinence. The favored sites are the inner aspect of the prepuce or the surface of the glans penis. Although the patches are usually erythematous and eroded, the initial lesion can be pustular or can exhibit white, macerated epithelium similar to that seen in some women. The

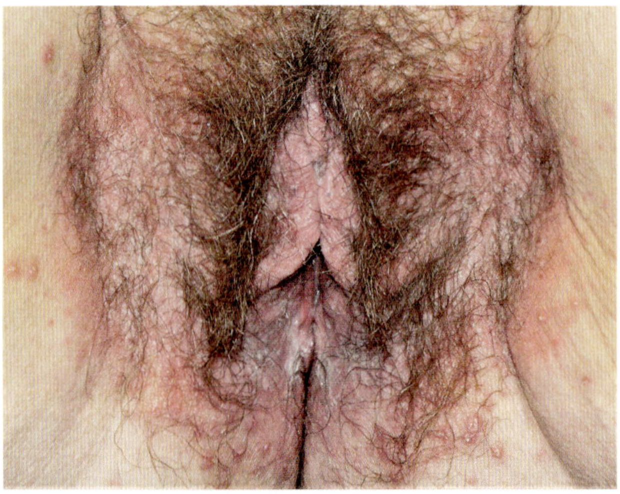

Fig. 8-47. The white surface of this red plaque of candidiasis is easily removable and shows sheets of mycelia on a fungal preparation.

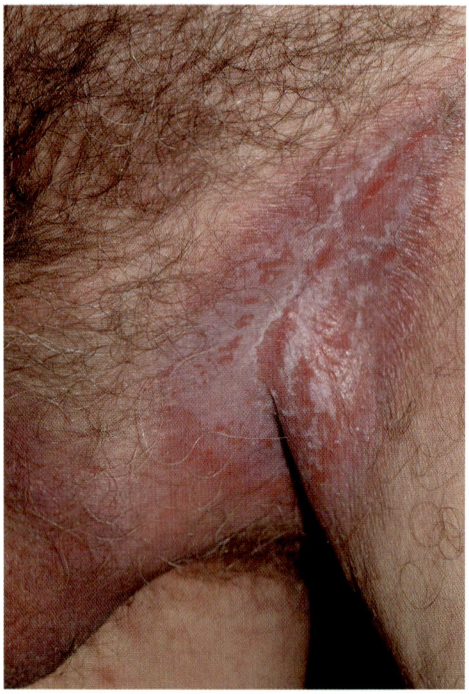

Fig. 8-48. Intertriginous candidiasis is often a factor in intertrigo dermatitis, and this white surface substance comprises both macerated epithelium and yeast in this man with diabetes.

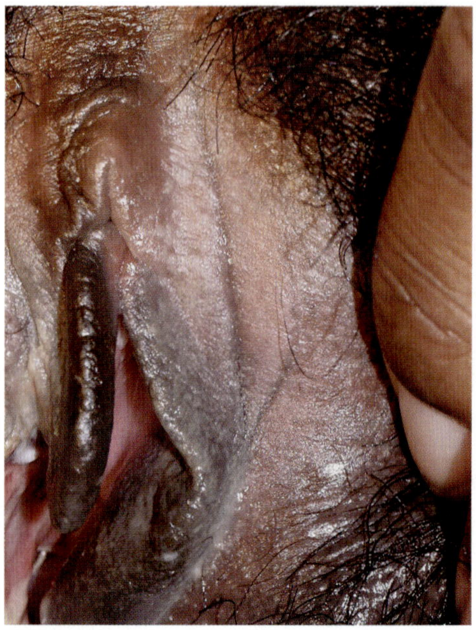

Fig. 8-49. This immunosuppressed patient with candidiasis shows a white nonadherent surface substance that consists of yeast microscopically

diagnosis generally is made by the identification of candidal pseudohyphae and hyphae on direct microscopy or by a fungal culture.

Many dermatoses can be mistaken for candidal vulvitis, particularly psoriasis, eczema/LSC, and Hailey-Hailey (benign familial pemphigus). The soft, hydrated epithelium of blisters and hyperkeratotic skin affected by pemphigus vegetans can resemble *Candida* infection. Occasionally, white erosions of herpes simplex virus infection are nearly indistinguishable from candidiasis.

Topical anticandidal agents, to include any azole cream and nystatin ointment, are effective therapies, but creams often burn with application. In addition, the vagina should be evaluated or treated empirically in women, since most premenopausal women have accompanying vagina candidiasis. Oral fluconazole is effective as well. Because intertriginous candidiasis is often recurrent due to predisposing factors of obesity, diabetes, incontinence, etc., patients may be provided with topical medication to use for recurrences or on a daily basis to prevent reappearance of candidiasis.

**CANDIDIASIS — Diagnosis**

- Red patches, sometimes with white exudate, particularly on mucous membrane or modified mucous membranes of the vulva, glans penis, prepuce, or skin folds
- Fungal preparation or culture showing yeast
- Biopsy not required

**CANDIDIASIS — Management**

- Oral fluconazole, or any topical azole, nystatin
- Control of any underlying process (antibiotics, immunosuppression, incontinence)

## Genital Warts

Genital warts most often present as skin-colored or brown tumors and are discussed primarily in Chapter 7, Skin-Colored Lesions. However, when occurring on damp skin, the hyperkeratotic surface of warts is often white due to hydration **(Figs. 8-50 and 8-51)**.

Anogenital warts (condylomata acuminata) are benign epidermal tumors produced by any of several human papillomavirus (HPV) types. HPV types 6 and 11 are responsible for most anogenital warts and are recognized as *low-risk* viruses as malignant transformation is rare. HPV types 16, 18, 31, and 33 are *high risk* and are involved in the genesis of intraepithelial neoplasia and squamous cell carcinoma. Therapies include physical destruction by liquid nitrogen, electrocautery, and laser; chemical destruction by trichloroacetic acid and podofilox; and promoting the local skin immunity with immune response–modulating creams such as imiquimod.

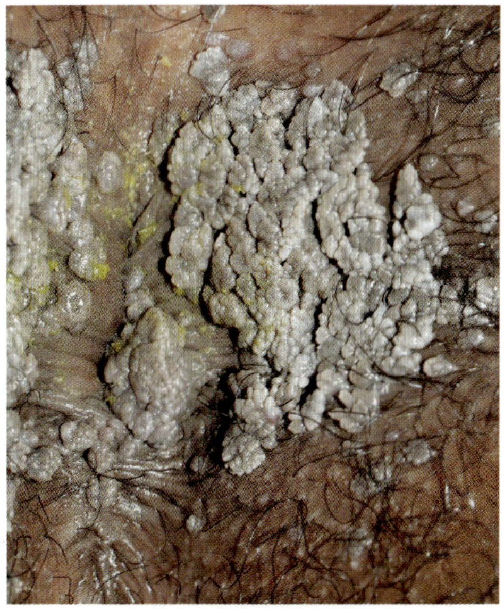

Fig. 8-50. The hyperkeratosis of anogenital warts causes them to appear white in occluded, moist areas such the perianal skin.

The new vaccines now available are a useful preventive measure.

## High-Grade Squamous Intraepithelial Lesions

High-grade squamous intraepithelial lesions (HSIL), previously called intraepithelial neoplasia, Bowenoid papulosis, and squamous cell carcinoma *in situ*, consists of full-thickness dysplasia of the epithelium produced by

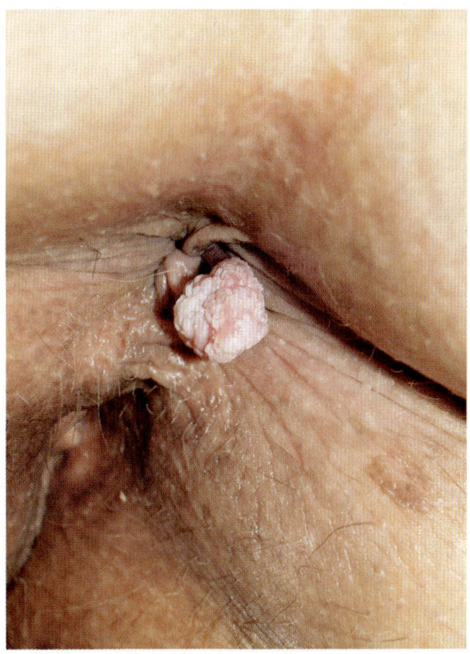

Fig. 8-51. Although warts are usually skin colored, their surface is white in wet areas.

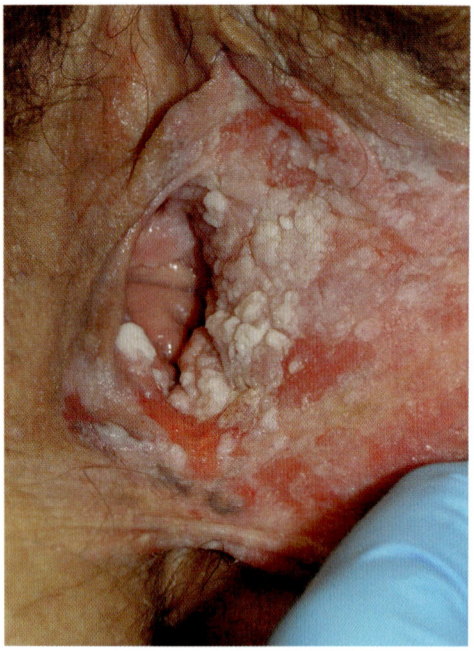

Fig. 8-52. As in warts, this HSIL, which is squamous cell carcinoma *in situ* on the basis of HPV infection, also appears white on wet skin.

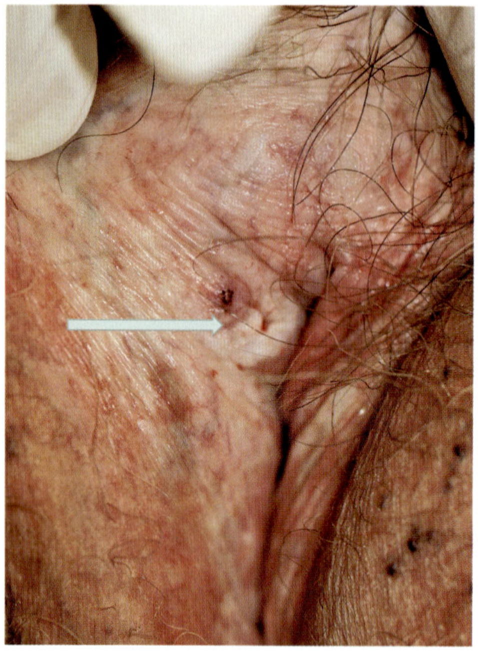

Fig. 8-53. This white nodule (*arrow*) represents dVIN, or squamous cell carcinoma *in situ* in a setting of lichen sclerosus; this is often an aggressive tumor.

HPV infection. This is discussed primarily in Chapter 7, Skin-Colored Lesions, but is also addressed in Chapters 5 and 9. As for anogenital warts, lesions of HSIL appear white when occurring on wet skin, so that the hydrated hyperkeratotic skin confers a white appearance (**Fig. 8-52**). However, these lesions are sometimes red, skin-colored, or brown.

## Differentiated Intraepithelial Neoplasia

Full-thickness epithelial dysplasia occurring in association with lichen sclerosus and lichen planus rather than HPV infection is currently termed differentiated intraepithelial neoplasia. This is discussed primarily in Chapter 7, Skin-Colored Lesions, but is also mentioned in Chapter 5. This presents as well-demarcated white, red, or skin-colored flat-topped papules and plaques (**Fig. 8-53**). The diagnosis of intraepithelial neoplasia is made by the morphologic appearance with confirmation on biopsy, which shows full-thickness dysplasia. The differential diagnosis for lesions of white intraepithelial neoplasia includes HSIL, lichen planus, lichen sclerosus, and basal cell carcinoma.

## Extramammary Paget Disease

Extramammary Paget disease (discussed primarily in Chapter 5) is a very uncommon malignancy of the anogenital skin, most often manifested by poorly demarcated red plaques in a setting of hypopigmented hyperkeratosis (**Fig. 8-54**). This disease is often mistaken for eczema lichen simplex

## Hailey-Hailey Disease (Benign Familial Pemphigus)

Hailey-Hailey disease, discussed primarily in Chapter 10, is an uncommon autosomal dominant condition that results in fragility of the skin, so that the epidermis separates easily from the dermis, producing superficial, delicate, small blisters that are generally not recognized as blisters. The confluent lesions and fragile skin result in plaques of white hydrated epithelium, with small, short linear fissures (**Fig. 8-55**). These form most easily in skin folds where there is friction, such as anogenital skin and the axillae.

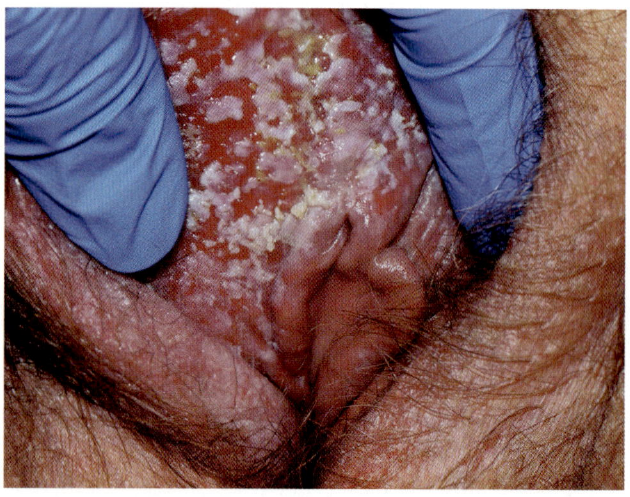

Fig. 8-54. Classic extramammary Paget disease is manifested by a red plaque covered with white islands of adherent white hyperkeratosis.

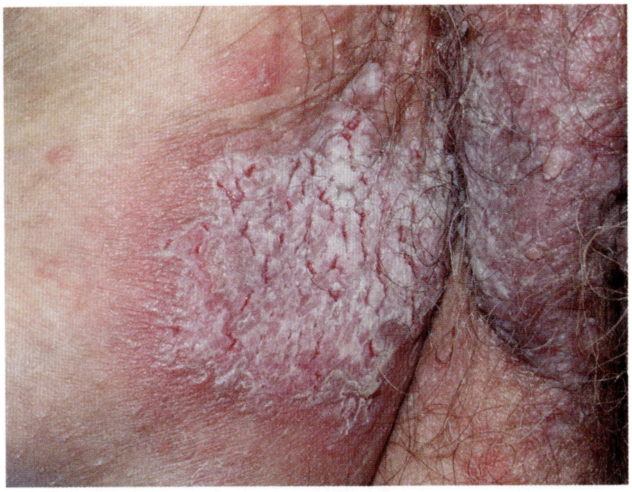

Fig. 8-55. Although Hailey-Hailey disease (benign familial pemphigus) is a condition produced by small blisters due to fragile skin, actual blisters are often not seen; the white, thick plaque consists of macerated blister roofs, and the multiple small, rather short, linear fissures are a classic hallmark.

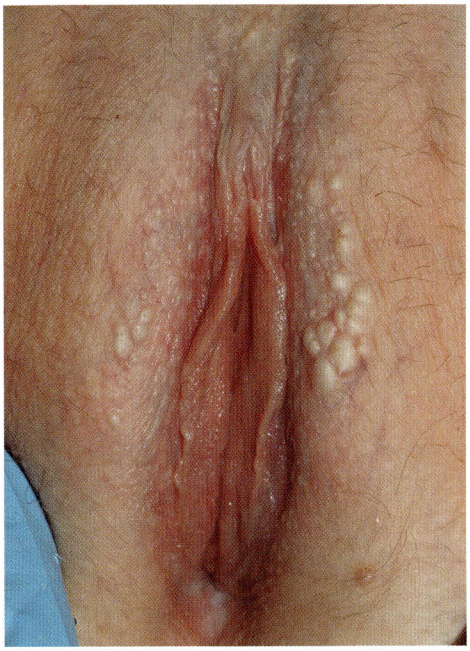

Fig. 8-56. Epidermal cysts (aka epidermoid cysts, "sebaceous" cysts) are common nodules produced by an occluded follicle that results in retained white (and odiferous) keratin trapped within the follicle. The vulva and scrotum are common areas for these to occur. The very small cysts are referred to as milia.

## White Papules and Nodules

### Epidermal (Epidermoid, Epidermal Inclusion, "Sebaceous") Cysts and Milia

Epidermal cysts are common benign nodules that occur when hair follicles become obstructed, and the deep portion of the follicle is gradually expanded by desquamated cells shed from the follicular epithelium (see also Chapters 6 and 7). These are so common as to be a normal finding. However, an occasional patient shows large numbers of cysts primarily on the scrotum or labia majora.

Epidermal cysts can occur at any age, but they arise most often in midlife and appear primarily on the labia majora, labia minora, penile shaft, scrotum, and perianal area. They do not occur in the vestibule and generally not on the glans penis. The cysts appear as dome-shaped, white, yellow, or skin-colored papules or nodules, often with a central plug **(Figs. 8-56 and 8-57)**. They are usually asymptomatic but can become inflamed and tender due to a foreign body reaction to keratin when a cyst ruptures. True infection is uncommon. Very small 1- to 2-mm papules are referred to as milia. Long-standing lesions can become calcified.

The diagnosis is made clinically, and it is easily confirmed if a lesion is pierced with a no. 11 scalpel blade, and cheesy material is expressed. Histologic features are a cyst wall composed of stratified squamous epithelium surrounding a cavity that contains lamellar birefringent keratin and hair.

White nodules that can mimic epidermal cysts include Fordyce spots, steatocystomata, vellus hair cysts, and lesions of molluscum contagiosum. Vestibular cysts should be considered, but these are usually bluish, skin colored, or more yellow, and they are located in the vulvar vestibule.

Therapy generally is not needed for most cases, but larger lesions that are troublesome can be excised and smaller cysts and milia can be extirpated, cauterized, or hyfrecated.

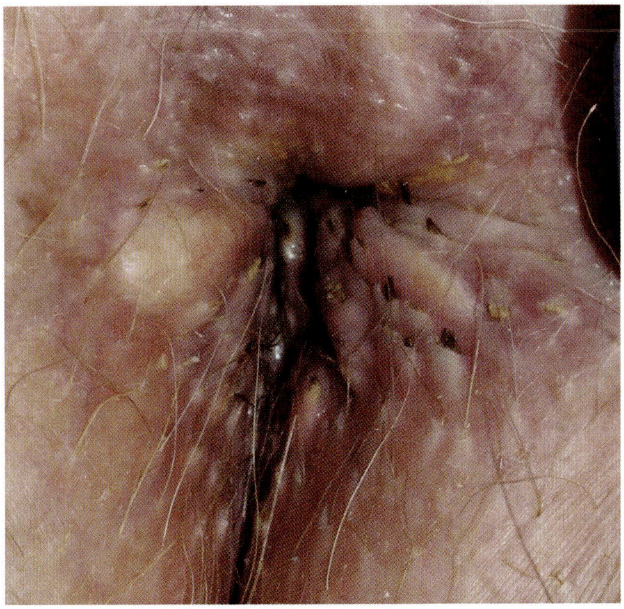

Fig. 8-57. Cysts are common on perianal skin as well; these can also occur as a result of chronic corticosteroid use that decreases the elasticity of the skin. These cysts began as open comedones, as seen by the black plug at the surface of many of the lesions.

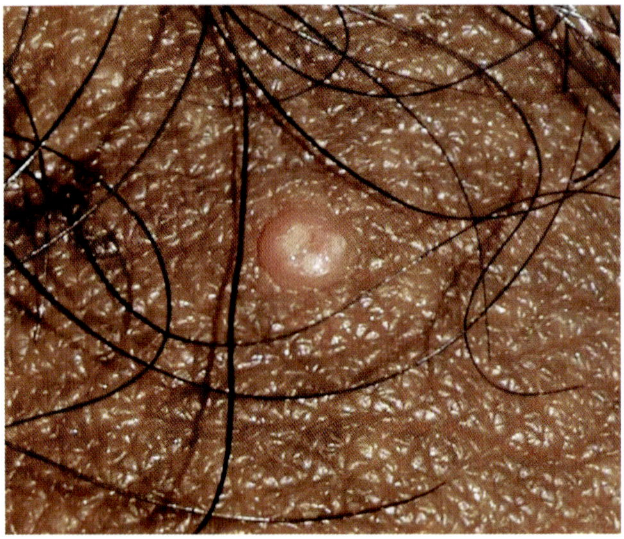

Fig. 8-58. Mollusca contagiosa are usually skin colored, but when white, they are sometimes difficult to differentiate from milia; this molluscum contagiosum on the shaft of the penis shows three white molluscum bodies within the papule.

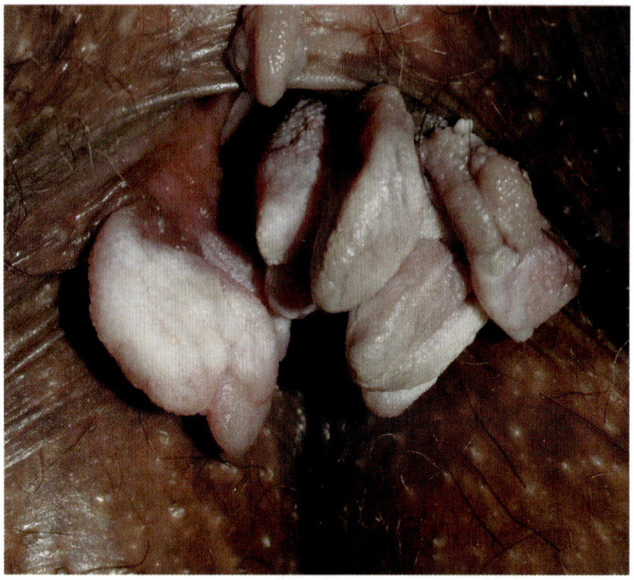

Fig. 8-59. Verrucous carcinomas are low-grade squamous cell carcinomas that mimic large anogenital warts; however, HPV has not been confirmed as an etiology.

## Molluscum Contagiosum

Mollusca contagiosa are skin lesions produced by a poxvirus and are usually sexually transmitted when they occur on the genitalia of adults. These are discussed primarily in Chapter 7, Skin-Colored Lesions. Mollusca can be skin-colored, pink, or white dome-shaped papules **(Fig. 8-58)**. Classically, at least some lesions have a central dell or depression. These are found on keratinized skin and, in immunocompetent people, are self-limited and self-resolving. These lesions involute spontaneously after any trauma, which includes extirpating with a sharpened orange stick or no. 21/22-gauge needle, curettage, light cryotherapy, hyfrecation, and cantharidin. The topical immune-modulating cream imiquimod (Aldara) is also effective in the treatment of extensive lesions, particularly in children who will not tolerate the other methods.

## Verrucous Carcinoma

### Clinical Presentation

This unusual tumor occurs in older patients, often in their eighth or ninth decade, but there are anecdotal cases described in younger patients. The lesion appears as a slowly growing warty or papillomatous nodule, most commonly sited on the labia majora **(Fig. 8-59)**, glans penis, or perianal skin. Verrucous carcinomas have also been described in the vagina, and on the cervix, penis, scrotum, rectum, and bladder, as well as in extragenital sites (ie, the nasopharynx and esophagus).

### Diagnosis

The diagnosis of verrucous carcinoma is often difficult in light of the rather banal histology, particularly in differentiating the lesion from a giant condyloma acuminatum. The histopathologic changes are undramatic and include marked hyperkeratosis and acanthosis with deeply penetrating, rounded, burgeoning rete ridges. The basal layer is intact and is clearly defined, and there is a striking lack of cellular atypia throughout the epithelium. A nonspecific inflammatory infiltrate is located around and beneath the tumor. A prominent granular layer with clear koilocytic cells is a frequent finding.

Other than a large wart, the main disease to be differentiated from verrucous carcinoma is typical squamous cell carcinoma. Histologic analysis should differentiate the two diseases.

**VERRUCOUS CARCINOMA — Diagnosis**

- Warty or papillomatous nodule
- Most often on the labia majora, glans penis, or perianal skin
- Biopsy required, but often banal and nonspecific, requiring a high index of suspicion and empiric diagnosis and therapy

### Pathophysiology

Verrucous carcinoma is now considered to be a variant of well-differentiated squamous cell carcinoma. Despite its deceptively benign histologic appearance, the tumor growth is destructive and invasive locally. In some cases, there has been evidence of HPV infection, a history of genital warts, and sometimes a background of lichen sclerosus. HPV is not regularly found in these lesions.

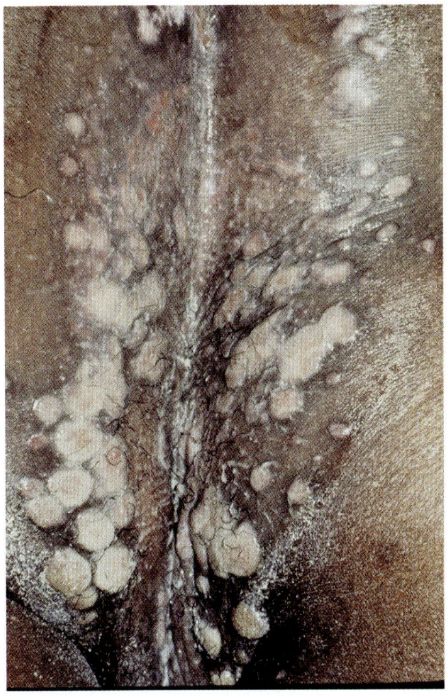

Fig. 8-60. These flat-topped papules exhibit a white surface due to the eroded surface and white fibrin debris.

### Management

Surgical excision is the treatment of choice, and lymphadenectomy is rarely indicated because metastases to lymph nodes are very uncommon.[60] Radiotherapy is not used because many tumors are not radiosensitive. Acitretin, an oral retinoid, has been used successfully in a few patients, with or without destruction.

| VERRUCOUS CARCINOMA | Management |
|---|---|
| • Surgical excision | |

## Condylomata Lata

Condylomata lata are lesions found primarily on mucous membranes or modified mucous membranes as a manifestation of secondary syphilis. This is also discussed in Chapter 7. The name "lata" alludes to the flat morphology, in contradistinction to condylomata acuminata, which describes one morphology of HPV infection, where the lesions are spiky (acuminate). The lesions are well-demarcated, skin-colored, flat-topped papules, which, on wet skin, exhibit a white surface (**Fig. 8-60**). Treatment consists of antibiotics for secondary syphilis.

## REFERENCES


1. Hans A, Reddy KA, Black SM, et al. Transcultural assessment of quality of life in patients with vitiligo. *J Am Acad Dermatol.* 2022;86(5):1114-1116. doi:10.1016/j.jaad.2021.03.118
2. Lambert JLW, De Schepper S, Speeckaert R. Cutaneous manifestations in biological-treated inflammatory bowel disease patients: a narrative review. *J Clin Med.* 2021;10(5):1040. doi:10.3390/jcm10051040
3. Wongvibulsin S, Pahalyants V, Kalinich M, et al. Epidemiology and risk factors for the development of cutaneous toxicities in patients treated with immune checkpoint inhibitors: a United States population-level analysis. *J Am Acad Dermatol.* 2022;86(3):563-572. doi:10.1016/j.jaad.2021.03.094
4. Maatouk I. Vitiligo-like lesions following imiquimod 5% application for condyloma acuminata: An additional case. *Indian J Dermatol Venereol Leprol.* 2016;82(5):572-574. doi:10.4103/0378-6323.182808
5. Alatabani M, Ghobara Y, Alissa A. Vitiligo-like depigmentation following treatment with Imiquimod 5% cream for Condylomata Acuminata. *Case Rep Dermatol.* 2021;13(1):36-41. doi:10.1159/000510736
6. García-Montero P, Repiso Jiménez JB, Fernández Morano MT, de Troya Martín M. Genital vitiligo-like hypopigmentation after treatment with 5% imiquimod. *Actas Dermosifiliogr.* 2017;108(4):378-380. doi:10.1016/j.ad.2016.10.007
7. Errichetti E, Stinco G. Dermoscopy in general dermatology: a practical overview. *Dermatol Ther (Heidelb).* 2016;6(4): 471-507.
8. Vinay N, Ranugha PSS, Betkerur JB, Shastry V, Ashwini PK. Non-venereal genital dermatoses and their impact on quality of life-A cross-sectional study. *Indian J Dermatol Venereol Leprol.* 2022;88(3):354-359. doi:10.25259/IJDVL_329_18
9. Morales-Sánchez MA, Vargas-Salinas M, Peralta-Pedrero ML, Olguín-García MG, Jurado-Santa Cruz F. Impact of vitiligo on quality of life. *Actas Dermosifiliogr.* 2017;108(7):637-642. doi:10.1016/j.ad.2017.03.007
10. Stinco G, Trevisan G, Buligan C, et al. Narrow band-ultraviolet B versus clobetasol propionate foam in the treatment of vitiligo: a retrospective study. *Dermatol Ther (Heidelb).* 2013;3(1):95-105. doi:10.1007/s13555-013-0028-8
11. Rokni GR, Golpour M, Gorji AH, Khalilian A, Ghasemi H. Effectiveness and safety of topical tacrolimus in treatment of vitiligo. *J Adv Pharm Technol Res.* 2017;8(1):29-33. doi:10.4103/2231-4040.197388
12. Guenther L, Lynde C, Poulin Y. Off-label use of topical calcineurin inhibitors in dermatologic disorders. *J Cutan Med Surg.* 2019;23(4_suppl):27S-34S. doi:10.1177/1203475419857668
13. Sharma CK, Sharma M, Aggarwal B, Sharma V. Different advanced therapeutic approaches to treat vitiligo. *J Environ Pathol Toxicol Oncol.* 2015;34:321-334.
14. Wada-Irimada M, Tsuchiyama K, Sasaki R, et al. Efficacy and safety of i.v. methylprednisolone pulse therapy for vitiligo: a retrospective study of 58 therapy experiences for 33 vitiligo patients. *J Dermatol.* 2021;48(7):1090-1093. doi:10.1111/1346-8138.15858.
15. Niu C, Xie HX, Aisa HA. Janus kinase inhibitors: a review of their application in the vitiligo. *Mini Rev Med Chem.* 2021;21(20):3203-3218. doi:10.2174/1389557521666210325120233
16. Mobasher P, Shiu J, Lentsch G, Ganesan AK. Comparing the efficacy of 2 different harvesting techniques for melanocyte keratinocyte transplantation in vitiligo. *Dermatol Surg.* 2021;47(5):732-733. doi:10.1097/DSS.0000000000002922
17. Doolan BJ, Weaich M, Mamo J, Gupta M. Autologous non-cultured epidermal cellular grafting in the surgical treatment of stable vitiligo: the skin hospital protocol. *Dermatology.* 2022;238(1):167-169. doi:10.1159/000515084

18. Asilian A, Kazemipour S, Mokhtari F, et al. Effectiveness of dermabrasion plus 5-fluorouracil vs suction blister in treating vitiligo: a comparative study. *Dermatol Ther.* 2021;34(2):e14750. doi:10.1111/dth.14750
19. Abd-Elazim NE, Yassa HA, Mahran AM. Microdermabrasion and topical tacrolimus: a novel combination therapy of vitiligo. *J Cosmet Dermatol.* 2020;19(6):1447-1455. doi:10.1111/jocd.13193
20. Bae JM, Hong BY, Lee JH, Lee JH, Kim GM. The efficacy of 308-nm excimer laser/light (EL) and topical agent combination therapy versus EL monotherapy for vitiligo: a systematic review and meta-analysis of randomized controlled trials (RCTs). *J Am Acad Dermatol.* 2016;74:907-915.
21. Whitton M, Pinart M, Batchelor JM, et al. Evidence-based management of vitiligo: summary of a Cochrane systematic review. *Br J Dermatol.* 2016;174(5):962-969. doi:10.1111/bjd.14356
22. Melnick LE, Steuer AB, Bieber AK, Wong PW, Pomeranz MK. Lichen sclerosus among women in the United States. *Int J Womens Dermatol.* 2020;6(4):260-262. doi:10.1016/j.ijwd.2020.05.001
23. Halonen P, Jakobsson M, Heikinheimo O, Gissler M, Pukkala E. Incidence of lichen sclerosus and subsequent causes of death: a nationwide Finnish register study. *BJOG.* 2020;127(7):814-819. doi:10.1111/1471-0528.16175
24. Kirtschig G. Lichen sclerosus-presentation, diagnosis and management. *Dtsch Arztebl Int.* 2016;113(19):337-343. doi:10.3238/arztebl.2016.0337
25. Lewis FM, Tatnall FM, Velangi SS, et al. British Association of Dermatologists guidelines for the management of lichen sclerosus, 2018. *Br J Dermatol.* 2018;178(4):839-853. doi:10.1111/bjd.16241
26. Dinh H, Purcell SM, Chung C, et al. Pediatric lichen sclerosus: a review of the literature and management recommendations. *J Clin Aesthet Dermatol.* 2016;9(9):49-54.
27. Kreuter A, Kryvosheyeva Y, Terras S, et al. Association of autoimmune diseases with lichen sclerosus in 532 male and female patients. *Acta Derm Venereol.* 2013;93(2):238-241.
28. Eberz, B, Berghold A, Regauer S. High prevalence of concomitant anogenital lichen sclerosus and extragenital psoriasis in adult women. *Obstet Gynecol.* 2008;111(5)1143-1147.
29. Errichetti E, Lallas A, Apalla Z, Di Stefani A, Stinco G. Dermoscopy of morphea and cutaneous lichen sclerosus: clinicopathological correlation study and comparative analysis. *Dermatology.* 2017;233(6):462-470.
30. Watchorn RE, van den Munckhof EHA, Quint KD, et al. Balanopreputial sac and urine microbiota in patients with male-genital lichen sclerosus. *Int J Dermatol.* 2021;60(2):201-207. doi:10.1111/ijd.15252
31. Doiron PR, Bunker CB Obesity-related male genital lichen sclerosus. *J Eur Acad Dermatol Venereol.* 2017;31(5):876-879. doi:10.1111/jdv.14035
32. Bunker CB, Shim TN. Male genital lichen sclerosus. *Indian J Dermatol.* 2015;60:111-117.
33. Hayden JP, Boysen WR, Peterson AC. Medical management of penile and urethral lichen sclerosus with topical clobetasol improves long-term voiding symptoms and quality of life. *J Urol.* 2020;204(6):1290-1295. doi: 10.1097/JU.0000000000001304
34. Kantere D, Löwhagen GB, Alvengren G, Månesköld A, Gillstedt M, Tunbäck P. The clinical spectrum of lichen sclerosus in male patients—a retrospective study. *Acta Derm Venereol.* 2014;94(5):542-546. doi:10.2340/00015555-1797
35. Lee A, Bradford J, Fischer G. Long-term management of adult vulvar lichen sclerosus: a prospective cohort study of 507 women. *JAMA Dermatol.* 2015;151:1061-1067.
36. Funaro D, Lovett A, Leroux N, Powell J. A double-blind, randomized prospective study evaluating topical clobetasol propionate 0.05% versus topical tacrolimus 0.1% in patients with vulvar lichen sclerosus. *J Am Acad Dermatol.* 2014;71:84-91.
37. Borghi A, Corazza M, Minghetti S, Virgili A. Topical tretinoin in the treatment of vulvar lichen sclerosus: an advisable option? *Eur J Dermatol.* 2015;25:404-409.
38. Ioannides D, Lazaridou E, Apalla Z, Sotiriou E, Gregoriou S, Rigopoulos D. Acitretin for severe lichen sclerosus of male genitalia: a randomized, placebo controlled study. *J Urol.* 2010;183(4):1395-1399. doi:10.1016/j.juro.2009.12.057
39. Kreuter A, Tigges C, Gaifullina R, Kirschke J, Altmeyer P, Gambichler T. Pulsed high-dose corticosteroids combined with low-dose methotrexate treatment in patients with refractory generalized extragenital lichen sclerosus. *Arch Dermatol.* 2009;145(11):1303-1308. doi:10.1001/archdermatol.2009.235
40. Cuellar-Barboza A, Bashyam AM, Ghamrawi RI, Aickara D, Feldman SR, Pichardo RO. Methotrexate for the treatment of recalcitrant genital and extragenital lichen sclerosus: a retrospective series. *Dermatol Ther.* 2020;33(4):e13473. doi:10.1111/dth.13473
41. Olejek A, Gabriel I, Bilska-Janosik A, Kozak-Darmas I, Kawczyk-Krupka A. ALA-Photodynamic treatment in Lichen sclerosus-clinical and immunological outcome focusing on the assessment of antinuclear antibodies. *Photodiagnosis Photodyn Ther.* 2017;18:128-132. doi:10.1016/j.pdpdt.2017.02.006
42. Kastner U, Altmeyer P. [Cryosurgery--the last resort or a surgical alternative in the treatment of lichen sclerosus et atrophicus of the vulva (LSAV)?]. *J Dtsch Dermatol Ges.* 2003;1(3): 206-211. doi:10.1046/j.1610-0387.2003.03517.x
43. Wu C, Zou M, Xiong Y, et al. Short- and long-term efficacy of focused ultrasound therapy for non-neoplastic epithelial disorders of the vulva. *BJOG.* 2017;124(Suppl 3):87-92. doi:10.1111/1471-0528.14747
44. Wu M, Reitamo S. Treatment of lichen sclerosus with carbon dioxide laser vaporization. *Br J Dermatol.* 1997;136(3):356-359.
45. Vyas KS, Saba ES, Tran N. Regenerative properties of autologous fat grafting in a complicated radiation-induced wound. *Wounds.* 2021;33(2):E20-E23.
46. Almadori A, Hansen E, Boyle D, et al. Fat grafting improves fibrosis and scarring in vulvar lichen sclerosus: results from a prospective cohort study. *J Low Genit Tract Dis.* 2020;24(3):305-310. doi:10.1097/LGT.0000000000000520
47. Goldstein AT, Mitchell L, Govind V, Heller D. A randomized double-blind placebo-controlled trial of autologous platelet-rich plasma intradermal injections for the treatment of vulvar lichen sclerosus. *J Am Acad Dermatol.* 2019;80(6):1788-1789. doi:10.1016/j.jaad.2018.12.060
48. Navarrete J, Echarte L, Sujanov A, et al. Platelet-rich plasma for male genital lichen sclerosus resistant to conventional therapy: first prospective study. *Dermatol Ther.* 2020;33(6):e14032. doi:10.1111/dth.14032
49. Eshtiaghi P, Sadownik LA. Fact or fiction? Adipose-derived stem cells and platelet-rich plasma for the treatment of vulvar lichen sclerosus. *J Low Genit Tract Dis.* 2019;23(1):65-70. doi:10.1097/LGT.0000000000000440
50. Balchander D, Nyirjesy P. Fractionated CO2 laser as therapy in recalcitrant lichen sclerosus. *J Low Genit Tract Dis.* 2020;24(2):225-228. doi:10.1097/LGT.0000000000000512

51. Bizjak Ogrinc U, Senčar S, Luzar B, Lukanović A. Efficacy of non-ablative laser therapy for lichen sclerosus: a randomized controlled trial. *J Obstet Gynaecol Can.* 2019;41(12):1717-1725. doi:10.1016/j.jogc.2019.01.023
52. Burkett LS, Siddique M, Zeymo A, et al. Clobetasol compared with fractionated carbon dioxide laser for lichen sclerosus: a randomized controlled trial. *Obstet Gynecol.* 2021;137(6):968-978. doi:10.1097/AOG.0000000000004332
53. Mitchell L, Goldstein AT, Heller D, et al. Fractionated carbon dioxide laser for the treatment of vulvar lichen sclerosus: a randomized controlled trial. *Obstet Gynecol.* 2021;137(6):979-987. doi:10.1097/AOG.0000000000004409
54. Ferrara F, Messori S, Abbenante D, Patrizi A, Bardazzi F. Fractional CO(2) laser therapy of lichen sclerosus in males: a new therapeutic opportunity? *J Dermatolog Treat.* 2022;33(2):941-945. doi:10.1080/09546634.2020.1793886
55. Preti M, Vieira-Baptista P, Digesu GA, et al. The clinical role of LASER for vulvar and vaginal treatments in gynecology and female urology: an ICS/ISSVD Best Practice Consensus Document. *J Low Genit Tract Dis.* 2019;23(2):151-160. doi:10.1097/LGT.0000000000000462
56. Smith SD, Fischer G. Childhood onset vulvar lichen sclerosus does not remit at puberty: a prospective case series. *Pediatr Dermatol.* 2009;26:725-729.
57. Kammire MS, Anderson K, Howell JO, McShane DB, Corley SB, Morrell DS. Pediatric vulvar lichen sclerosus: a survey of disease course. *J Pediatr Adolesc Gynecol.* 2021;34(5):597-602. doi:10.1016/j.jpag.2021.04.010
58. Micheletti L, Preti M, Radici G, et al. Vulvar lichen sclerosus and neoplastic transformation: a retrospective study of 976 cases. *J Low Genit Tract Dis.* 2016;20:180-183.
59. Errichetti E. Dermoscopy of inflammatory dermatoses (inflammoscopy): an up-to-date overview. *Dermatol Pract Concept.* 2019;9:169-180. doi:10.5826/dpc.0903a01
60. Fawaz B, et al. Surgical treatment of verrucous carcinoma: a review. *J Dermatolog Treat.* 2022;1-5. doi:10.1080/09546634.2021.1914312


## SUGGESTED READINGS

### *Vitiligo:*


Rashighi M, Harris JE. Vitiligo pathogenesis and emerging treatments. *Dermatol Clin.* 2017;35(2):257-265. doi:10.1016/j.det.2016.11.014


### *Lichen sclerosus:*


Kantere D, Löwhagen GB, Alvengren G, Månesköld A, Gillstedt M, Tunbäck P. The clinical spectrum of lichen sclerosus in male patients - a retrospective study. *Acta Derm Venereol.* 2014;94(5):542-546. doi:10.2340/00015555-1797.

Krapf JM, Mitchell L, Holton MA, Goldstein AT. Vulvar lichen sclerosus: current perspectives. *Int J Womens Health.* 2020;12:11-20. doi:10.2147/IJWH.S191200. eCollection 2020. Review.

Kwok R, Shah TT, Minhas S. Recent advances in understanding and managing Lichen Sclerosus. *F1000Res.* 2020;9:F1000 Faculty Rev-369. doi:10.12688/f1000research.21529.1. eCollection 2020. Review.

Singh N, Mishra N, Ghatage P. Treatment options in vulvar lichen sclerosus: a scoping review. *Cureus.* 2021;13(2):e13527. doi:10.7759/cureus.13527. Review.

# Dark-Colored Lesions: Brown, Blue, Gray, or Black Disorders 9

PETER J. LYNCH

Hyperpigmentation is commonly present on the skin of the genitalia. It may occur diffusely or as individual pigmented lesions. The basis for this hyperpigmentation includes physiologic (hormonal, racial, etc.) pigmentation, postinflammatory hyperpigmentation (PIH), some infections, and some benign or malignant neoplasms. Most dark colors arise as a result of melanin pigmentation. Melanin pigment is made within cytoplasmic organelles (melanosomes) in melanocytes that lie along the basement membrane of the epithelium. The amount of color in both normal skin and various lesions is determined by several factors: the density of melanocytes, the amount of melanin produced per melanocyte, and the transfer rate of the melanized melanosomes to the 30 or so keratinocytes that surround each melanocyte. The density of melanocytes does not vary appreciably in people of different racial backgrounds, but it does vary by site. Genital tissue, for instance, has about 50% more melanocytes per unit of area than does truncal skin. The development of increased pigmentation is dependent on genetic factors (variability in racial groups) and hormonal factors (especially in women). It is also dependent on acquired factors such as ultraviolet light (UVL), the presence of inflammation (particularly that involving basal layer damage), and some types of infection (notably HPV infection in the genital and perigenital areas). Increased pigmentation also occurs when there is proliferation in the number of normally melanized keratinocytes (epithelial hyperplasia) and/or when there is an increased retention of normally melanized keratinocytes in the stratum corneum. For a few disorders in this chapter, heme pigment rather than melanin explains the presence of the dark color.

## Physiological Hyperpigmentation

In physiological hyperpigmentation, deep tan, brown, dark-brown, or even black pigmentation occurs as symmetrical, flat, smooth-surfaced, asymptomatic darkening of the anogenital skin. The most commonly affected sites include the median raphe of the penis and scrotum in male patients and the labia majora and outer edges of the labia minora in female patients (**Figs. 9-1 and 9-2**).[1,2] The perianal skin in both genders usually displays some degree of physiologic hyperpigmentation. Appreciable variation in hue occurs across racial groups and also from person to person even within a given racial group. The degree of pigmentation can be so light as to be hardly noticeable or may be so dark as to be almost black in color.

The diagnosis of physiological hyperpigmentation is made on a clinical basis. Dermoscopy is nonspecific and may take on the characteristics of the condition that produced the hyperpigmentation. The differential diagnosis includes PIH, but this latter color change follows a history of inflammation, may have some residual red or red-brown hues, tends be patchier, and is generally less symmetrically distributed. If biopsy is carried out because of concern by either patient or the clinician, increased melanin will be found in both the melanocytes and keratinocytes, which line the basal layer of the epithelium. Physiological

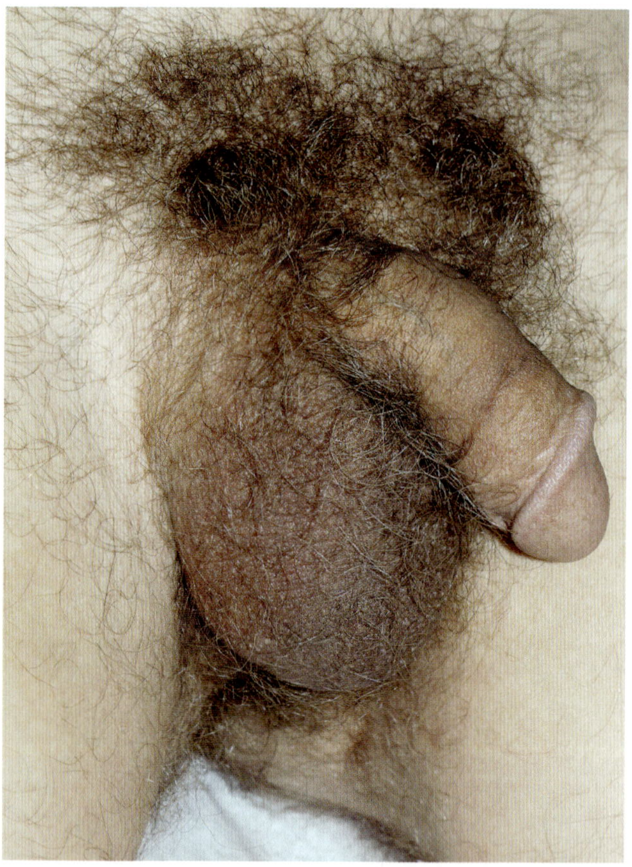

Fig. 9-1. Physiologic hyperpigmentation regularly occurs on the scrotum.

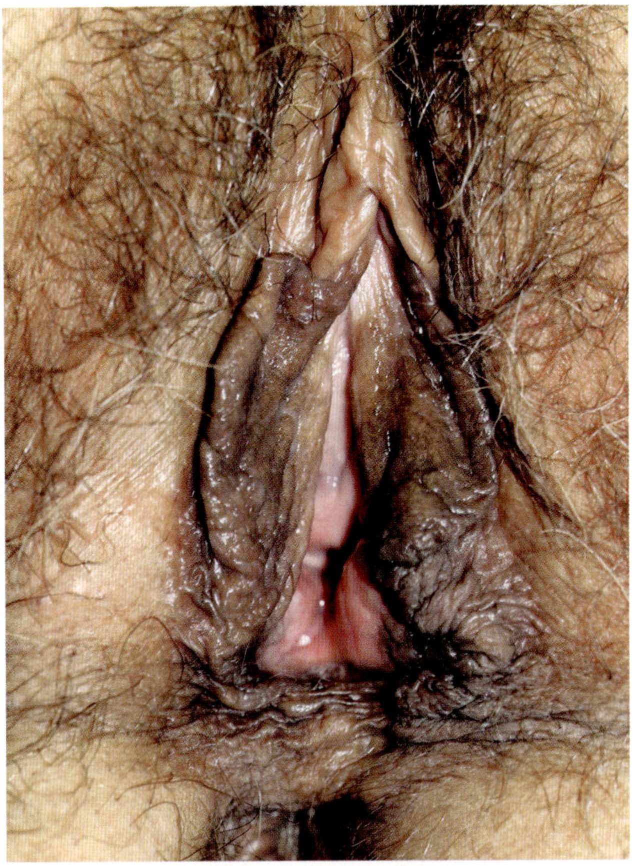

Fig. 9-2. Darker-complected women are likely to show hyperpigmentation of the labia minora and posterior fourchette, and perianal skin is often dark in both sexes.

hyperpigmentation of the genitalia occurs because of the greater density of melanocytes in the genitals compared to surrounding skin. These areas of hyperpigmentation will darken further under the influence of both endogenous and exogenous sex hormones. This darkening is particularly notable during pregnancy. Darkening will also occur due to the presence of increased melanocyte-stimulating hormone in neonates and in patients with disorders such as Addison disease due to the marked disturbance in pituitary-adrenal axis function.

Treatment of physiological hyperpigmentation is not necessary or even desirable. However, it is worth noting that patient obsession with anogenital hyperpigmentation has led to the provision of bleaching services by both licensed and unlicensed practitioners.

## Acanthosis Nigricans

The prevalence of acanthosis nigricans (AN) varies with skin color and race. It is present in about 20%-25% of African American, 20% of Hispanic, and 5% of Caucasian children and adolescents.[3] Acanthosis nigricans was an uncommon disorder 50 years ago, but it is found much more often in recent years due to the marked increase of obesity, especially in children. While acanthosis nigricans is most often found in those who are obese, it also occurs with various endocrinopathies, malignancies, the metabolic syndrome, and the use of some medications.

Acanthosis nigricans appears as poorly demarcated light brown to dark brown lesions around the neck, in the axillae, and in the crural folds (Fig. 9-3). Rarely, it develops in other folded areas of the body and on the genitalia. The hyperpigmentation initially is flat but gradually thickening occurs. Characteristically, there are elevated linear ridges running parallel to one another. The surface of the lesions is slightly "bumpy" and often feels either velvety or slightly rough on palpation. Skin tags are frequently present within well-developed lesions (Fig. 9-4). Acanthosis nigricans is asymptomatic or mildly pruritic, but it is troubling to the patient because it suggests the appearance of dirty skin.

Multiple classifications for the various forms of AN have been published, but they have not proven to be of much help clinically, and in any event, there is no agreement on which approach should be used. The same can be said about the many proposals for the determination of severity. The diagnosis is established clinically, but there is a characteristic dermoscopic appearance. There are brown dots in a linear configuration that corresponds to

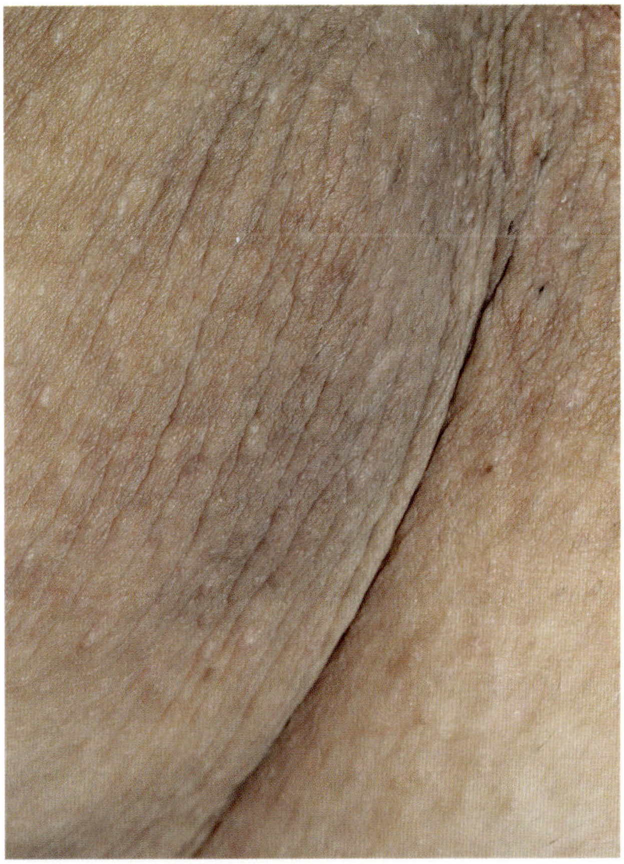

Fig. 9-3. The medial thigh is often affected by the linear folds of acanthosis nigricans, and this condition is common in overweight patients.

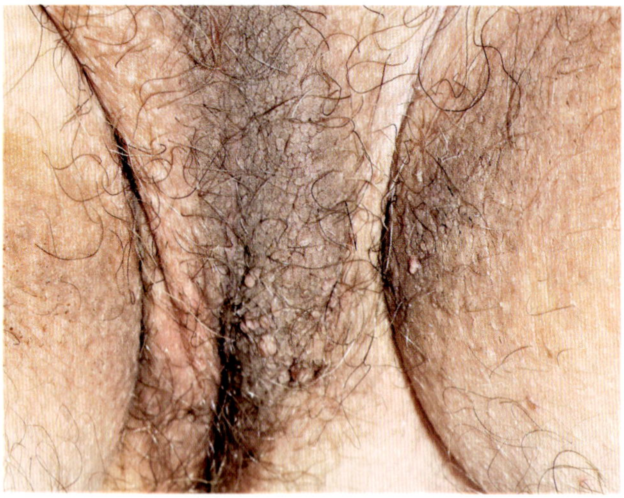

Fig. 9-4. Acanthosis nigricans is manifested by hyperpigmentation in skin folds caused by papillomatous changes in the skin, often associated with skin tags as has occurred on this man's perineum and medial thigh.

the parallel ridges of skin.[4] If biopsied for confirmation, a characteristic pattern can be found. This includes orthokeratotic hyperkeratosis, papillomatosis, and increased melanin in the epidermis and stratum corneum. Dermal inflammation, melanocytosis and surprisingly, given the name of the disorder, are even acanthosis, usually absent. The major condition to be considered in the list of differential diagnoses is atopic dermatitis/lichen simplex chronicus in which some degree of PIH has occurred.

Treatment of acanthosis nigricans is problematic. Topical retinoids and trichloroacetic acid peels can be tried, but often, the side effects are perceived as worse than the disorder. Oral retinoids and metformin may be helpful. However, the appearance can be improved through weight loss or effective treatment for any associated endocrinopathy or malignancy. Evaluation of patients with acanthosis nigricans is usually desirable because of the frequently associated presence of increased insulin levels, insulin resistance, abnormal glucose levels, hypertension, and elevated lipid levels.[3] Rarely in adults, acanthosis nigricans is associated with the development of malignancy, especially that involving the gastrointestinal tract. This association should be considered in those middle aged or older who lack endocrinopathy, are nonobese, have appreciable pruritus, or have a recent history of unintentional weight loss.

## Postinflammatory Hyperpigmentation

Inflammation affects melanocytes in two ways. First, *severely* damaged melanocytes discontinue the production of melanin with resulting hypopigmentation. Second, *mildly* damaged melanocytes react with increased melanin production and hyperpigmentation. PIH is an example of the second mechanism wherein hyperpigmentation

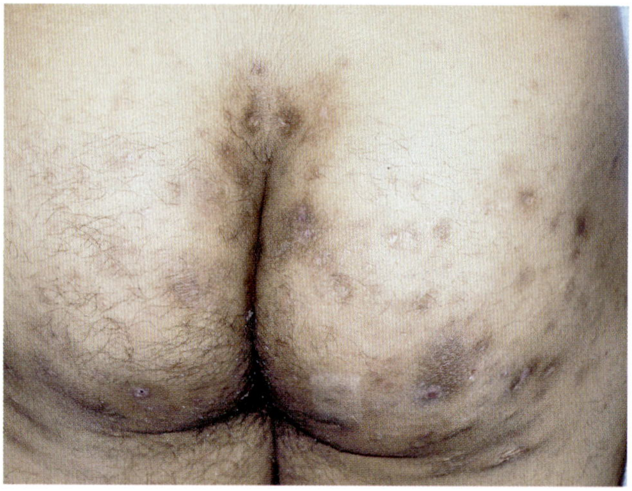

Fig. 9-5. This patient with hidradenitis suppurativa shows brown macules of postinflammatory hyperpigmentation from old inflamed cysts and eschars.

develops at the site of current or previous inflammation. Inflammation may be an inherent component of a skin disease or inflammation may develop at the site of trauma such as might occur following the use of liquid nitrogen, application of trichloroacetic acid, or following laser therapy. Even tanning after mild sunburn can be considered as an example of external PIH and dark color occurring with acne lesions would be an example of internal PIH. PIH is clinically recognized as light to dark brown, nonpalpable macules and patches occurring in fair-skinned individuals, whereas darker colors, sometimes displaying hues of gray, blue, or black, occur in darker-skinned individuals **(Fig. 9-5)**. The distribution and intensity of hyperpigmentation are dependent on the underlying cause of the preceding inflammation.

Diseases such as lichen sclerosus and lichen planus, in which inflammation preferentially damages the basal layer of the epithelium, with resultant take-up of melanin by dermal macrophages (melanophages), are more likely to be associated with darker gray or even black pigmentation than occurs with other inflammatory disorders **(Figs. 9-6 and 9-7)**. Not surprisingly, patients with naturally darker skin color more commonly develop PIH, and this observation appears to be independent of ethenicity.[5] Similarly, because normal genital color is generally darker than surrounding skin, inflammation in genital tissue is particularly likely to cause PIH. Pruritic skin disorders that lead to scratching and/or rubbing will usually develop more pigmentation than will nonpruritic conditions.

A history of prior trauma or previous inflammation is an important diagnostic clue but sometimes such a history cannot be obtained. This is particularly true in instances such as anogenital lichen planus and lichen sclerosus where extraordinarily long-lasting hyperpigmentation may first be noted a very long time after any clinical evidence of inflammation has resolved. In some

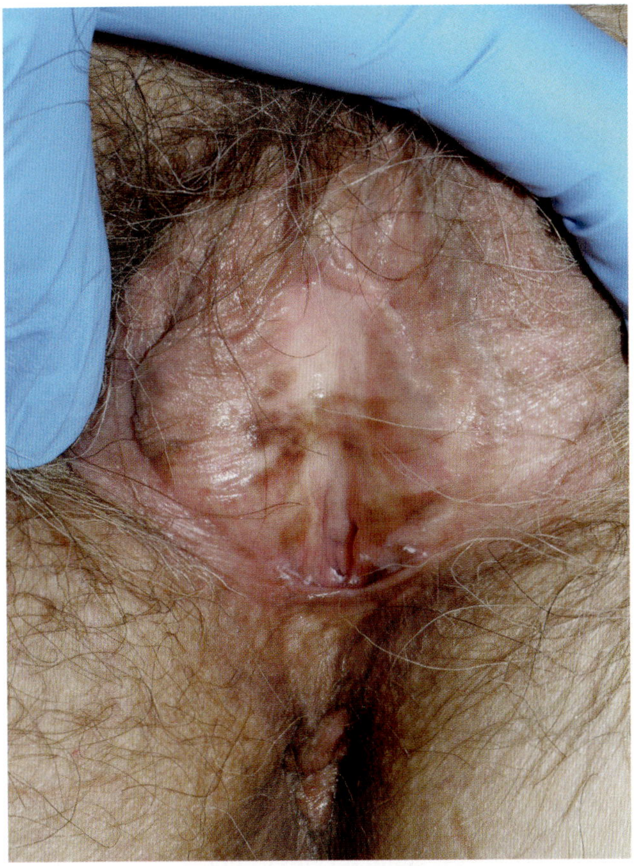

Fig. 9-6. Postinflammatory hyperpigmentation is fairly common in the setting of lichen sclerosus, where there is inflammation and disruption of the dermal epidermal junction, also the location of melanocytes.

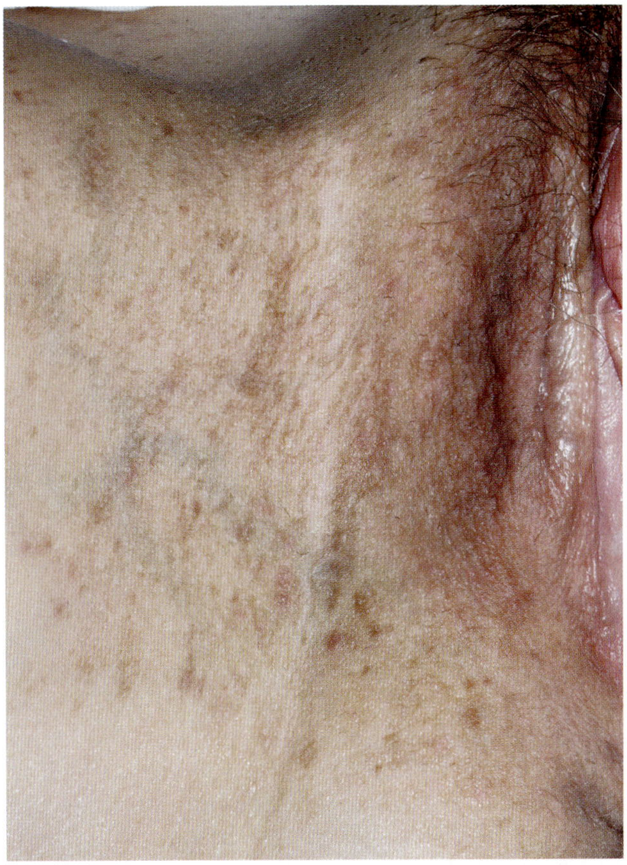

Fig. 9-7. Lichen planus is another disease that disrupts the dermal epidermal junction and produces marked, fairly long-lasting postinflammatory color change on dry, keratinized skin.

instances in which a history of previous inflammation cannot be obtained, a biopsy will be necessary to confirm a diagnosis of PIH. This is particularly true for pigmented macules or patches where the pigment density is variable or where gray or black hues are present. The histology usually demonstrates increased epidermal melanin, melanophages in the superficial dermis and a few nonspecific inflammatory cells around blood vessels in the papillary dermis.[5] Dermoscopy is often nonspecific but may show changes of the original cause of the underlying inflammation.[4]

Because PIH usually resolves over several to many months, treatment is most often unnecessary. However, the presence of pigmentation sometimes obscures continuing low-grade inflammation. Thus, if the pigmentation persists longer than expected, biopsy can be obtained to determine whether or not subclinical inflammation is present. If such is present, anti-inflammatory treatment, such as with topical steroids, should be administered. Topical fading agents, such as 4% hydroquinone, may improve pigmentation located in the epidermis but are of little or no use for pigment lying deeper in dermal melanophages. Other approaches for the treatment of PIH have been summarized in the 2018 review by Kaufman et al.[5]

## Seborrheic Keratosis (pl: Seborrheic Keratoses)

Seborrheic keratoses (SK) are extremely common, benign growths. Their prevalence increases with age. Most individuals over the age of 40 years have at least 1 or 2 lesions and often 50-100 may be present. Most are located on the trunk, but occasionally, they are noted on the proximal limbs and hair-bearing skin of the anogenital area. Seborrheic keratoses present as sharply marginated, square shouldered, tan, brown, gray, or black papules 8-15 mm wide and 2-10 mm tall **(Figs. 9-8 and 9-9)**. Rarely, very large seborrheic keratoses ("giant" SKs) are encountered **(Fig. 9-10)**. The sharp margination and square shoulders (clifflike transition to surrounding normal skin) contribute to a characteristic "stuck on" appearance. The surface often contains visible scale and is usually rough on palpation. However, in some instances, the surface has a smooth "waxy" feeling simulating a drop of candle wax on the surface of the skin **(Fig. 9-11)**. However, in these smooth lesions, the presence of scale can be identified if the surface is gently scraped with a blade held perpendicular to the top of the lesion.

The presence of scale is a very helpful point in distinguishing seborrheic keratoses from those of nevi, lentigines, and melanomas. Small, characteristic surface pits

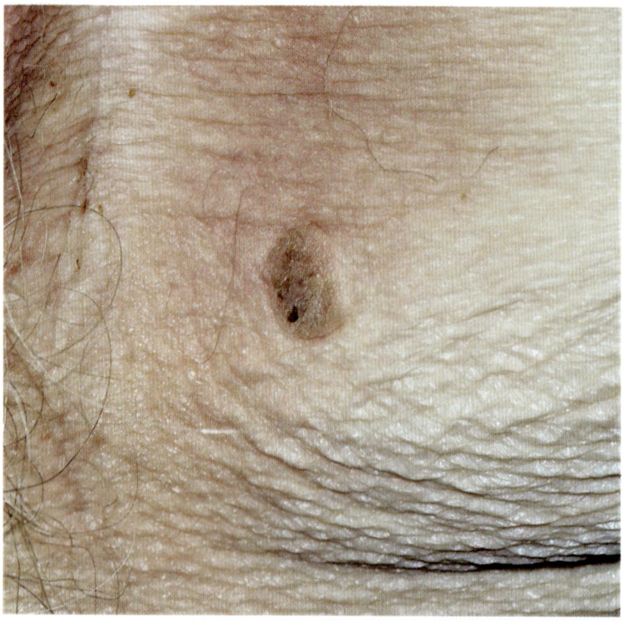

Fig. 9-8. A typical seborrheic keratosis is a tan, well-demarcated, flat-topped, rough, keratotic, or warty papule that can be mistaken for a wart.

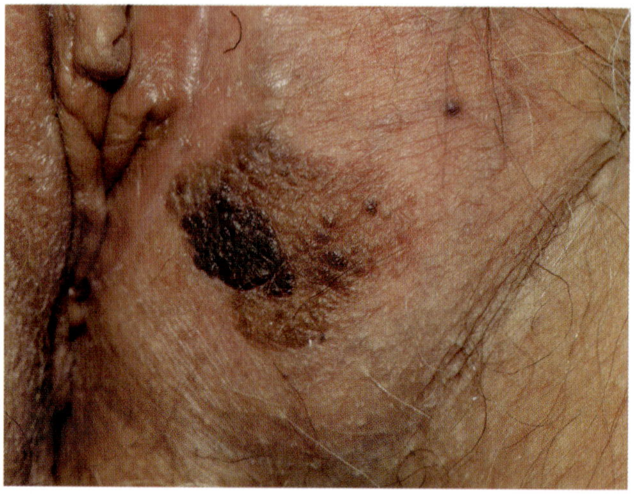

Fig. 9-10. An occasional seborrheic keratosis such as this one can be large, and show multiple colors, mimicking melanoma or HPV-associated squamous intraepithelial neoplasia, also called HSIL (high-grade squamous intraepithelial lesion). Although dermoscopy can be useful, a biopsy should be performed for any question.

may be found when magnification is used in the examination. Specifically, dermoscopy can be very helpful in recognizing these minute pits.[6] Genital seborrheic keratoses may also be quite difficult to differentiate from both pigmented genital warts and HPV-related intraepithelial neoplasia. They may also resemble pigmented basal cell carcinomas. Because differentiation of seborrheic keratosis from these lesions is so important, most genital seborrheic keratoses should be biopsied and all SKs exhibiting inflammation, erosion, ulceration, or bleeding must be biopsied.

The cause of seborrheic keratoses is unknown, but frequent familial patterns regarding age at onset and number of lesions suggest that both genetic and aging factors play a role. It is of considerable interest that somatic mutations in fibroblast growth factor receptor 3 (*FGFR3*) are found in 50%-75% of seborrheic keratoses. Mutations also occur in multiple other genes such as *PIK3CA*, *TERT*, and *DPH3*.[7] These same mutations may also be found in other lesions that behave in a malignant fashion, whereas malignancy rarely, if ever, develops in seborrheic keratoses; the reasons explaining this discrepancy are not completely known, but additional discussion of this topic can be found elsewhere.[8] Controversy exists as to whether or not human papillomavirus (HPV) infection plays any role in the development of anogenital seborrheic keratosis, and we doubt that it does. Others, however, disagree.[9]

Biopsy is desirable in any instance of uncertainty regarding the diagnosis. No therapy is necessary for

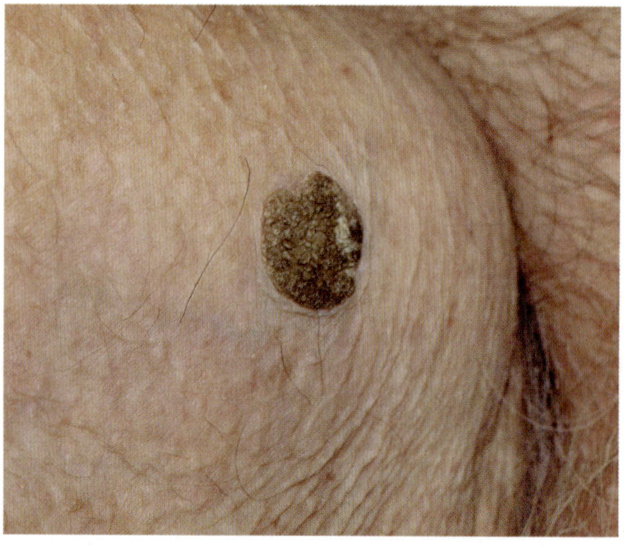

Fig. 9-9. Seborrheic keratoses are accompanied by similar seborrheic keratoses on other areas of the body, such as the trunk.

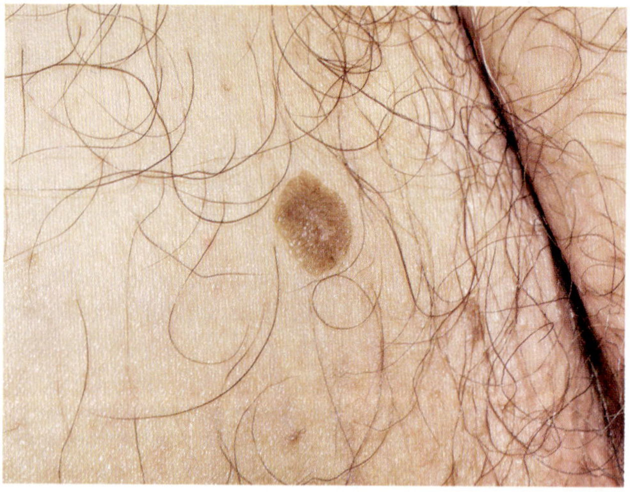

Fig. 9-11. The shine on the surface of this seborrheic keratosis demonstrates the smooth, waxy rather than rough texture of this lesion.

clinically typical, or histologically proven, seborrheic keratoses. Lesions that are irritated by clothing and those that are particularly bothersome to the patient may be treated with cryotherapy or with shave excision. The latter is preferred for anogenital SKs as it provides a specimen for histological examination. Recently, the U.S. Food and Drug Administration granted approval for medical therapy with 40% hydrogen peroxide (Eskata). It is moderately effective when used for thin seborrheic keratoses such as those that occur on the face, but it is not recommended for those that occur elsewhere on the body.

## Genital Varicosities

Varicosities may be small or large. Large dilated vessels are usually blue in color (Fig. 9-12). Such varicose veins occur on the vulva with appreciable frequency. In fact, they develop in about 10% of women who are pregnant, and this incidence increases with parity.[10] Fortunately, there is usually regression following parturition, but they are almost certain to recur with subsequent pregnancies. Vulvar varices also frequently can be observed in pregnant or nonpregnant women as part of the pelvic congestion syndrome, which is a pelvic chronic pain syndrome associated with pelvic varicosities.[11]

Varicosities are less common on the penis and scrotum. Scrotal varicocele is the analog of the female pelvic congestion syndrome. However, the varices that occur with varicocele are contained entirely within the scrotal sac, rather than within the skin of the scrotum, and while they are palpable (so-called bag of worms), their dusky blue color is somewhat muted, if visible at all.[12] Very small diameter dilated vessels ("spider veins") are more likely to be dusky or dark red (Fig. 9-13). Such telangiectasias occur commonly on the scrotum and often tiny angiokeratomas (see Chapter 6) overly these small telangiectatic vessels (Fig. 9-14).

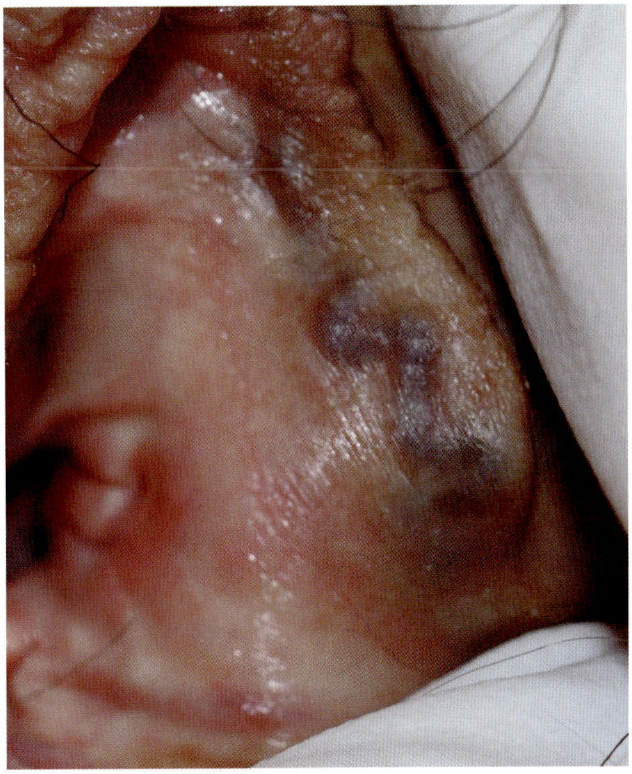

Fig. 9-12. Large dilated varicosities are most common during pregnancy or can occur in associated with pelvic congestion syndrome. These occur deep below the skin in men in varicoceles.

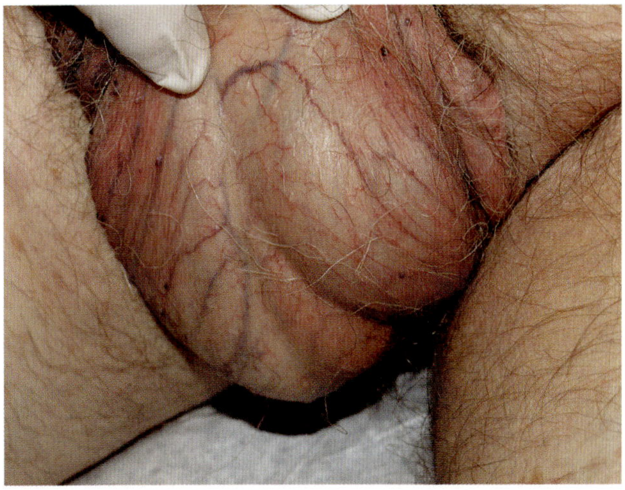

Fig. 9-13. More common in men are more superficial small and medium red vessels on the scrotum.

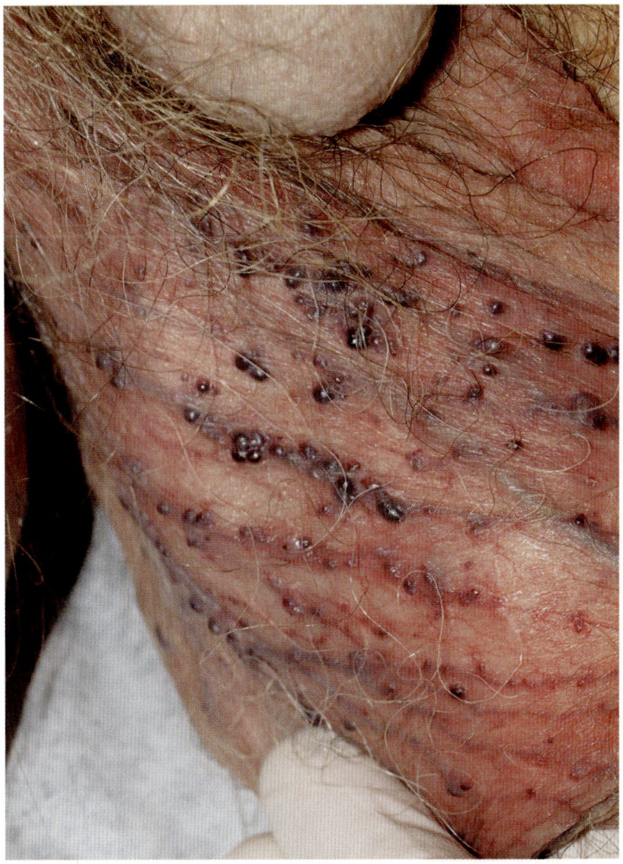

Fig. 9-14. Occasionally, angiokeratomas occur along the course of the superficial vessels.

Varicosities are identified by their disappearance following compression with a glass slide (diascopy). Treatment for large varicose veins lies outside the scope of this chapter. Therapy for small telangiectatic vessels is not ordinarily necessary, but when bleeding repeatedly follows trauma, they may require electrosurgical destruction.

## Genital Melanosis (Lentiginosis)

Genital melanosis and genital lentiginosis have been used interchangeably by clinicians, but, strictly speaking, the latter term is only applicable to those lesions that demonstrate a lentigolike histologic pattern on biopsy. Since this is not present in all cases, we prefer the term genital melanosis.

### Clinical Presentation

Pigmented lesions of melanocytic type are common on the genitalia with a prevalence estimated to be about 10%-15% in both men and women.[6] In women, about 60%-70% of all vulvar pigmented lesions are due to vulvar melanosis, and this is probably true for men as well.[6]

Genital melanosis consists of one or more nonpalpable, nonelevated macules and patches of pigmentation (**Figs. 9-15 to 9-17**). They develop mostly in midlife at an average age of about 40 years but can occur as early as the late teens or as late as age 80 years. This pigmentation occurs most often on mucous membranes or modified mucous membranes, but it can also arise on keratinizing skin. Specifically, in women, most of these pigmented patches are found on the labia minora, followed by the labia majora, and when multiple lesions are present, they frequently develop on both labia.[13] In men, most lesions occur on the glans penis and inner aspects of the prepuce, but penile shaft and urethral meatus involvement is also possible[6] (**Fig. 9-18**). Lesions may be either solitary or multifocal with the latter occurring slightly more frequently. There is a great deal of variation in the size and color of the pigmentation. Lesions are mostly small (5-10 mm), but many are considerably larger with up to 2 cm.[6,13,14] Asymmetry in distribution of multifocal lesions is common, and the configuration of individual lesions can be angular. The pigmentation color may be tan, brown, blue, or black, but when multiple lesions are present, the color is fairly consistent among all of the lesions. There is often pigment variegation ("speckling") within the lesions and occasionally small areas of hypopigmentation are noted. The borders may be either poorly or sharply marginated. For the first few years, there is usually some increase in the diameter of the lesions and/or darkening of the pigmentation, but with the passage of time, stabilization of size and color occurs.

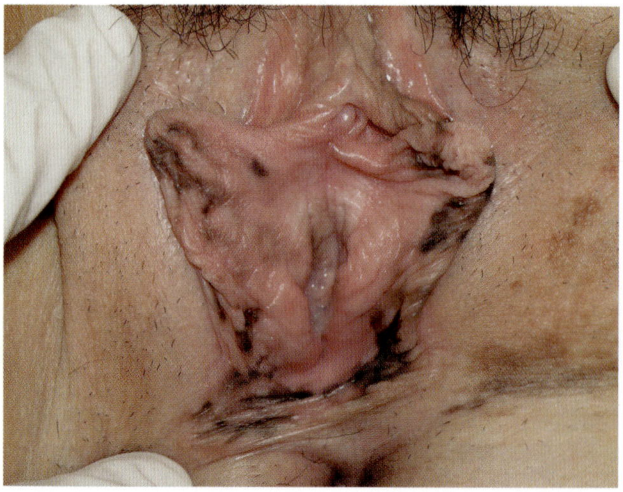

Fig. 9-15. These macules of genital lentiginosis are irregular in color, size, and shape and are indistinguishable from melanoma *in situ*. The encroachment of lesions onto dry, keratinized skin is unusual.

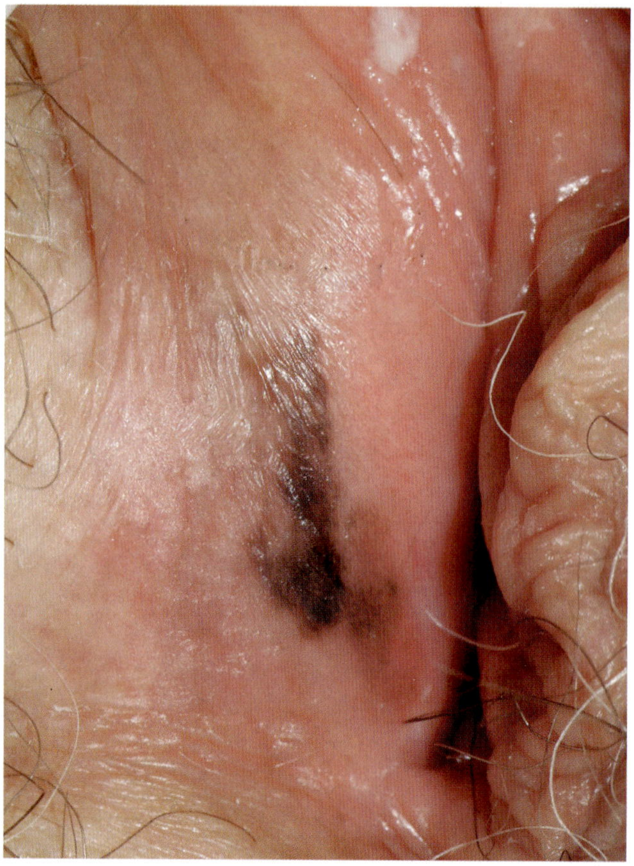

Fig. 9-16. This patient has only one area of lentiginosis, a patch of irregularly brown color ranging from tan to nearly black in the right vestibule and medial labium majus.

### Diagnosis

The correct diagnosis is often suggested, perhaps aided by dermoscopy, on clinical examination.[6,13] However, in the vast majority of instances, biopsy should be undertaken to

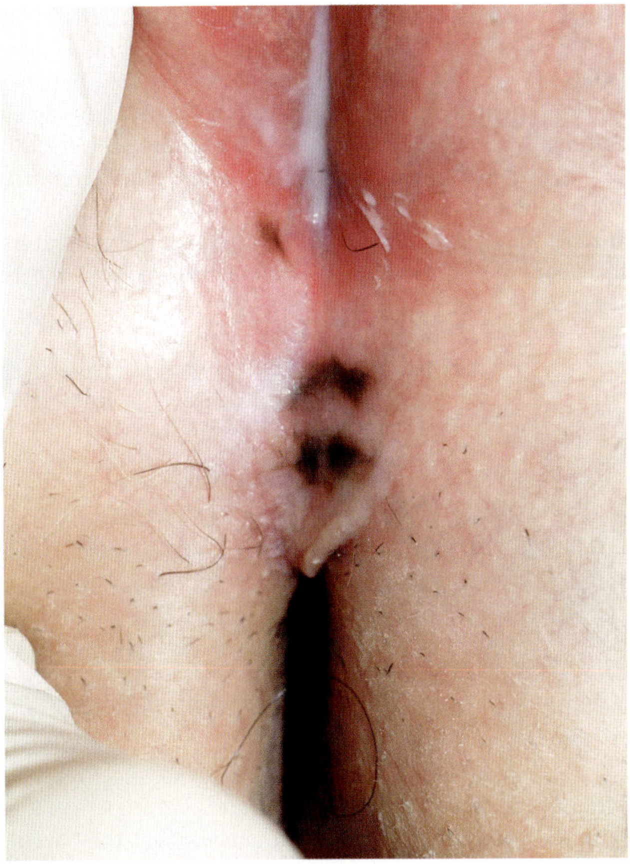

Fig. 9-17. These two nearly black macules of lentiginosis have occurred in a setting of lichen sclerosus.

rule out both benign conditions (eg, PIH) as well as malignancy (eg, superficial forms of melanoma). It cannot be emphasized enough how much genital melanosis clinically resembles melanoma and how little use simple guides for identifying melanomas (such as the widely publicized ABCDE approach) are in separating melanosis from melanoma. However, it is worth noting that patients with genital melanosis essentially never develop melanoma within

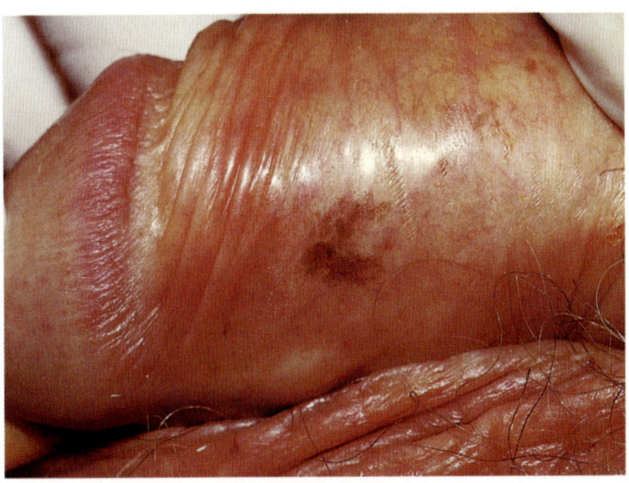

Fig. 9-18. Tan irregular macules of lentiginosis occur in men as well, most often on the glans or ventral prepuce, but also on the shaft.

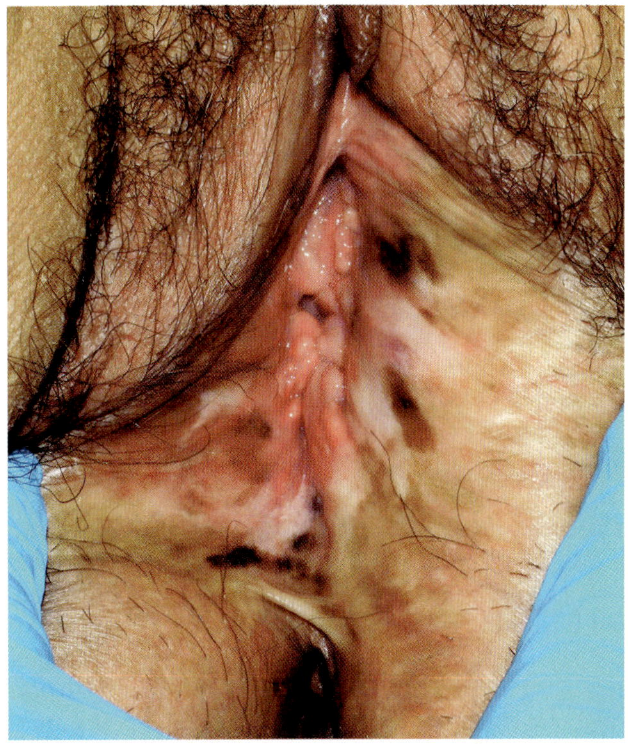

Fig. 9-19. This patient with lichen sclerosus shows discrete macules of variably dark brown color.

their melanosis lesions but nevertheless have a very interesting, complicated, and controversial relationship to melanoma. Specifically, patients with melanosis seem to have greater than chance possibility of a family history of melanoma, a past personal history of melanoma (almost always at a nongenital site) and, on follow up, development of a melanoma (again, at a nongenital site).[13,14]

Although it is reflected in only a few published studies, we believe that genital melanosis is particularly likely to arise from within an area of lichen sclerosus[13] **(Fig. 9-19)**. But note that when very young patients are diagnosed with genital melanosis, the oral mucous membranes should be inspected for the presence of similar lentiginous pigmentation. When this is found, consideration should be given to the possibility that any one of several rarely encountered conditions such as Peutz-Jeghers syndrome, Laugier-Hunziker syndrome, Bannayan-Riley-Ruvalcaba syndrome, LEOPARD syndrome, and the several syndromes with lentigines and cardiocutaneus myxomas may be present.[13]

**MELANOSIS — Diagnosis**

- Dark (usually black) flat, smooth, 5- to 25-mm patch
- Asymmetric or angular configuration
- Located primarily on nonkeratinizing (mucosal) tissue
- Unchanging appearance (if patient has previously been aware of the lesion)
- Incisional biopsy to rule out dysplasia and malignancy

Dermoscopy of lentiginosis requires an experienced dermoscopist, and there is no one pattern.[6] The parallel pattern with uniform linear and curved structures was found in 52.5% of lesions, with globular pattern in 32.5% of lesions, and a ringlike pattern in 50% of lesions, more in those with multiple lesions than those with a solitary lesion. A biopsy is imperative. Histologically most, but not all, specimens of genital melanosis demonstrate lentiginous elongation of the rete ridges with slight hyperproliferation of benign-appearing melanocytes within the basal layer. There are usually at least a few scattered pigmented macrophages ("melanophages") present within the dermis.

### Pathophysiology

The cause of genital melanosis is not known and the following is speculation. The uncommon, though greater than chance, presence of a family history of melanoma, the infrequent past personal history of melanoma, and the slight risk for the future development of a melanoma at a nongenital site makes one wonder about a genetic predisposition for the development of this pigmentary disorder. (And, as noted above, genital lentigines may occur in a number of heritable conditions, again suggesting a genetic etiologic component.) Finally, while there is usually no history of an associated dermatological problem in patients with melanosis, the development of melanosis in an area of lichen sclerosus raises the question of an immunological problem playing a role in the etiology of both disorders.

### Management

Genital melanosis, once it has stabilized in appearance, is believed to be a benign condition. There appears to be no tendency for the lesion, or lesions, to progress to melanoma in spite of their ominous clinical appearance. Once a diagnosis of genital melanosis is histologically confirmed, further therapy is not required. Essentially, all of the reported patients remained free of melanoma development within their lesions for as long as they were followed. However, because of the small number of reported patients and the relatively short duration of reported follow-up, one should probably conclude that the natural history of these melanosis lesions remains unclear. In any event, close follow-up is indeed strongly encouraged. This is particularly necessary regarding patients whose melanosis arose at the site of genital lichen sclerosus as it is possible that there is a relationship between lichen sclerosus and melanoma just as there is with another malignancy, squamous cell carcinoma. Thus, in a Finnish study, the authors found that women with lichen sclerosus of the vulva were much more likely to develop vulvar melanoma in their lichen sclerosus than were women without evidence of lichen sclerosus.[15] On the other hand, it should be acknowledged that there is considerable controversy regarding the differentiation of atypical genital nevi (AGNMT) from that of "true" genital melanomas in these quite young patients.[16] At any rate, long-term follow-up of patients with genital melanosis is advisable but periodic re-biopsy is not necessary unless either the patient reports a changed appearance or change is noted by the clinician at the time of examination. Having clinical photographs from the time at first diagnosis can be very helpful in this regard.

**MELANOSIS — Management**

- Depends on biopsy results:
  - If dysplasia or malignancy, excision of entire lesion.
  - If no dysplasia or malignancy, observation is appropriate.
- Benign course with little or no change is expected.
- But since data on the natural history are meager, periodic follow-up is appropriate.

## Melanocytic Nevus *("Mole," Pigmented Nevus, pl: Nevi)*

Melanocytic nevi are commonly found on the perigenital skin and on the genitalia of both genders, but they occur somewhat more often in women than in men. These nevi can be placed into four categories: common nevi, dysplastic nevi, atypical genital nevi, and nevi arising in lichen sclerosus. In addition, there are several other types of nevi (Spitz nevus, blue nevus, halo nevus, etc.) that occur too rarely in the genital region to warrant discussion in this chapter.

### Clinical Presentation

#### Common Nevus

"Common" nevi (having no abnormal clinical characteristics) account for the largest proportion of nevi in the anogenital region. These benign melanocytic nevi occur as symmetric macules (junctional nevi) or papules (compound nevi and intradermal nevi), smaller than 10 mm in diameter with well-demarcated borders and a homogenous tan or brown color (**Figs. 9-20 to 9-23**). (Note that some papular nevi of the intradermal type may be skin colored rather than tan or brown.) Papular nevi are somewhat soft on palpation, a feature that helps to distinguish them from more ominous, malignant neoplasms. Occasionally, a single atypical feature such as a notched border or slight pigment variegation may be present (**Figs. 9-24 and 9-25**). Common nevi may be located on either mucosal or hair-bearing skin, and they may be present at birth or acquired later in life. Congenital nevi are generally larger than acquired nevi, ranging from a centimeter to giant lesions (**Fig. 9-26**). An interesting subtype of common nevi is infrequently found on the penis in men, It is the so-called

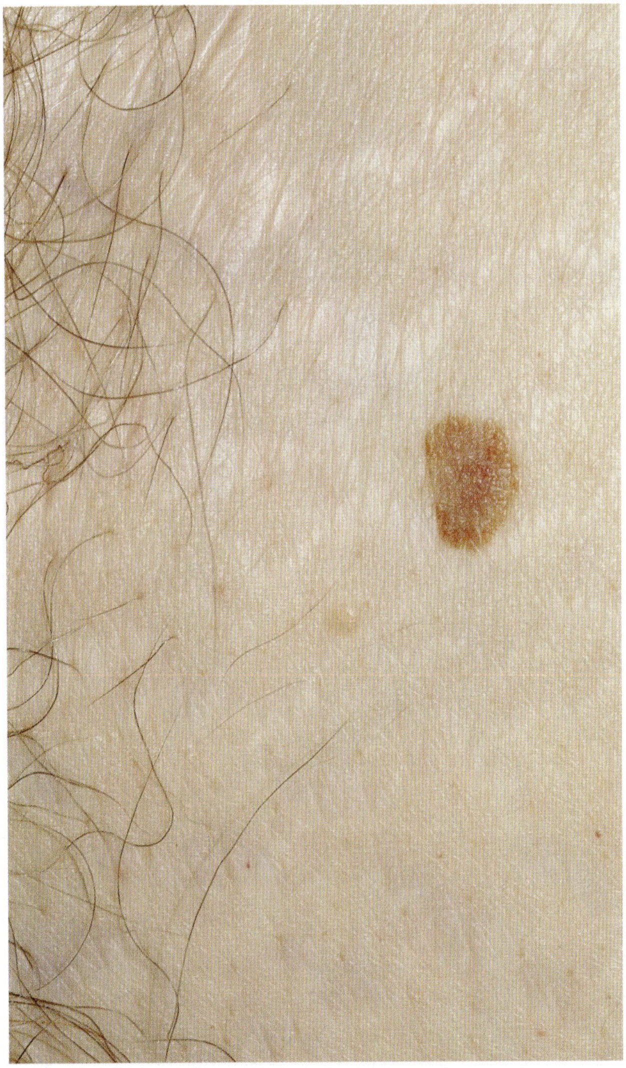

Fig. 9-20. A benign junctional nevus is an evenly pigmented brown, well-demarcated macule with regular smooth borders.

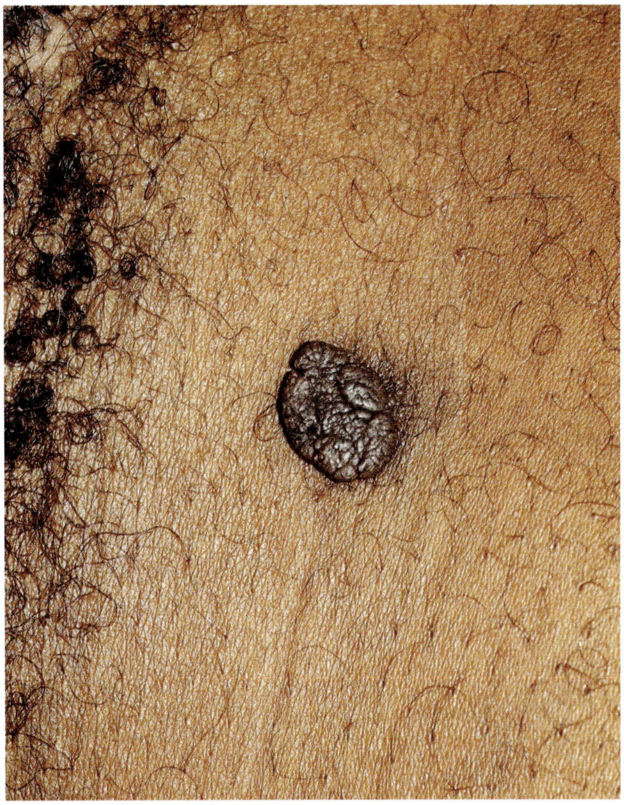

Fig. 9-21. A compound nevus is a well-demarcated, fleshy, brown papule with regular pigment.

divided nevus ("kissing nevus") that occurs on the corona of the glans with a mirror-image nevus being present on the underside of the prepuce (uncircumcised men) or on the shaft at the coronal sulcus (circumcised men).[17]

### Dysplastic Nevus

Dysplastic nevi occur in both men and women and account for about 5% of nevi occurring in the anogenital

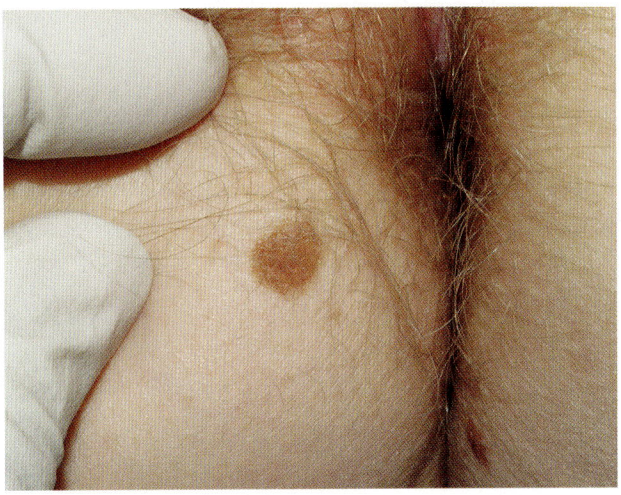

Fig. 9-22. This slightly raised papule is a normal compound papule; it has well-demarcated, regular borders and regular brown pigment.

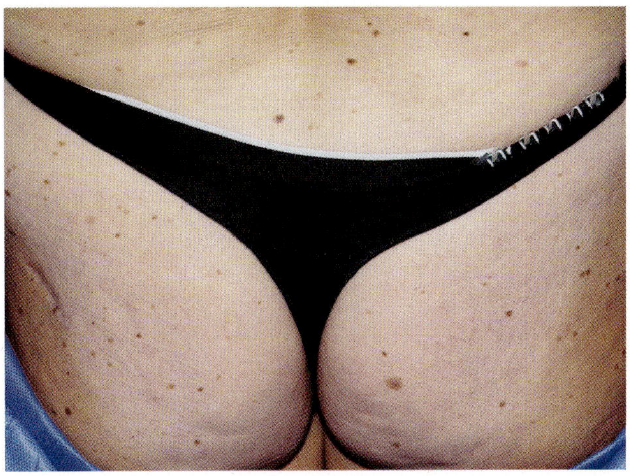

Fig. 9-23. Nevi are uncommon in the bathing trunk area; multiple nevi are a marker for tanning bed use. This woman also has small lentigines or "sun spots" that are indistinguishable from tiny junctional nevi.

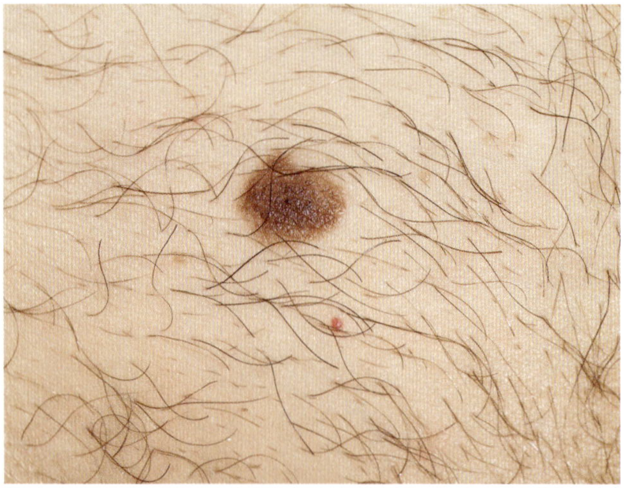

Fig. 9-24. This benign nevus shows reassuring signs of sharply demarcated borders and even pigmentation. The border is slightly notched; almost no nevus completely adheres to the ABCDE rules.

region. Nearly all of these lesions are located perigenitally rather than on the genitalia. Most often, these occur in individuals who have the dysplastic nevus syndrome in which the patient and other family members have large numbers (60-100) of nevi with clinically atypical features.

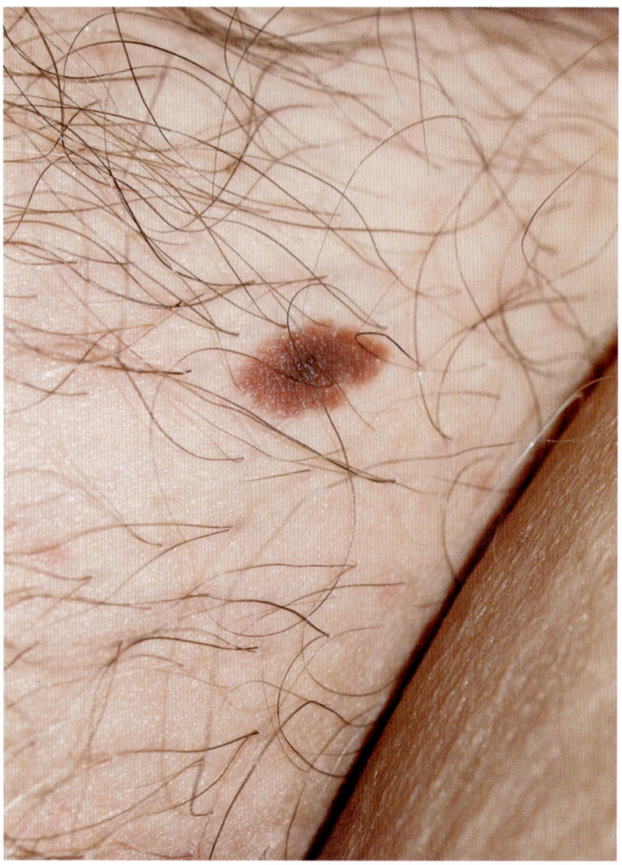

Fig. 9-25. The slightly irregular borders and darker center is exaggerated in this close-up photograph of this benign nevus. Different dermatologists have different threshold for concern, but few would worry about this lesion.

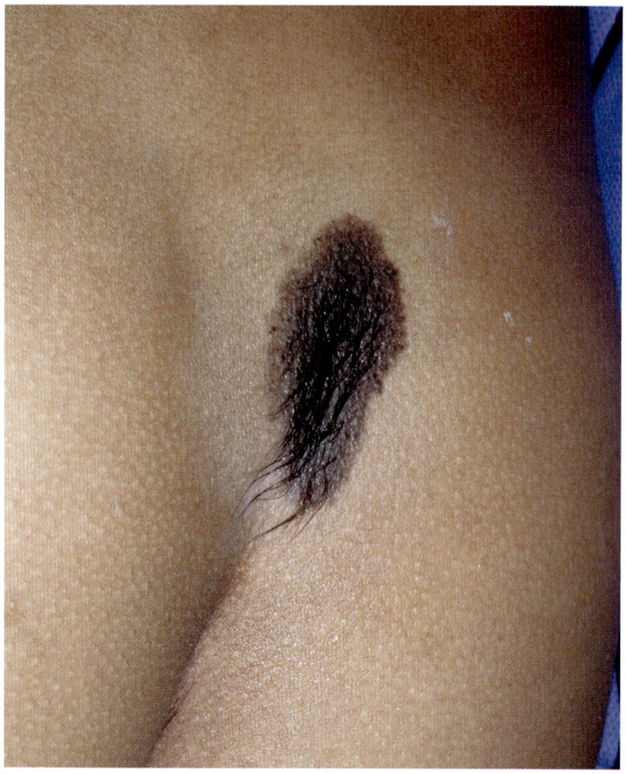

Fig. 9-26. Congenital nevi, as seen here, are often larger and, especially after puberty, tend to be thicker, often with terminal, dark hair. The risk of malignancy is slightly higher in these lesions, and any lesion that directly overlies the spine can be associated with overlying spinal or cord abnormalities.

Dysplastic nevi are flat or only slightly elevated and characteristically have some degree of asymmetry in configuration, indistinct margination, and variegation of pigment density. They are most often dark brown or even black with some degree of speckling. Red, white, and blue hues may also be present (**Figs. 9-27 to 9-30**). The most severely

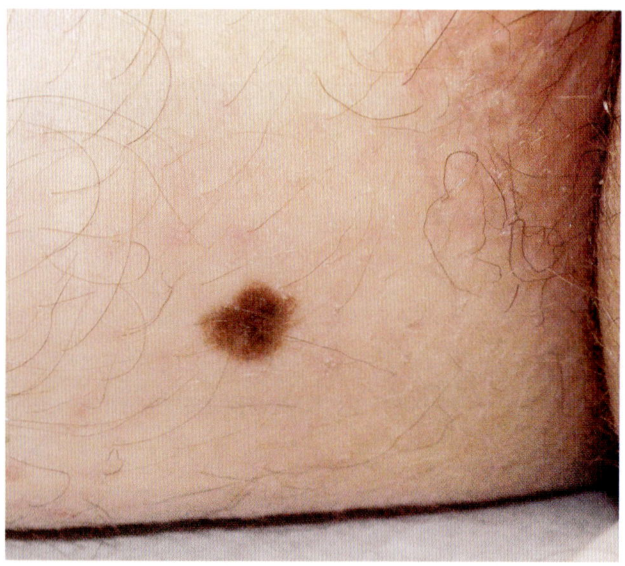

Fig. 9-27. Dysplastic nevi are characterized by their larger size and irregular shape and pigmentation.

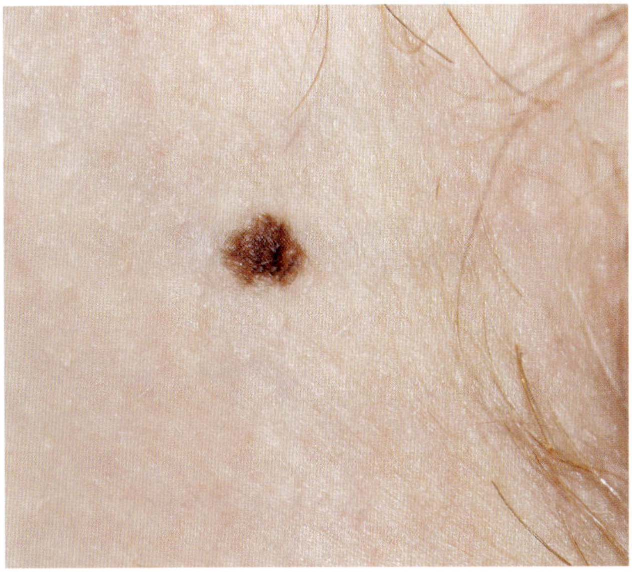

Fig. 9-28. A description of a dysplastic nevus, that of irregular border and irregular color, is similar to the description of melanoma. However, the abnormalities are less striking in an atypical nevus; experience and biopsies are important in differentiation of these tumors.

dysplastic lesions tend to be large (7-15 mm in diameter). When dysplastic nevi occur in the anogenital area, they may have clinical and histological features similar to the AMNGT nevi discussed in the paragraph below.[18]

### Atypical Melanocytic Nevus of Genital Type

Atypical melanocytic nevi of genital type (AMNGT) were identified as a specific subtype of nevus almost 50 years ago. Previously, these lesions were often mistakenly thought to be melanomas, and sometimes, they are still erroneously diagnosed as such.[6] In spite of their name, AMNGT are not restricted specifically to the genitalia and often occur along the anatomic milk line, most often in the axillae and on the breasts of women.[18,19] These lesions are

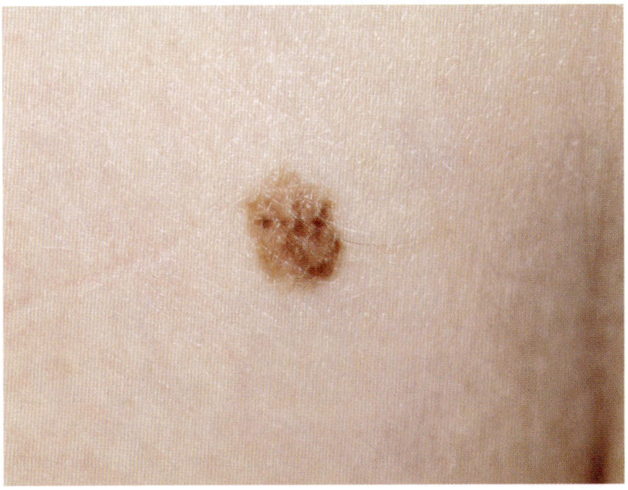

Fig. 9-29. Dysplastic nevi generally occur on dry, keratinized extragenital skin rather than genital skin.

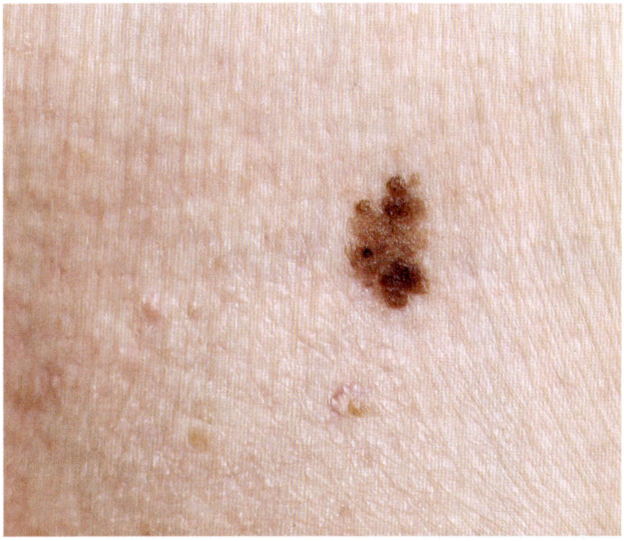

Fig. 9-30. This papule shows the same variegation of pigmentation and irregular borders as dysplastic nevi, but the irregularities are more striking, and a biopsy showed a melanoma.

far more often reported in women than they are in men.[18] In the anogenital region, they occur both on mucosal surfaces and hair-bearing skin. Most AMNGT are located on the labia minora and labia majora, but lesions may occur on the mons pubis, clitoris, and perineum. AMNGT develop primarily in girls and young women as early as childhood and continuing to about age 20 or 30 years. (Whereas anogenital melanomas, with which they may be confused, almost always occur in women who are 50 years or older.)[20] These nevi vary appreciably in size but most are about 6 mm in diameter. They are nearly always papular and may have a polypoid surface. Atypical clinical and histological features, as noted above for dysplastic nevi, are often present.[18,19]

### Nevi Arising in Lichen Sclerosus

Nevi have been reported to occur in association with the lesions of genital lichen sclerosus (**Fig. 9-31**). Most of these have been described with vulvar lichen sclerosus, but a few have also occurred in men.[16] The majority of the lesions have been described as small (3- to 6-mm) black macules, but a few larger ones have also been reported. The dark black color of these lesions and the type of histologic atypia (similar, or identical, to that found in AMNGT) suggest the possibility of melanoma.[16] This is particularly important as there has been a reported (possibly erroneously) association between lichen sclerosus and the development of melanoma.[15]

## Diagnosis

While "common" benign nevi can usually be identified as such clinically, the situation is different for the other three types of nevi (described above) where the need for biopsy is more controversial. Dermatologists may

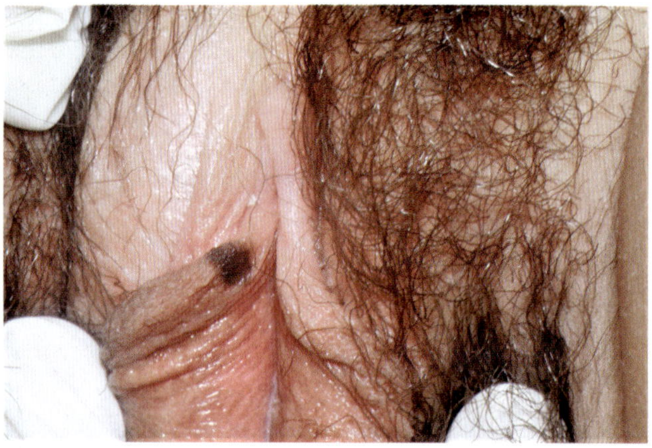

Fig. 9-31. Nevi arising in a setting of lichen sclerosus such as this lesion show especially atypical histology, as do atypical melanocytic nevi of genital type, which generally occur on the labia minora and tend to be very dark, with a polypoid surface. These lesions are easily misdiagnosed as melanoma.

be satisfied with a clinical diagnosis of lesions showing no clinical atypicality, whereas other clinicians will generally prefer to biopsy all anogenital pigmented lesions. For both types of clinicians, biopsy is mandatory for any lesion presenting with atypical clinical features and for all patients presenting with pigmented lesions arising within areas of lichen sclerosus. For those experienced with its use, dermoscopy may be of assistance in making a decision whether or not to biopsy "normal"-appearing nevi.[6]

Dermoscopy is useful for experienced dermoscopist, but even beginners can sometimes be reassured by classic findings of a seborrheic keratosis. Atypical melanocytic nevi of the genital type exhibit more than one pattern on dermoscopy, most often showing the globular or mixed pattern.[6] Dermoscopy of dysplastic nevi is characterized by irregularity and different patterns, but this is complicated specialty requiring experience and training. Biopsies are required for diagnosis. The histologic features of common nevi and dysplastic nevi are well understood by most pathologists, and therefore, biopsied lesions will be correctly diagnosed. However, the situation for atypical melanocytic genital nevi genital type (AMNGT) and those nevi arising in lichen sclerosus is different. The histology of AMNGT reveals many changes that are regularly present in melanoma such as appreciable junctional melanocytic proliferation (either in a lentiginous pattern or forming unusually large, oval nests), mild melanocyte spread into the mid epidermis, and varying degrees of cytological atypia.[18] A similar situation occurs with nevi arising in patients with genital lichen sclerosus, and in this situation, histologic atypicality similar to that occurring in AMNGT is usually present and may easily be misdiagnosed as melanoma.[16]

The differential diagnosis of nevi includes melanoma, pigmented intraepithelial neoplasia, mucosal melanosis, and PIH.

**MELANOCYTIC NEVUS — Diagnosis**

- **Common nevus**
  - Tan to brown, smooth-surfaced, 3- to 10-mm macule or papule.
  - Borders are sharp, color is even, shape is symmetrical.
- **Dysplastic nevus**
  - Brown, smooth-surfaced, 6- to 20-mm macule or papule
  - One or more other features include diffuse margination; speckling of color (additional red, white, or blue hues); asymmetry
- **Atypical nevus, genital type**
  - Similar to the common nevus but often larger (6-15 mm).
  - Surface may be polypoid (mammillated, "bumpy")
- **Nevus arising from a background of lichen sclerosus**
  - Black, smooth-surfaced, 5- to 20-mm macule, patch, or papule

## Pathophysiology

Nevi are thought to be developmental hamartomas, or benign proliferations, of melanocytes that possess some growth advantage over those of normal melanocytes. However, the exact reason why nevi arise is not known. Genetic factors appear to play a role in their development as there is often a familial pattern regarding the clinical appearance and number. UVL exposure plays an important role in nevi arising on sun-exposed surfaces, but this is clearly not the case for anogenital nevi. Hormonal factors are likely important especially for the development of AMNGT since these lesions arise almost mostly in young women and occur mainly within the milk line. Mutations in *BRAF*, which are commonly present in nevi and melanomas on sun-exposed skin, but which are less common in nevi and melanomas from non–sun-exposed sites, are found in genital nevi of both common and AMNGT types.[20] Lack of additional UVL-driven mutations probably explains why these BRAF mutations in genital nevi remain benign in nature.[20]

## Management

Biopsied nevi with a benign histology can appropriately be left in place as there is little or no likelihood of progression to melanoma. In fact, almost no genital melanomas, as opposed to melanomas on sun-exposed skin, develop from nevi. It is controversial whether or not dysplastic nevi with histological identification of atypicality should be excised. It seems more likely today that the association of dysplastic nevi and development of melanoma (as occurs on sun-exposed skin) is based on additional UVL-induced mutations. AMNGT, in spite of their suspicious histological appearance, have a low recurrence rate following excision and do not appear to progress to melanoma.[19,20] However, given the sparsity of follow-up information about them, excision with clear margins is recommended. Nevi arising in lichen sclerosus for the reasons discussed above should also be excised with clear margins.

## Melanoma

The frequency of melanoma arising in the anogenital region is very low. The incidence of vulvar melanoma in the Western world is under 2.0 per 1 000 000 individuals, whereas penile melanoma is about 10 times less common at about 0.2 per 1 000 000. Scrotal melanoma is even rarer. Anorectal melanoma, in both men and women, has an incidence of ~0.4 per 1 000 000 and is the only melanoma occurring in the anogenital region for which the incidence seems to be rising.[21] Nevertheless, these uncommon melanomas are discussed here because early recognition has quite a positive effect on what is otherwise a very dismal survival outcome.

Anogenital melanomas differ from cutaneous melanomas arising in sun-exposed skin in multiple ways. First, with the exception of anal melanoma, there is a stable, or possibly even a decreasing, incidence. Second, they occur in an appreciably older age group. Third, they are obviously not related to DNA damage secondary to UVL. Fourth, there is only rarely an association with a preceding nevus. Fifth, the proportion of melanomas that are amelanotic is higher. Sixth, in a very large proportion of cases, the histologic pattern is that of mucosal-type melanoma and is surprisingly similar to that occurring in acral lentiginous melanoma. Seventh, the outcome, no doubt related in part to delayed diagnosis, is appreciably worse. Eighth, cutaneous melanomas have a high frequency of mutations in the *BRAF* gene, whereas in mucosal melanomas, *KIT* is the gene that is most often mutated.[22]

Unfortunately, because of the infrequency with which anogenital melanomas occur, all of the published reports consider within a single group both those tumors arising on mucous membrane (mucosal melanoma) and those arising on hair-bearing, keratinizing skin (cutaneous melanoma). One might think it likely that there would be major differences between these two types of anogenital melanoma histologically, but the data indicate that no matter where melanomas occur in the anogenital region, they contain a mutational profile that is "mucosal melanoma" in type.[22] This probably happens because of the lack of UVL damage in anogenital tissue and thus the absence of UVL-related mutations.

### Clinical Presentation

#### Vulvar Melanoma

Melanoma is the second most common malignancy arising in the vulva, but even so, it only accounts for about 5% of all malignant vulvar neoplasms and <3% of all of the melanomas occurring anywhere in women.[23,24] While the incidence of melanoma occurring on sun-exposed skin is increasing fairly rapidly, the incidence of vulvar melanoma has been stable for the last 50 years.[23] It is disproportionally more common in the White population, and it occurs predominantly in older women with a mean age at diagnosis in the mid to late 60s.[23,24] Importantly, the few reported vulvar melanomas arising in children and very young women have been reported almost entirely in a setting of lichen sclerosus.[15] As mentioned above, however, do note that many, including the authors of this book, believe that these latter melanomas may have been atypical melanocytic nevi of the genital type (AMNGT) that were misdiagnosed as melanomas.[16]

Most vulvar melanomas have a clinical appearance similar both to AMNGT and to those melanomas that occur at other cutaneous sites. Features suggesting melanoma include large size (2-3 cm), dark brown or black pigmentation, dark speckling of pigment against a lighter background, color variegation with red, white, and blue hues, nonsharp margination, and a configuration that is angular or asymmetric[23,24] (**Figs 9-32 to 9-38**). In contrast to melanomas occurring on sun-exposed skin, ~20% of vulvar melanomas are multifocal, 5%-25% are amelanotic (**Fig. 9-39**), and 50%-75% occur on glabrous skin or mucosal tissue.[23-25] Most vulvar melanomas are asymptomatic, but, when symptoms and signs are present, they most commonly include pruritus, presence of a palpable lesion, bleeding, and/or visual change in a preceding lesion. Tumors are most often found on the labium majus and labium minus, but location on the clitoris and periclitoral area is also fairly common.[24,25] Reflecting their large size and presumed long duration before recognition, ulceration of the surface occurs with considerable frequency.[24] At the time of diagnosis, about 50% of the women have localized disease without evidence

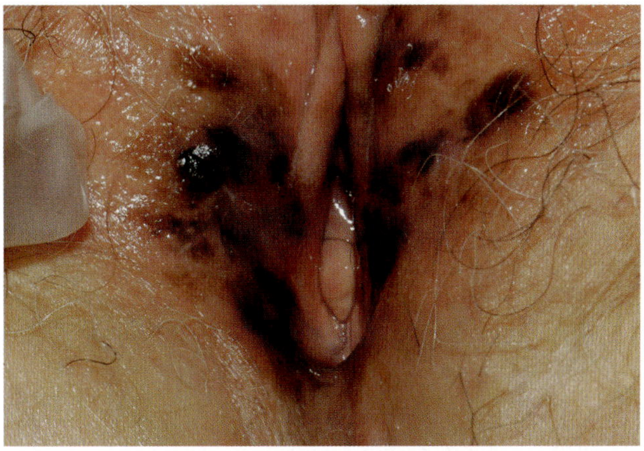

Fig. 9-32. The deep gray-black, irregular pigment on the vulva is a classic sign of either melanoma or genital lentiginosis—in this case, melanoma. The black nodule indicates the correct diagnosis. (Courtesy of Dr. Hope Haefner.)

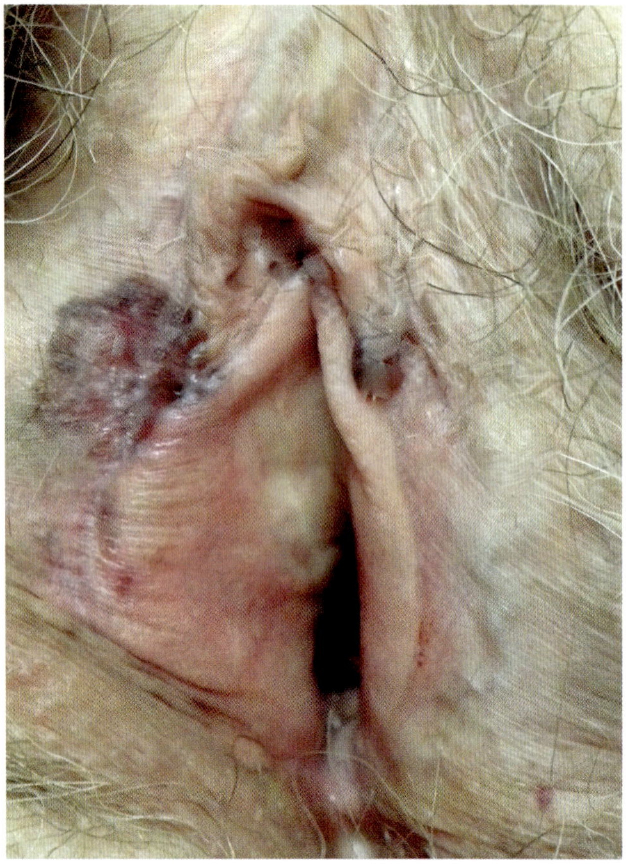

Fig. 9-33. Some melanomas show gray and red colors. Like many vulvar melanomas, this patient exhibits multifocal tumors. (Courtesy of Dr. Claudia Marchitelli.)

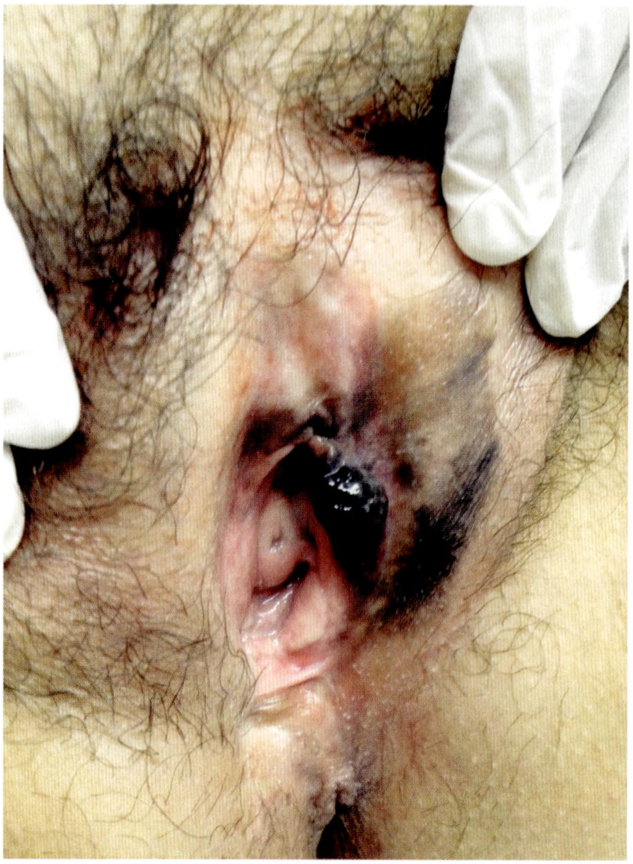

Fig. 9-34. A large, ill-defined black and gray patch with a central large nodular melanoma is indicative of the bad prognosis of most genital melanomas that are discovered late. (Courtesy of Dr. Claudia Marchitelli.)

of regional or distant spread.[23] Nodular and lentiginous types of melanoma are overrepresented among vulvar melanomas compared to the high frequency of superficial spreading melanomas found at other nonanogenital, cutaneous sites.[23,25]

### Penile and Scrotal Melanoma

Two, rather similar reviews from the U.S. Surveillance, Epidemiology, and End Results (SEER) data, provide most of the information about penile and scrotal melanomas.[26,27] As noted above, penile melanomas are very rarely encountered. The average age at diagnosis occurs in the seventh decade and is thus the age at onset is similar to that of vulvar melanoma. Most of these neoplasms occur on the glans and inner prepuce, but involvement of the penile shaft or the urethra is also possible.[27] Lesions may be flat patches or raised papules and nodules; many are polypoid. About 40% are ulcerated. As is true for vulvar melanoma, it appears that a larger than expected number of penile melanomas are amelanotic. The majority of patients have localized disease at the time of diagnosis.[27] Scrotal melanomas occur even more rarely. In a large review, scrotal melanomas were found only half as often as were penile melanomas.[26]

### Anal Melanoma

Anal melanomas occurs infrequently; the incidence (about 0.4 per million) lies between that of vulvovaginal melanoma and that of penoscrotal melanoma. The incidence of anorectal melanoma appears to be the only type of melanoma occurring in the anogenital region that is increasing. However, the number of tumors pertinent to most of our readers is somewhat uncertain because many of the published series do not separately identify those patients with *anal* melanoma from those with *rectal* melanoma. It appears that about two-thirds of the reported cases occur in the anus or anal canal and thus might be relevant to our clinicians.[28,29] Here, too, more anorectal melanomas occur in women than in men reversing the situation for melanomas arising on sun-exposed skin.[29] As is true for genital melanoma, anorectal melanoma occurs predominantly in an older population with a mean age in the seventh decade at the time of diagnosis.[28] The most frequent symptoms and signs present at presentation were rectal bleeding, anal pain, presence of a mass, and a change in bowel habits.[28] As is true for genital melanomas, a sizeable proportion (about 20%) of these melanomas is amelanotic.[21] Other information such as

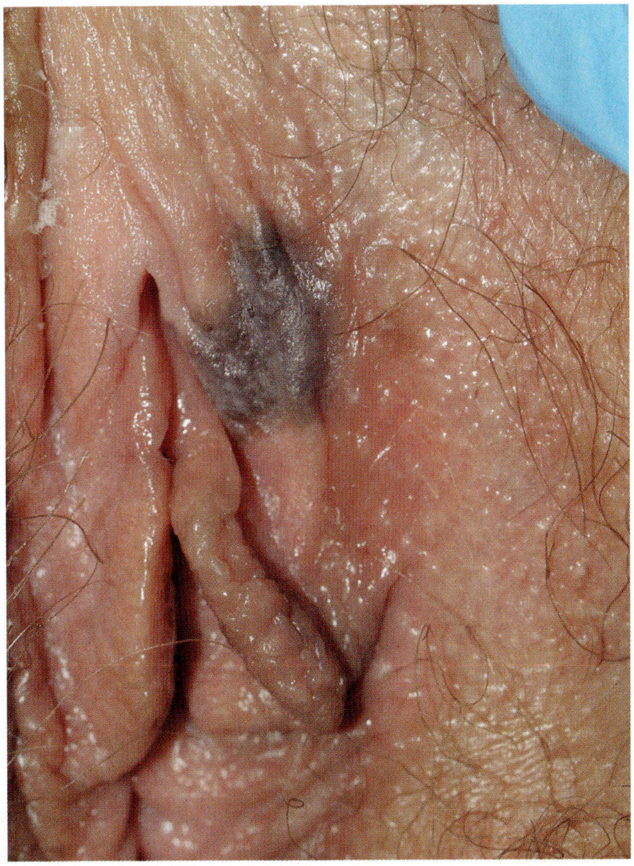

Fig. 9-35. This melanoma is gray and large, but well demarcated and uniform in color; but the overall morphology is not consistent with any usual lesion and deserves a biopsy.

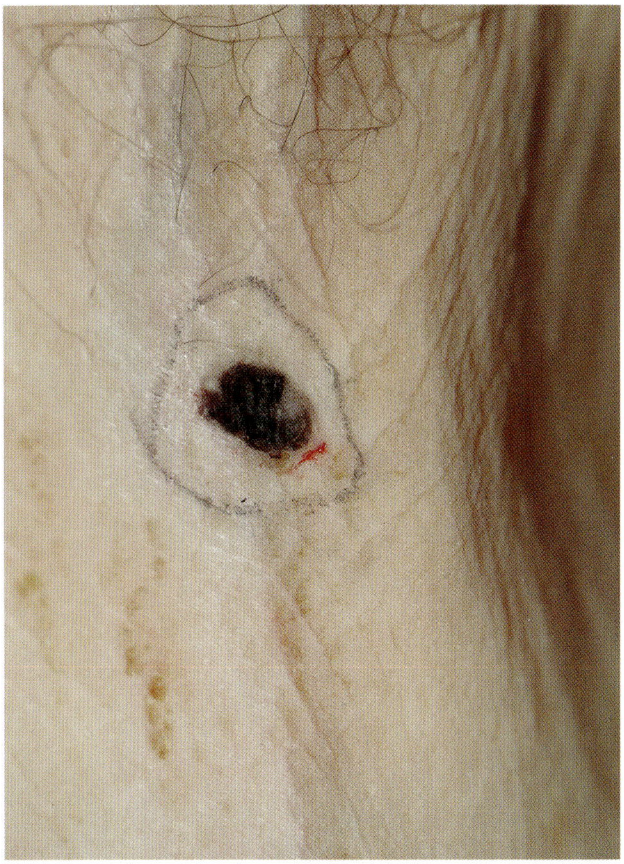

Fig. 9-37. One of us (LE) thought that this small, well-demarcated, black papule was probably a seborrheic keratosis, but the black color and very slight atypical nature prompted a biopsy. It proved to be a melanoma. Any pigmented lesion that is not absolutely typical for a benign lesion should be sampled.

the clinical appearance, size of the tumors, percentage that is ulcerated, etc., is not readily available in recently published reviews. Only a third of patients have localized disease at the time of presentation; the other two-thirds have nodal or distant metastases.[21]

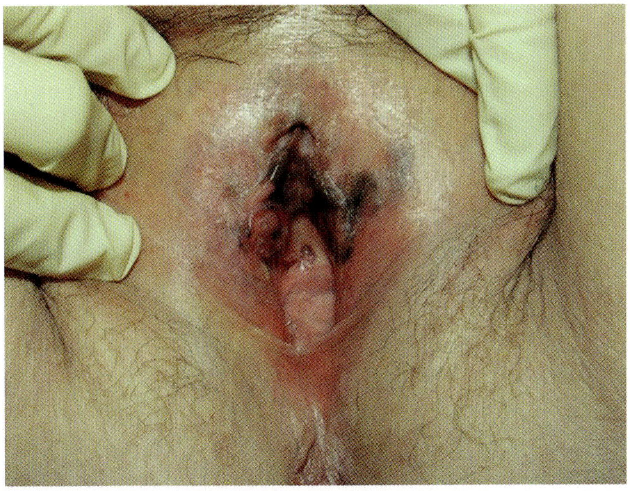

Fig. 9-36. This large poorly demarcated patch of variegate pigmentation that includes black and gray colors is classic for melanoma. (Courtesy of Dr. Sophie Berville-Levy.)

## Diagnosis of Anogenital Melanomas

Anogenital melanomas may be flat, plaquelike nodular or polypoid. A clinical diagnosis is often possible on the basis of an older person with dark, frequently variegated, pigmentation, which may be intermingled with other blue, gray, red, or white hues (Figs. 10-21 to 10-24). Dermatoscopic evaluation may be helpful in assisting clinicians in clinical diagnosis. Blue, gray, and white colors have high predictive value, as does a blue-white veil. White lines, peripheral black dots, blue-gray structureless area are important as well. However, amelanotic tumors, which account for about 20%-25% of anogenital melanomas, are more easily missed **(Fig. 9-39)**. With dermoscopy, amelanotic melanoma shows polymorphous vessels. Clearly, biopsy is crucial.

Diseases to be considered in the differential diagnosis include atypical nevi, lentiginoses, hemorrhoids, vascular thromboses, seborrheic keratoses, pigmented basal cell carcinomas, and both pigmented and nonpigmented forms of squamous cell carcinoma.

A suspected clinical diagnosis must, of course, be confirmed with biopsy. Excisional biopsy is preferred so that the entire lesion can be examined histologically. However,

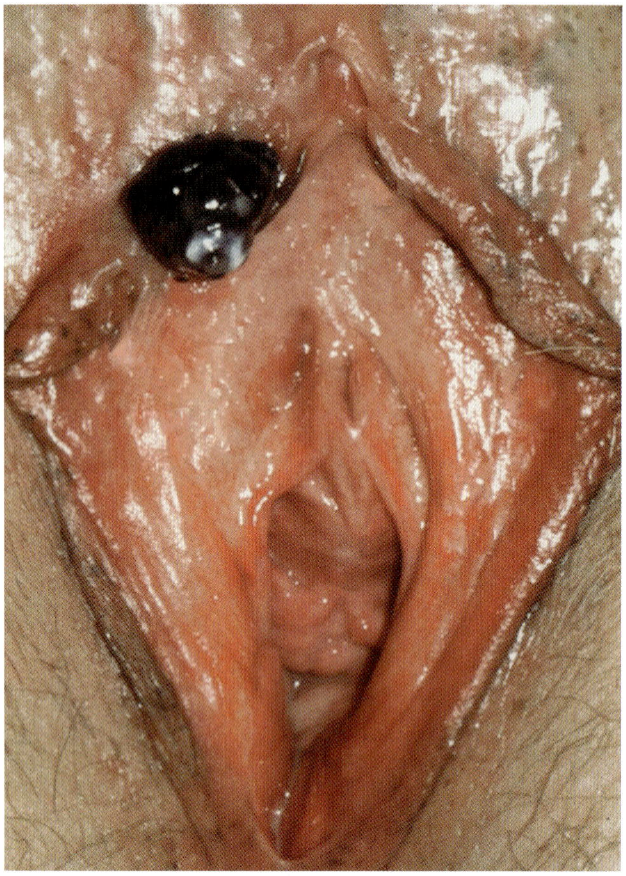

Fig. 9-38. Nodular melanomas do not display the classic ABCD signs of melanoma. (Credit Dr. Ron Jones.)

for large lesions, one or more incisional/punch biopsies may be appropriate. The diagnosis is usually apparent with routine hematoxylin and eosin (H&E) stain. However, in some cases, especially for amelanotic melanoma, special techniques can enhance the sensitivity and specificity of the diagnosis. The most common approach uses immunohistochemical (IHC) staining, which is available in most pathology laboratories and is relatively inexpensive.[30] Melanocytic markers are most often used, and they identify whether or not cells in question are melanocytes: melan-A/MART-1 and HMB-45 have high specificity, whereas S100 and SOX10 have somewhat better sensitivity.[30] Proliferation markers are also available, but currently, this aspect of identifying a melanoma is mostly determined by counting the number of mitoses/mm$^2$. Breslow depth and Clark levels are determined, as well, in an attempt to provided information about prognosis.[30] Interestingly, and in contrast to melanomas occurring on sun-exposed skin, a contiguous nevus is essentially never found in anogenital melanomas. This suggests that nearly all anogenital melanomas arise *de novo* rather than from existing nevi.

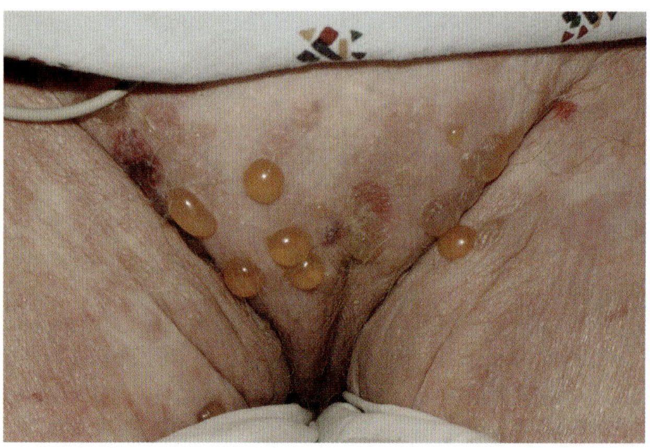

Fig. 9-39. Amelanotic melanomas are overrepresented in the anogenital areas; this mass at the posterior fourchette is primarily amelanotic, although there is a bit of pigment at the borders. (Courtesy of Dr. Ron Jones.)

MELANOMA — **Diagnosis**

- Older patient (50-80)
- Atypical features: basically black, some color variegation (red, white, or blue hues); consider amelanotic melanoma if color is pink or red.
- Surface may be friable or ulcerated.
- Symptoms (pruritus, pain) and signs (palpable mass, history of rapid growth) may or may not be present.
- Biopsy any lesions for which there is the slightest suspicion.

## Pathophysiology

Not a lot is known as to why anogenital melanomas develop. Certainly, it has nothing to do with sunlight damage, which is so clearly a major factor in the etiology of cutaneous melanomas. In fact, those anogenital melanomas that arise on non–sun-exposed tissue are part of the entirely different family of melanomas known as "mucosal-type melanomas" (MTM). Somewhat surprisingly, the pathophysiology for anogenital melanomas, at least as determined by gene mutations, appears to be the same for those melanomas that arise on glabrous or hair-bearing skin as for those that arise on "true" mucous membranes.[22] However, some genetic factors are shared with common cutaneous melanoma, while others are not. Clinical similarities with cutaneous-type melanomas include the development of multiple primary melanomas at nongenital sites at the same rate as for anogenital melanomas. The total number of skin nevi and also the rate of development of nonmelanoma skin cancers are the same in both groups. Clinical differences between the two groups include more frequent family history of melanoma in the MTM group, the older age, and greater preponderance of women in the MTM.

The other differences that also exist between the two groups perhaps can be partially explained by delayed diagnosis in those with anogenital MTM melanomas

These differences include greater likelihood of positive regional lymph nodes at time of diagnosis, greater mean Breslow depth, greater histologic likelihood of a lentiginous melanoma pattern vs a superficial spreading pattern, and more frequent death related to melanoma. The take away message is probably that we should separate melanomas into those with UVL damage signatures (eg, "cutaneous-type" melanomas) and those who lack UV damage signatures (eg, "mucosal-type" melanomas). This approach is supported by gene analysis demonstrating a high rate of *BRAF* V600 and *NRAS* mutations in the "cutaneous melanoma" group and those showing a high rate of *KIT* and *SF3B1* mutations in the MTM group.[22,31] But do note that there are also other types of melanoma (acral, desmoplastic, familial, etc.) that also have their own different mutational profiles.

As opposed to the known role that UVL plays in developing mutations for melanomas that occur on sun-exposed skin, the cause for the mutations in anogenital melanomas remains an enigma. There is not even a clear consensus regarding lifestyle risk factors that might be playing a role in the development of these melanomas. However, there is agreement that HPV infection and the presence of chronic inflammation, two factors important in the etiology of anogenital squamous cell carcinoma, play no role in the development of anogenital melanomas.

## Management

Management of anogenital melanoma is generally carried out by clinicians who specialize in melanoma therapy. Nevertheless, some general discussion regarding prognosis and therapy is warranted here. Staging represents the first step in management because it is important to determine the status of malignancy at a specific moment in time and then to stratify the morbidity and ultimate prognosis of these neoplasms. Staging also helps to determine the best approach to therapy.

Staging can be as simple and practical as the approach used by the U.S. Surveillance, Epidemiology, and End Results (SEER) database group, which uses a simple three stage system of localized disease, regional disease, and distant disease.[29] But this represents a rather simplistic guideline containing an insufficient number of variables to offer a complete and accurate approach. For that reason, increasingly authors at least in the United States and Canada are using the eighth edition of the American Joint Committee on Cancer (AJCC) melanoma staging system that was implemented in 2018.[32] Detailed discussion here is perhaps too arcane for the likely readers of this book but would be appropriate and necessary for those clinicians specializing in oncological care. Suffice it to say that the AJCC staging incorporates the tumor, node, and metastasis (TNM) approach and includes information for the tumor component (Breslow levels of tumor thickness and tumor ulceration) that most directly influence prognosis and therapy for localized disease (stages I and II). Interestingly, the mitotic rate was used in the seventh edition but was dropped for the eighth edition with the observation that it did not predict outcome as well as tumor depth and the presence or absence of ulceration.

Multiple studies have shown that wide local excision for all types of anogenital melanoma offers results at least as good as were previously obtained with the more radical procedures carried out in the past. And it is interesting that lymph node mapping and sentinel lymph node biopsy have almost completely replaced prophylactic lymphadenectomy for decisions about the management of regional lymph nodes. Some immunotherapy is also available for adjuvant treatment, but discussion of that approach is for advanced disease and thus lies beyond the scope of this book.

Despite therapy, the outcome for anogenital melanoma is still very poor. For women with vulvar melanoma (the most common of all the anogenital melanomas), the overall 5-year survival ranges from about 25% to 60%.[25] However, for patients with early, localized disease and no node involvement, it may be as high as 70%-75%.[23] But survival is related to the time since diagnosis and therapy. Thus, in one study, carried out more than a decade ago, the survival rates at 1, 5, and 10 years were 85%, 51%, and 30%, respectively. Survival for those with anorectal melanoma is even worse. In a recent publication, 5-year survival was given as 27% for stage I (localized) disease, 10% for stage II (regional node metastases) disease, and 0% for stage III (disseminated) disease.[28] Due to the infrequency with which it is encountered, data for men with penile and scrotal melanoma are limited. However, perhaps in part related to more easy visibility, survival appears to be a little better for these men than for patients with vulvar and anorectal melanoma.[26,27] In one fairly large retrospective review, patients with general (cutaneous and mucosal) penile and scrotal melanoma had a 5-year survival of 69%.[26]

**MELANOMA — Management**

- Carry out staging (see text).
- Consider sentinel node biopsy for lesions with more than 1-mm invasion.
- Wide local excision.
- Radical surgery seldom is indicated.

## Lichen Planus

The primary discussion of lichen planus (LP) can be found in Chapter 5 under the red patches and plaques. It is also briefly mentioned earlier in this chapter under PIH. It is now discussed here again to indicate that most

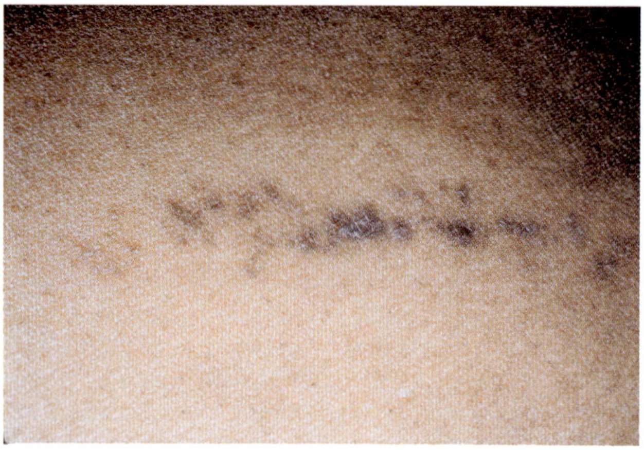

Fig. 9-40. Lichen planus sometimes is hyperpigmented rather than red or erosive when occurring on dry, keratinized skin, especially in patients of darker complexion. The linear configuration and shiny surface is suggestive of this diagnosis.

authors believe that while LP begins as erythematous papules and plaques, it progresses with the passage of time through a stage of violaceous (purple) lesions and eventually enters a darker, hyperpigmented stage. Eventually it spontaneously, or with treatment, does end up as gray or black PIH.[33] These stages are particularly apparent in patients of color where dark hyperpigmentation is observed earlier in many as 15% of the patients **(Fig. 9-40)**.[34]

## Prurigo Nodularis

The primary discussion of prurigo nodularis (PN) occurs in Chapter 6 in the section on red nodules. It is also mentioned here because it sometimes presents as a hyperpigmented nodule. Generally, it is described clinically as a pink to red nodule with a dark hyperpigmented, ringlike border. However, when photographs of patients appear in publications (and in clinical actuality), PN often appears as a red-brown, brown, or even black hyperpigmented nodule **(Fig. 9-41)**. This situation, as is true with other red nodules of long-standing duration, is particularly apparent in patients of color. In any event, the history of intense pruritus followed by incessant scratching and picking, generally allows for easy clinical diagnosis. Dermoscopy can be useful and shows a peripheral circular radially arranged white line or halo with some centrifugal coarse projections on a brownish and/or reddish background, the so-called white starburst pattern.[35]

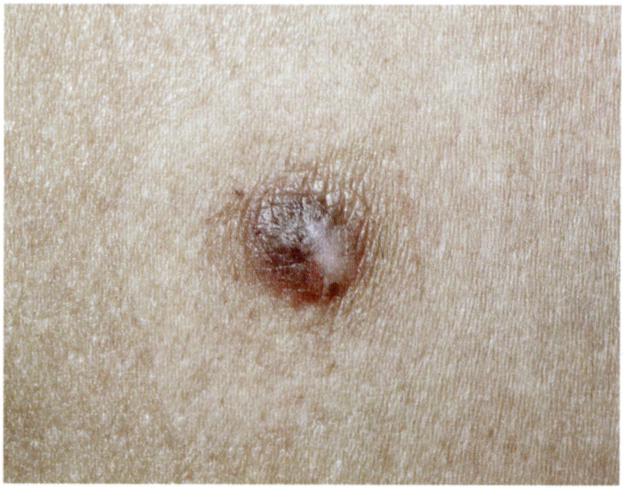

Fig. 9-41. A prurigo nodule, or picker's nodule, is produced by chronic picking that results in lichenification and postinflammatory hyperpigmentation, particularly in patients with a naturally darker skin color. The accentuation of skin markings that displays lichenification can be seen and the light area is scar; often the center shows an erosion/excoriation rather than scar.

## Pigmented Warts

Genital warts of the flat-topped type, which frequently develop in the anogenital area, are often tan, brown, brown-red, or black in color **(Figs. 9-42 and 9-43)**. These lesions are covered along with all other types of warts in Chapter 7.

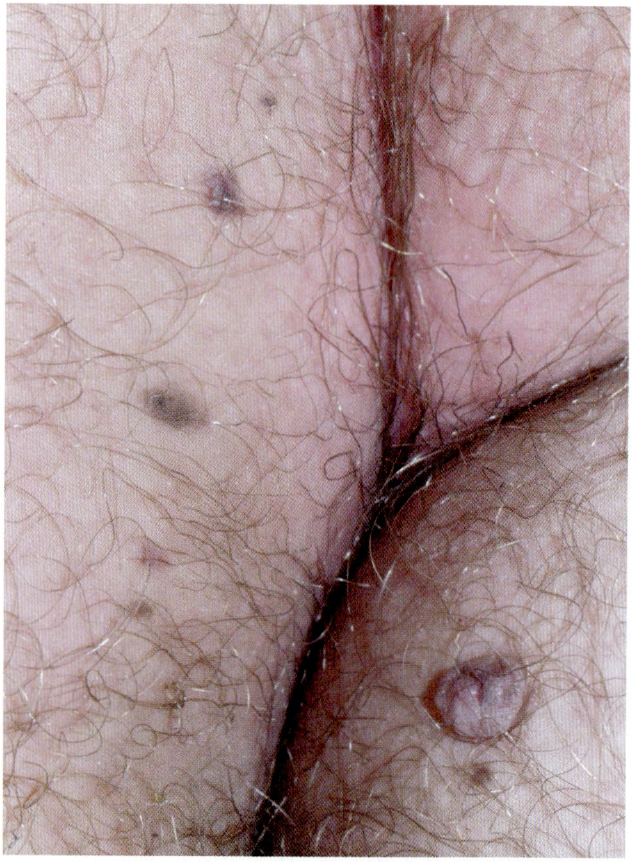

Fig. 9-42. Anogenital warts can be skin colored, brown, hypopigmented, or red.

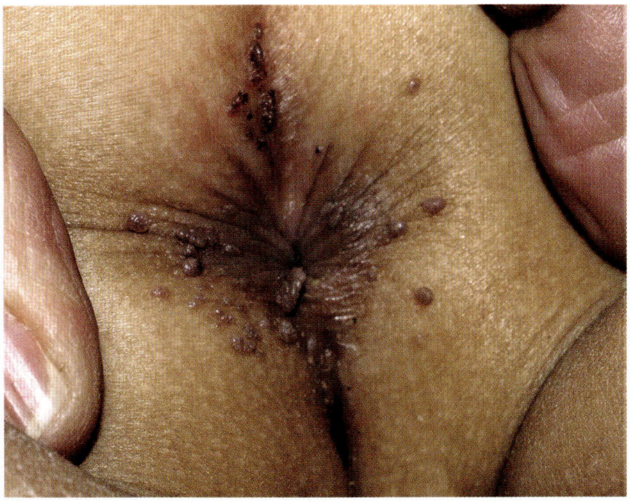

Fig. 9-43. Patients of color regularly exhibit hyperpigmented anogenital warts.

### Genital Intraepithelial Neoplasia

HPV-related vulvar, penile and scrotal intraepithelial neoplasia is frequently tan, brown, or black in color (Figs. 9-44 and 9-45). These disorders are discussed in Chapters 5 and 7.

### Pigmented Basal Cell Carcinomas

Basal cell carcinomas are normally skin colored, but a small proportion contain sufficient melanin to be at least partially brown, blue, or black in color (Fig. 9-46). These lesions are covered in Chapter 7.

### Angiokeratomas

Genital angiokeratomas are usually light to dusky red in color, but those occurring on the vulva are sometimes blue, purple, or black (Figs. 9-47 and 9-48). These lesions are covered in Chapter 6.

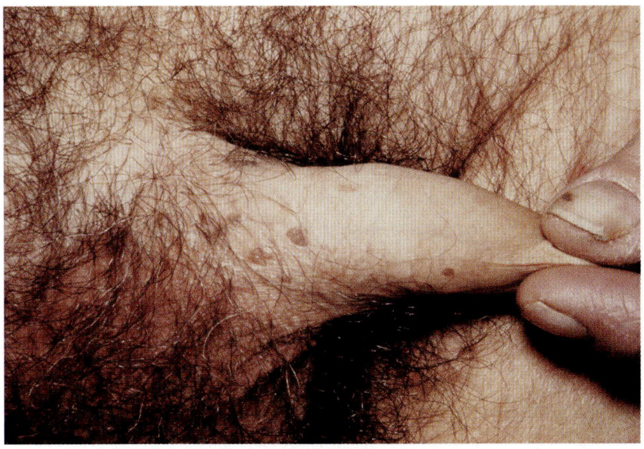

Fig. 9-44. Pigmented "warts" in light-complected patients are more likely to represent HPV-related intraepithelial neoplasia, also called HSIL, high-grade squamous intraepithelial lesions. This morphology is called Bowenoid papulosis.

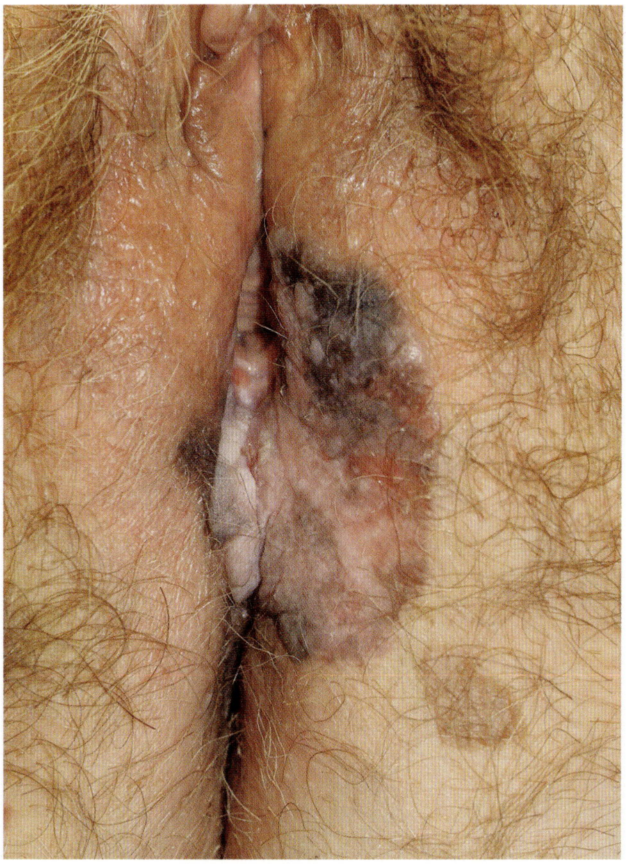

Fig. 9-45. This plaque of HSIL, or HPV-related intraepithelial neoplasia, shows hyperpigmented, hypopigmented, and red colors.

### Kaposi Sarcoma

The nodules and plaques of Kaposi sarcoma occurring on the trunk and genitalia are usually medium to dusky red in color. Less often they are darker in color and may have blue, purple, or even black hues (Fig. 9-49). This condition is also discussed in Chapters 6 and 15.

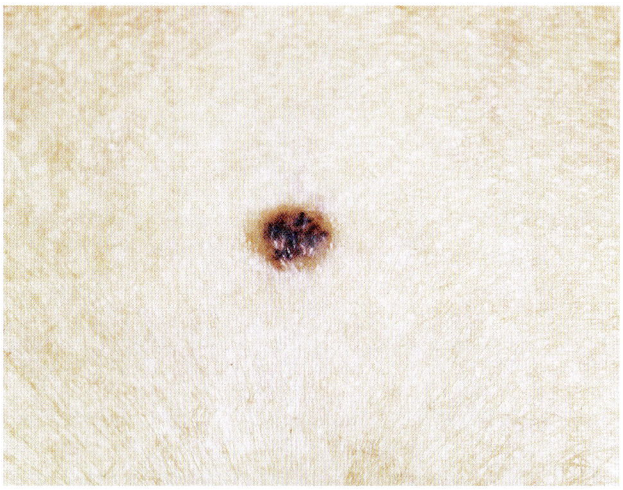

Fig. 9-46. Pigmented basal cell carcinomas classically appear translucent with flecks or tiny globules of black pigmented suspended within the papule.

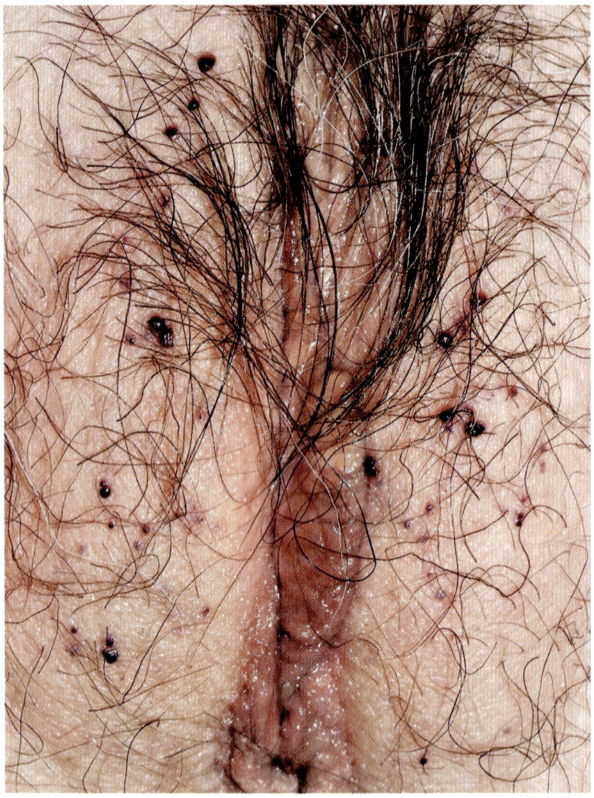

Fig. 9-47. Although angiokeratomas are vascular growths, they sometimes appear black. Dermoscopy shows the presence of tiny vessels, however.

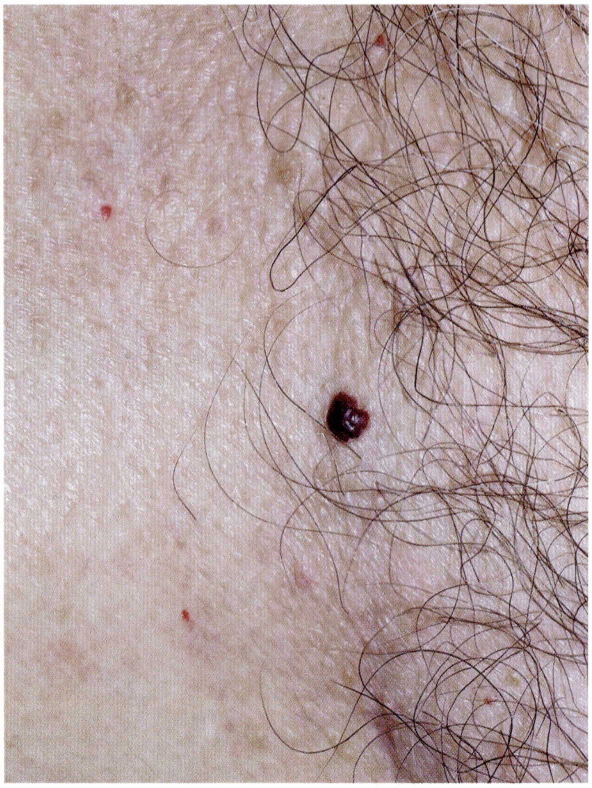

Fig. 9-48. A solitary angiokeratoma must sometimes be differentiated from a nodular melanoma.

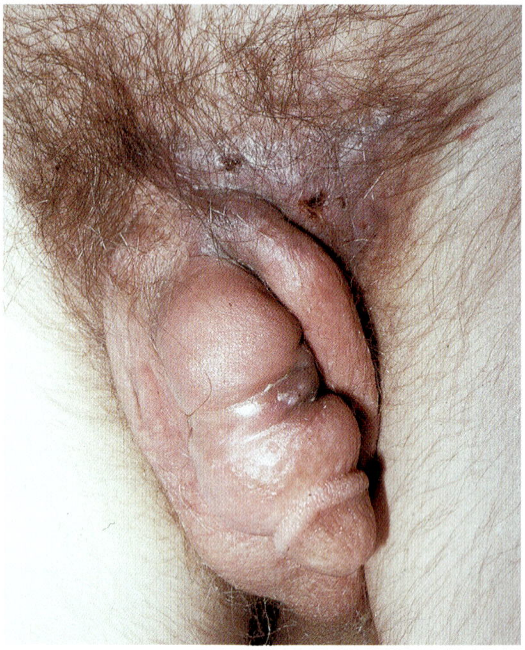

Fig. 9-49. Kaposi sarcoma is another vascular growth that can appear either purple or red brown; but this can sometimes simply present as hyperpigmented, especially in patients of color.

## REFERENCES


1. Venkatesan A. Pigmented lesions of the vulva. *Dermatol Clin.* 2010;28(4):795-805. doi:10.1016/j.det.2010.08.007
2. Gabrielson AT, Le TV, Fontenot C, Usta M, Hellstrom WJG. Male genital dermatology: a primer for the sexual medicine physician. *Sex Med Rev.* 2019;7(1):71-83. doi:10.1016/j.sxmr.2018.09.004
3. Maguolo A, Maffeis C. Acanthosis nigricans in childhood: a cutaneous marker that should not be underestimated, especially in obese children. *Acta Paediatr.* 2020;109(3):481-487. doi:10.1111/apa.15031
4. Sandhu S, Neema S, Radhakrishnan S. Dermoscopy of disorders of hyperpigmentation. *Pigment Int.* 2021;8:14-21.
5. Kaufman BP, Aman T, Alexis AF. Postinflammatory hyperpigmentation: epidemiology, clinical presentation, pathogenesis and treatment. *Am J Clin Dermatol.* 2018;19(4):489-503. doi:10.1007/s40257-017-0333-6
6. Cengiz FP, Emiroglu N, Wellenhof RH. Dermoscopic and clinical features of pigmented skin lesions of the genital area. *An Bras Dermatol.* 2015;90(2):178-183. doi:10.1590/abd1806-4841.20153294
7. Wollina U. Recent advances in managing and understanding seborrheic keratosis. *F1000Res.* 2019;8:F1000 Faculty Rev-1520. doi:10.12688/f1000research.18983.1
8. Karadag AS, Parish LC. The status of the seborrheic keratosis. *Clin Dermatol.* 2018;36(2):275-277. doi:10.1016/j.clindermatol.2017.09.011
9. Dasgupta S, van Eersel R, Morrel B, et al. Relationship of human papillomavirus with seborrheic keratosis of the female genital tract–a case-series and literature review. *Histol Histopathol.* 2021;36:1209-1218. doi:10.14670/HH-18-357
10. Kim AS, Greyling LA, Davis LS. Vulvar varicosities: a review. *Dermatol Surg.* 2017;43(3):351-356. doi:10.1097/DSS.0000000000001008

11. Basile A, Failla G, Gozzo C. Pelvic congestion syndrome. *Semin Ultrasound CT MR.* 2021;42(1):3-12. doi:10.1053/j.sult.2020.07.001
12. Xu C, Xia W, Sun Y, Chen H, Song T. Positive effects of the inclusion of open-mouth pressure for elimination of blood in microscopic subinguinal varicocelectomy. *Int Urol Nephrol.* 2019;51(11):1933-1939. doi:10.1007/s11255-019-02228-9
13. De Giorgi V, Gori A, Salvati L, et al. Clinical and dermoscopic features of vulvar melanosis over the last 20 years. *JAMA Dermatol.* 2020;156(11):1185-1191. doi:10.1001/jamadermatol.2020.2528
14. Haugh AM, Merkel EA, Zhang B, et al. A clinical, histologic, and follow-up study of genital melanosis in men and women. *J Am Acad Dermatol.* 2017;76(5):836-840. doi:10.1016/j.jaad.2016.11.003
15. Hieta N, Kurki S, Rintala M, et al. Association of vulvar melanoma with lichen sclerosus. *Acta Derm Venereol.* 2019;99(3):339-340. doi:10.2340/00015555-3103
16. Tekin HG, Skyum H, Spaun E, Juel J. Lichen sclerosus-associated nevus on glans penis mimicking melanoma. *JAAD Case Rep.* 2020;6(4):323-325. doi:10.1016/j.jdcr.2020.02.017
17. Savas S, Balı YY, Erdemir AV, Simsek H. Divided nevus of the penis. *Int J Dermatol.* 2018;57(6):724-726. doi:10.1111/ijd.13899
18. Xavier JCC Jr, Ocanha-Xavier JP, Camilo DJ Jr, D'ávilla SCGP, Mattar NJ. Series of 50 special-site nevi cases: is it a unique entity or only one variant of dysplastic nevi? *J Cutan Pathol.* 2020;47(7):664-666. doi:10.1111/cup.13670
19. Ahn CS, Guerra A, Sangüeza OP. Melanocytic nevi of special sites. *Am J Dermatopathol.* 2016;38(12):867-881. doi:10.1097/DAD.0000000000000568
20. Yélamos O, Merkel EA, Sholl LM, et al. Nonoverlapping clinical and mutational patterns in melanomas from the female genital tract and atypical genital nevi. *J Invest Dermatol.* 2016;136(9):1858-1865. doi:10.1016/j.jid.2016.05.094
21. Callahan A, Anderson WF, Patel S, et al. Epidemiology of anorectal melanoma in the United States: 1992 to 2011. *Dermatol Surg.* 2016;42(1):94-99. doi:10.1097/DSS.0000000000000579
22. Zarei S, Voss JS, Jin L, et al. Mutational profile in vulvar, vaginal, and urethral melanomas: review of 37 cases with focus on primary tumor site. *Int J Gynecol Pathol.* 2020;39(6):587-594. doi:10.1097/PGP.0000000000000636
23. Wohlmuth C, Wohlmuth-Wieser I, May T, et al. Malignant melanoma of the vulva and vagina: a US population-based study of 1863 patients. *Am J Clin Dermatol.* 2020;21(2):285-295. doi:10.1007/s40257-019-00487-x
24. Joste M, Dion L, Brousse S, et al. Vulvar and vaginal melanomas: a retrospective study spanning 19 years from a tertiary center. *J Gynecol Obstet Hum Reprod.* 2021;50(5):102091. doi:10.1016/j.jogoh.2021.102091
25. Tan A, Bieber AK, Stein JA, Pomeranz MK. Diagnosis and management of vulvar cancer: a review. *J Am Acad Dermatol.* 2019;81(6):1387-1396. doi:10.1016/j.jaad.2019.07.055
26. Sanchez A, Rodríguez D, Allard CB, et al. Primary genitourinary melanoma: epidemiology and disease-specific survival in a large population-based cohort. *Urol Oncol.* 2016;34(4):166.e7-166.e14. doi:10.1016/j.urolonc.2015.11.009
27. Vyas R, Thompson CL, Zargar H, Selph J, Gerstenblith MR. Epidemiology of genitourinary melanoma in the United States: 1992 through 2012. *J Am Acad Dermatol.* 2016;75(1):144-150. doi:10.1016/j.jaad.2015.10.015
28. Dodds TJ, Wilmott JS, Jackett LA, et al. Primary anorectal melanoma: clinical, immunohistology and DNA analysis of 43 cases. *Pathology.* 2019;51(1):39-45. doi:10.1016/j.pathol.2018.09.060
29. Zheng Y, Cong C, Su C, Sun Y, Xing L. Epidemiology and survival outcomes of primary gastrointestinal melanoma: a SEER-based population study. *Int J Clin Oncol.* 2020;25(11):1951-1959. doi:10.1007/s10147-020-01759-x
30. Davis LE, Shalin SC, Tackett AJ. Current state of melanoma diagnosis and treatment. *Cancer Biol Ther.* 2019;20(11):1366-1379. doi:10.1080/15384047.2019.1640032
31. Nassar KW, Tan AC. The mutational landscape of mucosal melanoma. *Semin Cancer Biol.* 2020;61:139-148. doi:10.1016/j.semcancer.2019.09.013
32. Keung EZ, Gershenwald JE. The eighth edition American Joint Committee on Cancer (AJCC) melanoma staging system: implications for melanoma treatment and care. *Expert Rev Anticancer Ther.* 2018;18(8):775-784. doi:10.1080/14737140.2018.1489246
33. Kaur H, Nikam BP, Jamale VP, Kale MS. Lichen planus severity index: a new, valid scoring system to assess the severity of cutaneous lichen planus. *Indian J Dermatol Venereol Leprol.* 2020;86(2):169-175. doi:10.4103/ijdvl.IJDVL_650_17
34. Diop A, Ly F, Ndiaye MT, et al. Epidemiology, clinical features, and associated factors in 78 cases of lichen planus on black skin. *Int J Dermatol.* 2020;59(2):137-142. doi:10.1111/ijd.14698
35. Errichetti E. Dermoscopy of inflammatory dermatoses (inflammoscopy): an up-to-date overview. *Dermatol Pract Concept.* 2019;9:169-180. doi:10.5826/dpc.0903a01


## SUGGESTED READINGS


Cengiz FP, Emiroglu N, Wellenhof RH. Dermoscopic and clinical features of pigmented skin lesions of the genital area. *An Bras Dermatol.* 2015;90(2):178-183. doi:10.1590/abd1806-4841.20153294

Davis LE, Shalin SC, Tackett AJ. Current state of melanoma diagnosis and treatment. *Cancer Biol Ther.* 2019;20(11):1366-1379. doi:10.1080/15384047.2019.1640032

De Giorgi V, Gori A, Salvati L, et al. Clinical and dermoscopic features of vulvar melanosis over the last 20 years. *JAMA Dermatol.* 2020;156(11):1185-1191. doi:10.1001/jamadermatol.2020.2528

Haugh AM, Merkel EA, Zhang B, et al. A clinical, histologic, and follow-up study of genital melanosis in men and women. *J Am Acad Dermatol.* 2017;76(5):836-840. doi:10.1016/j.jaad.2016.11.003

Tan A, Bieber AK, Stein JA, Pomeranz MK. Diagnosis and management of vulvar cancer: a review. *J Am Acad Dermatol.* 2019;81(6):1387-1396. doi:10.1016/j.jaad.2019.07.055

Tuma B, Sergio Yamada S, Atallah AN, Araujo FM, Hirata SH. Dermoscopy of black skin: a cross-sectional study of clinical and dermoscopic features of melanocytic lesions in individuals with type V/VI skin compared to those with type I/II skin. *J Am Acad Dermatol.* 2015;73:114-119. doi:10.1016/j.jaad.2015.03.043

# Blistering and Pustular Diseases 10

LIBBY EDWARDS

Blisters are skin lesions that are filled with fluid. Blisters larger than half a centimeter are called bullae, and those smaller are called vesicles. Certainly, there is overlap between bullae and vesicles, but most vesicular diseases have primarily small blisters, and most bullous diseases have prominent larger blisters. Pustules are blister that are filled with pus, and these are nearly always small. Sometimes the identification of blisters and pustules is not straightforward. When blisters occur on fragile skin such as the genital area or any mucous membrane, the blister is unroofed quickly, leaving erosions so that the original blistering nature is not appreciated. Also, some blistering lesions are superficial and thus innately fragile, with the blister split occurring within the epidermis. Erosions resulting from a blister are usually well demarcated and round, or arcuate when blisters coalesce before eroding. Often, there are blisters on surrounding or extragenital skin that provide a clue to the blistering nature. As an intact vesicle ages, the fluid can appear cloudy and mimic a pustule. However, if the lesion is pierced, the fluid is clear rather than thick pus, showing the true vesicular nature.

## Blistering Infections

### Herpes Simplex Virus Infection

The classic genital vesicular disease is herpes simplex virus (HSV) infection, a lifelong sexually transmitted disease that is often asymptomatic but, when symptomatic, manifested by recurrent painful blisters and erosions. There are two types of HSV, type 1, which primarily produces oral infection, and type 2, which accounts for the vast majority of genital HSV infection. The Center for Disease Control reports that there is an increasing proportion of HSV 1 occurring on genital skin,[1] presumably due to the frequency of oral sexual activity.

There are estimates of nearly half a billion people 0-49 years old worldwide with genital HSV infection in 2016, of whom only 122-192 million are caused by HSV 1.[2] In the United States, there was an estimated prevalence of 18.6 million people between 18 and 49 years with HSV-2, with two-thirds of infections occurring in women.[3] Older people are more likely to be seropositive than younger, and numbers are highest in Africa, with South Pacific, South Asia, and then the Americas next. In the United States, 12.1% of individuals age 14-49 were positive for HSV 2, down from 18% in 1999-2000.[2] Highest numbers were in non-Hispanic Black patients (34.6%), and lowest in non-Hispanic Asians (3.8%), with almost twice as many women affected as men.[2]

#### Clinical Presentation

Herpes simplex virus infection is especially likely in younger, sexually active individuals, and in those who have higher risks of contagion due to several lifetime sexual partners.

Most people with genital HSV are unaware of their disease and experience latent disease. HSV produces both primary and recurrent infections. Primary infection with HSV is often subclinical and unrecognized, estimated to occur in about 80% of cases. When a primary infection is recognized, the outbreak is much more severe than recurrent episodes. Primary genital HSV infection follows exposure by 2-7 days and generally exhibits associated fever, malaise, headache, and other constitutional symptoms. Regional lymphadenopathy is usual; pain and edema may cause urinary retention. The lesions present as 1 to 3 mm, scattered and grouped vesicles occurring typically on the mucous membrane and modified mucous membrane portion of the vulva, sometimes extending to keratinized skin, or the glans or shaft of the penis in men (**Figs. 10-1 through 10-9**). Often, well-demarcated, discrete, round, and arcuate erosions in addition to or instead of vesicles are seen, because the blisters are fragile and quickly rupture. Healing requires about 2 weeks but may be complicated by irritation from overwashing or topical agents used empirically by an anxious patient.

After a primary infection, HSV remains latent in neuronal cells located in the dorsal ganglia. Then, the virus may intermittently reactivate, producing recurrent disease that is usually milder, localized, and shorter in duration. These recurrences are generally not associated with constitutional symptoms. However, patients experience a prodrome of localized tingling, burning, or dysesthesias before the onset of skin lesions. Recurrent HSV is also often located on the mucous membranes and modified

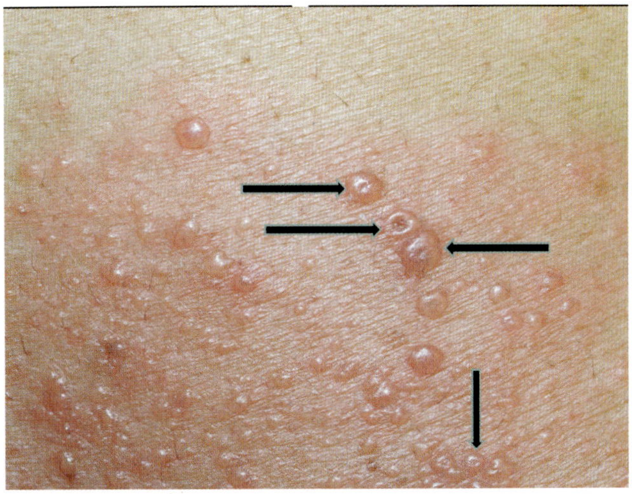

Fig. 10-1. Clustered vesicles are classic for a recurrent herpes simplex virus infection; a classic herpes vesicle, both herpes simplex and varicella zoster virus vesicle, collapses in the center as it ages. Several of these small blisters have small depressions, more or less obvious depending upon the degree of the collapse of the center (*arrows*).

mucous membrane portion of the vulva, or the glans and shaft of the penis, but lesions can occur on any epithelial surface, including the buttocks, sacral area, scrotum, perianal skin, and hair-bearing labia majora. Rather than scattered discrete vesicles, recurrent episodes are characterized by a small area of grouped vesicles that quickly develop into well-demarcated, round, and arciform erosions. Round crusts rather than erosion are common on dry, keratinized skin such as the shaft of the penis or the hair-bearing labia majora. Rarely, recurrent HSV outbreaks can occur as fissures, most often in skinfolds, such as the interlabial sulci of the vulva or within normal skin wrinkling of the penile shaft.

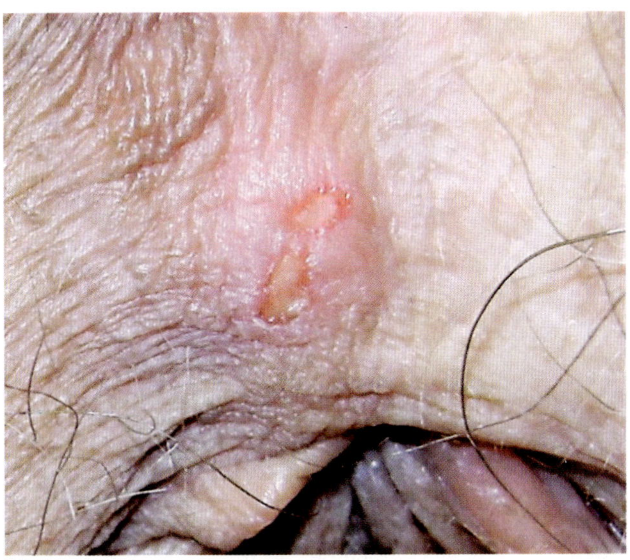

Fig. 10-2. These oval erosions are typical of the remains of the fragile vesicles of HSV on delicate skin.

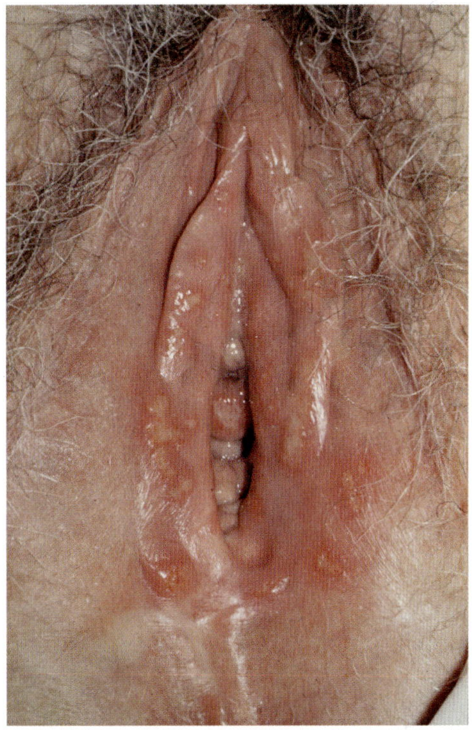

Fig. 10-3. Primary HSV is characterized by widespread discrete and coalescing erosions rather than a localized plaque of erosions or vesicles.

Usually, the first recognized episode of a genital HSV infection has a recurrent pattern and course, since the primary infection is most often subclinical and, therefore, unrecognized. Because the appearance of this nonprimary but first clinical episode is delayed, the time and

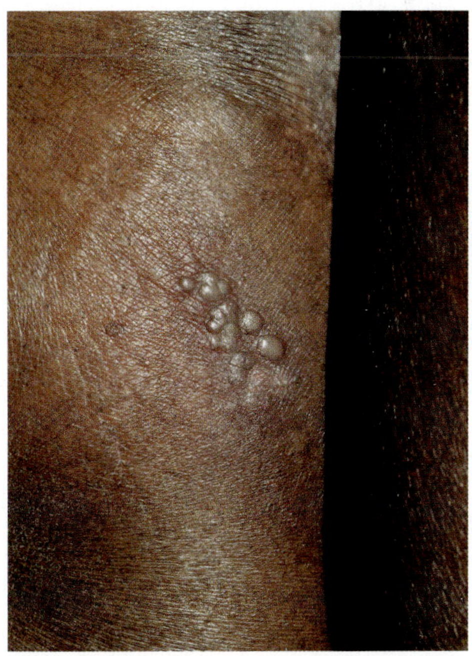

Fig. 10-4. These typical vesicles of recurrent HSV on the buttocks are on keratinized skin and tend to remain as blisters longer than those on thinner genital skin or mucosa.

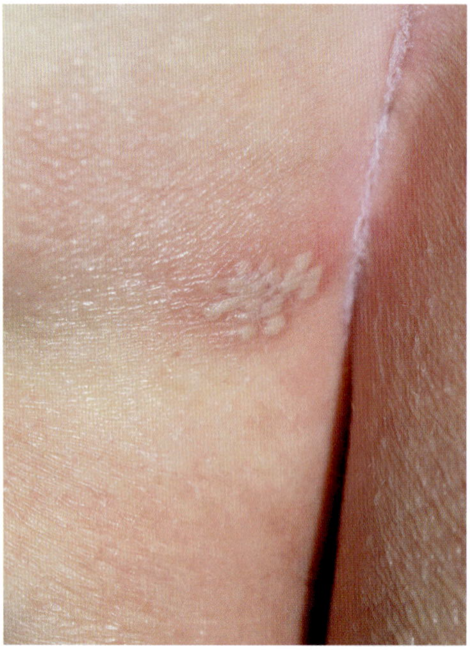

Fig. 10-5. Older vesicles often appear pustular; however, if these are pierced, clear fluid is expressed, showing the true vesicular nature.

circumstances of transmission cannot be determined; on occasion, this delay is years long.

Immunosuppressed patients sometimes are unable to contain their HSV infections. This is especially common in those with cell-mediated issues as occurs in human immunodeficiency virus disease and immunosuppressive medications (see Chapters 7 and 15). These patients are likely to experience chronic HSV that can become ulcerative rather than erosive, with ongoing enlargement of the area of involvement (**Fig. 10-10**). In addition, there is a synergistic effect of HSV and HIV, with the presence of HSV infection predisposing to HIV infection.

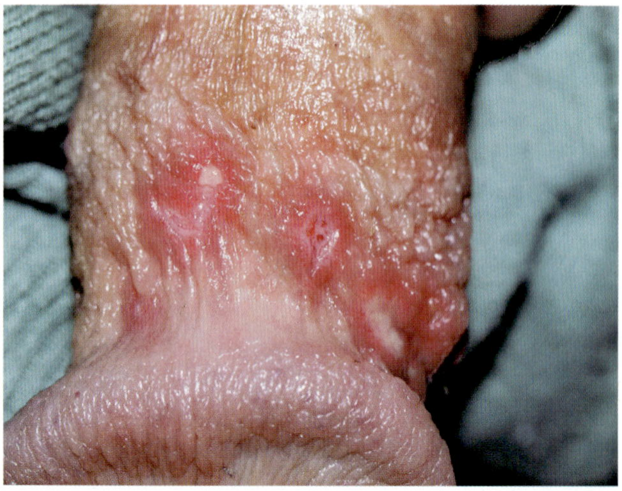

Fig. 10-6. Sometimes these superficial erosions become macerated and lose their sharp definition that otherwise normally displays round erosions of HSV.

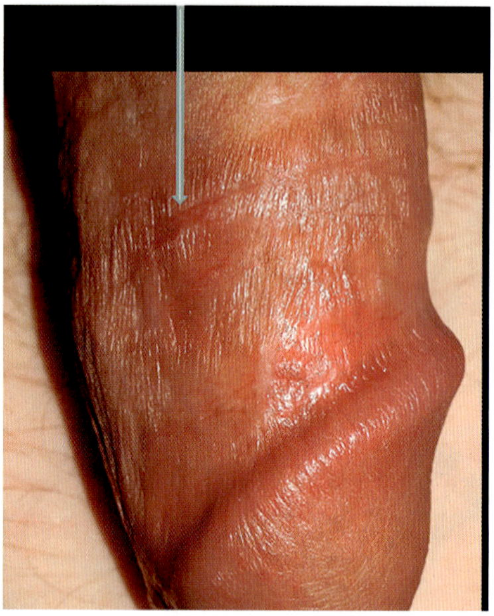

Fig. 10-7. Uncommonly, HSV produces fissures (*arrow*).

Also, HSV has been shown to be a risk factor for bacterial vaginosis in women. And, the association with depression, loss of self-esteem, and shame is well recognized. A recent study shows that depression associated with HSV may even be higher than that associated with HIV.[4]

## Diagnosis

The diagnosis of classic HSV is a clinical one, but laboratory confirmation is often important to the patient, since the diagnosis is psychologically crucial. The test of choice is polymerase chain reaction, with sensitivity of 80%-90%. A swab for direct fluorescent antibody is quick and is positive in 60%-70% of cases, but an ade-

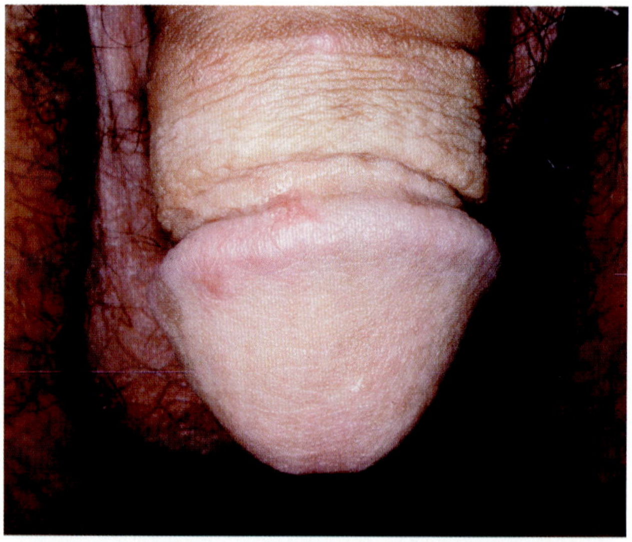

Fig. 10-8. Very mild or early HSV can be very subtle and show only red papules without clinical vesicles. However, a biopsy shows microscopic changes of HSV.

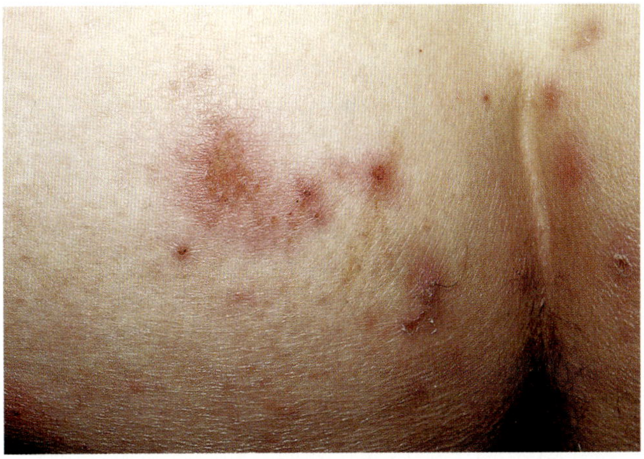

Fig. 10-9. Sacral HSV is often pruritic, and the resulting rubbing and scratching give it an eczematous rather than vesicular appearance. Only the recurrent nature and location indicate the diagnosis.

quate sample is of utmost importance.[5] Scraping the base of the ulcer with a number 15 blade usually suffices for an adequate cell sample, but the CDC reports that sensitivity is inadequate.[1] A viral culture is only positive in about 50% of patients with HSV. Very sensitive is a shave skin biopsy from the edge of an erosion or of an intact vesicle **(Fig. 10-11)**. However, a biopsy only diagnoses the presence of a herpes blister but does not differentiate HSV from VZV. That differentiation can generally be made clinically. The Tzanck preparation, although very quick, is less reliable, even in experienced hands, and again does not differentiate between HSV and VZV.[1] Serology is not an adequate means of diagnosing an episode of HSV. Positive IgG for HSV varies very widely according to the country, occurring in up to 80% of adults; this denotes exposure, but not current, active disease. Negative serology indicates no past infection, but does not rule out a primary episode, since about 6 weeks is required for conversion.

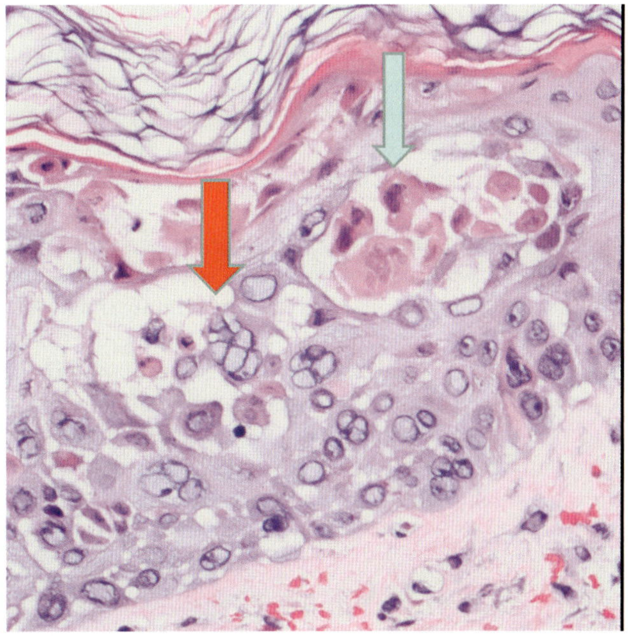

Fig. 10-11. The biopsy of HSV is a sensitive means to diagnose a herpes blister, although it cannot differentiate between herpes simplex and herpes zoster. Epidermal cells coalesce into multinucleate cells (*red arrow*) with the nuclei molded together into a cluster, and red cells are necrotic (*blue arrow*); this necrosis eventually leads to a vesicle as the necrotic cells fall apart.

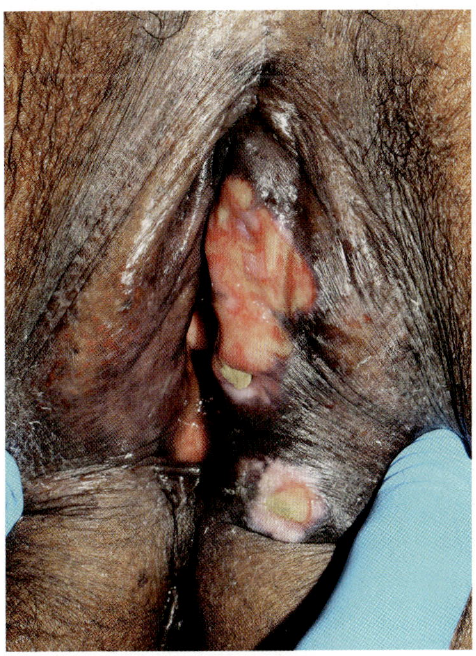

Fig. 10-10. HSV in an immunosuppressed patient sometimes is not self-limited, but rather enlarges relentlessly, losing all semblance of its original blistering nature as has occurred in this woman with a kidney transplant.

The histologic appearance of HSV includes an intraepidermal vesicular dermatitis formed by acantholysis. Individual keratinocytes show intracellular edema (ballooning) and reticular degeneration (intracellular edema causing cell walls to burst). Eosinophilic intranuclear inclusion bodies may be present. Multinucleated keratinocytes are pathognomic for herpes virus infections but do not distinguish between HSV and varicella-zoster virus (VZV) infections.

HSV must be differentiated from several other vesicular and pustular diseases. Occasionally, the differentiation of genital HSV infection from VZV infection can be difficult, because both exhibit grouped vesicles or erosions. However, genital VZV infection usually occurs in the older patient and presents in a dermatomal pattern, also affecting the medial thigh or buttock unilaterally. VZV infection occurs once in the immunocompetent patient, rather than recurrently, as is usual with HSV infection. The fragile pustule roofs of Candidiasis of the modified mucous membranes of the vulva or the uncircumcised glans penis sometimes mimic the erosions of HSV. A fungal smear is positive in that case. Scattered discrete red papules, pustules, or crusts of folliculitis, both irritant and staphylococcal, can resemble primary HSV. Erythema multiforme and Stevens-Johnson syndrome both mimic and sometimes follow HSV infection. A hypersensitivity reaction to HSV is the most common cause of recurrent erythema multiforme. These patients with blistering erythema multiforme usually exhibit both intraoral and genital erosions that are less well demarcated than those of HSV, and HSV does not occur inside the mouth, except for the initial primary outbreak. In addition, erythema multiforme generally also exhibits red, nonscaling, flat-topped papules or even blisters on the palms, soles, and sometimes other keratinized surfaces is common. Finally, a fixed drug eruption can mimic herpes simplex virus infection by producing same-site recurrent blisters or erosions, but the lesions are generally larger rather than showing small coalescing vesicles or erosions.

### HERPES SIMPLEX VIRUS INFECTION Diagnosis

- Presentation
- Primary, first episode HSV with scattered and grouped vesicles and round erosions on genital and perianal skin
- Recurrent with grouped vesicles or erosions
- Prodrome of tingling or burning
- Confirmation by polymerase chain reaction technique or biopsy

## Pathophysiology

Herpes simplex virus (HSV) types 1 and 2 are double-stranded DNA viruses (*Herpesvirus hominis*) capable of producing vesicular and erosive mucocutaneous disease. Genital HSV infection is usually produced by HSV type 2, while oral mucocutaneous and ocular disease are produced by HSV 1, despite the frequency of oral sexual activity. Essentially all HSV 2 is transmitted via genital-to-genital contact, whereas HSV 1 is transmitted by oral to genital contact, through saliva as well as direct contact with active oral lesions. Preexisting oral HSV 1 is protective against the acquisition of genital HSV 1, but not against contagion of HSV 2. Fortunately, genital disease produced by HSV 1 is less severe and less frequently recurrent that that produced by HSV 2, and neonatal HSV is less problematic in women with HSV 1.

Estradiol is known to be protective against the acquisition of HSV2, which is surprising since this infection is twice as common in men as women; a recent study suggest that the mechanism of action may be an enhanced establishment of antiviral memory T-cell responses in the presence of estradiol when exposed to HSV.[6] However, there is evidence that some hormonal contraceptives, especially depot medroxyprogesterone acetate, may increase the risk of HSV acquisition.[7]

## Management

The management of HSV infection involves far more than prescribing antiviral medication, and ideally would begin with prevention and education before exposure.[8] However, from a practical standpoint, this begins with the sensitive and nonjudgmental education and counseling of the patient. This is not a diagnosis that should be given by a nonmedical office worker or by email. These patients exhibit marked anxiety, depression, fear, and self-esteem issues. There are little data on the best means for the management of the psychological effects of the diagnosis of genital HSV infection, but counseling and support should be provided or arranged.

The patient should be informed regarding the infectivity of the disease, its recurrent nature, and the importance of avoidance of sexual intercourse when open lesions are present. However, patients also should be counseled that intermittent shedding of the virus occurs when there is no evidence of active HSV infection, and the infection can be transmitted even in the absence of blisters and erosions. In fact, most HSV infection is contracted during asymptomatic episodes. Shedding also occurs in those receiving long-term suppressive antiviral medication, albeit in smaller amounts. Circumcision and condoms have been shown to confer modest protection from infection. Therefore, the use of a condom, even when there are no obvious lesions, is wise and confers significant but not complete protection.[9] Neonatal transmission of HSV during delivery should be discussed to ensure the protection of future infants, although most neonatal HSV infections occur due to maternal primary infection, or at least recent acquisition.

HSV infections are shortened by prompt treatment with specific oral antiviral agents.[1] There are three very equally effective antiviral choices for HSV. Primary HSV infection can be treated with acyclovir 400 mg three times a day, valacyclovir 1 g twice a day, or famciclovir 250 mg twice a day for 7-10 days, and the duration can be extended if lesions have not healed. A mild initial infection does not predict mild recurrences, and some patents will experience severe future outbreaks. All patients should be prepared for recurrences, at least with prescriptions, and even better with prescriptions that have been filled. Medication should be started with the prodrome, or at least with the first sign of lesions. Recurrences can be treated with acyclovir 800 mg 3 times a day for 2 days or 800 mg 2 times a day for 5 days; famciclovir 1 g twice a day for 1 day or 500 mg once followed by 250 mg twice a day for 2 days, or 125 mg twice daily for 5 days; or valacyclovir 500 mg for 3 days or 1 g daily for 5 days. Side effects are minimal with each. Topical antiviral agents provide minimal benefit.

Suppressive therapy with chronic oral antiviral agents is often used for patients who experience frequent recurrences and to decrease shedding and to minimize, but not eliminate, the risk of transmission. Regimens for those with genital HSV 2 include acyclovir 400 mg twice daily, valacyclovir 500 mg or 1 g daily, or famciclovir 250 mg twice daily.[1] Recurrences with genital HSV 1 are much less frequent with genital HSV 1, and after the first year, asymptomatic shedding is far less, so that suppressive therapy is often not required.

Intravenous acyclovir 5-10 mg/kg every 8 hours until clinical resolution occurs is occasionally needed if disease is severe, or there is organ involvement, especially if the patient is immunosuppressed or if gastrointestinal absorption is a major problem, as can occur in the HIV-positive patient. Resistance of HSV to currently available oral medications is rare and occurs primarily in immunocompromised patients, and the following are alternative treatments.[1] Therapies include foscarnet 40-80 mg/kg IV every 8 hours until clinical resolution occurs is first-line therapy. Cidofovir 5 mg/kg IV weekly is also used. Both medications are nephrotoxic and should be administered by infectious disease specialists. Imiquimod 5% applied to the lesion for 8 hours 3 times/week has been reported to be effective as has compounded cidofovir gel 1% applied 2-4 times daily; however, cidofovir must be compounded at a pharmacy.

Therapeutic vaccines have been studied for years with many results in the literature, and COVID 19 has introduced new ideas and methods with use of mRNA vaccines. Some vaccines have shown promise, with high neutralizing titers and robust B-cell immune response.[10,11]

Some patients erroneously believe that HSV infection can be followed by postherpetic neuralgia. Fortunately, that is not a sequel to this infection; this only follows herpes zoster infection. Primary HSV infection can produce malaise and fever, and sometimes outbreaks can create radicular pain. Very rarely, HSV can cause HSV encephalitis.

**HERPES SIMPLEX VIRUS INFECTION Management**

- Patient education
- Antiviral therapy—primary
  - Acyclovir 400 mg tid for 7-10 days
  - Valacyclovir 1 g bid for 7-10 days
  - famciclovir 250 mg tid for 7-10 days
- Antiviral therapy—recurrences
  - Acyclovir 800 mg bid for 5 days, or 800 mg tid for 2 days
  - Valacyclovir 1 g daily for 5 days or 500 mg bid for 3 days
  - Famciclovir 1 g bid for 1 day, or 500 mg once, then 250 mg bid for 2 day, or 125 mg bid for 5 days
- Suppression of HSV 2:
  - Acyclovir 400 mg bid
  - Valacyclovir 500 mg to 1 g daily
  - Famciclovir 250 mg bid

## Herpes Zoster Infection (Varicella, Shingles)

Varicella zoster virus (VZV) is a virus that is related to HSV, produces blisters that are similar morphologically, and lies latent in nerve ganglia like HSV. However, this virus causes two diseases distinct from those produced by HSV; the primary infection of scattered discrete vesicles, varicella, and herpes zoster, with grouped vesicles along a dermatome. Both can affect the genitalia but present very differently. The first episode of VZV (varicella, chicken pox) is rare in Western countries because of the availability of a very effective vaccine and presents with generalized rash. The subsequent episode of VZV, herpes zoster, is localized and painful. Hopefully, with the availability of both the varicella and shingles vaccines, these conditions will become vanishingly rare.

### Clinical Presentation

The initial infection with VZV is varicella (chickenpox). This usually occurs in childhood and is extraordinarily infectious, so that in the past, nearly all adults had had varicella, whether or not it was remembered. Now, in most industrialized countries, adults over 30 years were vaccinated as children, and childhood varicella is rare. Varicella presents with fever and constitutional symptoms, then a generalized pruritic eruption of vesicles with a predilection for the genital skin and vagina. Lesions begin as small red papules, then evolve into vesicles that develop the central depression that is characteristic of a herpetic vesicle, and then a central crust. Multiple stages of these lesions simultaneously are characteristic (**Fig. 10-12**). Mucous membranes are often involved.

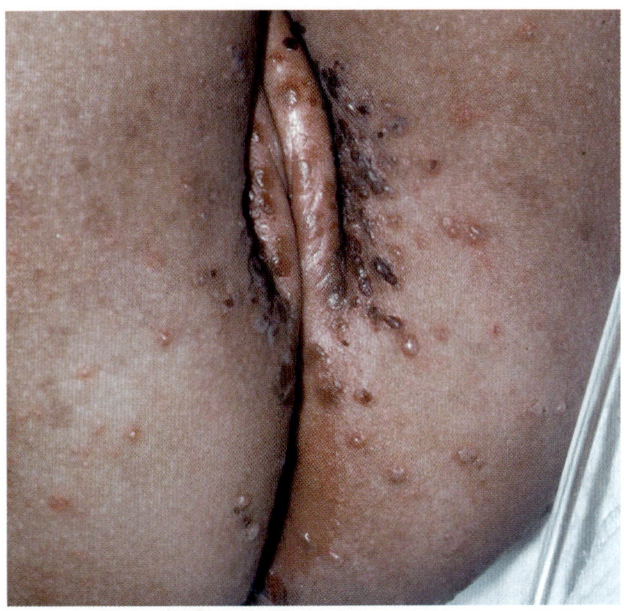

Fig. 10-12. Varicella is mostly a childhood disease and manifested by red papules, vesicles, and crusts that include both keratinized skin and mucous membranes.

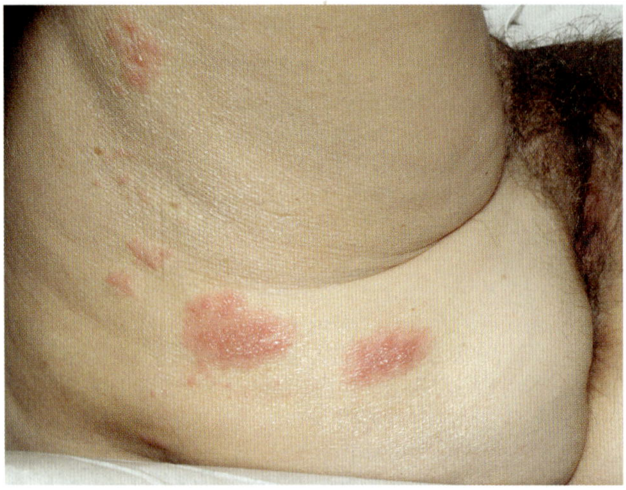

Fig. 10-13. Clustered and coalescing vesicles on a red base, distributed along a dermatome are characteristic of herpes zoster.

The reactivation of the latent varicella zoster virus, herpes zoster, occurs primarily in patients with immune deficiency by virtue of age, disease, or medications, but occasionally occurs in young and healthy individuals. Constitutional symptoms are minimal or absent compared to varicella, but many patients experience a localized prodrome of pain, itching, burning, or aching, followed in one or a few days by pink, nonscaling papules and plaques that resemble hives in a unilateral dermatomal distribution **(Figs. 10-13 and 10-14)** in the symptomatic area. Blisters they form on the pink plaques, and coalesce into larger blisters. Hemorrhage into the blisters later give a purple, purpuric color to some blisters **(Fig. 10-15)**. Then, the blisters crust and heal over the next 2 or 3 weeks. The surface of fragile blisters on mucous membranes and modified mucous membranes of the genitalia are quickly unroofed so that erosions usually predominate in those areas. Likewise, the friction from skinfolds and clothing often tears blister roofs even on the more keratinized genital skin. Herpes zoster can become disseminated, ulcerative, chronic, or hyperkeratotic in immunosuppressed patients (see Chapter 15).

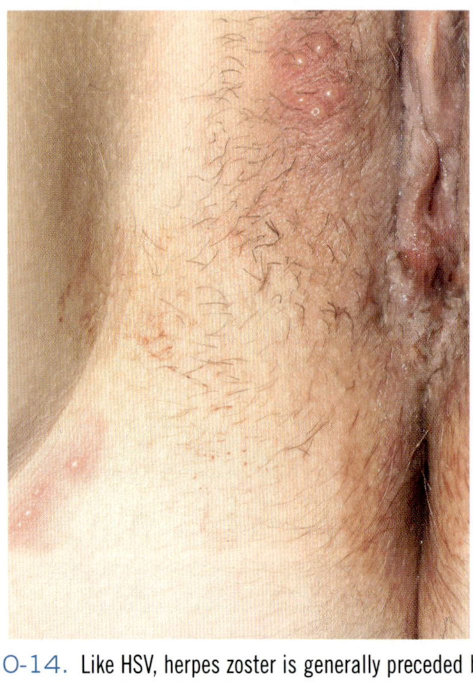

Fig. 10-14. Like HSV, herpes zoster is generally preceded by a prodrome of pain in the distribution of the skin lesions.

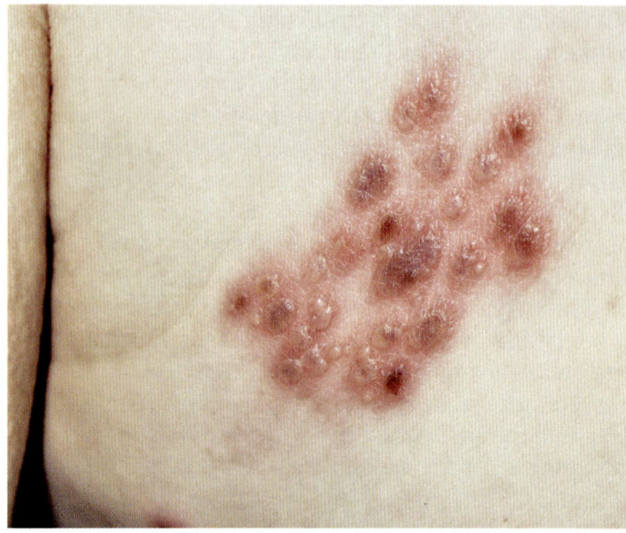

Fig. 10-15. The vesicles of herpes zoster arise from a deeper red base than those of HSV, and they often coalesce into a larger vesicle. Bleeding into the vesicles of herpes zoster sometimes gives them a gray or purple appearance.

Herpes zoster is sometimes associated with mild headache, malaise, and a low-grade fever. But, the primary complication of herpes zoster infection is the development of postherpetic neuralgia, in which chronic pain persists after the eruption resolves. This is most common in individuals over 60 years of age and in immunosuppressed people. Unlike HSV, VZV does not typically recur in immunocompetent patients, and most patients with "recurrent shingles" of the genitalia actually experience recurrent HSV. Although some providers believe that postherpetic neuralgia is responsible for vulvodynia, penodynia, and scrotodynia, historically herpes zoster rarely is reported as a preceding event. There is now a suggestion that vaccination with COVID 19 may precipitate the appearance of herpes zoster.[12]

### Diagnosis

The diagnosis of herpes zoster is usually made clinically, on the basis of plaques of blisters distributed along dermatomes. When necessary, this can be confirmed by the identification of viral DNA with the PCR technique. The virus is rather fastidious, so cultures are sometimes falsely negative, but the PCR technique is very sensitive and now easily available when performed in the first 48-72 hours. A Tzanck preparation is poorly validated and does not differentiate HSV from

VZV. A biopsy is extremely sensitive but also does not differentiate between HSV infection and herpes zoster, a distinction that can usually be made on clinical grounds.

The histologic appearance of herpes zoster infection is identical to that of HSV infection. Keratinocytes swell and burst, and some epithelial cells form giant cells. Occasionally, leukocytoclastic vasculitis underlies these epithelial changes, but this does not indicate a primary or possibly systemic problem of vasculitis.

Occasionally, genital herpes zoster can be difficult to differentiate from HSV. However, HSV is a recurrent disease, whereas herpes zoster is a one-time event, except in significantly immunosuppressed patients. Both diseases can be unilateral, and both are classically painful. Other blistering diseases should be considered, such as bullous impetigo, but these usually show larger blisters, are not generally grouped, are not especially painful, and not dermatomal in distribution.

**HERPES ZOSTER VIRUS INFECTION Diagnosis**

- Morphology of painful plaques of clustered vesicles in a dermatomal distribution
- Confirmation by PCR if needed

### Pathophysiology

Herpes zoster infection is a blistering disease that results from reactivation of VZV that has been latent in nerve ganglia since a remote episode of varicella. This condition occurs most often in older individuals whose immune system is less efficient or in immunocompromised patients.

### Management

Even more important than antiviral therapy is pain control for most patients. Narcotic pain analgesia is needed in some patient for the first few weeks. Only very early diagnosis and treatment (within 72, but especially 48 hours) with oral antiviral therapy somewhat reduces the duration of an acute infection. This improvement is not striking, so therapy is optional in younger, healthy patients. Treatment after this time does not affect the short-term or long-term course of the disease. However, immunosuppressed or elderly people should be treated. Some studies have shown an arguably significant reduction of postherpetic neuralgia in patients treated early.

Choices include acyclovir 800 mg five times a day for 7-10 days, famciclovir 500 mg three times daily for 7 days, and valacyclovir 1 g every 8 hours for 7 days. The advantage of valacyclovir and famciclovir is the less frequent dosing schedule.

Those patients who experience postherpetic neuralgia deserve medication for neuropathic pain, including amitriptyline, gabapentin, pregabalin, venlafaxine, or duloxetine, the same medications as used for genital pain syndromes and discussed in Chapter 13. Sometimes, referral to a pain clinic is necessary. These medications can be started early, since several weeks are required for onset of relief.

Otherwise, the best current management is prevention. A two dose effective vaccine for the prevention of herpes zoster is available, approved by the Food and Drug Administration for people over 60 years of age.

**HERPES ZOSTER VIRUS INFECTION Management**

- Patient education
- Antiviral therapy
    - Acyclovir 800 mg 5×/day for 7-10 days
    - Valacyclovir 1 g q8h for 7 days
    - Famciclovir 500 mg tid for 7days
- Pain control
- Attention to post herpetic neuralgia

## Impetigo

Impetigo is a bacterial infection of the superficial epidermis that produces blisters, crusting, and erosions. Some phage types of *Staphylococcus aureus* cause separation of the stratum corneum from the rest of the epidermis and very fragile blisters, with rapid loss of this fragile blister roof. Then, well-demarcated, superficial round erosions with collarettes are typical **(Fig. 10-16)**. When produced by α-hemolytic *Streptococcus* infection, the classic honey

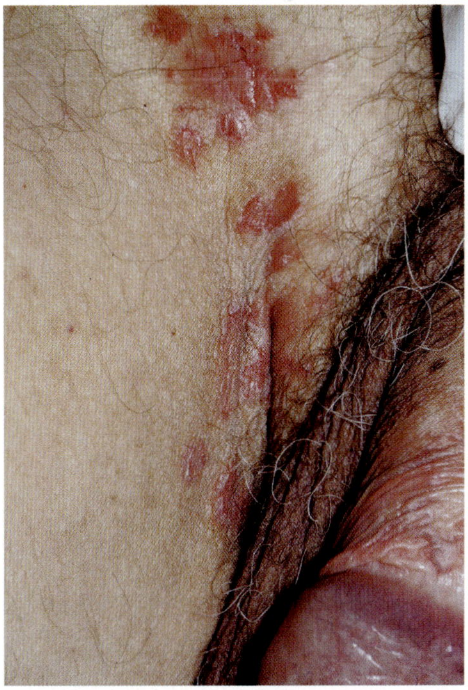

Fig. 10-16. Bullous impetigo consists of extremely fragile blisters, so that the blister roof desquamates quickly, leaving an extremely superficial erosion with a red base.

crusting and erosions commonly occur. Bacterial folliculitis often accompanies impetigo, where infection that has extended into nearby hair follicles, producing discrete red papules, pustules, and small erosions and crusts. The diagnosis is confirmed by a bacterial culture and response to therapy. A culture is important due to the frequency of resistant *S aureus*. Treatment consists of an antibiotic effective against both *S aureus* and *Streptococcus* species while awaiting culture results, such as cephalexin, clindamycin, and trimethoprim-sulfamethoxazole. Despite prompt response to therapy, lesions sometimes recur after therapy. This occurs most often in patients who are nasal carriers of *S aureus*, and these patients benefit from the administration of intranasal mupirocin cream or ointment four times a day, for 1 week each month for several months to minimize this carrier state.

## Noninfectious Blistering Eruptions

Blisters that are not produced by infection are usually caused by autoimmune disease, hypersensitivity reactions, or chemical or thermal burns, but Hailey-Hailey disease results from a genetic abnormality in the structure of the skin.

In autoimmune blistering diseases, autoantibodies are directed against target antigens that are involved in helping epithelial cells adhere to each other or to the basement membrane. Such antibodies fix to the target antigen and trigger complement activation that eventuates in destruction of the adherence of these structures to each other, resulting in blisters. The fragile blisters of the mucous membranes and modified mucous membranes are so transient as to be unnoticed, and the usual presentation is that of erosion. However, the round shapes of the erosions and the frequent accompanying blisters on nearby keratinized skin often declare the underlying blistering nature of the disease.

A biopsy is important for the correct diagnosis of noninfectious blistering diseases. The best site for biopsy is the edge of a blister on nonmucous membrane skin, so that both normal skin and the blister are visualized, and the location of the blister within the skin is seen. The sample is placed in formalin for a routine biopsy. The edge of an erosion often gives the diagnosis if an intact blister is not present. If there are no intact blisters on keratinized skin, then the edge of an erosion or mucous membrane blister can be sampled. When an immunobullous disease is considered, nearby normal skin should be sampled and placed in transport media for direct immunofluorescent testing.

### Pemphigus

#### Clinical Presentation

Pemphigus comprises a group of associated autoimmune superficial blistering diseases that affect the skin and mucous membranes. There are three major types of pemphigus; pemphigus vulgaris, making up about 70% of all patients with pemphigus; pemphigus foliaceous, which does not exhibit mucous membrane involvement; and paraneoplastic pemphigus. This discussion is directed toward pemphigus vulgaris. Pemphigus vulgaris (vulgaris, meaning common) occurs most often between the ages of 30 and 60 years, most frequently in women, and more common in the Ashkenazi Jewish population and Mediterranean descendants.[13] Childhood cases are rare.

Most patients with pemphigus vulgaris present with painful oral erosions that are not recognized as blisters. Blisters on extramucosal skin may not follow for several months. Nearly all patients with pemphigus vulgaris experience mucosal disease at some point. Forty-one percent of patients experience genital involvement, and 35% of women exhibit Pap smears that report acantholysis and inflammation consistent with but not diagnostic of pemphigus,[14] and genital blisters and erosions are common.

Pemphigus vulgaris occurs on keratinized skin, as well as on all squamous mucous membrane and modified mucous membrane sites. Blisters of pemphigus are notoriously superficial and fragile, so that clinical bullae are rarely recognized mucous membranes. Instead, rather bland, nonspecific erosions are often the lesions first noted (**Fig. 10-17 through 10-19**). Pemphigus is classically a nonscarring disease, but the vulva scars easily so that resorption of the labia minora is common, and clitoral phimosis can occur, and the end stage mimics lichen planus, lichen sclerosus, and mucous membrane pemphigoid.

Pemphigus vulgaris of the penis is less common than pemphigus of the vulva, and when present it occurs most often on the glans, but the distal shaft and corona also

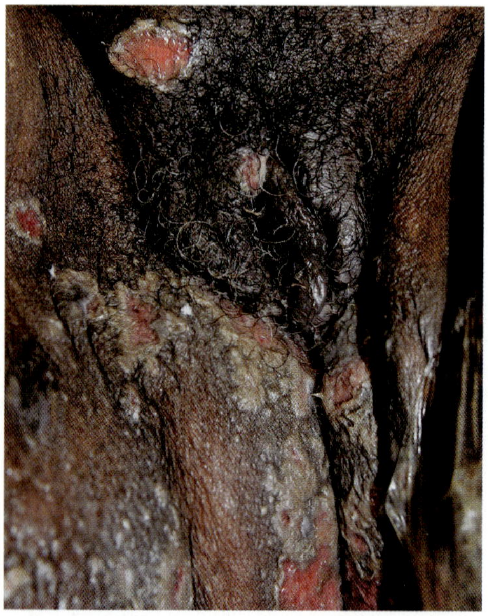

Fig. 10-17. The blisters of pemphigus vulgaris are fragile, so that intact fluid-filled bullae are often not seen. Here, there are collapsed lesions with flaccid necrotic blister roofs and erosions.

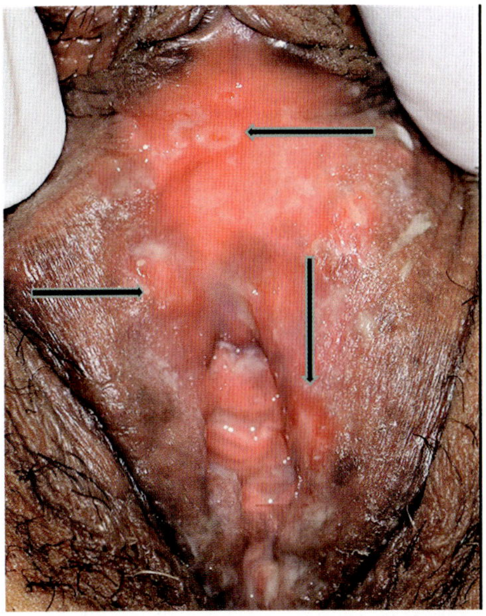

Fig. 10-18. These fragile blisters of pemphigus vulgaris on mucous membranes and modified mucous membranes have eroded into superficial erosions that appear annular and arcuate due to the white border of macerated epithelium from the edge of the blisters (*arrows*).

are sites that are affected. Scarring of the penis can occur, with blunting of the corona in circumcised men and phimosis in uncircumcised individuals. The oral mucosa is usually affected in both men and women **(Fig. 10-20)**.

The blisters of pemphigus on keratinized skin are superficial and flaccid. Gentle traction on a blister extends the blister by shearing the tenuous adherence of the upper epidermis to underlying tissue, producing the Nikolsky

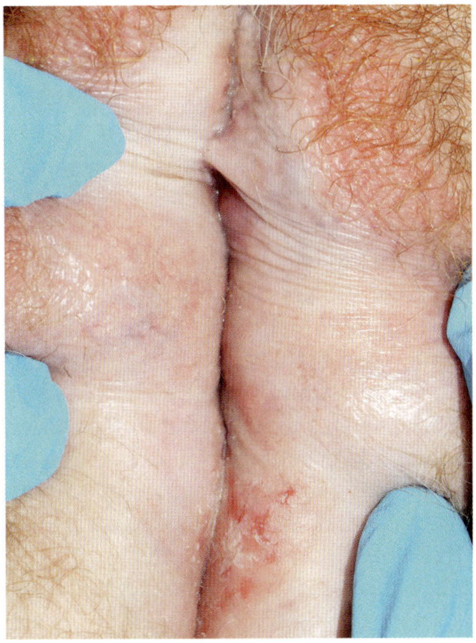

Fig. 10-19. Although pemphigus vulgaris is generally considered to be a nonscarring condition due to its very superficial nature, scarring definitely occurs on anogenital skin. The white skin can mimic lichen sclerosus, with loss of architecture and hypopigmentation.

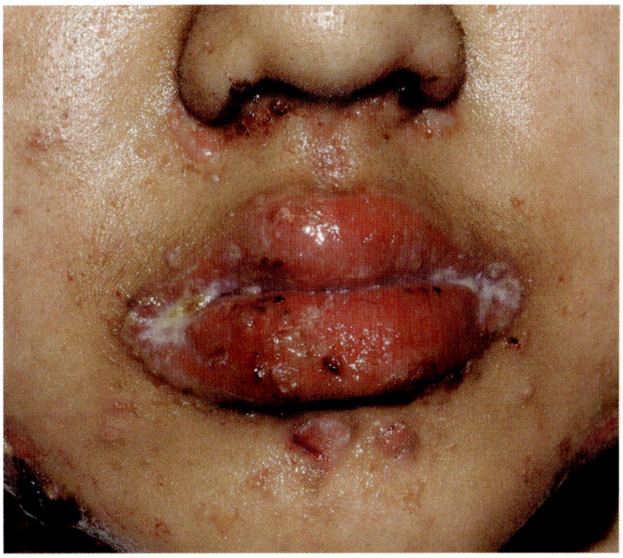

Fig. 10-20. Pemphigus regularly affects the mouth as well, and like the genital skin, erosions rather than intact blisters are the rule. However, small vesicles can be seen around the nose.

sign. These very superficial blisters rupture easily to leave large eroded areas, but they normally heal without scarring except on the genitalia.

Pemphigus vegetans is a variant of pemphigus vulgaris characterized by erosions, often with peripheral pustules in the early phases of the disease. Later, large, thickened, and frequently verrucous plaques occur **(Fig. 10-21)**.

Pemphigus foliaceous is a rare condition that generally begins on the chest, scalp, and face, and not recognized as a blistering condition because of the very superficial nature and tiny size of the blisters. These do not generally affect mucous membranes. Paraneoplastic pemphigus has many different clinical presentations but typically presents with painful mucosal erosions and dusky patches on the skin that later desquamate. Severe widespread disease

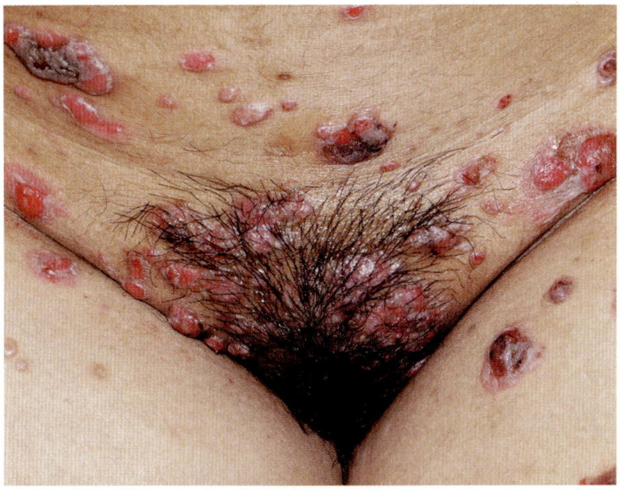

Fig. 10-21. Pemphigus vegetans is an uncommon manifestation of pemphigus, where erosions are covered with thickened hyperkeratotic plaques.

can result in dehydration requiring intensive care management or a burn center, and genital involvement is a relatively minor issue. This disease is often systemic rather than affecting only epithelial surfaces, generally fatal, and is usually associated with lymphoproliferative neoplasms.[15]

## Diagnosis

All variants of pemphigus are diagnosed by skin biopsy, although the clinical morphology of fragile bullae in a setting of mucous membrane erosions is highly suggestive. The skin biopsy shows a superficial blister within the epidermis **(Fig. 10-22)**. Pemphigus vulgaris and early pemphigus vegetans exhibit a blister located just above the basal cell layer. The basal cells adhere to the basement membrane, but not to each other or to overlying cells, thus producing a picture similar to that of a row of tombstones. In addition, within the blister cavity are detached epidermal cells that, with loss of cohesion to surrounding cells, appear round and are called acantholytic cells. Direct immunofluorescence biopsies obtained from normal-appearing skin near a blister or erosion show immunoglobulin G (IgG) deposition in the epidermal intercellular substance. In addition, indirect immunofluorescence of patients' serum showing IgG autoantibodies that bind to the epidermal cell surface occur in 70%-90% of patient with PV.[13]

Biopsies of pemphigus vegetans often show, in addition, neutrophilic inflammation producing intraepithelial abscesses. In its later, hyperkeratotic form, pemphigus vegetans reveals squamous hyperplasia and pseudoepitheliomatous hyperplasia on biopsy, in addition to the characteristic suprabasilar blister. Pemphigus foliaceus shows a very superficial blister formed by acantholysis in the uppermost epidermis.

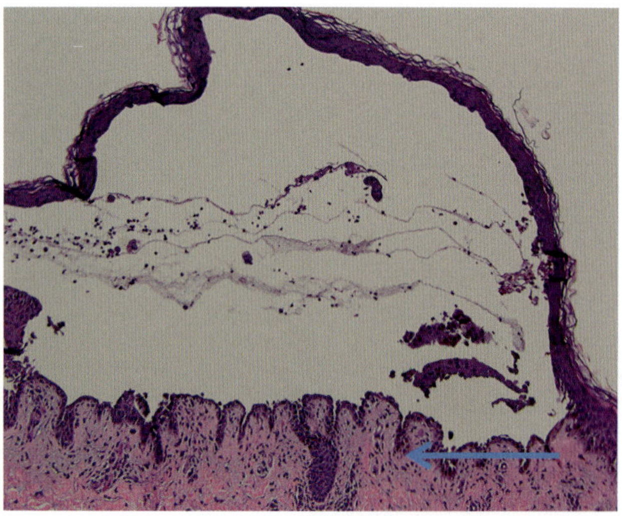

Fig. 10-22. The histology of pemphigus vulgaris explains the fragility of the blisters; the roof of the blister is only part of the epidermis, with the base of the blister composed of basal cells still attached to basement membrane (*arrow*). (Courtesy of Jason Reutter, MD.)

Most other blistering diseases can mimic PV. Pemphigus vulgaris often begins with mucosal erosions indistinguishable from erosive lichen planus. Routine biopsies usually differentiate the two diseases, and pemphigus vulgaris progresses to produce blisters and erosions on keratinized skin, unlike lichen planus. Pemphigus vulgaris resembles mucous membrane pemphigoid early on, with both producing nonspecific mucosal erosions. The milder and intermittent occurrence of a fixed drug eruption and the explosive onset of blistering forms of erythema multiforme, Stevens-Johnson syndrome, and toxic epidermal necrolysis usually distinguish these diseases from pemphigus.

**PEMPHIGUS VULGARIS — Diagnosis**

- Morphology of mucosal erosions, flaccid blisters of dry, keratinized skin
- More gradual onset compared to Stevens-Johnson syndrome and toxic epidermal necrolysis
- Confirmation by routine and direct immunofluorescent biopsies

## Pathophysiology

Pemphigus is a group of autoimmune intraepidermal bullous diseases produced by IgA autoantibodies to the surface of epidermal cells. The IgG is directed primarily against desmogleins 1 and 3, proteins that function in the attachment of squamous cells to each other, but other autoantibodies are often present as well, perhaps providing a synergistic effect.[13]

This ultimately produces a loss of adhesion of these cells, leading a superficial blister within the epidermis. The most common form of pemphigus, pemphigus vulgaris, is produced by loss of adhesion of the basal cells from the upper epidermis.

There is a genetic component to PV also, with certain major histocompatibility complex (MHC) class II molecules occurring more frequently in individuals with PV. These are the same MHC seen more often in the Jewish population and in countries of the eastern Mediterranean and the Middle East and borne out in the epidemiology of the disease. Like pemphigus vulgaris, pemphigus vegetans is produced by a split in the epidermis just above the basal cell layer, but it is characterized by the later development of thickened, hyperkeratotic skin.

In some cases, medications can precipitate pemphigus. The most common medication is penicillamine, and other offenders are captopril, tiopronine and related drugs, as well as nonsteroidal anti-inflammatory medications, and calcium channel blockers.[16] As many as 7% of patient taking penicillamine for 6 months can develop

PV.[17] Injury has also precipitated pemphigus at times. One form of pemphigus, benign familial pemphigus (also called Hailey-Hailey disease), is of autosomal dominant rather than autoimmune origin, and it is discussed later in this chapter.

### Management

Pemphigus generally is rarely controlled with topical therapy, although the genitalia benefit from local care. This widespread disease is treated systemically, falls in the prevue of a dermatologist, and ideally includes careful evaluation of the patients' overall health, and recruitment of a primary care provider, with availability of other specialists such as dentists and ophthalmologists to aid with management of common issues with the disease and side effects of medications.[18] Comorbidities of hypertension, diabetes, obesity, osteoporosis, etc. are common due to therapy, and these should be anticipated and managed.[19]

Specific first-line therapy for pemphigus is now systemic corticosteroids and CD20 inhibitors, specifically, rituximab infusions, now approved by the Food and Drug Administration for pemphigus. The advent of systemic corticosteroids has been lifesaving in these patients who generally died before the use of corticosteroids.[20] Now, the cause of death in patients with pemphigus now is primarily pneumonia and septicemia due to therapy.[21] Initial therapy is prednisone or its equivalent, beginning at about 40-80 mg/d, and adjusting the dose up or down as needed. Pemphigus is not a disease that is curable, so control is the goal. This condition is chronic, and patients generally are on prolonged courses of systemic corticosteroids. However, the newer use of rituximab has been a remarkable addition to the management of pemphigus, often allowing patients to discontinue prednisone. This medication eliminates the antibodies to desmogleins by depleting B cells, and it may be more effective if begun early in the course of the disease. After initial dosing, patients are usually maintained with semiannual infusions.

Second-line therapy consists of the steroid-sparing agents azathioprine and mycophenolate mofetil, followed by intravenous immunoglobulin infusions, cyclophosphamide and immunoadsorption.[13,18,19]

Local care of the genital area is important for comfort and to prevent scarring that interferes with sexual functioning and micturition. Topical corticosteroid therapy in addition to systemic therapy may be useful. Intralesional corticosteroids are a time-honored safe and cost-effective therapy for persistent erosions (see Chapter 4). Intralesional rituximab also has been reported as useful.[22] One study of 11 patients treated recalcitrant pemphigus with two intralesional injections of biosimilar rituximab.[23] There was a decrease in serum antibodies and B cells with this intralesional therapy, as well as healing of lesions, and there was a safer profile compared to intravenous infusions. One trial reported equivalent results of intralesional triamcinolone acetonide compared to intralesional rituximab.[24]

Measures to prevent secondary infection of genital skin, especially Candidal, are also important. Women especially who are on systemic corticosteroids should be monitored for this, and perhaps treated with weekly fluconazole, particularly when antibiotics are added or they are diabetic. Unlike many skin diseases in men, pemphigus is not cleared with circumcision and requires medical therapy. Women with vaginal involvement should insert dilators regularly to prevent vaginal adhesions, and uncircumcised men should retract the foreskin daily and apply petroleum jelly to prevent phimosis.

Although the prognosis of pemphigus vulgaris has improved remarkably since the use of corticosteroids and now rituximab, recurrence or low level persistence is common.

**PEMPHIGUS VULGARIS — Management**

- Prednisone 40-80 mg/d initially and rituximab infusions
- Steroid-sparing adjuvant medications in addition when needed
- Mycophenolate mofetil
- Azathioprine
- IVIG
- Cyclophosphamide
- Immunoadsorption
- Local care to prevent scarring

## Bullous Pemphigoid

### Clinical Presentation

Although bullous pemphigoid is the most common autoimmune blistering disease, it does not generally affect mucous membranes or modified mucous membranes, so does not present primarily as a genital dermatosis. It occurs equally in men and women and is most common in individuals over 60 years of age, with no racial predilection. However, bullous pemphigoid rarely occurs in childhood. About 10% of patients experience genital involvement, primarily of keratinized epithelium rather than the mucous membranes.

Patients regularly complain of itching, and this often precedes the blisters, sometimes by months. The pruritic skin sometimes mimics urticaria, and eventually small vesicles and then bullae arise. The genital areas most likely to be involved are the hair-bearing areas of inner thighs, inguinal crease, and perineum. Blisters are tense and filled with straw-colored and, occasionally, hemorrhagic fluid (**Figs. 10-23 through 10-25**). Scarring does not occur in the absence of a complicating event such as secondary infection, since bullous pemphigoid does not affect mucous membranes.

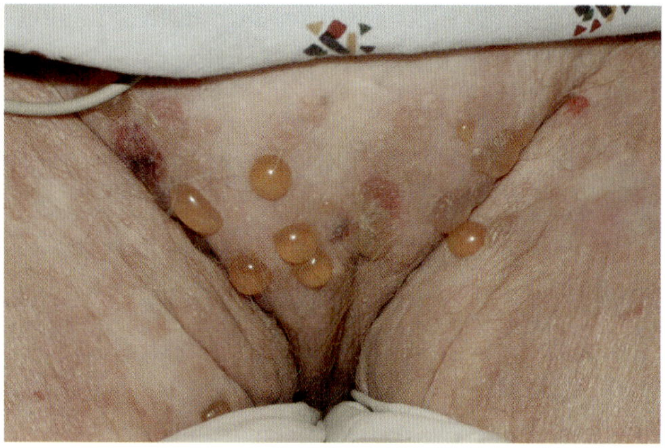

Fig. 10-23. Unlike pemphigus vulgaris, bullous pemphigoid exhibits tense blisters. (Courtesy of Errol Craig, MD.)

An association of bullous pemphigoid with neurologic disease, especially dementia and Parkinson disease, has been described,[25] but the long debated association of malignancy with bullous pemphigoid seems to be losing favor. There is a controversial association of bullous pemphigoid with underlying malignancy.[26,27]

## Diagnosis

The clinical presentation of bullous pemphigoid allows for a provisional diagnosis, but confirmation by biopsy for routine histology and direct immunofluorescence is mandatory. Biopsy of an intact new blister shows characteristic histology; subepidermal blistering with a variable dermal inflammatory infiltrate including eosinophils is usual **(Fig. 10-26)**. Direct immunofluorescent biopsy of perilesional skin shows deposition of IgG and complement components along the basement membrane zone (BMZ). A direct immunofluorescent examination of salt-split skin shows that the binding is epidermal, to the roof of the blister. This differentiates bullous pemphigoid from epidermolysis bullosa acquisita, in which the binding is to the base or dermal side of the blister. Indirect immunofluorescent studies of the sera of patients with bullous pemphigoid show the presence of IgG directed toward the pemphigoid target antigens in the lamina lucida of the BMZ.

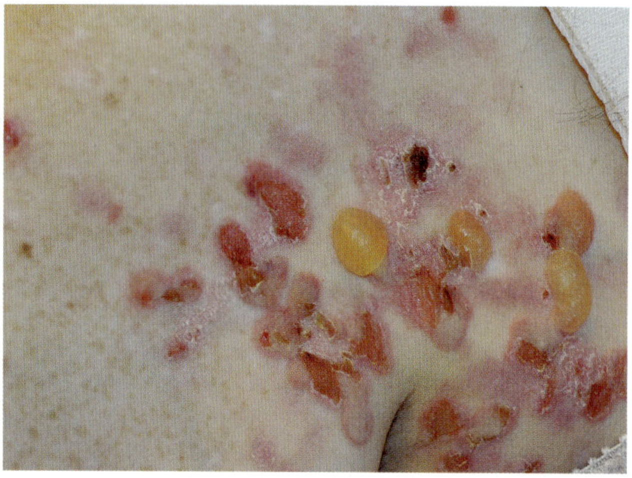

Fig. 10-25. The blisters of bullous pemphigoid occur from a deeper cleft in the skin, under the epidermis, resulting in tense, straw-colored blisters, rather than flaccid lesions.

Most other blistering disease can be differentiated by the morphology and onset, but epidermolysis bullosa acquisita and linear IgA dermatosis can be difficult to distinguish without biopsies. Other blistering diseases to consider include Stevens-Johnson syndrome and toxic epidermal necrolysis, but these essentially always exhibit mucosal lesions, and the onset is generally more abrupt. Pemphigus vulgaris, unlike bullous pemphigoid, generally affects mucous membranes prominently and is characterized by erosions and flaccid bullae, rather than by

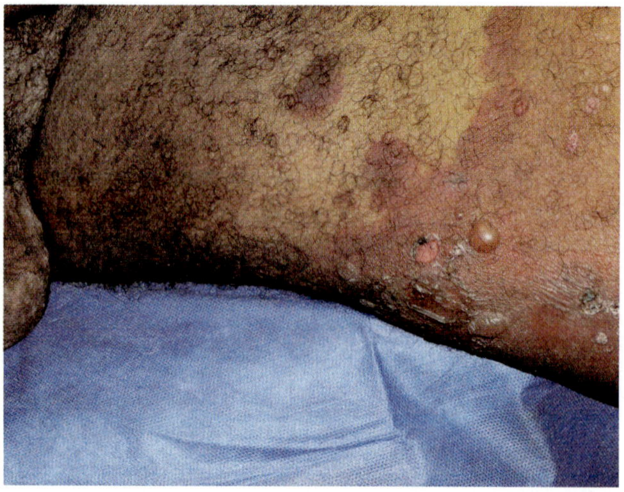

Fig. 10-24. Bullous pemphigoid affects the keratinized skin, generally sparing the mucous membranes and modified mucous membranes of the genitalia.

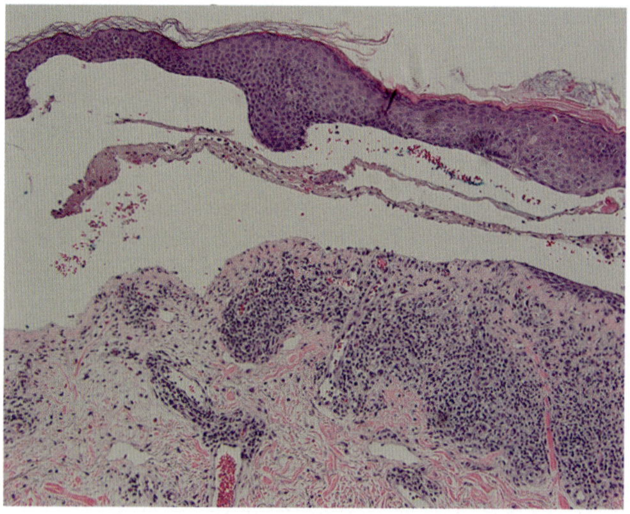

Fig. 10-26. A biopsy of bullous pemphigoid shows the loss of adhesion of the epidermis from the dermis, so that the blister roof is thicker, and the blister less fragile. (Courtesy of Jason Reutter, MD.)

tense blisters. Less often, bullous impetigo can mimic bullous pemphigoid. However, blisters are usually few in number and flaccid and of sudden and recent onset. Mucous membranes are spared.

### Pathophysiology

The blisters of bullous pemphigoid are produced by autoantibodies directed basal keratinocyte hemidesmosomal proteins BP antigen 230 (BPAG1) and BP antigen 180 (BPAG2 or type XVII collagen), which are crucial in the adhesion of the epithelium to the dermis. The binding of these autoantibodies is followed by inflammation and complement activation, ultimately with damage to the dermal-epidermal junction and detachment of the epidermis.[28] Although usually occurring spontaneously and without an identifiable precipitating factor, bullous pemphigoid is sometimes associated with specific drugs, such as loop diuretics, aldosterone antagonists, dipeptidyl dipeptidase inhibitors, and PD1 and PDL-1 inhibitors.[29]

The mRNA vaccines for COVID 19 appear to be linked to the development of bullous pemphigoid, with a boost in severity of the disease with the second vaccination also reported.[30,31]

### Management

For localized and prebullous disease, treatment with potent topical steroids sometimes is sufficient, especially in the elderly and those for whom systemic corticosteroids are especially dangerous. For generalized bullous pemphigoid, systemic steroids are first-line therapy. However, the doses required are generally from 40 to 60 mg/d, tapered according to response. Steroid-sparing immunosuppressive agents, whose effect is more delayed and less effective, are usually added; these include azathioprine, cyclophosphamide, or minocycline with nicotinamide. Methotrexate has also been used as a steroid-sparing agent. More recently, the biologic medications, including omalizumab, have been used and appear more beneficial.[32,33] Rituximab has shown efficacy, but less than for pemphigus, and one study suggests that it is equivalent to omalizumab.[33,34] Especially interesting seems the efficacy of dupilumab, which is only FDA approved in the United States for atopic dermatitis but has been shown useful in a number of reports for bullous pemphigoid and has a very good safety profile.[35,36]

The lesions in bullous pemphigoid are nonscarring, and the course of bullous pemphigoid is self-limiting, with remission in treated patients usually occurring in months to 6 years. Partly because bullous pemphigoid occurs primarily in the elderly, and because of the toxicity of therapy, the overall mortality of bullous pemphigoid in the first year or two after diagnosis is about 7 times the reference population.[37] Although treatment does not significantly improve mortality, it improves the quality of life, which can be ruined by the intractable and miserable pruritus. The condition may recur, but recurrences are usually milder than the initial bout.

## Mucous Membrane Pemphigoid (Cicatricial Pemphigoid)

According to a guideline on mucous membrane pemphigoid (MMP) by the Task Force for Autoimmune Blistering Diseases of the European Academy of Dermatology and Venereology, mucous membrane pemphigoid is a group of autoimmune skin and mucous membrane blistering diseases, characterized by a chronic course and by predominant involvement of the mucous membrane.[38] Mucous membrane pemphigoid should be considered a disease phenotype, with different conditions producing different autoantibodies targeting different autoantigens. Although histologically mucous membrane pemphigoid mimics bullous pemphigoid, this condition exhibits characteristic mucous membrane disease and very prominent scarring. Although rare, genital involvement is prominent and management can be challenging.

### Clinical Presentation

Mucous membrane pemphigoid is much less common than bullous pemphigoid, but this phenotypic form of pemphigoid affects the mucous membrane of the genitalia, and it is often more difficult to diagnose. Many patients exhibit no intact blisters on extramucosal skin, and the prompt erosion of the mucous membrane blisters belie the underlying blistering nature of the condition. The age of onset of mucous membrane pemphigoid is between 60 and 80 years and is more common in women.[38]

Mucous membrane pemphigoid affects the genitalia in 28%-38% in two series.[39,40] It affects keratinized skin only in about 20%-35% of cases.[38] Because the diagnosis is difficult in the absence of intact blisters on hair-bearing skin, it may be delayed or sometimes missed. Mucous membrane pemphigoid usually starts with irritation, mild blisters, and erosions of the mouth, the eye, and the genitalia. Men report penile lesions, dysuria, and difficulty retracting the foreskin. Women report pain, pruritus, and dysuria. Morphologically, genital mucous membrane pemphigoid is characterized by painful erosions and scarring **(Figs. 10-27 and 10-28)**. These mucous membrane erosions may progress rapidly to produce scarring with considerable morbidity. The initial, nonspecific, enlarging erosions produce scarring in more developed disease. Men may develop meatal stenosis and phimosis, and women may experience urethral stenosis, fusion of the labia, clitoral burial, and introitus stenosis.

Painful erosions in the mouth are usual **(Fig. 10-29)**. Erythema and erosions of the gingiva may lead to scarring and retraction with resulting secondary dental disease. The esophagus can be involved as well. Nasal mucosa, larynx, and pharynx may also be affected, and stridor,

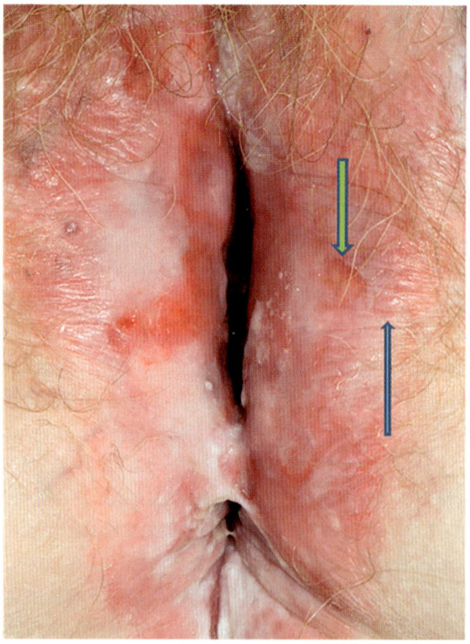

Fig. 10-27. At first glance, this patient could have lichen planus; however, there are round erosions indicating ruptured blisters (*green arrow*), and an intact blister on the left medial labium majus (*blue arrow*). Both routine and direct immunofluorescent biopsies are required for diagnosis.

dysphonia, or dysphagia may result. The eye, despite feeling dry and gritty, may appear normal initially, but an ophthalmologic examination detects early abnormalities: reduced lacrimation or adhesions of the bulbar to

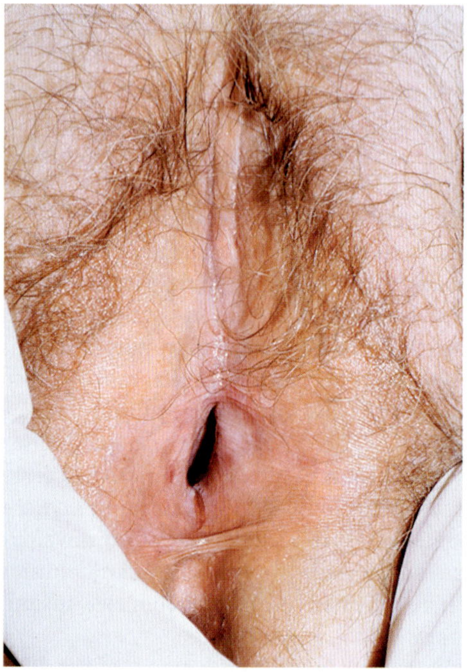

Fig. 10-28. The scarring from mucous membrane pemphigoid can be indistinguishable from lichen sclerosus and lichen planus, but the presence of other mucous membrane disease, lack of typical texture change of lichen sclerosus, and, often, blisters on extragenital skin help to differentiate the diseases.

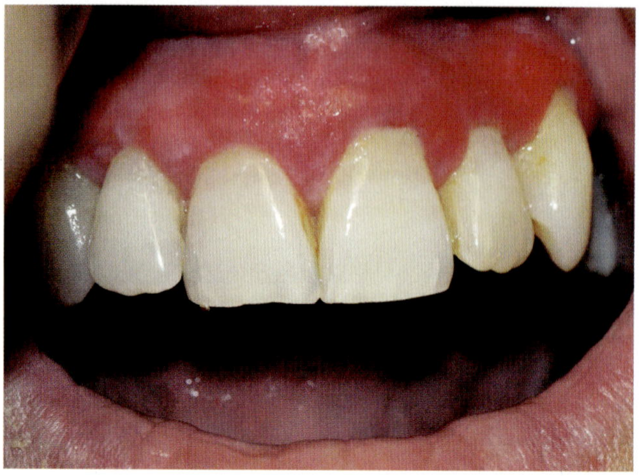

Fig. 10-29. Erosive gingivitis indistinguishable from that of pemphigus vulgaris and erosive lichen planus is regularly seen in patients with mucous membrane pemphigoid.

the palpebral conjunctivae (**Fig. 10-30**). Later, more extensive scarring may cause severe adhesions, entropion, and corneal scarring with blindness. Nonmucous membrane lesions, when present, are very helpful by demonstrating the underlying blistering nature of the process. Lesions are small, straw-colored blisters that may scar.

## Diagnosis

The diagnosis is suspected by the constellation of ocular, oral, and genital irritation and erosions and a high index of suspicion and confirmed by the identification of anti-basement membrane zone antibodies in nearby normal skin. There is linear deposition of IgG, IgA, and C3 at the BMZ. The diagnosis is often delayed, with resultant scarring. A biopsy for routine histology can be useful as well but is less sensitive and less specific. In the absence of a

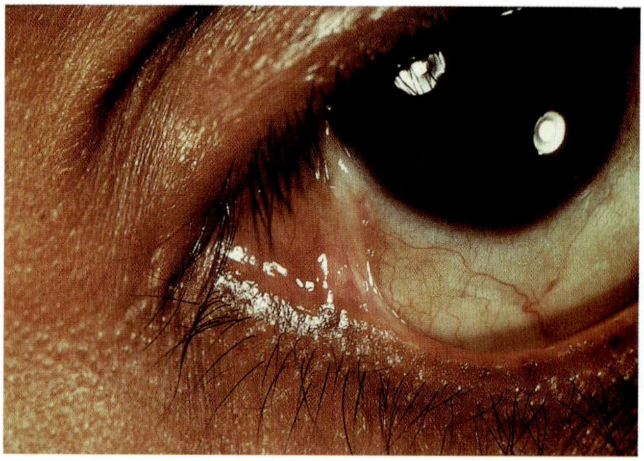

Fig. 10-30. A pathognomonic hallmark of mucous membrane pemphigoid is scarring of the conjunctivae, with early synechiae between the palpebral and bulbar conjunctivae. This can advance to produce blindness, but subtle early signs can require specialized equipment for detection.

blister, the edge of an erosion should be sampled. Histology shows a subepidermal blister, a mixed inflammatory infiltrate, and dermal scarring. Immunofluorescent studies of salt-split skin show the antibodies to be in the roof (epidermal) portion of the blister, although some are located in the floor (dermal) aspect of the blister.

All mucous membrane erosive diseases must be considered initially in patients with mucous membrane pemphigoid. Blistering diseases that can mimic mucous membrane pemphigoid include pemphigus vulgaris and epidermolysis bullosa acquisita. Although the two diseases are clinically different, mucous membrane pemphigoid and bullous pemphigoid appear identical histologically, and some target antigens in mucous membrane pemphigoid are identical to those in bullous pemphigoid. However, as noted above, mucous membrane pemphigoid is a heterogenous group of diseases that target different antigens, even within this phenotypic group.[38] Because blisters are often not apparent in patients with mucous membrane pemphigoid, other scarring diseases such as erosive lichen planus or erosive lichen sclerosus are in the differential diagnosis for genital mucous membrane pemphigoid.

**MUCOUS MEMBRANE PEMPHIGOID Diagnosis**

- Blisters, erosions of mucous membranes
- Often, tense blisters of dry, keratinized skin
- Confirmation by routine and direct immunofluorescent biopsies

### Pathophysiology

Mucous membrane pemphigoid is a phenotype of a group of immunochemically distinct autoimmune subepidermal blistering diseases. As occurs with the closely related bullous pemphigoid, antibodies are directed against various components of the basement membrane, resulting in a loss of adhesion of the epidermis to the dermis and subsequent blistering.

### Management

Mucous membrane pemphigoid is often difficult to control; treatment modifies the disease but generally does not completely suppress it. However, recent biologic therapies report patients with complete remissions of disease.[41] Various accepted guidelines for the management of mucous membrane pemphigoid vary among countries.[42-46]

A primary goal of therapy is comfort of the patient and the avoidance of scarring of the eye and blindness, as well as scarring of the genitalia, airways, and esophagus. Although superpotent topical corticosteroids are often used, these frequently are not sufficient for control, even less efficacious and poorly tolerated is as is tacrolimus ointment applied twice daily. Data for topical therapy are limited to case reports. Intralesional corticosteroids can be useful for mucosal erosions (see Chapter 4).

Most patients by far require systemic therapy. Those with milder disease may respond to antibiotics that have anti-inflammatory effects; primarily dapsone and tetracyclines, with or without nicotinamide.[43,44] Doxycycline or minocycline at 100 mg twice daily with food to minimize gastritis with or without nicotinamide has been shown to be useful. Dapsone, starting at about 25 mg a day and increasing as high as 100 mg twice a day, can be used, with careful attention to the hematologic side effects, risk of hemolysis of red cells, methemoglobinemia, and neuropathy. Patients with more severe oral, or pharyngeal, esophageal, laryngeal, or ocular involvement in danger of scarring should begin systemic corticosteroids early. Systemic prednisone or its equivalent at about 50-80 mg/d and reduced according to response. Systemic corticosteroids are regularly accompanied by steroid-sparing drugs. Common historical choices include oral or pulse cyclophosphamide, azathioprine, mycophenolate mofetil, and methotrexate.

More recently, biologics have been used in mucous membrane pemphigoid. A recent survey of the literature evaluated trials that included 154 patients treated with intravenous immunoglobulin (IVIG), 112 patients receiving rituximab, and 7 patients treated with a tumor necrosis alpha blocker.[41] Of those receiving IVIG, 61.7% experienced complete remission, with a recurrence rate of 22.7%. 70.5% of patients treated with rituximab achieved complete remission, with 35.7% experiencing recurrence. Five of seven treated with a tumor necrosis alpha inhibitor achieved remission, and none experienced recurrence.

Local care of genital erosions are important, both for patient comfort and to minimize scarring.

Potent topical steroids are useful. Tacrolimus ointment is reported as useful, but we rarely find it to be tolerated. Tacrolimus solution can be used as a douche, with the dissolving a 1 mg capsule in 500 cc of water, a cost effective medication. There are no data on this preparation. In addition, local care of the mucous membranes by multiple specialties and prevention of secondary infection are essential. The use of a dilator to prevent the development of vaginal synechiae is important with there are vaginal and introital erosions. Uncircumcised men should regularly lubricate and retract the prepuce to prevent phimosis, and be observant for meatal involvement and stenosis. Surgery should only be performed when the disease is controlled or there is urgent obstruction.

Mucous membrane pemphigoid is a chronic disease, although activity may fluctuate. Continuing care is necessary. There is no proven link with internal malignancy, but carcinoma of involved has been reported, possibly from chronic erosion and immunosuppressive treatment.

**MUCOUS MEMBRANE PEMPHIGOID Management**

- Topical and intralesional corticosteroids for mild disease
- Doxycycline/minocycline 100 mg bid with food with or without nicotinamide, or dapsone 50-100 mg bid
- Oral corticosteroids, prednisone 50-80 mg/d or equivalent initially for mucous membrane disease of eyes, pharynx, larynx, esophagus, or severe of other mucous membranes, with
- Cyclophosphamide, azathioprine, methotrexate, mycophenolate mofetil or
- Doxycycline or minocycline 100 mg bid
- If needed, add rituximab, or
- IVIG, or
- tumor necrosis alpha inhibitors
- Local care to prevent scarring

## Linear IgA Bullous Dermatosis

### Epidemiology and Clinical Morphology

Linear IgA bullous dermatosis (LAD) is a rare immunobullous dermatosis that presents at any age, with the peak incidence at more than 60 years. About a third of cases occur in children, when it is called "chronic bullous disease of childhood."

The initial presentation of LAD consists of tense blisters that resemble bullous pemphigoid (Fig. 10-31). However, annular, erythematous, nonscaling, red plaques with peripheral blistering occur, and blisters are characteristically annular, but can be linear or sausage shaped (Fig. 10-32). These plaques gradually become more generalized. Mucosal involvement occurs in about 80% of adults.[29] Children present with genital and perioral blisters, suggesting the possibility of sexual abuse. When medication induced, the disease can be severe, even mimicking toxic epidermal necrolysis.

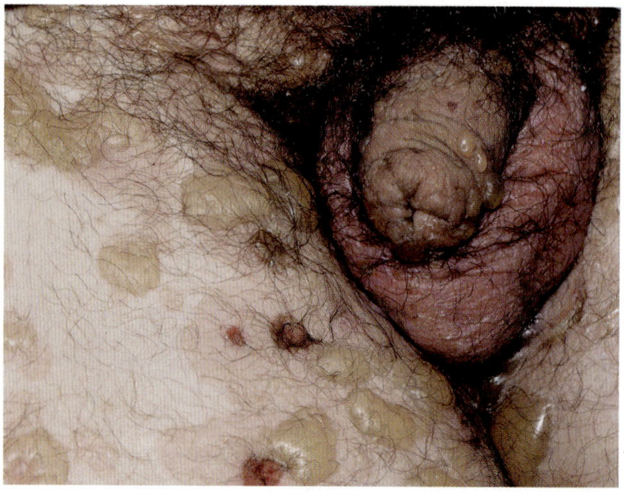

Fig. 10-31. The individual lesions of linear immunoglobulin A disease resemble those of bullous pemphigoid, with tense, straw-colored blisters.

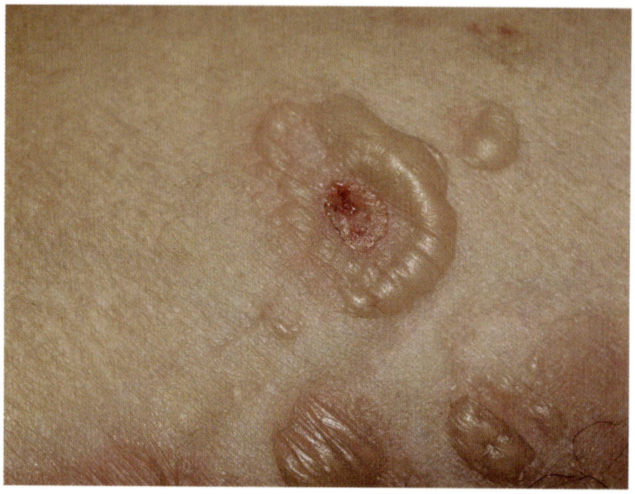

Fig. 10-32. Characteristic blisters of linear IgA disease are annular, showing a central collapse and crust and peripheral bulla.

### Diagnosis

This disease is suspected by the characteristic annular morphology of the skin lesions, and it is confirmed by the direct immunofluorescent biopsy of normal skin near a blister that shows a linear band of IgA deposition at the basement membrane zone. Immunofluorescent studies of salt-split skin show the IgA deposition to be epidermal, and indirect immunofluorescent assays of serum show IgA antibodies in all children and most adults. However, particularly with drug-induced LAD, immunofluorescent studies may be negative. An extremely rapid response to dapsone therapy is a less-sophisticated diagnostic test. A routine biopsy shows a subepidermal blister with a neutrophilic infiltrate.

Initial, annular pink plaques can be confused with urticaria, and once blistering occurs, bullous pemphigoid, Stevens-Johnson syndrome, and toxic epidermal necrolysis must be considered. However, the classic annular blistering plaques are unique to LAD.

### Pathophysiology

Linear IgA disease is an acquired autoimmune blistering disease reacting to multiple target antigens and resulting tissue damage.[29] This disease is sometimes produced by medications, most notably vancomycin, amiodarone, diclofenac, captopril, ceftriaxone-metronidazole, naproxen, piroxicam, and phenytoin.[29] Hormonal changes may alter the ability of the IgA to bind antigen, and although pregnancy improves the disease, a relapse is common 3 months postpartum. There are multiple reports of ulcerative colitis associated with linear IgA bullous dermatosis.[47] Occasionally, localized LAD may occur at sites of cutaneous trauma such as a burn. There may be an increased incidence after infection or antibiotic administration.

### Management

Systemic therapy is required for the control of LAD. Treatment with dapsone or sulfonamides produces improvement in most patients with LAD within 48 hours. For those allergic to sulfa, systemic corticosteroids are generally used but colchicine, thalidomide, cyclosporine, and niacinamide have been reported useful at times. Minocycline with nicotinamide, or azathioprine with dapsone, has been tried, sometimes successfully in those recalcitrant or combinations of dapsone and systemic corticosteroids. IVIG, rituximab, and omalizumab have been shown in case reports to be useful as well.[29,48,49] Care of the mucous membranes, prevention of secondary infection, and use of topical steroids are also important in management.

Sixty percent of adults experience remission, usually within 3 years. The immune deposits are lost from the skin. The disease is self-limiting in children, with most experiencing remission before puberty. Mucous membrane lesions may be more recalcitrant.

Those patients with unusually severe disease may be more likely to have the antiepiligrin type of disease. This may be important because the immunosuppressive medications used for mucous membrane pemphigoid may accelerate the activity of any underlying adenocarcinoma that is more likely to occur with this form of pemphigoid.

## Benign Familial Pemphigus (Hailey-Hailey Disease)

### Clinical Presentation

Hailey-Hailey is autosomal dominant condition occurring in about 1 in 50 000 people, and presenting in the 20s or 30s with variable severity.[50] Although it is a blistering condition, the vesicles are so small and superficial, that the blistering nature is often not recognized, and the skin becomes macerated. The skin lesions of Hailey-Hailey disease are characterized by recurrent, small, usually subtle blisters and crusted erosions occurring on an erythematous base, largely in intertriginous zones and perianal skin (**Figs. 10-33 through 10-35**). These eventuate into thickened, macerated red plaques that exhibit characteristic, short, irregular, linear fissures. Exudation is common, and vesicles may become pustules. There may be expanding erythematous plaques with peripheral scaling in the axillae, groin, and perineum that resemble a fungal infection. Mucous membrane lesions do not occur.

### Diagnosis

The diagnosis is made on the basis of morphology, family history, and a routine biopsy. A skin biopsy shows loss of adhesion between squamous cells above the basal layer, so that there are clefts in the epithelium and areas of intraepidermal separation (**Fig 10-36**). Immunofluorescence is negative.

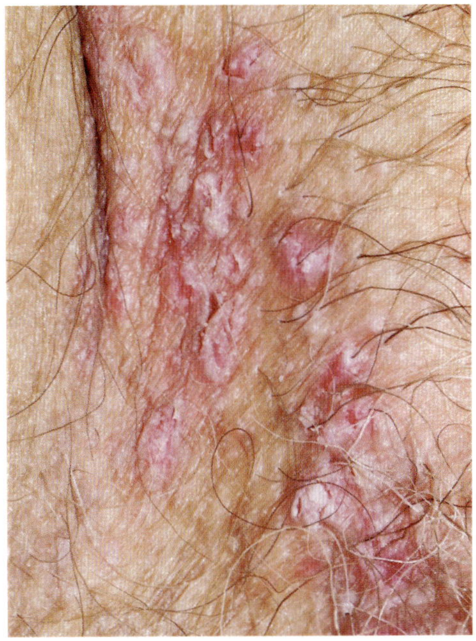

Fig. 10-33. Soft, superficial, moist coalescing vesicles of Hailey-Hailey disease show the typical white surface due to hydration of the necrotic epithelium.

The most common morphology, which of exudative red, scaling plaques, can resemble tinea cruris, eczema, and psoriasis. When pustules are present, candidiasis as a diagnosis or complicating factor should be considered. In addition, HSV can mimic the tiny erosions within the plaques. At times, HSV infection can secondarily infect Hailey-Hailey disease (Kaposi varicelliform eruption), so refractory disease should be evaluated for this possibility. However, the erosions of candidiasis and HSV

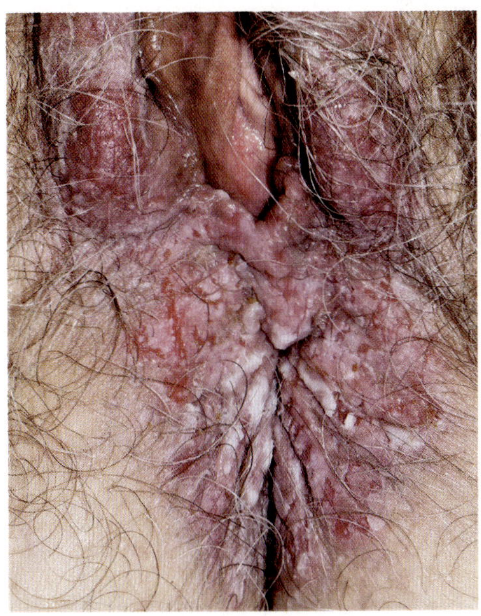

Fig. 10-34. Hailey-Hailey consists of fragile skin that, in areas of friction such as skinfolds, produces erosions and detached white necrotic epithelium, sparing mucous membranes.

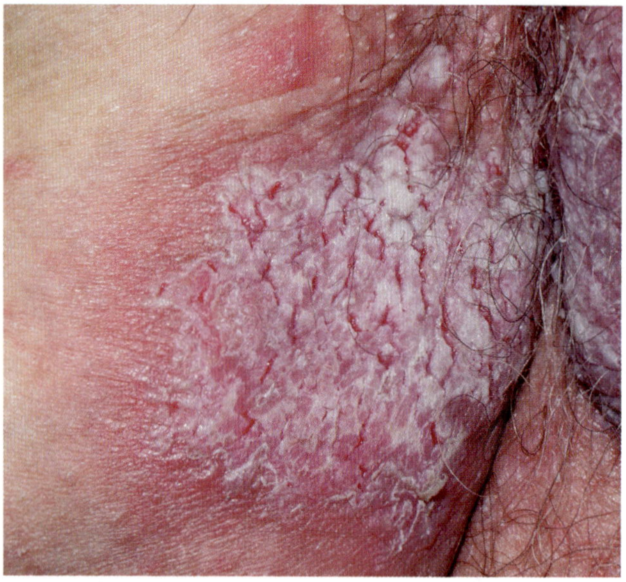

Fig. 10-35. Hailey-Hailey often develops into red plaques of white, macerated epithelium with characteristic linear cracks due to fractured epithelium.

are generally round or arcuate from coalescing blisters, whereas the small erosions from Hailey-Hailey disease are characteristically linear and angular.

**HAILEY-HAILEY DISEASE** **Diagnosis**

- Moist, usually white plaques with short linear fissures in skinfolds such as perianal skin and crural creases
- Family history of similar skin conditions
- Confirmed by routine biopsy if no family history

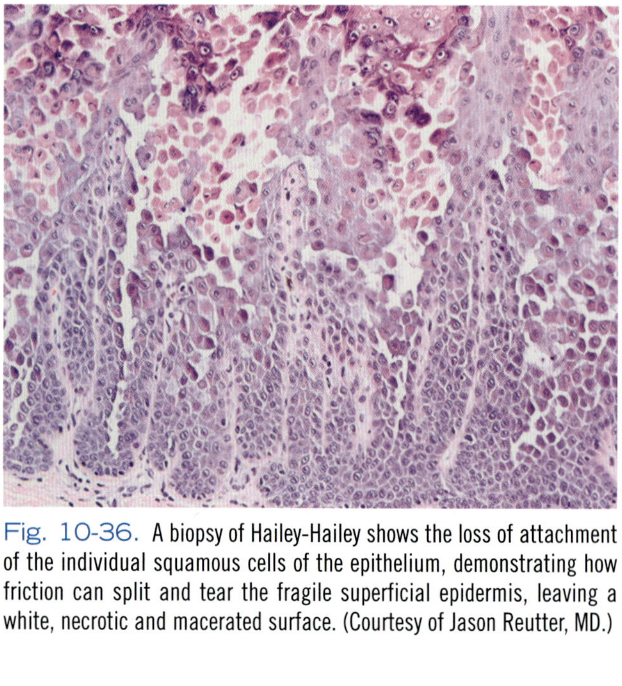

Fig. 10-36. A biopsy of Hailey-Hailey shows the loss of attachment of the individual squamous cells of the epithelium, demonstrating how friction can split and tear the fragile superficial epidermis, leaving a white, necrotic and macerated surface. (Courtesy of Jason Reutter, MD.)

### Pathophysiology

Hailey-Hailey disease is an autosomal dominant disease resulting in a defect in normal adhesion between keratinocytes. This condition is associated with various mutations in the *ATP2C1* gene. The friction, heat, perspiration, bacterial and yeast colonization, and infection most marked in skinfolds precipitate separation of the epidermis from the dermis and resulting erosions. HSV infection sometimes plays a role as well.

### Management

There is no satisfactory, specific therapy for Hailey-Hailey disease. Supportive care is important, including the prompt treatment of secondary infection. Blistering can be minimized by the suppression of cutaneous bacteria by long-term administration of topical antibiotics such as clindamycin or erythromycin solutions, or oral medication such as doxycycline or clindamycin. In addition, an antiperspirant can reduce the friction that worsens with sweating, and the subsequent blistering and maceration. However, antiperspirants can produce remarkable stinging and irritation when they are applied to eroded or macerated skin, so these agents should be used only as maintenance therapy on relatively well-controlled skin. If "clinical strength" over-the-counter potent antiperspirants up to 12% are not adequately effective, prescription-strength aluminum chloride can be used. Mid-potency topical corticosteroids such as triamcinolone ointment (applied very very sparingly to avoid adding to the moistness of the area) can be useful for the inflammation caused by the chronic erosions. Tacrolimus ointment is generally too irritating and stings with application.

A time-honored, effective, but painful therapy is ablative $CO_2$ therapy.[51] This treatment disrupts sweat glands. Dapsone, methotrexate, photodynamic therapy, dermabrasion, Er:YAG laser, vascular laser, radiofrequency, and electron beam are therapies that are supported only by case reports and small open series and recently reviewed.[51]

More recent, open label trials report remarkable results with intralesional botulinum toxin type A, 50-100 IU per site in patients with Hailey-Hailey disease, presumably because of elimination of sweating.[52,53] Results in my patients have not been as impressive. Recent reports of low-dose naltrexone have been promising as well.[54,55] Very recent, solitary case reports have reported good results with dupilumab and apremilast.[56,57] The advantage of these recent strategies is the lack of pain and tissue damage, but the disadvantage is the financial cost, and the disadvantage of all is the lack of data.

The course of the disease is one of spontaneous exacerbations and remissions. It is usually worse in hot summer months when sweating worsens the condition. There is no tendency to improve with age.

**HAILEY-HAILEY DISEASE — Management**

- Control of sweat
- Antiperspirants
- Botulinum toxin A
- Destructive therapies that disrupt sweating, such as $CO_2$ laser, photodynamic therapy
- Topical antibiotics such as clindamycin to minimize irritation from colonizing organisms
- Topical corticosteroids such as triamcinolone oint or cream 0.1% bid prn

## Stevens-Johnson Syndrome, Toxic Epidermal Necrolysis

Stevens-Johnson syndrome (SJS) and toxic epidermal necrolysis (TEN) are dangerous medication-induced hypersensitivity reactions that exist on a spectrum and produce widespread blistering reactions that include mucous membranes.

### Clinical Presentation

Stevens-Johnson syndrome and toxic epidermal necrolysis are blistering medication reactions that are differentiated by severity and the surface area involved. These affect mucous membranes, often including the genitalia, and are slightly more common in females. Both often are preceded by fever, sore throat, cough, myalgias, followed by rash and skin pain. About 15% of patients have no history of a medication producing the eruption. Much more often, an offending medication was begun in a naïve patient from 2 weeks to 3 months prior to onset of the illness, or a previously taken medication was recently restarted. Discrete, red flat papules or plaques coalesce and slough or form blisters, or large areas or erythema detach (**Figs. 10-37 through 10-43**). If <10% of the surface of the skin is involved, the condition is termed Stevens-Johnson syndrome; if more than 30% is affected, the patient has toxic epidermal necrolysis. Between 10% and 30% is overlap. The prognosis is dependent upon the extent of the disease with widespread disease associated with a very high mortality rate.

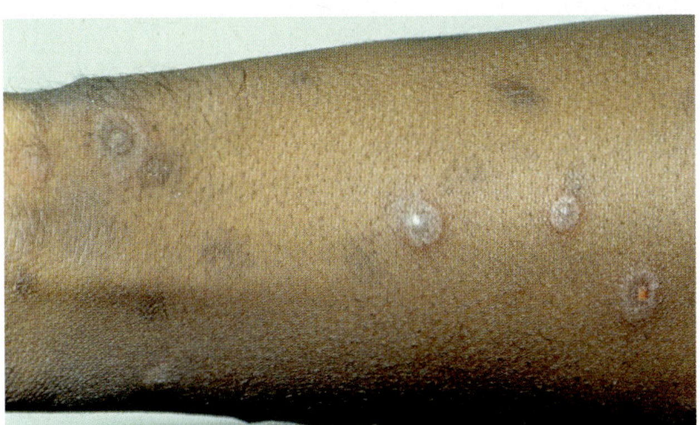

Fig. 10-37. Stevens-Johnson syndrome presents as red papules with central blistering or erosions in a setting that includes mucous membrane erosions.

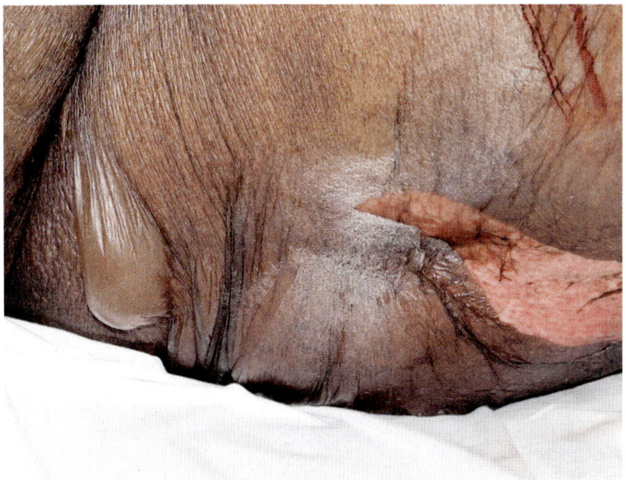

Fig. 10-38. Toxic epidermal necrolysis represents a severe end of the spectrum, in which more than 40% of the skin is involved and sheets of red, painful epithelium become detached. Because this is a patient of color, the erythema is subtle.

SJS/TEN generally involve multiple mucous membranes, and, like other blistering disorders, the blisters on mucous membrane and modified mucous membrane rupture almost instantly, producing erosions rather than recognized intact blisters.

Patients with widespread lesions are toxic, exhibit a marked risk of secondary infection, dehydration, electrolyte deviations, and temperature instability, and generally experience the same complications as burn patients. When cutaneous involvement is widespread, mortality

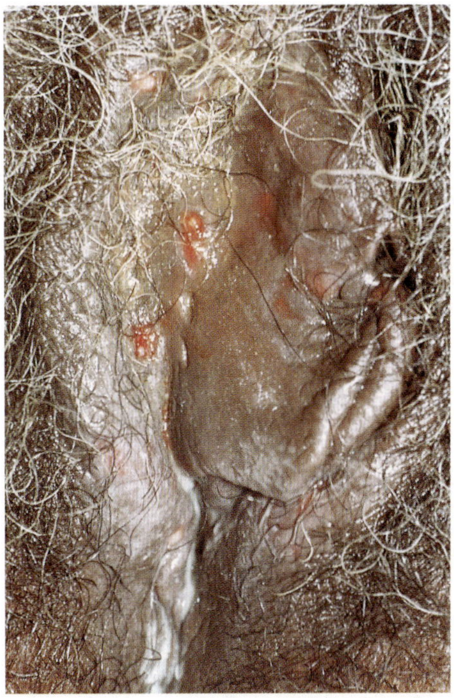

Fig. 10-39. Discrete erosions on the modified mucous membranes and mucous membranes are typical of milder forms of the SJS/TEN spectrum.

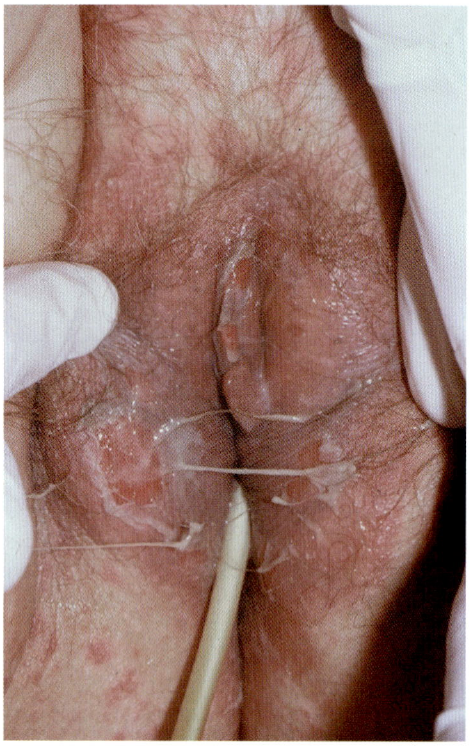

Fig. 10-40. This patient experienced generalized blistering and sloughing, including her keratinized skin, vagina, mouth, and eyes, as a result of an allergy to a nonsteroidal anti-inflammatory medication. Women can develop vaginal synechiae as a result of erosions associated with SJS and TEN.

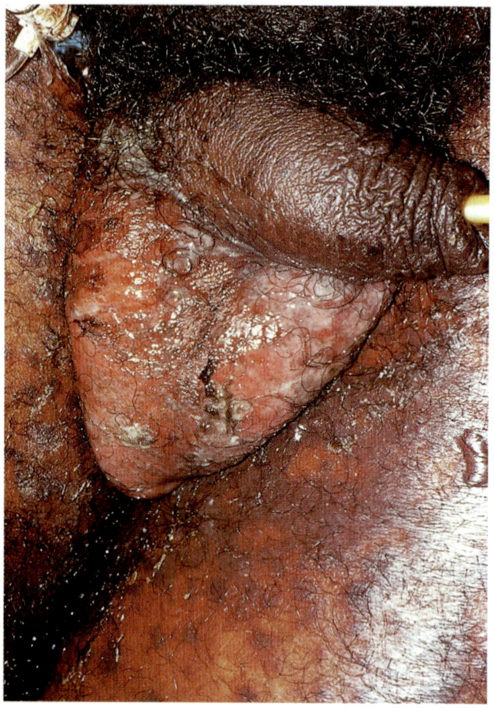

Fig. 10-42. The scrotal sloughing was only a minor part of this patient's generalized blistering and erosive reaction to sulfa. He developed phimosis as a result of erosions of the glans and the ventral aspect of the prepuce, and lack of local care.

can be high. Because of this, mucous membrane care if often neglected. Even though skin lesions can heal quickly after the inciting agent is withdrawn or treated, scarring of the genitalia and eyes can be severe. Vaginal lesions occasionally result in synechiae, and uncircumcised men can experience phimosis and paraphimosis.

A recent retrospective review of 149 women with SJS/TEN showed that 12.7% experienced vulvovaginal involvement, and there was no specific protocol for management.[58] Only 3 of 19 affected patients were seen in follow-up, and one experienced vaginal agglutination, which was managed in the office with blunt dissection. Others report up to 77% of vulvovaginal involvement.[59] The frequency in men is less known.

## Diagnosis

The diagnosis of SJS/TEN is made by the clinical picture of the abrupt onset of cutaneous blisters with mucous membrane erosions in an ill patient, usually in someone who is receiving a medication known to produce this reaction. The diagnosis should be confirmed by biopsy to rule out other diseases such as pemphigus vulgaris or

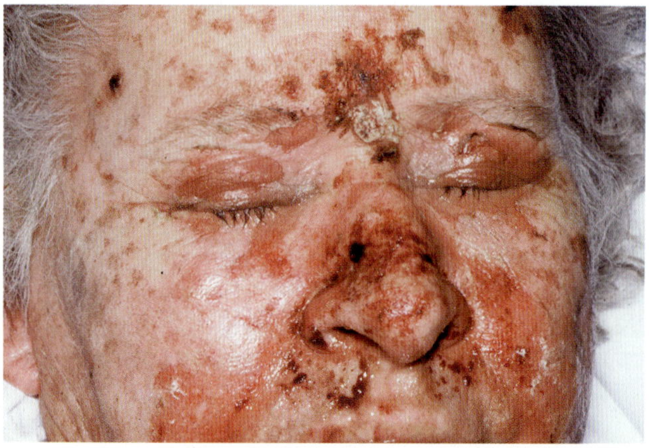

Fig. 10-41. The patient from **Fig 10-40**; she ultimately required a corneal transplant due to scarring from corneal scarring due to TEN.

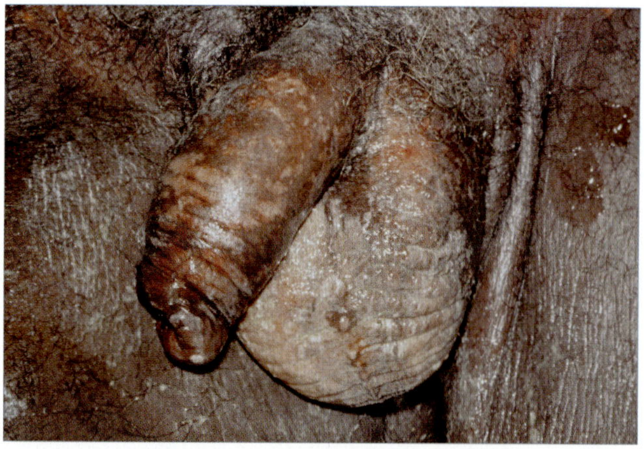

Fig. 10-43. The keratinized surfaces of the genitalia were preferentially affected compared to other areas of keratinized skin in TEN. This man succumbed to his allergy to phenytoin.

mucous membrane pemphigoid, which nearly always are much more indolent, but are treated differently.

The most striking histologic abnormalities of blistering forms of SJS/TEN are epidermal. Early lesions show groups of necrotic keratinocytes, and more advanced disease shows liquefaction degeneration of the basal cell layer with extensive epidermal necrosis. Dermal chronic perivascular mononuclear inflammation is usual.

Pemphigus vulgaris can be almost indistinguishable from widespread toxic epidermal necrolysis, although it is usually slower in onset. Erythema multiforme major (EMM) not only can be confused with SJS, but used to be felt to be synonymous. EMM shows red papules with blisters and oral erosions, sometimes with other mucous membrane lesions, produced either by medications or infections (primarily HSV or mycoplasma). Newer data suggest that these are distinct conditions, without catastrophic progression and sequalae.[60] Bullous pemphigoid can be similar, but usually spares mucous membranes, and mucous membrane pemphigoid characteristically produces similar genital lesions but generally does not display widespread cutaneous blisters. Staphylococcal scalded skin syndrome is a rare condition that used to be named toxic epidermal necrolysis of the Ritter type; this is an unrelated disease produced by a toxin elaborated by a phage type of *S aureus*, causing this very superficial stratum corneum to separate from the surface of the epidermis. Sheets of stratum corneum slough, but although dramatic, this is not dangerous unless the *S aureus* infection is dangerous, and does not affect mucous membranes.

**TABLE 10-1**

**Common Medications Causing Stevens-Johnson Syndrome and Toxic Epidermal Necrolysis**

- Antibiotics
  - Penicillins
  - Sulfonamides
  - Fluoroquinolones
  - Cephalosporins
- Anticonvulsant medications
  - Carbamazepine
  - Barbiturates
  - Phenytoin
  - Lamotrigine
  - Phenobarbital
  - Valproic acid
- Cardiovascular medications
  - Hydrochlorothiazide
  - Furosemide
  - Procainamide
- Other
  - Allopurinol
  - All nonsteroidal anti-inflammatory medications
  - Acetaminophen
  - Immune checkpoint inhibitors

**STEVENS-JOHNSON SYNDROME, TOXIC EPIDERMAL NECROLYSIS — Diagnosis**

- Explosive onset of mucous membrane erosions
- Red flat papules coalescing into plaques with bullae or generalized sloughing
- Confirmed by biopsy

### Pathophysiology

SJS/TEN are believed to be T-cell–mediated, type IV hypersensitivity reactions to medications, but beyond this, the pathophysiology is not well understood. HLA genotype appears to have a significant association with the risk of SJS/TEN. Although nearly every available medication has been reported to produce blistering medication reactions, allopurinol, nonsteroidal anti-inflammatory medications, acetaminophen, sulfas, anticonvulsants, and immune checkpoint inhibitors are medications most associated with this event (**Table 10-1**).

### Management

Treatment includes, obviously, stopping the offending drug. Supportive care is the second most important aspect of therapy. The aggressive identification and treatment of any secondary infection and replacement of fluid loss are essential. Referral to a burn unit for those with widespread disease is required in many people. The use of systemic corticosteroids, cyclosporine, IVIG, and tumor necrosis alpha inhibitors are used variously by providers in early disease, but there are no controlled trials for these medications.

Local care of affected mucous membranes is essential, especially the eyes, and early consultation with an ophthalmologist is crucial.

Those who are caring for these very ill patients are generally unaware of the measures needed to prevent long-term sequelae of erosions on genital skin. These are better described in women than men and include loss of vulvar architecture, vaginal adhesions, including complete occlusion of the vagina with trapping of menstrual blood proximally.[61] Urethral strictures could occur, and there have been reports or vulvar and vaginal adenosis and rare reports of malignant transformation.[61] There can be loss of elasticity, pigment changes. Men can experience urethral strictures and, when uncircumcised, phimosis.

When erosions are present, the genitalia should be covered with generous lubrication, and petroleum jelly is adequate, and regular retraction of the glans in uncircumcised men can help to prevent scarring, as can the insertion of a small vaginal dilator daily in women with vaginal involvement. The goal is to prevent scarring, not to reverse and dilate narrowing. The application of a superpotent topical corticosteroid such as clobetasol propionate 0.05 ointment twice daily may useful, and this can be used on a vaginal dilator as well.

Local yeast infections in women and uncircumcised men are especially common in this setting of frequent concomitant immunosuppressive and antibiotic use. Weekly fluconazole at 150 or 200 mg can control this complication.

**STEVENS-JOHNSON SYNDROME, TOXIC EPIDERMAL NECROLYSIS — Management**

- Discontinuation of offending medication
- Infection, pain, and fluid control
- Burn unit when severe
- Possibly systemic corticosteroids/IVIG/Cyclosporine/ TNF alpha inhibitors
- Local care of genitalia
- Superpotent topical steroid ointment twice a day
- Lubrication with petroleum jelly
- Vaginal dilation daily
- Suppression of menses
- Retraction of foreskin daily
- *Candida* suppression

## Fixed Drug Eruption

### Clinical Presentation

A fixed drug eruption is a peculiar reaction to a medication consisting of recurrent same-site skin lesions, occurring in any sensitized individual, independent of gender or age. Following exposure to the causative medication, the patient notes a single or a few lesions, with most patient having fewer than five lesions. The lips and upper extremities are common locations, and about 90% of men experience penile lesions.[62]

On keratinized skin, these present as well-demarcated, round, edematous, erythematous plaques that may blister. Lesions on mucous membranes such as the oral mucosa, the modified mucous membrane skin of the vulva, or the glans penis normally blister but quickly erode before the blister is recognized (**Figs. 10-44 through 10-46**). On this thinner, moist epithelium, the individual lesions are often more irregular in shape. These lesions are often accompanied by a burning sensation. Further exposures to the causative medication produce subsequent fixed drug reaction lesions at previously affected sites, although each exposure may be associated with new lesions as well. The lesions disappear when the drug is withdrawn, although residual postinflammatory hyperpigmentation is common.

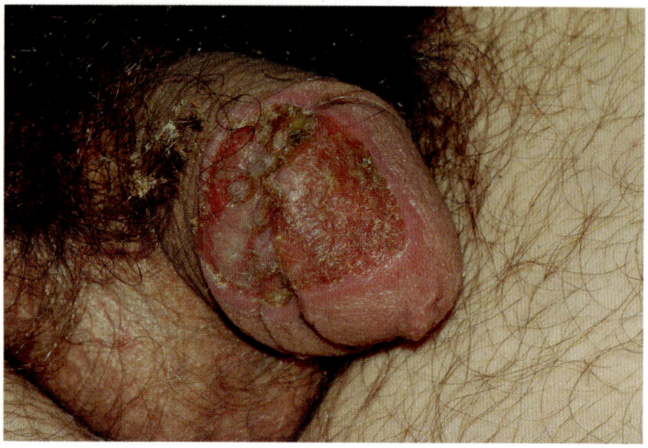

Fig. 10-44. A fixed drug eruption presents as one or a few blisters that, on fragile skin, immediately erode, recurring with each exposure to the medication; these can easily be misdiagnosed historically as recurrent herpes simplex virus infection, but the size of the erosions are too large for classic HSV. (Courtesy of Errol Craig, MD.)

### Diagnosis

The diagnosis of a fixed drug eruption is made by the abrupt onset of oral and/or genital erosions, often with blisters or edematous round plaques of keratinized skin, in the presence of a history of recent ingestion of a medication known to cause this skin eruption. Usually, the history also reveals that recurrent lesions in the same location have occurred in the past. Although mucous membrane erosions of a fixed drug eruption generally are nonspecific, keratinized skin lesions are often very helpful when pres-

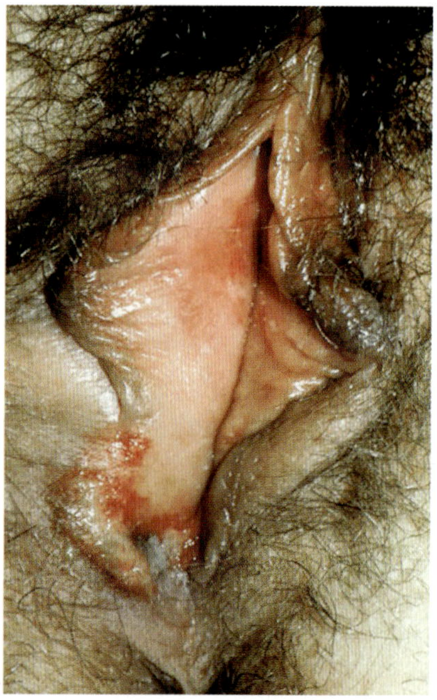

Fig. 10-45. The recurrent erosion of a fixed drug eruption occurs in the exact same spot, as on posterior right vulva. Although these are usually round due to the original shape of the blister, on fragile mucous membranes or modified mucous membranes, friction can erode the lesion and change the shape.

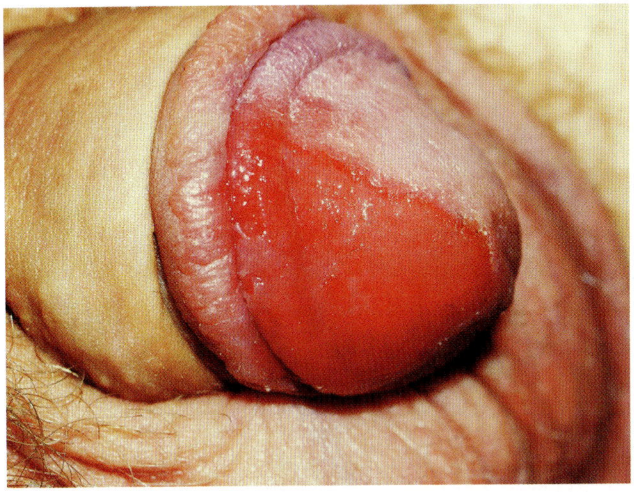

Fig. 10-46. This well-demarcated erosion is classic for a fixed drug eruption to doxycycline taken for acne.

ent, and round, well-demarcated patches of deep postinflammatory hyperpigmentation from past episodes are pathognomonic. When needed, a biopsy is usually characteristic. Histologic findings include liquefaction degeneration of the basal cell layer, with upper dermal pigment incontinence. Dyskeratotic keratinocytes and separation of the epidermis from the dermis produce bullae. Epidermal necrosis with neutrophils is characteristic.

The history of recurrent genital and oral erosions in the same locations often suggests a diagnosis of recurrent HSV infection, but the morphology does not suggest a coalescence of small erosions of vesicles. The size of the lesions is more consistent with those of an immunobullous blistering disease or trauma. Individual lesions are suggestive of blistering erythema multiforme, but the numbers of lesions is usually many fewer.

**FIXED DRUG ERUPTION — Diagnosis**

- Recurrent same-site blisters/erosions, often strikingly round
- Likely offending medication identified
- Confirmatory biopsy if needed

### Pathophysiology

Fixed drug eruptions are uncommon, peculiar hypersensitivity reactions to any of several possible medications. This eruption appears to be mediated by CD8+ memory T cells that reside in the basal layer of the epidermis. More common medications include the antibiotics amoxicillin, levofloxacin, and doxycycline, as well as nonsteroidal anti-inflammatory medications and antiseizure medications (**Table 10-2**). Foods have also been implicated, to include cashew nuts, almonds, and walnuts; seafoods such as shell fish and crab; fruits including strawberries and kiwi; and lentils have been shown to cause fixed drug eruption.[62] Quinine in tonic water, yellow food color additives such as tartrazine and quinoline yellow that are commonly found in foods and medications, have been implicated in so-called "fixed food-and-drug eruption."[62] Occasionally, an offending agent cannot be identified.

**TABLE 10-2**

**Common Medications Producing Fixed Drug Eruptions**

| |
|---|
| Acetaminophen |
| Allopurinol |
| Barbiturates |
| Carbamazepine |
| Furosemide |
| Griseofulvin |
| Metronidazole |
| Nonsteroidal anti-inflammatory medications |
| Oral contraceptive medications |
| Penicillins |
| Phenytoin |
| Tetracyclines |
| Sulfonamides |

### Management

The most important aspects of treatment are the identification and elimination of the offending medication. Otherwise, therapy is supportive only. Soaks, infection control, and pain medication are mainstays.

**FIXED DRUG ERUPTION — Management**

- Discontinuation of offending medication
- Bland emollients, barrier pastes

## Trauma and Iatrogenic and Artifactual Disorders

### Clinical Presentation

Injury is a well-known cause of blisters, and the protected site of the genitalia makes this a relatively uncommon cause, except for medications and genital hygiene measures (**Fig. 10-47**). The morphology of the trauma blisters and the degree and timing of discomfort depend on the insult, with many producing immediate pain. Liquids often produce a drip pattern, and blisters produce a round erosion.

### Diagnosis

The diagnosis is often made easily because the injury is immediately painful. In addition, the shape of the erosion is suggestive of the diagnosis.

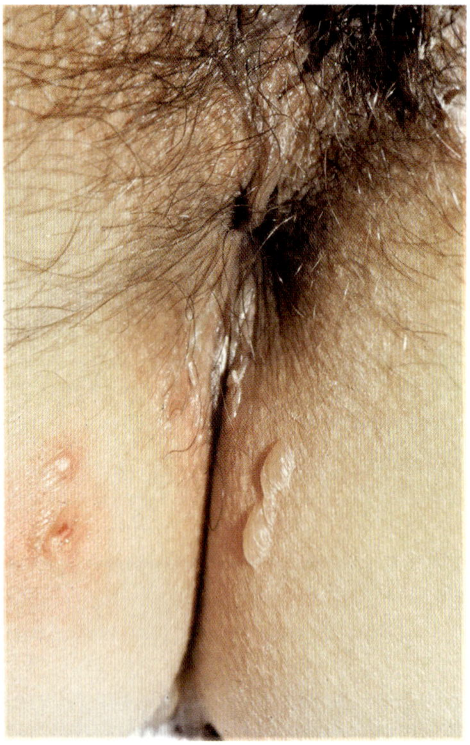

Fig. 10-47. Cantharidin was applied to destroy mollusca contagiosa and produced these blisters.

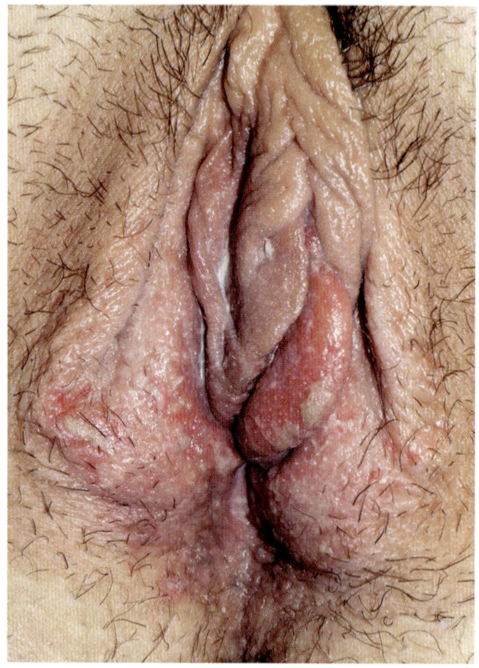

Fig. 10-48. Eutectic mixture of local anesthesia (EMLA) was applied before a biopsy and produced blistering with immediate sloughing due to acute irritant contact dermatitis.

Autoimmune blistering diseases are occasionally mistaken for traumatic lesions. However, an examination of other areas usually shows evidence of these other diseases, and a biopsy can be helpful in difficult cases.

### Pathophysiology

Erosions and blisters from trauma can occur from many different types of insults. A common cause of genital erosions is a chemical burn, particularly from wart therapies such as podophyllin, trichloroacetic and bichloroacetic acids, and fluorouracil. Less often, patient-applied podofilox or imiquimod produces erosions. Thermal burns can occur in this area, but these are uncommon, whereas blisters and erosions from cryotherapy for warts or dysplasia are usual reactions to treatment. Other traumas inflicted for medical purposes that cause erosions include laser surgery and electrocautery.

### Management

Bland emollients, soaks, pain medication, and infection control are important. The prognosis depends upon the cause of the trauma.

## Contact Dermatitis

Blisters can occur from acute contact dermatitis produced by contact with a caustic irritant or a specific strong allergen. Normally, that substance was applied directly to the area of the dermatitis. However, sometimes, the offending agent is carried by unsuspecting fingers accidently. A tiny amount of medication left on fingers following application to another area is wiped onto genital skin following urination. Then, the genital skin becomes pruritic, and more medication is carried there by scratching fingers throughout the day.

Irritant contact dermatitis is produced by a substance that directly and nonimmunologically damages the skin. An irritant reaction sufficient to produce erosions or blisters is generally called a chemical burn (see the above discussion of trauma) **(Fig. 10-48)**.

Allergic contact dermatitis is a cell-mediated type IV allergic reaction to a specific allergen, occurring at the point of contact. Although most allergic contact dermatitis presents as red, scaling, pruritic plaques, some allergens are so potent that they cause blisters, the most well-known of which is the allergen in plants such as poison ivy and poison oak. More common allergens that cause blisters relevant to the genitalia include topical creams containing the antibiotic neomycin (triple antibiotic ointment, Neosporin) and the local anesthetics benzocaine (Vagisil) and diphenhydramine (Benadryl). The patient must be sensitized to the allergen. One or two days following a subsequent exposure to the allergen, the rash develops. An acute, strong allergic contact dermatitis consists of confluent small, firm, and pruritic vesicles within an area of erythema. On the genitalia, this often presents as erosions and blisters on a background of erythema **(Figs. 10-49 and 10-50)**. Patients should be quizzed about the specific use of these medications on any area of the body. Previous use without incident does not rule out contact dermatitis

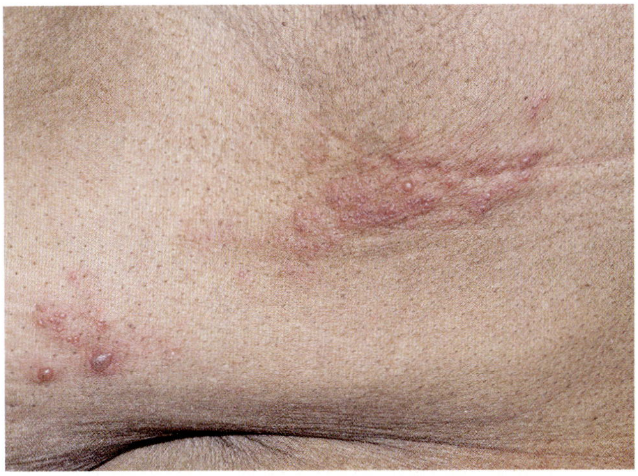

Fig. 10-49. This man inadvertently carried neomycin ointment from insect bites on his arms to his medial thighs and experienced this allergic contact dermatitis.

to that agent. This eruption may persist in the form of erythema and pruritus for several weeks after discontinuation of the medication.

The diagnosis can generally be made by the appearance and the history of a contactant. Rarely, confirmation of allergic contact dermatitis requires confirmation by patch testing normal skin with the suspected allergen. Treatment involves the elimination of responsible causative substances. The use of ointment emollients and cooling with ice packs are most soothing for irritant contact dermatitis. Allergic contact dermatitis is more responsive to corticosteroids. A superpotent topical ointment such as a tiny amount of clobetasol propionate or halobetasol propionate (15 g no refills) applied twice daily and covered with petroleum jelly is useful. For those with more severe disease, intramuscular triamcinolone acetonide 40 mg (small person) to 80 mg (large person) is appreciated, provides an automatic 1-month taper, with almost no effect on blood pressure, blood sugar, etc.

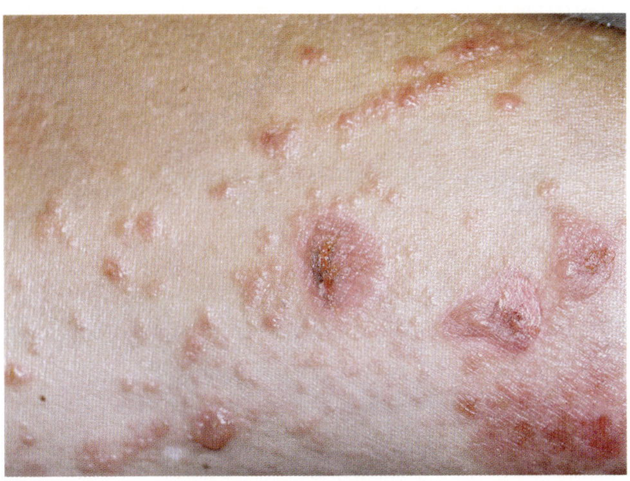

Fig. 10-50. A camping trip was responsible for exposure to poison ivy and small vesicles of allergic contact dermatitis.

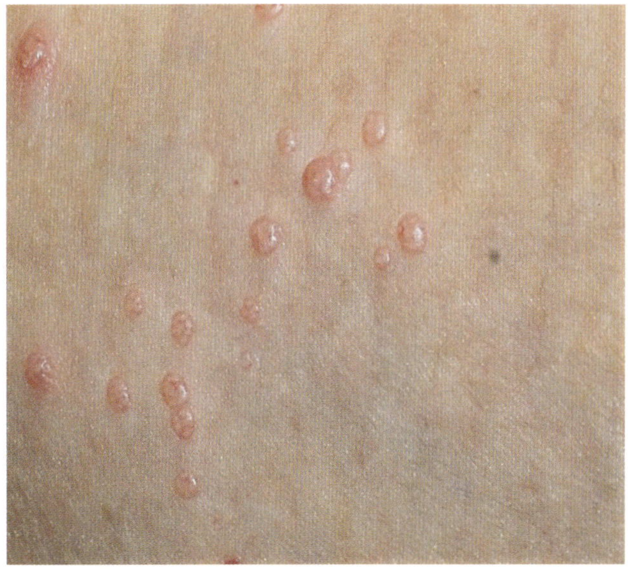

Fig. 10-51. Mollusca contagiosa are sometimes dubbed "water warts" because of their resemblance to a vesicle.

## Pseudovesicular Conditions

There are several skin conditions that can appear to be vesicular when, in fact, they are solid. Usually, that distinction can be made by touch the lesion. Occasionally, the lesion must be pierced by a needle.

### Mollusca Contagiosa

Mollusca contagiosa most often appear white or skin-colored and solid, but, true to their moniker "water wart" these lesions are sometimes sufficiently shiny that they appear vesicular (**Fig. 10-51**). This condition is discussed primarily in Chapters 7, 8, and 15.

### Hidradenoma Papilliferum

Hidradenoma papilliferum is a small cystic tumor that occurs primarily on the vulva and may appear vesicular with intermittent drainage of clear mucoid material from an overlying punctum (**Fig. 10-52**). However, these are solid to the touch. See also Chapters 6 and 7.

### Mucous Cysts/Vestibular Cysts

Mucous cysts of the vulva are relatively common cysts that arise from the obstruction of the minor vestibular glands. Often, they are translucent, and, if ruptured, these lesions emit clear mucus (**Fig. 10-53**). These are generally asymptomatic and therapy is rarely necessary.

### Lymphangiectasias and Lymphangioma Circumscriptum

Lymphangiectasias and lymphangioma circumscriptum (also discussed in Chapter 12) occur when lymphatic vessels protrude above the epithelium, producing blebs filled with lymphatic fluid. This occurs in two settings.

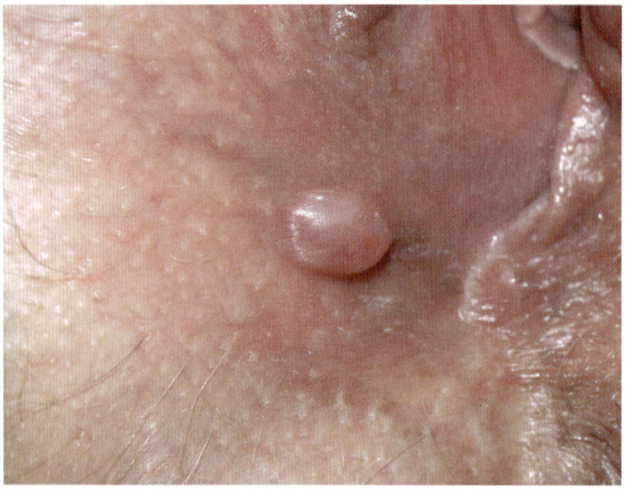

Fig. 10-52. Hidradenoma papilliferum is an uncommon tumor found most often on the vulva that sometimes mimics a blister.

The most common is in a setting of chronic; the edema obstructs lymphatic return, and dilated lymphatic vessels distend, then the overlying epithelium, and bulge above it (Fig. 10-54). This is termed lymphangiectasia or secondary lymphangioma circumscriptum. This occurs mostly on the vulva and scrotum, primarily as a result of surgery and radiation for malignancy but also from hidradenitis suppurativa, Crohn disease, and infection, especially mycobacterial. The second condition is primary lymphangioma circumscriptum, a vascular malformation of the lymphatics that produces the same surface clinical appearance. Often, a deep malformation results in fairly widely scattered, grouped multiloculated bulging lymphatics protruding though the surface. These abnormalities not only mimic vesicles but also can resemble raspberry-shaped genital warts.

The diagnosis can be made by the appearance and, usually, by the history of surgery/radiation and presence of edema, but sometimes the degree of edema can be surprisingly subtle. Rarely, a biopsy is required, but is diagnostic, showing superficial dilated lymphatic vessels.

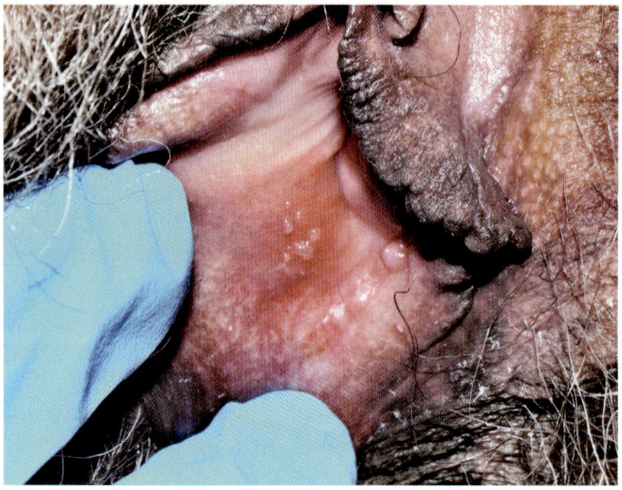

Fig. 10-53. Mucous cysts mimic blisters as well.

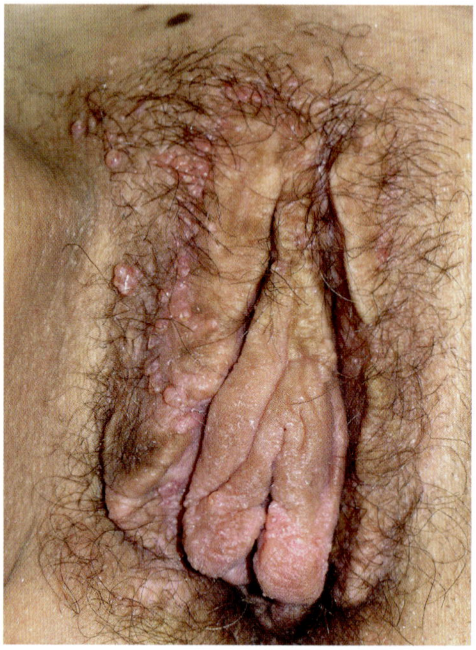

Fig. 10-54. Lymphangiectasias, also called secondary lymphangioma circumscriptum, appear as vesicles in this woman with long-standing edema of both the vulva and legs.

Dermoscopy shows lesions presented well-demarcated red-orange lacunae surrounded by white lines.[63]

There are very little data on management, but these blebs sometimes rupture and drain. Unlike true blisters, the draining can be continuous, since these connect to the entire lymphatic system, causing continuous wetness, irritant contact dermatitis, and discomfort. Laser cauterization of the surface of the blebs has been reported as successful,[64] as has vulvectomy in women.[65,66] Recurrence is usual, and repeat surgeries are required. I have found that electrocautery is often useful. This office procedure is less elegant than laser and produces a thicker surface scar, possibly allowing for a longer duration between needed treatments compared to laser.

## Basal Cell Carcinoma

Basal cell cancers usually are associated with sites of sun exposure, but 10% occur on nonexposed sites and account for 5% of genital cancers (see Chapter 7). They occur more frequently in fair individuals. The nodular type of basal cell carcinoma is sometimes described as "pearly" or "translucent," giving it the appearance of a blister (Fig. 10-55). However, these are clearly solid to the touch.

## Pustules and Pseudopustules

Pustules are vesicles filled with pus. Long-standing vesicles can appear white and mimic pustules but, if pierced, the contents are visibly clear. On occasion, desquamated, hydrated stratum corneum that obstructs or distends follicles form milia that appear somewhat yellow and mimic pustules or mucous containing cysts show a yellowish color.

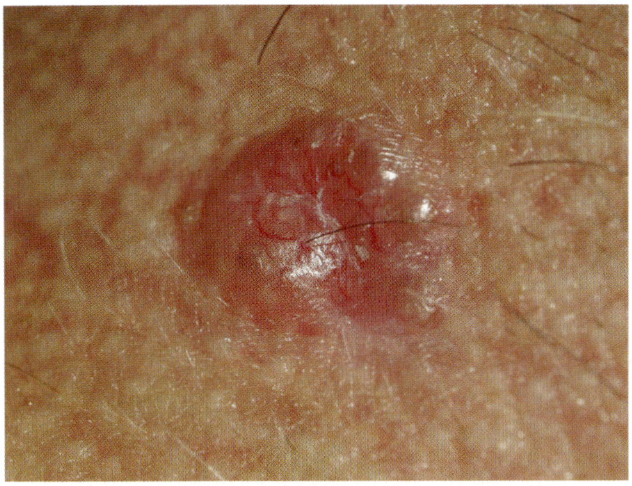

Fig. 10-55. Basal cell carcinomas often have a translucent appearance that resembles a blister, but these are firm and solid.

## True Pustular Diseases

### Folliculitis

Folliculitis refers to inflammation of hair follicles, resulting in red papules, pustules, and crusts. This is also discussed in Chapter 6. This can be bacterial, fungal, or irritant.

#### Clinical Presentation

Folliculitis occurs in all age groups, and the affected population depends on the underlying etiology **(Figs. 10-56 and 10-57)**. Irritant folliculitis occurs most often in women who shave the area and in overweight individuals at risk for prominent pressure, friction, and chronic moisture. Staphylococcal folliculitis occurs is all groups, whereas hot tub folliculitis is found in individuals exposed to inadequately treated hot tubs, or those who bathe or shower with washcloths or sponges that do not completely dry between uses. Fungal folliculitis occurs primarily in middle-aged or older men, especially those with fungal toenail infection **(Fig. 10-58)**.

Noninfectious, irritant folliculitis is most often asymptomatic, but sometimes a cosmetic issue. Scattered small pustules or red papules characterize these almost ubiquitous lesions. These occur most often on those areas of friction and pressure, such as the medial thighs and the buttocks. Shaving folliculitis (also called pseudofolliculitis barbae) is a very common form of irritant folliculitis, as increasing numbers of women shave the vulva **(Fig. 10-59)**. This consists of follicular papules, pustule, and/or crust and with magnification, hairs can often be seen curving back and into the skin **(Fig. 10-60)**.

*Staphylococcus aureus* folliculitis usually presents with symptoms of mild tenderness and pruritus. On examination, there are red papules and variable numbers of small yellow pustules from 1 to 3 mm in size with a surrounding red flare. The pustule is short lived and leaves a residual red papule with crust or a fine collarette of scale. Individual lesions heal within 7-10 days. Some patients have associated furunculosis, representing a deeper infection of the follicle. These tender, red nodules often suppurate and drain. Frequent sites include the mons pubis, buttocks, and thighs.

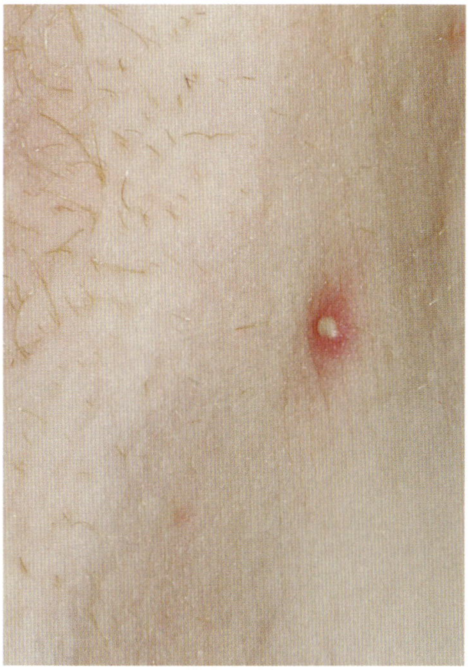

Fig. 10-56. Although folliculitis classically exhibits a hair from the center from each pustule, these are often inapparent; folliculitis is most often bacterial (especially *S aureus*) or irritant.

Pseudomonas folliculitis presents as tender, red, nonscaling papules and occasional pustules concentrated in areas where contaminated water has been held against the skin, such as intertriginous skin and under wet swimsuits.

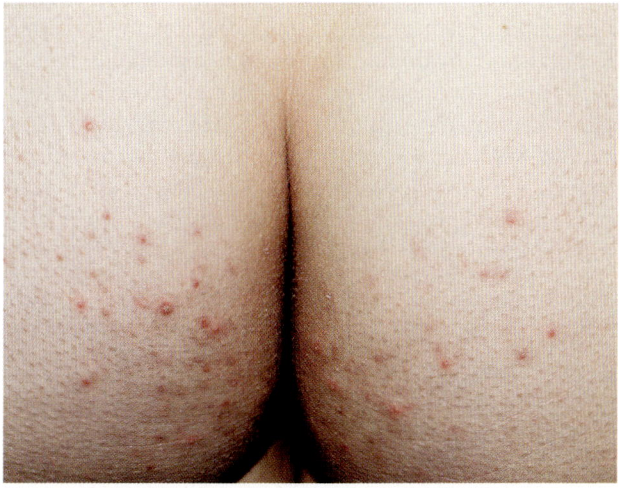

Fig. 10-57. Red papules and pustules are characteristic of folliculitis; the buttocks is a common place for irritant folliculitis due to occlusion from sitting.

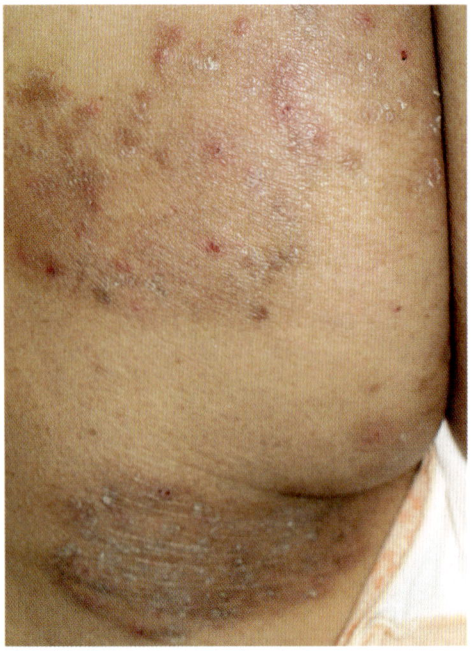

Fig. 10-58. Fungal folliculitis usually occurs as crusted papules or pustules within a plaque of scaling tinea.

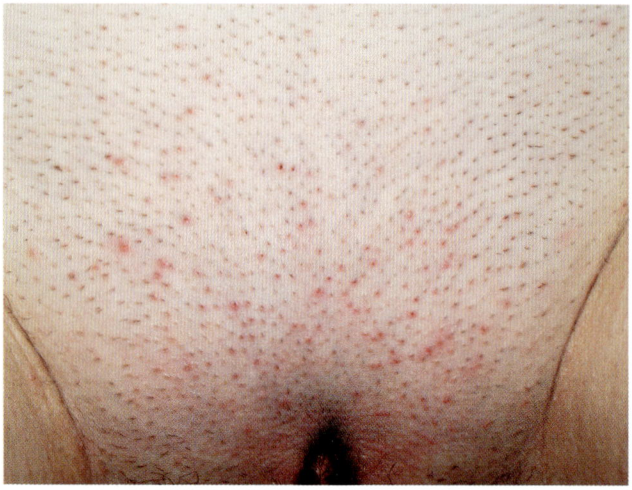

Fig. 10-59. Shaving folliculitis is a common occurrence as young women regularly shave genital hair. These are mostly manifested by red papules and erosions rather than pustules.

Sometimes, patients exhibit constitutional symptoms such as fever, malaise, ear pain, and sore throat.

Fungal folliculitis occurs within red, scaling plaques of tinea. Small nodules or follicular crusts and pustules within scaly, annular, pink-red plaques of tinea cruris characterize fungal folliculitis. However, women with tinea pedis sometimes develop scattered discrete papules or pustules of fungal folliculitis on their lower legs and thighs by inoculating fungi into follicles when they shave their legs.

## Diagnosis

The diagnosis of folliculitis is usually made clinically. A bacterial or fungal culture is often helpful to identify a causative organism and to guide the treatment course. A potassium hydroxide preparation sometimes reveals hyphae in dermatophyte folliculitis. Histopathology shows neutrophils within the hair follicle with abscess formation. Special stains may reveal the causative organism.

Folliculitis can be confused with scabies, pustular miliaria, *Candida* infection, arthropod bites, keratosis pilaris, and herpes simplex virus (HSV) infection.

**FOLLICULITIS** — **Diagnosis**

- Morphology of red papules, pustules, and crusts, sometimes with a hair piercing an occasional lesion
- Culture showing causative organism, or fungal preparation showing branching hyphae should reveal infectious causes

## Pathophysiology

Bacterial folliculitis is most often caused by *S aureus*, but it can be caused by gram-negative bacteria, especially *Pseudomonas aeruginosa*, the cause of hot tub folliculitis. Folliculitis may also be caused by dermatophytes and is most often seen in men in association with tinea cruris. Irritant folliculitis results from occlusion from pressure, friction, and moisture, so this can be exacerbated by overweight and occlusive clothing. Shaving folliculitis occurs when the shaved, short, curly hair curves back and pierces the skin, producing an inflammatory reaction or the prominent tips of follicles are removed by the razor, again causing an irritant reaction.

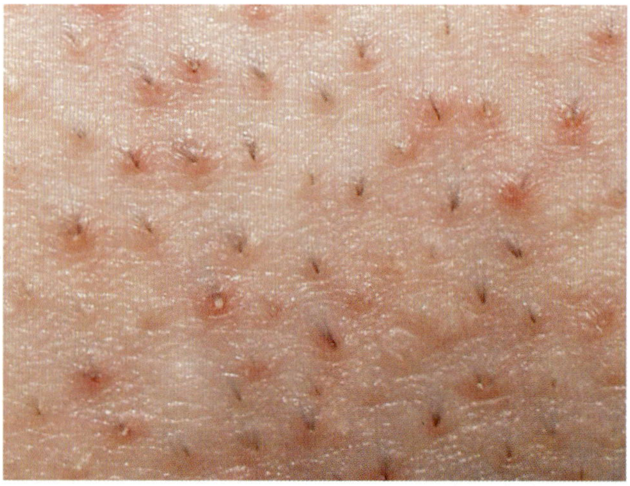

Fig. 10-60. Shaving actually produces pseudo-folliculitis when curly hair arcs back and pierces the skin, causing ingrown hairs and inflammation.

## Management

The treatment of folliculitis depends upon the etiology. Staphylococcal folliculitis can be treated with oral and topical antibiotics, with treatment guided by antibiotic sensitivities in this day of resistant organisms. Doxycycline and trimethoprim-sulfamethoxazole are nearly always effective. Mupirocin cream and ointment are extremely effective for the first week of use but resistance occurs quickly.

Recurrence of staphylococcal folliculitis is common. Nasal staphylococcal carriage is an explanation in some of these individuals with chronic and recurrent folliculitis. These patients benefit by the application of mupirocin ointment to the anterior nares twice a day for 5 days. Because carriers often have recurrent colonization of *S aureus* within their nares, some clinicians recommend that these patients apply the mupirocin treatment for 5 days every 1 to 6 months indefinitely to prevent recurrent folliculitis.

Pseudomonas folliculitis (hot tub folliculitis) requires no treatment because it resolves when exposure ceases. Therefore, identification of the source of the organism and avoidance of reinoculation are most important. Emptying and cleaning the spa or hot tub and proper maintenance of bactericidal chemicals is also important. However, those patients who exhibit constitutional symptoms may improve more rapidly if they receive oral ciprofloxacin at 500 mg twice a day or levofloxacin 500 mg/d. Patients should be advised to allow washcloths and sponges in the shower or bath to completely dry between uses to minimize the growth of pseudomonas.

Fungal folliculitis requires oral therapy because the organism extends into the follicle where topical antifungal creams cannot penetrate. Oral terbinafine at 250 mg/d until the skin is clear is effective, and it is an inexpensive solution. Alternatively, oral fluconazole or itraconazole may also be prescribed at doses of 100 mg/d orally for 15 days or until the skin is clear. Fluconazole 100-200 mg daily, itraconazole 200 mg daily, as well as griseofulvin 500 mg twice daily with fatty food twice daily until the eruption resolves are effective as well. After treatment, the daily use of an antifungal cream or powder to the groin area helps to prevent recurrences.

Irritant folliculitis can be improved by minimizing irritants. Avoiding shaving clears shaving folliculitis; permanent laser hair removal may be preferable. Cool, nonocclusive clothing, weight loss, and powders may prevent chronic moisture, pressure, and friction. Otherwise, the chronic administration of anti-inflammatory antibiotics such as doxycycline or minocycline 100 mg bid or clindamycin 150 mg bid can improve irritant folliculitis, although improvement generally requires about a month and entails ongoing administration.

**FOLLICULITIS — Management**

- Depends on the underlying cause:
  - Bacterial folliculitis: treat according to culture results. For suspected staphylococcal folliculitis, oral doxycycline 100 mg bid, clindamycin 150 mg bid, trimethoprim-sulfamethoxazole double strength bid.
  - Fungal folliculitis: terbinafine 250 mg daily, fluconazole 100-200 mg daily, or itraconazole 200 mg a day, or griseofulvin 500 mg bid until clear
  - Irritant folliculitis: minimize irritants. Discontinue shaving, add powders to reduce friction and moisture. When required, chronic anti-inflammatory antibiotics such as doxycycline 100 mg bid can be taken chronically

## Sebaceous Adenitis (Vulvar Fordyce Adenitis)

Sebaceous adenitis is a recently described idiopathic condition of red papules, pustules, nodules, and pitted scars on the vulva, primarily on the labia minora and medial labia majora **(Fig. 10-61)**. An evaluation of 45 women reported 17 of 26 for who information was available also had acne, and the age range was 16-60 years.[67] Four biopsies performed showed neutrophilic inflammation around sebaceous glands. There are vestigial hair follicles in this area of the vulva, and I have seen biopsy proven folliculitis here as well. Without a biopsy, I suspect that these two conditions could be indistinguishable. Chronic tetracyclines, often with antiandrogens such as spironolactone, are generally effective in controlling vulvar sebaceous adenitis.[68]

## Furunculosis

While folliculitis is characterized by inflammation of the superficial portion of the hair follicle, furunculosis is a

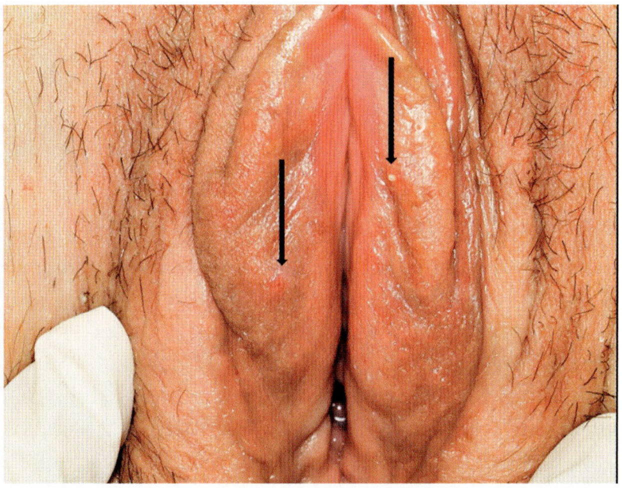

Fig. 10-61. Sebaceous adenitis is indistinguishable from folliculitis except for its location; on the modified mucous membranes of the vulva, especially the medial labia minora. This is manifested by pustules and red papules/erosions (*arrows*), and often depressed scars are present.

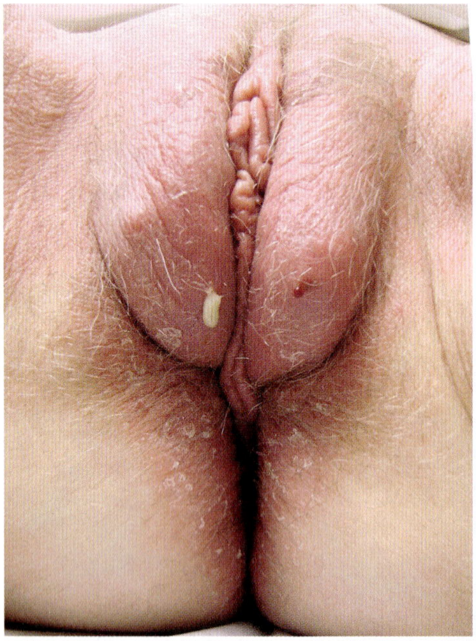

Fig. 10-62. Furuncles consist of bacterial infection, nearly always *S aureus*, that occurs in deeper portions of the follicle, producing abscesses and deep nodules. The very sudden onset at age 42, the association with psoriasis, and a culture showing *S aureus* differentiated these nodules from hidradenitis suppurativa.

bacterial infection that involves the deeper follicle, producing a red "boil" (see Chapter 6).

### Clinical Presentation

Furunculosis occurs in all patient populations. It is somewhat more common in patients who are immunosuppressed, diabetic, or who exhibit scaling dermatoses that are likely to be colonized with *S aureus*.

A furuncle is a red, usually painful nodule that typically suppurates and drains **(Fig. 10-62)**. Patients experience evolving lesions, with some appearing as others heal. Often, there is associated staphylococcal folliculitis or even surrounding cellulitis. Uncommonly, patients develop associated fever and malaise.

### Diagnosis

The diagnosis is made on clinical grounds, and it is confirmed by a culture that usually yields *S aureus*. A biopsy is generally not performed, but it reveals a dermal and subcutaneous abscess with surrounding cellulitis. Special stains show organisms consistent with *S aureus*.

A furuncle occurring in the genital area is indistinguishable from an inflamed epidermal ("sebaceous") cyst. Cysts of the genital area, when recurrent, are due to hidradenitis suppurativa (HS), which is a form of deep cystic acne. However, furuncles are not confined to the genital and axillary area as is HS, and hidradenitis suppurativa usually also exhibits comedones and scarring from recurrent draining abscesses. Cultures of hidradenitis suppurativa usually show normal skin organisms or a multitude of bacteria including enteric organisms. Additional diagnostic confusion can occur with other inflamed cysts, such as an inflamed Bartholin gland duct cyst or a vestibular cyst. Occasionally, inflamed tumors such as a basal cell carcinoma can mimic a furuncle.

### Pathophysiology

Furunculosis represents a bacterial infection, usually with *S aureus*, of the deep portion of the follicle, with a resulting inflammatory nodule.

### Management

Oral antistaphylococcal antibiotics are effective in clearing furunculosis. Previous first-line medications such as cephalexin, dicloxacillin, and methicillin are often ineffective due to the increase in community-acquired methicillin *S aureus*. Trimethoprim-sulfamethoxazole double strength, doxycycline, or antibiotics according to culture results are preferable. Unfortunately, recurrent disease after discontinuation of medication sometimes occurs. A rare patient requires prolonged oral therapy, in addition to the insertion of mupirocin ointment to the anterior nares twice a day for the first 5 days of therapy to reduce the carrier state. Washing with antiseptics such as povidone-iodine solution or chlorhexidine can decrease the recurrence rate as well, but these are often very irritating.

## Hidradenitis Suppurativa (Acne Inversa) (Discussed Primarily in Chapter 6)

This relatively common eruption is often misdiagnosed as furunculosis but actually represents cystic acne of skinfolds rather than an infectious process.

### Clinical Presentation

Hidradenitis suppurativa (HS) is an inflammatory condition of skinfolds that presents with a remarkable variability of severity, ranging from a rare inflamed nodule to coalescing ulcerated nodules with chronic foul-smelling, painful draining sinus tracts and firm fibrotic scars **(Figs. 10-63 to 10-65)**.

Hidradenitis suppurativa generally occurs after puberty, and this condition is worse in overweight individuals. There is a strong association with smoking as well. Painful, firm, red nodules occur in the axillae and/or the genital area, including the crural creases, proximal inner thighs, scrotum, buttocks, and vulva. Occasionally, the lower abdomen can be involved. These nodules become fluctuant and drain, with some draining tracts become chronic. A careful examination usually yields some comedones and follicles with more than one outlet to the surface. HS is

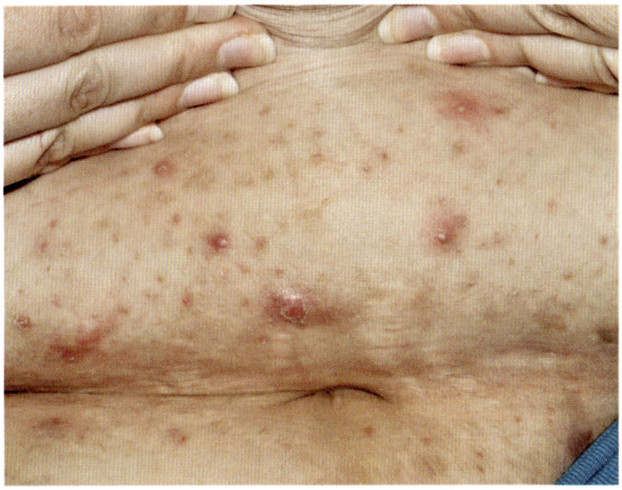

Fig. 10-63. Often mistaken for furunculosis, hidradenitis suppurativa is chronic, shows negative cultures, and does not clear with antibiotics.

graded according to severity. In communicating with providers, the most common grading scale is Hurley staging. Hurley stage I is one or more discrete nodules without sinus tracts or scarring. Hurley stage II consists of multiple cysts with sinus tracts and scarring, but these are fairly spaced. Hurley stage III occurs when inflamed cysts with sinus tracts are connected and cover large areas.

This disease is more than a skin condition. Most patients are obese, and HS is very strongly associated with the metabolic syndrome.[69] There are additional comorbidities sufficiently common that the Canadian and U.S. HS Foundations recommend specific screening; acne, dissecting cellulitis of the scalp, pilonidal disease, pyoderma gangrenosum, depression, generalized anxiety disorder, suicide, smoking, substance use disorder, polycystic ovary syndrome, obesity, dyslipidemia, diabetes mellitus, hypertension, cardiovascular disease, inflammatory bowel disease, spondyloarthritis, and sexual dysfunction.[70] It should not be surprising that hidradenitis

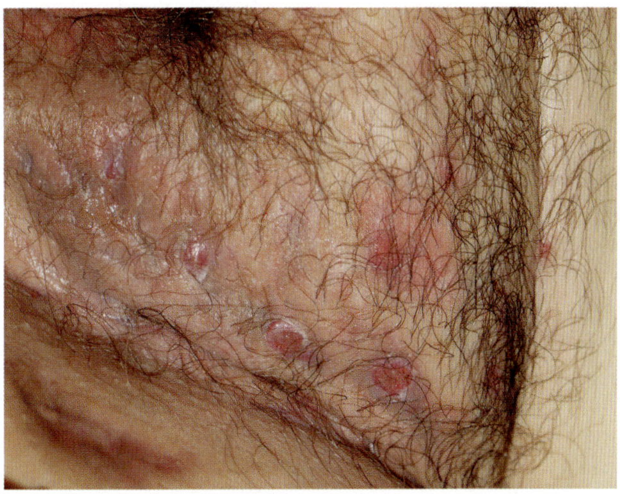

Fig. 10-64. The inflamed cysts of hidradenitis suppurativa often rupture, and then form chronic draining sinus tracts to the surface.

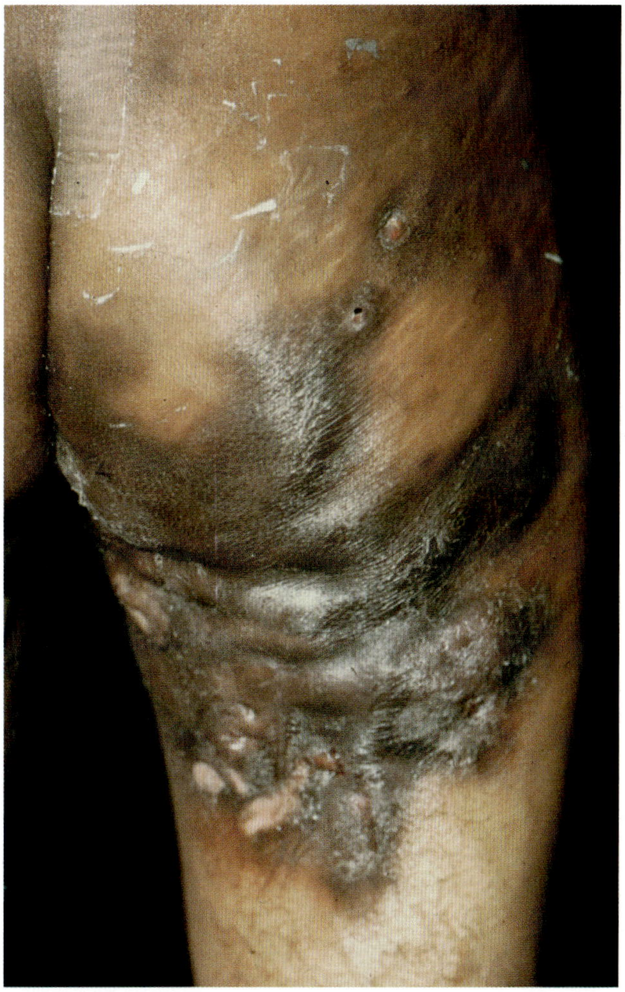

Fig. 10-65. With severe HS, cysts not only drain to the surface, but interconnect into coalescing plaques with purulent drainage.

suppurativa produces depression and issues with body image, self esteem, and sexual dysfunction.[71] Pain is often prominent, and HS at times seems to precipitate pain out of proportion to that expected from the degree of the disease present, and this has been postulated to occur from central sensitization precipitated by HS.[72]

Rarely, long-standing disease can eventuate into squamous cell carcinoma (SCC). A review of 95 patients with SCC showed that the mean time from onset of HS to diagnosis of SCC was 25.5 years of disease activity.[73] Most reports were in men, with the most common sites being, in this order, the gluteal area, perianal skin, and genital skin, so careful surveillance of these areas is indicated in long-standing disease. The mortality rate was 58.7%.

## Diagnosis

The diagnosis is made on the basis of the presence of chronic or recurrent draining nodules localized to the anogenital skin, axillae, buttocks, medial thighs, abdomen, and the presence of comedones. A biopsy, which is not indicated, reveals a distended follicle with surrounding inflammation consisting of neutrophils, lymphocytes, and histiocytes. Abscesses form and destroy pilosebaceous units, with resulting granulation tissue and epithelialized sinus tracts.

Staphylococcal furunculosis is the disease most easily confused with hidradenitis suppurativa. However, furunculosis is acute, usually not limited to the axillae and groin, yields a pure growth of a pathogen on culture, and responds quickly to appropriate antibiotics. In addition, comedones are not seen in association with furunculosis. A solitary inflamed epidermal cyst can mimic mild HS and may, in fact, represent mild HS.

**HIDRADENITIS SUPPURATIVA — Diagnosis**

- Morphology of inflamed nodules, comedones, and scarring
- Location of the groin, buttocks, medial thighs, vulva, scrotum, lower abdomen, breast areas, and/or axillae
- Chronic or recurrent
- Cultures that show normal skin flora or mixed bacteria and enterics
- Incomplete response to antibiotics

### Pathophysiology

HS is a condition that is multifactorial in origin, and the pathogenesis is poorly understood and has evolved over the years. Recent manuscripts discuss different factors in detail and are available as free articles.[74,75] These factors are only briefly acknowledged here.

Lifestyle is important. Obesity is a known important risk factor, and weight loss alone sometimes produces remarkable improvement in HS. Many more than back ground patients with HS smoke. Genetics plays a role, with about a third of patients reporting a family history. Although HS is not an infectious disease, the presence of bacteria, fungi, and viruses on the skin may play a role in the inflammatory response of this disease. Sex hormones are likely to play a role, as evidenced by age of onset after puberty, changes in severity during pregnancy, premenstrual flaring, and improvement with antiandrogens. Clearly, the follicle is important, and histology shows hyperkeratosis of the follicular epithelium and inflammation of the follicle, followed later by rupture of the follicle. There are also alterations of the innate immune system, and a role for the cytokine milieu. The efficacy of TNF alpha blockers in therapy suggests a role for TNF alpha in the pathogenesis of HS, and interferon $\gamma$ is found in wound drainage, and there is evidence for the interleukins as factors.

### Management

Patient education, as is usual, is paramount. A discussion regarding the presence of the metabolic syndrome is important, and support for the coexistent very common depression and pain can be crucial. Weight loss is often the single most important specific intervention, and weight loss in a very obese patient alone sometimes produces a remarkable improvement in the disease. However, aggressively addressing weight loss is a difficult task while also offering psychological support to a patient who is already depressed and suffering from a poor body image. Whereas smoking cessation may be lifesaving in a patient with the metabolic syndrome, it does not improve HS, although it may provide enhanced improvement with adalimumab.

Time honored prevention of the development of inflammatory nodules consists of topical and oral antibiotics used both to decrease surface bacteria that may irritate the skin, and for the anti-inflammatory effects of some antibiotics.[76] Usual choices include the tetracyclines doxycycline or minocycline at 100 mg twice a day with food, clindamycin 150 mg twice a day, sometimes with rifampin, or trimethoprim-sulfamethoxazole double strength twice daily, ongoing. Fluoroquinolones have been reported useful but are more expensive and with more side effects. Because these antibiotics are used for their anti-inflammatory effects rather than curative antimicrobial effects, a month or longer are required for improvement, and discontinuation results in relapse. The older medication dapsone, at 50-150 mg a day, has been reported as useful both alone and in combination with oral antibiotics,[77] and colchicine, at 1 mg a day, has shown variable results.[78,79]

Triamcinolone acetonide injected into a very early nodule (see Chapter 4) can prevent almost overnight evolution of the lesion into an abscess, so that the patient with an occasional lesion can be controlled with only intralesional corticosteroids. And, for those with frequent new or recurrent lesions, intralesional corticosteroids represent good adjuvant therapy. However, large fluctuant nodules are not good candidates for intralesional therapy, as the medication is simply diluted in the middle of the abscess. Patients can even inject their own nodules. Although incision and drainage of tense, fluctuant lesions make the patient more comfortable, this approach provides only temporary improvement of individual lesions.

The advent of biologic therapy for hidradenitis suppurativa has changed the face of management of the disease. Tumor necrosis factor (TNF) alpha blockers are useful for HS, and adalimumab (Humira) has FDA indication approval at a dose of 40 mg weekly. Trials are ongoing with infliximab. Ustekinumab (Stelara) has shown promise for the management of HS as well.[76] As with antibiotics, improvement is slow, requiring up to 3 months for significant improvement. Although this is an immunosuppressant, the side effect profile has proven to be very acceptable as long as tuberculosis exposure is monitored and care is taken in patients with preexisting malignancy.[80] Interestingly, neither adalimumab nor ustekinumab during COVID-19 for inflammatory diseases including HS has been associated with an increased risk of contracting the disease, or with a worsened COVID-19 outcome.[81]

Other therapies that have been used include oral retinoids, such as isotretinoin, which are primarily used for cystic acne of the face and trunk. Although a 4- to 5-month course of isotretinoin normally induces long-term remission of acne, incomplete clearing and prompt relapse of hidradenitis suppurativa is usual. A relatively new safe but expensive oral medication for psoriasis, apremilast, has been reported in several trials as useful for HS.[82] Women with hidradenitis sometimes derive benefit from hormonal therapy. High-estrogen oral contraceptives such as those with ethinyl estradiol 0.035 mg or higher and antiandrogens such a spironolactone can sometimes be useful. Dairy has been implicated by at least one expert in the treatment of hidradenitis.

Although successful medical therapy prevents the appearance of new cysts and abscesses, it does not heal draining sinus tracts. When disease is recalcitrant, surgical removal of the affected skin should be considered when practical. Excision is a common mode of removal, but hidradenitis suppurativa occurring in the groin can be too expensive for excision. Alternatives include carbon dioxide laser ablation with healing by secondary intention, excision of only the most involved areas, and excision of individual fistulas. Also, de-roofing of individual chronic cysts and sinus tracts is performed by some and is a successful office procedure for limited areas. This procedure is explained and pictured in Chapter 4.

**HIDRADENITIS SUPPURATIVA — Management**

- Life-style changes: weight loss, discontinuation of smoking
- Management of metabolic syndrome
- Mild disease
  - Oral anti-inflammatory antibiotics: doxycycline or minocycline 100 mg bid, clindamycin 150 mg bid, trimethoprim-sulfamethoxazole double strength bid
  - Topical antibiotics, clindamycin solution twice a day
  - Intralesional corticosteroid injection into new individual inflamed cysts
  - High-estrogen oral contraceptives (women)
  - Spironolactone 50-200 mg as anti-androgen (women)
  - Unroofing of sinus tracts, unroofing or excision of chronic cysts
- Moderate and severe disease, add
  - Adalimumab 40 mg SQ weekly
  - Aggressive surgical excision

## Mucocutaneous Candidiasis (see Chapters 5 and 13)

Cutaneous candidiasis occurs in women with severe vaginal candidiasis, but also in men and women who are overweight, diabetic, and/or incontinent so that there is a warm, wet environment. Immunosuppression can be a major factor.

Because the pustules are extremely fragile, with the split in the skin occurring just at the top of the epithelium, intact pustules are not commonly seen (**Figs. 10-66 through 10-68**). More often, the typical presentation is that of collarettes, the circle of scale from the ruptured pustule and superficial erosions. *Candida* vaginitis usually accompanies the skin disease in women. In men, intertriginous candidiasis presents with red, well-demarcated plaques in the crural crease, and multiple satellite 1- to 3-mm papulopustules, erosions, or collarettes at the periphery. Eventually,

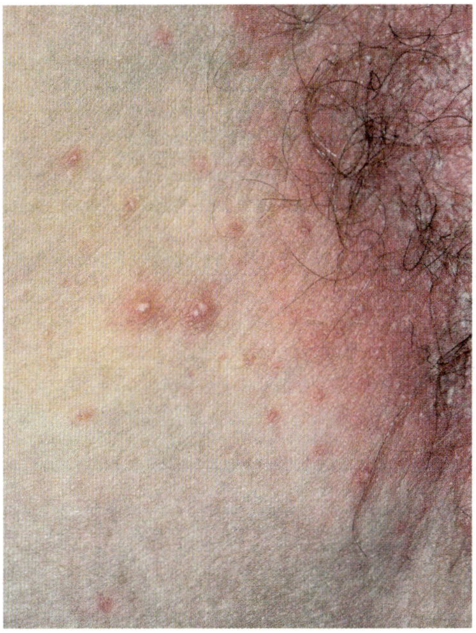

Fig. 10-66. *Candida intertrigo* is manifested by a moist red plaque in skinfolds, here with white maceration. Although classic, intact pustules as seen here are uncommon because of the fragility of these pustules.

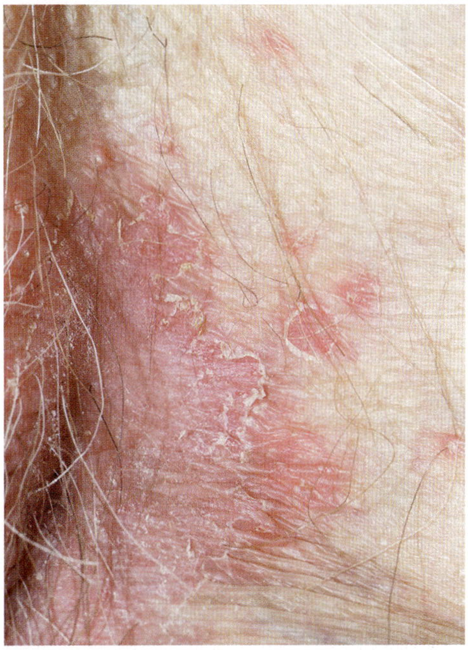

Fig. 10-67. More common than intact pustules are flaccid collarettes of empty blisters and peripheral remains of ruptured pustules around the intertrigo.

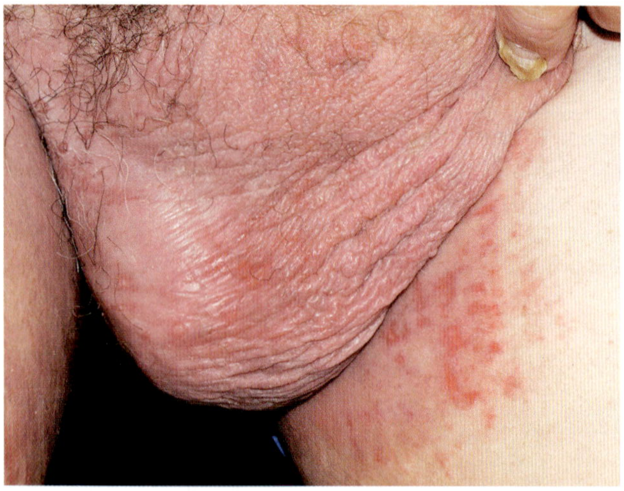

Fig. 10-68. Most commonly found in pustular candidiasis are the erosions from broken pustules rather than the pustules themselves.

the disease may spread to the scrotum and the proximal, medial thighs. Uncircumcised men may develop balanitis or balanoposthitis with flat, delicate, white-yellow, discrete 1-mm pustules, and surface erosions on the glans penis.

The diagnosis of candidiasis is confirmed by direct microscopic examination of the skin scrapings or purulent exudate, using potassium hydroxide, by a fungal culture, or by response to therapy after a clinical diagnosis.

Intertriginous candidiasis can be indistinguishable from inverse psoriasis. Other conditions that can be confused with cutaneous candidiasis include seborrheic dermatitis, tinea cruris, and folliculitis. Intertrigo dermatitis can mimic and coexist with candidiasis.

When severe, maceration and exudation are initially managed with cool soaks. Tap water is adequate for this, is inexpensive, and contains no allergens or irritants. Although topical azoles such as miconazole, clotrimazole, terconazole, econazole, and ketoconazole are the most commonly prescribed anticandidal agents, those patients who exhibit pustules, erosions, or crusting may experience local irritation or burning with these topical, alcohol-containing creams. Nystatin is available in a more soothing ointment form.

Fluconazole 150 mg once is the only oral medication that has indication approval by the United States Food and Drug Administration for the treatment of vulvovaginal candidiasis. Patients with prominent involvement of keratinized skin may require more than single-dose therapy, and 100 mg daily for several days until the skin is clear or healed sufficiently so that a topical therapy can be substituted is a common regimen. Acute inflammation and pruritus can be rapidly improved by the addition of topical hydrocortisone ointment 1% or 2.5% twice daily for the first 2 or 3 days.

Treatment of recurrent intertriginous candidiasis requires drying of the skin by minimizing occlusion, applying drying antifungal powders, and separating skinfolds of obese patients with soft cloth. Oral fluconazole given weekly can also help to control this problem in those with recalcitrant disease. Once clear, antiperspirants help to maintain dryness in skinfolds, and antifungal powders minimize recurrences.

## Pustular Psoriasis

Psoriasis is a disease that exhibits several very disparate morphologies. This disease is discussed primarily in Chapter 5; the pathogenesis and therapies are similar for all varieties of psoriasis.

Pustular psoriasis occurs when the neutrophilic inflammation is sufficiently marked as to aggregate into clinically apparent, small abscesses, changing the morphologic character from the classic red, scaling, well-demarcated plaques into plaques of pustules. This form of psoriasis is rare on genital skin. Crops of pustules within well-demarcated red plaques occur, but these rupture quickly to produce small, well-demarcated, coalescing erosions with scale or crust **(Figs. 10-69 and 10-70)**.

On dry, keratinized skin, ruptured pustules become plaques of crust with yellow scale. Macerated lesions also occur on the glans of the uncircumcised penis, whereas scaling occurs on the circumcised glans. On occasion, arcuate white/yellow papules occur on the glans, mimicking balanitis circinata of the very closely related disease, reactive arthritis (Reiter disease). In skinfolds, red plaques occur, with satellite papules and pustules that mimic Candidiasis.

Psoriasis is associated with obesity, anxiety and depression, alcoholism, arthritis, and metabolic syndrome, particularly in those individuals who exhibit widespread or severe disease.

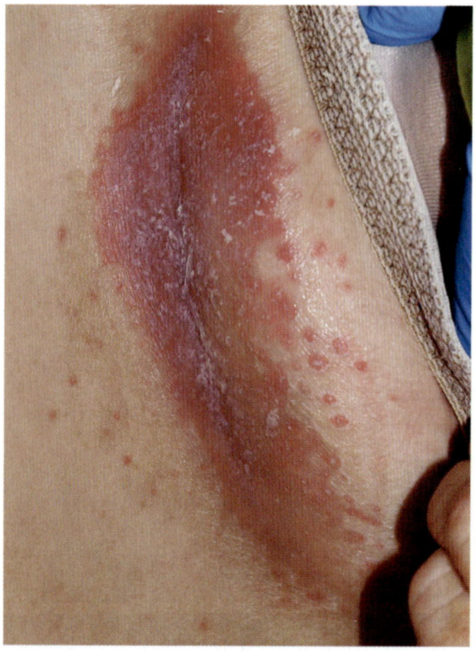

Fig. 10-69. This plaque of inverse psoriasis with satellite pustules is indistinguishable from intertriginous Candidiasis; negative fungal cultures, a high index of suspicion, and a response to topical corticosteroids confirmed the diagnosis of psoriasis.

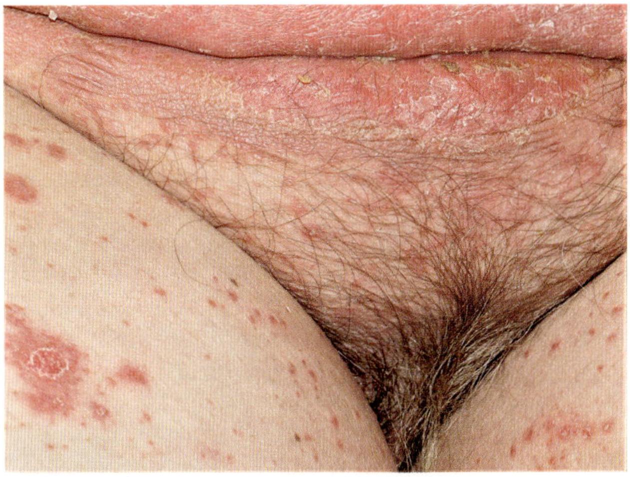

Fig. 10-70. This patient shows both scattered intact pustules and yellow scale/crust consistent with ruptured pustules in the scaling plaques of psoriasis.

The diagnosis is usually suspected from the clinical appearance, and it is confirmed by microscopic smears and cultures that are negative for infection, and by biopsy. A biopsy shows neutrophils that collect in the tips of the papillary dermis and migrate into the epidermis to form spongiform degeneration with numerous neutrophils. Neutrophilic abscesses collect just under the stratum corneum. Psoriasiform acanthosis is usual in developed disease.

Localized pustular psoriasis often cannot be distinguished morphologically or histologically from the very closely related reactive arthritis. Differentiation rests with the more common occurrence of arthritis, inflammatory eye changes, and urethritis in patients with reactive arthritis. However, these abnormalities can occur with pustular psoriasis as well, and these closely related diseases exist on a spectrum. Localized pustular psoriasis also must be distinguished from tinea cruris with pustular follicular involvement, impetigo, and acute candidiasis. Subcorneal pustular dermatosis resembles pustular psoriasis and may, in fact, represent a form of psoriasis. Discrete larger pustules with "lakes of pus" that exhibit a fluid-pus level characterize subcorneal pustular dermatosis.

Tinea cruris with follicular involvement and candidiasis can be differentiated by the identification of fungal organisms on microscopic smears or culture and by complete resolution with therapy.

Patients with localized, mild disease can be treated with a mid-potency or high-potency topical corticosteroid ointment such as triamcinolone 0.1% or fluocinonide 0.05% with a variable measure of prompt improvement. However, satisfactory and long-lasting benefit of significant pustular psoriasis from topical corticosteroids is rare, and specific systemic therapy is generally required. Topical calcipotriene (Dovonex) cream and calcipotriol (Vectical) ointment, applied twice a day, can improve the skin, and the combination medication calcipotriene and betamethasone dipropionate ointment applied daily can be useful. Other standard antipsoriasis topical therapies including tars, retinoids, and anthralin are too irritating for use in the genital area.

There are several systemic therapies for pustular psoriasis. These medications are quite effective, but because they exhibit important adverse reactions, they should be used only with great care and by physicians knowledgeable about their use and necessary monitoring. Cyclosporine is a short-term rescue medication for those with severe disease. Acitretin (Soriatane) is an oral aromatic retinoid that is very useful for many patients with erythrodermic or pustular psoriasis. This medication produces rapid cessation of new pustules with substantial clearing of the skin within a few weeks. However, this potent medication has several major adverse reactions. It is a formidable teratogen that can be stored for years in body fat if it is ingested with alcohol. In addition, retinoids raise serum triglyceride levels and they sometimes produce exostoses. More common and sometimes incapacitating but reversible symptoms are skin fragility, dryness, and arthralgias. The usual dose of acitretin is 0.5-1.0 mg/kg/d, generally given as 25-50 mg once a day. Methotrexate and biologics as well as apremilast are additional systemic agents used for recalcitrant psoriasis.

## Reactive Arthritis (Reiter Syndrome)

Originally called Reiter syndrome, this eponymous term was changed to reactive arthritis because Reiter is believed to have been the director of the Kaiser Wilhelm Institute of Experimental Therapy in Nazi Germany.[83] Reactive arthritis is a relatively rare, immune-mediated inflammatory spondylarthritis that occurs following a genitourinary or gastrointestinal infection. See also Chapter 15.

### Clinical Presentation

Reactive arthritis is defined as a triad of conjunctivitis, nongonococcal urethritis, and oligoarthritis, although most patients present without all three signs, and the picture becomes complete over time. This condition is often associated with skin lesions identical to those of pustular psoriasis. Reactive arthritis affects men over women in a ratio of 20:1 and occurs most often in those who are human leukocyte antigen (HLA)-B27 positive.[83] The most commonly affected ages are the second and third decade. Those patients with disease triggered by diarrhea usually report diarrhea about 3 weeks earlier, which has resolved by the time of presentation, and those triggered by sexually transmitted disease report dysuria, penile discharge and testicular pain (men), and bleeding and pelvic pain (women). The arthritis can be short lived, recurrent, or continuous, and about 20% of affected individuals develop chronic joint, eye, and heart disease.

Skin lesions appear as well-demarcated, red, scaly, crusted, or pustular papules or plaques on the palms and soles and on dry, hair-bearing, keratinized genital skin.

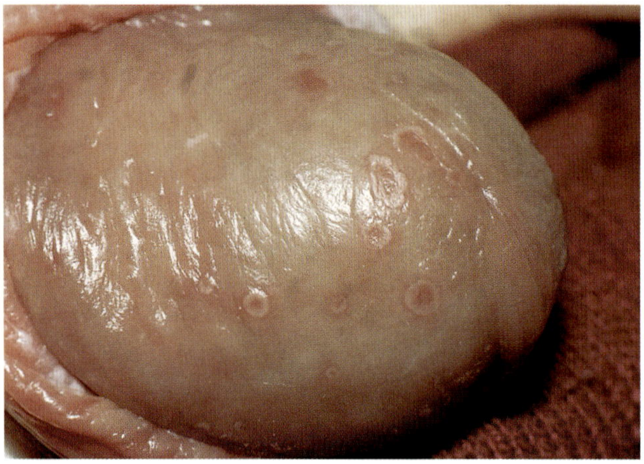

Fig. 10-71. Circinate balanitis of reactive arthritis in an uncircumcised man consists of small, annular white papules.

As palm and sole plaques become chronic, hyperkeratosis occurs, resulting in the typical lesions of keratoderma blennorrhagicum.

The uncircumcised glans penis typically shows circinate balanitis, which appears as white, circinate, well-demarcated papules and superficial red erosions (**Fig. 10-71**). In the rare case of reactive arthritis in women, the hydrated skin of the labia minora and vestibule can exhibit similar erosions or white solid, annular, or arcuate papules. Hair-bearing vulvar skin and the dry skin of the penis exhibit well-demarcated, crusted, red, scaly papules, and plaques. Other genitourinary features include urethritis, prostatitis, seminal vesiculitis, hemorrhagic cystitis, and urethral stricture. The cervix may demonstrate white, arcuate, interlacing papules.

The arthritis of reactive arthritis is an asymmetric arthritis of the large, weight-bearing joints such as the back, knee, or ankle. Heel pain from inflammation at the insertion of the Achilles tendon is also characteristic. Patients may develop anterior uveitis, conjunctivitis, and iritis necessitating close ophthalmologic management.

## Diagnosis

The diagnosis of reactive arthritis is a clinical one. A combination of genitourinary symptoms, metatarsophalangeal joint involvement, elevated C reactive protein, and positive HLA-B27 renders a 69% sensitivity and 93.5% specificity to the diagnosis of reactive arthritis.[84] However, a high degree of suspicion is required to make the diagnosis of reactive arthritis, because patients usually do not develop all the defining clinical features at the outset.

Infectious causes of symptoms, especially gonorrhea, must be ruled out. Radiographs of joints can show periarticular osteoporosis and enthesopathy, a combination of erosions around the insertion of tendons and ligaments, bone lucency, and new bone formation to include spurs. Serum studies for HLA typing typically reveal the presence of the HLA-B27 antigen in patients with reactive arthritis.

A biopsy of skin lesions does not differentiate from pustular psoriasis. The skin diseases to be differentiated from reactive arthritis are candidiasis and pustular psoriasis. Psoriasis is a closely related disease that exists on a spectrum with reactive arthritis, and these two diseases cannot always be distinguished. *Candida* can be eliminated by culture or microscopic smear, as well as by nonresponse to therapy. Tinea cruris, impetigo, and superinfected eczema can also be occasionally confused with the genital lesions of reactive arthritis.

**REACTIVE ARTHRITIS** — **Diagnosis**

- Accompanying chronic arthritis, conjunctivitis, urethritis, or cervicitis. Negative microscopic examinations and cultures
- Identification of red plaques of superficial pustules, scale, crusting on hands, feet, and genitalia; uncircumcised glans penis with annular, white, coalescing papules

## Pathophysiology

Reactive arthritis results from a reactive immune response that is triggered in a genetically susceptible individual. The most common infections reported to precipitate reactive arthritis are with those organisms that cause dysentery or urethritis such as *Yersinia enterocolitica*, *Shigella flexneri*, *Neisseria gonorrhoeae*, *Chlamydia trachomatis*, *Ureaplasma urealyticum*, *Campylobacter fetus*, and, more recently, *Borrelia burgdorferi* and HIV. It is not known whether HIV directly provokes the disease or whether the immune changes associated with the human immunodeficiency syndrome causes an individual to become more susceptible to reactive arthritis. Reactive arthritis and pustular psoriasis share many common features and exist on a spectrum. Reactive arthritis syndrome has occasionally been reported to be familial, and HLA-B27 positivity is common.

More recently, additional organisms and viruses, including infections of other areas of the body and COVID-19, have been implicated in the pathogenesis of reactive arthritis.[85] However, the definition of reactive arthritis seems to be expanding to include those that are a less specific group of individuals with arthritis triggered by infection.

## Management

Reactive arthritis is a chronic and difficult disease to treat. The management of joint disease falls under the purview of the rheumatologist, with help from the ophthalmologist and, at times, the cardiologist. Mild genital skin disease can be treated with topical corticosteroid ointments such as clobetasol propionate and halobetasol propionate ointment daily with careful follow-up to monitor for improvement and side effects. Those that do not sufficiently improve can be treated with methotrexate or the biologics as are used for psoriasis.

**REACTIVE ARTHRITIS** **Management of skin disease**

- Mild disease
  - Treatment of any underlying infection
  - Topical corticosteroid ointment
- Moderate to severe disease
  - Add oral methotrexate or cyclosporine, or
  - Add a biologic (infliximab, etanercept, adalimumab)

## Solid Lesions That Sometimes Appear Pustular

### Keratosis Pilaris

Keratosis pilaris is a common condition consisting of superficial keratin plugs occurring primarily on the lateral arms and buttocks (see Chapter 6 for full discussion). However, the anterior thighs and even the cheeks are sometimes affected. This problem is generally asymptomatic, but it produces a rough, sandpapery texture to the skin. Most often, individual lesions are small, skin-colored acuminate papules (Fig. 10-72). However, associated follicular erythema occurs in some patients, and this finding with an associated keratin plug sometimes resembles a pustule. In addition, patients sometimes experience significant secondary inflammation and actual pustules (Fig. 10-73).

Therapy is not needed, and it is unsatisfactory. Patients who want treatment for cosmetic reasons can soften keratin plugs by soaking in warm water, and they can subsequently scrub them out with an abrasive sponge. Lactic acid 12% lotion, salicylic lotions, or tretinoin cream 0.025% may help to dissolve these plugs in some patients, but these can also be irritating.

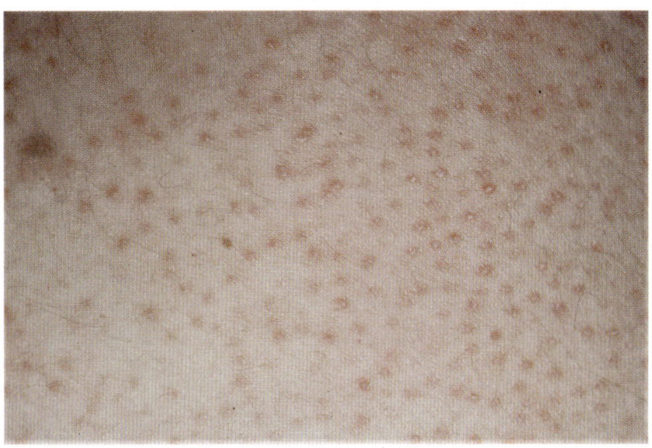

Fig. 10-72. Keratosis pilaris consists of tiny follicular papules with a central keratin plug that can mimic a pustule.

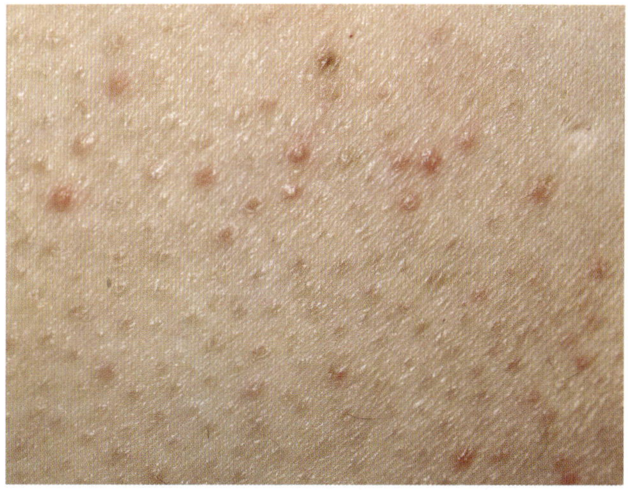

Fig. 10-73. Sometimes, individual lesions of keratosis pilaris can become inflamed and produce a pustule.

### Fordyce Spots (Ectopic Sebaceous Glands)

Numerous ectopic sebaceous glands appear on the medial aspect of the labia minora and less commonly on the lateral surface of the labia minora, the labia majora, the prepuce of the clitoris, or the prepuce and the shaft of the penis. See also Chapters 1 and 7. They appear as pinpoint, lobular, and/or flat, irregular, yellowish to skin-colored papules that may be discrete or confluent (Figs. 10-74 and 10-75). The abundance of large sebaceous glands, called Fordyce condition, is a normal variant and is asymptomatic, although this finding was once believed to produce pruritus.

The diagnosis is made on the basis of the location and the morphologic appearance. A biopsy is rarely necessary.

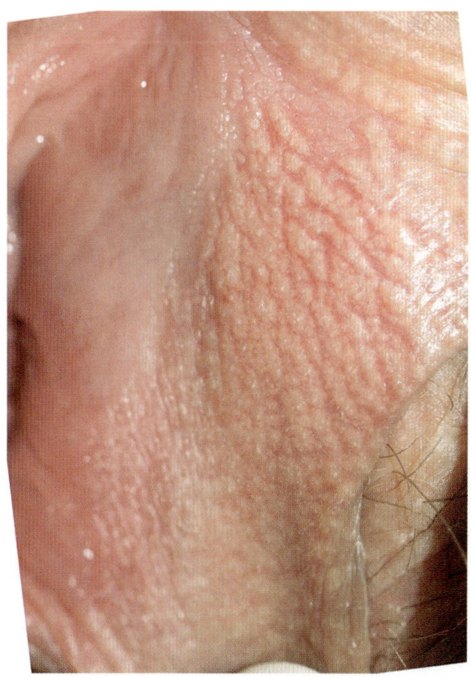

Fig. 10-74. The yellow papules of Fordyce spots or ectopic sebaceous glands vaguely resemble pustules at times.

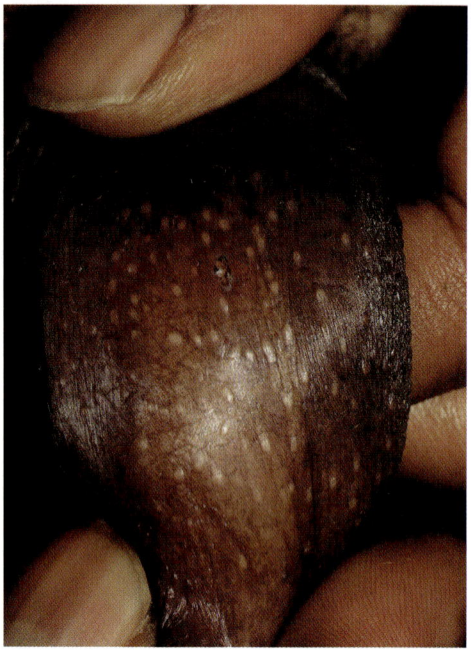

Fig. 10-75. Yellow sebaceous glands sometimes occur on the penile shaft as well as the vulva.

If Fordyce spots are examined by biopsy inadvertently, histology reveals enlarged but normal sebaceous glands. Normally, sebaceous glands are associated with and secrete into hair follicles, yet on the labia minora where hairs are scant, they open freely on the surface.

Fordyce spots may be easily confused with condylomata acuminata, tiny epidermal cysts or milia, and mollusca contagiosa. Unlike warts, Fordyce spots are yellowish rather than skin colored and are distributed symmetrically. Milia are usually more white than yellow, more discrete, fewer in number, and firmer. In addition, unlike milia, individual Fordyce spots are often subtly multilobular. Mollusca contagiosa are more discrete, less symmetrical, shiny, and more nodular and dome shaped.

These ectopic sebaceous glands are normal structures, but the larger size may be related to hormonal influences. Visible Fordyce spots on the female genitalia rarely occur before puberty or after several years following the climacteric. Ectopic sebaceous glands are a normal anatomic variant, and medical or surgical treatment is unwarranted.

## Inflamed Molluscum Contagiosum (see also Chapters 7 and 15)

These highly infectious papules are seen in two major populations: young children and young sexually active individuals. Children exhibit lesions on any skin surface, but when occurring on the genitalia, lesions do not imply sexual contact. Mollusca contagiosa of adults is most often a sexually transmitted disease, with lesions found primarily on the vulva, penis, scrotum, proximal, medial thighs, and perineal skin. Individual mollusca are usually skin-colored or white, dome-shaped papules, some with a tiny central depression. However, they can occasionally appear slightly yellow or even become inflamed and frankly pustular (Fig. 10-76). Although mollusca contagiosa are generally asymptomatic, inflamed, pustular lesions are often pruritic.

The diagnosis is usually made on the basis of the clinical appearance, but when the diagnosis is not clear, a microscopic examination of a curetted lesion with Tzanck smear usually demonstrates the typical Henderson-Patterson inclusion bodies, also called molluscum bodies. Mollusca contagiosa can mimic tumors, Fordyce spots, milia, or genital warts. When inflamed, mollusca can be confused with folliculitis, but the usual presence of surrounding typical lesions generally indicates the correct diagnosis.

Molluscum contagiosum is caused by a DNA poxvirus. Mollusca contagiosa in an immunocompetent person resolves spontaneously within a year or 2. The presence of pustular lesions can indicate a host immunological response to the infection with imminent eradication of the virus. Otherwise, cryotherapy, curettage, podophyllin resin, podofilox, trichloroacetic acid, cantharidin, and salicylic acid preparations have been used successfully. Imiquimod has been reported to be beneficial as well. Even pulse-dye laser has been reported as useful. Many clinicians believe that daily application of tretinoin cream 0.05% helps to minimize recurrences and gradually eliminate small lesions.

## Epidermal Cysts

Epidermal cysts, sometimes erroneously called sebaceous cysts, are extremely common on the labia majora and scro-

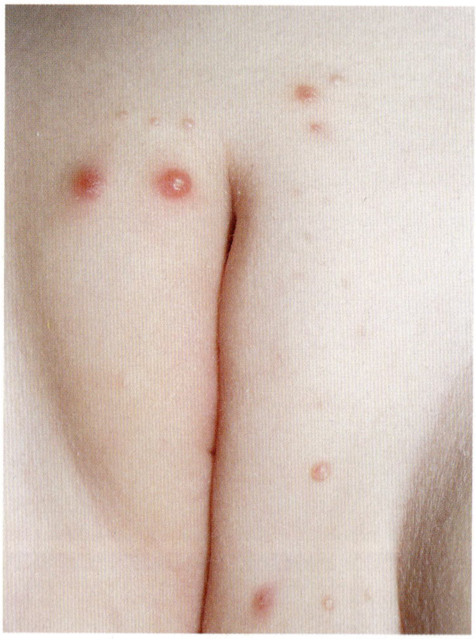

Fig. 10-76. The inflammatory response to mollusca contagiosa often produce red pustules that can be mistaken for infection.

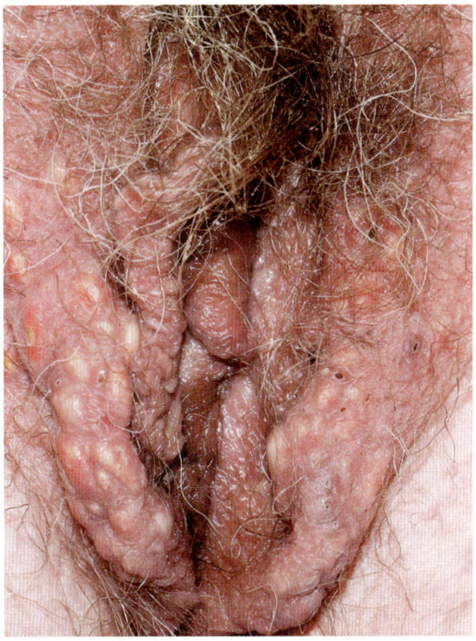

Fig. 10-77. Epidermal cysts can sometimes appear yellow and erroneously suggest pustulation.

tum (see also Chapters 1, 6, and 8). Epidermal cysts arise from hair follicles that become obstructed and distended with keratin. The hydrated keratin within the cyst gives the lesion its white-yellow color (Fig. 10-77). This hydrated keratin is a tallowy, cheesy, crumbly, malodorous material. Many of these cysts demonstrate a follicular opening that manifests as a small punctum or black dot centrally on the surface of the cyst. If the cyst is traumatized, keratin leaks through its capsule of follicular epithelium into the dermis, thus producing a brisk inflammatory response. The nodule becomes red, painful, and purulent as a result of this foreign body response rather than from infection. Sometimes, especially on the modified mucous membranes of the vulva, multiple tiny epidermal cysts (milia) occur and can be frequently and recurrently inflamed.

An inflamed epidermal cyst is most often confused with furunculosis, a deep follicular infection with *S aureus*. However, an inflamed cyst is usually an isolated inflammatory lesion, and, unlike in bacterial furunculosis, erythema generally is limited to the nodule and does not extend far onto surrounding skin. Multiple chronic or recurrently inflamed cysts represent hidradenitis suppurativa. Patients with frequent inflammation of milia are easily misdiagnosed as having suppurative folliculitis. Epidermal cysts do not require therapy except for cosmetic reasons or if there is inflammation. Inflamed cysts are best treated with 0.1-0.3 mL of triamcinolone acetonide, 3-5 mg/mL injected intralesionally before they become fluctuant. After they are fluctuant, incision and drainage can provide some comfort for the patient, but recurrence is common. Definitive therapy consists of excision, but cysts should not be excised while inflamed. When inflamed, cyst borders are indistinct and edematous, requiring a larger excision and more scarring than would occur in the absence of inflammation. Antibiotics are generally unhelpful acutely. However, patients with recurrently inflamed cyst nodules (hidradenitis suppurativa) or frequently inflamed milia benefit from the long-term administration of anti-inflammatory antibiotics such as twice-daily administered doxycycline or minocycline 100 mg, clindamycin 150 mg, or double-strength trimethoprim-sulfamethoxazole.

## Vestibular Cysts

Vestibular or mucous cysts of the vulva are relatively common cysts that arise from persistent urogenital sinus epithelium or from the obstruction of the minor vestibular glands (see also Chapter 7). Vestibular cysts are nodules, 2 mm to 2 cm, that can be skin colored, yellow, or bluish (Fig. 10-78). Often, they are translucent, and, if ruptured, these lesions emit clear mucus. These cysts are generally asymptomatic, although if large they rarely cause dyspareunia or urinary tract obstruction. The diagnosis is usually made clinically, with the differential diagnosis primarily containing only other types of benign cysts. The differentiation of vestibular cysts from other local cysts is unimportant. Therapy is rarely necessary, but vestibular cysts can be surgically excised if they are symptomatic.

## Other Diseases That Can Appear Yellow or Produce Crusting

Any diseases that cause ulceration, erosion, or blistering can, when occurring on dry skin, cause crusting. These are generally the same diseases that produce erosions

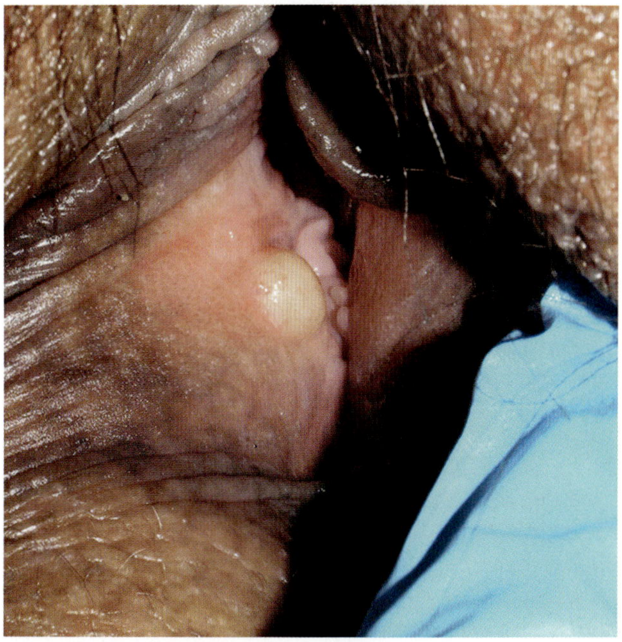

Fig. 10-78. Vestibular cysts are sometimes yellow.

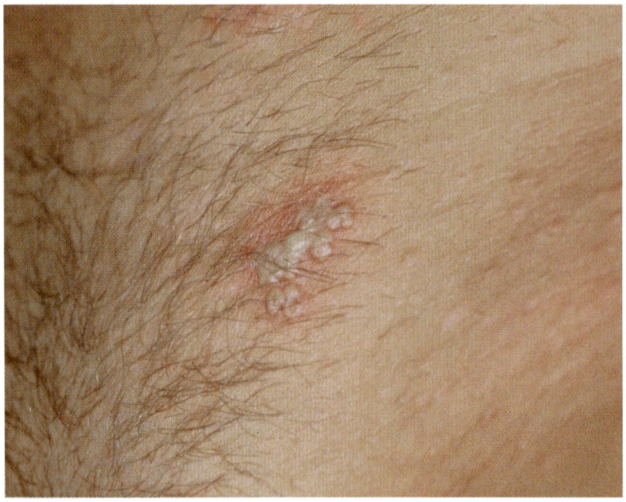

Fig. 10-79. Any blistering disease, including these vesicles from herpes simplex virus, appears pustular after they have been present for several days. However, piercing the blister reveals serous fluid rather than thick pus.

when occurring on more fragile mucous membrane epithelium, such as the vagina, or on modified mucous membrane, such as the glans penis and clinically non–hair-bearing skin of the vulva. Erosions on these epithelial surfaces often exhibit a yellow fibrin base.

HSV infections are usually classified as vesicular or erosive. However, like any vesicular eruption, this viral infection can exhibit a yellow morphology in several settings **(Fig. 10-79)**. First, as vesicles on keratinized skin break, exudation and drying produce a yellow crust that can mimic impetigo. In addition, the vesicles of HSV infections often become secondarily cloudy when they occur on keratinized skin, where the skin is less fragile and vesicles do not quickly disintegrate. Finally, ulcers frequently develop a yellowish coagulum at the base **(Fig. 10-80)**. Immunosuppressed patients are especially likely to acquire papular HSV infection, as adherent, coalescing papules of yellow fibrin form on erosions.

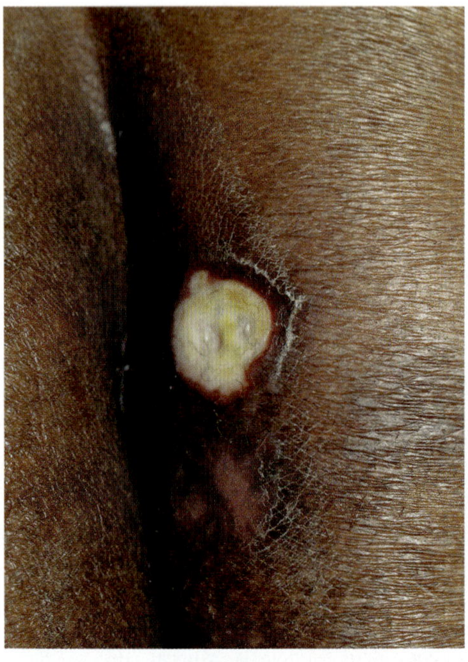

Fig. 10-80. An ulcer often exhibits a yellow/white fibrin base that can be confused with purulence, but this is a nonspecific finding for any ulcer, as it is for this immunosuppressed patient with an ulcer from herpes simplex virus infection.

## REFERENCES


1. Center for Disease Control and Prevention. *Genital Herpes Treatment and Care. Treatment Guidelines and Updates.* July 22, 2021. https://www.cdc.gov/std/treatment-guidelines/herpes.htm
2. James C, Harfouche M, Welton NJ, et al. Herpes simplex virus: global infection prevalence and incidence estimates, 2016. *Bull World Health Organ.* 2020;98(5):315-329. doi:10.2471/BLT.19.237149
3. Spicknall IH, Flagg EW, Torrone EA. Estimates of the prevalence and incidence of genital herpes, United States, 2018. *Sex Transm Dis.* 2021;48:260-265. doi:10.1097/OLQ.0000000000001375
4. Ginieri-Coccossis M, et al. Quality of life and depression in chronic sexually transmitted infections in UK and Greece: the use of WHOQOL-HIV/STI BREF. *Psychiatriki.* 2018;29(3):209-219. doi:10.22365/jpsych.2018.293.209
5. Majewska A, Romejko-Wolniewicz E, Zareba-Szczudlik J, Kilijańczyk M, Gajewska M, Młynarczyk G. [Laboratory diagnosis of genital herpes--direct immunofluorescence method]. *Ginekol Pol.* 2013;84:615-619.
6. Bagri P, et al. Estradiol enhances antiviral CD4+ tissue-resident memory T cell responses following mucosal herpes simplex virus 2 vaccination through an IL-17-mediated pathway. *J Virol.* 2020;95:e01206-e01220. doi:10.1128/JVI.01206-20
7. McCarthy KJ, Gollub EL, Ralph L, van de Wijgert J, Jones HE. Hormonal contraceptives and the acquisition of sexually transmitted infections: an updated systematic review. *Sex Transm Dis.* 2019;46:290-296.
8. Workowski KA, et al. Sexually transmitted infections treatment guidelines, 2021. *MMWR Recomm Rep.* 2021;70:1-187.
9. Magaret AL, et al. Effect of condom use on Per-act HSV-2 transmission risk in HIV-1, HSV-2-discordant couples. *Clin Infect Dis.* 2016;62:456-461.
10. Stanfield BA, Kousoulas KG, Fernandez A, Gershburg E. Rational design of live-attenuated vaccines against herpes simplex viruses. *Viruses.* 2021;13:1637.
11. Awasthi S, Knox JJ, Desmond A, et al. Trivalent nucleoside-modified mRNA vaccine yields durable memory B cell protection against genital herpes in preclinical models. *J Clin Invest.* 2021;131(23):e152310. doi:10.1172/JCI152310
12. Koumaki D, et al. Herpes zoster viral infection after AZD1222 and BNT162b2 coronavirus disease 2019 mRNA vaccines: a case series. *J Eur Acad Dermatol Venereol.* 2022;36(2):e85-e86. doi:10.1111/jdv.17720
13. Costan V-V, Popa C, Hâncu MF, Porumb-Andrese E, Toader MP. Comprehensive review on the pathophysiology, clinical variants and management of pemphigus (Review). *Exp Ther Med.* 2021;22(5):1335. doi:10.3892/etm.2021.10770

14. Kavala M, Topaloğlu Demir F, Zindanci I, et al. Genital involvement in pemphigus vulgaris (PV): correlation with clinical and cervicovaginal Pap smear findings. *J Am Acad Dermatol.* 2015;73(4):655-659.
15. Kappius RH, Ufkes NA, Thiers BH. Paraneoplastic pemphigus. In: *StatPearls [Internet]*. Treasure Island, FL: StatPearls Publishing; 2021. Review.
16. Pile HD, Yarrarapu SNS, Jonathan S, Crane JS. Drug induced pemphigus. In: *StatPearls [Internet]*. Treasure Island, FL: StatPearls Publishing; 2021.
17. Brenner S, Goldberg I. Drug-induced pemphigus. *Clin Dermatol.* 2011;29(4):455-457.
18. Murrell DF, et al. Diagnosis and management of pemphigus: recommendations of an international panel of experts. *J Am Acad Dermatol.* 2020;82(3):575-585.e1. doi:10.1016/j.jaad.2018.02.021
19. Askin O, Ozkoca D, Kutlubay Z, Mat MC. A retrospective analysis of pemphigus vulgaris patients: demographics, diagnosis, co-morbid diseases and treatment modalities used. *North Clin Istanb.* 2020;7:597-602. doi:10.14744/nci.2020.37039
20. Lernia VD, Casanova DM, Goldust M, Ricci C. Pemphigus vulgaris and bullous pemphigoid: update on diagnosis and treatment. *Dermatol Pract Concept.* 2020;10:e2020050. doi:10.5826/dpc.1003a50
21. Kridin K, Sagi SZ, Bergman R. Mortality and cause of death in patients with pemphigus. *Acta Derm Venereol.* 2017;97:607-611. doi:10.2340/00015555-2611
22. Vinay K, Kanwar AJ, Mittal A, Dogra S, Minz RW, Hashimoto T. Intralesional rituximab in the treatment of refractory oral pemphigus vulgaris. *JAMA Dermatol.* 2015;151:878-882. doi:10.1001/jamadermatol.2014.3674
23. Mazloom E, et al. Intralesional injection of biosimilar rituximab in recalcitrant mucocutaneous lesions of patients with pemphigus vulgaris: a pilot study. *Dermatol Ther.* 2020;33:e14407. doi:10.1111/dth.14407
24. Iraji F, et al. Comparison between the efficacy of intralesional rituximab versus intralesional triamcinolone in the treatment refractory Pemphigus Vulgaris lesions: a randomized clinical trial. *Int Immunopharmacol.* 2019;73:94-97. doi:10.1016/j.intimp.2019.04.031
25. Kridin K, Hübner F, Recke A, Linder R, Schmidt E. The burden of neurological comorbidities in six autoimmune bullous diseases: a population-based study. *J Eur Acad Dermatol Venereol.* 2021;35:2074-2078. doi:10.1111/jdv.17465
26. Wright B, Halper K, Worswick S. Bullous Pemphigoid and malignancy in two different hospital populations: a retrospective cohort review. *Oncology.* 2020;98:318-320. doi:10.1159/000506055
27. Kridin K, Hammers CM, Ludwig RJ, Cohen AD. Risk of solid malignancies in bullous pemphigoid: a large-scale population-based cohort study. *J Dermatol.* 2021;48:317-323. doi:10.1111/1346-8138.15685
28. Baigrie D, Nookala V. Bullous pemphigoid. In: *StatPearls [Internet]*. Treasure Island, FL: StatPearls Publishing; 2021. Review.
29. Montagnon CM, Tolkachjov SN, Murrell DF, Camilleri MJ, Lehman JS. Subepithelial autoimmune blistering dermatoses: clinical features and diagnosis. *J Am Acad Dermatol.* 2021;85:1-14. doi:10.1016/j.jaad.2020.11.076
30. McMahon DE, et al. Clinical and pathologic correlation of cutaneous COVID-19 vaccine reactions including V-REPP: a registry-based study. *J Am Acad Dermatol.* 2022;86(1):113-121. doi:10.1016/j.jaad.2021.09.002
31. Schmidt V, Blum R, Möhrenschlager MJ. Biphasic bullous pemphigoid starting after first dose and boosted by second dose of mRNA-1273 vaccine in an 84-year-old female with polymorbidity and polypharmacy. *J Eur Acad Dermatol Venereol.* 2022;36(2):e88-e90. doi:10.1111/jdv.17722
32. Balakirski G, Alkhateeb A, Merk HF, Leverkus M, Megahed M. Successful treatment of bullous pemphigoid with omalizumab as corticosteroid-sparing agent: report of two cases and review of literature. *J Eur Acad Dermatol Venereol.* 2016;30:1778-1782. doi:10.1111/jdv.13758
33. Kremer N, Snast I, Cohen ES, et al. Rituximab and omalizumab for the treatment of bullous pemphigoid: a systematic review of the literature. *Am J Clin Dermatol.* 2019;20:209-216.
34. Bishnoi A, De D, Handa S, Mahajan R. Biologics in autoimmune bullous diseases: current scenario. *Indian J Dermatol Venereol Leprol.* 2021;87:611-620. doi:10.25259/IJDVL_886_19. Review.
35. Abdat R, et al. Dupilumab as a novel therapy for bullous pemphigoid: a multicenter case series. *J Am Acad Dermatol.* 2020;83:46-52. doi:10.1016/j.jaad.2020.01.089
36. Saleh M, Reedy M, Torok H, Weaver J. Successful treatment of bullous pemphigoid with dupilumab: a case and brief review of the literature. *Dermatol Online J.* 2021;27:13030/qt0dv3f9h6.
37. Försti AK, Jokelainen J, Timonen M, Tasanen K. Risk of death in bullous pemphigoid: a retrospective database study in Finland. *Acta Derm Venereol.* 2016;96:758-761. doi:10.2340/00015555-2347
38. Rashid H, et al. European guidelines (S3) on diagnosis and management of mucous membrane pemphigoid, initiated by the European Academy of Dermatology and Venereology—Part I. *J Eur Acad Dermatol Venereol.* 2021;35:1750-1764. doi:10.1111/jdv.17397
39. Setterfield J, Theron J, Vaughan RW, et al. Mucous membrane pemphigoid: HLA-DQB1*0301 is associated with all clinical sites of involvement and may be linked to antibasement membrane IgG production. *Br J Dermatol.* 2001;145:406-414.
40. Bernard P, Antonicelli F, Bedane C, et al. Prevalence and clinical significance of anti-aminin 332 autoantibodies detected by a novel enzyme-linked immunosorbent assay in mucous membrane pemphigoid. *JAMA Dermatol.* 2013;149:533-540.
41. Lytvyn Y, et al. Biologic treatment outcomes in mucous membrane pemphigoid: a systematic review. *J Am Acad Dermatol.* 2022;87(1):110-120. doi:10.1016/j.jaad.2020.12.056
42. Patel PM, Jones VA, Murray TN, Amber KT. A review comparing international guidelines for the management of bullous pemphigoid, pemphigoid gestationis, mucous membrane pemphigoid, and epidermolysis acquista. *Am J Clin Dermatol.* 2020;21:557-565. doi:10.1007/s40257-020-00513-3
43. Schmidt E, et al. European Guidelines (S3) on diagnosis and management of mucous membrane pemphigoid, initiated by the European Academy of Dermatology and Venereology—Part II. *J Eur Acad Dermatol Venereol.* 2021;35:1926-1948. doi:10.1111/jdv.17395
44. Alkeraye S, AlZamil LR, Alenazi S. Dapsone in the management of pemphigus and pemphigoid: rediscovery of its long-lost efficacy. *Cureus.* 2020;12:e8805. doi:10.7759/cureus.8805
45. Montagnon CM, Lehman JS, Murrell DF, Camilleri MJ, Tolkachjov SN. Subepithelial autoimmune bullous dermatoses disease activity assessment and therapy. *J Am Acad Dermatol.* 2021;85:18-27. doi:10.1016/j.jaad.2020.05.161

46. Santi CG, et al. Consensus on the treatment of autoimmune bullous dermatoses: bullous pemphigoid, mucous membrane pemphigoid and epidermolysis bullosa acquisita—Brazilian Society of Dermatology. *An Bras Dermatol.* 2019;94(2 Suppl 1):33-47. doi:10.1590/abd1806-4841.2019940207
47. Kanda N, Nakadaira N, Otsuka Y, Ishii N, Hoashi T, Saeki H. Linear IgA bullous dermatosis associated with ulcerative colitis: a case report and literature review. *Australas J Dermatol.* 2020;6:e82-e86. doi:10.1111/ajd.13121
48. Shin L, Gardner JT II, Dao H Jr. Updates in the diagnosis and management of linear IgA disease: a systematic review. *Medicina (Kaunas).* 2021;57:818. doi:10.3390/medicina57080818
49. Vale ECSD, Dimatos OC, Porro AM, Santi CG. Consensus on the treatment of autoimmune bullous dermatoses: dermatitis herpetiformis and linear IgA bullous dermatosis—Brazilian Society of Dermatology. *An Bras Dermatol.* 2019;94(2 Suppl 1):48-55. doi:10.1590/abd1806-4841.2019940208
50. Ben Lagha I, Ashack K, Khachemoune A. Hailey-Hailey disease: an update review with a focus on treatment data. *Am J Clin Dermatol.* 2020;21:49-68. doi:10.1007/s40257-019-00477-z
51. Farahnik B, Blattner CM, Mortazie MB, Perry BM, Lear W, Elston DM. Interventional treatments for Hailey-Hailey disease. *J Am Acad Dermatol.* 2017;76(3):551-558.e3. doi:10.1016/j.jaad.2016.08.039
52. Dreyfus I, et al. Botulinum toxin injections as an effective treatment for patients with intertriginous Hailey-Hailey or Darier disease: an open-label 6-month pilot interventional study. *Orphanet J Rare Dis.* 2021;16:93. doi:10.1186/s13023-021-01710-x
53. Martina E, Diotallevi F, Radi G, Campanati A, Offidani A. Therapeutic use of botulinum neurotoxins in dermatology: systematic review. *Toxins (Basel).* 2021;13:120. doi:10.3390/toxins13020120
54. Lim D, Belisle A, Davar S. Improvement in Hailey-Hailey disease with a combination of low-dose naltrexone and oral magnesium chloride: a case report. *SAGE Open Med Case Rep.* 2020;8:2050313X20984121. doi:10.1177/2050313X20984121
55. Sousa Gomes M, Araújo Pereira J, Trocado V, Prata JP, Teixeira V, Pinheiro P. Vulvar Hailey-Hailey disease treated with low-dose naltrexone: case report and literature review. *Arch Gynecol Obstet.* 2020;302:1081-1086. doi:10.1007/s00404-020-05705-0
56. Alzahrani N, et al. Hailey-Hailey disease treated with dupilumab: a case series. *Br J Dermatol.* 2021;185:680-682. doi:10.1111/bjd.20475
57. Di Altobrando A, Sacchelli L, Patrizi A, Bardazzi F. Successful treatment of refractory Hailey-Hailey disease with apremilast. *Clin Exp Dermatol.* 2020;45:604-605. doi:10.1111/ced.14173
58. Crowder CA, Jeney SES, Kraus CN, Bernal N, Lane F. Vulvovaginal involvement in Stevens-Johnson syndrome and toxic epidermal necrolysis: management and techniques used to reduce gynecologic sequelae. *Int J Dermatol.* 2022;61(2):158-163. doi:10.1111/ijd.15676. Epub 2021 May 26.
59. Frantz R, Huang S, Are A, Motaparthi K. Stevens-Johnson syndrome and toxic epidermal necrolysis: a review of diagnosis and management. *Medicina (Kaunas).* 2021;57:895. doi:10.3390/medicina57090895
60. Soares A, Sokumbi O. Recent updates in the treatment of erythema multiforme. *Medicina (Kaunas).* 2021;57:921. doi:10.3390/medicina57090921
61. O'Brien KF, et al. Vulvovaginal manifestations in Stevens-Johnson syndrome and toxic epidermal necrolysis: prevention and treatment. *J Am Acad Dermatol.* 2021;85:523-528. doi:10.1016/j.jaad.2019.08.031
62. Anderson HJ, Lee JB. A review of fixed drug eruption with a special focus on generalized bullous fixed drug eruption. *Medicina (Kaunas).* 2021;57:925. doi:10.3390/medicina57090925. Review.
63. Silvestre-Torner N, Imbernón-Moya A, Martínez-García M, Burgos-Lázaro F. Acquired cutaneous lymphangiectasia: dermoscopic evidence from white-yellowish lacunae. *Dermatol Pract Concept.* 2021;11:e2021062. doi:10.5826/dpc.1103a62
64. Huilgol SC, Neill S, Barlow RJ. CO(2) laser therapy of vulval lymphangiectasia and lymphangioma circumscriptum. *Dermatol Surg.* 2002;28:575-577.
65. Vignes S, Arrault M, Trévidic P. Surgical resection of vulva lymphoedema circumscriptum. *J Plast Reconstr Aesthet Surg.* 2010;63:1883-1885. doi:10.1016/j.bjps.2009.11.019
66. Ghaemmaghami F, Karimi Zarchi M, Mousavi A. Surgical management of primary vulvar lymphangioma circumscriptum and postradiation: case series and review of literature. *J Minim Invasive Gynecol.* 2008;15:205-208. doi:10.1016/j.jmig.2007.09.005
67. Poizeau F, Plantier F, Bell H, Moyal-Barracco M. Vulvar Fordyce adenitis: a cohort of 45 women. *Ann Dermatol Venereol.* 2021;148(4):221-227. doi:10.1016/j.annder.2021.04.001
68. Dixit S, Olsson A, Fischer G. A case series of 11 patients with hormone-responsive sebaceous adenitis of the labia minora. *Australas J Dermatol.* 2014;55(1):80-83. doi:10.1111/ajd.12066
69. Mintoff D, Benhadou F, Pace NP, Frew JW. Metabolic syndrome and hidradenitis suppurativa: epidemiological, molecular, and therapeutic aspects. *Int J Dermatol.* 2021. 2021 Sep 16. doi: 10.1111/ijd.15910. Online ahead of print.
70. Garg A, et al. Comorbidity screening in hidradenitis suppurativa: evidence-based recommendations from the US and Canadian Hidradenitis Suppurativa Foundations. *J Am Acad Dermatol.* 2022;86(5):1092-1101. doi:10.1016/j.jaad.2021.01.059
71. Tugnoli S, Agnoli C, Silvestri A, Giari S, Bettoli V, Caracciolo S. Anger, emotional fragility, self-esteem, and psychiatric comorbidity in patients with hidradenitis suppurativa/acne inversa. *J Clin Psychol Med Settings.* 2020;27:527-540. doi:10.1007/s10880-019-09640-4
72. Sachdeva M, et al. Squamous cell carcinoma arising within hidradenitis suppurativa: a literature review. *Int J Dermatol.* 2021;60:e459-e465. doi:10.1111/ijd.15677
73. Aarts P, Aitken JJ, van Straalen KR. Prevalence of central sensitization in patients with hidradenitis suppurativa. *JAMA Dermatol.* 2021;157:1209-1212. doi:10.1001/jamadermatol.2021.2918
74. Rosi E, et al. Insights into the pathogenesis of HS and therapeutical approaches. *Biomedicines.* 2021;9:1168. doi:10.3390/biomedicines9091168
75. Scala E, et al. Hidradenitis suppurativa: where we are and where we are going. *Cells.* 2021;10:2094. doi:10.3390/cells10082094
76. Goldburg SR, Strober BE, Payette MJ. Hidradenitis suppurativa: current and emerging treatments. *J Am Acad Dermatol.* 2020;82(5):1061-1082. doi:10.1016/j.jaad.2019.08.089
77. López-Llunell C, Riera-Martí N, Gamissans M, Romaní J. Dapsone in hidradenitis suppurativa: a case series of 56 patients. *Dermatol Ther.* 2021;34(6):e15161. doi:10.1111/dth.15161

78. Liakou AI, et al. Colchicine improves clinical outcomes and quality of life in hidradenitis suppurativa patients: a retrospective study. *J Clin Med*. 2021;10:4742. doi:10.3390/jcm10204742
79. van der Zee HH, Prens EP. The anti-inflammatory drug colchicine lacks efficacy in hidradenitis suppurativa. *Dermatology*. 2011;223:169-173. doi:10.1159/000332846
80. Holcomb ZE, Porter ML, Kimball AB. A safety review of biologic therapies for the management of hidradenitis suppurativa and unmet needs. *Expert Opin Drug Saf*. 2021;20:1147–1161. doi:10.1080/14740338.2021.1924147
81. Jones ME, Kohn AH, Pourali SP, et al. The use of biologics during the COVID-19 pandemic. *Dermatol Clin*. 2021;39(4):545-553. doi:10.1016/j.det.2021.05.010
82. Kerdel FR, Azevedo FA, Kerdel Don C, Don FA, Fabbrocini G, Kerdel FA. Apremilast for the treatment of mild-to-moderate hidradenitis suppurativa in a prospective, open-label, phase 2 study. *J Drugs Dermatol*. 2019;18:170-176.
83. Cheeti A, Chakraborty RK, Ramphul K. Reactive arthritis. In: *StatPearls [Internet]*. Treasure Island, FL: StatPearls Publishing; 2021.
84. Selmi C, Gershwin ME. Diagnosis and classification of reactive arthritis. *Autoimmun Rev*. 2014;13:546-549.
85. Zeidler H, Hudson AP. Reactive arthritis update: spotlight on new and rare infectious agents implicated as pathogens. *Curr Rheumatol Rep*. 2021;23:53. doi:10.1007/s11926-021-01018-6

## SUGGESTED READINGS

Baigrie D, Nookala V. Bullous pemphigoid. In: *StatPearls [Internet]*. Treasure Island, FL: StatPearls Publishing; 2021. Review.

Ben Lagha I, Ashack K, Khachemoune A. Hailey-Hailey disease: an update review with a focus on treatment data. *Am J Clin Dermatol*. 2020;21(1):49-68. doi:10.1007/s40257-019-00477-z

Center for Disease Control and Prevention. *Genital Herpes Treatment and Care. Treatment Guidelines and Updates*. July 22, 2021. https://www.cdc.gov/std/treatment-guidelines/herpes.htm

Cheeti A, Chakraborty RK, Ramphul K. Reactive arthritis. In: *StatPearls [Internet]*. Treasure Island, FL: StatPearls Publishing; 2021.

Costan V-V, Popa C, Hâncu MF, Porumb-Andrese E, Toader MP. Comprehensive review on the pathophysiology, clinical variants and management of pemphigus (Review). *Exp Ther Med*. 2021;22(5):1335. doi:10.3892/etm.2021.10770

Crowder CA, Jeney SES, Kraus CN, Bernal N, Lane F. Vulvovaginal involvement in Stevens-Johnson syndrome and toxic epidermal necrolysis: management and techniques used to reduce gynecologic sequelae. *Int J Dermatol*. 2021. doi:10.1111/ijd.15676

Frantz R, Huang S, Are A, Motaparthi K. Stevens-Johnson syndrome and toxic epidermal necrolysis: a review of diagnosis and management. *Medicina (Kaunas)*. 2021;57:895. doi:10.3390/medicina57090895

# Erosions and Ulcers 11

LIBBY EDWARDS AND PETER J. LYNCH

Many clinicians do not distinguish erosions from ulcerations, but to a dermatologist, these represent separate differential diagnostic categories. An erosion is a superficial defect, with only the epithelium lost from the surface. An ulcer is deeper, with the defect extending into or even through the dermis. Erosions generally are red, and there is no discernible depression in the skin to the touch (Fig. 11-1). Ulcers on mucous membranes most often have a white or yellowish fibrin base and have palpable tissue loss (Fig. 11-2). On dry, keratinized skin, the base of extramucosal ulcers are often red, frequently with adherent yellow fibrin remnants, and erosions and ulcers on dry skin can be covered with a crust (scab) of blood and fibrin. Of course, there is overlap; an ulcer begins as an erosion and becomes an erosion as it heals. An erosion can deepen into an ulcer due to infection, irritating medications, or manipulation.

## SECTION A: EROSIONS

Many erosions occur when a blister roof sloughs; therefore, all blistering diseases should be considered in the differential diagnosis when erosions are seen (see Chapter 10).

Usually, when an erosion is produced by a blister, the erosion is round or arcuate (Fig. 11-3), and often some intact blisters can be seen. When produced by trauma, erosions are generally irregular, linear or angular.

Erosive skin diseases can be infectious, immune-mediated, or malignant, or traumatic, such as excoriation from scratching.

### Erosive Lichen Planus

Lichen planus (LP) exhibits widely differing morphologies, with erosive lichen planus being the most common noninfectious erosive disease of the vulva. Erosive lichen planus is less common on the penis. Red papules (see Chapter 6) are more common than erosions in men, and wet skin often exhibits white skin lesions (see Chapter 8). Some patients exhibit several morphologies, such as white striae surrounding erosions. There are few studies on genital lichen planus, but data on oral lichen planus are more abundant and relative to anogenital lichen planus, so is often referenced in this chapter.

#### Clinical Presentation

Erosive vulvovaginal lichen planus does not occur in children, is rare in young adults, and, in women, is primarily a postmenopausal disease. Erosive genital LP is by far more common in women, especially in the dermatoses, lichen planus of the penis occurs primarily in uncircumcised males.[1] A series of 89 patients with penile lichen planus showed that very few of these were the erosive variant.[2] The vast majority of women with erosive vulvovaginal lichen planus have no involvement of extragenital, extramucosal sites. Patients often report genital pruritus, but rubbing and scratching are often painful, and burning, irritation, rawness, dysuria, dyspareunia, and postcoital bleeding are predominant symptoms. Both men and women with erosive genital LP often report oral symptoms of rawness and pain, especially with hard food such as chips, and spicy and acidic foods. Two-thirds to three-

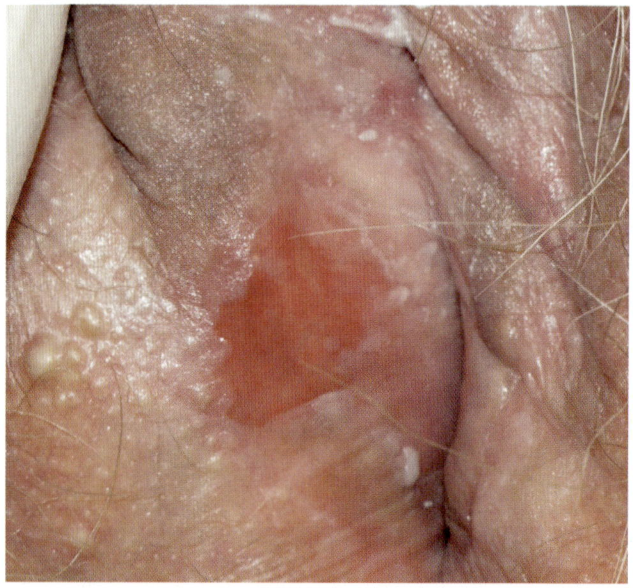

Fig. 11-1. An erosion represents a loss of the epidermis, which is very thin, so that the erosion is nearly flush with the surrounding skin; on a mucous membrane, an erosion is usually red.

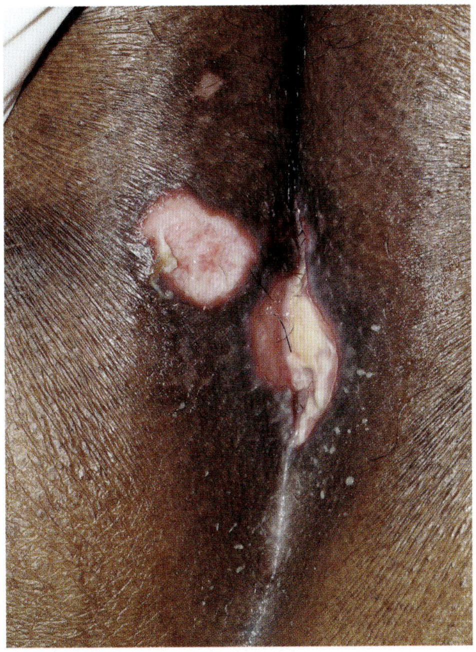

Fig. 11-2. Tissue loss that extends into or through the dermis translates into a palpable defect. The base of an ulcer on wet skin usually exhibits a white fibrin base, but sometimes is red.

quarters of women with erosive vulvar lichen planus have oral involvement, but the frequency in men is less well documented.[3] A series of men with penile LP, mostly nonerosive, had no extragenital involvement including no oral disease in 88.8%.[2]

The classic lesions of lichen planus on extramucosal skin are pruritic, violaceous, flat-topped papules (see Chapter 5), but these are rare in patients with erosive genital LP. The most common morphologies of mucous membrane LP are white lacy or fernlike striae, especially in the mouth, or erosions, particularly on the non–hair-bearing skin of the vulva and the glans and the ventral

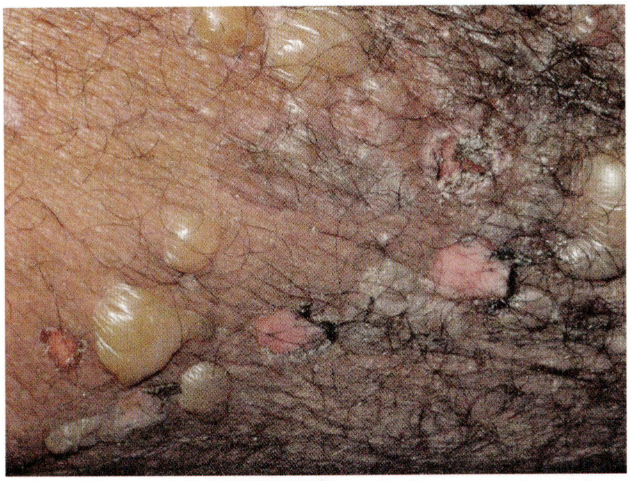

Fig. 11-3. Blisters become erosions when the blister roof is shed. This is a prompt event on thin mucosa that does not sport a stratum corneum, but even on keratinized skin such as this medial thigh it is inevitable. The erosions are roughly round, and the periphery shows remnants of the edge of the blister.

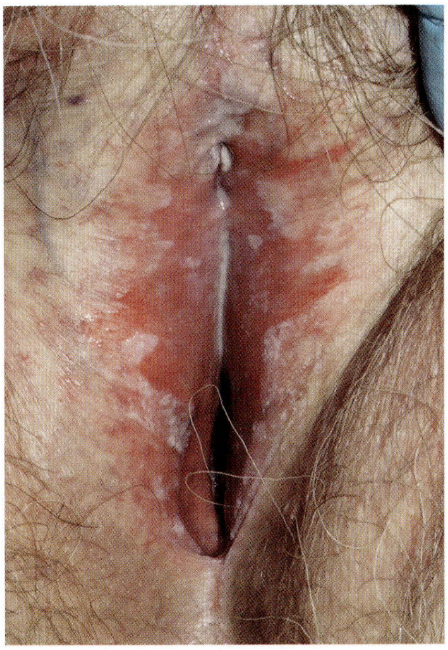

Fig. 11-4. Erosive lichen planus is manifested by bland, nonspecific erosions, characteristically in the vestibule and extending to the medial labia majora, having obliterated the labia minora.

prepuce of the uncircumcised penis. White morphology is discussed in Chapter 8.

Erosive LP typically affects the modified mucous membranes of the vulva is usual, with bright red, thin epithelium and erosions often most marked in the true mucous membranes of the vestibule, but frequently include the labia minora (**Figs. 11-4 through 11-6**).

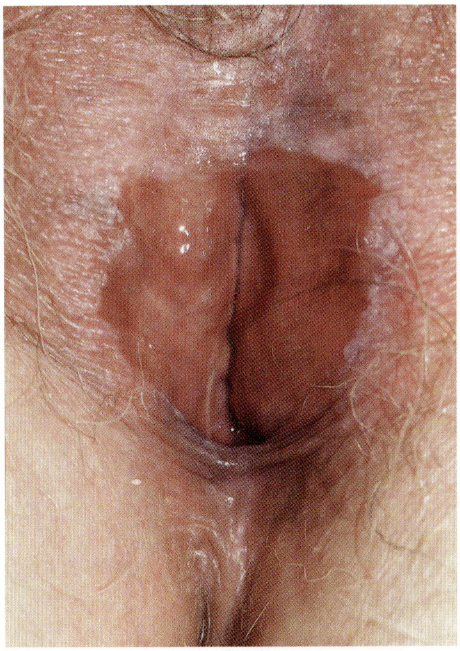

Fig. 11-5. Again, erosive lichen planus shows nonspecific erosions in a typical location with eradication of all vulvar architecture. This appearance is indistinguishable from pemphigus vulgaris and mucous membrane pemphigoid, and these diseases also characteristically affect the mouth and vagina. However, there are no keratinized skin lesions, and routine and direct immunofluorescent biopsies rule out immunobullous diseases.

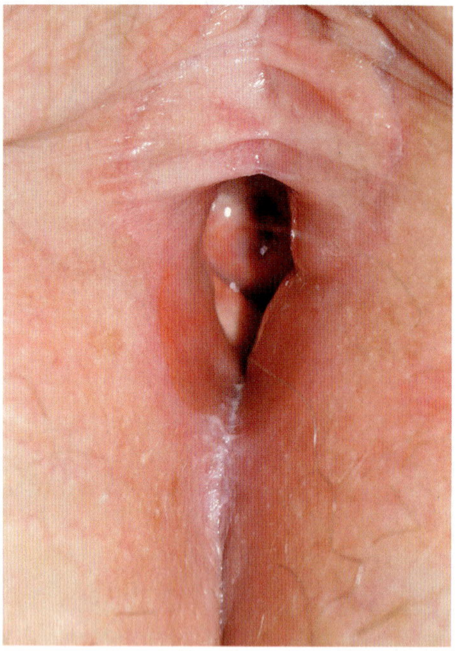

Fig. 11-6. Not all erosive lichen planus is dramatic; this patient shows limited erosions in the posterior vestibule extending to the perineum. Still, even though the erosions are fairly limited, the labia minora have resorbed.

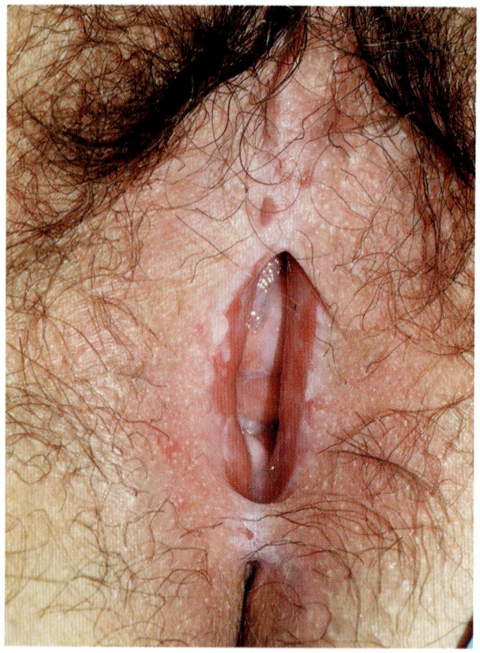

Fig. 11-8. Another erosion with a rim of white hyperkeratosis; a biopsy of this area showed changes consistent with LP.

Normally, these are nonspecific and indistinguishable from pemphigus vulgaris, mucous membrane pemphigus, or an acute irritant contact dermatitis. Sometimes, the erosions are surrounded by white epithelium that can represent the white morphologic variant of LP **(Figs. 11-7 and 11-8)**. However, any mucous membrane erosion is likely to produce a white border due to nonspecific inflammation of adjacent denuded skin. However, when nearby reticulate white lacy plaques are present, the diagnosis is clearly that of lichen planus **(Figs. 11-9 and 11-10)**. In 1982, Pelisse and associates described the vulvovaginal-gingival syndrome, introducing erosive lichen planus as a common subgroup in women.[4] Char-

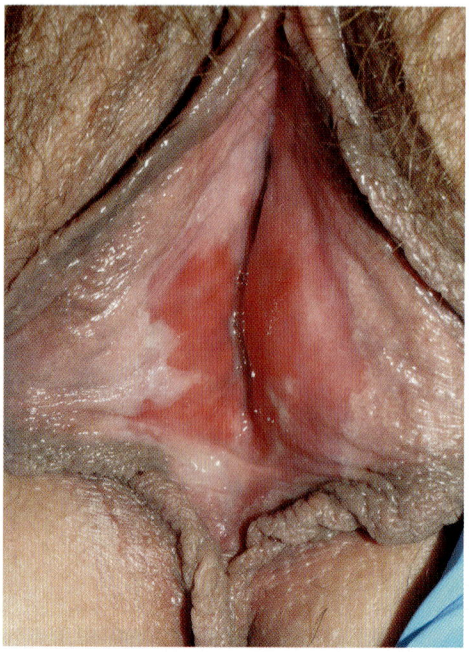

Fig. 11-7. At times, the erosions of lichen planus are surrounded by white epithelium. Sometimes, this white epithelium represents the white, papular form of LP. At other times, this white change is a nonspecific reaction to the inflammation.

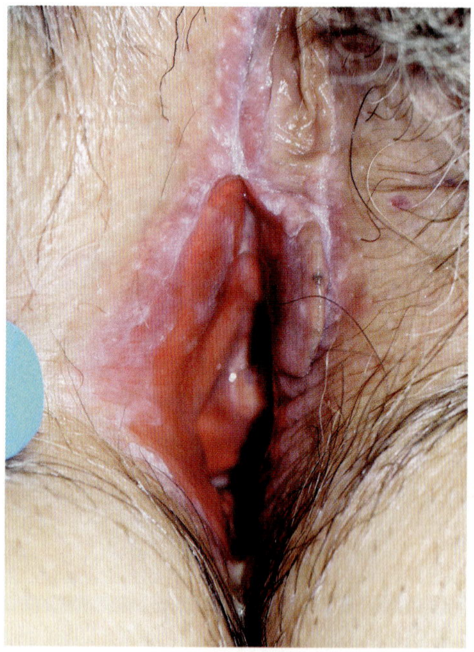

Fig. 11-9. This large erosion of modified mucous membrane is surrounded by not only white epithelium but white striae that demonstrate the diagnosis of lichen planus so that a biopsy is not needed.

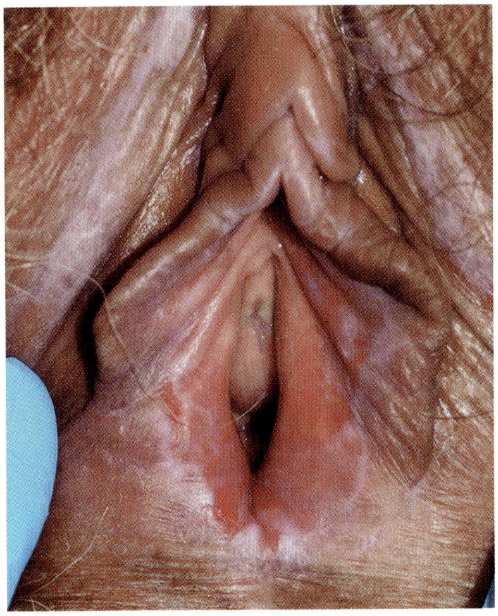

Fig. 11-10. White arcuate and linear papules both at the edge of the vestibule and on the hair-bearing labia minora are classic for LP. Even apparently uninvolved skin such as the labia minor and clitoral hood show marked edema.

acteristically, these patients suffer erosions of the vulva, vagina, and oral mucosa, especially the gingivae, which otherwise is not a common location for LP **(Figs. 11-11 and 11-12)**. The peno-gingival syndrome is less common but recognized as well **(Figs. 11-13 and 11-14)**.[5]

Erosive lichen planus often produces remarkable scarring, even when activity of the disease seems low **(Fig. 11-15)**. Labial resorption and scarring of the clitoral hood over the clitoris are common. Narrowing of the introitus is also a frequent complication that can result eventually in urinary retention.

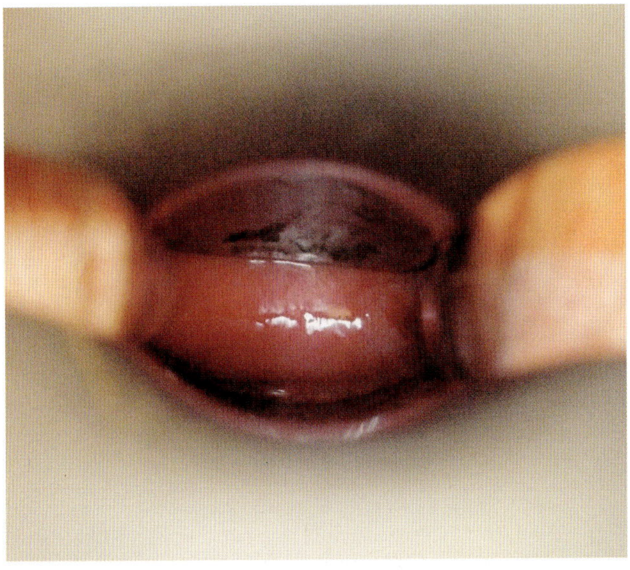

Fig. 11-11. The vagina is often involved in women with erosive vulvar LP; this woman has the vulvovaginal-gingival syndrome, a distinct group of women with involvement of all three areas.

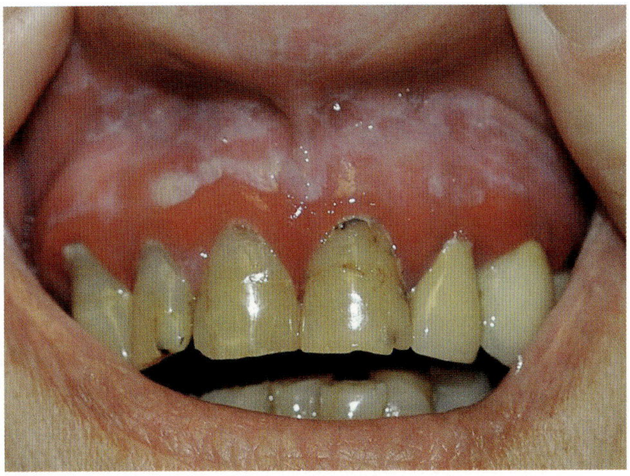

Fig. 11-12. The patient pictured in Fig. 11-11 also displayed very painful gingival erosive and hyperkeratotic LP. Treatment of gingival lichen planus is very difficult, owing largely to the difficulty of keeping topical therapies on the epithelium. Clearly, her teeth are suffering from the gingival disease, and hygiene is a painful and difficult affair.

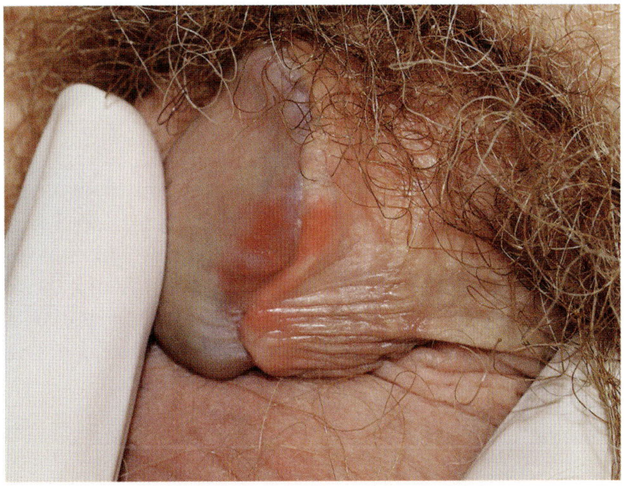

Fig. 11-13. The peno-gingival syndrome is much less common, which is not surprising considering that erosive penile LP is much less common in general. This nonspecific erosion of erosive LP has begun obvious early scarring of the glans to the prepuce.

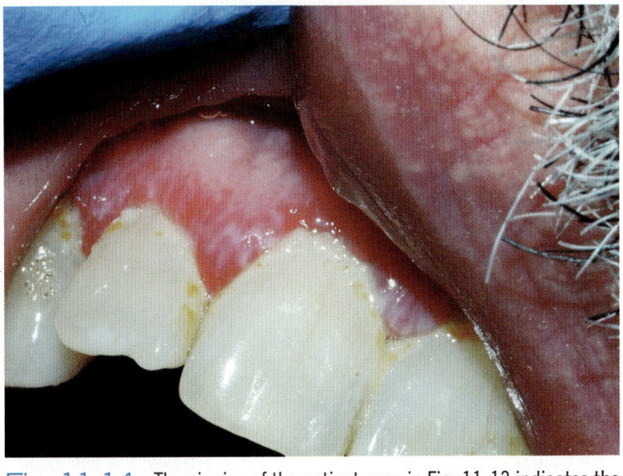

Fig. 11-14. The gingiva of the patient seen in Fig. 11-13 indicates the diagnosis of LP, with both erosion and pathognomonic white linear striae.

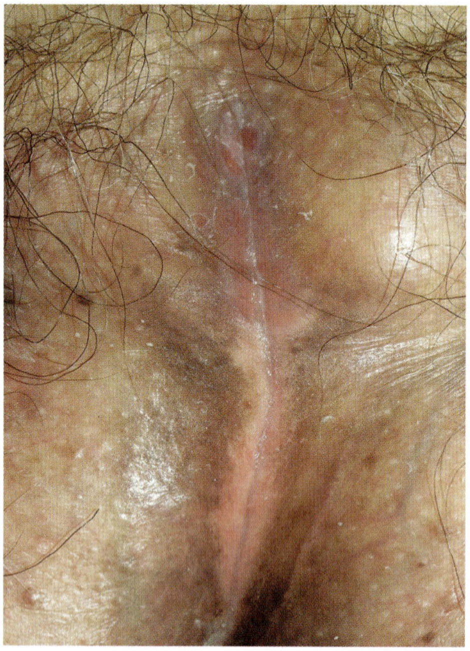

Fig. 11-15. The scarring associated with erosive LP occurs early, and it often happens with skin disease that is not especially dramatic. That scarring can be extraordinary so that early intervention can be important. The introitus here consists of several 1 mm openings that are so small that the vulva appears completely sealed shut.

Vaginal involvement is very common in women with erosive vulvar lichen planus. This is discussed further in Chapter 14, Vaginitis and Balanitis. This ranges from discrete erosions to generalized erythema, both accompanied by an inflammatory vaginitis **(Figs. 11-11, 11-16, and 11-17)**. Rarely, vaginal lichen planus occurs in the absence of vulvar involvement, when the diagnosis is much more easily missed. Erosive vaginal lichen planus produces purulent vaginal secretions that incite an irritant contact dermatitis in the vestibule and worsen the symptoms of vestibular lichen planus. Vaginal adhesions occur with severe disease, sometimes producing obliteration of the vaginal space that makes sexual intercourse or the introduction of a speculum impossible.

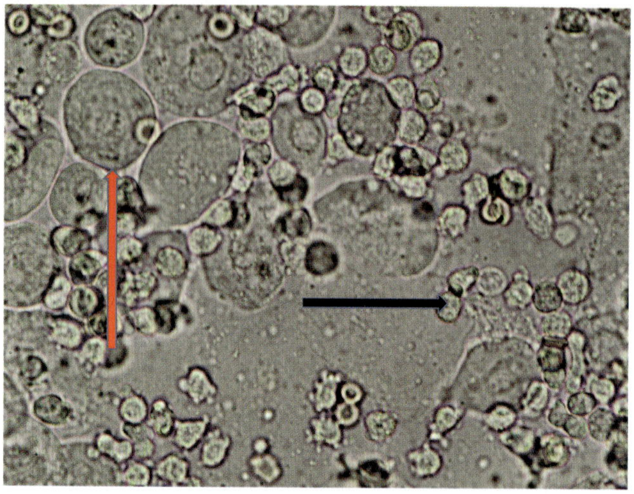

Fig. 11-17. A characteristic wet mount for erosive lichen planus shows large round parabasal cells (*red arrow*) and increase in lymphocytes (*black arrow*).

Penile lichen planus is less often erosive, but when erosions occur, they can be very painful **(Figs. 11-13, 11-18, and 11-19)**. These erosions may be associated with oral lesions and run

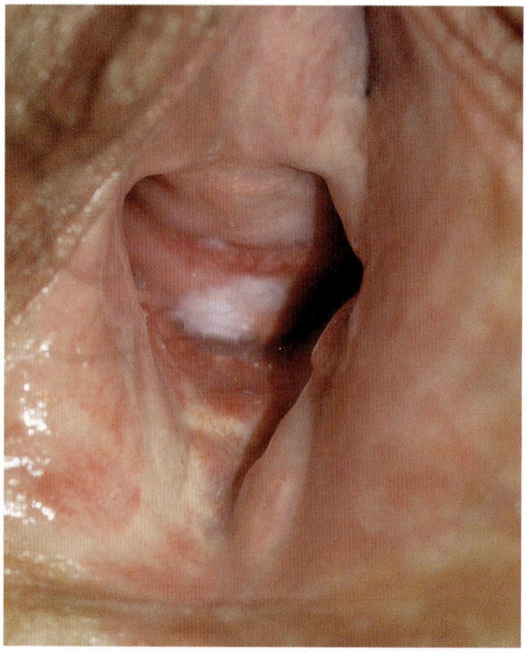

Fig. 11-16. The distal vagina is exposed here; there are erosions surrounding a white hyperkeratotic plaque. Sometimes, there is diffuse redness, and at other times, there are discrete erosions.

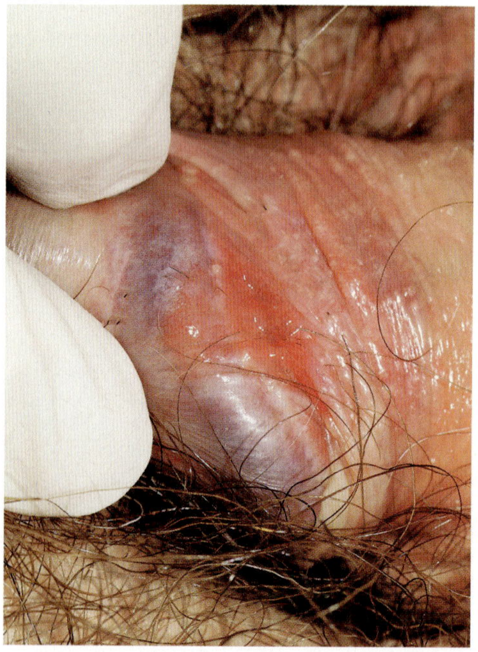

Fig. 11-18. This uncircumcised man has a nondiagnostic erosion on the corona extending to the ventral aspect of the prepuce. The diagnosis will depend upon more specific findings on other surfaces such as the oral mucosa, or a consistent biopsy from the edge of the erosion.

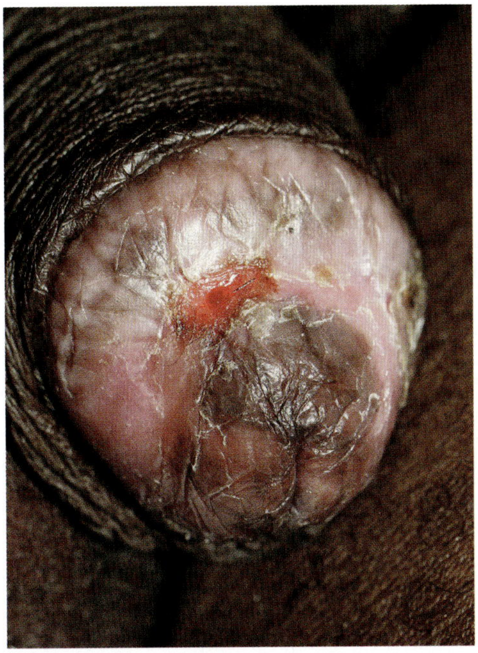

Fig. 11-19. When an erosion is not covered by a foreskin, as has occurred in this circumcised man with erosive lichen planus, there is crusting and surrounding scale.

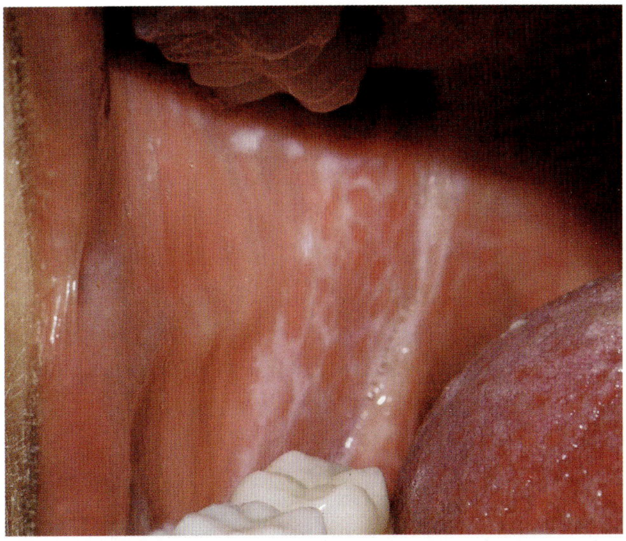

Fig. 11-21. The classic, pathognomonic sign of lichen planus is the lacy or fernlike pattern of white papules on the posterior buccal mucosa, which is very common in patients with erosive genital lichen planus. This patient also has small erosions within the annular white papules.

a similar prolonged clinical course to that seen in women.[2] Men with erosive penile lichen planus also experience scarring, with phimosis if uncircumcised, or obliteration of the sharp distinction of the glans from the shaft in the circumcised penis. Perianal lesions sometimes occur in both genders, but erosive disease of this area can be subtle and the area should be specifically examined **(Fig. 11-20)**.

Gingival lesions can be localized or generalized, primarily manifested by tender erosions and desquamative gingivitis, sometimes with surrounding solid or reticulate white papules **(Figs. 11-11 and 11-13)**. Classic and more common are linear reticulate papules or erosions on the buccal mucosa, and the tongue is often affected as well **(Figs. 11-21 and 11-22)**. Esophageal lichen planus is increasingly recognized and is likely more common than the literature suggests. Strictures producing dysphagia and weight loss are suggestive of this involvement, and squamous cell carcinoma (SCC) of the esophagus is a rare but serious complication.[6] Esophageal scarring predisposes to reflux disease, and reflux worsens esophageal lichen planus, confounding the diagnosis and biopsies at times. Conjunctival

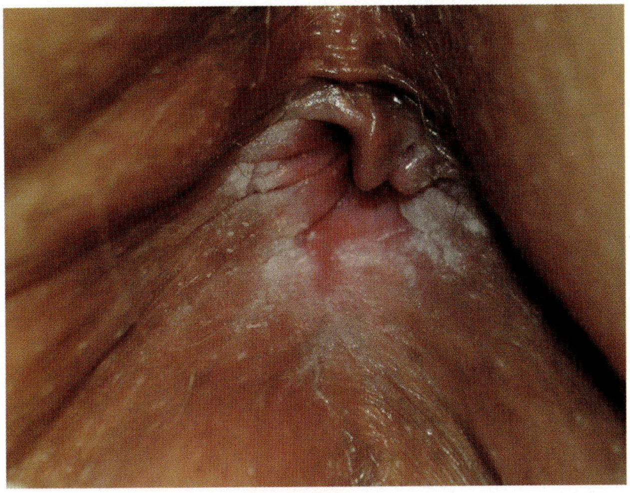

Fig. 11-20. Perianal erosive lichen planus can occur in both genders. Because it can be subtle, the area should be examined carefully and the rectal skin gently everted for better visualization.

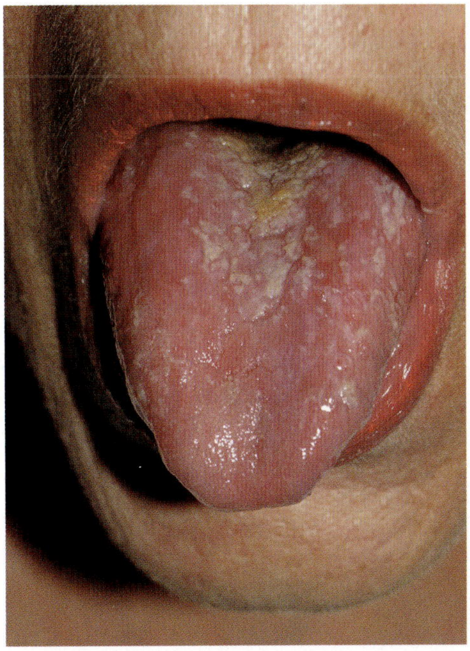

Fig. 11-22. The tongue is involved in some patients, ranging from erosions and hyperkeratosis as seen here, to nonspecific erosions on the lateral tongue, to a shiny dorsal tongue surface from loss of papillae due to chronic gradual scarring.

involvement and lacrimal duct scarring can occur.[7] Much less common is involvement of the extra-auditory canals, primarily manifested by otorrhea and hearing loss, and rarely resulting in obliteration of the canal.[8]

Squamous cell carcinoma (SCC) sometimes occurs in oral, vulvar, and penile lichen planus. Recent information suggests that vulvar SCC is less common that previously believed.[9] A survey of 13 100 women with all forms of lichen planus showed twice as many vulvar and esophageal malignancies as expected, but no increase in the risk of vaginal cancer.[10] Cancer of the lip was increased 5-fold, the tongue 12-fold, and the oral cavity 8-fold.[10] Although probably less common than in lichen sclerosus, SCC is an event we also have seen in women with severe, long-standing lichen planus, so clinicians should be aware. Malignancy in the setting of penile lichen planus certainly occurs and is reported only in case reports and very small series.

There have been reports for many years of lichen planus occurring more often in patients with hepatitis C as well as and reports discounting this association. A recent survey of over 2000 patients with lichen planus of all types showed the incidence of hepatitis C to be 1.8%, significantly increased over 0.6% incidence in controls, but still uncommonly present.[11] The incidences of hepatitis B and cirrhosis were twice that of controls.[11] More recently, a study has noted an association of oral lichen planus and hypothyroidism.[12] The metabolic syndrome appears to be more common with lichen planus in general, but there are no reports of this association specifically with erosive mucosal LP.[13] There also appears to be an association of lichen planus with lichen sclerosus, named an LP/LS overlap. This refers to both diseases occurring in the same patient, most often oral lichen planus and vulvar lichen sclerosus, but sometimes one biopsy-proven genital disease evolving into the other.[14] This is a combination that I see frequently.

Finally, unreported but generally recognized by vulvologists is the development of residual pain, both following the successful management of erosive vulvar lichen planus and on uninvolved areas of the vulva in women with erosive lichen planus. In a chart review in the office of one of us (LE) of 114 women with erosive vulvar or vulvovaginal lichen planus, 44 patients experienced clinical clearing of the vulva and vagina. However, 10 of those women reported persistent pain. There were even more patients with residual LP who reported pain in unaffected areas, but these were not included. (Coombs A, Edwards L, presented at XXI World Congress ISSVD, Paris, 2011.) So, in this small review, at least 23% of women with successfully managed LP met the criteria for vulvodynia. I am unaware of this finding being discussed in relation to men with erosive LP, and my numbers of men with erosive LP are small.

## Diagnosis

Erosions with accompanying white striae are diagnostic of lichen planus; however, this finding is usually absent on the genitalia. When white striae are seen in the mouth of patients with chronic nonspecific genital erosions, this usually indicates that the genital disease is lichen planus as well. However, the clinician should take care because of the occurrence of LP/LS overlap as noted above.

For practical purposes, chronic, nonspecific vulvar erosions without signs of blisters are nearly always lichen planus. And, when accompanied by oral disease, this is especially true. Similarly, chronic erosions of the glans penis without signs of blistering disease are likely erosive lichen planus. Although a biopsy is useful in ruling out other diseases, many genital specialists report that, on mucous membranes or modified mucous membranes, they rarely have a biopsy of erosive lichen planus returned as diagnostic. The histology generally is interpreted as "lichenoid dermatitis" consistent with but not diagnostic of lichen planus. Lichen planus and a lichenoid medication reaction can produce identical clinical and histologic picture, and even contact dermatitis and some phases of lichen sclerosus and immunobullous diseases can show similar nonspecific findings. The biopsy should be taken from the edge rather than the center of an erosion, and it should be submitted for routine histology. If the biopsy is nonspecific or is suggestive of an autoimmune blistering disease, an additional biopsy of nearby noneroded skin can be submitted in transport media rather than formalin for direct immunofluorescence.

The classic biopsy of erosive lichen planus shows a dense, lymphocytic, dermal bandlike infiltrate extending to and damaging the basal layer (Fig. 11-23). A prominent granular cell layer, hyperkeratosis, and acanthosis are common, but erosive mucous membrane lichen planus often exhibits epithelial thinning and flattening. A biopsy that does not include epithelium cannot provide a diagno-

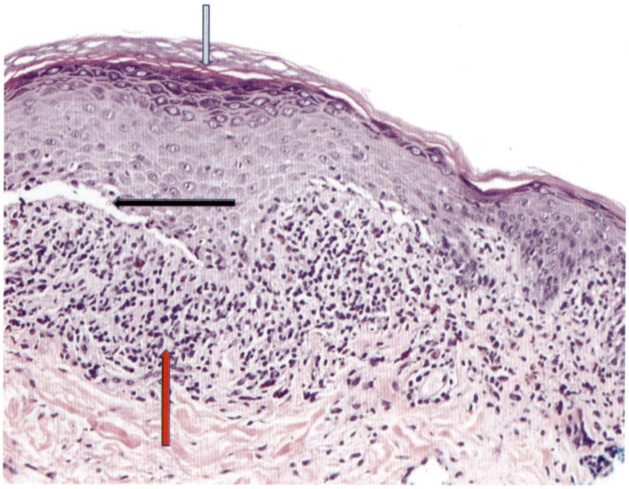

Fig. 11-23. This uncharacteristically characteristic photomicrograph shows a dense lymphocytic infiltrate in the upper dermis (*red arrow*) that has destroyed the basement membrane and allowed the epidermis to lift from the dermis (*black arrow*). There is also wedge-shaped hypergranulosis (*blue arrow*). (Courtesy of Jason Reutter, MD.)

sis of LP. Colloid and Civatte bodies are frequently seen in the lower epidermis and upper dermis, and a direct immunofluorescent biopsy makes these more easily visualized.

Most chronic erosive/blistering skin diseases are in the differential diagnosis of erosive genital lichen planus. Pemphigus vulgaris and benign mucous membrane pemphigoid can be nearly indistinguishable, but these are far, far less common and usually more easily diagnosed by routine and direct immunofluorescent biopsy. Sometimes, white epithelium can resemble lichen sclerosus, but the texture of this white epithelium does not have the characteristic crinkled texture of LS. Toxic epidermal necrolysis, severe erosive candidiasis, and an irritant contact dermatitis to an agent such as podophyllum resin can mimic erosive lichen planus, but these are acute rather than chronic in onset. Like erosive lichen planus, plasma cell mucositis also exhibits red, moist, glistening papules, and plaques that may appear erosive. The histology usually white, lacy striae of genital skin are pathognomonic for genital lichen planus. Unfortunately, this differentiates lichen planus from plasma cell vulvitis or balanitis, but many feel that LP and plasma cell mucositis are at least related if not the same disease. Chronic graft vs host disease is indistinguishable clinically and histologically from lichen planus, but the history is clearly the differentiating feature.

**EROSIVE LICHEN PLANUS** **Diagnosis**

- Nonspecific chronic erosions of mucous membranes or modified mucous membranes statistically indicate the diagnosis
- White lacy striae of the mouth strongly suggest the diagnosis by association
- Pathognomonic lacy, white surrounding striae on anogenital skin confirm diagnosis
- A biopsy of the edge of an erosion reporting lichenoid mucositis or dermatitis gives presumptive diagnosis in the appropriate clinical setting

## Pathophysiology

Although the etiology of lichen planus is not well understood, autoimmune T-cell–mediated destruction of basal cell keratinocytes is believed to be a major factor. Rarely, lichen planus or a nearly identical lichenoid medication reaction is produced by medications, most often from gold, antimalarial drugs, β-blockers and angiotensin-converting enzyme inhibitors. Recent observations included associations with novel drugs such as biologics (eg, tumor necrosis factor antagonists) and immune checkpoint inhibitors.[15]

## Management

Erosive genital lichen planus usually responds fairly well to superpotent topical corticosteroids, local care, and, in postmenopausal women, estrogen replacement (**Figs. 11-24 and 11-25**). Occasionally, genital erosive lichen planus can be severe and recalcitrant. Erosive oral disease is often more challenging, as are the less common esophageal and rare eye and ear disease. Where topical corticosteroids cannot be applied or where they do not adhere well, such as in the mouth, intralesional or systemic therapy with antimetabolites or immunosuppressive drugs is sometimes used for persistent disease.

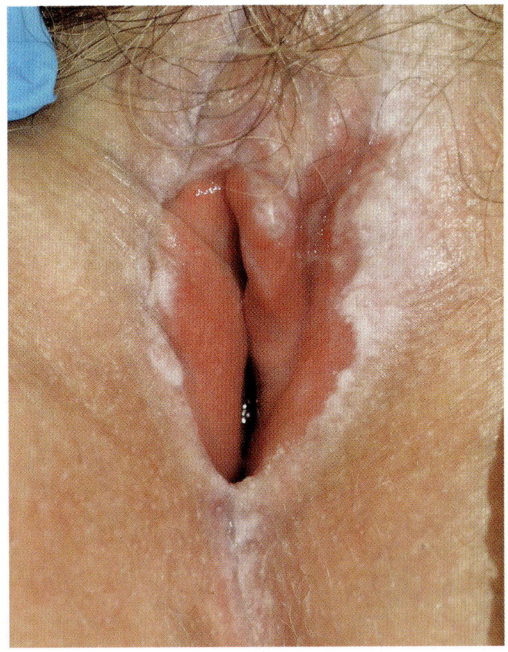

Fig. 11-24. Vulvar erosive lichen planus at baseline before therapy.

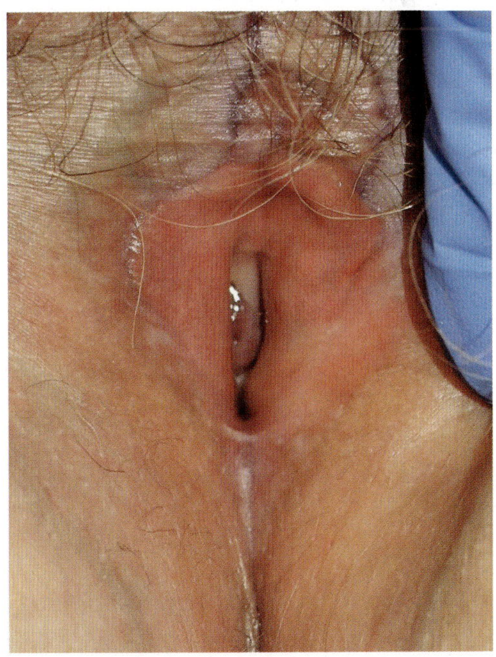

Fig. 11-25. Six weeks after initiation of a tiny amount of halobetasol ointment applied twice a day and covered with a touch of petroleum jelly initially, the vulva has improved remarkably.

Data regarding the benefit of therapy are poor. A Cochrane Database review showed no convincing evidence for benefit of any therapies[16]; however, clinicians see very significant improvement in patients with some therapies, especially corticosteroids. Although medications do not cure the disease, lichen planus in most patients is managed quite well with topical corticosteroid therapy. Circumcision is sometimes curative in men.

**EROSIVE LICHEN PLANUS** **Management**

Topical therapy
- Superpotent corticosteroid ointment twice daily
- Calcineurin inhibitors (tacrolimus or pimecrolimus) twice daily
- Local supportive care—dilators, infection control, avoidance of irritants
- For postmenopausal women with vaginal lichen planus—estrogen replacement

Intralesional corticosteroids
- Triamcinolone acetonide 10 mg/cc into recalcitrant lesions

Systemic therapy occasionally (poor data)—added to topical, intralesional therapy
- Hydroxychloroquine 200 mg orally twice daily
- Methotrexate up to 25 mg orally weekly
- Mycophenolate mofetil up to 1500 mg twice daily
- Many other immunosuppressives and antimetabolites from case reports

### Nonspecific Therapy

Avoidance of irritants such as soap and overwashing, panty liners, and unnecessary topical medications is useful. Topical emollients such as petrolatum are soothing, as are measures such as air-drying rather than towel-drying. Because vulvovaginal lichen planus occurs primarily in the postmenopausal age group, topical or systemic estrogen replacement can be crucial, avoiding an additional and easily corrected cause for mucosal thinning. Estrogen replacement is discussed in Chapter 14, Vaginitis and Balanitis. Women with vaginal lichen planus or with introital narrowing should be counseled in the use of vaginal dilators to use several times a week to prevent continued tightening of the vaginal canal, and men should be encouraged to retract the prepuce daily to minimize the risk of phimosis.

### Topical Therapy

The overwhelming first-line therapy for genital lichen planus is topical corticosteroid therapy. Superpotent topical corticosteroid ointments (eg, clobetasol propionate 0.05%, halobetasol propionate 0.05%) applied to vulvar or penile lesions twice daily and covered with a small amount of petroleum jelly can be beneficial. Because occlusion enhances the potency of medication, recalcitrant lichen planus of the circumcised glans can be treated carefully with corticosteroids under condom occlusion for short periods with careful follow-up. Ointments are by far the vehicle of choice; creams, gels, lotions, and solutions are to be avoided because of the irritation induced by the additives regularly contained in these vehicles.

There are no corticosteroids formulated for the vagina. However, small amounts of a corticosteroid ointment can be inserted with a vaginal applicator intravaginally overnight. Alternatively, a commercially available 25-mg hydrocortisone acetate rectal suppository can be inserted vaginally, or hydrocortisone acetate foam designed for hemorrhoids can be inserted into the vagina with a finger. However, these preparations are very low potency. More potent vaginal suppositories can be compounded, with hydrocortisone acetate 100-300 mg suppositories sometimes used, or with insertion of superpotent corticosteroids into the vagina. However, significant absorption can occur, and there are no safety data on vaginal administration. I obtain cortisol stimulation on women using intravaginal superpotent corticosteroids more often than thrice weekly, because I have seen clinically cushingoid features occur in women using daily superpotent vaginal corticosteroids. Also, intravaginal corticosteroids sometimes precipitate vaginal candidiasis, so weekly fluconazole, twice or thrice weekly insertion of a topical antifungal cream, or a warning to the patient to call if sudden itching occurs is important.

The mouth should be addressed as well. I often find oral lichen planus to be a greater challenge than genital lichen planus, and dentists in general do not aggressively treat this miserable condition. There are several suboptimal options for the delivery of a corticosteroid to the mouth. Dexamethasone elixir can be used in a swish, hold as long as possible, and spit fashion. Because topical corticosteroids in the mouth increase the occurrence of Candidiasis, mixing the dexamethasone half and half with nystatin oral solution decreases that risk but also decreases the potency of the corticosteroid. The patient should not eat or drink for 30 minutes after use. Alternatively, clobetasol gel 0.05% can be applied to affected areas of the mouth. Covering the gel with a wet paper towel can hold the medication again the mucosa for longer and increase the effect. Both of these methods of use are started at about four times a day, and then decreased when the disease is better controlled to the least frequent use that maintains comfort.

Some have advocated the use of dental trays to hold medication against the affected gingivae. Dentists who make mouth guards from individualized molds for patients can do this and then leave intact rather than trim the edge that covers the gingivae from the guard. When the disease is better controlled, the frequency of application is decreased to the least frequent use that maintains comfort.

Second-line therapy for erosive mucosal lichen planus consists of the topical calcineurin inhibitors pimecrolimus 1% cream and, especially, tacrolimus 0.1% ointment.[17] Tacrolimus suppositories for the vagina can be compounded as well, and compounding pharmacies have these recipes. However, these medications are not approved by the U.S. Food and Drug Administration (FDA) for lichen planus, and although generally well tolerated in the mouth, usually produce unacceptable and long-lasting burning when applied to inflamed genital skin. In addition, improvement is delayed when compared to topical corticosteroids, and they are black-boxed by the FDA for a risk of producing skin cancer and lymphoma, worrisome to patients who are already at risk for transformation to SCC. The occurrence of these malignancies does not seem to have actually appeared in response to use of topical calcineurin inhibitors. However, these authors and many of our colleagues have not found these medications to be particularly useful for genital erosive lichen planus.

### Intralesional Therapy

Corticosteroids injected into recalcitrant mucosal lesions often prompt excellent healing when topical corticosteroids fail (see Chapter 4). Triamcinolone acetonide 10 mg/cc is the usual preparation, using about 0.1 cc/cm$^2$. The oral epithelium can be anesthetized with an oral anesthetic compounded by dentists to produce prompt and complete anesthesia, resulting in a painless injection. However, this topical anesthetic should be avoided on genital skin, where it sometimes produces sloughing. Compounded tetracaine 6%/lidocaine 6% applied for 15-30 minutes is far better tolerated and affords fairly good anesthesia on genital skin.

Intralesional corticosteroids can be used by gastroenterologists during endoscopy, and often in combination with dilation, for chronic recalcitrant esophageal disease as well.[18]

### Systemic Therapy

The only predictably beneficial systemic therapy for erosive lichen planus is systemic corticosteroid therapy, especially prednisone or prednisolone. Dosing of prednisone 40-60 mg/d effects significant and rapid improvement in most patients, but the condition recurs when the medication is stopped. Clearly, the toxicity of chronic systemic corticosteroid therapy prevents this treatment for anything except brief use for flares of disease. Prednisone can be used initially in patients with severe erosions to clear skin sufficiently before transitioning to topical therapy. Alternatively, corticosteroids can be administered by intramuscular injection with triamcinolone acetonide, 40-80 mg. One regimen consists of a monthly injection for 3 months in an attempt to interrupt the disease process and trigger long-lasting benefit (personal communication, Lynnette Margesson, MD).

However, other immunosuppressive medications that are safer for chronic use sometimes appear to produce modest improvement in lichen planus, although the data from controlled trials are lacking. The onset of benefit of these treatments is slow, requiring at least 3 months to produce full effect, and these therapies improve lichen planus less predictably. Hydroxychloroquine 200 mg twice a day is a time-honored inexpensive therapy with minimal laboratory monitoring, and a recent letter reported that 60% of 15 patients experienced an undefined good response.[19] Methotrexate 25 mg weekly is another cost-effective therapy, but again with very little data. A letter describing a comparison between methotrexate and mycophenolate mofetil in the treatment of vulvar lichen planus in 44 patients showed comparable benefit using doses of methotrexate mostly <25 mg/wk (70% responded) and mycophenolate mofetil up to 2500 mg/d (64% responded). The degree of response was not reported.[3] There are allusions to benefit from oral retinoids such as isotretinoin 40-80 mg/d and acitretin at about 25 mg/d including a recent case report of benefit in penile LP,[20] but side effects including teratogenicity require careful monitoring. Other systemic treatments used historically include oral griseofulvin, azathioprine, cyclophosphamide, azathioprine, dapsone, and metronidazole with anecdotal benefit in some patients; clinician familiarity with these medications for appropriate monitoring is important. Thalidomide was shown in a small open trial to be as effective as topical steroids for oral lichen planus, but this has not been repeated.[21] There are several case reports of oral cyclosporine being used for lichen planus, and topical cyclosporine swish and spit for oral LP. An unusually well-designed 2013 open label trial examined the effect of apremilast, an oral medication for psoriasis, on LP. Ten patients with moderate to severe LP (only one with mucosal disease) showed significant improvement in 30% of patients.[22] However, there have been only six positive case reports since that time and no studies. The JAK inhibitor tofacitinib has been reported in several case reports of lichen planopilaris (LP of hair follicles) and LP of nails, and I have treated four patients with recalcitrant and life-ruining disease with tofacitinib 5 mg twice daily; three cleared by at least 95%, and one patient experienced no improvement. Obtaining this prohibitively expensive medication for LP when not approved for use for any dermatologic indications has proved to be nearly impossible. Potential side effects include intestinal perforation, immunosuppression, and thrombosis. However, trials on other skin diseases are showing good effects, and other systemic and topical JAK inhibitors are available and in development. A large randomized study on the systemic JAK inhibitor ruxolitinib for graft vs host disease, a condition with clinically and histologically identical skin findings, showed robust data showing benefit.[23] And, the JAK inhibitor ruxolitinib has just been released as a cream for atopic dermatitis. The current price is about $2000 for a large tube. There have been reports of some of the biologic agents, primarily adalimumab and ustekinumab, providing some relief for patients with lichen planus, but there are also reports of these medications producing paradoxical lichenoid skin reactions. Other than systemic corticosteroids, there are no systemic therapies known at this time to produce consistent good improvement in resistant erosive genital lichen planus, but trial and error treatment often yields therapies that improve disease when added to good topical and intralesional corticosteroid therapy and local care.

### Surgery

Circumcision is the only surgical procedure that sometimes improves the mucosal lichen planus. However, surgery is occasionally needed to separate vaginal adhesions, reverse tightening of the introitus, or to uncover a buried clitoris. Narrowing of the vaginal introitus occasionally progresses to complete closure, resulting in urinary retention requiring urgent surgery. Skin disease should be controlled as well as possible before surgery is contemplated, and great care has to be taken postoperatively to prevent rapid scar reformation. Use of topical steroids and dilators is advisable.

Erosive anogenital lichen planus is chronic and painful, and there are no standard treatment measures that help all patients. Nor are there any high level controlled trials that evaluate therapy for anogenital lichen planus. However, experience suggests that there are various therapies that help some patients. Occasionally, erosive anogenital lichen planus remits, but this is the exception. Also, because of the risk of SCC, patients should be checked regularly throughout the course of the disease. Indurated erosions and ulcers should be biopsied, as should chronic hyperkeratotic areas.

In summary, most patients do well simply with superpotent topical corticosteroid ointments applied twice daily, covered with petroleum jelly, and tapering the frequency of application when skin disease improves. Adjunctive therapies are added to corticosteroids rather than replacing them. Local care is important, such as insertion of a dilator in women with vaginal involvement or introital narrowing to minimize scarring, and careful daily retraction of the prepuce in men to prevent phimosis. Estrogen replacement in postmenopausal women is imperative, and infection control in both sexes is key as well. Those with prominent pruritus should receive bedtime sedation to prevent nighttime scratching. Careful follow-up for early signs of malignant change and side effects of medication is crucial.

Vulvologists have noted residual pain in many women successfully treated for erosive vulvovaginal lichen planus, showing that lichen planus can trigger vulvodynia. Therefore, those patients who continue to report burning and rawness should be re-evaluated for active lichen planus rather than simply treated for this LP more aggressively. Often, medication for neuropathic pain and physical therapy directed at management of vulvodynia precipitated by lichen planus should be the next step, while continuing to medications that control the underlying erosive LP.

## Plasma Cell Balanitis and Vulvitis (Zoon Balanitis/Vulvitis)

Zoon mucositis is discussed primarily in Chapter 5. Zoon balanitis or vulvitis (also called balanitis or vulvitis circumscripta plasmacellularis, inflammatory erythroplasia) is a characteristic nonblanching deep red, rusty/orange, or brown red patch on a mucous membrane that shows increased plasma cells on biopsy. The cause is unknown, but the similarity in appearance and histology causes some to suspect a relationship to lichen planus.

Plasma cell vulvitis and balanitis present as a usually solitary plaque on the glans penis or vulva. Although this often appears erosive, the epithelium generally is atrophic but intact **(Figs. 11-26 and 11-27)**. Zoon is most often uncomfortable, with patients describing burning or irritation, and less often itching or no discomfort.

In men, circumcision generally is curative. Otherwise, potent topical corticosteroids are standard first-line therapy that offers some symptomatic relief and improvement in appearance in many patients. As for other dermatoses, relapse is the rule on discontinuation of treatment. Topical tacrolimus, pimecrolimus, and masoprocol have been useful in some, but reported results of therapy are conflicting and I find tacrolimus/pimecrolimus to be

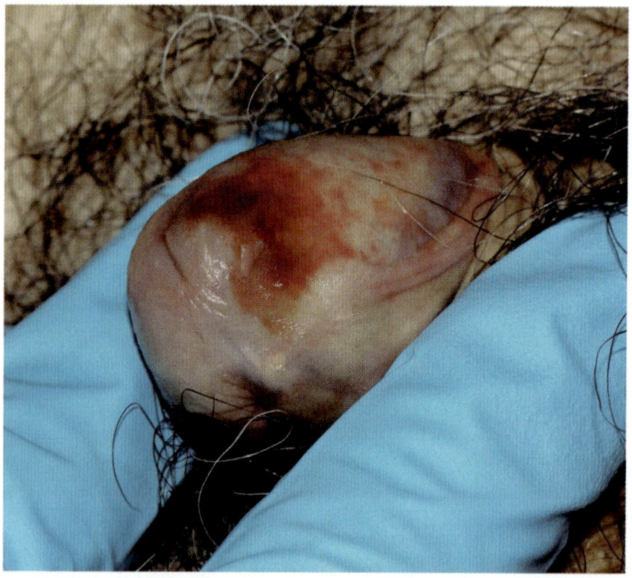

Fig. 11-26. Plasma cell balanitis is characterized by deep red, purpuric well-demarcated patches on the glans.

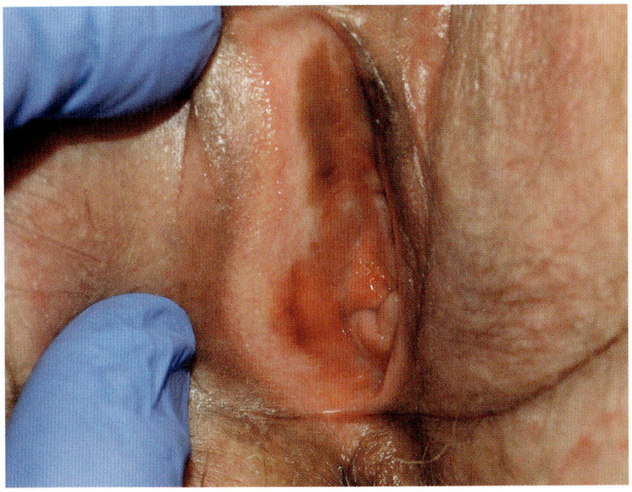

Fig. 11-27. The iron from the extravasated blood in the dermis gives established lesions a brown or rust color.

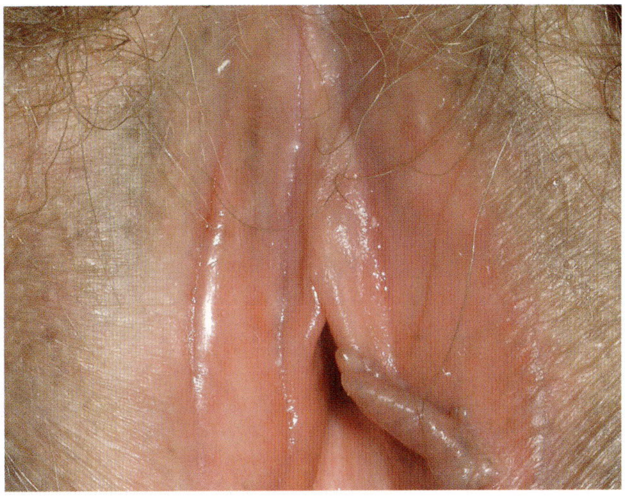

Fig. 11-28. There are very fine red streaks representing skinfold fissures, here produced by Candidiasis that is also causing erythema and puffiness of the modified mucous membranes.

poorly tolerated due to local burning with application. Topical corticosteroids mixed with fusidic acid, imiquimod, intralesional corticosteroids, and $CO_2$ laser have been reported beneficial at times. Although a differentiating feature from lichen planus is sometimes said to be lack of scarring, I have had patients with Zoon vulvitis experience loss of labia minora and clitora phimosis. Also, there are several reports of SCC *in situ* (intraepithelial neoplasia) in a setting of plasma cell balanitis, so that ongoing surveillance is recommended.

## Genital Skinfold Fissures

Genital skinfold fissures are a physical finding rather than a disease; these are a common nonspecific feature of several inflammatory genital diseases, seen primarily on the vulva and perianal skin. Patients sometimes describe these fissures as "paper cuts," and the clinician has the task of finding the cause and management.

### Clinical Presentation

These linear erosions occur within skinfolds, especially the interlabial folds and edges of the clitoral hood in women, in the coronal sulcus and skin wrinkling of the penile shaft, and within the normal skin markings of the perineal body and perianal skin of both men and women (**Figs. 11-28 through 11-32**). They often are transient so that the diagnosis is made by the history in association with thin, red lines in the areas of fissuring, or by having the patient return as soon as fissures recur. Sometimes, magnification is required for identification. At other times, the fissures are so deep as to actually represent ulcers.

Patients report irritation as well as stinging that is accentuated when urine, semen, medicated creams, or sometimes even water touches the area.

### Diagnosis

The recognition of skinfold fissures is made by visualization of the finding. The diagnosis of the underlying cause is sometimes obvious, but sometimes difficult and occasionally no cause is found. When acute, Candidiasis is the most common underlying diagnosis. Herpes simplex virus is an uncommon cause of an acute fissure in men and women and, rarely, a bacterial infection, either *Staphylococcus aureus* or, less often, *Streptococcus* spp. cause fissures. Although infection with group B *Streptococcus* has been reported, this is usually *Streptococcus pyogenes*, and this is often in association with inflammatory vaginitis.

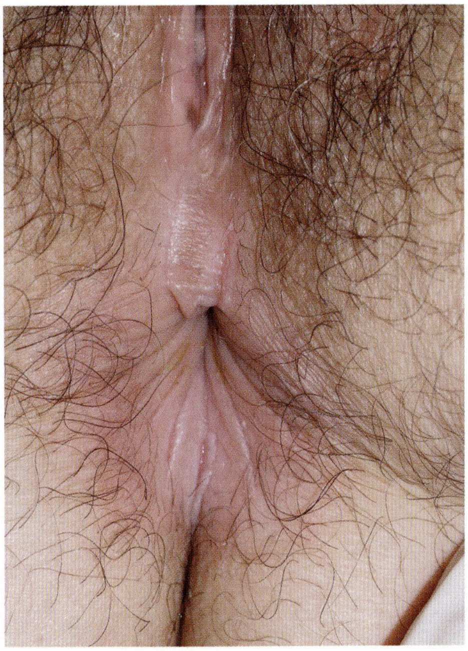

Fig. 11-29. The lichenification of lichen simplex chronicus is also often associated with skinfold fissures on the perineum and perianal skin.

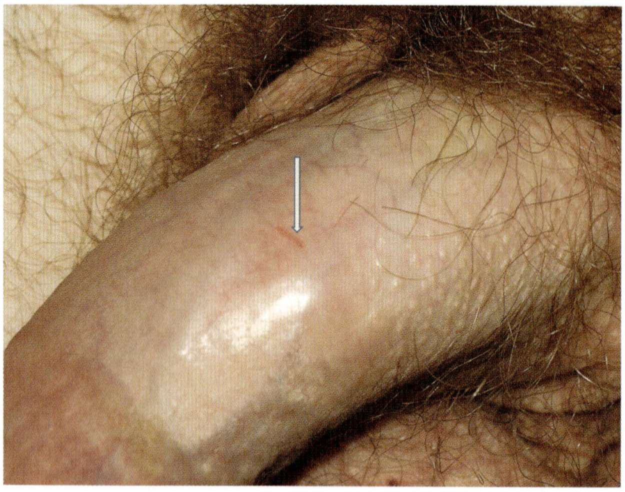

Fig. 11-30. Skinfold fissures are seen in men as well, but much less often (*arrow*).

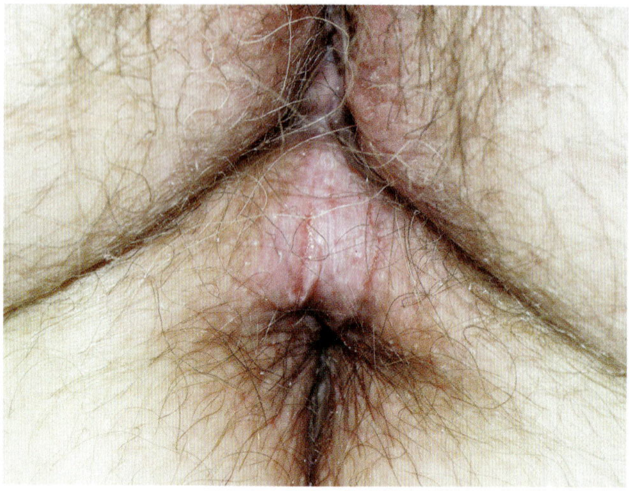

Fig. 11-32. Lichen sclerosus is even more likely to fissure when rubbing is prominent.

When chronic, noninfectious inflammatory dermatoses are most likely, especially lichen simplex chronicus and lichen sclerosus, although contact dermatitis, psoriasis and any other cause of inflammation can cause fissures less often. Intraepithelial neoplasia and high-grade squamous intraepithelial lesions have been associated with fissure. Maddeningly, at times there is no accompanying skin disease, and cultures, molecular studies and cultures are negative.

### Pathophysiology

Presumably, delicate genital skin becomes even more friable when the skin becomes inflamed, and rather than bending in folds, the epithelium cracks. Chronic inflammation often prompts skin to thicken so that it bends less easily, and breaks. Also, many people experience itching with inflammation and resulting rubbing can produce fissures.

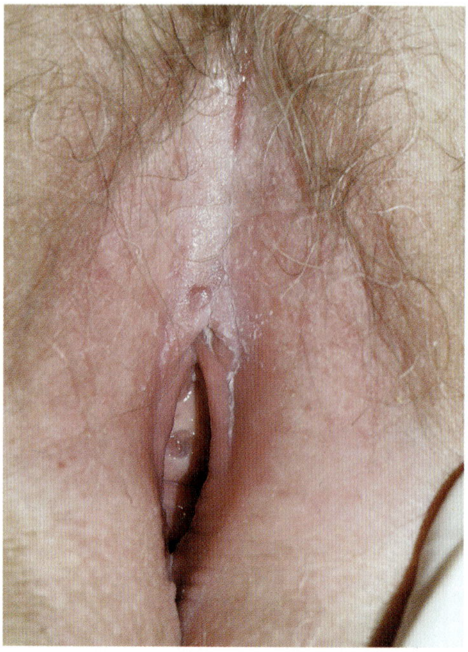

Fig. 11-31. The fragility of lichen sclerosus is a factor in the cause of skinfold fissures.

### Management

For skinfold fissures, the identification, treatment, and then suppression of the underlying condition usually eliminate the fissures. When no underlying factors are identified, an empiric trial of a topical corticosteroid ointment such as clobetasol or halobetasol, covering with fluconazole 150-200 mg every 4-7 days for several weeks, manages most causes of fissures. After the skin has healed, the medications can be gradually discontinued, although recurrence is common.

## Mechanical Vulvar Fissures

Mechanical fissures consist of splits occurring at the introitus, usually at the posterior fourchette and primarily with coitus.

### Clinical Presentation

Mechanical fissures occur most often in premenopausal women and almost exclusively in sexually active individuals. The onset is usually sudden, without preceding trauma or infection; stinging and splitting of the posterior fourchette occurs during sexual intercourse. Semen, water, and urine burn on contact. The area usually heals quickly but recurs with most acts of intercourse.

On clinical examination, there is a linear erosion at the midline posterior fourchette that may be thin and subtle, or relatively wide, obvious, and nearly ulcerative

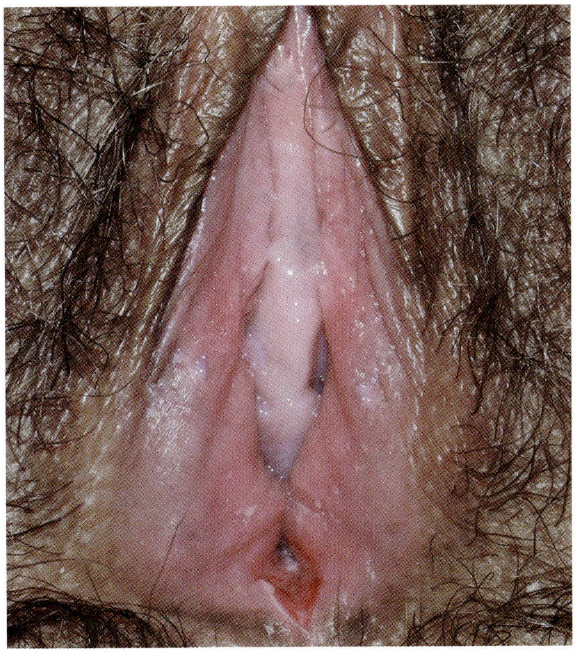

Fig. 11-33. Mechanical fissures are usually located at the posterior fourchette, occurring primarily with coitus.

(**Figs. 11-33 through 11-35**). Some patients exhibit fairly long-lasting erythema of the area after healing. Posterior fourchette fissuring is easily seen when the patient presents within a day or two following sexual intercourse. Rarely, women experience erosions or ulcerations that are not at the 6 o'clock position, and in my experience, these are usually at 3 or 9 o'clock. These may be linear fissures, or a small, recurrent, punctate ulcer (**Fig. 11-36**).

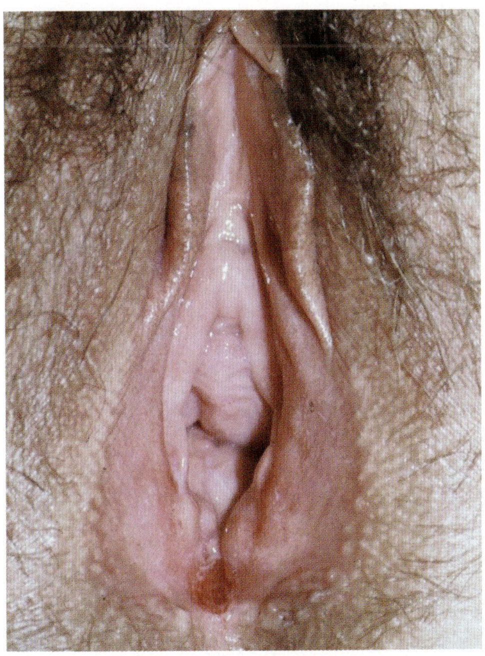

Fig. 11-34. Most women with posterior fourchette fissures have no surrounding skin abnormalities or other cause for the recurrent splitting with sexual activity.

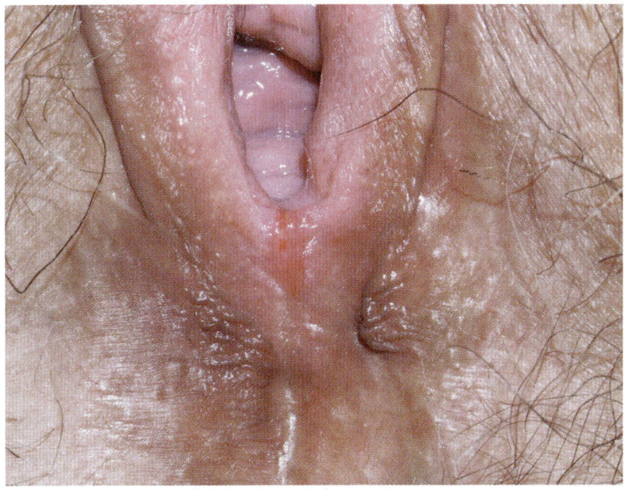

Fig. 11-35. Some mechanical fissures are superficial as seen here, or very thin so that they heal almost overnight.

Some women report associated pain distinct from the fissure but within the vestibule. Some clinicians postulate that fissuring occurs in association with vulvodynia or vestibulodynia (previously called the vulvar vestibulitis syndrome) (Chapter 13).

## Diagnosis

The diagnosis of a recurrent posterior fissure is easily made by the morphology and history. However, the clinician should take care to visualize the fissure either in the office or by photograph. Some patients with vulvodynia/vestibulodynia describe fissuring with intercourse, but when seen following sexual activity in the office, the patient and provider learn that although the pain feels like splitting, there is no actual tearing. The diagnosis is not that of a mechanical fissure, but rather vestibulodynia. Additional diseases to consider include HSV infection because of the same-site erosions. However, this should

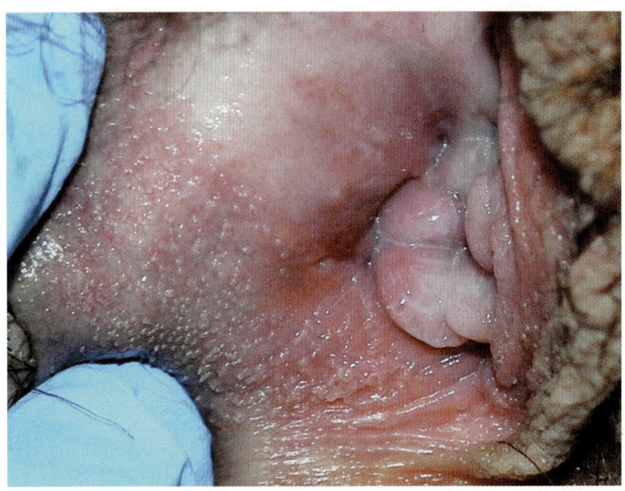

Fig. 11-36. Occasionally, mechanical fissures are located just adjacent to the hymeneal ring rather than at the posterior fourchette.

not occur with each act of coitus, and molecular studies for HSV will be negative.

**MECHANICAL VULVAR FISSURES — Diagnosis**

- Both history and visualization of a same-site fissure immediately following sexual activity

### Pathophysiology

The cause of mechanical fissures is not known. Although some clinicians have implicated low estrogen levels as a cause of posterior fourchette fissuring, there are no clinical signs of this, and the addition of oral or topical estrogen replacement is not helpful. Some believe that pelvic floor abnormalities may contribute to both vestibulodynia and posterior fourchette fissuring, helping to explain a possible association of these two conditions. Lichen sclerosus predisposes to posterior fourchette fissuring, and this fissuring resolves with treatment of the lichen sclerosus. Most women simply and relatively suddenly experience the onset of posterior fourchette fissuring with no known cause or accompanying abnormalities. Interestingly, a condition termed a perineal groove is seen rarely in newborn girls, and it generally heals in the first year or two.[24] This is described as a wet, red groove from the posterior fourchette to the anus at 12 o'clock, and this can be the entire length or partial length. This is postulated to be a self-healing congenital malformation; perhaps there is a relationship.

### Management

Liberal lubrication during sexual activity, topical anesthetics such as lidocaine jelly 2%, and woman on-top positioning minimizes fissuring for some women, but this does eliminate the problem. Avoiding sexual activity to allow the area to heal well is not useful. Primary excision with suture closure generally worsens the fissuring by narrowing the vaginal opening.

One management option consists of the patient applying a topical anesthetic such as lidocaine or, more effective, compounded tetracaine 6%/lidocaine 6%, then produce the fissure with sexual activity. Then, keep the fissure open with the frequent use of dilators, so that re-epithelialization occurs across the surface of the erosion (Hope Haefner, MD, personal communication).

Otherwise, definitive management consists of a perineoplasty. The skin surrounding the posterior fourchette is surgically excised, and vaginal epithelium is advanced to cover the defect. The success of the procedure depends largely on patient selection. Women should be evaluated for the likely presence of vestibulodynia before surgery, since their pain does not totally remit unless the entire vestibule is removed, or unless they receive medical treatment and/or physical therapy for vestibulodynia in addition to surgery.

**MECHANICAL VULVAR FISSURES — Management**

- Careful visual evaluation for underlying skin disease such as lichen sclerosus
- Replace estrogen if atrophic wet mount
- Lubrication before sexual activity
- Patient produces the fissure, then keep it open with careful perineal massage with petroleum jelly and dilators, to allow the fissure to re-epithelialize and heal in the open position
- If unsuccessful, perineoplasty; avoid simple excision with suture closure

## Erosive Lichen Sclerosus (Lichen Sclerosus et Atrophicus, Hypoplastic Dystrophy)

Lichen sclerosus is a chronic fragile dermatosis characterized by atrophic white plaques, occurring most commonly on the genital skin of both sexes, although there is a female preponderance of 10:1 (see Chapter 8 for primary discussion). Although lichen sclerosus is not primarily an erosive disease, intense itching with resulting rubbing of this fragile skin often produces erosions and purpura. There is fissuring of the anterior midline, as well as vestibular erosions following sexual activity.

The usual presenting symptom of lichen sclerosus is severe pruritus, often leading to painful erosions as this fragile skin is scratched (Fig. 11-37). These excoriations and other erosions resulting from fragility of the skin can be very painful and can predispose to secondary infection.

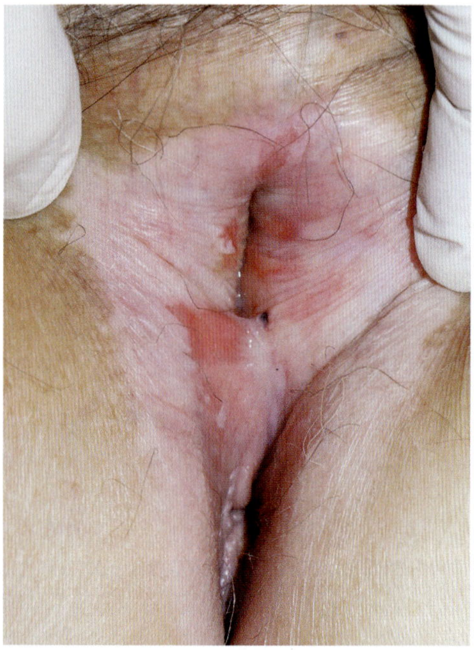

Fig. 11-37. The fragility of lichen sclerosus and rubbing of this pruritic skin can produce erosions.

The atrophic skin fissures more easily, so patients may present with pain on intercourse, and young girls often experience constipation resulting from pain of fissures with defecation.

Eroded lichen sclerosus is sometimes indistinguishable from erosive lichen planus, benign mucous membrane pemphigoid and pemphigus vulgaris, so biopsy and examination of other mucous membranes and skin surfaces may be necessary to make the diagnosis of lichen sclerosus.

Eroded lichen sclerosus is more likely than noneroded disease to develop bacterial or candidal superinfection when a superpotent topical corticosteroid is added for treatment. Early detection and treatment is appreciated, and I sometimes prophylax these women with cephalexin and weekly fluconazole the first week until healing begins.

## Lichen Simplex Chronicus (Eczema, Atopic Dermatitis, Neurodermatitis)

This excruciatingly pruritic condition exhibits erosions only secondarily, as a result of rubbing and scratching (see Chapter 5 for primary discussion). Erosions from scratching (excoriations) and fissures occur in many patients **(Fig. 11-38)**. The diagnosis is generally recognized by the history of scratching and the observation of irregular or linear erosions consistent with excoriations on the vulva or scrotum. Therapy includes topical corticosteroids, infection control, and nighttime sedation to minimize scratching during sleep.

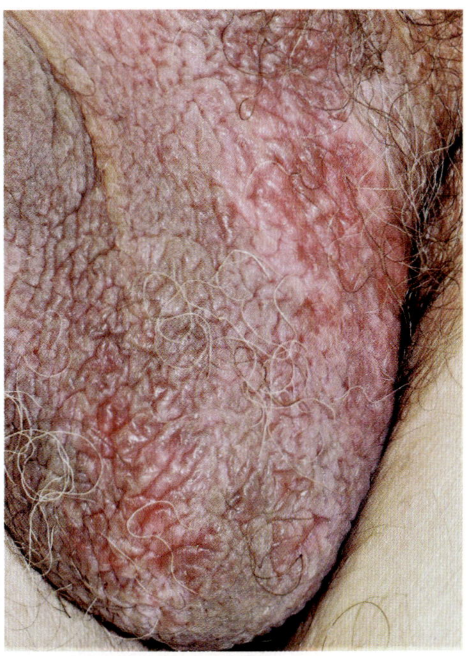

Fig. 11-38. Lichen simplex chronicus is produced by rubbing and scratching; erosions here have been caused by rubbing that removed the surface. Scratching is more likely to produce linear erosions or excoriations.

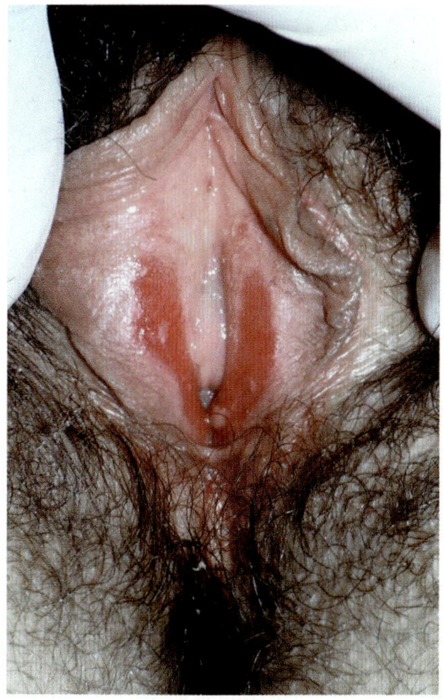

Fig. 11-39. Fluorouracil applied to genital warts produced this miserable erosive irritant contact dermatitis.

## Contact Dermatitis

Contact dermatitis sometimes presents with erosion on genital skin; this is often preceded by blistering that is evanescent and unnoticed (see Chapter 10). The most common contact dermatitis to produce genital erosions is a strong irritant contact, which is a chemical burn that can either blister or erode. The erosions are in the distribution of contact with the irritant, usually with surrounding erythema **(Fig. 11-39)**. Because the irritant is strong, the original agent and burning with contact most often is remembered.

## Fixed Drug Eruption

A fixed drug eruption, discussed primarily in Chapter 10, is a peculiar allergic reaction to a medication that produces same-site blisters that erode into well-demarcated, often round lesions **(Fig. 11-40)**.

## Necrolytic Migratory Erythema

This is a very rare condition that is caused by a glucagonoma, an α-cell tumor of the pancreas, which is usually malignant. Serum levels of glucagon are elevated. Patients are usually ill with weight loss, diarrhea, malabsorption, and diabetes. This rash can also be seen with liver disease, inflammatory bowel disease, pancreatitis, malabsorption disorders (ie, celiac sprue), and other malignancies, when the eruption is termed pseudoglucagonoma syndrome.

The rash begins as erythematous papules around orifices and flexures, including those of the genitalia. These

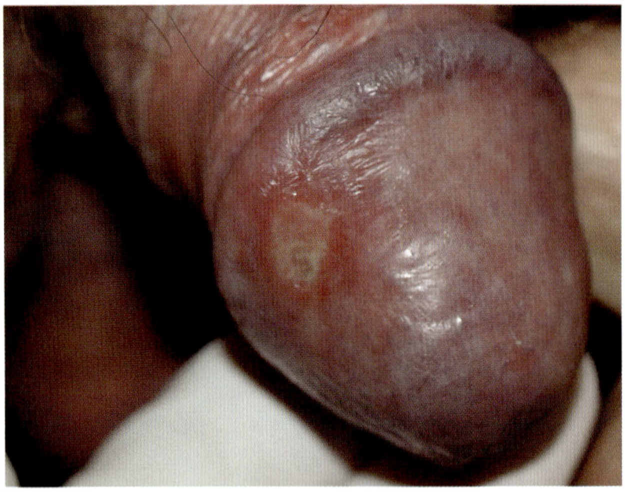

Fig. 11-40. A fixed drug eruption is a blistering medication reaction that occurs at the same site each time the medication is taken.

papules coalesce into plaques, and central erosions occur and crust, eventually producing a circinate migratory erythema. Histology of the skin shows superficial necrolysis and infiltration with lymphocytes. Treatment consists of removal of the tumor, if possible, or correction of the underlying cause of the pseudoglucagonoma syndrome. Topical corticosteroids may improve symptoms of the rash, but they do not clear it.

## Malignancies Presenting as Erosions

### Basal Cell Carcinoma

Basal cell cancers are associated, classically, with sites of sun exposure, but 10% occur on nonexposed sites and account for 5% of genital cancers (see Chapter 7). The lesions often display the typical pearly, rolled edge, with a central depression or necrotic erosion (**Fig. 11-41**). The tumors are more fragile than normal, nonneoplastic skin, and the skin erodes as they outgrow their blood supply, especially in this area of friction. They invade locally, but almost never metastasize. The diagnosis is made by biopsy, and management consists of conservative local excision. Those in more difficult sites may be amenable to radiotherapy.

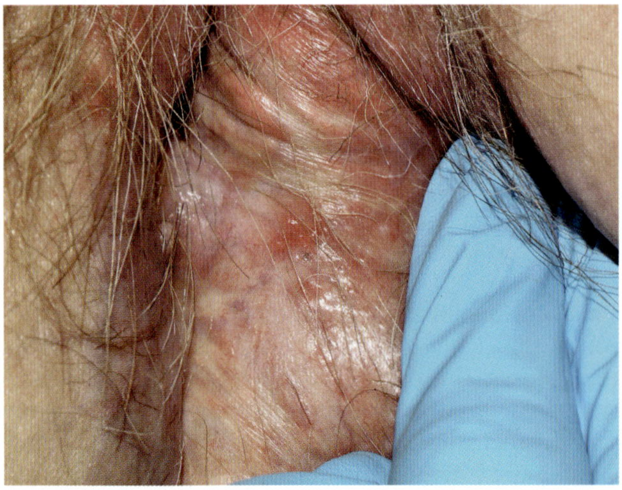

Fig. 11-41. Skin cancers are well recognized as fragile, and the surface of this basal cell carcinoma is eroded.

### Invasive Squamous Cell Carcinoma

Squamous cell cancers account for more than 90% of genital cancers and often arise in the site of chronic scarring or inflammation such as lichen sclerosus and lichen planus (see Chapter 7 for primary discussion) or as a result of high risk human papillomavirus infection (**Fig. 11-42**). The lesions present as red or skin-colored plaques or nodules that erode and eventually ulcerate as they enlarge. The diagnosis is made by biopsy, and therapy initially is managed by a surgical oncologist.

### Intraepithelial Carcinoma (Differentiated Vulvar/Penile/Scrotal/Anal Intraepithelial Neoplasia, High-Grade Squamous Intraepithelial Lesion, Bowen Disease, Bowenoid Papulosis, Squamous Cell Carcinoma *In Situ*, Erythroplasia of Queyrat)

Histologic SCC *in situ* is termed differentiated intraepithelial neoplasia when associated with lichen sclerosus or lichen planus or high-grade squamous intraepithelial lesion when associated with human papilloma virus infection. See Chapters 5 and 7 for primary discussion. These conditions can present with multiple morphologies, including skin-colored, white, or brown papules and

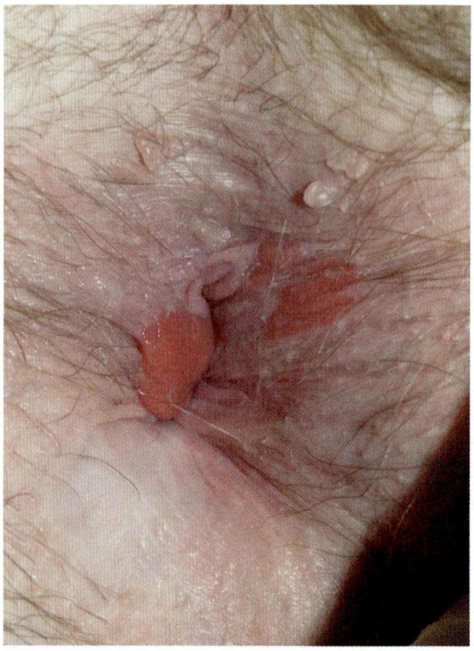

Fig. 11-42. The perianal squamous cell carcinoma in this man (here produced by multifocal human papillomavirus infection) also frequently erodes.

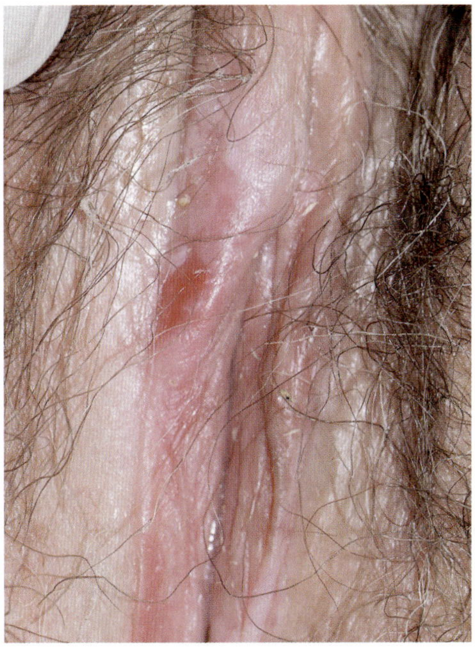

Fig. 11-43. d-VIN (histologic squamous cell carcinoma *in situ*) associated with LS as seen here can erode, as can HSIL (*in situ* squamous cell carcinoma associated with HPV infection).

plaques. The appearances illustrated here are erosive and ulcerative (Fig. 11-43).

### Extramammary Paget Disease (See Chapter 5 for Primary Discussion)

Extramammary Paget disease is a rare adenocarcinoma found primarily on anogenital skin.

This condition presents as a chronic red plaque with erosions and white islands of hyperkeratosis, often mistaken for eczema/lichen simplex chronicus (Fig. 11-44).

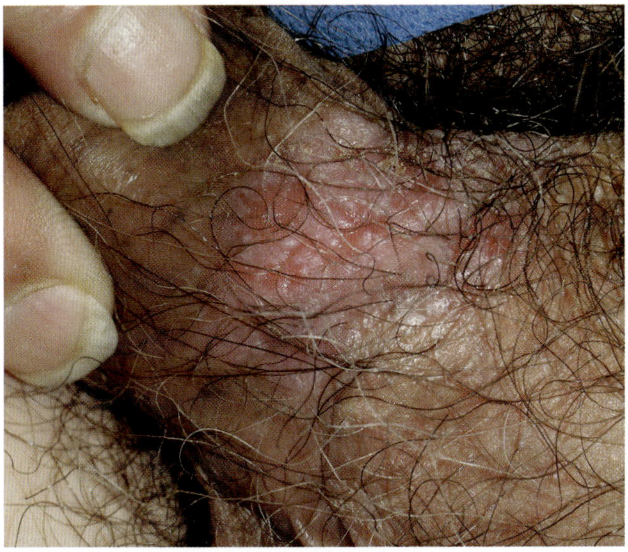

Fig. 11-44. Red plaques of Paget disease typically exhibit erosions, and the overall appearance can resemble rubbed and scratched eczema/LSC.

The diagnosis is by biopsy, and treatment is by surgical wide excision and investigation for underlying tumor. Local recurrences requiring repeated excisions are usual.

## SECTION B: ULCERS

Erosions and ulcers occur when tissue is lost from the surface of the skin or mucous membrane. Erosions and ulcers are differentiated on the basis of depth. Tissue loss limited to the epithelium produces erosions, whereas tissue loss that extends into, or through, the dermis results in ulcers. The base of an erosion may be either red or covered by a loosely adherent yellow crust. The base of an ulcer, on the other hand, may be red or may be covered with a crust that has red, blue, or black heme pigment due to damage or destruction of blood vessels within the dermis. On wet mucous membranes or modified mucous membranes, the fibrin base is often yellow. The crusts covering ulcers may also have considerable fibrin in them and for this reason are adherent and tenacious; this is sometimes termed eschar formation. (See this Chapter, Part A for coverage of erosive disorders.)

## Infectious Ulcers

### Syphilis

Syphilis is a sexually transmitted infection that is characterized by asymptomatic periods of varying duration, interrupted by three stages of clinical disease. In primary syphilis, a painless and nontender ulcer ("chancre") develops, most often in or around the genitalia. The major discussion of syphilis will be found in this chapter with brief mention made of secondary syphilis elsewhere. Congenital syphilis and neurosyphilis will not be discussed at all. Although syphilis is a global problem, the data in this chapter refer primarily to sexually acquired syphilis in Western countries.

#### Clinical Presentation

The rate of primary and secondary syphilis in the United States declined 90% from 1990 to 2000 at which point it reached its nadir. Since then the rate has been steadily increasing. Most of this increase has been in men and in 2018 men accounted for about 85%-90% of patients. Half or more of these men acknowledged having sex with men (MSM).[25,26] The rate for women has also increased though not as rapidly. In 2017, the overall incidence of syphilis was about 9.5 per 100 000 in the United States.[26] The rate is somewhat higher in Hispanic men and African-American men and women.[26] Worldwide, the incidence

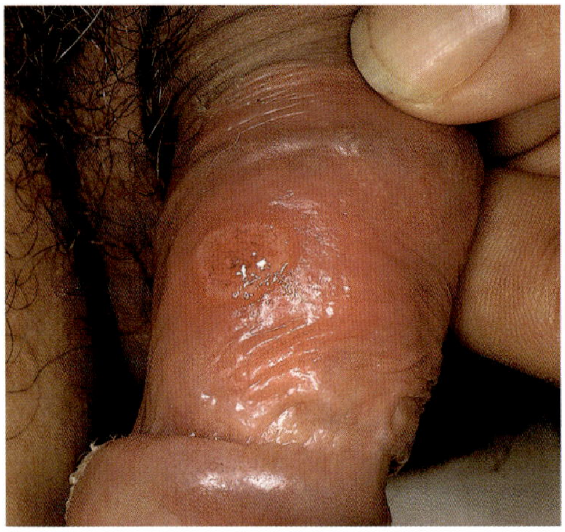

Fig. 11-45. A chancre of primary syphilis is firm, well demarcated, and nontender.

of syphilis is even higher with as many as 150 per 100 000 population infected.[26] Syphilis occurs most frequently between the ages of 20-30 in men; women tend to be a little younger than men when they become infected. Coinfection with human immunodeficiency virus (HIV) is encountered fairly frequently.

After an incubation period of 5-90 days (average of 21 days), the primary lesion occurs at the original site of inoculation. It begins as a small red papule that quickly enlarges and ulcerates to form a painless, usually nontender, ulcer ("chancre") that may be up to 2 cm in diameter. A chancre has a clean (little or no crust), red, glistening base (**Figs. 11-45 through 11-46**). A small amount of nonpurulent, watery exudate may be present. The ulcer borders are sharply demarcated and are characteristically raised and indurated. The base feels firm on palpation. Most patients present with a solitary ulcer, but two or even multiple lesions are possible. Chancres are most often located at the distal tip of the penis in men and on the labia majora or vestibule in women. However, since chancres occur at the site of initial inoculation, they may develop on the fingers, in or around the mouth, or at less apparent sites such as the vagina or on the cervix. And those individuals who have anal intercourse may develop chancres within or around the anus. When chancres occur in these semi-hidden sites, the first clinical sign of syphilis may be the secondary stage of the disorder. Secondary bacterial infection of chancres, though uncommon, may distort the clinical presentation causing tenderness and purulent discharge. Within about 1 week of chancre formation, regional lymphadenopathy generally develops. Thus for chancres located in the anogenital area, unilateral or bilateral inguinal lymphadenopathy with nontender, firm, rubbery, mobile lymph nodes may be palpable. Even in the absence of treatment, chancres heal spontaneously, without scarring, within a matter of weeks.

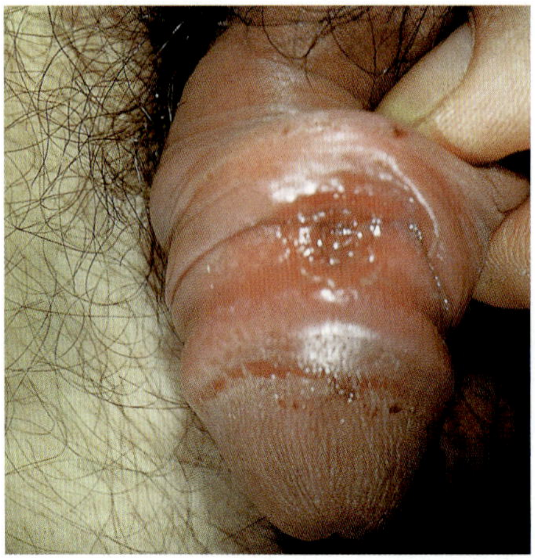

Fig. 11-46. This typical chancre shows clean borders and a base without purulent exudate.

The incubation period after exposure to *Treponema pallidum* is quite variable but averages about 3 weeks. Unfortunately, before the end of the incubation period and, therefore, before the development of a chancre, spirochetes may have already gained access to the regional lymph nodes and the central nervous system.[25] For this reason, syphilis can be viewed as a systemic infection from its earliest inception.

If untreated, a chancre undergoes spontaneous, nonscarring resolution within 6-12 weeks. This may lead the patient to the misconception that the process has healed and that it is not necessary to seek medical attention. However, as indicated, syphilis becomes a systemic infection soon after the initial inoculation such that after a short latent period, the generalized lesions of secondary syphilis are highly likely to appear. Rarely, secondary lesions appear, without a latent period, while the chancre is still present. If the symptoms and signs of secondary syphilis are unrecognized and the patient remains untreated, the patient enters the late latent period, leading some years later to the possibility of late (tertiary) syphilis.

## Diagnosis

The presence of a solitary, nontender ulcer with a clean, firm base is highly likely to represent primary syphilis. Nevertheless, a clinical diagnosis must be confirmed by laboratory means and most of what follows in this section on diagnosis is based on information contained in a recent review.[27] Direct detection of *T pallidum*, the cause of syphilis, provides quite good sensitivity and specificity. Of note, as of the time this was written, the U.S. Centers for Disease Control and Prevention (CDC) had only accepted two methods for detecting these spirochetes: dark-field microscopy and polymerase chain reaction (PCR). Unfortunately, there are problems associated with both of these. In years past, the quickest confirmation could be obtained by a dark field examination carried out on-site by the clinician. Unfortunately, this test has almost completely disappeared due to the lack of dark-field microscopes in clinicians' offices and declining skills in carrying out this test. Besides, even under the best of circumstances, the sensitivity and specificity of this approach were far from perfect. PCR examination from smears is much better in this regard (about 90% sensitivity and >95% specificity), but no commercial sources for this assay are currently available. Nevertheless, some highly specialized labs do have this technique available. Alternatively, one can biopsy the lesion and have the lab use special stains to identify the presence of spirochetes, but, here too, there are problems with sensitivity and specificity. And, of course, having a biopsy meets very appreciable patient resistance!

Because of the difficulties mentioned in the paragraph above, confirmation of a clinical diagnosis usually depends on serological testing. There are two types of serologic tests: treponemal and nontreponemal. The nontreponemal tests measure antibody reactivity to cardiolipin and other substances that are released when human cells are attacked by treponemes; these tests, if reactive, are titered. Examples most commonly include the Venereal Disease Research Laboratory (VDRL) and the rapid plasma regain (RPR) tests. On the other hand, treponemal tests measure antibodies specific for *T pallidum* proteins and are reported as reactive or nonreactive; the results are not titered. Examples of treponemal tests include the fluorescent treponemal absorption (FTA-ABS) test, the *T pallidum* particle agglutination (TP-PA) test, and the *T pallidum* hemagglutination (TP-HA) test; in addition, newer tests such as the enzyme immunoassay (EIA) and the chemiluminescence immunoassay (CLIA) are also used in some labs.

The use of both nontreponemal and treponemal tests is necessary for diagnosis and there are two algorithms for which type is used first. Most often the older algorithm (nontreponemal tests first) is preferred but as the sensitivity of treponemal tests is better and their costs have come down, some labs prefer to use the "reverse sequence" algorithm (treponemal tests first). Unfortunately there are several drawbacks to these tests: (1) the test may not become positive until 1 or 2 weeks after the chancre has appeared; (2) false-positive tests occur with some frequency; (3) false-negative tests may occur due to the prozone phenomenon especially in those patients who are coinfected with HIV; and (4) treponemal tests, unlike the nontreponemal tests, usually remain positive after previous effective treatment and thus cannot be used for determining a response to therapy. And, of course, patients with syphilis are likely to have been exposed to other sexually transmitted diseases. For this reason, patients should be examined and tested for other infections when a diagnosis of syphilis has been established.

There are several considerations in the list of differential diagnoses. Perhaps most troublesome are aphthous ulcers and genital herpes (HSV) infection in the immunosuppressed population. Genital herpes occurring in those who are immunosuppressed may present with fairly deep, persistent and relatively less painful ulcers rather than the more typical, transient, painful erosions seen in immunocompetent persons. Individual aphthous ulcers (as occur in complex aphthosis and Behçet disease) are similar in appearance to a chancre but, in contrast, several ulcers are usually present, they are extremely painful and they tend to occur mostly in children and adolescent women. Chancroid is extremely uncommon in Western countries and is associated with a crusted base, softer feel of the base on palpation along with considerable pain and tenderness. Anogenital ulcers occur with Crohn disease, hidradenitis suppurativa, and granuloma inguinale, but the morphology is different as is the histopathology.

**PRIMARY SYPHILIS — Diagnosis**

- One or two relatively painless genital ulcers
- Ulcer base is clean without crust or eschar
- Base of the ulcer is firm and nontender on palpation
- Positive RPR or VDRL; confirmed by positive FTA-ABS
- If serology is negative, repeat tests in 1 week or biopsy

## Pathophysiology

Syphilis is caused by the spirochete, *Treponema pallidum*, which is a spiral-shaped bacterium. The level of contagion for syphilis is very high; it has been estimated that about one-third of individuals having direct contact with infectious lesions of syphilis such as chancres, mucous patches, and the nodules of condyloma lata will develop syphilis. The likelihood of becoming infected is further enhanced when there are even minor breaks in the skin as well as in a setting of immunosuppression such as occurs with HIV infection. (The reverse is also true as there is an increased risk for the acquisition of HIV in patients with chancres.) Many, but not all, studies suggest that circumcision in males reduces the likelihood of acquiring syphilis during intromission.[28]

## Management

Most clinicians in the United States follow the treatment guidelines recommended by the Centers for Disease Control (CDC). Benzathine penicillin G (Bicillin L-A) 2.4 million units, administered intramuscularly in a single dose, is the recommended therapy for primary and secondary syphilis in men and in pregnant or nonpregnant women.[25] Note that Bicillin L-A (containing only benzathine penicillin) is to be used rather than Bicillin C-R, which contains a combination of benzathine penicillin and the short-acting procaine penicillin. No penicillin resistance has yet been noted. Guidelines that are similar to those of the CDC have been developed for Europe.[29]

Because of their similarity to the CDC guidelines, they will not be reviewed here.

For those who are allergic to penicillin, the CDC recommends desensitization rather than use of a second-line treatment with a nonpenicillin product. However, where desensitization is not very feasible (as it is in most circumstances), it is appropriate to use alternative antibiotics such as doxycycline (100 mg orally twice daily, or 200 mg once daily, for 14 days) or ceftriaxone (1 g IM or IV daily for 10 days).[25] Azithromycin was also used in the past; however, because of some reports of azithromycin resistance, it is no longer recommended. The CDC recommendation for desensitization stems from a relative lack of published experience with all three of these agents. Moreover, patients who are pregnant must be treated with penicillin even if that requires desensitization. There is really no evidence suggesting that in HIV-infected persons the response to therapy may be diminished. Nevertheless, some clinicians choose to repeat the 2.4 million units of benzathine penicillin weekly once or twice. The CDC does not recommend examination of the spinal fluid for patients with early (primary or secondary) syphilis.

The Jarisch-Herxheimer reaction is an acute febrile reaction that may occur within 24 hours of treatment for syphilis, regardless of the treatment regimen used. Symptoms include headache, malaise, myalgia, arthralgia, and fever. This transient reaction occurs most commonly after treatment for early syphilis and requires only reassurance, bed rest, and antipyretics for management.

Patients who are treated for primary or secondary syphilis require follow-up documentation of adequate response. This is done by determining the titer of RPR or VDRL antibodies at periodic intervals until at least a fourfold drop in titer is observed. Note that although either the RPR or the VDRL can be used, the same test must be used consistently as the titer levels differ between the two tests. Nearly all patients with early syphilis will eventually develop a negative RPR or VDRL test. However, this is not true for the treponemal specific tests (see above) where life-long positivity usually continues.

**PRIMARY SYPHILIS — Management**

- Benzathine penicillin (Bicillin L-A) single dose 2.4 million units IM
- Consider repeating the dose if patient is HIV positive
- Desensitize if patient is allergic to penicillin
- Or, doxycycline 100 mg bid × 14 days
- Follow RPR or VDRL titer until negative

## Chancroid

Chancroid is seldom encountered in Western societies. Only about 10 cases per year are reported in the United States and as a result there have been no major reviews of this disorder since 2016.[30] Even in less developed countries, where chancroid had been epidemic, there has been a marked decline in prevalence. The few infections seen today generally occur in the setting of risky sexual behavior such as occurs with drug use and with involvement of a great many sexual partners. This is particularly true for men who have sex with men (MSM) where coinfection with HIV also frequently occurs. In any event, reports suggest that chancroid develops more often in men than in women, but this may be partly an artifact related to the semi-hidden, thus less often discovered, location of chancroid ulcers in the vagina and on the cervix of women.

### Clinical Presentation

After a short incubation period of 3-7 days, a small red papule or pustule appears at the site of inoculation. This inflammatory lesion is rarely encountered in a clinical setting because it quickly evolves into a painful, deep, shaggy ulcer with ragged and undermined margins (Figs. 11-47 and 11-48). In contrast to the chancre of syphilis, firm induration of the ulcer base is not typically present. Moreover, the base of the ulcer is often covered with a yellow-gray, foul-smelling, necrotic exudate. Most patients present with one or two ulcers, but multiple or giant ulcer formation is also possible. Fifty percent of patients develop painful, most often unilateral, inguinal lymphadenitis. Massively enlarged nodes (bubo formation) develop in 25% of cases and when untreated these may become fluctuant with spontaneous rupture and chronic drainage.

### Diagnosis

There are no easily available diagnostic tests for chancroid. The causative bacterium, *Haemophilus ducreyi*, is difficult to identify on smears taken from the ulcer even when Giemsa stain is used. And *H ducreyi* can only be

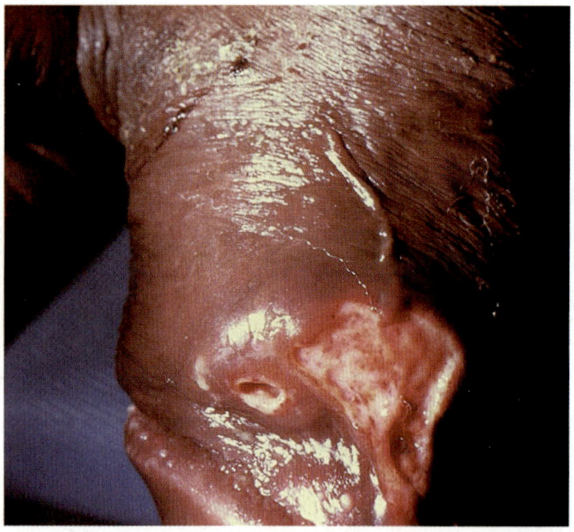

Fig. 11-47. The classic chancroid ulcer exhibits a shaggy border and a base that shows purulence. (Courtesy of Dr. Jack Mosley.)

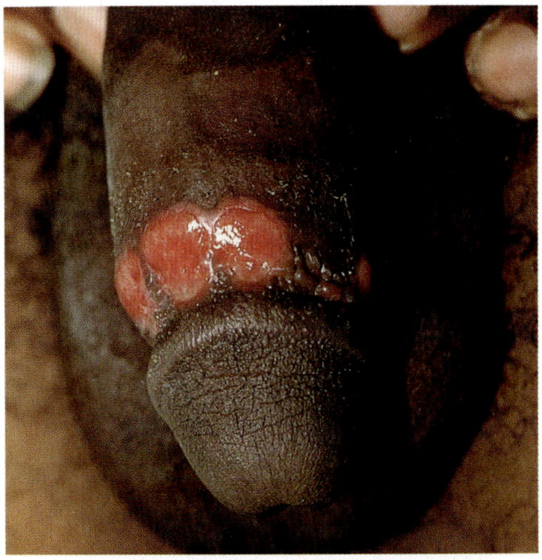

Fig. 11-48. The diagnosis of a sexually transmitted ulcer cannot be made on the basis of morphology alone; these ulcers represent chancroid, despite the smooth round borders.

cultured on special media, and unfortunately these media are not available commercially. As a result, most laboratories cannot culture this bacterium. Biopsy does reveal a fairly characteristic pattern consisting of three separate horizontal zones with distinctive vascular changes where the floor of the ulcer shows necrosis, red blood cells, neutrophils, and fibrin. Underlying this top layer is a wide area of new vessel formation with proliferating endothelial cells that sometimes obstruct the lumina. The deepest portion of the ulcer demonstrates an inflammatory infiltrate of plasma cells and lymphoid cells.

The CDC indicates that a presumptive clinical diagnosis can be made if all of the following criteria are met: (1) the ulcers are painful and tender; (2) a serological test for syphilis, taken at least 7 days after the ulcer has appeared, is negative; (3) the clinical presentation, including lymphadenopathy, is typical for chancroid; and (4) a test for herpes simplex virus (HSV) performed on the ulcer is negative.[31] Fortunately, a more sensitive and specific approach to diagnosis using the polymerase chain reaction (PCR) has been developed, but this is not available in very many laboratories.[30] In the differential diagnosis of chancroid, the following disorders should be considered: primary syphilis, genital HSV infection, lymphogranuloma venereum, granuloma inguinale, ulcerated carcinoma, and secondarily infected traumatic lesions.

**CHANCROID — Diagnosis**

- Single, sometimes two or three, painful ulcers
- Base of ulcer is covered with purulent crust
- Base is soft and very tender on palpation
- Inguinal lymphadenopathy is usually present
- Biopsy if confirmation of the diagnosis is needed

### Pathophysiology

Chancroid is caused by the fastidious, gram-negative, aerobic, or facultative anaerobic bacterium, *Haemophilus ducreyi*. It is highly contagious such that autoinoculation and experimental transfer from human to human is fairly easily carried out. In fact, clinical autoinoculation was once a legitimate diagnostic tool for chancroid.

### Management

Untreated, the ulcer of chancroid lasts about 2 months before spontaneous healing, generally with scarring, takes place. Ulceration and drainage from the enlarged nodes, if present, lasts even longer. The CDC indicates that all of the following can be used for treatment: azithromycin (1 g orally in a single dose), ceftriaxone (250 mg IM in a single dose), ciprofloxacin (500 mg orally twice a day for 3 days), and erythromycin base (500 mg orally three times a day for 7 days).[32] With any of these treatments, healing of the ulcer occurs in about 1 week with lymph node response occurring much more slowly. Greatly enlarged, fluctuant nodes may require needle aspiration or incision and drainage.

**CHANCROID — Management**

- Azithromycin 1 g orally in a single dose or
- Ceftriaxone 250 mg IM as a single dose
- Incise and drain if lymph node is fluctuant
- Follow to ensure complete healing

## Genital Herpes in the Immunosuppressed

Herpes simplex virus (HSV) infection in those with normal immune status causes blisters that quickly evolve into shallow, self-healing genital *erosions*. This presentation of genital herpes in immunocompetent individuals is covered in Chapter 10. However, in those who are immunosuppressed, HSV infection becomes locally more severe as reflected by the development of chronic *ulcers* rather than transient erosions. Less often these immunocompromised patients can also develop ulcerated exophytic nodular lesions.

### Clinical Presentation

In normal circumstances, control of HSV infection depends in large part on the presence of an intact cell-mediated immune system. For this reason, it is not surprising that evidence of genital HSV infection becomes prolonged and more severe in patients who are chronically immunosuppressed due to disorders such as, most commonly, HIV infection, but also malignancy (especially of hematopoietic origin) and those receiving long-term immunosuppressant medication for reasons such as organ or bone marrow transplantation. Genital and perigenital HSV infection is usually due to HSV type 2, but infection with HSV type 1 occurs as well; it then quickly transforms from an erosive to an ulcerative disease.[33]

In immunosuppressed patients, the lesions of HSV most often arise from reactivation of preexisting disease rather than from a primary infection and careful questioning usually reveal prior, more typical recurrent episodes of genital herpes. As is true for HSV infection occurring in immunocompetent patients, immunosuppressed patients describe accompanying pain though it is often less severe.

HSV outbreaks in immunosuppressed patients start as grouped vesicles on an erythematous base. The roofs of these vesicles disintegrate almost immediately leaving well-demarcated, discrete erosions. However, unlike the situation in immunocompetent patients, the erosions may not heal, but rather coalesce, enlarge in diameter and deepen to form well-demarcated ("punched out"), somewhat painful, nonhealing ulcers (**Figs. 11-49 to 11-51**).[34] These ulcers may not be very deep initially but regularly deepen as they become more chronic (**Fig. 7-5**). Secondary bacterial infection is possible but does not occur frequently. The configuration of the ulcers may be round but arcuate shapes are common due to coalescence of centrifugally expanding ulcers (**Fig. 7-6**). In men, chronic HSV ulcers are commonly found in a perianal distribution but also occur on the penis, scrotum, or in the groin. In women, ulcers may involve the mucosal portion of the vulva but also may extend to the labia majora and minora and even to the groin or inner thighs. As for men, HSV infection in women may also occur in a perianal location. Less frequently, HSV lesions in immunocompromised individuals appear as eroded or ulcerated papules or exophytic nodules.[35] These latter tumorlike lesions are, not surprisingly, often clinically believed to represent malignancy especially SCC.

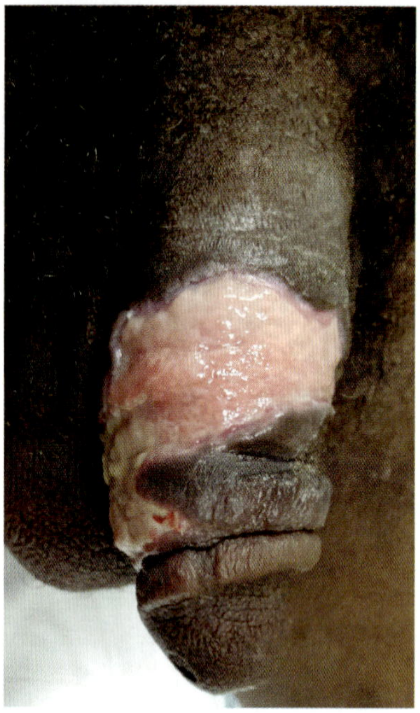

Fig. 11-50. A genital ulcer in an immunosuppressed patient is most likely herpes simplex virus infection; however, the possibility of other infections and tumors should be investigated.

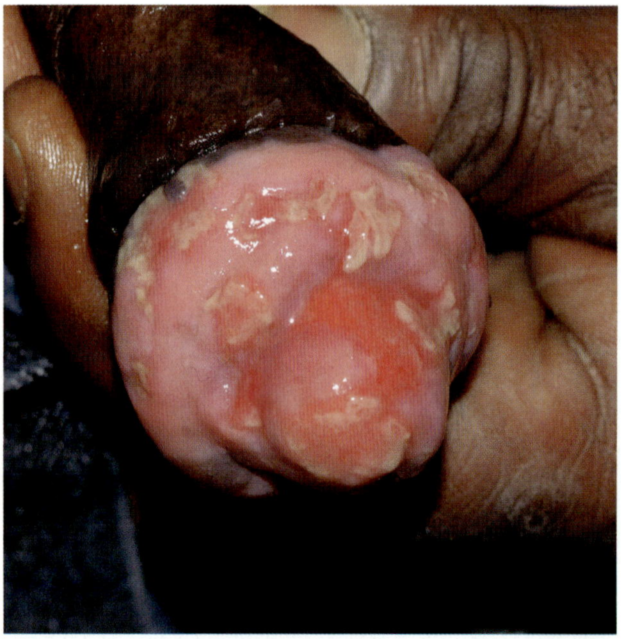

Fig. 11-49. Herpes simplex virus infection is a blistering and then erosive disease, but this infection progresses into ulcers with scarring in the immunosuppressed patient.

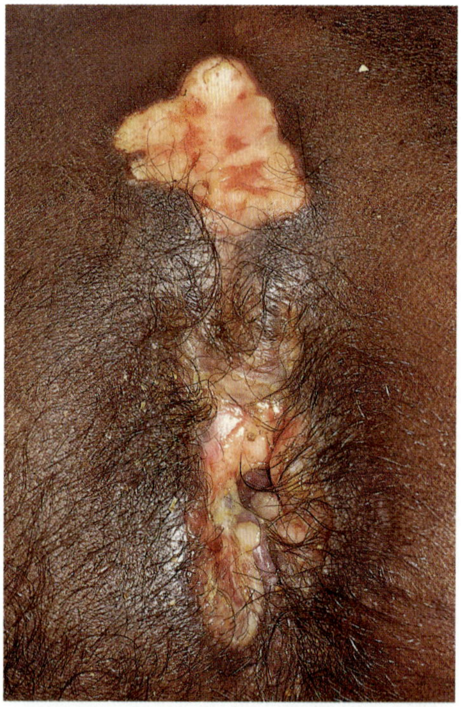

Fig. 11-51. This large ulcer with arcuate borders connects to the rectal mucosa where the original cutaneous HSV infection began.

### Diagnosis

A high index of suspicion should be present for HSV infection in any chronic, nonhealing ulcer in an immunosuppressed patient. A viral culture will usually confirm a clinically suspected diagnosis, but viral growth may be slow and results may be delayed for a week or more. Examination of a stained smear taken from the base of the lesion (a Tzanck preparation) is less reliable for the diagnosis of a chronic ulcerative herpetic infection than is true for HSV infection in immunocompetent patients. Direct immunofluorescent antibody testing is available in most labs and offers a rapid diagnosis. This test is carried out by scraping the base of the ulcer with a number 15 blade and smearing the material collected on a microscope slide. The slide is then submitted to the laboratory, and the results may be available within an hour or two. However, when it is available, nucleic acid amplification such as by polymerase chain reaction (PCR) is the single best diagnostic tool because it offers almost 100% sensitivity and specificity.

Biopsy should be strongly considered for any nonhealing ulcer or exophytic nodule in an immunocompromised patient in order to rule out malignancy and assist in the diagnosis of HSV infection. The characteristic histologic features found in HSV infection include ballooning degeneration of keratinocytes, reticular degeneration, and formation of multinucleated keratinocytic giant cells. Multinucleated keratinocytes are nearly pathognomonic for herpes virus infections, but they do not distinguish between HSV and varicella-zoster virus infection.

Although the presence of multiple well-demarcated, painful, chronic ulcers is clinically highly suggestive of HSV infection, several other ulcerating infections must be considered in the list of differential diagnoses. Syphilis produces one or more relatively short-lived, firm, painless, noncrusted ulcers. Chancroid causes a painful, ragged crusted ulcer and may cause massive painful inguinal adenitis. Granuloma inguinale consists of one or more genital ulcers often linear ("knifelike"), in configuration, containing exuberant granulation tissue. Rarely cytomegalovirus (CMV) has been reported to cause large, deep, necrotic ulcers in immunosuppressed patients, particularly in those with acquired immunodeficiency syndrome (HIV/AIDS). Biopsy confirmation for CMV infection may be needed because HSV infection can occur concomitantly with CMV and may overgrow CMV in viral culture. Noninfectious causes such as malignancy, aphthous ulcers, and Crohn disease should also be considered.

**HSV IN IMMUNOSUPPRESSED — Diagnosis**

- Patient is significantly immunosuppressed
- Punched out ulcers or ulcerated nodules
- Arcuate configuration when confluence of ulcers occurs
- Lesions are variable in terms of pain
- HSV PCR, immunofluorescent smear, or biopsy to confirm

### Management

Left untreated, HSV ulcers in immunosuppressed patients may persist indefinitely. However, complete response to conventional medical therapy is usually quite good. Acyclovir, famciclovir, and valacyclovir are the recommended medications; all three utilize the same pathway and block HSV polymerase after they are phosphorylated.[33] Many dosage schedules are possible. They include, for example, acyclovir 400 mg orally three to five times daily, famciclovir 500 mg orally twice daily, or valacyclovir 500 mg orally twice daily. They can be used for 10 days or until the lesions heal. Rarely, intravenous administration of acyclovir may be necessary if there is inadequate response to oral therapy.

Viral resistance to acyclovir occurs in up to 5%-10% of immunocompromised individuals and acyclovir-resistant strains are resistant to valacyclovir and famciclovir as well.[33] The currently recommended treatment for acyclovir-resistant anogenital herpes is intravenous cidofovir or foscarnet, but assistance from an infectious disease specialist is recommended if this is necessary. For HIV/AIDS patient not already receiving highly active retroviral therapy (HAART), starting such a regimen can lead to improvement to the HSV infection though there is also some risk of exacerbation of latent HSV infection as part of the immune reconstitution inflammatory syndrome (IRIS) when HAART is administered.[35]

**HSV IN IMMUNOSUPPRESSED — Management**

- Start HAART therapy if not already underway
- Acyclovir 400 mg orally 5 times per day until ulcers are healed or
- Famciclovir 500 mg bid or
- Valacyclovir 500 mg bid
- Foscarnet or cidofovir if ulcer is acyclovir resistant

## Granuloma Inguinale (Donovanosis)

Granuloma inguinale is a chronic, mildly contagious gram-negative bacterial infection, with a slowly progressive and destructive course. Four different clinical variants of the disease exist, and this variability can result in an array of difficult-to-diagnose clinical presentations. These four types include ulcerovegetative (the most common), hypertrophic (nodular), necrotic, and cicatricial forms of the disease.[36] All of these lesions tend to be nonpainful. A fairly extensive review of the disease was published in 2020 and much of what follows is supported by information contained in it.[37]

Granuloma inguinale is very rarely encountered in North America and Europe, but it has been endemic, especially in lower socioeconomic classes, in some lesser developed tropical and subtropical areas. Overall, its prevalence appears to be decreasing worldwide. The majority of cases are found in adults, where transmission is due to sexual activity, but nonvenereal transmission is possible and may account for most of the uncommon cases reported in babies and children. Its continued presence today may relate, at least in part, to an increase in unprotected sexual activity owing to better treatment options and medicinal prophylaxis for HIV infection.[37] The incubation period is unknown but seems to vary greatly in length. Typically, the median time from contact to lesion development is given as about 2 months.

## Clinical Presentation

The ulcerovegetative form of the disease is by far the most common clinical presentation. In this type of granuloma inguinale, the onset is insidious with formation of solitary or multiple ulcers that frequently involve skinfolds (**Figs. 11-52 and 11-53**). In these sites, the ulcers characteristically have a linear ("knife cut") morphology. The base of the ulcers is usually noncrusted with beefy-red granulation tissue that bleeds easily. The ulcer margins are sharp without undermining and the edges may be flat or rolled. The configuration may be serpiginous and sometimes there is enlargement of a portion of the ulcer while other areas are undergoing healing with scarring. In the second, less often encountered nodular variant of the disease, soft red papules, and/or nodules develop and subsequently ulcerate. The ulcers on the surface of these lesions also contain appreciable amounts of granulation tissue. The third type, the necrotic form of granuloma inguinale consists of large vegetating masses that are undergoing foul-smelling necrosis. Lastly, in the cicatricial variant, the ulcers are almost obliterated with expanding plaques of fibrotic scar tissue.

Lesions in men most often occur in the anal and perianal area but also can be found on the penis in the coronal sulcus or on the inner aspect of the foreskin in uncircumcised individuals. In women, the vulva is most often

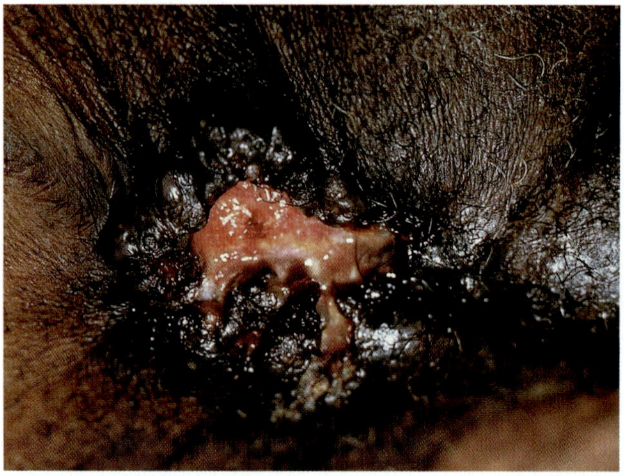

Fig. 11-52. The heaped up borders of this ulceration are typical of granuloma inguinale.

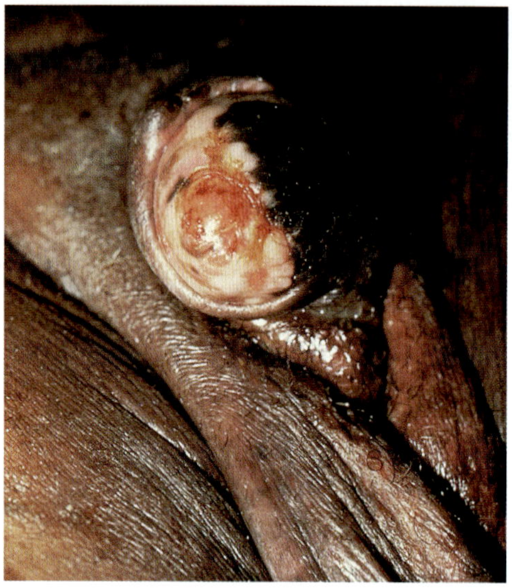

Fig. 11-53. Keratotic ulcerations can occur with granuloma inguinale as well.

involved but occasionally lesions occur in the vagina or on the cervix. Perianal ulcers also occur in women. And, in both sexes lesions are fairly frequently found in the intertriginous folds of the perigenital skin. Typically, lymphadenopathy does not occur but spread of the granuloma inguinale lesions to areas around the inguinal lymph nodes may cause swelling and ulceration. This condition is termed pseudobubo. The general lack of lymph node enlargement is characteristic enough to be a helpful clue in clinical diagnosis.

Complications of chronic disease include architectural distortion and destruction of the genitalia as well as phimosis, lymphedema, and elephantiasislike swelling of the vulva.

## Diagnosis

Clinically suspicious lesions can be confirmed by a histological demonstration of clustered bacteria (Donovan bodies) located within macrophages. This can be carried out using a swab, or preferentially a snip, of granulation tissue taken from the base of the ulcers. This tissue is crushed between two glass slides. The material is then fixed and stained with Wright or Giemsa stain after which the characteristic Donovan bodies can usually be identified within the cytoplasm of mononuclear inflammatory cells.

The causative bacterium is very hard to culture. For this reason, biopsy is appropriate if tissue smears are negative in patients with clinically suspicious lesions. Histology of the lesion shows acanthosis and an extensive dermal infiltrate composed of plasma cells and histiocytes. Warthin-Starry or Giemsa stain reveals large macrophages with cytoplasmic vacuoles containing bacteria (Donovan bodies).

Syphilis, chancroid, genital herpes in the immunosuppressed, amebiasis, and lymphogranuloma venereum are infections that may be confused with granuloma inguinale. Noninfectious conditions to be considered are cutaneous Crohn disease, hidradenitis suppurativa, Langerhans cell histiocytosis, and SCC. It should be noted that occasionally the marked epithelial hyperplasia seen on histopathologic examination has been misinterpreted as suggesting SCC.

**GRANULOMA INGUINALE — Diagnosis**

- One or more very slowly enlarging ulcers
- Configuration may be arcuate or linear
- Linear "knife cut" ulcers in skinfolds is characteristic
- Ulcer borders are rolled; base has granulomatous appearance
- Confirm by the presence of bacteria in macrophages on crushed smear or biopsy

### Pathogenesis

The cause of granuloma inguinale is the bacterium *Klebsiella granulomatis*, which was previously termed *Calymmatobacterium granulomatis*. This is a gram-negative, short intracellular bacterium. As indicated above, it is not a particularly contagious process but the likelihood of infection appears to be enhanced in the presence of poor hygiene and/or breaks in the skin.

### Management

Left untreated, the ulcers of granuloma inguinale slowly heal over months to years leaving residual scar formation and genital architectural distortion or destruction. Chronic massive edema (elephantiasis) of the genitalia frequently develops. This is particularly likely to involve the vulva. Rare cases of SCC have been reported to have developed in ulcers of long-standing duration. Current treatment guidelines suggest that one of several types of antibiotics is highly likely to be effective. These include azithromycin (1000 mg once weekly for 3 weeks), doxycycline (100 mg bid for 21 days), ciprofloxacin (750 mg bid for 21 days), or trimethoprim-sulfamethoxazole (400/800 mg bid for 21 days).[37] Note that treatment must be for at least 3 weeks but should be continued after that, if necessary, to achieve complete healing.[37]

**GRANULOMA INGUINALE — Management**

- Doxycycline 100 bid for 21 days
- Azithromycin 1.0 g weekly for 3 weeks
- Ciprofloxacin 750 mg bid for 21 days
- Treat until the ulcers are healed but for at least 3 weeks

## Lymphogranuloma Venereum

Lymphogranuloma venereum is a sexually transmitted disease that is caused *Chlamydia trachomatis*. The initial lesion may be a papule or an ulcer, but these lesions quickly heal spontaneously. Instead, almost all patients present with impressive lymphadenopathy or proctitis rather than an ulcer.[38] For this reason, the primary discussion of this disease will be found in Chapter 7, The Skin Colored Disorders.

## Epstein-Barr Virus and Cytomegalovirus-Associated Ulcers

Even though these ulcers are associated with infectious disease, they are discussed in the next section because their clinical appearance is identical to that of aphthous ulcers and it is likely that these viral infections simply trigger the development of aphthae rather than causing the ulcers by direct infection of the skin.

## Noninfectious Ulcers

## Genital Aphthous Ulcers and Complex Aphthosis (Synonyms: Lipschütz Ulcer, Ulcus Vulvae Acutum, Reactive Nonsexually Related Acute Genital Ulcers)

(See also aphthouslike ulcers associated with viral infections later in this section.)

Discussion in this paragraph relates to terminology often used for aphthous ulcers. Aphthous ulcers in the oral cavity (synonyms: aphthae, aphthous stomatitis, "canker sores") are extremely common, but similar ulcers are encountered much less frequently on the genitalia. The adjectives "minor" (<1 cm; shallow; heal without scarring), "major" (>1 cm; deep; may heal with scarring), and "herpetiform" (10 or more, very small clustered) are often used for the morphological description of aphthous ulcers.[39] The term "complex aphthosis" is used for either of two groups of patients: (1) individuals with three or more, almost constantly present, oral aphthae and (2) those with recurrent oral and genital aphthae in the absence of Behçet disease.[39] Complex aphthosis may be "primary" (idiopathic and not occurring in direct association other conditions) or "secondary" (associated with some other medical disorder more often than would be expected by chance).[39] There is no difference in clinical or histological appearance between primary and secondary form of aphthous ulcers. Since many, though not all, patients with genital aphthous ulcers also have a history of, or the concomitant presence of, oral aphthae, they can be said to have complex aphthosis

Aphthous ulcers of the genitalia and perigenital area were originally described as occurring only in females, but it is now known that they also occur, though a lot less frequently, in males.[40] Moreover, it has become apparent that the condition previously described as "juvenile gangrenous vasculitis of the scrotum" is in actuality a form of aphthous ulceration occurring in men.[41,42]

Based on the similarity of clinical morphology and course of disease, many of us also believe that "Lipschütz ulcer" and "ulcus vulvae acutum" are synonyms for primary aphthous ulcers of the vulva (**Fig. 7-14**).[14,15] Thus, one can say that while Lipschütz was the first to describe these ulcers, his name remains associated with them in many publications to this day. Unfortunately, his name became associated with a quite narrow definition of these ulcers: nonrecurrent, large, deep, gangrenous ulcers, which developed only in young girls who were not yet sexually active. This led to the belief that it was a rare disorder. It was not until the publication of Vieira-Baptista et al in 2016 that it became accepted that the definition should also include recurrent idiopathic vulvar ulcers of all sizes and depths as well as those occurring in sexually active women of any age.[43] Subsequently, we and others support this broadened definition.[44,45]

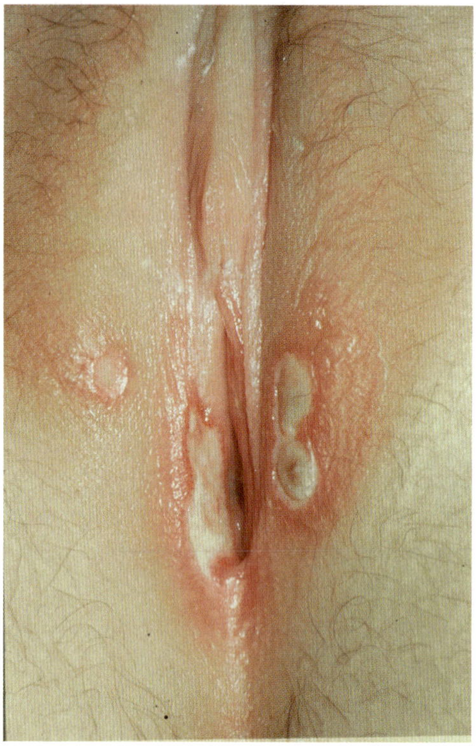

Fig. 11-54. The classic vulvar aphthous ulcer has well demarcated borders and a white fibrin base, and most often occurs on the mucous membrane or modified mucous membrane.

## Clinical Presentation

The lifetime incidence of primary *oral* aphthae is usually given as about 20%-30%, but some estimates are as high as 60%. Data regarding the incidence of primary *genital* aphthous ulcers are not available, but it is probably <1% given the relatively few published studies of this disorder. Two relatively recent systematic reviews of women with so-called Lipschütz ulcer are available.[45,46] However, most of the reported cases in these two reviews came from before 2016 and thus included descriptions of ulcers using the restricted original definition. Examining the cases published after 2016 (diagnoses mostly using the expanded definition), we believe that a more realistic picture can be assembled. Doing so suggests that, while a substantial proportion of instances still involve sexually inactive girls and adolescents who have nonrecurrent ulcers, there are many sexually active, somewhat older women, who also have (or have had) oral aphthae, and have recurrent genital ulcers. However, it is recognized that the incidence of both oral and genital aphthous ulcers does gradually decreases with age.

Aphthous ulcers of the vulva primarily occur within the vulvar vestibule, but lesions can also develop on the outer labia minora, on the labia majora, on the perineum, and at the vaginal introitus (**Figs. 11-54 through 11-58**). The diameter (up to 2 or 3 cm) and depth (up to 1 cm) of these genital ulcers tends to be greater than those occurring in the mouth. Intravaginal, especially introital, ulcers are also possible though the frequency and appearance of such lesions is not well described in the published reports. Interestingly, and, in complete contrast to oral aphthae, those developing on the genitalia often develop on hair-bearing, keratinizing epithelium (**Fig. 11-59**), as well as on mucosal epithelium.

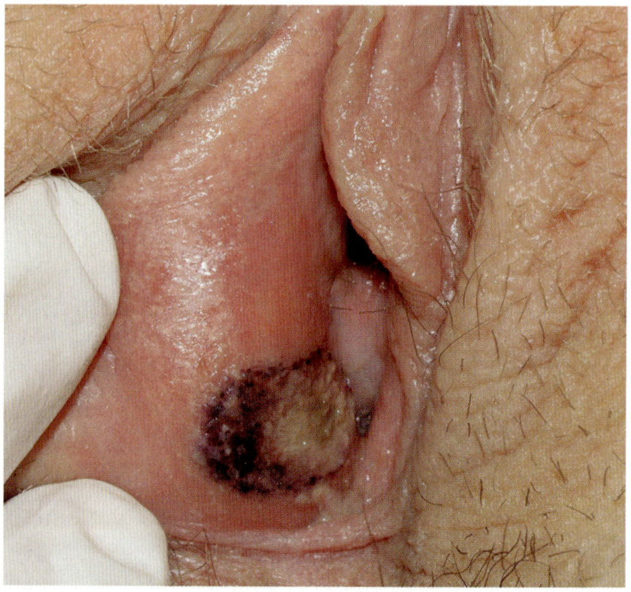

Fig. 11-55. Although often missed, the aphthous ulcer begins with a painful, purple purpuric plaque that evolves into a black eschar.

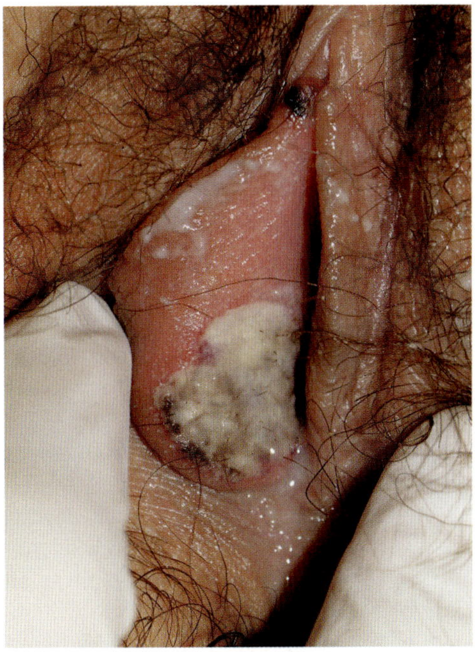

Fig. 11-56. The black eschar then sloughs, leaving the ulcer.

Genital aphthous ulcers in men tend to occur more often on the scrotum than on the penis but are otherwise similar to those that occur in women. The few genital aphthous ulcers that I have personally encountered in men have represented *secondary* complex aphthosis occurring in the setting of Behçet disease, hidradenitis suppurativa, or inflammatory bowel disease. This experience is supported by the notable infrequency of published reports of *primary* aphthous ulcers involving male genitalia.[40]

The majority of patients have two or more round ulcers, but, when multiple, confluent growth may occur leading to very large (2-3 cm) ulcers with gyrate borders. The base of the ulcers can be bright red or may be covered with either gray, necrotic material or heme-colored eschar. Genital ulcers are extremely painful and their

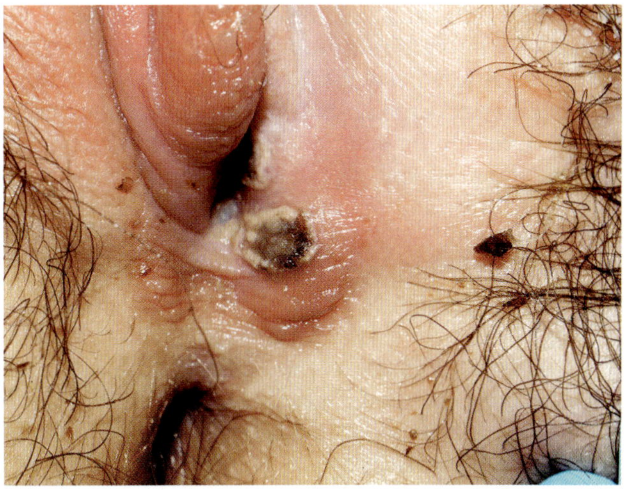

Fig. 11-58. This black eschar surrounded by edema is about to shed, and another is just inside the introitus.

appearance is sometimes preceded by, or accompanied by, low-grade fever, malaise, gastrointestinal, and/or respiratory symptoms. Many of these women also have dysuria and palpable inguinal lymphnodes.[45]

Most genital aphthous ulcers heal spontaneously within about 3 weeks. Small, shallow ulcers heal without scarring but larger, deeper lesions may heal with scarring. Just as is true for oral lesions, genital ulcers can recur at periodic intervals though the recurrence rate seems to be less frequent than for oral aphthae.

## Diagnosis

The diagnosis is made on a clinical basis as there are no characteristic histologic or laboratory abnormalities. Some patients do have an associated infection most notably with Epstein-Barr virus (EBV) and cytomegalovirus (CMV) but also with many other infectious agents

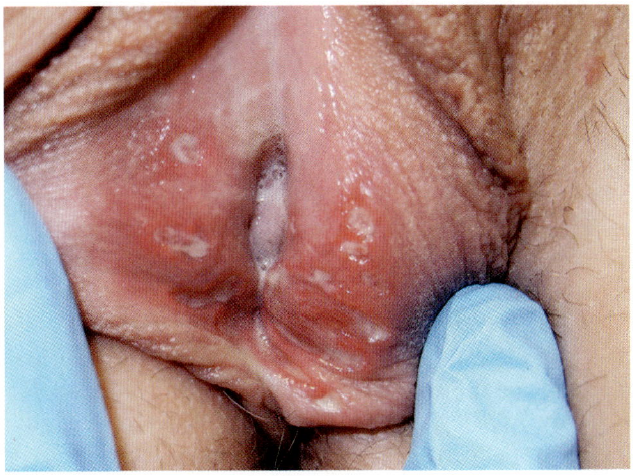

Fig. 11-57. One morphologic type of aphthae is the herpetiform morphology, because the many small ulcers resemble a herpetic outbreak even though there is no relationship.

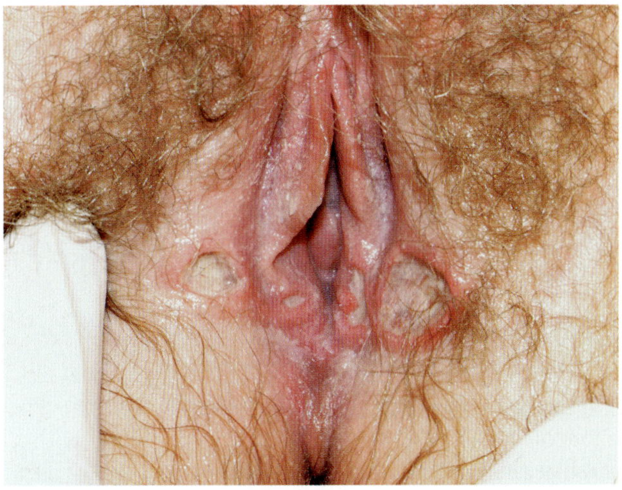

Fig. 11-59. Not all aphthae are on mucous membrane or modified mucous membrane skin; a large aphthous ulcer here extends to the keratinized surface of the left labium majus.

including caronavirus.[47] However, what, if any, role these viruses play in the direct cause of these genital ulcers is controversial (see below). Biopsy reveals only nondiagnostic acute and chronic but may be desirable or even necessary, to rule out other causes of genital ulceration.

Most clinicians initially, and incorrectly, believe that patients with genital aphthous ulcers have HSV infection.[40] However, HSV infection in *immunocompetent* patients leads only to erosions, not the deeper ulcers usually found in genital aphthous ulcers. Nevertheless, it is appropriate to obtain HSV cultures or immunofluorescent antibody studies so as not to miss this common and easily treatable infection. Primary syphilis and chancroid cause ulcers but these are unlikely to be confused with aphthae because of lack of pain in the former and impressive lymphadenopathy in the latter.

It may be hard to distinguish primary from secondary aphthous ulcers because the appearance of aphthae may precede evidence for the development of an associated disease by months or even years. The disease that most often needs to be considered in a list of potentially linked secondary disorders is Behçet disease. Oral and genital ulcers are the two most common findings in both complex aphthosis and in Behçet disease and they have an identical clinical appearance in both of these settings. Unfortunately, there are no laboratory tests that definitively identify Behçet disease. Thus, making this diagnosis generally depends on the patient meeting established diagnostic criteria. (See Behçet disease below.) Unfortunately, these criteria are rather broad and some of us believe that their use leads to overdiagnosis of Behçet disease. However, since the symptoms and signs of Behçet disease usually evolve over a considerable period of time, patients with complex aphthosis need to be followed on a regular basis as a few such individuals may eventually develop Behçet disease. But in my experience, and that of others, this happens only rarely in Western countries.[39]

Secondary aphthous ulcers occur with several other conditions, most commonly inflammatory bowel disease and HIV/AIDS. Rare disorders that may be accompanied by aphthae include cyclic neutropenia, lupus erythematosus, and the MAGIC (mouth and genital ulcers with inflamed cartilage) and PFAPA (periodic fever, aphthae, pharyngitis, and adenitis) syndromes.

**APHTHOUS ULCERS — Diagnosis**

- Occurrence primarily in girls and young women
- Several, punched out, very painful ulcers
- Flulike prodrome may precede or accompany ulcers
- Arcuate configuration when ulcers become confluent
- Rule out HSV, syphilis and chancroid
- Look for associated systemic disease especially Behçet disease and inflammatory bowel disease

## Pathophysiology

The cause and pathophysiology of oral and genital aphthous ulcers are not well understood. We and others believe that aphthae can be considered as a nonspecific immunological reactive inflammatory response triggered by a large variety of underlying factors. These factors include nutrient deficiency, poor eating habits, lack of sleep, psychological problems, genetic susceptibility, hematological disorders, allergens, medications (nicorandil, foscarnet, etc.), trauma (pathergy), and a large variety of infections.[39,48,49] As regards the latter, many authors consider these infections a direct etiology; whereas we and others prefer to think of these infections as "triggers" rather than as a direct cause. This thinking is based on (1) the similar, but nonspecific histology, of the ulcers regardless of which infectious agent was involved and (2) the relative rarity with which culturable agents can be recovered from the ulcers. In this sense, these aphthous ulcers could be thought of as analogous to inflammatory conditions such as erythema nodosum, erythema multiforme, urticaria (hives), etc. that can occur in a variety of situations.

No matter what the initiating events are, the end result is the development of a brisk influx of inflammatory cells with elaboration of vast array inflammatory cytokines such as interleukin 2, tumor necrosis factor alpha (TNF-α), vascular cell adhesion molecules (VCAM), vascular endothelial growth factor (VEGF), endocan, etc.[48] The resultant severe inflammation leads to vascular destruction, induction of localized tissue necrosis, and subsequently, ulcer formation.

## Management

With the obvious exception of "swish and swallow" approaches, the treatment of genital aphthae is similar to that employed for oral aphthous ulcers.[50] Symptomatic treatment is possible with topically applied anesthetics such as 5% lidocaine ointment applied several times per day. If pain is not controlled with this approach, the nerve ending in the ulcer can be destroyed chemically using the application of a standard silver nitrate stick.[50] Topically applied steroids such as 0.05% clobetasol ointment may be somewhat helpful in mild cases but, depending on a patient's tolerance, intralesional injections of triamcinolone (Kenalog) 10 mg/mL directly into each ulcer base is appreciably more effective.

A topical approach used alone for genital ulcers is seldom completely successful. For that reason, I usually initiate oral prednisone therapy (40 mg each morning for 7-10 days) at the first visit. This leads to satisfactory healing in most patients and can be repeated as necessary with recurrent episodes of ulceration. Systemic steroids used for what is considered to be a benign disorder are, however, controversial; some clinicians value their use while others are at least somewhat opposed.[45-47] As an alternative to oral prednisone, nonsteroidal anti-inflammatory therapy can be offered with oral medications such as doxycycline or minocycline (100 mg twice daily), pentoxifylline (400 mg tid), colchicine (0.6 mg bid to tid), dapsone (100-150 mg/d), or any one of several anti-inflammatory "biological." These and other agents have been recently reviewed.[51] For the minority of patients who fail to respond to these relatively safe approaches, the therapies described in the next section on Behçet disease can be considered.

When those patients with recognized associated disease are excluded, it can be said that patients with primary complex aphthosis have an excellent prognosis. It is certainly true that a few patients with primary complex aphthosis might go on to develop associated illness, especially Behçet disease, but this appears to happen only rarely in Western countries. For this reason I believe that it is undesirable and even inappropriate, to indicate that American and Western European patients who fail to meet rigorous diagnostic criteria for Behçet diseases at the time of first evaluation, have, or are likely to develop, this disorder in the future.

**APHTHOUS ULCERS** **Management**

- Topical 5% lidocaine ointment
- Light application of silver nitrate sticks
- Prednisone 40 mg orally for 7-10 days
- If frequently recurrent, suppression with
  - Colchicine 0.6 mg bid or tid and/or
  - Dapsone 100-150 mg/d
  - TNF alpha blockers

## Aphthouslike Ulcers Associated With Infections

Flulike symptoms and signs have been reported to precede, or occur with, ulcers that are identical in every way with genital aphthous ulcers in about 60%-80% of patients.[45,46] When such patients have been evaluated, testing most often revealed evidence of a viral infection. Epstein-Barr viral (EBV) infection in the form of infectious mononucleosis was the most often identified followed by cytomegalovirus. Other viral infections have also been occasionally reported including, recently, coronavirus (COVID 19).[47] Bacterial and other types of infectious agents have rarely been identified as triggers. In the vast majority of instances, the viral infection was detected on the basis of serology rather than being found in the ulcers. The exception to this observation occurred in a few patients with EBV infection where occasionally the virus was identified within cells located in the ulcer.[45]

The relationship of these infections to the development of genital aphthouslike ulcers is controversial. As noted in the discussion of genital aphthous ulcers in the section above, many authors consider these infections a direct etiology; whereas, we and others think of these infections as "triggers" rather than as a direct cause. This thinking is based on (1) the similar, but nonspecific histology, of the ulcers regardless of which infectious agent was involved and (2) the relative rarity with which culturable agents can be recovered from the ulcers. In this sense, these aphthous ulcers could be thought of as analogous to inflammatory conditions such as erythema nodosum and urticaria (hives) that can occur as a result of multiple etiologies. This explanation would also be analogous to the triggering of erythema multiforme in some patients with HSV infection or the development of Gianotti-Crosti syndrome with any one of several viral diseases.

## Behçet Disease

Behçet disease is a rare disorder first described in Turkey in 1937 as a triad of oral aphthous ulcers, genital aphthous ulcers, and uveitis. It is now considered a multisystem disease with potential development of problems in many organs such as the mucocutaneous tissues, eyes, joints, cardiovascular system, central nervous system, and gastrointestinal tract. Since it is a disease that will rarely be encountered by the audience for whom this book is intended, only a brief discussion emphasizing the presence of oral and genital aphthae is included in this section.[52]

The prevalence of this disease is fairly high in the Mediterranean, Middle East, and Japan. Turkey has the highest prevalence with a rate of up to 400 per 100 000 individuals, but in most Western countries, it much less common with reported prevalence rates of <1-5 per 100 000 in the United States, Germany, Sweden, Portugal, and the United Kingdom.[53] Note, however, that migration of people from areas of high prevalence to countries with low prevalence is gradually narrowing some of these differences. In most, but not all, countries, the disease occurs slightly more frequently, and with somewhat greater severity, in men.[52] In both sexes, the usual age of onset is between 20 and 40 and it uncommonly develops after mid-adult life.[52,53]

Recurrent oral and genital aphthous ulcers are, in general, both the earliest clinical signs and the overall most common lesions in patients with Behçet disease.[53] They are essentially identical with those seen in primary complex aphthosis though they may be larger, deeper, more painful, and more frequently recurrent **(Fig. 11-60)**. Because of these clinical similarities and the lack of pathognomonic laboratory findings, it is difficult, and sometimes impossible, to determine with certainty whether the correct diagnosis is that of primary complex aphthosis or Behçet disease.

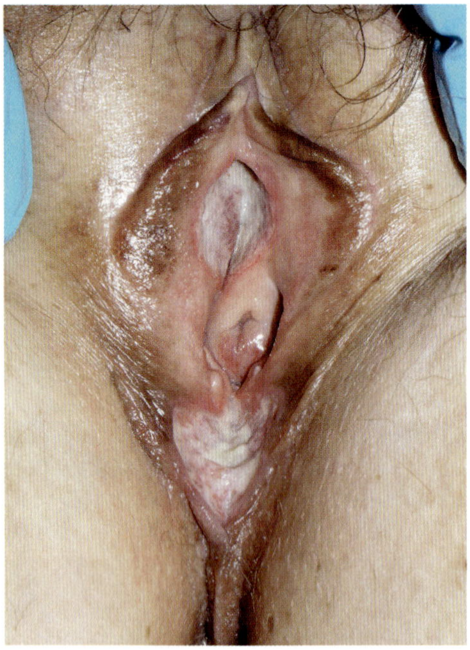

Fig. 11-60. Although classic Behçet disease is rare in Western industrialized countries, the aphthae of Behçet's are much more common in the East, and far, far more common in men than in women.

The majority of clinicians use either the 1990 International Study Group (ISG) criteria for the diagnosis of Behçet disease or the 2014 (revised) International Conference of Behçet Disease (ICBD) criteria.[53] The ISG criteria require recurrent oral ulcerations plus any two of the following: recurrent genital ulceration, uveitis (or other listed orbital abnormalities), evidence of pathergy, or certain skin disorders such as erythema nodosum, pseudofolliculitis, papulopustular lesions, and acneiform nodules. On the other hand, the 2014 ICBD criteria require 4 points taken from this list: oral aphthosis (2 points), genital aphthosis (2 points), ocular manifestations (2 points), vascular manifestations (1 point), neurological manifestations (1 point), skin manifestations such as pseudofolliculitis, erythema nodosum, or cutaneous ulcers (1 point) and positive pathergy test (1 point).

Unfortunately, from a dermatological standpoint, these criteria are flawed. Young western patients with genital aphthous ulcers regularly have had or will develop recurrent oral aphthosis and often have one or another of the listed skin manifestations. Thus, strictly speaking, they meet the ISG and the ICBD criteria for a diagnosis of Behçet disease even though almost all of them neither have, nor will develop, the classical other findings of this severe, life-threatening disorder. It seems to me that labeling these patients as having Behçet disease, rather than terming what they have as primary complex aphthosis, is clearly a disservice to the patients and their families. It seems most appropriate instead to work with a diagnosis of complex aphthosis until, and if, a diagnosis of Behçet disease can be subsequently established indisputably. Many other sets of criteria have been suggested but few add sufficient specificity or are too complicated and cumbersome, to be used in the typical office clinical setting.

Material covering the extracutaneous clinical manifestations, list of differential diagnoses, and pathogenesis of Behçet disease can be found in review articles such as those by Davatchi et al., Scherrer et al., and Tong et al.[52-54] Treatment of the mucocutaneous ulcers is similar to that described in the section on complex aphthosis above. Basically glucocorticoids and colchicine represent the first-line treatment with azathioprine and tumor necrosis factor alpha (TNF $\alpha$) inhibitors (infliximab, etanercept, adalimumab, etc.) suggested as second-line therapies.[55] It is also worth noting that the U.S. Food and drug administration has recently approved apremilast (documented as an effective, safe treatment) for oral ulcers occurring in Behçet disease. Additional systemic therapy is available for those patients with more severe or treatment-resistant disease.[55]

## Crohn Disease

The term inflammatory bowel disease encompasses both ulcerative colitis and Crohn disease (CD). These two disorders are somewhat similar clinically inasmuch as both are regularly associated with chronic diarrhea, abdominal pain, and weight loss. Somewhat less often there is also fever and malaise; there may also be blood and/or mucus mixed in with the diarrhea. Moreover, both conditions frequently have associated extraintestinal manifestations involving the eyes, joints, and hepatobiliary tract. They differ, however, in that Crohn disease is frequently associated with cutaneous involvement of the anogenital area, whereas ulcerative colitis is not. For this reason, we have restricted our discussion to Crohn disease.

Crohn disease is a chronic granulomatous inflammatory process that may affect any region of the intestinal tract from the mouth to the anus but occurs most commonly in the ileum and the colon. It has an incidence of ~10 per 100 000 persons each year and a prevalence of about 250 per 100 000 persons in the United States.[56] The orocutaneous conditions that occur in CD are generally classified as *specific* (share the histopathological features of the bowel disease), *reactive* (share the pathogenesis of the bowel disease but not the histopathology), *associated* (no shared pathogenesis or histopathology but occurring more commonly than expected by chance), and *treatment related* (precipitated by therapy of the CD).[56-59] In spite of the widespread use of this classification, we find that the pathogenesis of the various orocutaneous conditions occurring in CD is too uncertain to allow for dependable separation of the *reactive* and *associated* disorders. Accordingly, in what follows I have combined these two categories into a single *reactive and/or associated* group. Note that the conditions in this group are not specific for inflammatory bowel disease and can also occur with other underlying problems. Note also that these conditions usually develop following the diagnosis of CD, but in about 15%-25% of instances, they may precede the diagnosis of CD.

## Clinical Presentation

The disorders that are described below have been the subject of several recent reviews and for that reason will not be extensively referenced.[56-59]

### Specific Orocutaneous Disorders

The conditions in this category (lesions containing Crohn-type granulomas) can be divided into those that are contiguous with the bowel disease and those that are separated by normal tissue (ie, are noncontiguous) from the bowel disease.

### Contiguous Cutaneous Crohn Disease

Technically, these would only include perianal and peristomal fistulous lesions containing Crohn-type granulomas. However, determining whether or not lesions actually connect to the intestinal tract (ie, are really fistulas) can be quite difficult. Moreover, generally all perianal disease is considered "contiguous" even if there is a "skip area" of normal appearing rectum between the perianal disease and Crohn disease elsewhere in the gastrointestinal tract. Note that for convenience those pustules, papules, plaques, nodules, abscesses, and ulcers of the tissue in close proximity to the anus and stoma are considered as contiguous Crohn disease if they contain Crohn-type granulomas.

### Noncontiguous Cutaneous Crohn Disease

Noncontiguous ("metastatic") Crohn disease involving the vulva, penis, scrotum, perineum, inguinal folds, perineum, and other skin in the anogenital region is believed to be quite uncommon. A recent review concludes that fewer than 250 cases in children and adults have been published.[60] We, and others, however, believe that it occurs more often than has been reported. This difference in opinion, I believe, revolves around the question of what constitutes "specific" evidence of Crohn disease occurring outside of the bowel. Is the identification of granulomas on biopsy a hard and fast requirement? Consider the fact that such granulomas are frequently absent in resected bowel segments of patients clinically assessed to have Crohn disease.[61] Thus, we believe that the absence of granulomas in biopsy specimens of the edema, abscesses, ulcers, and other lesions of patients carrying a diagnosis of Crohn disease does not exclude placing these lesions in the category of "metastatic" Crohn disease.

Edema, of the vulva with or without granulomatous change on biopsy, is the most common cutaneous clinical finding in women and this is probably also true for

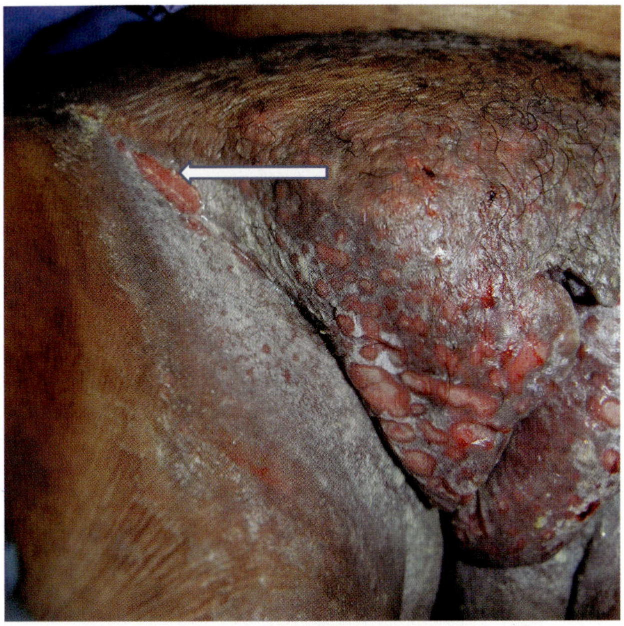

Fig. 11-61. A common early sign of Crohn disease is edema; massive edema is present here, as well as the classic "knife-cut" ulcer in the right inguinal crease (*arrow*). Less often, round erosions and ulcers occur.

men **(Fig. 11-61)**. This edema may precede, occur concomitantly with, or follow a diagnosis of intestinal disease. In women, the edema may be unilateral or bilateral and, in some instances, small areas of "out pouching" edema may give the labia a somewhat characteristic, "multinodular" shape. Biopsy of this edematous tissue is rarely performed and for that reason it is not possible to state the frequency with which the edema is simply passively present vs its association with granulomatous inflammation. It should be noted, however, that nonspecific granulomatous changes are generally present in the edematous vulvas of women with the condition known as Melkersson-Rosenthal disease (see Chapter 12), and it has been hypothesized that this condition represents a *forme fruste* of Crohn disease.[62]

Linear fissures and deeper linear ("knife-cut") ulcers, usually occurring in intertriginous folds, are among the most characteristic cutaneous lesions in anogenital Crohn disease (**Figs. 11-62 to 11-64**). They appear to be more common in women than in men. In Western countries where granuloma inguinale is rare, these linear ulcers are nearly pathognomonic of Crohn disease. Perianal fistulas (when cutaneous ulcers can be demonstrated to connect to the rectum) are also highly characteristic of CD **(Fig. 11-65)**. Erythematous and violaceous nodules (that frequently develop into abscesses, and eventually into ulcers) are also frequently found in the anogenital region of patients with Crohn disease **(Fig. 11-66)**.

### Reactive and/or Associated Orocutaneous Disorders

Two of these (erythema nodosum and oral aphthous ulcers) are common but not terribly serious conditions,

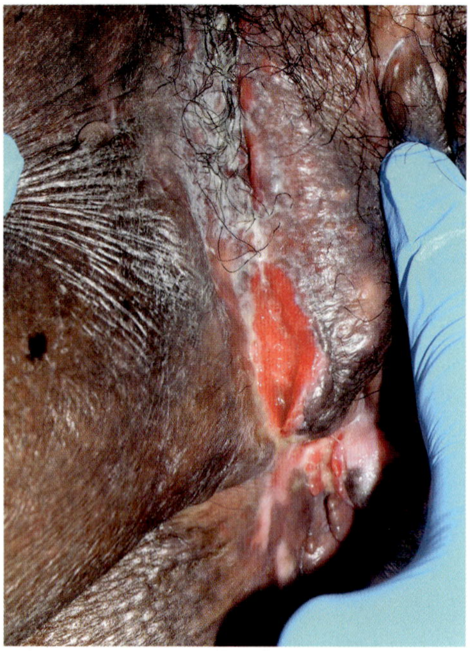

Fig. 11-62. This deep linear ulcer in the inguinal crease is pathognomonic of Crohn disease in Western countries where granuloma inguinale is nearly unknown.

and, on the other hand, two (pyoderma gangrenosum and hidradenitis suppurativa) are less common but can be severe and debilitating. These four disorders are covered in the paragraphs that follow, whereas other associated disorders will simply be listed.

### Erythema Nodosum

Erythema nodosum (EN) consists of erythematous to violaceous, tender or painful, nodules, which range in size from 1 to 5 cm in diameter.[56] EN develops in 5%-15% of patients with CD; less often in those with ulcerative colitis (UC). They typically occur in clusters of lesions on the anterior aspects of the lower extremity, especially over the

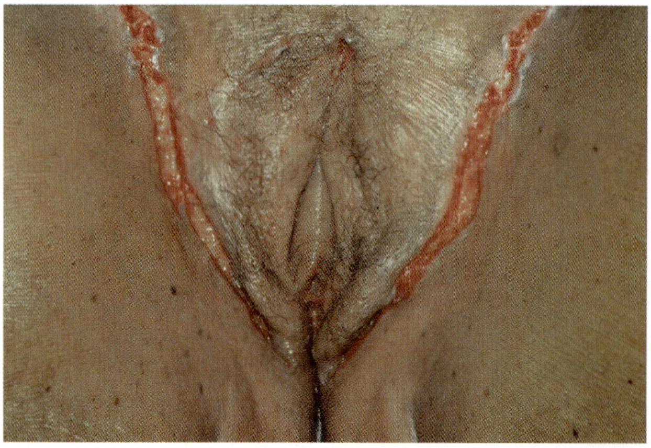

Fig. 11-63. These extensive linear ulcerations of Crohn disease are associated with edema of the clitoral hood and ulcers that occurred under the pannus and in the interlabial folds.

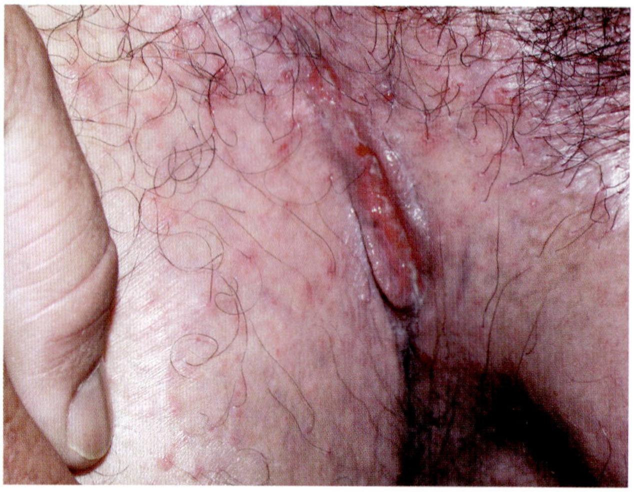

Fig. 11-64. The linear ulcer in this man's inguinal crease exhibits exophytic skin growth along the sides of the ulcer, a relatively common finding.

shins, and develop more often in women than in men. Because of the clinical distinctiveness of EN, biopsy is rarely needed. EN also occurs in a variety of settings other than inflammatory bowel disease; these include infections, lymphomas, sarcoidosis, Behçet disease, pregnancy, and as a part of some medication reactions. Generally, EN requires only pain relief and heals spontaneously without scarring within 4-8 weeks.

### Oral Aphthous Ulcers

Oral aphthous ulcers occur in ~10% of patients with either CD or UC. They usually develop on the buccal, labial, and gingival mucous membranes and frequently precede the signs and symptoms of the inflammatory bowel disease.

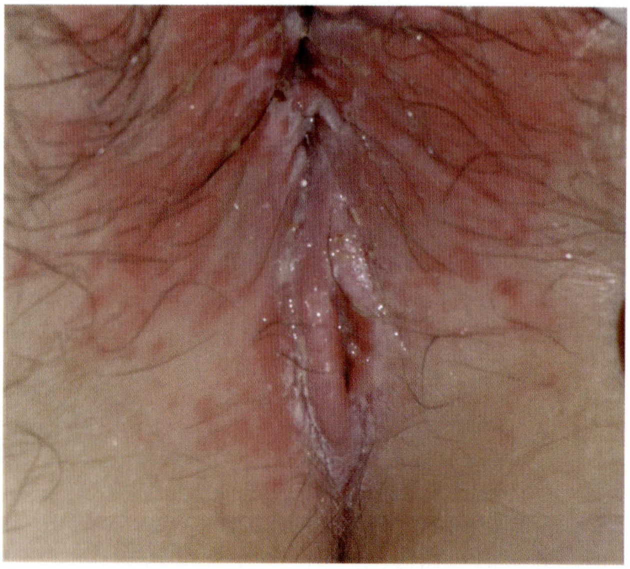

Fig. 11-65. This man with contiguous Crohn disease has a linear perianal ulcer at 6 o'clock; this ulcer represented a perianal fistula. There is perianal dermatitis due to chronic drainage from rectal disease.

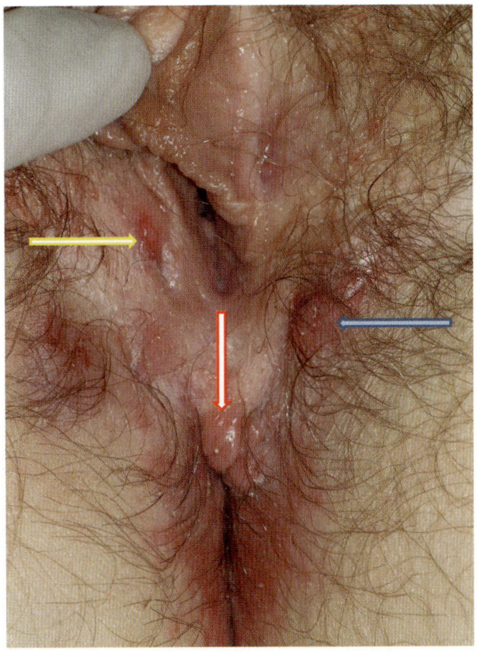

Fig. 11-66. Nodules (*arrows*) are seen in some patients with Crohn disease, and occasionally are eroded (*yellow and blue arrows*); these patients could be confused as having hidradenitis suppurativa.

Aphthous ulcers, albeit those found in the anogenital region rather than in the mouth, are discussed earlier in this chapter (q.v.) and for that reason this discussion will not be repeated here.

## Pyoderma Gangrenosum

Pyoderma gangrenosum (PG) occurs in about 1%-2% of patients with inflammatory bowel disease; it develops slightly more often in patients with UC than in those with CD.[58,59] The initial lesion is a pustule or an erythematous papule or nodule which quickly develops into an expanding, deep ulcer. Either single or multiple ulcers may be present. The base of the ulcer is purulent (though sterile) and the border is violaceous and undermined. Most often these ulcers are located on the lower legs but may be located in the anogenital region. This subject is extensively covered later in this chapter (q.v.) and for that reason will not be further discussed here.

## Hidradenitis Suppurativa

Hidradenitis suppurativa (HS) occurs more often than would be expected by chance in inflammatory bowel disease and, because of the similarity of lesions occurring in the anogenital region, distinguishing between the two disorders can be difficult at times especially when the diagnosis of Crohn disease has not otherwise been well established **(Fig. 11-67)**.[63] HS is extensively covered in Chapter 6 with the red nodules (q.v.) and for this reason further discussion is not warranted here.

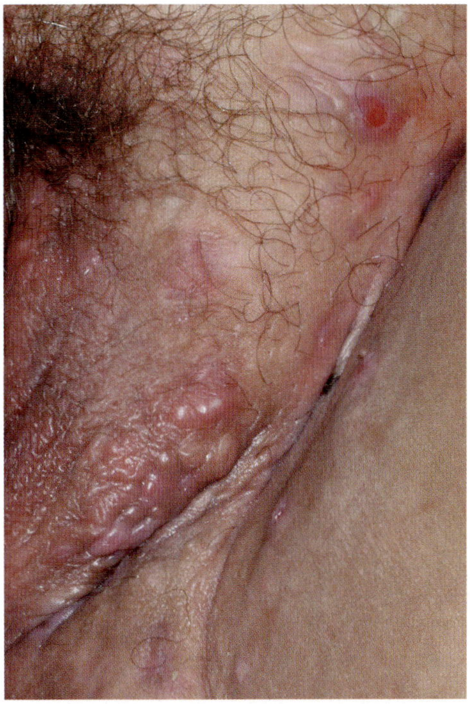

Fig. 11-67. These nodules and scattered ulcerations due to ruptured nodules represent hidradenitis suppurativa; the differentiation from Crohn disease can be difficult, and HS sometimes occurs in patients with Crohn disease.

## Miscellaneous Disorders Associated With Crohn Disease

Numerous conditions have been reported to occur in patients with Crohn disease and/or ulcerative colitis. None of these is particularly likely to involve the anogenital region, so they are simply listed: Sweet syndrome, psoriasis, epidermolysis bullosa acquisita, bowel-associated dermatitis-arthritis syndrome, pyodermatitis-pyostomatitis vegetans, SAPHO syndrome (synovitis, acne, pustulosis, hyperostosis, and osteitis), and PAPA syndrome (pyogenic arthritis, pyoderma gangrenosum, and acne).[59]

## Treatment-Related Conditions

Several medications used to treat inflammatory bowel disease are sometimes associated with the development of skin disease. In particular, the tumor necrosis factor alpha antagonists (TNF-α antagonists), such as infliximab, adalimumab, and certolizumab, can cause psoriasiform and eczematous reactions in about 5%-10% of treated patients.[56,59] The pathogenesis of these paradoxical reactions remains speculative but, thankfully, they are usually mild, and even though they respond to cessation of treatment, ongoing therapy is often possible.

# Diagnosis

In the setting of previously diagnosed *intestinal* Crohn disease, it is usually possible to make a clinical diagnosis of *cutaneous* Crohn disease especially when anogenital fistulae and/or linear skinfold ulcers are present. With less characteristic clinical lesions, or in the absence of diagnosed intestinal Crohn disease, a biopsy is necessary. Unfortunately, the granulomatous inflammation in cutaneous Crohn disease seems to occur less often than these histologic changes occur within the intestinal lesions. This often results in a hedged pathology report and in this situation the diagnosis will have to be determined by clinical-pathologic correlation. Please note that when there is no established diagnosis of intestinal Crohn disease, radiological and/or endoscopic examination should be strongly considered because intestinal Crohn disease may be present in some, otherwise asymptomatic patients. And, of course, in a small percentage of cases, cutaneous lesions may precede any evidence, whatsoever, of intestinal Crohn disease.

Several disorders need to be considered in the differential diagnosis of Crohn disease. As indicated above, genital edema with histological evidence of granulomatous inflammation similar to that of CD occurs in the condition termed Melkersson-Rosenthal disease. It is not clear whether or not this disease is a distinct entity or is a forme fruste of Crohn disease.[62]

Hidradenitis suppurativa (HS) is the disease most often confused with cutaneous Crohn disease. Patients with anogenital HS may present with abscesses and fistulas that are very similar to those found in Crohn disease. On biopsy, these lesions of HS generally show nonspecific granulomatous inflammation making differentiation between the two disorders very difficult. The presence of abscesses in the axillae (or anywhere along the milk line) together with the presence of atypical comedones in any of these locations will correctly identify HS. However, it should be noted that these two diseases have been reported to occur concomitantly more often than chance alone would suggest.[63]

Linear ulcers like those in Crohn disease also occur in granuloma inguinale and Langerhans cell histiocytosis. Biopsy will allow for correct identification of these two diseases. Behçet disease, herpes genitalis in an immunosuppressed patient, syphilis, chancroid, traumatic ulcerations, and ulcerated carcinoma cause anogenital ulcers, but these disorders are less likely to cause confusion with Crohn disease.

**CROHN DISEASE — Diagnosis**

- History of intestinal symptoms and signs
- Perianal tags and/or genital edema
- Abscesses and/or fistulas
- Linear "knife-cut" ulcers in skinfolds
- Biopsy to confirm

## Pathophysiology

The cause of Crohn disease is unknown. CD is certainly multifactorial, and it is probably best to consider the pathogenesis as an interaction between genetic and environmental factors. Much of what follows is based on an extensive and thorough review published in 2018.[64] More detailed reviews are also available, but they extend beyond the needs of the audience for whom this book is intended.[65,66]

### Genetic Factors

Approximately 15% of CD patients have a family history of the disorder and the concordance rate for the development of CD in monozygotic twins can be as high as 50%. The best studied mutations have included those occurring in the *NOD2 (CARD15)*, *IL23R*, *IRGM*, and *ATG16L1* genes; the most important of which are believed to be those occurring in the *NOD2* gene. Two things should be noted: first, mutations in these genes occur in some, but not all, patients with CD; second, the *IL23R* gene plays a role in the development of TH-17 lymphocytes which in turn elaborate interleukin-17 (IL-17) an important mediator of inflammation in CD. Other inflammation provoking interleukins that are increased in Crohn disease include IL-12 and IL-23.

### Environmental Factors

Inhaling cigarette smoke, actively or second-hand, is a risk factor for the development of CD. It fosters early onset of the disorder as well as increasing the frequency of recurrences following surgical therapy. Dietary deficiency of fiber, especially fruit-related fiber, increases the risk of CD by way of enhancing inflammatory mediators. Vitamin D3 deficiency is another deficiency that seems to be problematic in this regard. Lifestyle stress that provokes anxiety, depression, and sleep deprivation has long been recognized as a precipitating determinant for CD. (On the other hand, physical activity lowers the risk for this condition.) Appendectomy for appendicitis is another risk factor though it seems likely that the inflammation associated with appendicitis, rather than the actual surgery, is responsible for this higher risk.

## Gastrointestinal Bacteria

There are three changes in gut bacteria that probably play a role in the development of CD. These include (1) a decreased diversity in the normal GI microbiota; (2) an increase in adherent-invasive *Escherichia coli*, a bacterial species which promotes gut inflammation; and (3) a decrease in *Faecalibacterium prausnitzii*, a bacterial species that protects against the development of inflammation.

These changes may occur for a variety of reasons among which may be the influence of dietary factors.

### Management

The cutaneous manifestations of Crohn disease generally occur, and are worsened, with bowel disease activity. The major exception to this generality is pyoderma gangrenosum; treatment for which can be found in the following separate section on this disorder. Treatment for other forms of cutaneous involvement is covered in the following paragraphs. Not surprisingly, the first step is to modify, where possible, the environmental factors that may have been playing a role in the development of the CD. For the most part, this means the discontinuation of any smoking that had been in place and an attempt to reduce lifestyle stress.

When intestinal disease is inactive or not present, local therapy can be implemented. Fluctuant abscesses should be incised and drained. Smaller, solid inflammatory lesions and small ulcers can be intralesionally injected with triamcinolone acetonide (Kenalog) in a concentration of 10-20 mg/mL. Localized areas of persistent edema can be similarly treated with intralesional triamcinolone injections. (Surgery, which is beyond the scope of this book, will be required for intestinal complications such as fistulas.)

If intestinal disease is active, therapy should be directed toward it. Detailed discussion of therapy lies outside of the purview of this textbook and for this reason will only be outlined. Therapy generally occurs in two steps: induction of remission and maintenance of control.[67] Historically, remission was attempted, and was usually achieved, with a variety of high-dose systemic steroids. Today, the steroid of choice is orally administered budesonide as it acts primarily in the gut due to significant first-pass liver metabolism, thus reducing adverse steroid effects. The average dose in adults is 9 mg (3 capsules of three mg each), which is tapered as remission occurs. A biological agent such as an anti-TNF-α, anti-IL-12/23, or anti-integrin α4β7 is usually started at the same time as the steroid therapy and is continued on for maintenance once remission is obtained. The steroid is tapered and eventually discontinued. Alternatively, a trial of immune modulators such as azathioprine, 6-mercaptopurine, or methotrexate can be instituted for maintenance or can be used along with the biologics mentioned above.

The biological agents mentioned in the paragraph above, though quite costly, have revolutionized the treatment of inflammatory bowel disease. As of this writing, a half dozen or so biologics have been approved by the U.S. Food and Drug Administration (FDA) for the treatment of CD. They include those directed against TNF-α (adalimumab [Humira], certolizumab [Cimzia], infliximab [Remicade]), against IL-12/IL-23 (ustekinumab [Stelara]), and against integrins (vedolizumab [Entyvio], natalizumab [Tysabri]). In addition, a number of biosimilar (generic) agents have also been approved.

Finally, the ulcers, abscesses, and fistulas are very destructive and cause appreciable scarring and architectural distortion. As is true for several other genital chronic inflammatory diseases, such as lichen sclerosus, lichen planus, and hidradenitis suppurativa, a possibility exists that SCC may develop in nonhealing or scarred lesions.[68]

**CROHN DISEASE — Management**

- Control-associated bowel disease; refer if necessary
- Intralesional triamcinolone 10 mg/mL for solid lesions
- Incise and drain fluctuant lesions
- Consider oral prednisone or biologics
- Observe for the possible development of squamous cell carcinoma

## Pyoderma Gangrenosum

Pyoderma gangrenosum (PG) belongs to the group of diseases known as the neutrophilic dermatoses. It is the most commonly encountered member of this family, but it is rarely reported to involve the anogenital area. Nevertheless, because pyoderma gangrenosum is associated with Crohn disease (albeit usually occurring on the legs) and because it can be serious, even life threatening, it is discussed in this chapter.

### Clinical Presentation

The overall annual incidence of pyoderma gangrenosum is about 1 per 100 000 persons. Approximately half of the patients with PG have an underlying disorder. The most common of these include inflammatory bowel disease (both CD and UC), inflammatory arthritis, or malignancy, especially of the hematological type.[69] PG can occur in people of any age from childhood to the elderly though it most often develops in early to mid adult life. It develops slightly more often in women. The ulcers of pyoderma gangrenosum usually occur on the lower legs but lesions in other sites such as peristomal skin, female breasts, face, and dorsal hands. Lesions occasionally develop in the anogenital region especially in the perineal and perianal area.[70,71] Only about 50 cases of genital involvement have been reported.[72,73]

Pyoderma gangrenosum occurs as one of four morphological types of lesions: (1) ulcerative, (2) pustular, (3) bullous, and (4) vegetative.[69] The most common of these by far is the ulcerative form and, since it is the only one that seems to have been reported as occurring in the anogenital region, it is the only type that is discussed here. It usually starts as a pustule that very rapidly (within a

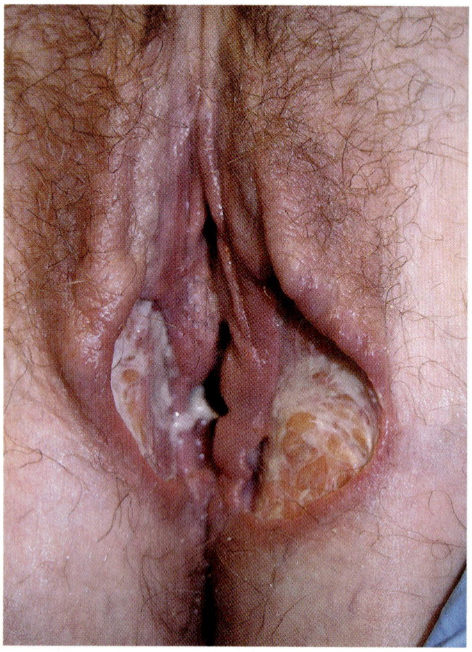

Fig. 11-68. This ulcer of pyoderma gangrenosum shows classic red, undermined borders.

matter of days) becomes violaceous and subsequently undergoes necrosis to form an ulcer. Occasionally, the initial lesion is a papule or nodule rather than a pustule. Over the next week or two, the ulcer expands in diameter, usually in a polycyclic manner, such that the margins are serpiginous when viewed from above. The ulcer edges are typically undermined and deeply violaceous in color; a red 5-10 mm inflammatory rim generally surrounds the ulcer (**Figs. 11-68 to 11-70**). Most often only a solitary ulcer is present but occasionally multiple lesions occur.

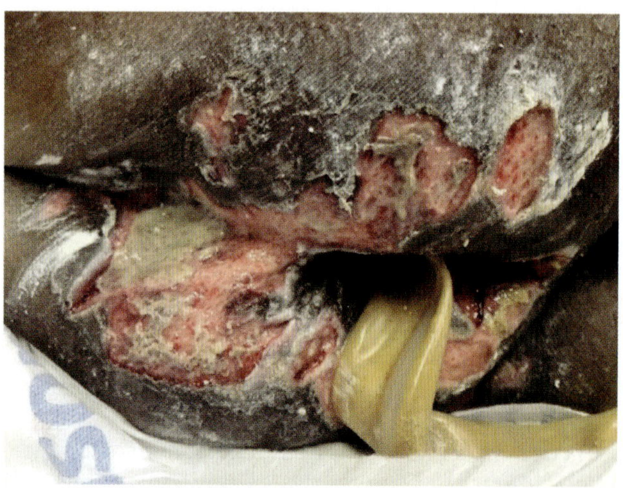

Fig. 11-69. Because this patient with pyoderma gangrenosum is dark complexioned, the erythema of the edges of the ulcer is not remarkable. However, the sharp edges and, in some areas, the overhanging borders, as well as negative cultures and lack of response to antibiotics, suggest this diagnosis. The diagnosis was confirmed by rapid healing with prednisone.

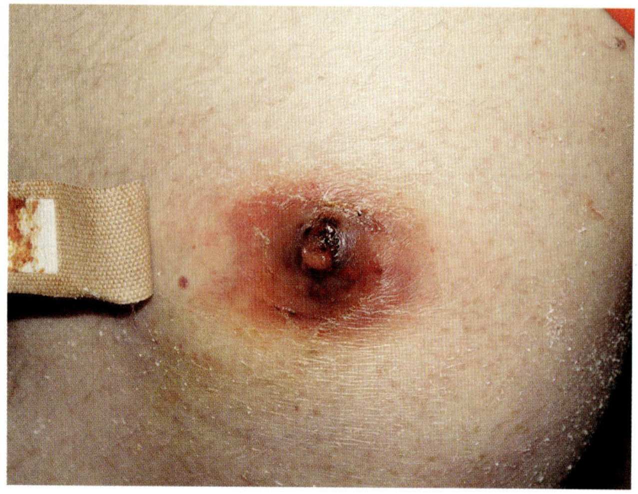

Fig. 11-70. The clinical appearance of this early ulcerating nodule of PG is not diagnostic, but the clinical setting and a nearby classic ulcer of PG indicated the correct diagnosis **(Fig. 11-70)**.

Pathergy, the development of a lesion at a site of trauma, may account for the location of the ulcer. The ulcer is typically quite painful, often out of proportion to its size and appearance. Ulcers eventually heal spontaneously usually with a cribriform pattern of fibrosis prior to completer re-epithelialization. Recurrences, often at the same site, are common.

## Diagnosis

If the lesion is classical in appearance, especially when it occurs in setting of inflammatory dowel disease, a clinical diagnosis is possible. If the ulcer is not classical in appearance, biopsy should be carried out from tissue located 5-10 mm from the edge of the ulcer. If a dense infiltrate of neutrophils is present, clinicopathologic correlation can lead to the correct diagnosis. However, often in older ulcers, only nonspecific inflammation may be found in which case a diagnosis can only be established by ruling out other diseases described on the list of differential diagnoses; that is, sometimes PG is a diagnosis of exclusion. Disorders on the list of differential diagnoses are numerous; we have only included those likely to occur in the anogenital area. They include bacterial, viral, and fungal infections (including multiple sexually transmitted infections), ulcerating malignancies, genital aphthous ulceration, Behçet disease, and cutaneous Crohn disease. Please note that necrotizing fasciitis (termed Fournier gangrene when the anogenital area is involved) mimics very closely the appearance of pyoderma gangrenosum and is an especially strong consideration if fever, malaise, and an elevated white blood cell count are also present.[74,75]

Over the years, several papers have been published suggesting that the diagnosis of PG is best established through the use of diagnostic algorithms. The two most often used appear to be those from the Mayo clinic and from the University of California, Davis.[76,77] These algorithms can be quite in clinical research but we have found them to be somewhat cumbersome for use in a standard office setting.

**PYODERMA GANGRENOSUM — Diagnosis**

- Rapid development of painful ulcer with purpuric borders
- Classical ulcer is deep with undermined margins
- Bullous hemorrhagic form is shallow with purpuric blister roof over part or all of the ulcer
- Biopsy to confirm
- Look for associated disease, especially Crohn disease, LE, rheumatoid arthritis, hidradenitis suppurativa, and hematopoietic malignancy

### Pathogenesis

The cause of pyoderma gangrenosum is unknown though it appears to be a reactive neutrophilic autoinflammatory reaction that involves neutrophil dysfunction, immune dysregulation, and genetic susceptibility.[78] Early studies focused on neutrophils because of the density of these cells at the necrotic margins of the ulcers. These neutrophils are present even though infection is not part of PG pathophysiology and there is a lack of true neutrophilic vasculitis. The abnormalities in PG that have been found relate to abnormal cell migration, chemotaxis, and phagocytosis.[69]

However, with the realization that PG was part of the autoinflammatory disorders, attention turned to defects in the immune system. T cells were noted to be numerous in biopsies from the edges of PG ulcers. These T cells produce numerous chemokines, which influence the trafficking of neutrophils. Some of the most important of these include tumor factor alpha (TNF-α) and interleukins 8 (IL-8), 17 (IL-17), and 23 (IL-23). Also notable is an increase in Th-17 cells and a decrease in regulatory T cells.[69] The Th-17 cells produce the IL-17 that recruits neutrophils. IL-1β is also increased and it leads to the development of inflammasomes (typically found in the autoinflammatory disorders) that also increase the elaboration of inflammatory cytokines.

There is also a genetic component for PG involving several genes, including *PSTPIP* genes, that account for the occurrence of several rare syndromes such as PAPA (pyogenic arthritis, PG, and acne), SAPHO (synovitis, acne, pustulosis, hyperostosis, and osteitis), and PAPASH (pyogenic arthritis, PG, acne, and hidradenitis suppurativa). All of the material in this section on pathogenesis has been simplified. For a much more detailed description, the interested reader is referred to the recent reviews by Ahn et al. and Maverakis et al.[78,79]

### Management

Pyoderma gangrenosum is a chronic condition in which spontaneous healing is unlikely or, at least, is significantly delayed. Therapy is difficult as might be supposed given the paucity of randomized, controlled trials and the numerous medications that have been recommended. However, a detailed algorithm for the treatment of PG has recently been published.[79] Almost all approaches suggest a trial of topical or intralesional corticosteroids for mild ulceration; we generally use either topical halobetasol, or its equivalent, clobetasol, along with intralesional injections of triamcinolone acetonide (Kenalog) in a concentration of 10-20 mg/mL.

For more severe ulceration, systemic corticosteroids represent the first line of treatment. Prednisone is administered in a dose of 60 mg/d until healing begins. At that time, the dose can be tapered but it is likely that even if a good response is observed, a steroid sparing medication (such as cyclosporine, thalidomide, mycophenolate mofetil, etc.) or a biologic agent should be initiated. Biologics and their biosimilars are increasingly being recommended in spite of their high cost partly because of their relative safety. They are especially helpful when PG occurs in the setting of Crohn disease because most of the biologics can improve, or even clear, both disorders.[69,80] Treatment of other underlying disease associated with PG is useful but does not necessarily lead to resolution of the PG.

The prognosis for patients with PG is not good. Healing, most often with scarring, of any single ulcer occasionally occurs spontaneously but overall recurrences are common and even fatality is higher for all patients with the disorder whether or not the individual also has an underlying disorder associated with PG.[69]

**PYODERMA GANGRENOSUM — Management**

- Prednisone 60 mg orally QAM; taper as healing occurs
- Intralesional triamcinolone 10 mg/mL as adjuvant therapy
- Oral antibiotics and dapsone for their anti-inflammatory effect
- Cyclosporine and/or TNF alpha inhibitors if necessary
- Treat any underlying disease that is present

## Ulcers Due to External Trauma

External trauma can lead to the development of ulcers. A clue suggesting a traumatic etiology often is related to the presence of a linear or an angular ulcer configuration. Traumatic ulcers arise in several contexts: (1) deep excoriation ("gouging"), (2) unintentional induction by the patient or the clinician; and (3) intentional, but unacknowledged, self-induction by the patient.

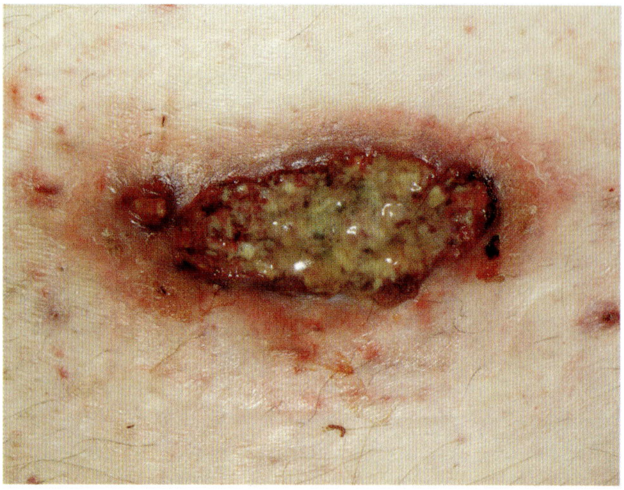

Fig. 11-71. The red/purple arcuate border of this very painful ulcer is typical for PG.

## Deep Excoriation

Chronic scratching, sometimes to the point of "gouging," represents the most common cause of traumatic genital ulcers. This is most properly named "excoriation disorder" but has also been termed "neurotic excoriations."[81,82] These deep excoriations may occur independently or may be found in the setting of prurigo nodularis or lichen simplex chronicus (**Figs. 11-71 and 11-72**). Such excoriation ulcers are most commonly found on the face, forearms, and legs but sometimes are located on the scrotum in men and on the labia majora and pubic region in women. Perianal and buttock lesions can develop in both genders. Excoriation disorder is classified with the obsessive-compulsive disorders (OCD) in the 2013 Diagnostic and Statistical Manual of Mental Disorders (DSM-5).

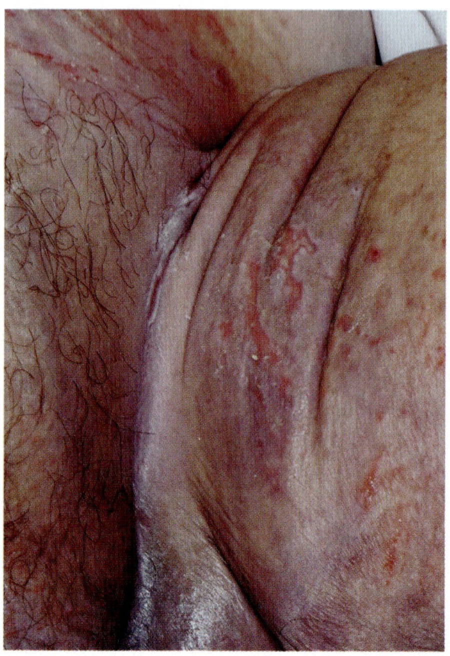

Fig. 11-72. Linear and irregular angular ulcerations on the medial thigh of this man were produced by scratching, in a setting of irritant contact dermatitis and eczema associated with incontinence.

Patients generally acknowledge that their scratching is causing ulcers, but in some instances (when the habitual scratching occurs at a subconscious level or while the patient is asleep), the patient may be of unaware of the role he or she is playing in the ulcer etiology. Whether aware of the scratching or not, patients are unable to discontinue the scratching of their own volition. For this reason, admonition by the clinician to stop scratching cannot be complied with and is usually counterproductive. Ulcers due to chronic scratching can almost always be recognized clinically by an angular and/or linear configuration; in fact, this morphology is essentially pathognomonic of external trauma. In the differential diagnosis, skin-centered body dysmorphic disorder should be considered.[81] In this latter condition, patients, when they are directly confronted, will usually acknowledge that their scratching or picking is directed toward their erroneous belief that there is a serious defect in the appearance of their body tissue and that their scratching is an attempt to modify this appearance.

In addition to the standard therapy for pruritus (see Chapters 3, 5 and 14), use of a selective serotonin reuptake inhibitor (SSRI) for these disorders is almost always warranted.[81,82] Most of these agents are approved for treatment of OCD and for this reason can reasonably be used in the setting of habitual, destructive excoriation. The normal or usual starting dose should be used but often an increase in that amount will be required. These medications can be taken in the morning or in the evening. I prefer the former as in almost all cases hydroxyzine 25-75 mg or doxepin 25-75 mg should be administered 2 hours before bedtime (see Chapters 3, 5 and 14). There is some potential for drug-drug interaction between the SSRIs and the tricyclics, so care should be taken when maximizing the dose of either agent. Onset of action may be slow and a period of 4 to 6 weeks must be allowed to determine the level of effectiveness. If the patient is still gouging at that time, in my opinion, the use of an antipsychotic agent should be considered as these medications are quite valuable for the therapy of SSRI-resistant OCD, including that of chronic excoriation.

## Acknowledged Nonscratching, External Trauma

Clinicians may prescribe, or apply, medications that potentially can cause either erosions or ulcers. The three medications most often responsible are clinician-applied

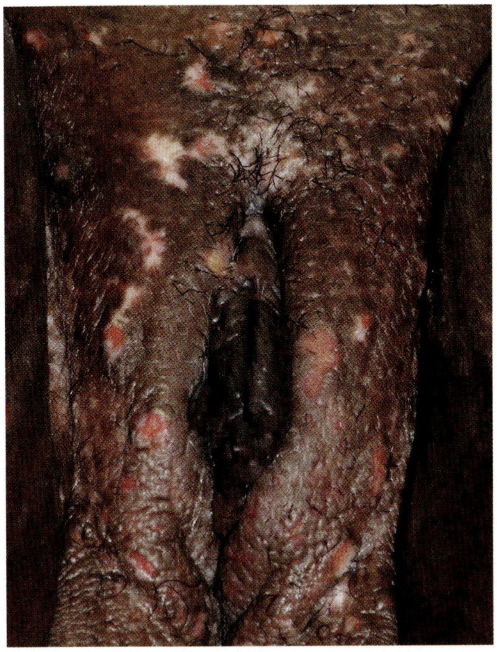

Fig. 11-73. Both active irregular ulcers and healed hypopigmented scars speak to the chronicity of excoriations on the vulva of this woman with lichen simplex chronicus.

trichloroacetic acid and patient-applied fluorouracil or imiquimod **(Figs. 11-73 and 11-74)**. The caustic reaction to these latter two agents is not immediate and tissue destruction may not occur for days or even a week after treatment has been initiated. When patients are given prescriptions for imiquimod or fluorouracil, they should be warned to stop the applications if inflammation becomes more than

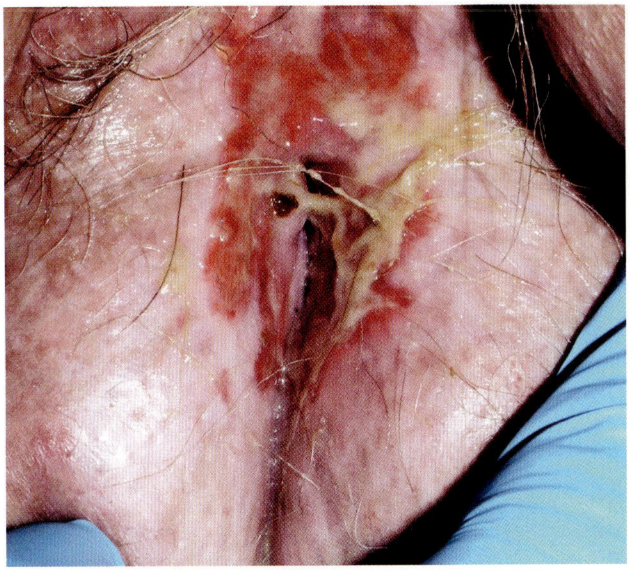

Fig. 11-74. Imiquimod applied to differentiated vulvar intraepithelial neoplasia in a setting of lichen sclerosus produced this painful purulent ulcer.

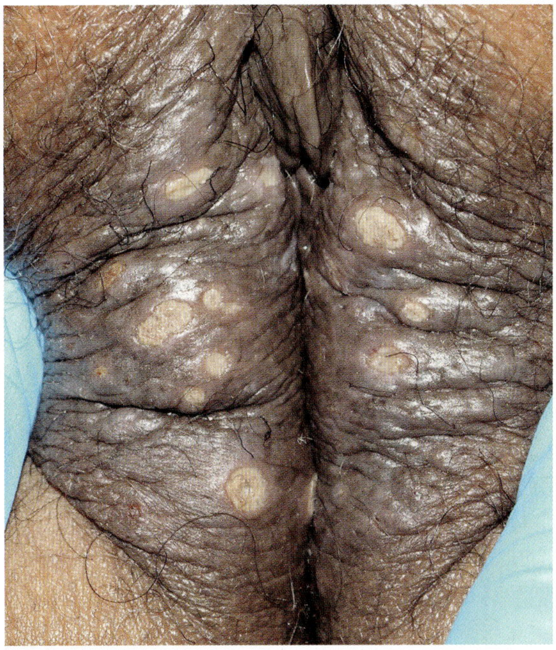

Fig. 11-75. These ulcers were produced by the application of sinecatechins for genital warts.

moderately severe. Similarly, and not unexpectedly, ulcers can also occur following the use of liquid nitrogen and ablative electrosurgical and laser therapy.

Patients, especially women, sometimes have the perception that the anogenital area is "dirty" and for that reason, extraordinary approaches to hygiene may be used. They might then scrub with a stiff brush, apply bleach, or overuse cleansers that were never designed for application to the anogenital skin **(Fig. 11-75)**. Patients who are incontinent or have chronic vaginal discharge may persistently occlude the anogenital area with diapers or panty liners. The chronic presence of moisture can then lead to breakdown of the skin and the formation of erosions and ulcers (see also Chapter 5).

Genital ulcers may develop as a result of ritualistic female mutilation used either for proof of virginity or to reduce libido. This is still practiced in some African societies but can also occasionally be encountered in Western countries.[83] Considerable controversy exists as to whether or not male circumcision is also a form of genital mutilation.[84]

## Unacknowledged External Trauma

Patients with psychiatric disorders may mutilate the skin by way of unacknowledged burning, cutting, gouging, or other forms of self-mutilation. This may occur because they fear that something is abnormally present in the skin (delusions of parasitosis, Morgellons disease) and they then feel compelled to physically remove these perceived bugs or fibers. They often deny that any behavior on their part is responsible for the repeated and persistent ulceration. Alternatively, traumatic self-abuse can represent a psychiatrically abnormal behavior pattern in adolescents, particularly young women. Most such self-mutilation will occur on easily accessible parts of the body such as the arms and legs. This behavior is generally reported using the terms *dermatitis artefacta* or *factitial dermatitis*.[85] Since most such self-mutilation will occur at body sites outside of the anogenital region, we will instead only cover only genital self-mutilation.

Genital self-mutilation ranges from relatively minor practices such as genital cutting (seemingly more common in adolescent and young adult women) as was vividly portrayed in the highly rated 2001 movie *The Piano Teacher* to much more serious mutilation (probably more common in adult men) such as penile implantations, glans amputations, and castrations.[86,87] These patients who self-mutilate their genitalia almost always have extremely serious psychological problems and are at appreciable risk of suicide. As such, they require rapid referral to psychiatrists with only minor, but necessary, supportive treatment by other clinicians.

## Miscellaneous Ulcers

Pressure ulcers are generally recognized easily when they occur on the buttocks or sacrum of bedridden individuals. More challenging are pressure ulcers of other areas in patients with neurologic compromise preventing pain with pressure in more unusual areas **(Fig. 11-76)**. Ulcers also can arise at the site of what originally were erosions. Thus, ulcers may sometimes occur in erosive lesions of lichen sclerosus and lichen planus **(Fig. 11-77)**. Hidradenitis suppurativa patients generally present with abscesses (which may undergo ulceration) and fistulas **(Fig. 11-78)**. When tumor growth outstrips its blood supply, the surface may undergo necrosis resulting in the development of an ulcer **(Fig. 11-79)**.

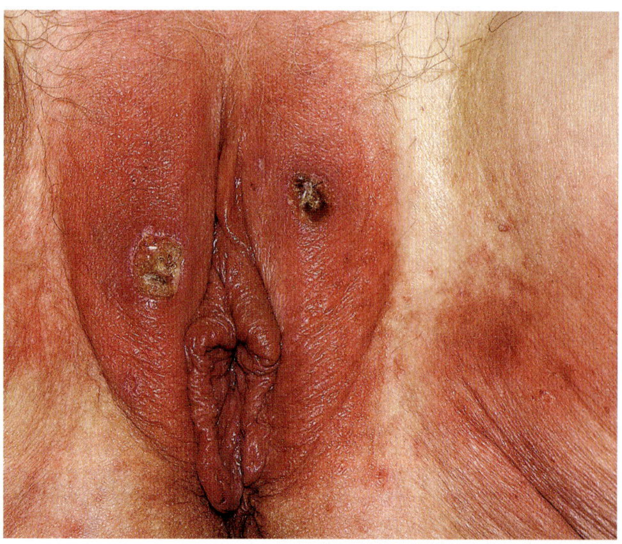

Fig. 11-76. Ulcers have occurred in a background of redness, caused by frequent, compulsive scrubbing with antiseptic solutions.

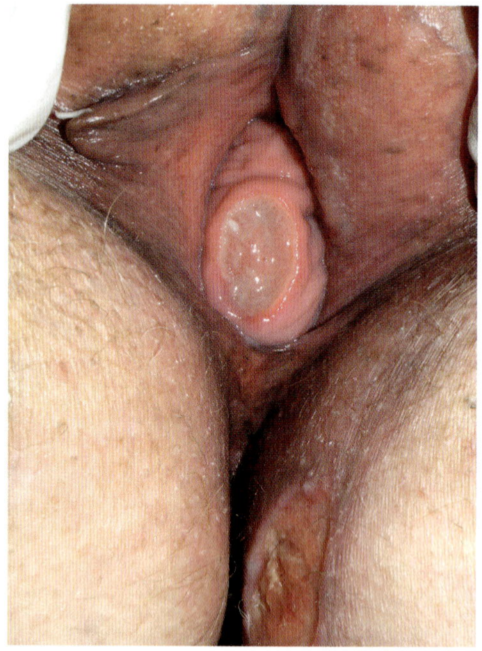

Fig. 11-77. This paraplegic patient experienced a large asymptomatic pressure ulcer of the vagina proper as well as the proximal, medial thigh medial thigh from sitting all day in one position in a chair without shifting.

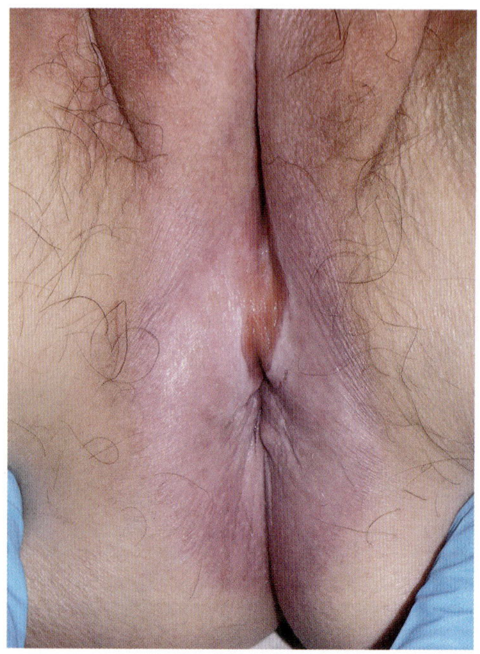

Fig. 11-78. Lichen sclerosus is not primarily an ulcerative condition, but the skin of this disease is so fragile that erosions and ulcers sometimes occur.

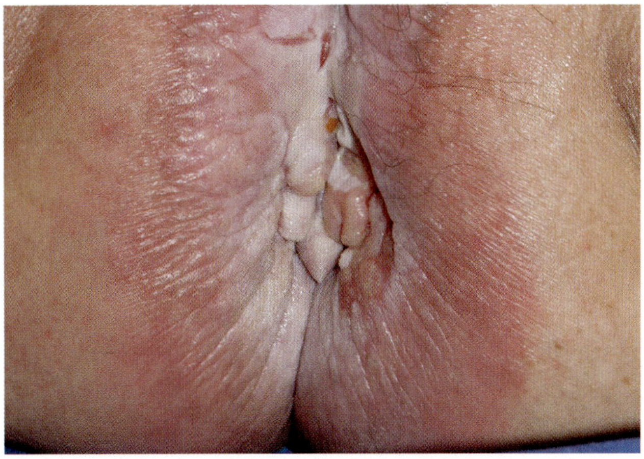

Fig. 11-79. This large ulcer in a patient with lichen sclerosus has occurred within a nodule of squamous cell carcinoma.

## REFERENCES


1. Elakis JA, Hall AP. Skin disease of penis and male genitalia is linked to atopy and circumcision: caseload in a male genital dermatology clinic. *Australas J Dermatol.* 2017;58:e68-e72. doi:10.1111/ajd.12485
2. Amsellem J, Skayem C, Duong TA, Bagot M, Fouéré S, Dauendorffer JN. Male genital lichen planus: A retrospective study of 89 cases. *Ann Dermatol Venereol.* 2022;149(1):28-31. doi:10.1016/j.annder.2021.04.007
3. Hrin ML, Bowers NL, Feldman SR, Huang WW, Pichardo RO. Mycophenolate mofetil versus methotrexate for vulvar lichen planus: a 10-year retrospective cohort study demonstrates comparable efficacy and tolerability. *J Am Acad Dermatol.* 2021:S0190-9622(21)02434-8. doi:10.1016/j.jaad.2021.08.061
4. Pelisse M. The vulvo-vaginal-gingival syndrome. A new form of erosive lichen planus. *Int J Dermatol.* 1989;28:381-384.
5. Petruzzi M, De Benedittis M, Pastore L, Grassi FR, Serpico R. Peno-gingival lichen planus. *J Periodontol.* 2005;76:2293-2298. doi:10.1902/jop.2005.76.12.2293
6. Thomas M, Makey IA, Francis DL, Wolfsen HC, Bowers SP. Squamous cell carcinoma in lichen planus of the esophagus. *Ann Thorac Surg.* 2020;109:e83-e85.
7. Webber NK, Setterfield JF, Lewis FM, Neill SM. Lacrimal canalicular duct scarring in patients with lichen planus. *Arch Dermatol.* 2012;148:224-227.
8. Sartori-Valinotti JC, Bruce AJ, Krotova Khan Y, Beatty CW. A 10-year review of otic lichen planus: the Mayo Clinic experience. *JAMA Dermatol.* 2013;149:1082-1086.
9. Day T, Otton G, Jaaback K, Weigner J, Scurry J. Is vulvovaginal lichen planus associated with squamous cell carcinoma? *J Low Genit Tract Dis.* 2018;22:159-165.
10. Halonen P, Jakobsson M, Heikinheimo O, Riska A, Gissler M, Pukkala E. Cancer risk of Lichen planus: a cohort study of 13,100 women in Finland. *Int J Cancer.* 2018;142:18-22.
11. Wang JH, Hung SJ. Lichen planus associated with hepatitis B, hepatitis C, and liver cirrhosis in a nationwide cohort study. *J Am Acad Dermatol.* 2021;84:1085-1086.
12. Dave A, Shariff J, Philipone E. Association between oral lichen planus and systemic conditions and medications: Case–control study. *Oral Dis.* 2021;27:515-524.
13. Ying J, Xiang W, Qiu Y, Zeng X. Risk of metabolic syndrome in patients with lichen planus: a systematic review and meta-analysis. *PLoS One.* 2020;15:e0238005.
14. Day T, Moore S, Bohl TG, Scurry J. Co-morbid vulvar lichen planus and lichen sclerosus. *J Low Genit Tract Dis.* 2017;21:204-208.
15. Merk HF, Vanstreels L, Megahed M. [Lichenoid drug reactions]. *Hautarzt.* 2018;69:116-120. Review. German.
16. Cheng S, Kirtschig G, Cooper S, et al. Interventions for erosive lichen planus affecting mucosal sites. *Cochrane Database Syst Rev.* 2012;(2):CD008092.
17. Lodi G, Manfredi M, Mercadante V, Murphy R, Carrozzo M. Interventions for treating oral lichen planus: corticosteroid therapies. *Cochrane Database Syst Rev.* 2020;(2):CD001168.
18. Acar S, Koksal AS, Tozlu M, Gonullu E, Eminler AT. Treatment of esophageal stricture due to lichen planus with intralesional triamcinolone injection. *Eur J Gastroenterol Hepatol.* 2021;33:1611.
19. Vermeer HAB, Rashid H, Esajas MD, Oldhoff JM, Horváth B. The use of hydroxychloroquine as a systemic treatment in erosive lichen planus of the vulva and vagina. *Br J Dermatol.* 2021;185:201-203.
20. Poon F, De Cruz R, Hall A. Acitretin in erosive penile lichen planus. *Australas J Dermatol.* 2017;58:e87-e90.
21. Wu Y, Zhou G, Zeng H, Xiong CR, Lin M, Zhou HM. A randomized double-blind, positive-control trial of topical thalidomide in erosive oral lichen planus. *Oral Surg Oral Med Oral Pathol Oral Radiol Endod.* 2010;110:188-195.
22. Paul J, Foss CE, Hirano SA, Cunningham TD, Pariser DM. An open-label pilot study of apremilast for the treatment of moderate to severe lichen planus: a case series. *J Am Acad Dermatol.* 2013;68:255-261.
23. Zeiser R, et al. Ruxolitinib for glucocorticoid-refractory chronic graft-versus-host-disease. *N Engl J Med.* 2021;385:228-238.
24. Naji H, Ali Hassan R. Perineal groove: is it more common than we think? Clinical characteristics of four cases and review of literature. *Pediatr Rep.* 2021;13:490-494.
25. Ghanem KG, Ram S, Rice PA. The modern epidemic of syphilis. *N Engl J Med.* 2020;382(9):845-854. doi:10.1056/NEJMra1901593
26. Forrestel AK, Kovarik CL, Katz KA. Sexually acquired syphilis: historical aspects, microbiology, epidemiology, and clinical manifestations. *J Am Acad Dermatol.* 2020;82(1):1-14. doi:10.1016/j.jaad.2019.02.073
27. Forrestel AK, Kovarik CL, Katz KA. Sexually acquired syphilis: laboratory diagnosis, management, and prevention. *J Am Acad Dermatol.* 2020;82(1):17-28. doi:10.1016/j.jaad.2019.02.074
28. Morris BJ, Wamai RG, Krieger JN, Banerjee J, Klausner JD. Male circumcision to prevent syphilis in 1855 and HIV in 1986 is supported by the accumulated scientific evidence to 2015: response to Darby. *Glob Public Health.* 2017;12(10):1315-1333. doi:10.1080/17441692.2015.1104371
29. Janier M, Unemo M, Dupin N, Tiplica GS, Potočnik M, Patel R. 2020 European guideline on the management of syphilis. *J Eur Acad Dermatol Venereol.* 2021;35(3):574-588. doi:10.1111/jdv.16946
30. Lewis DA, Mitjà O. Haemophilus ducreyi: from sexually transmitted infection to skin ulcer pathogen. *Curr Opin Infect Dis.* 2016;29(1):52-57. doi:10.1097/QCO.0000000000000226
31. Copeland NK, Decker CF. Other sexually transmitted diseases chancroid and donovanosis. *Dis Mon.* 2016;62(8):306-313. doi:10.1016/j.disamonth.2016.03.016

32. Cologne KG, Hsieh C. Nonviral sexually transmitted diseases. *Clin Colon Rectal Surg.* 2019;32(5):358-363. doi:10.1055/s-0039-1687831
33. Karagounis TK, Pomeranz MK. Viral venereal diseases of the skin. *Am J Clin Dermatol.* 2021;22(4):523-540. doi:10.1007/s40257-021-00606-7
34. Sirka CS. Clinical features of a large chronic ulcer on the genital and perianal region in HIV-infected patients can be a strong clinical clue for the diagnosis of herpes simplex infection. *Indian J Sex Transm Dis AIDS.* 2020;41(2):192-195. doi:10.4103/ijstd.IJSTD_140_15
35. Sasso BM, Florence MEB, Magalhaes RF, et al. Herpes simplex virus mucocutaneous tumoural lesions—systematic review. *J Clin Virol.* 2020;123:104246. doi:10.1016/j.jcv.2019.104246
36. Maliyar K, Mufti A, Syed M, et al. Genital ulcer disease: a review of pathogenesis and clinical features. *J Cutan Med Surg.* 2019;23(6):624-634. doi:10.1177/1203475419858955
37. Belda Junior W. Donovanosis. *An Bras Dermatol.* 2020;95(6):675-683. doi:10.1016/j.abd.2020.07.002
38. Arandes-Marcocci J, Collgros H, Serra-Pladevall J, Vall-Mayans M. Primary genital lymphogranuloma venereum in the HIV pre-exposure prophylaxis era. *J Eur Acad Dermatol Venereol.* 2020;34(8):e427-e429. doi:10.1111/jdv.16374
39. Stewart KMA. Challenging ulcerative vulvar conditions: Hidradenitis Suppurativa, Crohn Disease, and Aphthous Ulcers. *Obstet Gynecol Clin North Am.* 2017;44(3):453-473. doi:10.1016/j.ogc.2017.05.009
40. Saxena S, Tandon S, Sardana K, Bajaj S. Herpetiform aphthous genital ulcers misdiagnosed as herpes genitalis in a young male and their effective response to colchicine therapy. *Int J STD AIDS.* 2019;30(13):1340-1343. doi:10.1177/0956462419870672
41. Chen W, Plewig G. Lipschütz genital ulcer revisited: is juvenile gangrenous vasculitis of the scrotum the male counterpart? *J Eur Acad Dermatol Venereol.* 2019;33(9):1660-1666. doi:10.1111/jdv.15598
42. Jimenez-Cauhe J, Gil-Redondo R, Dominguez-Santas M, et al. Juvenile gangrenous vasculitis of the scrotum: the male counterpart of Lipschütz ulcer? *J Eur Acad Dermatol Venereol.* 2019;33(12):e459-e461. doi:10.1111/jdv.15778
43. Vieira-Baptista P, Lima-Silva J, Beires J, Martinez-de-Oliveira J. Lipschütz ulcers: should we rethink this? An analysis of 33 cases. *Eur J Obstet Gynecol Reprod Biol.* 2016;198:149-152. doi:10.1016/j.ejogrb.2015.07.016
44. Schindler Leal AA, Piccinato CA, Beck APA, Gomes MTV, Podgaec S. Acute genital ulcers: keep Lipschütz ulcer in mind. *Arch Gynecol Obstet.* 2018;298(5):927-931. doi:10.1007/s00404-018-4866-6
45. Vismara SA, Lava SAG, Kottanattu L, et al. Lipschütz's acute vulvar ulcer: a systematic review. *Eur J Pediatr.* 2020;179(10):1559-1567. doi:10.1007/s00431-020-03647-y
46. Sadoghi B, Stary G, Wolf P, Komericki P. Ulcus vulvae acutum Lipschütz: a systematic literature review and a diagnostic and therapeutic algorithm. *J Eur Acad Dermatol Venereol.* 2020;34(7):1432-1439. doi:10.1111/jdv.16161
47. Christl J, Alaniz VI, Appiah L, Buyers E, Scott S, Huguelet PS. Vulvar aphthous ulcer in an adolescent with COVID-19. *J Pediatr Adolesc Gynecol.* 2021;34(3):418-420. doi:10.1016/j.jpag.2021.02.098
48. Mahmoud EA, Moneim WA, Shaker OG, Ghalwash DM. Expression of endocan and vascular endothelial growth factor in recurrent minor aphthous ulcers. *J Clin Exp Dent.* 2019;11(6):e534-e541. doi:10.4317/jced.55695
49. Wang Z, Cao H, Xiong J, et al. Recent advances in the aetiology of recurrent aphthous stomatitis (RAS). *Postgrad Med J.* 2022;98(1155):57-66.. doi:10.1136/postgradmedj-2020-139421
50. Saikaly SK, Saikaly TS, Saikaly LE. Recurrent aphthous ulceration: a review of potential causes and novel treatments. *J Dermatolog Treat.* 2018;29(6):542-552. doi:10.1080/09546634.2017.1422079
51. Sánchez-Bernal J, Conejero C, Conejero R. Recurrent aphthous stomatitis. *Actas Dermosifiliogr (Engl Ed).* 2020;111(6):471-480. English, Spanish. doi:10.1016/j.ad.2019.09.004
52. Scherrer MAR, Rocha VB, Garcia LC. Behçet's disease: review with emphasis on dermatological aspects. *An Bras Dermatol.* 2017;92(4):452-464. doi:10.1590/abd1806-4841.20177359.
53. Davatchi F, Chams-Davatchi C, Shams H, et al. Behcet's disease: epidemiology, clinical manifestations, and diagnosis. *Expert Rev Clin Immunol.* 2017;13(1):57-65. doi:10.1080/1744666X.2016.1205486
54. Tong B, Liu X, Xiao J, Su G. Immunopathogenesis of Behcet's disease. *Front Immunol.* 2019;10:665. doi:10.3389/fimmu.2019.00665.
55. Alibaz-Oner F, Direskeneli H. Advances in the treatment of Behcet's disease. *Curr Rheumatol Rep.* 2021;23(6):47. doi:10.1007/s11926-021-01011-z
56. Greuter T, Navarini A, Vavricka SR. Skin manifestations of inflammatory bowel disease. *Clin Rev Allergy Immunol.* 2017;53(3):413-427. doi:10.1007/s12016-017-8617-4
57. Garber A, Regueiro M. Extraintestinal manifestations of inflammatory bowel disease: epidemiology, etiopathogenesis, and management. *Curr Gastroenterol Rep.* 2019;21(7):31. doi:10.1007/s11894-019-0698-1
58. Alvarez-Payares JC, Ramírez-Urrea S, Correa-Parra L, Salazar-Uribe D, Velásquez-López M. Mucocutaneous manifestations of inflammatory bowel disease. *Cureus.* 2021;13(8):e17191. doi:10.7759/cureus.17191
59. Antonelli E, Bassotti G, Tramontana M, et al. Dermatological manifestations in inflammatory bowel diseases. *J Clin Med.* 2021;10(2):364. doi:10.3390/jcm10020364
60. Ickrath F, Stoevesandt J, Schulmeyer L, Glatzel C, Goebeler M, Kerstan A. Metastatic Crohn's disease: an underestimated entity. *J Dtsch Dermatol Ges.* 2021;19(7):973-982. doi:10.1111/ddg.14447
61. Johnson CM, Hartman DJ, Ramos-Rivers C, et al. Epithelioid granulomas associate with increased severity and progression of Crohn's disease, based on 6-year follow-up. *Clin Gastroenterol Hepatol.* 2018;16(6):900-907.e1. doi:10.1016/j.cgh.2017.12.034
62. Haaramo A, Kolho KL, Pitkäranta A, Kanerva M. A 30-year follow-up study of patients with Melkersson-Rosenthal syndrome shows an association to inflammatory bowel disease. *Ann Med.* 2019;51(2):149-155. doi:10.1080/07853890.2019.1591634
63. Deckers IE, Benhadou F, Koldijk MJ, et al. Inflammatory bowel disease is associated with hidradenitis suppurativa: results from a multicenter cross-sectional study. *J Am Acad Dermatol.* 2017;76(1):49-53. doi:10.1016/j.jaad.2016.08.031
64. Gajendran M, Loganathan P, Catinella AP, Hashash JG. A comprehensive review and update on Crohn's disease. *Dis Mon.* 2018;64(2):20-57. doi:10.1016/j.disamonth.2017.07.001
65. Guan Q. A Comprehensive review and update on the pathogenesis of inflammatory bowel disease. *J Immunol Res.* 2019;2019:7247238. doi:10.1155/2019/7247238

66. Petagna L, Antonelli A, Ganini C, et al. Pathophysiology of Crohn's disease inflammation and recurrence. *Biol Direct.* 2020;15(1):23. doi:10.1186/s13062-020-00280-5
67. Cushing K, Higgins PDR. Management of Crohn disease: a review. *JAMA.* 2021;325(1):69-80. doi:10.1001/jama.2020.18936
68. Kotsafti A, Scarpa M, Angriman I, Castagliuolo I, Caruso A. Fistula-related cancer in Crohn's disease: a systematic review. *Cancers (Basel).* 2021;13(6):1445. doi:10.3390/cancers13061445
69. Barbe M, Batra A, Golding S, et al. Pyoderma gangrenosum: a literature review. *Clin Podiatr Med Surg.* 2021;38(4):577-588. doi:10.1016/j.cpm.2021.06.002
70. Sousa M, Campos MA, Sousa AC, Lopes J, Rodrigues A, Carvalho J. Extensive refractory perineal pyoderma gangrenosum treated with infliximab, fecal diversion, and negative-pressure wound therapy. *GE Port J Gastroenterol.* 2020;27(2):128-131. doi:10.1159/000502982
71. Gracia-Cazaña T, Padgett E, Sánchez-Salas P, Borao E. Perianal pyoderma gangrenosum. *Cir Esp (Engl Ed).* 2021;99(8):613. doi:10.1016/j.cireng.2021.07.002.
72. Sadowsky LM, Clark MA, Schlosser BJ. Pyoderma gangrenosum of the vulva treated with mycophenolate mofetil and infliximab. *Dermatol Ther.* 2019;32(3):e12905. doi:10.1111/dth.12905
73. Loloi J, MacDonald SM. Pyoderma gangrenosum of the penis. *Can J Urol.* 2021;28(1):10560-10564.
74. Slocum AMY. A surgeon's nightmare: pyoderma gangrenosum with pathergy effect mimicking necrotising fasciitis. *BMJ Case Rep.* 2017;2017:bcr2017222145. doi:10.1136/bcr-2017-222145
75. Flynn RL, Chowdhury MH, Rudolph J, Einstein S. Rare presentation of postsurgical pyoderma gangrenosum presenting as necrotizing soft tissue infection. *Adv Skin Wound Care.* 2019;32(11):507-511. doi:10.1097/01.ASW.0000579692.74662.bb
76. Su WP, Davis MD, Weenig RH, Powell FC, Perry HO. Pyoderma gangrenosum: clinicopathologic correlation and proposed diagnostic criteria. *Int J Dermatol.* 2004;43(11):790-800. doi:10.1111/j.1365-4632.2004.02128.x
77. Maverakis E, Ma C, Shinkai K, et al. Diagnostic criteria of ulcerative pyoderma gangrenosum: a Delphi consensus of international experts. *JAMA Dermatol.* 2018;154(4):461-466. doi:10.1001/jamadermatol.2017.5980
78. Ahn C, Negus D, Huang W. Pyoderma gangrenosum: a review of pathogenesis and treatment. *Expert Rev Clin Immunol.* 2018;14(3):225-233. doi:10.1080/1744666X.2018.1438269
79. Maverakis E, Marzano AV, Le ST, et al. Pyoderma gangrenosum. *Nat Rev Dis Primers.* 2020;6(1):81. doi:10.1038/s41572-020-0213-x
80. Partridge ACR, Bai JW, Rosen CF, Walsh SR, Gulliver WP, Fleming P. Effectiveness of systemic treatments for pyoderma gangrenosum: a systematic review of observational studies and clinical trials. *Br J Dermatol.* 2018;179(2):290-295. doi:10.1111/bjd.16485
81. McDonald KA, Jafferany M, Rohani K. Excoriation disorder vs skin-centered body dysmorphic disorder: a clinical and therapeutic update. *Dermatol Ther.* 2020;33(6):e13994. doi:10.1111/dth.13994
82. Torales J, Díaz NR, Barrios I, et al. Psychodermatology of skin picking (excoriation disorder): a comprehensive review. *Dermatol Ther.* 2020;33(4):e13661. doi:10.1111/dth.13661
83. Adam B. The physical, mental, and emotional harm of female genital mutilation. *J Am Acad Child Adolesc Psychiatry.* 2021;60(7):801-803. doi:10.1016/j.jaac.2020.12.022
84. Piontek EA, Albani JM. Male circumcision: the clinical implications are more than skin deep. *Mo Med.* 2019;116(1):35-37.
85. Ferri JVV, de Araujo DB. Dermatitis artefacta mimicking cutaneous vasculitis: case report and literature overview. *Reumatologia.* 2019;57(2):106-108. doi:10.5114/reum.2019.84816
86. Veeder TA, Leo RJ. Male genital self-mutilation: a systematic review of psychiatric disorders and psychosocial factors. *Gen Hosp Psychiatry.* 2017;44:43-50. doi:10.1016/j.genhosppsych.2016.09.003
87. Lupu S, et al. Genital self-mutilation: a challenging pathology (Review). *Exp Ther Med.* 2021;22(4):1130. doi:10.3892/etm.2021.10564


## SUGGESTED READINGS


Amsellem J, Skayem C, Duong TA, Bagot M, Fouéré S, Dauendorffer JN. Male genital lichen planus: a retrospective study of 89 cases. *Ann Dermatol Venereol.* 2022;149(1):28-31.. doi:10.1016/j.annder.2021.04.007

Barbe M, Batra A, Golding S, Hammond O, Higgins JC, O'Connor A, Vlahovic TC. Pyoderma Gangrenosum: a literature review. *Clin Podiatr Med Surg.* 2021;38(4):577-588.

Fahy CMR, Torgerson RR, Davis MDP Lichen planus affecting the female genitalia: a retrospective review of patients at Mayo Clinic. *J Am Acad Dermatol.* 2017;77(6):1053-1059. doi:10.1016/j.jaad.2017.07.030

Forrestel AK, Kovarik CL, Katz KA. Sexually acquired syphilis: Historical aspects, microbiology, epidemiology, and clinical manifestations. *J Am Acad Dermatol.* 2020;82(1):1-14. doi:10.1016/j.jaad.2019.02.073

Forrestel AK, Kovarik CL, Katz KA. Sexually acquired syphilis: laboratory diagnosis, management, and prevention. *J Am Acad Dermatol.* 2020;82(1):17-28. doi:10.1016/j.jaad.2019.02.074

Foss MG, Ferrer-Bruker SJ. Necrolytic migratory erythema. In: *StatPearls [Internet].* StatPearls Publishing; 2021.

Halonen P, Jakobsson M, Heikinheimo O, Riska A, Gissler M, Pukkala E. Cancer risk of Lichen planus: a cohort study of 13,100 women in Finland. *Int J Cancer.* 2018;142(1):18-22. doi:10.1002/ijc.31025

Krapf JM, Cavallo K, Saleeb M, Goldstein AT. Plasma cell vulvitis: a systematic review. *J Low Genit Tract Dis.* 2021;25(4):312-317. doi:10.1097/LGT.0000000000000617

Maliyar K, Mufti A, Syed M, Selk A, Dutil M, Bunce PE, Alavi A. Genital ulcer disease: a review of pathogenesis and clinical features. *J Cutan Med Surg.* 2019;23(6):624-634. doi:10.1177/1203475419858955

Vismara SA, Lava SAG, Kottanattu L, Simonetti GD, Zgraggen L, Clericetti CM, Bianchetti MG, Milani GP. Lipschütz's acute vulvar ulcer: a systematic review. *Eur J Pediatr.* 2020;179(10):1559-1567. doi:10.1007/s00431-020-03647-y

# Edema 12

PETER J. LYNCH AND LIBBY EDWARDS

Edema consists of increased subcutaneous interstitial tissue fluid. Acute edema is generally related to plasma and termed angioedema, whereas chronic edema is associated with lymph and termed lymphedema. When lymphedema is extraordinary so that hardening and disfigurement occurs, the result is termed elephantiasis. This secondary change is sometimes accompanied by firm nodules and even hyperkeratosis, resulting in elephantiasis nostras verrucosa. At times, angioedema can transition into lymphedema, especially when inflammation is operative, so that the distinction is not always straightforward.

Although both forms of edema are characterized by swelling, acute edema is generally softer and usually exhibits pitting (Fig. 12-1). Chronic lymphedema, however, is usually firm, more stable, and nonpitting (Fig. 12-2). Edema of both types are often asymptomatic, although acute edema associated with an allergic reaction tend to itch, and there are often symptoms associated with the underlying cause of the edema, such as infection or skin disease.

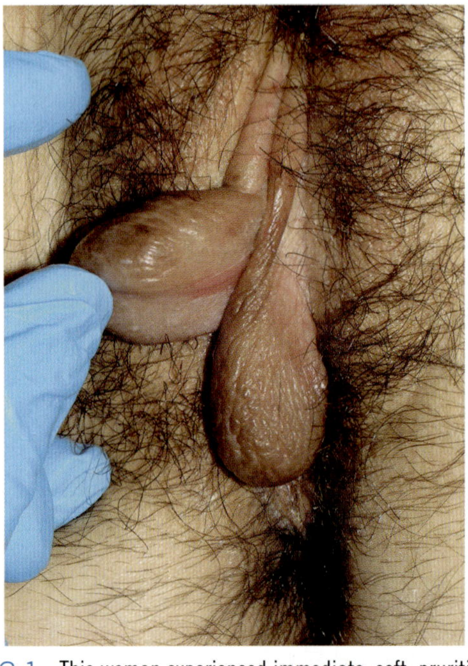

Fig. 12-1. This woman experienced immediate, soft, pruritic angioedema of the labia minora during sexual activity, with no systemic symptoms.

## Acute Genital Edema (Angioedema)

Genital edema is most often associated with an allergic reaction, either to a topically applied agent or to a systemic allergen in a sensitized patient. Genitalia affected with angioedema related to an allergic reaction normally begins quickly and then resolves over hours to days, returning to normal between each episode.

### Immunoglobulin E–Mediated Acute Edema

Type I hypersensitivity reactions are the most dangerous and important cause of acute genital edema. Patients with these immunoglobulin E (IgE)-mediated reactions risk the possibility of a systemic response and anaphylaxis. Latex and semen are the most common causes of this reaction in the genitalia.

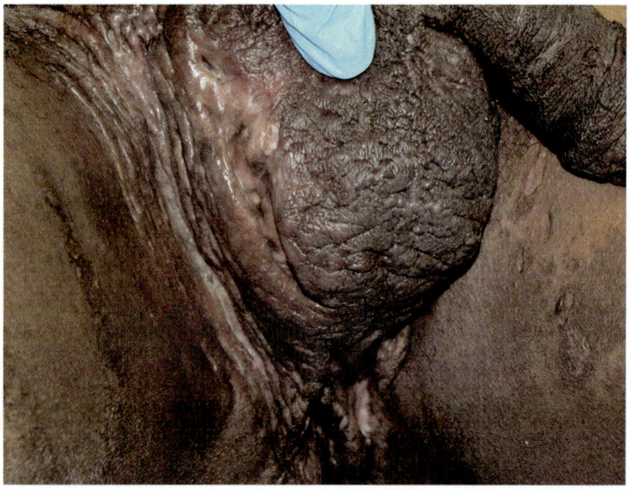

Fig. 12-2. Firm, nonpitting, stable, asymptomatic lymphedema is often associated with hidradenitis suppurativa.

### Latex Allergy

Latex has become a well-known cause of important allergic reactions, fortunately leading to near elimination of latex gloves and other latex sources in most health care environments. Up to 7.6% of the general population has a latex allergy, depending upon frequency of exposure and the presence of atopy.[1]

Although contact dermatitis with scaling and eczematous change is the most common skin reaction to latex in a sensitized patient, contact urticaria with edema and itching can also occur, and is relevant to this discussion. Occasionally, these patients can develop systemic reactions including anaphylaxis. Often, patients with type I hypersensitivity reaction to latex also report sensitivities to fruit, including banana and avocado.

The diagnosis is made on the basis of prick skin tests and serologic measurement of specific IgE. These patients should be managed by an allergist. Patient education and avoidance of latex is paramount; these patients should be aware of the possibility of latex in condoms, diaphragms, and other genital devices. Immunotherapy has been used, and the biologic omalizumab has shown promise.[2]

### Semen Allergy

IgE-mediated hypersensitivity to semen (seminal plasma) is probably an underdiagnosed condition, affecting as many as 40 000 women in the United States.[3] Hypersensitivity to the prostate-associated antigen has been reported as the culprit.[4]

Women can experience either localized or systemic reactions, with systemic reactions due to IgE hypersensitivity and localized due to a different immunologic phenomena.[5] Symptoms begin with vaginal discomfort and, in the case of a systemic reaction, are followed by wheezing, urticaria, shortness of breath, angioedema, gastrointestinal symptoms, and sometimes anaphylaxis.[4] Interestingly, about half of cases of localized reactions occur at first coitus. One study has noted cross-reactivity of an antigen found in male dog dander with the prostate-associated antigen, perhaps explaining this.[6]

The diagnosis is made clinically, when symptoms occur soon after intercourse, and are prevented with use of a condom. Edema following sexual activity can also occur in a setting of candidiasis, even very mild subclinical candidiasis, and following prolonged or traumatic intercourse causing an irritant reaction.

### Other Allergic Reactions

Genital edema that occurs as a result of most other IgE-mediated allergic reactions is accompanied by systemic signs, including, at times, anaphylaxis. Other than antihistamines and epinephrine, these require input and management by an allergist.

Genital edema sometimes is related to topically applied agents as a result of a type IV cell–mediated immune response. Although this usually produces a contact dermatitis with eczematous morphology, rare cases of anaphylaxis have been reported with some topical medications including neomycin and bacitracin. Unlike immediate IgE-mediated reactions, these are delayed by many hours following exposure, show more redness, and are accompanied by eczematous change. Contact dermatitis and its causes are discussed primarily in Chapter 5.

## Bradykinin Pathway–Mediated Acute Edema

Bradykinin-mediated angioedema is a rare disease, due to vasodilation and increased vascular permeability resulting from bradykinin. There is no urticaria or skin rash, and neither antihistamines nor corticosteroids are useful. This most commonly affects the abdominal and upper airways, and genital involvement occurs in only a small number of patients. This condition occurs due to an excess of bradykinin, occurring most often in patients receiving angiotensin-converting enzyme inhibitors but also in patients with C1 inhibitor deficiency leading to hereditary angioedema.[7] Management consists, obviously, of discontinuation of any causative medication, and perhaps icatibant, a bradykinin B2 receptor antagonist, in angiotensin-converting enzyme–associated disease. Recent literature does not support its use in hereditary disease.[8]

## Acute Genital Edema Related to Infection

Infection can produce genital edema. The most common infections to do this include bacterial infection, especially cellulitis, candidiasis in women, and epididymitis in men. Cellulitis is characterized by edema, erythema, and pain, often accompanied by fever and an elevated white blood count (Fig. 12-3). Risk factors include immunosuppression,

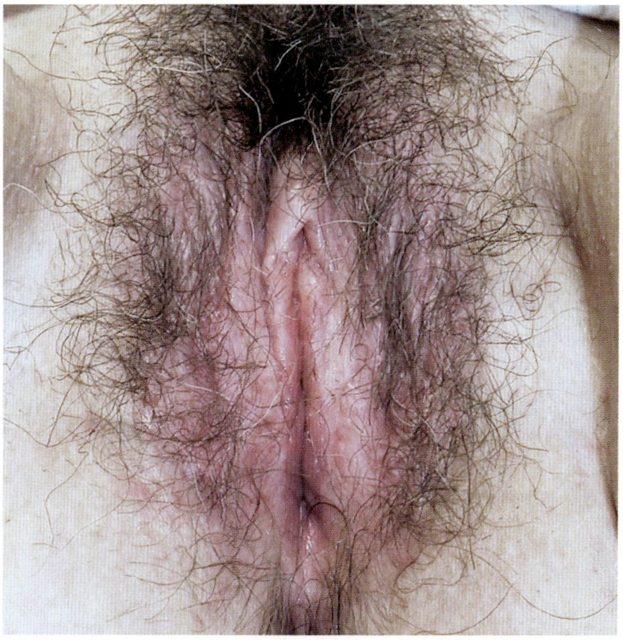

Fig. 12-3. This woman has developed cellulitis, manifested by the acute onset of edema, erythema, and pain.

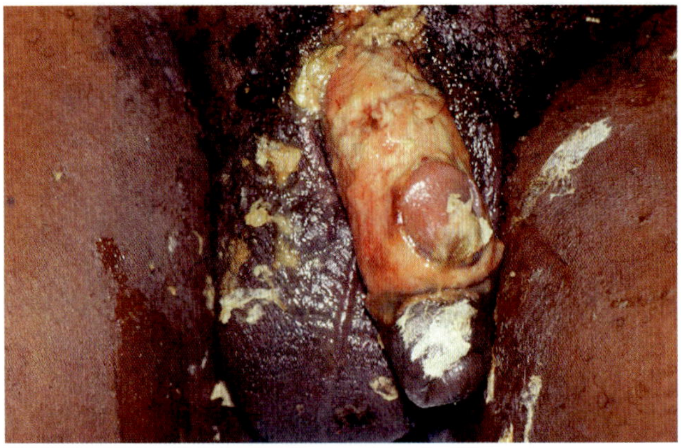

Fig. 12-4. Fournier gangrene (necrotizing fasciitis) refers to bacterial infection that has progressed to deep tissue necrosis, obliterating blood vessels and interrupting the blood supply to the area; this causes edema and sloughing, generally resulting in a catastrophic outcome without early intervention.

skin diseases that produce fissures and erosions, diabetes, and liver/kidney disease. The diagnosis is made clinically and confirmed by blood cultures, wound cultures when there are appropriate sites to culture, and response to treatment. Patients who are ill with more severe constitutional should be evaluated for a necrotizing deep tissue infection (Fournier gangrene, necrotizing fasciitis). This necrosis prevents the delivery of antibiotics to the area of infection, and this is a life-threatening emergency requiring urgent surgical debridement **(Fig. 12-4)**.

Candidiasis often produces puffiness of the modified mucous membranes of the vulva, but rarely, subclinical candidiasis is responsible for immediate and remarkable immediate edema with intercourse. Occasionally, even a culture is negative but ongoing suppression with once or twice weekly fluconazole prevents the edema.

Epididymitis is characterized by redness, pain, and edema of the scrotum, usually one-sided. This is most likely produced by gonorrhea or chlamydia in young men, or spread from a urinary tract infection or prostatitis in older men.

### Acute Genital Edema Related to Trauma

Clearly, trauma can produce edema or deep contusions, but these are usually recognized. However, hair can rarely twist around the clitoris or glans penis and gradually produce strangulation and edema. Long-distance bicycle riding can produce unrecognized trauma and edema. Peritoneal dialysis and paracentesis are sometimes associated with acute edema, and vulvar edema is well known to occur during late pregnancy and following delivery.

### Idiopathic Acute Scrotal Edema

This condition occurs primarily in boys and adolescents, with 60%-90% younger than 10 years of age.[9] Children present with sudden painless edema and redness of the scrotum, bilateral or unilateral. The main diseases to be considered in the differential diagnosis are epididymitis and testicular torsion. The condition clears without treatment over 2 or 3 days. Diagnosis consists of the exclusion of more important diseases; Doppler shows equal blood supply to both testicles, and ultrasound shows homogeneity of the testicular parenchyma.[9] Although rare, this can occur in adults as well, and ultrasound and a careful examination may avoid unnecessary surgery.[10]

## Chronic Genital Edema (Elephantiasis)

Chronic edema occurs when there is disruption of lymphatic drainage; this can occur as a result of tumor, surgery, infection, radiation, infection, structural abnormalities, etc. Occasionally, there is no known cause. Although lymphedema of some areas of the body, such as the legs, can be somewhat managed with compression, chronic edema of the genital area is rarely successfully treated.

### Chronic Edema Related to Congenital Abnormalities

Primary lymphangioma circumscriptum is a congenital vascular abnormality of lymphatic vessels manifested by grouped, sturdy vesicles that represent lymphatic vessels pushing up through the skin. These usually contain clear fluid but occasionally bloody fluid where the underlying lymphatic vessels connect with blood vessels. This malformation may or may not be associated with local edema. Treatment is difficult, since destruction or removal of the superficial vesicles is regularly followed by recurrence because the underlying malformation persists. There have been some recent case reports of benefit from topical sirolimus 0.1%, an inhibitor of angiogenesis.[11]

### Chronic Edema Secondary to Surgery and Radiation Therapy

Surgery, particularly when extensive for malignant tumors or the pelvis, lower abdomen, anogenital skin, and inguinal areas, can result in scarring that promotes edema **(Fig. 12-5)**. Radiation also can result in scarring and edema, but the combination is even especially problematic. Then, the resulting edema is a focus for recurrent cellulitis, which results in increasing scarring and edema with each occurrence (see below).

A well-recognized complication occurring in some of these patients with chronic edema associated with surgery and radiation for malignancy is the development of secondary lymphangioma circumscriptum (more properly called lymphangiectasias). In this condition, the pressure of the edema obstructs lymphatic drainage, which then distend and push above the surface of the skin, again

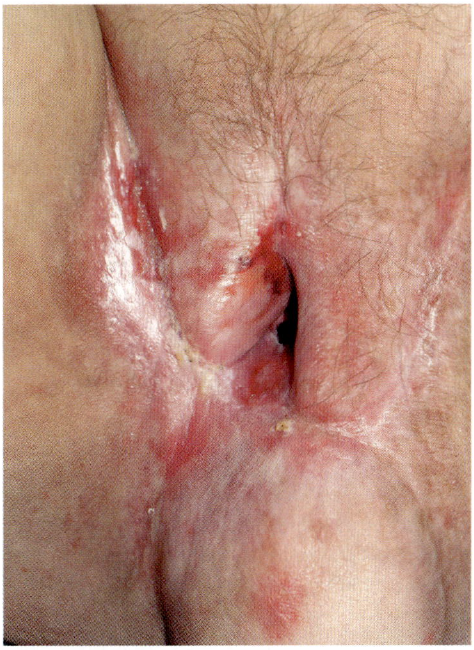

Fig. 12-5. Edema and scarring have been caused by repeated surgery as well as radiation for vulvar squamous cell carcinomas associated with lichen sclerosus.

appearing as vesicles, as seen with primary lymphangioma circumscriptum (Fig. 12-6). Although most common in this group, it can occur in any patient with chronic edema, especially that produced by with Crohn disease and hidradenitis suppurativa (Figs. 12-7 and 12-8). Although these vesicles are fairly tough and not easily denuded, they thin as they enlarge and are sometimes ruptured by

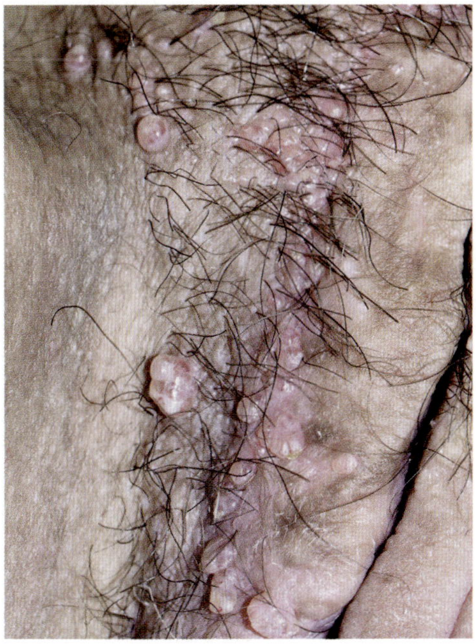

Fig. 12-6. Past surgery and radiation for cervical carcinoma have produced edema that has obstructed lymphatic return, so that lymph vessels have become distended and protruded above the surface of the skin, forming lymphangiectasias that mimic vesicles.

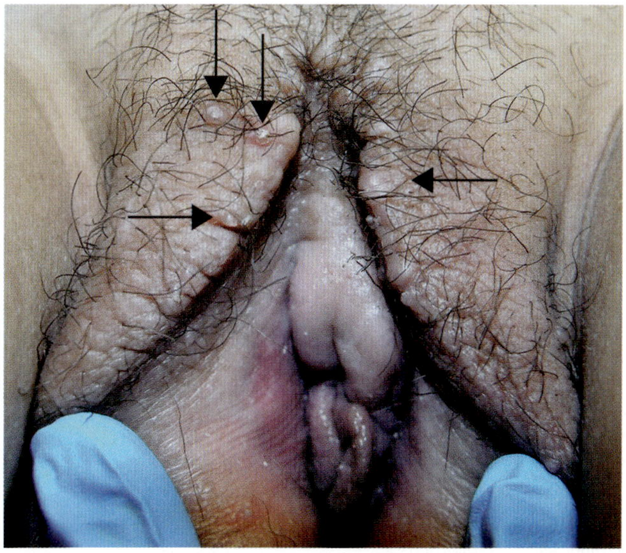

Fig. 12-7. This patient with Crohn disease shows marked edema that includes the clitoral hood, and there are lymphangiectasias on the hair-bearing verge of the labia majora (*arrows*).

the friction that normally occurs on genital skin, resulting in annoying and irritating drainage. Unlike usual blisters, these lesions are extensions of lymphatic vessels, so there is endless weeping. As is true for primary lymphangioma circumscriptum, treatment regularly results in recurrence. However, electrocautery or laser destruction can produce temporary ablation. In the author experience, the less elegant electrocautery may be more useful, perhaps by producing thicker surface scar that impedes the prompt recurrence of lymphangiectasias. Sclerotherapy and excision are sometimes used as well. In the past 3 years, there have been case reports of resection of these genital lymphangiectasias in combination with lymphaticovenous anastomosis decreasing the recurrence rate.[12] This surgical method redirects excess lymphatic fluid into

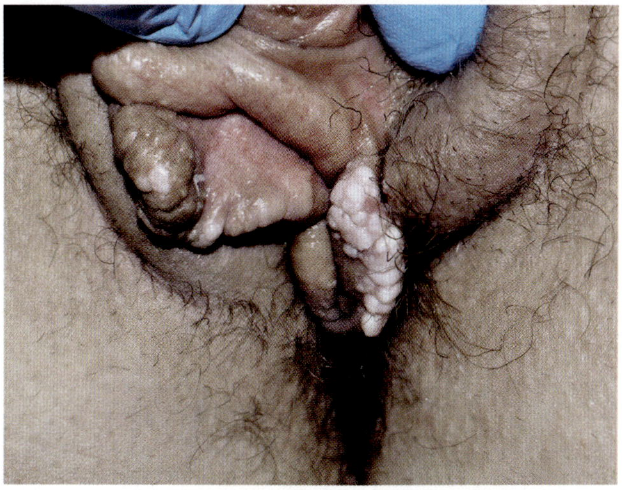

Fig. 12-8. Chronic edema has resulted in lymphangiectasias (also called secondary lymphangioma circumscriptum), here filled with cloudy white lymph fluid).

the venous system, relieving the pressure within lymphatics. Obviously, any control of the underlying cause of the edema is also important when possible.

## Chronic Edema Related to Infection

A patient who experiences genital (and leg) cellulitis, whether as a result of surgery, skin disease, or risk factors, is at risk for recurrent infection and increasing permanent edema with each episode **(Figs. 12-9 and 12-10)**. At times, cellulitis occurs with no obvious precipitating factors or portal of entry. And, the presence of preexisting lymphedema is known to be a risk factor for cellulitis.[13] There is some evidence that edema interferes with the immune response,[14] and the cellulitis and its attendant inflammation cause more sclerosis, more edema, and subsequent higher risk of infection, so that a vicious cycle ensues. These infections are regularly produced by group A *Streptococcus*, and there is evidence that *Streptococcus* can sequester within cells, possibly an additional explanation for the high rate of recurrence of cellulitis.[15] The area becomes red and somewhat tender, but constitutional signs are often mild and the patient may not be aware of the infection initially. The infection often cannot be documented, as blood cultures are generally negative and there is no open wound to culture. The infection usually responds quickly to antibiotics, but further damage and sclerosis has already occurred. Suppressive antibiotics have long been used for prophylaxis of recurrent cellulitis. A recent Cochrane review reported that studies evaluating oral erythromycin or penicillin as antibiotic prophylaxis in patients with cellulitis of the arms or legs found a decreased risk of cellulitis recurrence by 69%; the certainty of evidence was rated as moderate.[16] When antibiotics were discontinued, patients again experienced recurrence of their cellulitis. Oral or intramuscular long-acting benzathine G penicillin as prophylaxis is substantiated by data extrapolated from recurrent cellulitis of the extremities and our own experience.[17]

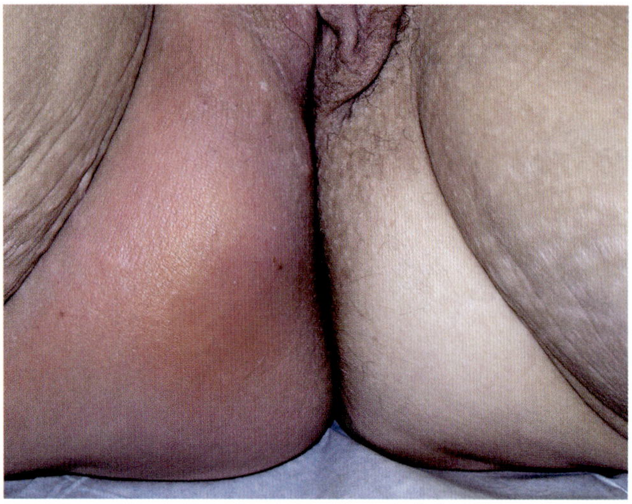

Fig. 12-10. This woman has chronic lymphedema, which is worsened with each episode of recurrent cellulitis, occurring at least partly due to her selective immunoglobulin deficiency.

Although streptococcus is the usual cause of infectious edema in Western countries, other infections should be considered in different parts of the world **(Fig. 12-11)**. Filariasis is a classic cause of elephantiasis of the legs and male genitalia in tropical areas, produced by the nematode *Wuchereria bancrofti*. Lymphogranuloma venereum, produced by *Chlamydia trachomatis*, and granuloma inguinale, caused

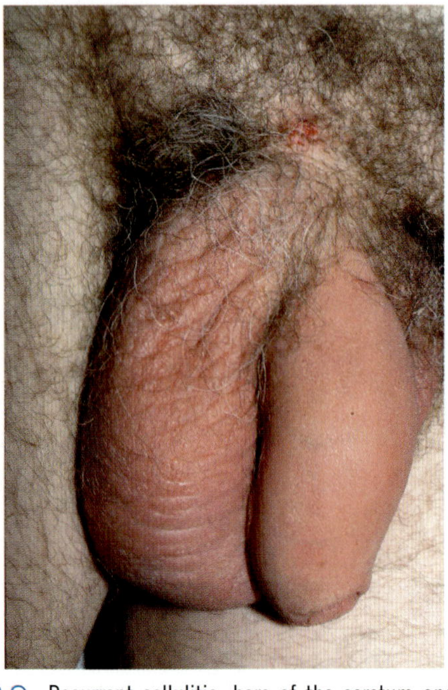

Fig. 12-9. Recurrent cellulitis, here of the scrotum and penis, is usually due to *Streptococcus pyogenes*.

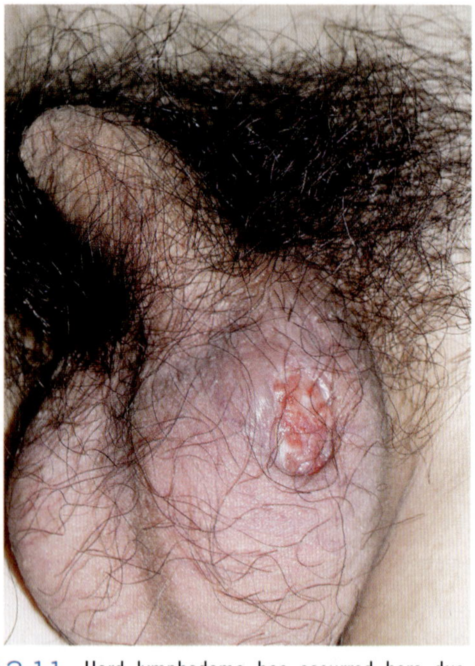

Fig. 12-11. Hard lymphedema has occurred here due to long-standing infection with tuberculosis.

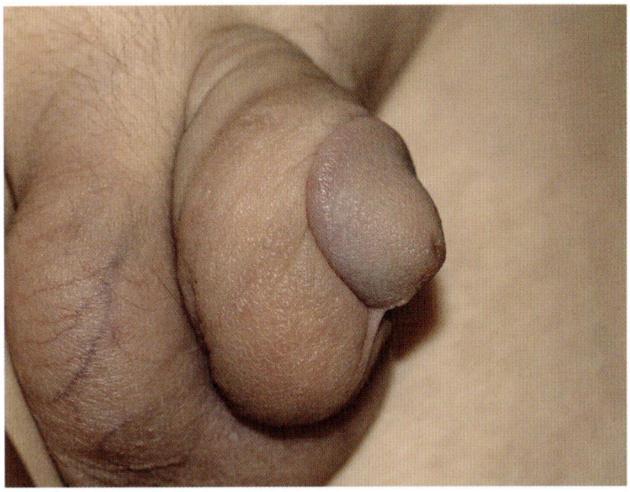

Fig. 12-12. Soft, chronic edema associated with Crohn disease that worsens just before each infliximab infusion, with short-term partial resolution after the treatment.

by *Klebsiella granulomatis*, are also well known but rare causes of chronic genital edema in Western countries.

## Chronic Edema due to Noninfectious Inflammation

Although any chronic or recurrent inflammation can theoretically produce edema, Crohn disease and hidradenitis suppurativa (**Figs. 12-12 to 12-15**) are relatively common diseases famous for causing this finding, likely because each is associated with inflammation that affects the deeper tissues (see Chapters 11 and 6). Sarcoidosis also causes chronic edema, but this condition is rarely found in anogenital skin. However, a biopsy shows granulomas that could be confused with the granulomas of Crohn disease. Ruptured inflamed cysts of hidradenitis suppurativa also sometimes show a granulomatous foreign body reaction to keratinous cyst contents. Finally, orofacial granulomatosis (Melkersson-Rosenthal syndrome), yet another condition associated with chronic oral and, rarely, genital edema, is also associated with histologic findings of granulomatous inflammation (see below). These conditions must be differentiated on clinical grounds and findings other than histology.

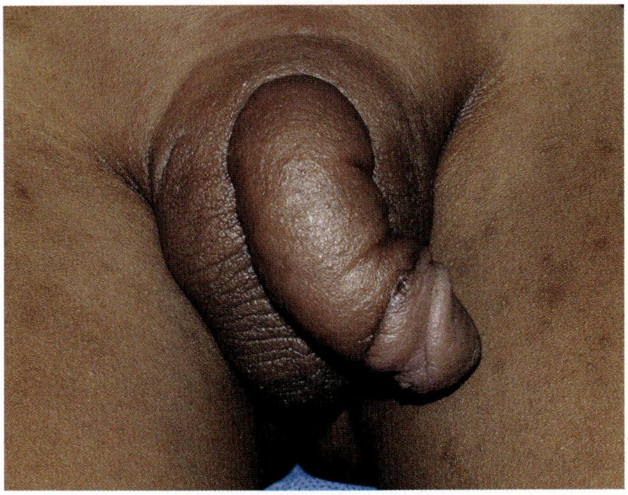

Fig. 12-13. Crohn disease is a classic cause of genital edema; this is sometimes disfiguring, and this child has undergone debulking and plastic surgery of the penis, with recurrence of the edema.

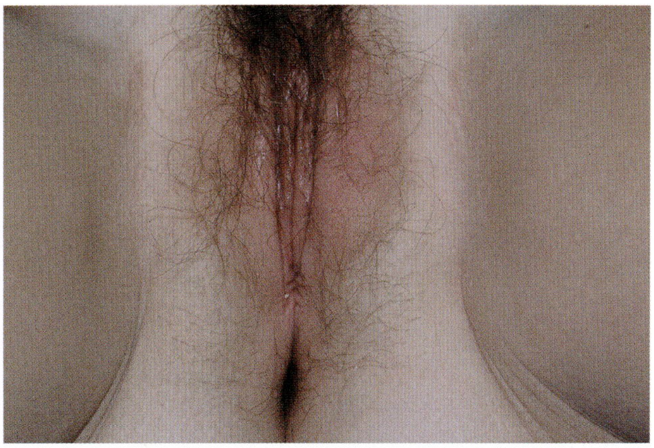

Fig. 12-14. The edema of Crohn disease can be subtle.

We have also seen chronic edema uncommonly associated with lichen simplex chronicus, psoriasis, and lichen planus.

## Idiopathic Chronic Genital Edema

### Orofacial Granulomatosis (Melkersson-Rosenthal Syndrome)

At times, there is no obvious underlying, definable condition producing the chronic edema. Melkersson-Rosenthal syndrome is such a disease of unknown cause that occasionally affects genital skin. This disease was originally described as a syndrome involving the triad of granulomatous swelling of the lip (usually unilateral), lingua plicata (fissured or folded tongue), and facial nerve palsy. When only the granulomatous swelling of the lip is present, the finding is termed *Miescher cheilitis*. Melkersson-Rosenthal syndrome and Miescher cheilitis are very rare, and even more rare is

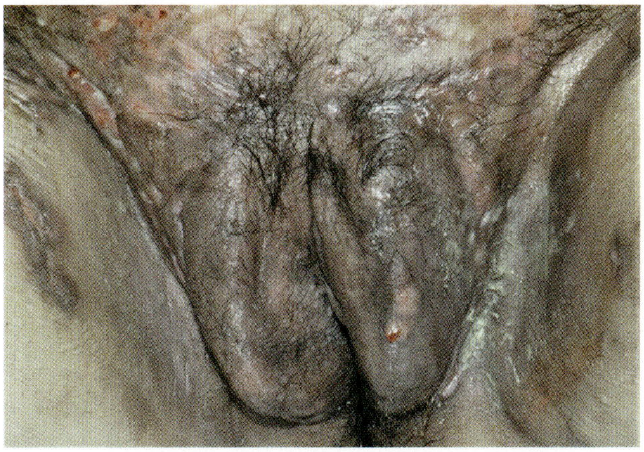

Fig. 12-15. Chronic, draining cysts have resulting in severe lymphedema of the vulva in this patient with hidradenitis suppurativa. Even mild HS occasionally produces marked edema.

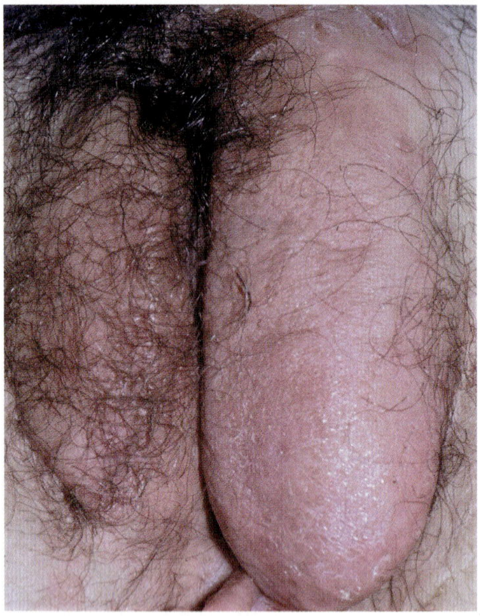

Fig. 12-16. This 14-year-old girl was asymptomatic with her very firm edema and was diagnosed with Melkersson-Rosenthal syndrome when an evaluation for inflammatory bowel disease was negative. Two years later, she developed severe Crohn disease.

an identical picture of granulomatous edema of the genitalia.[18] There are very few reported cases of idiopathic genital granulomatous inflammation, and most have developed Crohn disease.[19,20] Therefore, idiopathic genital edema that shows granulomatous changes on biopsy should be evaluated for Crohn disease and sarcoidosis, and followed with subsequent evaluations for these conditions in the event of negative results **(Fig. 12-16)**. In the meantime, the diagnosis of Melkersson-Rosenthal syndrome can be assigned.

There is no good treatment for Melkersson-Rosenthal. Corticosteroids are useful, but the benefit of topical therapy is limited. Intralesional triamcinolone (Chapter 4) can be useful in orofacial granulomatosis, and 1-week bursts of prednisone with 2 weeks of tapering are used for facial disease as well. Doxycycline, methotrexate, hydroxychloroquine, clofazimine, dapsone, and metronidazole have also been used.[21] More recently, anti-tumor necrosis factor alpha biologic agents adalimumab and infliximab have been used for facial disease according to case reports.[21]

## Localized Lymphedema

Localized lymphedema was originally described as massive localized lymphedema and was regularly associated with obesity.[22] This occurs on the genitalia and on the lower legs and is described as elephantiasis **(Fig. 12-17)**. More recently, smaller lesions, particularly in the genital area, have been described.[23,24] These have been mostly on the vulva but also on the scrotum and penis, and range from 1 to 30 cm, but mostly between 2 and 5 cm. The appearance is variable and often described as nodular,

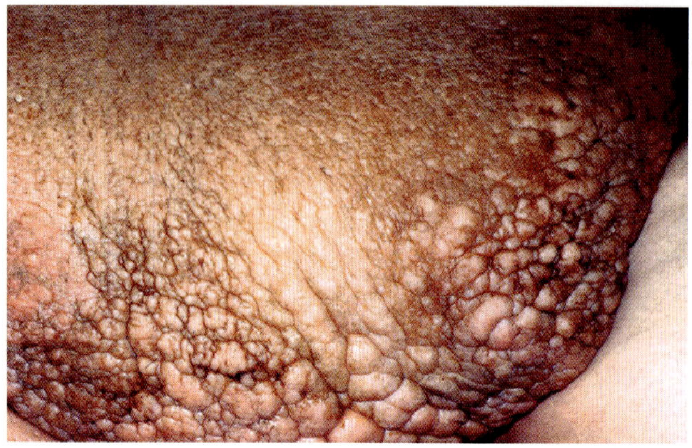

Fig. 12-17. This obese man has massive localized lymphedema, with the typical verrucous changes.

warty, hyperkeratotic, or with cauliflowerlike masses that can be mistaken for genital warts.

Although the cause is unknown, most patients, like those with massive localized lymphedema, are obese, often morbidly obese. Crohn disease was present in some, and cellulitis was operative in a minority, likely contributing to a lymphedema-associated immune suppression **(Figs. 12-18 and 12-19)**.[14]

Microscopically, tissue shows dermal edema, dilated lymphatics, and fibroplasia, with acanthosis and hyperkeratosis generally also present. The cause is unknown, but some postulate that fat lobules produce obstruction to lymphatic flow. The primary management is surgical, with recurrence surprisingly low.

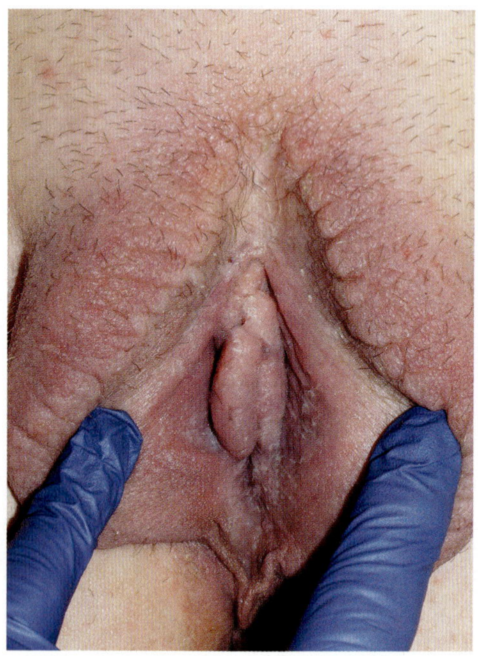

Fig. 12-18. Smaller lesions of localized lymphedema are fairly common, and although these are most common in obese patients, they can occur with other causes of edema, as in this patient with Crohn disease who has developed nodules of localized lymphedema at the hair-bearing verge of the labia minora.

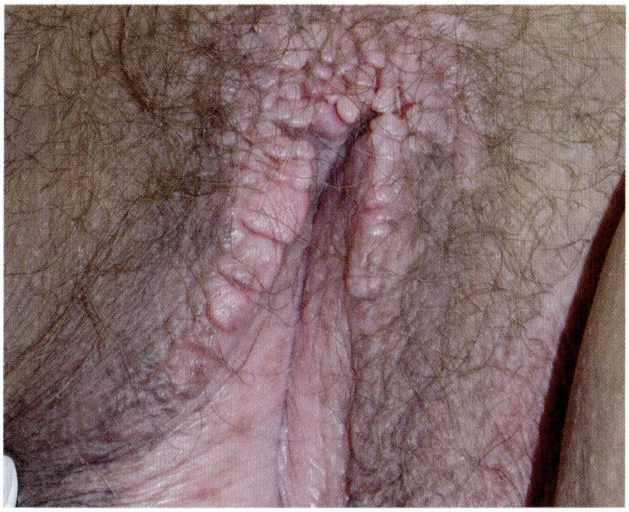

Fig. 12-19. These nodules of localized lymphedema are associated with lichen planus.

## REFERENCES


1. Kahn SL, Podjasek JO, Dimitropoulos VA, Brown CW. Natural rubber latex allergy. *Dis Mon.* 2016;62:5-17.
2. Parisi CAS, et al. Update on latex allergy: new insights into an old problem. *World Allergy Organ J.* 2021;14:100569. doi:10.1016/j.waojou.2021.100569
3. Sublett JW, Bernstein JA. Seminal plasma hypersensitivity reactions: an updated review. *Mt Sinai J Med.* 2011;78:803-809.
4. Konradsen JR, Borres MP, Nilsson C. Unusual and unexpected allergic reactions can be unraveled by molecular allergy diagnostics. *Int Arch Allergy Immunol.* 2021;182:904-916. doi:10.1159/000515708
5. Lavery WJ, Stevenson M, Bernstein JA. An overview of seminal plasma hypersensitivity and approach to treatment. *J Allergy Clin Immunol Pract.* 2020;8:2937-2942. doi:10.1016/j.jaip.2020.04.067
6. Basagana M, Bartolome B, Pastor C, et al. Allergy to human seminal fluid: cross-reactivity with dog dander. *J Allergy Clin Immunol.* 2008;121:233-239.
7. Lepelley M, Bernardeau C, Defendi F, Crochet J, Mallaret M, Bouillet L. Update on bradykinin-mediated angioedema in 2020. *Therapie.* 2020;75:195-205. doi:10.1016/j.therap.2020.02.011
8. Cai G, Barber C, Kalicinsky C. Review of icatibant use in the Winnipeg Regional Health Authority. *Allergy Asthma Clin Immunol.* 2020;16:96. doi:10.1186/s13223-020-00493-3
9. Patoulias D, Rafailidis V, Feidantsis T, Kalogirou M, Rafailidis D, Patoulias I. Fountain's sign as a diagnostic key in acute idiopathic scrotal edema: case report and review of the literature. *Acta Medica (Hradec Kralove).* 2018;61:37-39. doi:10.14712/18059694.2018.22
10. Tan LR, Liu Z, Leow JJ, Chong YL. Acute idiopathic scrotal edema in the adult: a case report. *Urol Case Rep.* 2019;28:101014. doi:10.1016/j.eucr.2019.101014
11. Leducq S, et al.; Groupe de Recherche de la Société Française de Dermatologie Pédiatrique. Topical sirolimus 0.1% for treating cutaneous microcystic lymphatic malformations in children and adults (TOPICAL): protocol for a multicenter phase 2, within-person, randomized, double-blind, vehicle-controlled clinical trial. *Trials.* 2019;20:739. doi:10.1186/s13063-019-3767-8
12. Hara H, Mihara M. Treating and preventing recurrence of recurrent genital acquired lymphangiectasia using lymphaticovenous anastomosis at genital area: a case report. *Microsurgery.* 2020;40:399-403. doi:10.1002/micr.30552
13. Vignes S, Poizeau F, Dupuy A. Cellulitis risk factors for patients with primary or secondary lymphedema. *J Vasc Surg Venous Lymphat Disord.* 2022;10:179-185.e1. doi:10.1016/j.jvsv.2021.04.009
14. Carlson JA. Lymphedema and subclinical lymphostasis (microlymphedema) facilitate infection, inflammatory dermatoses, and neoplasia; a locus minoris residentiae. *Clin Dermatol.* 2014;32:599-615.
15. Jendoubi F, Rohde M, Prinz JC. Intracellular streptococcal uptake and persistence: a potential cause of erysipelas recurrence. *Front Med (Lausanne).* 2019;6:6. doi:10.3389/fmed.2019.00006
16. Dalal A, et al. Interventions for the prevention of recurrent erysipelas and cellulitis. *Cochrane Database Syst Rev.* 2017;(6):CD009758. doi:10.1002/14651858.CD009758.pub2
17. Olszewski WL, Zaleska MT. Long-term benzathine penicillin prophylaxis lasting for years effectively prevents recurrence of dermato-lymphangio-adenitis (cellulitis) in limb lymphedema. *Lymphat Res Biol.* 2021;19:545-552. doi:10.1089/lrb.2020.0051
18. Chu Z, Liu Y, Zhang H, Zeng W, Geng S. Melkersson-Rosenthal syndrome with genitalia involved in a 12-year-old boy. *Ann Dermatol.* 2016;28:232-236.
19. Murphy MJ, Kogan B, Carlson JA. Granulomatous lymphangitis of the scrotum and penis. Report of a case and review of the literature of genital swelling with sarcoidal granulomatous inflammation. *J Cutan Pathol.* 2001;28:419-424.
20. Lloyd DA, Payton KB, Guenther L, Frydman W. Melkersson-Rosenthal syndrome and Crohn's disease: one disease or two? Report of a case and discussion of the literature. *J Clin Gastroenterol.* 1994;18:213-217.
21. Dhawan SR, Saini AG, Singhi PD. Management strategies of Melkersson-Rosenthal Syndrome: a review. *Int J Gen Med.* 2020;13:61-65.
22. Maclellan RA, Zurakowski D, Grant FD, Greene AK. Massive localized lymphedema: a case-control study. *J Am Coll Surg.* 2017;224:212-216.
23. Lu S, Tran TA, Jones DM, et al. Localized lymphedema (elephantiasis): a case series and review of the literature. *J Cutan Pathol.* 2009;36:1-20.
24. Plaza JA, Requena L, Kazakow DV, et al. Verrucous localized lymphedema of genital areas: clinicopathologic report of 18 cases of this rare entity. *J Am Acad Dermatol.* 2014;71:320-326.


## SUGGESTED READINGS


Dhawan SR, Saini AG, Singhi PD. Management strategies of Melkersson-Rosenthal syndrome: a review. *Int J Gen Med.* 2020;13:61-65.

Kokcu A, Sari S, Kefeli M. Primary vulvar lymphangioma circumscriptum: a case report and review of literature. *J Low Genit Tract Dis.* 2015;19:e1-e5.

Parisi CAS, et al. Update on latex allergy: new insights into an old problem. *World Allergy Organ J.* 2021;14:100569.

# Pruritus and Pain 13

PETER J. LYNCH AND LIBBY EDWARDS

## Pruritus

Pruritus (itch) is an uncomfortable sensation that provokes the urge to scratch. This does not necessarily mean that the patient is actively scratching; pruritus only provokes the urge to scratch. This depends upon the cause of itching, which exists on a spectrum, as well as the genetic and psychological makeup of the person involved. Atopic dermatitis/eczema is regularly associated with scratching; scratching produces intense pleasure, and the skin findings of atopic dermatitis are produced by the rubbing and scratching. Urticaria/hives is often associated with only modest scratching; scratching is not pleasurable, and scratching produces immediate worsening of the hives. And, aquagenic pruritus produces more of a prickling, stinging itch that generally does not induce scratching. There are several common mistakes made in describing and writing about pruritus. First, the correct spelling is prurit***us***, not prurit***is***, because this sensation does not indicate inflammation. Second, many confuse the word "itch" with the word "scratch." One scratches his skin, one does not itch it. Pruritus specific to the anogenital region has been recently reviewed.[1]

Pruritus is generally classified into four groups based on neuropathophysiology: (1) *pruriceptive pruritus* (itching arising in the context of recognizable skin disorders); (2) *neuropathic pruritus* (itching occurring due to damage of neurons of the peripheral or central nervous system by orthopedic issues such as entrapment, metabolic factors such as diabetes, neurogenerative factors, infections such as herpes zoster, and malignant tumors); (3) *neurogenic pruritus* (itching arising as a result of central stimulation secondary to systemic disease and occurring in the absence of skin disease); and (4) *psychogenic pruritus* (itching arising as a result of psychological factors). However, there may be considerable overlap; psychological factors can at least exacerbate if not serve as a primary factor in each of these groups, and there seems to be interactions between the immune system and cutaneous nerves in neurogenic itching.[2-5]

Pruritus, of course, is a symptom, not a disease, but it is discussed below for the convenience of the clinician as though it is one condition, in the patient who presents with the complaint of itching.

### Clinical Presentation

*Pruriceptive* itching is covered with the individual mucocutaneous disorders as they are discussed throughout this book. *Neuropathic* itching is localized mostly to areas outside the anogenital areas (eg, notalgia paresthetica, brachioradial pruritus), but pruritus can occur in the genital region with disorders such as postherpetic neuralgia, other small fiber neuropathies, and itching within scars as a result of reinnervation of the scar tissue. *Neurogenic* pruritus tends to be generalized and therefore may affect the anogenital region. This type of pruritus often occurs with medications such as opiates and with disorders such as Hodgkin lymphoma, chronic hepatobiliary diseases (especially in the presence of cholestasis), polycythemia vera, and other myeloproliferative disorders. *Psychogenic* pruritus occurs in patients with conditions such as obsessive-compulsive disorders and those with prurigo nodularis and delusions of parasitosis.

Regardless of cause, the presence of pruritus (especially if it is accompanied by scratching) leads to a greatly diminished quality of life (QoL), disturbance of sleep patterns, and very often leads to the development of, or worsening of, depression and anxiety.[6,7] Scratching while the person is unaware of doing so is common during daytime scratching and is also common during scratching that occurs at night, especially in the lighter stages of non-REM sleep.[8]

### Diagnosis

Identifying the cause of pruritus occurring in the *presence* of skin lesions depends on the clinician's morphologic identification of the associated cutaneous disorder. The general approach to doing so is described in Chapter 3. When the abnormality is identified, the clinician can locate it within the pages of this or other similar textbooks, and take necessary steps to confirm the diagnosis.

However, the identification of the cause of itching in the *absence* of skin disease is much more difficult. A detailed patient history, a complete physical examination, and appropriate laboratory testing is required. This process is nicely detailed in the 2016 excellent review article by Pereira et al.[9] Since most of the readers of this text will primarily be treating patients who have skin lesions, and since the material on history, examination, and laboratory testing is long and detailed, I will refer the reader who requires this information directly to their publication.

## Pathophysiology

Neurogenic and psychogenic pruritus, itching of central origin, is poorly understood, whereas the mechanisms of itching occurring at the peripheral level (pruritoceptive and neuropathic pruritus) are better known. For these latter types of pruritus, there are many similarities (and, of course, some dissimilarities) between the pathophysiology of pruritus and pain.[2,3] Most of the material on pathophysiology contained in the paragraphs that follow is based on a recent comprehensive review article.[3]

### Peripheral Nerve Pathways

Nociceptors are cutaneous nerves that receive and transmit pain, made up of narrow diameter, lightly myelinated type Aδ fibers. However, pruriceptors are cutaneous nerves that receive and transmit itching, made of very thin diameter, unmyelinated type C fibers. The pruriceptor fibers represent a quite small subset of the nociceptor fibers. Whether or not there are specific C fibers that carry itch, but not pain, remains controversial. The cell bodies of these pain and itch-related nerves are located in the dorsal root ganglia of the spinal cord and their axons terminate in the papillary dermis and intercalate in between the cells of the epidermis.

### Mediators and Receptors

Approximately 20 mediators and mediator-receptors have been identified. The best known mediator is histamine, which acts on H1 and H4 receptors. The remainder of the mediators are nonhistamine dependent and some of the better known include proteases, substance P, calcitonin gene-related peptide, and bradykinin. The opioids are a special case. They act on μ and κ receptors; opioids that are μ antagonists and those that are κ agonists decrease itching whereas μ agonists increase itching. An increase in mast cells, which elaborate histamine in addition to other mediators, have been identified in central and peripheral causes of pruritus as well as in itching associated with specific skin diseases.[4]

## Central Pathways

The peripheral C fibers terminate in the dorsal root ganglia and the itch sensation is then transmitted to neurons expressing gastrin-releasing peptide receptors (GRPRs) that cross over to the contralateral side and ascend the spinothalamic tract to the thalamus. Interestingly, there are also itch-inhibiting neurons in the spinal cord. From the thalamus, neuronal signaling is transmitted to cortical and subcortical sensory regions of the brain. Chronicity of pruritus is believed to be related to impairment of the itch-inhibitory pathways as well as to the development of central sensitization in a manner similar to that which occurs in chronic pain.

## Management

The management of pruritus is much the same for all itching, no matter whether *pruriceptive, neuropathic, neurogenic, or psychogenic pruritus.* The basic principles of this approach are given detailed coverage in the section on eczematous and lichenified disease (see Chapter 5). However, there are several additional modalities for use in patients with noneczematous cutaneous disorders and for pruritus occurring in the absence of skin lesions.[3,8,10] In the *pruriceptive* group, greater emphasis can be placed on the use on both sedating and nonsedating antihistamines for urticaria and other itching disorders mediated by histamine. In the *neuropathic* group, the antiepileptics, pregabalin and gabapentin, can be used in the treatment of the itching that sometimes occurs with diabetic and postherpetic neuropathies. In the *neurogenic* group, mirtazapine, naltrexone, naloxone, aprepitant, and ultraviolet light phototherapy may be considered for the itching associated with chronic renal disease, hepatobiliary disease, polycythemia vera, leukemia, and lymphoma. In the *psychogenic* group, much can be gained with clinical psychological intervention as well as with placement of earlier and greater emphasis on psychotropic medications.

# Anogenital Pain

Generally, patients who present with a chief complain of genital itching suffer from different diseases than those who describe primarily pain. Of course, scratching can produce pain, but those individuals usually describe pruritus as their primary symptom and report that they scratch to the point of pain. Interestingly, some patients deny the presence of pain, but rather insist they have burning, rawness, irritation, stinging, tearing, soreness, stabbing, aching, or throbbing. For the purposes of this chapter, all of these characterizations of discomfort are discussed under the umbrella of pain. Also, some people report itching that does not produce a desire to scratch; with more questioning, they sometimes describe this as a tingling, prickling, or stinging itch. These sensations are usually characterized under pain as well, since the definition of itching is an unpleasant sensation *that provokes a desire to scratch.*

True itching is generally not included in the same differential diagnosis as pain, although there are several exceptions, notably lichen planus and atypical pain syndromes/neuropathy. Most *chronic* itching with scratching results from dermatoses. Chronic superficial burning,

**TABLE 13-1**

**Causes of Chronic Genital Pain**

*Infection*, especially herpes simplex infection, rubbed/scratched yeast infection, trichomonas, fissures with Candidiasis
*Dermatoses* (noninfectious skin disease), especially lichen planus, excoriated/eroded lichen simplex chronicus or lichen sclerosus, irritant contact dermatitis, benign mucous membrane pemphigoid, pemphigus vulgaris, desquamative inflammatory vaginitis, atrophic vaginitis, fissures unassociated with infection
*Malignancy*—most often squamous cell carcinoma, but also high-grade squamous intraepithelial neoplasia, differentiated intraepithelial neoplasia, Paget disease
*Trauma,* including surgical
*Estrogen deficiency* in women
*Neuropathy*, including diabetic neuropathy, postherpetic neuralgia, multiple sclerosis, pudendal neuralgia, herniated disc disease
*Vulvodynia, penodynia, scrotodynia, anodynia*—multifactorial pain syndromes

soreness, and pain, as distinct from pelvic pain, most often occurs from the anogenital pain syndromes vulvodynia, penodynia, scrotodynia, and anodynia, but erosive skin diseases, malignancy, neuropathy, and, in women, estrogen deficiency occur regularly (**Table 13-1**).

Vulvodynia, penodynia, scrotodynia, and anodynia represent chronic discomfort in the absence of relevant clinical abnormalities. Whereas there is abundant literature on vulvodynia, there is little written about male genital pain syndromes, so that most of what we know is extrapolated from experience with vulvodynia.

The evaluation of the patient with chronic anogenital pain is quite easy and straightforward, requiring only a few carefully chosen questions of history, a careful examination of the skin and, in women, a wet mount (see **Table 13-2**). The skin should be examined using simple magnification if needed. The patient with pain and visible erosions does not present a diagnostic dilemma. However, erosions can be subtle at times; vaginal and introital erosions can be missed in women, and fissures are overlooked easily in both men and women.

Many patients who report symptoms of burning, irritation, or rawness also report redness, and, often, edema. Men especially frequently describe texture changes or stickiness. Redness that is mild, poorly demarcated, and without scaling or thickening is frequently within the range of normal, but patients are not generally in agreement and insist that this is new for them (**Figs. 13-1 and 13-2**).

**TABLE 13-2**

**Evaluation of the Patient With Genital Pain**

History
- Symptoms—pain vs itch
- Presence of characteristic comorbidities, other pain syndromes
- Neurologic history; diabetic neuropathy, herpes zoster in the genital distribution
- Local care; agents applied to the genital skin include soaps, medications, pads/liners washing frequency, cleansers, etc.

Physical examination
- Evaluation of affect
- Gross neurologic examination for allodynia, numbness, paresthesias of the anogenital skin and proximal medial thighs.
- Examination of the external genitalia with magnification if required for subtle fissures, erosions, signs of any skin disease, scarring/agglutination, or other specific lesions
- Assessment of vaginal mucosa with small Pederson speculum for redness, erosions

Microscopic examination of vaginal secretions for signs of infection, inflammation, and estrogen deficiency (in addition to yeast forms, evaluation for white blood cells, parabasal cells, lack of lactobacilli)
Culture if examination is suspicious for infection
Biopsy of any specific skin lesion only; no biopsy required for nonspecific redness alone or of painful area in normal-appearing skin

Those patients who have no *relevant* observable skin disease other than unimportant redness, no infection, and no specific neurologic abnormality fall into the category of a genital pain syndrome: vulvodynia, penodynia, scrotodynia, or anodynia. Abnormalities that do not produce pain, such as anogenital warts or *Candida glabrata*, are not relevant and can be disregarded. Sometimes patients have an abnormality that can cause symptoms, such as lichen sclerosus, but discomfort is not in the area of the lichen sclerosus; this person may have lichen sclerosus and vulvodynia. Also, at times, patients present with objective skin disease or infection, but their discomfort is disproportionate to the degree of skin disease noted, or pain persists after the infection or skin disease is cleared. These patients have an underlying pain syndrome that is either unassociated with the skin disease or triggered by it. For example, lichen sclerosus and lichen planus are recognized by vulvologists as initiators for the development of vulvodynia (Presented at ISSVD World Congress, Paris, 2011). Therefore, the skin disease or

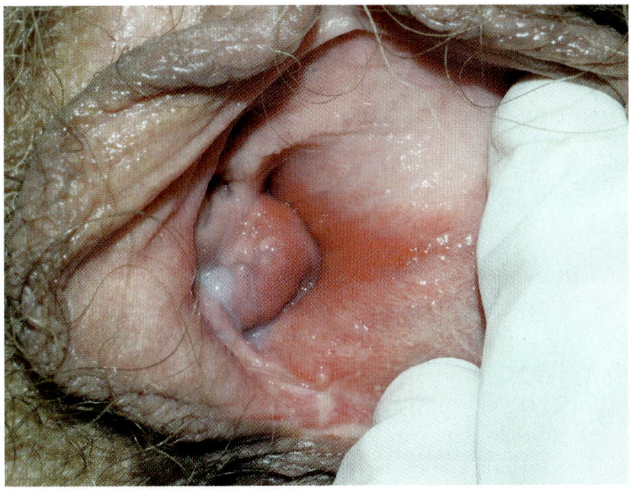

Fig. 13-1. The red patch in the vestibule, extending to the hymeneal caruncles, is characteristic of vestibulodynia and does not represent inflammation when compared to biopsies of the vestibule of asymptomatic women.

infection should be controlled, but a pain syndrome can be diagnosed and treated concomitantly.

Infection, skin disease, malignancy, trauma, estrogen deficiency (in women), neuropathy and pain syndromes are the usual causes of chronic genital pain (**Table 13-1**).

Many clinicians and most patients initially assume that genital pain (or itching) without obvious skin findings is due to *infection*, including yeast, bacterial vaginosis, or sexually transmitted disease. Chronic pain almost never occurs from infection in immunocompetent patients, and negative cultures and a lack of response to antimicrobial therapy also signifies a different diagnosis. Yeast, the most common cause implicated by patients and providers, usually is a pruritic rather than painful condition, and *C. albicans* clears, at least briefly, with therapy. Some postulate that an inflammatory response to low levels of yeast may cause pain.[11] Nonalbicans Candida is nearly always asymptomatic. Sexually transmitted diseases generally either do not cause superficial genital pain other than dysuria (gonorrhea, Chlamydia, warts) or they produce intermittent symptoms with visible skin findings (herpes simplex virus infection). However, trichomonas, particularly in women, certainly produces irritation and burning, although more often itching. These infections can be ruled out easily by molecular studies.

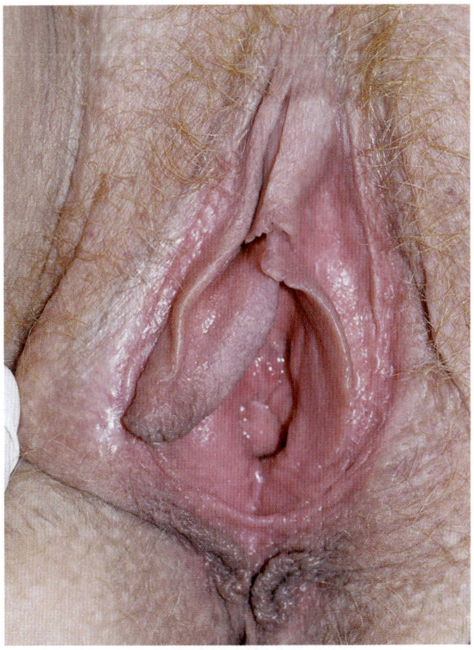

Fig. 13-2. The erythema of the modified mucous membranes of this red-headed woman is normal for her complexion but often is perceived as new and abnormal in women with vulvodynia.

Irritant contact dermatitis is the most common *skin disease* that causes symptoms of pain with irritation, rawness, or burning. Overwashing and medications (see Chapters 5 and 10) or strong irritants such as destructive therapies for warts that cause a chemical burn are common contactants. Allergic contact dermatitis produces itching more than burning and irritation. Lichen planus is an erosive skin disease, and one of the few that causes both itching and pain (Chapter 11). The blistering diseases pemphigus vulgaris and mucous membrane pemphigoid are painful (see Chapter 10). In women, erosive vaginal skin diseases produce a purulent vaginal discharge that causes an irritating contact dermatitis in the vestibule; these include lichen planus and mucosal immunobullous diseases (see Chapter 14). Abnormalities can be visualized.

*Malignancies* can produce ulcerations, especially late squamous cell carcinomas and melanoma, but squamous cell carcinoma *in situ* (high-grade squamous intraepithelial lesion, differentiated intraepithelial neoplasia, Bowenoid papulosis, squamous cell carcinoma *in situ*) can produce itching or pain symptoms, as can Paget disease. These can be seen.

*Trauma* regularly produces pain, whether it is surgical, overlapping with irritant contact dermatitis (application of acid for treatment of anogenital warts), accidental, etc. These can be seen in the office.

*Estrogen deficiency* in women can produce discomfort as well, by causing thinning and dryness of the vaginal mucosa. Because the vaginal mucosa can be difficult to visualize, especially in the patient with pain, a wet mount can be crucial to rule out these vaginal diseases.

The most common *specific neurologic disease* causing anogenital pain is pudendal neuralgia. This can be difficult to diagnose, at least partly because there are several types and causes, and there is considerable individual variation in the anatomy and course of this nerve.[10] There is no one standard evaluation and diagnostic regimen. This condition is suggested by sensory abnormalities in the saddle distribution of the pudendal nerve. There is pain or numbness of the genitalia and adjacent buttock, the proximal, medial thigh, and/or rectal area. Classically, the pain is worst when sitting and minimized by standing or lying. The diagnosis can be implicated further by a careful physical examination, magnetic resonance imaging examination performed by specialists in this disease, and magnetic resonance neurography. Management consists of physical therapy, medications for neuropathic pain and nerve block, behavioral modifications, surgical pudendal nerve decompression, radiofrequency, and spinal cord stimulation.[12] Other causes of specific neuropathic pain are uncommon and history is required for diagnosis. Postherpetic neuralgia only follows herpes zoster, not herpes simplex virus infection; the intake of all patients of one of us (LE) includes a question regarding past shingles of this area, and not one of several thousand patients with chronic pain or itching has had herpes zoster as a possible factor. And, this is an obvious diagnosis as shingles rarely occurs unnoticed. Diabetes can be associated with peripheral neuropathy, but far, far more common of the feet, and multiple sclerosis is sometimes associated with pain syndromes.

Patients with normal genital skin, to include the vagina, no specific diagnosable neuropathy, and, for women, a normal wet mount, are diagnosed as *vulvodynia, penodynia, scrotodynia, penodynia, or anodynia.*

## Vulvodynia

Vulvodynia is defined as chronic vulvar discomfort in the absence of relevant clinical abnormalities. Rarely, discomfort extends to anal skin or even solely affects the perianal area. The discomfort is most often described as burning, stinging, rawness, irritation, aching, stabbing, soreness, or throbbing. Itching is not a prominent symptom. Although most vulvologists believe that this is a symptom rather than a specific disease, others, including me (LE), feel that this is a specific condition. Vulvodynia is common, with a great deal of data available, including characteristic epidemiology, comorbidities, and reported management strategies.

Vulvodynia is the most common cause of chronic vulvovaginal pain. This is not a diagnosis of exclusion and can be diagnosed fairly reliably by a validated questionnaire; a study reported in 2006 shows that history alone is prognostic for vulvodynia.[13] Characteristic vulvar pain in the presence of recognized associated comorbidities is highly predictive of this diagnosis. Since then, we know that the finding of an abnormal pelvic floor examination confirms the diagnosis.

Vulvodynia is very, very common, although uncommonly recognized. From 10% to 28% of premenopausal women experience this at some point, but only 30%-48% sought care in one study, and fewer than 50% of those who did were given a diagnosis.[14] This condition appears to occur more often in those of Hispanic background than White,[14] and although recognized much less often in Black patients, this may be because of a difference in words used to describe symptoms.[15] It is truly amazing that women generally are unaware of a condition this common, and experience isolation, believing that they are the only individuals suffering from this vulvar pain.

### Clinical Manifestations

Vulvodynia often begins in young women, in their third and fourth decade, but occurs in all age groups, including in postmenopausal women and, rarely, in children and adolescents.[16,17] A common presentation is entry dyspareunia and self-described "vaginal" burning, irritation, redness, and rawness. Usually, they categorically deny itching that produces a desire to rub and scratch, and report that they do not scratch. Patients very often also have background discomfort as well, and irritation with tampons, tight clothing, exercise, and sitting for long periods. Often, they have consulted previous clinicians who have diagnosed and treated yeast, with incomplete improvement, and many women have been treated repeatedly for yeast and bacterial vaginosis, sometimes for years, and nearly always without laboratory confirmation.

Patients with vulvodynia exhibit typical comorbidities.[18] Nearly all patients with vulvodynia have a "positive review of systems" with anxiety, depression, insomnia, constipation, diarrhea, heartburn, urinary frequency, urgency, dysuria, headaches, arthralgias, and myalgias. Diagnoses including fibromyalgia, irritable bowel syndrome, migraine headaches, temporomandibular joint disorder, chronic fatigue syndrome, and interstitial cystitis are common. Many report multiple medication allergies, which are actually intolerances.

On examination, many patients are anxious and tearful. When asked to touch where they experience pain, most women indicate the vestibule, and they usually report vestibular redness and sometimes feel swelling of this area **(Fig. 13-1)**. The clinician may also see redness, but this is usually within the realm of normal (see Chapter 1). Redness is classically around the ostia of the vestibular glands and formerly was thought to be associated with inflammation of these glands, but this is seen in some asymptomatic women as well. A significant minority of women experience discomfort in other areas of the vulva, and many report redness in other areas as well **(Fig. 13-2)**.

If the skin is otherwise normal, the examination should include gently probing the vulva with the soft end of a cotton-tipped applicator. If the patient has pain in the vestibule with this probing, and only in the vestibule, as well as a history of pain limited to the vestibule, and a wet mount showing no infection, no inflammation, and no parabasal cells, then the diagnosis of the vestibulodynia subset of vulvodynia can be made with confidence. Previous names for this condition include the vulvar vestibulitis syndrome, vestibulitis, vestibular adenitis, and infection of the minor vestibular glands. The name has been changed to eliminate "itis," since clinical and histologic inflammation is lacking when compared to the normal vestibule. This is a quick and simple examination requiring no further testing. If there is discomfort to q-tip probing that extends beyond the vestibule or the patient reports that pain occurs in areas outside the vestibule, the patient has generalized vulvodynia, termed dysesthetic vulvodynia in the past. Uncommonly, patients have no pain to touch.

An examination of the pelvic floor is characteristic in women with vulvodynia. Pressure to the levator ani muscles with an inserted finger generally produces pain in addition to pressure, and asking the patient to squeeze that finger with her pelvic floor muscles produces minimal contraction and poor endurance.

Many years ago, the ISSVD divided vulvodynia into additional subsets beyond vestibulodynia and generalized vulvodynia, with the premise that different subsets had different epidemiology and different underlying etiologies. However, recent data increasingly show a lack of evidence-based information that these subsets represent distinct categories.[19] However, at least distinguishing vestibulodynia from generalized vulvodynia remains crucial for at least one reason. Excision of the vestibule is a treatment of choice only for women with vestibulodynia, due to the location of the discomfort. The ISSVD, the International Society for the Study of Women's Sexual Health, and the International Pelvic Pain Society revised the academic terminology and classification of persistent vulvar pain and vulvodynia in 2015 based on not only on location but also on the role of touch/pressure/friction (provocation), temporal onset, and pattern.[20] These basically are unimportant to the clinician in the diagnosis and management of vulvodynia.

Once believed to be a chronic condition with severity that waxes and wanes, vulvodynia now is reported to be characterized by remissions and recurrences, with persistence being the exception rather than the rule.[21,22] However, this is not my (LE) experience; my patients very rarely experience spontaneous remission, although waxing and waning of severity of symptoms is common. I suspect that the nature of these studies, where the patients did not seek care but rather received unsolicited surveys, selected for those with milder symptoms than those who fight their way to a specialty clinic. In addition, another study suggests that primary vulvodynia, those patients with dyspareunia since first coitus, are less likely to experience remission,[23] and these patients are known to be more resistant to treatment as well.

### Diagnosis

The diagnosis of vulvodynia is simple. The presence of pain in the absence of visible relevant abnormalities, no history consistent with a specific neuropathy, and a normal wet mount to include no signs of infection, inflammation, or signs of estrogen deficiency are all that is required to make this diagnosis; the presence of several characteristic comorbidities and a consistent pelvic floor are usually associated. Women who have discomfort out of proportion to their relevant abnormalities and who have these comorbidities and a suspicious pelvic floor examination are likely to have coexisting vulvodynia and may benefit from brief education regarding the existence of vulvodynia as well as careful follow-up to ensure that their symptoms resolve with treatment of their objective condition.

Conditions occasionally confused with vulvodynia include desquamative inflammatory vaginitis (see Chapter 14), in which a purulent vaginitis produces an irritant contact dermatitis in the vestibule. This is identified by a wet mount that shows sheets of white blood cells and parabasal cells. Occasionally, lichen planus shows vestibular erosions or erythema that is painful (see Chapter 11). The vestibular erythema of lichen planus is generally well demarcated and a deeper red than found with vestibulodynia/vulvodynia and accompanied by oral and/or vaginal abnormalities. When in doubt, a biopsy shows inflammation.

### Pathophysiology (Table 13-3)

Earlier reports referred to this condition as "psychosomatic vaginitis." In the 1980s, chronic yeast, hypersensitivity to colonizing Candida, and "subclinical human

**TABLE 13-3**

**Etiologic Factors in Vulvodynia**

Pelvic floor muscle abnormalities
- Increased muscle tone
- Muscle irritability
- Weakness
- Myofascial pain

Neuropathic pain
- Central sensitization (probably far most common)
- Regional pain referred from bladder or intestinal origin
- Peripheral neuropathy
- Complex regional pain syndrome

Psychological factors
- Depression of chronic pain, endogenous, or situational
- Anxiety
- Psychosexual issues, either primary or secondary from pain-induced sexual dysfunction

Other possible factors
- Inflammatory mediators
- Estrogen influences on pain
- Pain susceptibility genes

papillomavirus infection" were implicated. More recently, there have been increasing numbers of studies exploring neuropathy, pelvic floor abnormalities, anxiety and depression, as well as suggestions of proinflammatory cytokines and proliferation of cutaneous nerve fibers.

Neuropathic pain appears to be a major factor in the pain of vulvodynia as well. Although complex regional pain syndrome was a leading theory early, now most vulvologists believe that vulvodynia results from central sensitization, a systemic condition wherein there is a generalized lowered pain threshold, explaining the accompanying tendency toward headaches, fibromyalgia, temporomandibular joint disorder, etc.[24-26] Studies that measure pain threshold in women with vulvodynia compared to normal controls demonstrates this decreased pain threshold.[27] On the other hand, peripheral factors may be operative as well; increased numbers of nerve fibers have been reported in the vestibule, but this may be precipitated by immunologic mechanisms, or whether the hyperinnervation causes hypersensitivity or results from pain is not known.[28,29]

Pelvic floor muscle abnormalities are recognized as a crucial factor.[30] Originally, introital tightness and pain to insertion of a speculum, finger, penis, or tampon was assumed to be solely an expected reflex to pain and tenderness. However, this tightness, which is sometimes misinterpreted as weakness when tight muscles cannot be further contracted on examination, now is known to be a constitutional abnormality that predisposes to vulvodynia. Hypertonicity, irritability, and poor endurance are typical findings in vulvodynia. This observation is confirmed by the good response of vulvodynia to pelvic floor physical therapy.[31]

Anxiety and depression are prominent factors in vulvodynia.[32-34] A recent study found that almost half of patients with vestibulodynia exhibited pain-related anxiety and almost a third experienced pain-related depression, many with both.[35] And, anxiety and depression can exacerbate discomfort, possibly magnified when the cause cannot be seen, measured, or easily explained to others. The additional impact of pain with sexual activity on isolation, relationships, and self-image is considerable. A significant minority of vulvodynia clinicians, including Peter Lynch, believe that psychosexual dysfunction is the overwhelming or only etiologic factor, and report that equal improvement described in women with vulvodynia who were treated with pelvic floor physical therapy, biofeedback, or cognitive-behavioral therapy helps to confirm this.[36] Whether psychosexual dysfunction is the entire cause of pain, one aspect present at varying degrees in the pathogenesis, or is a result of unremitting and unexplained pain is fiercely debated, and there is evidence that antecedent anxiety and depression increase the risk of vulvodynia, and vulvodynia increases the risk of psychopathology.[37] Most vulvologists believe that anxiety and depression are but a piece of the vulvodynia picture, although a very large and important one that requires attention.

Hormonal issues are believed by some to be operative in vulvodynia. Clearly, patients with estrogen deficiency as the sole factor in pain do not have vulvodynia, but rather atrophic vagina/vaginitis. Some believe that abnormalities of estrogen effect even in women who appear well estrogenized may be important, but variable reports and a general lack of improvement with treatment with estrogen in premenopausal women with vulvodynia has led most to look elsewhere for causes of vulvodynia.

Inflammation has not been found histologically or clinically in women with vulvodynia when compared to controls, and treatment with anti-inflammatory medications including topical corticosteroids is not useful. This was the motivation for changing the terminology from vulvar vestibulitis syndrome to vestibulodynia, reflecting the lack of histologic inflammation. However, recent data, performed almost entirely on the vestibulodynia subset, suggest that there may be inflammatory components to vulvodynia at the proinflammatory mediator level.[38-41] Mast cells have been found variably to be increased and normal.[42,43] Some have postulated that a difference in microbiomes may prompt an inflammatory response in women with vulvodynia, but other surveys do not confirm this.[44,45] There are variable reports of increased numbers of macrophages and mast cells.

Previous theories of etiologies for vulvodynia have been generally discredited; these include chronic yeast infection, subclinical human papillomavirus infection,[28] and oxaluria.[29] Critical and common exacerbating factors in many women with vulvodynia include irritant (and, less so, allergic) contact dermatitis to overwashing, topical medications, lubricants, and panty liners/pads and estrogen deficiency.

## Management

The management of vulvodynia requires careful patient education for these women who have never heard of this condition, many of whom are confident that they have discomfort on the basis of an infection. The treatments for vulvodynia sound senseless to the patient who does not understand the basic causes of vulvodynia. A short explanation of this condition as a pain syndrome associated with pelvic floor tightness, neuropathy, and anxiety/depression is crucial. Then, supplying her with a handout such as the one in the appendix of this book and a warning to avoid social media populated by unhappy patients is helpful. Written information helps to confirm the very real existence of this condition and helps to minimize the sense of isolation patients feel when they believe they are the only ones with these symptoms. Patients often require reassurance that they have no sexually transmitted disease, premalignant condition, or abnormality that results in infertility or pregnancy.

Although up to 22% of patients in a 2-year study experienced spontaneous resolution of symptoms in one study, most women have ongoing symptoms and require therapy.[22] They should be told that there is no cure for vulvodynia, but symptoms can be managed, and most patients experience remarkable improvement, although not quickly and often after trial and error therapy.

There are three areas that require attention; pelvic floor muscle dysfunction, neuropathy, and anxiety/depression (see **Table 13-4**). In addition, women with the vestibulodynia pattern of vulvodynia resistant to these first-line therapies can be treated with a vestibulectomy, surgical removal of the area of pain, generally with excellent results. Also, there are nonspecific, general therapies that are important for all patients, including topical anesthetics, avoidance of irritants, and management of any coincidental issues such as estrogen deficiency or Candidiasis. Finally, there are alternative, anecdotal therapies that may be useful for the patient who is intolerant or unresponsive of standard therapies. There are few sufficiently large, double-blind, controlled studies evaluating treatments for vulvodynia; however, overall experience shows that treatment is very useful for vulvodynia.

Nearly all patients experience anxiety and/or depression to some degree associated with their discomfort, and psychosexual factors are universal. This must be acknowledged, and most patients require therapy, although patients often respond best if these issues are discussed toward the end of a visit, after a relationship is achieved. This can be achieved by referral for *professional counseling, sex therapy, and antidepressants* that double as medication for neuropathic pain (see below). Both traditional and mindfulness-based cognitive-behavioral therapy have been shown to be useful for vulvodynia.[46,47] Vulvovaginal pain that produces painful sexual activity is not the woman's problem alone, but also affects her partner.[48] Also, her partner's response to her pain affects her benefit with therapy. Involvement of therapy with her partner can be beneficial for both.[49]

*Pelvic floor physical therapy* is an exceptionally useful therapy for patients with vulvodynia.[50,51] This treatment not only treats the pelvic floor hypertonicity but also provides desensitization for patients who are afraid of the pain that occurs with touch and serves as emotional support for the patient who is depressed, anxious, frightened, and isolated. The goal of physical therapy includes strengthening the pelvic floor muscles that, in turn, produce a background of relaxed and quiet muscles that lack the irritability of that found in women with vulvodynia. Individual therapists use different methods for achieving these goals, with individualization of therapy depending upon the patient's needs and the therapist's training and experiences. Some women exhibit sufficient muscle rigidity that therapy begins with relaxation techniques of the hips and other joints even before the pelvic floor muscles are addressed. Other procedures include pelvic floor exercises to strengthen the pelvic floor, which also helps train these muscles to relax. Also, soft tissue mobilization and myofascial release of the pelvic girdle, pelvic floor, and associated structures are used by most. Bowel and

TABLE 13-4

**Therapy of Vulvodynia/Penodynia/Scrotodynia/Anodynia**

| |
|---|
| General, nonspecific measures |
| Patient education, handouts |
| Elimination of irritants, unnecessary topical cleansers, medications, etc. |
| Counseling for most |
| Evaluation for and correction of coincidental abnormalities; irritant contact dermatitis, estrogen deficiency, infections, etc. |
| Topical lidocaine 2% jelly, 5% ointment (variable burning with application) |
| Pelvic floor evaluation and physiotherapy (not studied in men) |
| Neuropathic pain/pain syndrome, oral (see individual patient handouts) |
| Duloxetine, beginning at 20 mg titrating up to 60 mg/day. |
| Venlafaxine sustained/extended release, beginning at 37.5 mg, titrating up to 150 mg qd |
| Tricyclic medications beginning at 5-10 mg, titrating as high as 150 mg hs |
| Gabapentin beginning at 100 mg, titrating as high as 1200 mg tid |
| Pregabalin beginning at 25 mg, titrating as high as 300 mg bid |
| Topiramate beginning at 50 mg twice daily, increasing up to 200 mg bid |
| Lamotrigine, beginning at 25 mg twice daily. Increasing up to 100 mg bid |
| Counseling |
| Cognitive-behavioral therapy |
| Psychological counseling |
| Sex therapy |
| Antidepressant therapy |
| Vestibulectomy in women with vestibulodynia (pain strictly localized to the vestibule) |
| Other therapies (only reported in women) |
| Topical therapies |
| Amitriptyline 2%/baclofen 2% compounded |
| Amitriptyline 2%/baclofen 2%/ketamine 2% compounded |
| Nitroglycerin 0.2% compounded, three times a week and 5-10 minutes before sexual activity |
| Gabapentin 4% or 6% compounded (botulinum toxin, hypnotherapy, acupuncture used for vulvodynia by some) |

bladder retraining is used in some patients. The importance of meeting with a compassionate physical therapist on a regular basis for psychological benefit is enormous. Many women are unwilling to seek formal psychological counseling because of expense, stigma, and the implication that their pain is not real but rather psychosomatic. But the psychological benefit through physical therapy is usually acceptable to the patient and very useful.

*Oral therapy for neuropathic factors* is a mainstay of therapy, but firm data from quality trials are lacking, not only for vulvodynia but for neuropathic pain in general. These medications either belong to the antidepressant or to the anticonvulsant class of medications (see Table 13-4). Because women with vulvodynia tend to tolerate medications poorly, doses of each should be started very low and titrated up as tolerated. And, a common mistake is the use of an ultimate dosage that is too low to be effective. Patients need to be advised that improvement is delayed with these medications, as they do not function as pain suppressants, but rather from management of neuropathy. Improvement may require 2-4 weeks after reaching an optimal dose. Partial improvement with one medication often can be maximized by the addition of a medication of a different class.

I generally begin with a medication from the antidepressant rather than anticonvulsant class for several reasons. First, this class of medications addresses not only neuropathic pain but also the anxiety component, and it is also useful for the often-present depression. Second, dosing is once daily rather than the twice or thrice daily dosing of antileptics. Also, the titrating schedule for the widely used gabapentin is unwieldy, with its low dose of 100 mg a day to start gradually increasing to 2400-3600 mg/day. An easily used medication from the antidepressant class for pain is the serotonin norepinephrine reuptake inhibitor duloxetine (Cymbalta).[52,53] It is approved by the United States Food and Drug Administration (FDA) for neuropathic pain and fibromyagia as well as anxiety and depression; patients often appreciate this formal endorsement for neuropathic discomfort to avoid to stigma of taking an antidepressant for their problem, since this smacks of pain that is "all in their head." It is generally well tolerated, inexpensive, and can be titrated to an effective dose quickly; 20 mg daily for a week, then 40 mg daily for a week, then the target dose of 60 mg each day. The related venlafaxine (Effexor) is also useful; it has been shown useful for neuropathy, including complex regional pain syndromes, and is used for fibromyalgia.[54] A titrating dose is 37.5 mg of the extended release once a day for a week, then 75 mg once a day for a week, then 112.5 once a day for a week, and finally 150 mg daily. Withdrawal syndrome is more common with venlafaxine than duloxetine and other medications used for pain syndromes, and these medications are best discontinued by taper than abruptly.[55,56] Milnacipran (Savella) is another medication from this class of antidepressants that may theoretically be beneficial for vulvodynia, as it has indication approval for fibromyalgia.

The tricyclic medications, to include amitriptyline, desipramine, nortriptyline, and imipramine, have the longest history of use for peripheral neuropathy and for vulvodynia.[57,58] Evaluation of pain relief from data is extremely difficult, since the dosing of tricyclic medications in various studies range from 10 to 150 mg. In addition, different individuals metabolize tricyclic medications at variable rates due to differences in genotypes, so that the effective dose is often unknown.[59] But, as noted in a Cochrane review, the lack of unbiased clinical evidence for efficacy should be weighed against decades of observed successful benefit.[60] Side effects are very common and annoying; these include dry mouth and eyes, sedation, constipation, increased appetite; less often, free-floating anxiety, palpitations, tremor, and sleeplessness occur. Amitriptyline exhibits the most sedating effects and highest likelihood of increased appetite. Desipramine is most likely to produce tremor and anxiety. Imipramine is available in a sustained released preparation that is well tolerated. These medications, for vulvodynia patients, are generally started at a very low dose. I begin patients at half of a 10 mg tablet 2 hours before bedtime, because of the long-lasting sedation, and increase by 5 mg nightly as tolerated until discomfort is relieved, the patient reaches 150 mg, or until there are limiting side effects. Often, if the titration is slow, the patient acclimates. Mirtazapine is a tetracyclic antidepressant used widely for interstitial cystitis that is a theoretically possible choice for vulvodynia.[61]

Although, in the past, selective serotonin re-uptake inhibitors have not been used for neuropathic pain, recent publications suggest these medications as possible options.[62]

Many women object to being on antidepressants "on principle." Careful explanation for the reasons for these medications (for neuropathic pain as the primary objective and the fortuitous secondary effects as an antidepressant) most often reassures patients that the clinician is not using the tricyclic medication because the pain if believed to be due to depression. Therefore, I refer to these medications as "tricyclic medications" rather than "tricyclic antidepressants," and I refer to the other medications in the antidepressant class by their specific name rather than by their function as an antidepressant.

The medications from the antiseizure class that have FDA indication approval for neuropathic pain are gabapentin (Neurontin) and pregabalin (Lyrica). More recently, gabapentin is even used for postsurgical pain and other acute and chronic pain that is not of neuropathic origin, although there are little data to show efficacy.[63] There is evidence for efficacy of gabapentin for neuropathy at doses of 1800-3600 mg/day, higher doses than many providers use for pain.[64] Gabapentin is a medication regularly used for vulvodynia as well, with only low-level supportive data although clinicians find benefit in many patients.[57] A recent double blind placebo controlled study has shown no benefit in vulvodynia, but dosing was as low as 1200 mg.[65] Side effects include fatigue and dependent edema, but generally it is much better tolerated than the tricyclic medications. Again, because vulvodynia patients often do not tolerate medications well, I begin patients with lower doses than most clinicians, but titrate up as high as 3600 mg/day. I prescribe 100 mg of gabapentin a day initially and increase by 100 mg a day in three divided doses as tolerated up to 1200 mg three times a day, until the patient is comfortable, or until there are limiting side effects, whichever is first.

Closely related to gabapentin, pregabalin is regularly used for vulvodynia as well, with data limited to benefit found in a case report and in one retrospective survey.[66,67] Pregabalin has similar side effects, but is taken only twice a day, and begun with 50 mg a day, increasing to 150-300 mg twice a day.

Two medications from the anticonvulsant class used less often for neuropathic pain and with even less data for vulvodynia include topiramate and lamotrigine. Topiramate has been shown useful for migraine headaches and polyneuropathy, and clinicians informally report benefit in vulvodynia.[68] Lamotrigine was reported useful in an open label pilot study for vulvodynia.[69] These can interfere with the action of oral contraceptives, and lamotrigine in particular can produce especially severe Steven's Johnson syndrome/toxic epidermal necrolysis. Topiramate can be started at 50 mg twice daily and titrated up to 200 mg twice daily, while lamotrigine was begun at 25 mg and titrated up to 200 mg twice daily. Side effects of topiramate include blurred vision, burning, prickling, or tingling sensations, clumsiness, or unsteadiness and memory issues, while side effects of lamotrigine include blurred vision, double vision, clumsiness, unsteadiness, dizziness, and drowsiness.

In a completely different area, there are data that show cannabis and cannabinoids have analgesic properties, and a preliminary trial showing benefit in vulvodynia.[70,71]

*Topical medications* are used for vulvodynia. These are less well studied but have the advantage of avoidance of systemic adverse reactions so common in patients with vulvodynia. Topical therapies that have shown efficacy data include amitriptyline, gabapentin, lidocaine, baclofen, and hormones.[57] Lidocaine 5% ointment applied nightly (initial burning with application can be limiting), amitriptyline 2%/baclofen 2% compounded in an aqueous base and applied two or three times a day, and gabapentin 2%-8% applied several times a day are all used regularly by practitioners. Most recently, compounded diazepam vaginal suppositories 5-10 mg to induce pelvic floor relaxation is believed by some clinicians and physical therapists to be useful, although a recent review shows inconsistent results.[72] These can be inserted an hour before physical therapy, or on a nightly basis. There are no published reports as to the risk of systemic absorption, addiction, or safety for driving after use of these, but diazepam serum levels 1 hour after insertion of diazepam 10 mg in my office have all shown undetectable levels.

Topical corticosteroids are not useful, and topical testosterone generally is not used, although Dr Andrew Goldstein feels strongly that topical testosterone in combination with estradiol is very beneficial in women whose pain began while on oral contraceptives (personal communication).[73]

*Local injectable therapy* is used in several situations. First, a rare patient who has reproducible point tenderness to touch or pressure, a trigger point, may benefit from an intralesional injection of a corticosteroid such as triamcinolone acetonide (Kenalog), about 0.2-0.3 cc into the center of the painful area with a 30-g needle. If comfort is achieved, a follow-up consolidation dose can be useful. Second, nerve blocks/pudendal blocks administered by an experienced gynecologist or pain clinic can produce relief for some women, and impar ganglion blocks have recently been reported useful.[74] Finally, botulinum toxin A injected into pelvic floor muscles is used for relaxation of pelvic floor muscles by some clinicians. This medication has a long record of use for pain, and there are a number of reports of benefits for vulvodynia, although a recent controlled study showed no effect.[75,76] The wide range of doses and methods used make comparisons among reports difficult to interpret.

A *vestibulectomy* has long been felt to be the most predictable effective therapy available for women with vestibulodynia, vulvodynia that is strictly localized to the vestibule, with improvement occurring in 56%-85% of patients.[77] This surgery consists of excision of the area of pain in the vestibule, often to include the hymeneal ring, with advancement of the vagina to cover the defect. From these studies, primary (lifelong) vestibulodynia responds less well to surgery, and surgical technique does not seem crucial. A recent survey comparing a very small number of patients who were treated with both conservative therapy and surgery to those receiving conservative therapy alone; there was a lower pain score in the surgical group postoperatively, but 3 years later, there was no statistical difference in the improvement score between the two groups; the surgical group changing from 9 preoperatively to 2, and the conservatively treated group from 7 to 4.[78] Fortunately, surgery is not usually required, as the therapies discussed above usually produce sufficient pain control.

Two other surgical procedures have been used. A vestibuloplasty removes only the area of pain mapped before administration of anesthesia, and this may be a small or large area. Failures are generally due to pain in an area not removed. Or a vestibuloplasty may consist of incisions without tissue removal, and undercutting the skin to denervate the area, a procedure that is not effective. Perineoplasties were performed more in the past, where the perineum was removed in addition to the vestibule.

There are therapies that have been used for vulvodynia, which, over time, have been found to be ineffective. These include oral and topical corticosteroids, systemic and intralesional interferon alpha, oral and topical antifungal medications in the absence of documented yeast infections, laser ablation, therapies for human papillomavirus, and the low oxalate diet. There have been limited studies using fractional $CO_2$ laser, and early pilot studies or retroactive chart reviews were promising.[79,80] However, later studies have shown no benefit.[81,82] The International Society for the Study of Vulvodynia has expressly criticized laser therapy for vulvodynia and other vulvar conditions as unproven.[83]

When women with vulvodynia experience a flaring of symptoms, prescribing therapy for yeast or bacterial vaginosis is the easiest path for the provider. However, these additional irritants are not needed, and this only reinforces the patient's impression that her underlying problem is one of resistant or recurrent infection. Rather, evaluation for factors such as infection or contact dermatitis followed by reassurance, bland emollients such as petroleum jelly, cool compresses, and topical lidocaine should be advised. And, if the worsening of discomfort continues, then a change in therapy for the underlying vulvodynia is indicated.

## Penodynia/Scrotodynia

Although there is very little data on pain syndromes in men, one report notes that the second most common condition seen in a male genital dermatology clinic was "dysesthesia."[84] And, informal discussions with dermatologists find that most dermatologists have cared for men with penile and scrotal discomfort with no visible cause. This addresses discomfort that is perceived as skin discomfort, and should be distinguished from orchialgia, or scrotal contents pain. The following consists of what little is found in the literature, extrapolation from what is known of vulvodynia, and the experience of the authors.

We consider scrotodynia and penodynia to be male equivalents of vulvodynia. The presentation is similar, and most men respond to therapy otherwise used for vulvodynia. Like vulvodynia, scrotodynia, penodynia, and anodynia are defined as pain symptoms in the absence of relevant skin disease, infection, trauma, malignancy, or definable neuropathy such as postherpetic neuralgia or diabetic neuropathy. Sometimes the term "red scrotum syndrome" is used synonymously for scrotodynia, but others define red scrotum syndrome as redness from corticosteroid overuse, also called steroid addiction.

### Clinical Manifestations

Although penile and scrotal discomfort in the face of normal skin or modest redness alone seems uncommon, the frequency of male genital pain is probably underrecognized. Penodynia and scrotodynia have been reported only in adult men. Patients complain of penile or scrotal pain or swelling, often with a perception of redness and burning **(Fig. 13-3)**. Although erythema is a common normal finding on the scrotum, patients (and providers) generally do not notice the redness until symptoms occur. Within this area of little data, what exists deals almost entirely with scrotal rather than penile symptoms, although more of our patients present with penile than scrotal symptoms.

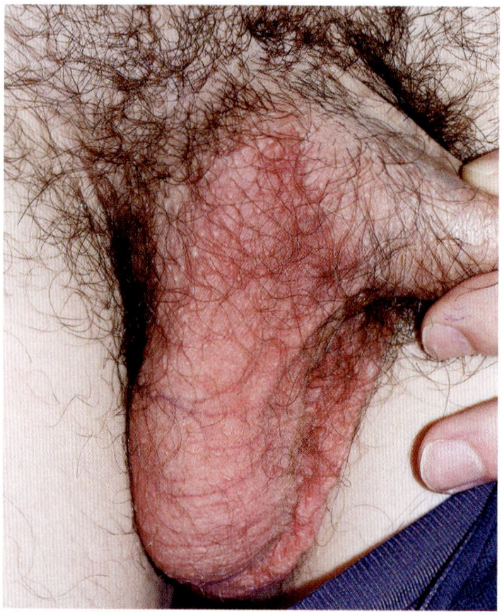

Fig. 13-3. Scrotal redness is often reported in scrotodynia, but sometimes is a normal finding in men without symptoms, as is true here.

The quality of the discomfort is that of burning, stinging, soreness, aching, or hypersensitivity, but usually not itching. These men sometimes report changes in the texture of their skin. This generally interferes with sexual activity and exercise. Often, the patient has consulted multiple clinicians and, like women with vulvodynia, has been treated with many topical antifungal therapies. At times, topical corticosteroids have been used, sometimes producing redness of steroid dermatitis or atrophy, which exacerbates symptoms.

Peter Lynch feels strongly that scrotodynia and penodynia are accompanied by, and produced by, psychosexual dysfunction (see discussion in Chapter 15). He reported a series of 13 men who displayed an unusual degree of psychosexual dysfunction. These men ranged from 35 to 70 years, with an average of 50 years. Eight had never been married, but three of four of the older men were married. When pain was associated with a precipitating event, the event was most often a sexual contact that produced feelings of guilt or anxiety. Nine men had only penile pain, whereas two had only scrotal pain; two had both. The penile pain was either solely or primarily of the glans in all patients. All patients perceived redness, although most exhibited normal degrees of erythema on examination; several who showed greater redness were using topical steroids. Patients improved but did not clear with antidepressants, including amitriptyline. I have seen 21 men in the past 15 years, and my patients followed a similar epidemiologic pattern, with all having been seen by multiple physicians, and most having penile pain.

### Diagnosis

The diagnosis of scrotodynia and penodynia is, like vulvodynia, made by the presence of chronic discomfort in the absence of objective, definable causes of pain. Background redness is sometimes present, and this should be differentiated from irritant contact dermatitis. Deeper genital pain can be due to testicular abnormalities, prostatitis, or an inguinal hernia, requiring evaluation by a urologist.

### Pathophysiology

The pathophysiology is unknown. I (LE) operate on the theory that these male genital pain syndromes are analogous to vulvodynia, with neuropathic pain in the form of central processing dysfunction, pelvic floor hypertonicity, and anxiety/psychosexual issues as primary causes. Peter Lynch is confident that the underlying etiology is somatoform, and psychologically based. Various additional etiologies include over use of corticosteroids,[85,86] psychosexual dysfunction,[87] neuropathic pain,[88,89] a form of erythromelalgia,[85] abnormalities of the cutaneous biofilm,[90] and rosacea. Although a longstanding theory is "steroid addiction," my patients have not had a history of prolonged use of a topical corticosteroid.

The issue of pelvic floor abnormalities as a cause of penodynia and scrotodynia has not been reported although pelvic floor dysfunction is known to be a factor in pelvic pain and chronic prostatitis symptoms in men.[91]

### Management

Treatment, as is true for diagnosis, is extrapolated from our information on vulvodynia, and details can be obtained from that preceding section (**Table 13-4**). Patient education, discontinuation of irritants, and psychological support are crucial. Then, medications for neuropathic pain are my first-line therapy, with duloxetine first choice due to its effectiveness for both neuropathic pain and the psychological factors of anxiety and depression. Tricyclic medications can be useful as well, but have more annoying side effects. Pregabalin is the easiest to use of the medications for neuropathic pain from the antileptic class, and there is anecdotal corroboration.[92,93]

Further medications reported useful in case reports or small series include chronic doxycycline (presumably due to resemblance to rosacea), tricyclic medications,[86] gabapentin,[89] the beta blockers carvedilol and topical timolol,[89,94,95] and one report of response to indomethacin.[96]

Topical medications have not been reported, and although I sometimes refer for pelvic floor physical therapy is awkward, as most therapists work in women's pelvic floor rehabilitation facilities, and the physical therapists are women. I use these medications as well as duloxetine and venlafaxine as well as pelvic floor physical therapy.

As for women with vulvodynia, most of these patients should be referred for counseling. Genital pain syndromes can be life ruining and careful and compassionate care of these patients can remarkably improve their quality of life and, at least theoretically, improve symptoms in some patients.

## Anodynia

Like scrotodynia, penodynia, and vulvodynia, anodynia is a pain syndrome. However, anodynia has a second definition, namely, the absence of pain in a previously painful area.

Unreported, anal discomfort is seen most often in combination with vulvodynia or scrotodynia. The causes and treatment must be extrapolated from information derived from experience with vulvodynia; women should be treated as for vulvodynia, and men as for penodynia/scrotodynia.

## REFERENCES


1. Swamiappan M. Anogenital pruritus—an overview. *J Clin Diagn Res*. 2016;10(4):WE0-WE3.
2. Liu T, Ji R-R. New insights into the mechanisms of itch: are pain and itch controlled by distinct mechanisms? *Pflugers Arch*. 2013;465(12):1671-1685.
3. Chuquilin M, Alghalith Y, Fernandez KH. Neurocutaneous disease. Cutaneous neuroanatomy and mechanisms of itch and pain. *J Am Acad Dermatol*. 2016;74:197-212.
4. Siiskonen H, Harvima I. Mast cells and sensory nerves contribute to neurogenic inflammation and pruritus in chronic skin inflammation. *Front Cell Neurosci*. 2019;13:422. doi:10.3389/fncel.2019.00422
5. Nakashima C, Ishida Y, Kitoh A, Otsuka A, Kabashima K. Interaction of peripheral nerves and mast cells, eosinophils, and basophils in the development of pruritus. *Exp Dermatol*. 2019;28:1405-1411. doi:10.1111/exd.14014
6. Altunay İK, Özkur E, Uğurer E, Baltan E, Aydın Ç, Serin E. More than a skin disease: stress, depression, anxiety levels, and serum neurotrophins in lichen simplex chronicus. *An Bras Dermatol*. 2021;96:700-705. doi:10.1016/j.abd.2021.04.011
7. Podder I, Mondal H, Kroumpouzos G. Nocturnal pruritus and sleep disturbance associated with dermatologic disorders in adult patients. *Int J Womens Dermatol*. 2021;7:403-410. doi:10.1016/j.ijwd.2021.02.010
8. Lavery MJ, Stull C, Kinney MO, Yosipovitch G. Nocturnal pruritus: the battle for a peaceful night's sleep. *Int J Med Sci*. 2016;17. Pii: E425. doi:10.3390/ijms17030425
9. Pereira MP, Kremer AE, Mettang T, Ständer S. Chronic pruritus in the absence of skin disease: pathophysiology, diagnosis and treatment. *Am J Clin Dermatol*. 2016;17:337-348. doi:10.1007/s40257-016-0198-0
10. Patel P, Patel K, Pandher K, Tareen RS. The role of psychiatric, analgesic, and antiepileptic medications in chronic pruritus. *Cureus*. 2021;13:e17260. doi:10.7759/cureus.17260

11. Luesma MJ, Galé I, Fernando J. Diagnostic and therapeutic algorithm for pudendal nerve entrapment syndrome. *Med Clin (Barc)*. 2021;157:71-78. doi:10.1016/j.medcli.2021.02.012
12. Soon-Sutton TL, Feloney MP, Antolak S. Pudendal neuralgia. In: *StatPearls* [Internet]. StatPearls Publishing; 2021.
13. Reed BD, Haefner HK, Harlow SD, et al. Reliability and validity of self-reported symptoms for predicting vulvodynia. *Obstet Gynecol*. 2006;108:906-913.
14. Harlow BL, Kunitz CG, Nguyen RH, Rydell SA, Turner RM, MacLehose RF. Prevalence of symptoms consistent with a diagnosis of vulvodynia: population-based estimates from 2 geographic regions. *Am J Obstet Gynecol*. 2014;210(1):40.e1-40.e8.
15. Brown CS, Foster DC, Bachour CC, et al. Presenting symptoms among black and white women with provoked vulvodynia. *J Womens Health (Larchmt)*. 2015;24:831-836. doi:10.1089/jwh.2014.5164
16. Vieira-Baptista P, Donders G, Margesson L, Edwards L, Haefner HK, Pérez-López FR. Diagnosis and management of vulvodynia in postmenopausal women. *Maturitas*. 2018;108:84-94. doi:10.1016/j.maturitas.2017.11.003
17. Dunford A, Rampal D, Kielly M, Grover SR. Vulval pain in pediatric and adolescent patients. *J Pediatr Adolesc Gynecol*. 2019;32(4):359-362. doi:10.1016/j.jpag.2019.03.005
18. Graziottin A, Murina F, Gambini D, et al. Vulvar pain: the revealing scenario of leading comorbidities in 1183 cases. *Eur J Obstet Gynecol Reprod Biol*. 2020;252:50-55. doi:10.1016/j.ejogrb.2020.05.052
19. Reed BD, Sen A, Harlow SD, Haefner HK, Gracely RH. Multimodal vulvar and peripheral sensitivity among women with vulvodynia: a case–control study. *J Low Genit Tract Dis*. 2017;21:78-84. doi:10.1097/LGT.0000000000000267
20. Bornstein J, Goldstein AT, Colleen K, et al. 2015 ISSVD, ISSWSH, and IPPS consensus terminology and classification of persistent vulvar pain and vulvodynia. *J Low Genit Tract Dis*. 2016;20:126-130. doi:10.1097/LGT.0000000000000190
21. Reed BD, Harlow SD, Plegue MA, Sen A. Remission, relapse, and persistence of vulvodynia: a longitudinal population-based study. *J Womens Health (Larchmt)*. 2016;25:276-283. doi:10.1089/jwh.2015.5397
22. Reed BD, Haefner HK, Sen A, Gorenflo DW. Vulvodynia incidence and remission rates among adult women: a 2-year follow-up study. *Obstet Gynecol*. 2008;112:231-237.
23. Nguyen RH, Mathur C, Wynings EM, Williams DA, Harlow BL. Remission of vulvar pain among women with primary vulvodynia. *J Low Genit Tract Dis*. 2015;19(1):62-67. doi:10.1097/LGT.0000000000000041
24. Basha ME, Kellogg-Spadt S, Burrows LJ, et al. Thermal and mechanical pain thresholds of women with provoked localized vulvodynia: a pilot study. *J Am Osteopath Assoc*. 2019;119:164-172. doi:10.7556/jaoa.2019.027
25. Gupta A, Woodworth DC, Ellingson BM, et al. Disease-related microstructural differences in the brain in women with provoked vestibulodynia. *J Pain*. 2018;19:528.e1-528.e15. doi:10.1016/j.jpain.2017.12.269
26. Torres-Cueco R, Nohales-Alfonso F. Vulvodynia-it is time to accept a new understanding from a neurobiological perspective? *Int J Environ Res Public Health*. 2021;18:6639. doi:10.3390/ijerph18126639
27. Phillips N, Brown C, Bachmann G, et al. Relationship between nongenital tender point tenderness and intravaginal muscle pain intensity: ratings in women with provoked vestibulodynia and implications for treatment. *Am J Obstet Gynecol*. 2016;215:751.e1-751.e5.doi:10.1016/j.ajog.2016.06.047
28. Liao Z, Chakrabarty A, Mu Y, et al. A local inflammatory renin-angiotensin system drives sensory axon sprouting in provoked vestibulodynia. *J Pain*. 2017;18:511-525. doi:10.1016/j.jpain.2016.12.008
29. Barry CM, Matusica D, Haberberger RV. Emerging evidence of macrophage contribution to hyperinnervation and nociceptor sensitization in vulvodynia. *Front Mol Neurosci*. 2019;12:186. doi:10.3389/fnmol.2019.00186
30. Fontaine F, Dumoulin C, Bergeron S, et al. Pelvic floor muscle morphometry and function in women with primary and secondary provoked vestibulodynia. *J Sex Med*. 2018;15:1149-1157. doi:10.1016/j.jsxm.2018.06.001
31. Bardin MG, Giraldo PC, Martinho N. Pelvic floor biometric changes assessed by 4D translabial ultrasound in women with vulvodynia submitted to physical therapy: a pilot study of a randomized controlled trial. *J Sex Med*. 2020;17:2236-2246. doi:10.1016/j.jsxm.2020.07.020
32. Govind V, Krapf JM, Mitchell L, et al. Exploring pain-related anxiety and depression in female patients with provoked vulvodynia with associated overactive pelvic floor muscle dysfunction. *Sex Med*. 2020;8:517-524. doi:10.1016/j.esxm.2020.05.009
33. Chisari C, Monajemi MB, Scott W, Moss-Morris R, McCracken LM. Psychosocial factors associated with pain and sexual function in women with Vulvodynia: a systematic review. *Eur J Pain*. 2021;25:39-50. doi:10.1002/ejp.1668
34. Tribó MJ, Canal C, Baños JE, Robleda G. Pain, anxiety, depression, and quality of life in patients with vulvodynia. *Dermatology*. 2020;236:255-261. doi:10.1159/000503321
35. Goldfinger C, Pukall CF, Thibault-Gagnon S, McLean L, Chamberlain S. Effectiveness of cognitive-behavioral therapy and physical therapy for provoked vestibulodynia: a randomized pilot study. *J Sex Med*. 2016;13:88-94.
36. Lynch PJ. Vulvodynia as a somatoform disorder. *J Reprod Med*. 2008;53:390-396.
37. Khandker M, Brady SS, Vitonis AF, et al. The influence of depression and anxiety on risk of adult onset vulvodynia. *J Womens Health (Larchmt)*. 2011;20(10):1445-1451. doi:10.1089/jwh.2010.2661
38. Zanotta N, Campisciano G, Scrimin F, et al. Cytokine profiles of women with vulvodynia: identification of a panel of pro-inflammatory molecular targets. *Eur J Obstet Gynecol Reprod Biol*. 2018;226:66-70. doi:10.1016/j.ejogrb.2018.05.035
39. Falsetta ML, Foster DC, Woeller CF. Toll-like receptor signaling contributes to proinflammatory mediator production in localized provoked vulvodynia. *J Low Genit Tract Dis*. 2018;22:52-57. doi:10.1097/LGT.0000000000000364
40. Baker DA, Peresleni T, Kocis C. Inflammatory markers in vestibulodynia [4]. *Obstet Gynecol*. 2016;127(Suppl 1):1S-2S.
41. Falsetta ML, Wood RW, Linder MA. Specialized pro-resolving mediators reduce pro-nociceptive inflammatory mediator production in models of localized provoked vulvodynia. *J Pain*. 2021;22(10):1195-1209. doi:10.1016/j.jpain.2021.03.144
42. Regauer S, Eberz B, Beham-Schmid C. Mast cell infiltrates in vulvodynia represent secondary and idiopathic mast cell hyperplasias. *APMIS*. 2015;123:452-456.
43. Papoutsis D, Haefner HK, Crum CP, Opipari AW Jr, Reed BD. Vestibular mast cell density in vulvodynia: a case-controlled study. *J Low Genit Tract Dis*. 2016;20:275-279.
44. Park SY, Lee ES, Lee SR, Kim SH, Chae HD. Vaginal microbiome is associated with vulvodynia, vulvar pain syndrome: a case–control study. *Sex Med*. 2021;9:100314. doi:10.1016/j.esxm.2020.100314

45. Bedford L, Parker SE, Davis E, et al. Characteristics of the vaginal microbiome in women with and without clinically confirmed vulvodynia. *Am J Obstet Gynecol.* 2020;223:406.e1-406.e16. doi:10.1016/j.ajog.2020.02.039
46. Brotto LA, Bergeron S, Zdaniuk B, Basson R. Mindfulness and cognitive behavior therapy for provoked vestibulodynia: mediators of treatment outcome and long-term effects. *J Consult Clin Psychol.* 2020;88:48-64. doi:10.1037/ccp0000473
47. Dunkley CR, Brotto LA. Psychological treatments for provoked vestibulodynia: integration of mindfulness-based and cognitive behavioral therapies. *J Clin Psychol.* 2016;72:637-650. doi:10.1002/jclp.22286
48. Sadownik LA, Smith KB, Hui A, Brotto LA. The impact of a woman's dyspareunia and its treatment on her intimate partner: a qualitative analysis. *J Sex Marital Ther.* 2017;43:529-542. doi:10.1080/0092623X.2016.1208697
49. Rosen NO, Bergeron S, Sadikaj G, Delisle I. Daily associations among male partner responses, pain during intercourse, and anxiety in women with vulvodynia and their partners. *J Pain.* 2015;16:1312-1320.
50. Ghaderi F, Bastani P, Hajebrahimi S, Jafarabadi MA, Berghmans B. Pelvic floor rehabilitation in the treatment of women with dyspareunia: a randomized controlled clinical trial. *Int Urogynecol J.* 2019;30:1849-1855.
51. Jahshan-Doukhy O, Bornstein J. Long-term efficacy of physical therapy for localized provoked vulvodynia. *Int J Womens Health.* 2021;13:161-168. doi:10.2147/IJWH.S297389
52. Dhaliwal JS, Spurling BC, Molla M. Duloxetine. In: *StatPearls* [Internet]. StatPearls Publishing; 2021.
53. Lunn MP, Hughes RA, Wiffen PJ. Duloxetine for treating painful neuropathy, chronic pain or fibromyalgia. *Cochrane Database Syst Rev.* 2014;(1):CD007115. doi:10.1002/14651858.CD007115.pub3.
54. Singh D, Saadabadi A. Venlafaxine. In: *StatPearls* [Internet]. StatPearls Publishing; 2021
55. Fava GA, Benasi G, Lucente M, Offidani E, Cosci F, Guidi J. Withdrawal symptoms after serotonin-noradrenaline reuptake inhibitor discontinuation: systematic review. *Psychother Psychosom.* 2018;87(4):195-203. doi:10.1159/000491524
56. Gong H, Du X, Wu L, et al. Discontinuation syndrome of extended-release venlafaxine during the COVID-19 epidemic. *Psychiatr Danub.* Spring 2021;33(1):121-122.
57. Loflin BJ, Westmoreland K, Williams NT. Vulvodynia; a review of the literature. *J Pharm Technol.* 2019;35:11-24. doi:10.1177/8755122518793256
58. Reed BD, Caron AM, Gorenflo DW, Haefner HK. Treatment of vulvodynia with tricyclic antidepressants: efficacy and associated factors. *J Low Genit Tract Dis.* 2006;10:245-251.
59. Hicks JK, Sangkuhl K, Swen JJ, et al. Clinical pharmacogenetics implementation consortium guideline (CPIC) for CYP2D6 and CYP2C19 genotypes and dosing of tricyclic antidepressants: 2016 update. *Clin Pharmacol Ther.* 2017;102:37-44. doi:10.1002/cpt.597
60. Moore RA, Derry S, Aldington D, Cole P, Wiffen PJ. Amitriptyline for neuropathic pain in adults. *Cochrane Database Syst Rev.* 2015;2015:CD008242. doi:10.1002/14651858.CD008242.pub3
61. Miki K, Murakami M, Oka H, et al. Efficacy of mirtazapine for the treatment of fibromyalgia without concomitant depression: a randomized, double-blind, placebo-controlled phase IIa study in Japan. *Pain.* 2016;157(9):2089-2096. doi:10.1097/j.pain.0000000000000622
62. Patetsos E, Horjales-Araujo E. Treating chronic pain with SSRIs: what do we know? *Pain Res Manag.* 2016;2016:2020915. doi:10.1155/2016/2020915
63. Hah J, Mackey SC, Schmidt P, et al. Effect of perioperative gabapentin on postoperative pain resolution and opioid cessation in a mixed surgical cohort: a randomized clinical trial. *JAMA Surg.* 2018;153:303-311. doi:10.1001/jamasurg.2017.4915
64. Wiffen PJ, Derry S, Bell RF, et al. Gabapentin for chronic neuropathic pain in adults. *Cochrane Database Syst Rev.* 2017;6(6):CD007938. doi:10.1002/14651858.CD007938.pub4
65. Brown CS, Bachmann GA, Wan J, Foster DC; Gabapentin (GABA) Study Group. Gabapentin for the treatment of vulvodynia: a randomized controlled trial. *Obstet Gynecol.* 2018;131:1000-1007. doi:10.1097/AOG.0000000000002617
66. Jerome L. Pregabalin-induced remission in a 62-year-old woman with a 20-year history of vulvodynia. *Pain Res Manag* 2007;12:212-214.
67. van Beekhuizen HJ, Oost J, van der Meijden WI. Generalized unprovoked vulvodynia; a retrospective study on the efficacy of treatment with amitriptyline, gabapentin or pregabalin. *Eur J Obstet Gynecol Reprod Biol.* 2018;220:118-121. doi:10.1016/j.ejogrb.2017.10.026
68. Nazarbaghi S, Amiri-Nikpour MR, Eghbal AF, Valizadeh R. Comparison of the effect of topiramate versus gabapentin on neuropathic pain in patients with polyneuropathy: a randomized clinical trial. *Electron Physician.* 2017;9:5617-5622. doi:10.19082/5617
69. Meltzer-Brody SE, Zolnoun D, Steege JF, Rinaldi KL, Leserman J. Open-label trial of lamotrigine focusing on efficacy in vulvodynia. *J Reprod Med.* 2009;54:171-178.
70. Mücke M, Phillips T, Radbruch L, Petzke F, Häuser W. Cannabis-based medicines for chronic neuropathic pain in adults. *Cochrane Database Syst Rev.* 2018;(3):CD012182. doi:10.1002/14651858.CD012182.pub2
71. Barach E, Slavin MN, Earleywine M. Cannabis and vulvodynia symptoms: a preliminary report. *Cannabis.* 2020;3:139-147. doi:10.26828/cannabis.2020.02.001
72. Stone RH, Abousaud M, Abousaud A, Kobak W. A systematic review of intravaginal diazepam for the treatment of pelvic floor hypertonic disorder. *J Clin Pharmacol.* 2020;60(Suppl 2):S110-S120. doi:10.1002/jcph.1775
73. Burrows LJ, Goldstein AT. The treatment of vestibulodynia with topical estradiol and testosterone. *Sex Med.* 2013;1:30-33. doi:10.1002/sm2.4
74. Hong DG, Hwang SM, Park JM. Efficacy of ganglion impar block on vulvodynia: case series and results of mid- and long-term follow-up. *Medicine (Baltimore).* 2021;100:e26799. doi:10.1097/MD.0000000000026799
75. Pelletier F, Parratte B, Penz S, et al. Efficacy of high doses of botulinum toxin A for treating provoked vestibulodynia. *Br J Dermatol.* 2011;164:617-622.
76. Haraldson P, Mühlrad H, Heddini U, Nilsson K, Bohm-Starke N. Botulinum toxin A as a treatment for provoked vestibulodynia: a randomized controlled trial. *Obstet Gynecol.* 2020;136:524-532.
77. Swanson CL, Rueter JA, Olson JE, Weaver AL, Stanhope CR. Localized provoked vestibulodynia: outcomes after modified vestibulectomy. *J Reprod Med.* 2014;59:121-126.
78. Aalto AP, Huhtala H, Mäenpää J, Staff S. Combination of treatments with or without surgery in localized provoked vulvodynia: outcomes after three years of follow-up. *Biores Open Access.* 2019;8(1):25-31. doi:10.1089/biores.2018.0044

79. Murina F, Karram M, Salvatore S, et al. Fractional $CO_2$ laser treatment of the vestibule for patients with vestibulodynia and genitourinary syndrome of menopause: a pilot study. *J Sex Med.* 2016;13:1915-1917.
80. Leclair CM, Goetsch MF, Lee KK, et al. KTP-nd:YAG laser therapy for the treatment of vestibulodynia: a follow-up study. *J Reprod Med.* 2007;52:53-58.
81. Trutnovsky G, Bliem B, Greimel E, Tamussino K, Gold D. Microablative erbium: YAG laser therapy for vulvodynia—a report on efficacy, safety, and treatment satisfaction. *Sex Med.* 2021;9(6):100432. doi:10.1016/j.esxm.2021.100432
82. Lev-Sagie A, Kopitman A, Brzezinski A. Low-level laser therapy for the treatment of provoked vestibulodynia-A randomized, placebo-controlled pilot trial. *J Sex Med.* 2017;14:1403-1411.
83. Preti M, Vieira-Baptista P, Digesu GA, et al. The clinical role of LASER for vulvar and vaginal treatments in gynecology and female urology: an ICS/ISSVD best practice consensus document. *J Low Genit Tract Dis.* 2019;23:151-160.
84. Elakis JA, Hall AP. Skin disease of penis and male genitalia is linked to atopy and circumcision: caseload in a male genital dermatology clinic. *Australas J Dermatol.* 2017;58(3):e68-e72. doi:10.1111/ajd.12485
85. Khalil S, Kurban M, Abbas O. Red scrotum syndrome: An update on clinicopathologic features, pathogenesis, diagnosis, and management. *J Am Acad Dermatol.* 2020 Jun 1; S0190-9622(20)30988-9. doi:10.1016/j.jaad.2020.05.113. Online ahead of print
86. Narang T, Kumaran MS, Dogra S, Saikia UN, Kumar B. Red scrotum syndrome: idiopathic neurovascular phenomenon or steroid addiction? *Sex Health.* 2013;10:452-455.
87. Hosthota A, Bondade S, Monnappa D, Basavaraja V. Scrotodynia: diagnostic and therapeutic challenge. *Skinmed.* 2016;14:237-238.
88. Raef HS, Elmariah SB. Treatment of male genital dysesthesia with botulinum toxin. *JAAD Case Rep.* 2021;10:60-62. doi:10.1016/j.jdcr.2021.01.018
89. Mizes A, Bunimovich O, Bunimovich YL. Combined carvedilol and gabapentin treatment induces a rapid response in red scrotum syndrome. *Dermatol Online J.* 2021;27(5). doi:10.5070/D327553619
90. Perry TW. Cutaneous microbial biofilm formation as an underlying cause of red scrotum syndrome. *Eur J Med Res.* 2021;26:95. doi:10.1186/s40001-021-00569-9
91. Burzynski B, Jurys T, Burzynski K, Cempa K, Paradysz A. Physiotherapeutic assessment and management of chronic pelvic pain syndrome: a case report. *Medicine (Baltimore).* 2021;100(15):e25525. doi:10.1097/MD.0000000000025525
92. Cardenas-de la Garza JA, Villarreal-Villarreal CD, Cuellar-Barboza A, et al. Red scrotum syndrome treatment with pregabalin: a case series. *Ann Dermatol.* 2019;31:320-324. doi:10.5021/ad.2019.31.3.320
93. Miller J, Leicht S. Pregabalin in the treatment of red scrotum syndrome: a report of two cases. *Dermatol Ther.* 2016;29:244-248. doi:10.1111/dth.12354
94. Merhi R, Ayoub N, Mrad M. Carvedilol for the treatment of red scrotum syndrome. *JAAD Case Rep.* 2017;3:464-466. doi:10.1016/j.jdcr.2017.06.021
95. Pyle TM, Heymann WR. Managing red scrotum syndrome (RSS) with topical timolol. *Int J Dermatol.* 2019;58(8):e162-e163. doi:10.1111/ijd.14463
96. Hwang AS, Costello CM, Yang YW. Rapid improvement of burning scrotum syndrome with indomethacin. *JAAD Case Rep.* 2021;12:32-33. doi:10.1016/j.jdcr.2021.03.050

## SUGGESTED READINGS

Bergeron S, Reed BD, Wesselmann U, Bohm-Starke N. Vulvodynia. *Nat Rev Dis Primers.* 2020;6(1):36. doi:10.1038/s41572-020-0164-2

Buteau A, Reichenberg J. Psychogenic pruritus and its management. *Dermatol Clin.* 2018;36(3):309-314. doi:10.1016/j.det.2018.02.015

Khalil S, Kurban M, Abbas O. Red scrotum syndrome: an update on clinicopathologic features, pathogenesis, diagnosis, and management. *J Am Acad Dermatol.* 2020 Jun 1; S0190-9622(20)30988-9. doi:10.1016/j.jaad.2020.05.113. Online ahead of print

Loflin BJ, Westmoreland K, Williams NT. Vulvodynia; a review of the literature. *J Pharm Technol.* 2019;35(1):11-24. doi:10.1177/8755122518793256

Patel P, Patel K, Pandher K, Tareen RS. The role of psychiatric, analgesic, and antiepileptic medications in chronic pruritus. *Cureus.* 2021;13(8):e17260. doi:10.7759/cureus.17260

Pereira MP, Wiegmann H, Agelopoulos K, Ständer S. Neuropathic itch: routes to clinical diagnosis. *Front Med (Lausanne).* 2021;8:641746. doi:10.3389/fmed.2021.641746

Roh YS, Choi J, Sutaria N, Kwatra SG. Itch: epidemiology, clinical presentation, and diagnostic workup. *J Am Acad Dermatol.* 2022;86:1-14. doi:10.1016/j.jaad.2021.07.076

Satoh T, et al. 2020 guidelines for the diagnosis and treatment of cutaneous pruritus. *J Dermatol.* 2021;48(9):e399-e413. doi:10.1111/1346-8138.16066

Szok D, Tajti J, Nyári A, Vécsei L. Therapeutic approaches for peripheral and central neuropathic pain. *Behav Neurol.* 2019;2019:8685954. doi:10.1155/2019/8685954

# Vaginitis and Balanitis 14

LIBBY EDWARDS

The terms vaginitis and balanitis simply refer to inflammation of the vagina and the glans penis and are not specific diseases. Often noninflammatory conditions that produce vaginal discharge, such as bacterial vaginosis, or neoplasms, such as pseudoepitheliomatous, micaceous, and keratotic balanitis, are lumped into these categories, which will be discussed here also. Vaginitis and balanitis refer to location rather than etiology, so there is considerable overlap with other conditions discussed in more detail earlier in this book. For example, lichen planus (LP) causes vaginitis and balanitis and is pictured in the chapter, but because LP usually affects other genital skin surfaces as well, it is discussed primarily in other sections of this book. Irritating or infectious vaginal secretions often produce concomitant vulvitis **(Fig. 14-1)**.

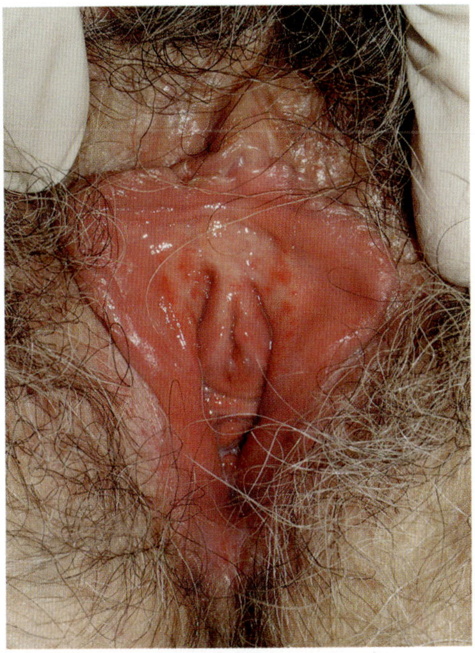

Fig. 14-1. Irritating or infectious vaginal fluid associated with vaginitis often produces vulvar inflammation as well, manifested by nonspecific erythema and, sometimes, edema of the modified mucous membranes.

## Vaginitis

Vaginitis is characterized by one or more of the following: excess discharge, odor, and/or introital irritation and itching. Vaginitis is divided into one of two overlapping categories: true vaginitis or vaginosis. Vaginitis is manifested by signs of inflammation, such as yellow vaginal secretions and redness of the vagina and vestibule. Vaginosis specifically lacks signs of inflammation; there is no erythema, and the discharge is not clinically or microscopically purulent. Bacterial vaginosis is the most common and universally agreed upon example. Although *Candida albicans* is the most common cause of vaginitis, this infection is sometimes unaccompanied by visible erythema or increased numbers of white blood cells on wet mount. In addition, patients with the controversial conditions of cytolytic vaginosis and *Lactobacillus* vaginosis characteristically report symptoms of inflammation, particularly itching, despite no clinical signs of inflammation.

In recent years, very sensitive molecular testing for pathogens and vaginal flora has become available. Many providers assume all vaginitis to be caused by infection and use these probes rather than a wet mount. However, although yeast, trichomoniasis, chlamydia, and gonorrhea are best diagnosed by these probes, all other causes of vaginal discharge and symptoms are best or only diagnosed by wet mount. Unfortunately, more and more clinics are without a microscope.

The diagnosis of vaginitis cannot be made on the basis of symptoms. Evaluation with a physical examination is sometimes useful, but crucial is objective testing for infection and evaluation of a wet mount in many patients. Second best to actually seeing the patient, and far better than diagnosing by telephone, is an examination or laboratory submission of a self-collected swab for those patients with a history of problematic vaginitis.[1]

Before the vagina and vaginal secretions can be evaluated, the examiner must be aware of the appearance of normal vaginal epithelium and normal vaginal secretions (see Chapter 4). The normal estrogenized vestibule and vagina are pink and wet, with prominent folds, or rugae.

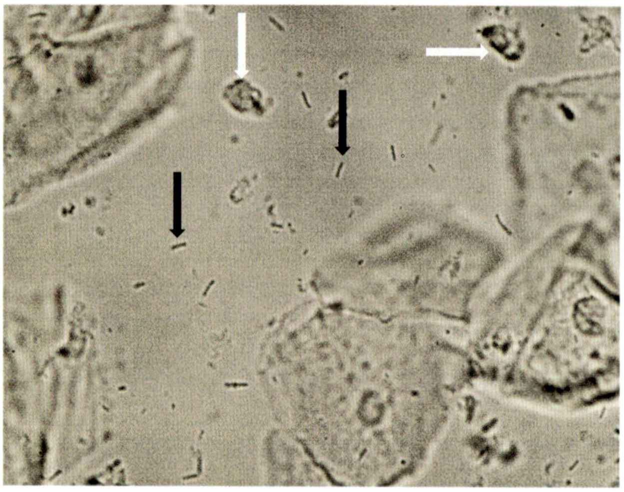

Fig. 14-2. A wet mount of normal vaginal secretions of a premenopausal woman shows large, flattened mature squamous cells and abundant lactobacilli (*black arrows*). There are one or fewer white blood cells (*white arrows*) per squamous cell.

This normal erythema is often perceived by patients as abnormally red. Prepubertal girls and postmenopausal women normally exhibit pale, smooth vaginal epithelium with a loss of these rugae.

A normal wet mount in a well-estrogenized vagina shows mature, large, flat, folded epithelial cells shed from the surface of the epithelium (Fig. 14-2). Rods representing lactobacilli are present, providing an acid pH lower than 5. White blood cells are regularly present, and they should number about one for each epithelial cell.

## Infectious Vaginitis

Most patients and clinicians generally assume that the term *vaginitis* refers to a vaginal infection. In fact, many generalize further and expect all vulvovaginal symptoms, especially when accompanied by abnormal secretions, to be caused by yeast or bacterial vaginosis. These may be the most common and easily diagnosable forms of vaginitis, but other less well-described processes also occur.

### *Candida* Vaginitis

Vulvovaginal candidiasis (VVC), particularly that produced by *C albicans*, is extremely common. VVC also generally takes the initial blame for any vulvovaginal itching or burning, whether or not yeast actually is identified on microscopic smears or cultures. The Center for Disease Control and Prevention reports that at least 75% of women experience at least one episode of candidiasis in their lifetime, with 40%-45% having additional episodes, and 10%-20% experiencing complicated yeast requiring special diagnostic and therapeutic considerations.[2] Candidiasis is not a reportable disease, so the true prevalence is unknown, relying on self-reporting, a notoriously unreliable measure that overestimates the frequency.[3] Most patients referred to this author arrive with a diagnosis of frequent candidiasis, but only rarely is this the cause for patients' chronic symptoms.

#### *Clinical Presentation*

*C albicans* and *Candida tropicalis* usually present with symptoms of itching, sometimes with burning and vulvar dysuria as well. Although *C albicans* vaginitis classically is accompanied by a white, clumped, cottage cheese–like discharge that is often not particularly copious, vaginal secretions frequently appear normal clinically. Vestibular erythema is usual, and some patients develop more extensive erythema, skinfold fissures, and scale, as well as peripheral satellite pustules, erosions, or collarettes (Fig. 14-3). VVC classically occurs or flares during menses and following sexual activity. Rarely, remarkable, immediate edema occurs with sexual intercourse.

Vaginitis produced by non-*albicans* yeast, including *Candida glabrata*, *Candida parapsilosis*, *Candida krusei*, and *Saccharomyces cerevisiae*, comprise about 15% of all yeast infections.[4] These are overwhelmingly asymptomatic. If symptoms occur, women generally report irritation and burning more than itching. Vaginal secretions in women with non-*albicans Candida* infections are clinically unremarkable, and redness, fissures, and satellite pustules are absent.

Complicated VVC is defined as severe non*albicans Candida* infection or recurrent VVC. Four or more episodes of documented *Candida* infections identify recurrent VVC.

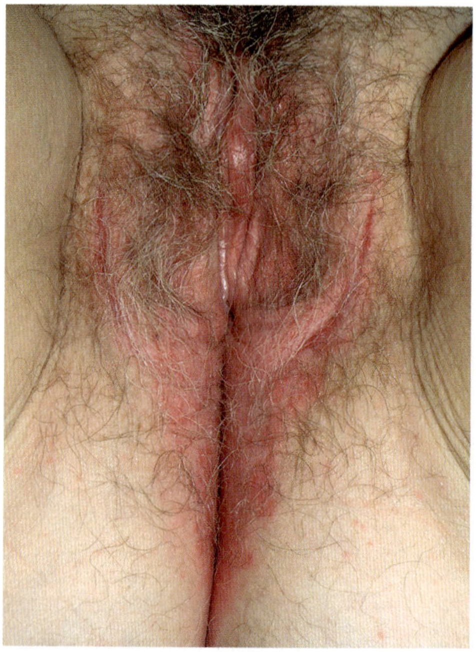

Fig. 14-3. Vaginal candidiasis sometimes extends to the vulva, where it classically shows erythema, fissures, and puffiness of the labia minora and clitoral hood.

### Diagnosis

The diagnosis of a *C albicans* infection requires identification of the organism on a microscopic examination of vaginal secretions, a positive culture or positive molecular studies. The diagnosis cannot be made by history alone, and erythema, fissures, and satellite pustules or collarettes can be caused by other conditions such as inverse psoriasis. The organism can be identified on a microscopic smear, where a drop of vaginal fluid is placed on the microscope slide, and a drop of KOH is added to dissolve skin cells, leaving the buds, hyphae, and pseudohyphae. However, the ease of this examination is generally underestimated by the nondermatologist; when the index of suspicion is high but a smear is negative or a smear is positive but the patient does not improve as expected, a vaginal culture or molecular studies should be performed.

The identification of non-*albicans Candida* on microscopic smear is much more difficult the first time an examiner finds it on wet mount or fungal preparation, since only buds are seen. Only *C albicans* and *C tropicalis* exhibit hyphae, pseudohyphae, and budding yeasts that are normally seen with the 10× objective (**Fig. 14-4**). Non-*albicans Candida* infections reveal only small, budding yeasts that can be seen best with the 40× objective (**Fig. 14-5**). However, a non-*albicans Candida* infection usually exhibits multiple budding yeasts, so nearly every field shows at least one yeast form. This author finds presence of non-*albicans Candida* far more easily identified on a wet mount rather than a smear treated with potassium hydroxide. Debris from the lysis of cells by potassium hydroxide obscures the small budding yeasts.

Molecular testing with a screen for vaginal organisms also confirms this diagnosis and often yields the species, but the cost is generally significantly higher. A culture provides the most information, with sensitivity and speciation in the case of non-*albicans Candida*.

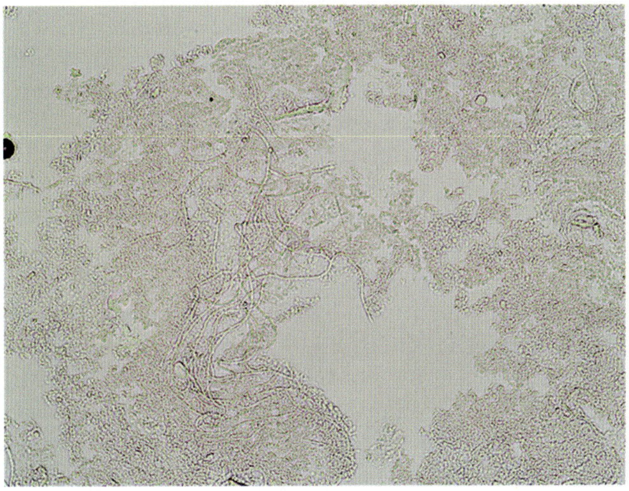

Fig. 14-4. A fungal preparation of *Candida albicans* of the vagina shows branching hyphae and pseudohyphae.

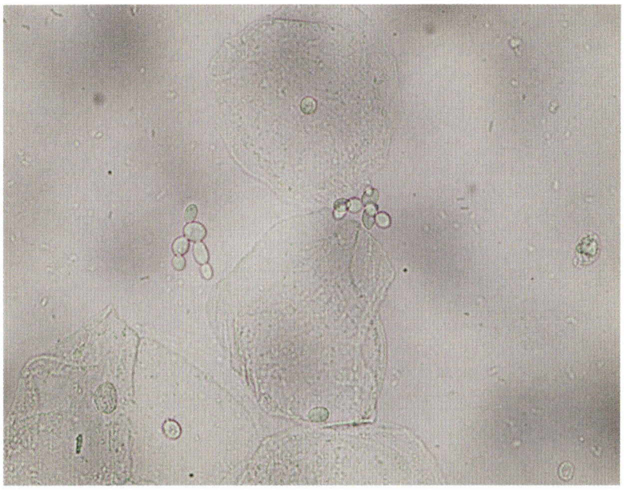

Fig. 14-5. Non-*albicans Candida* shows only budding yeast without mycelia. This wet mount exhibits the fairly large round buds of *Saccharomyces*.

Biopsies of yeast vaginitis are performed only if the diagnosis is not suspected by the clinician, because less expensive and less painful methods of diagnosis are usual. However, a typical tissue sample of acute vaginal candidiasis reveals inflammation consisting primarily of lymphocytes with some plasma cells and neutrophils, as well as stromal edema and spongiosis. Fungal elements are often seen within the most superficial portions of the vaginal epithelium. Less inflammation is seen in chronic candidiasis.

*C albicans* vaginitis often coexists with, precipitates, and drives eczema. Therefore, *C albicans* vaginitis should be considered in the differential diagnosis of eczema or any other itchy vulvovaginal disease. Vulvar psoriasis, contact dermatitis, and lichen sclerosus are other pruritic dermatoses that are often misdiagnosed as and often coexist with *Candida* vulvovaginitis.

Non-*albicans Candida* infection is nearly always asymptomatic. This rarely produces irritation or burning, so vulvodynia is often mistaken for non-*albicans* candidiasis. However, documented non-*albicans* candidiasis is generally coincidental rather than causative, and when the infection clears, symptoms persist.

**CANDIDA VULVOVAGINITIS — Diagnosis**

- Usually, introital pruritus, irritation
- Vaginal and introital erythema, sometimes extending to the vulva, with skinfold fissures, pustules
- Hyphae/pseudohyphae on microscopy
- Positive fungal culture
- Positive molecular studies showing yeast

| RECURRENT OR RESISTANT *CANDIDA* VULVOVAGINITIS | Diagnosis |
|---|---|

- Positive fungal culture
- Positive molecular studies
- Confirmatory sensitivities for diagnosis of resistant *Candida albicans*

| NON-*ALBICANS CANDIDA* | Diagnosis |
|---|---|

- Usually, no physical findings or symptoms
- Budding yeast on wet mount or apparently normal wet mount/fungal preparation
- Confirmed, speciated with culture when needed

### *Pathophysiology*

The most common cause of vulvovaginal yeast infections is *C albicans*, representing about 85% of yeast infections.[4] Most U.S. providers do not find that non-*albicans Candida* infections represent this large proportion of yeast infections, but the fact that non-*albicans Candida* is usually asymptomatic leads to underdiagnosis. In Europe, *C albicans* accounts for 95% of yeast species.[5]

The simple presence of *C albicans* does not provide a diagnosis of *Candida* vaginitis. Nonculture testing for *Candida* shows the presence of yeast in more than 60% of premenopausal, nonpregnant women, with cultures positive in about 20% of immunocompetent women and 30% of immunocompromised patients.[5] A yeast infection generally is produced by higher numbers of organisms and an inflammatory response to these organisms. Cutaneous vulvar candidiasis is associated with superficial invasion of the epithelium by yeast.

Risk factors for VVC, in addition to virulence factors of the yeast organisms, include immunosuppression by virtue of illness or medications, poorly controlled diabetes mellitus, sexual activity, oral sex, spermicides, condoms, and high estrogen states to include high estrogen oral contraceptives, pregnancy, and estrogen replacement. The oral sodium-glucose cotransporter-2 (SGLT-2) inhibitors for diabetes, empagliflozin (Jardiance), canagliflozin (Invokana), dapagliflozin (Farxiga), and ertugliflozin (Steglatro) have been associated with an increase in genital candidiasis in both men and women, because these medications produce glycosuria. Antibiotics increase both colonization and infection with yeast, but the reason is not clear.[6] It does not appear that the cause is elimination of lactobacilli, since candidiasis occurs primarily in the presence of lactobacilli. Women with abundant lactobacilli have a four times higher likelihood of a *Candida* infection.[7]

Recently, the role of the vaginal biofilm produced by *Candida* has become recognized as a factor in virulence of the yeast, and protection of the yeast leading to poor responses to antifungal therapy, unrelated to specific drug resistance.[8]

### *Management*

There are multiple effective, inexpensive, well-known, and safe options, both oral and topical, for treating *C albicans* vaginitis. These include over-the-counter and prescription medications, both off-label and approved for candidiasis by the Food and Drug Administration (FDA). These medications are roughly equal in effectiveness for *C albicans* and differ by price, convenience, patient preference, and tolerability. Both the Centers for Disease Control and Prevention (CDC)[9] and the Vulvovaginal Yeast App developed by the International Society for the Study of Vulvovaginal Disease ($4.99 at the App store) are convenient and detailed sources for the treatment of uncomplicated and complicated vulvovaginal yeast infections. The latter discusses management for each of the major non-*albicans Candida* species.

Topical antifungal medications are available over the counter. Miconazole and clotrimazole are topical agents available over the counter as creams or tablets, ranging from a one dose formulation up to 7-day dosing. Tioconazole is available over the counter as a one dose cream or ointment. Butoconazole (1- and 3-day vaginal cream) and terconazole (3- and 7-day cream and 3-day suppositories) are topical agents available by prescription. The topical creams, especially those that are 1-day or 3-day formulations, may be irritating for those women who are especially inflamed, so either nystatin ointment or oral therapy is preferred in those patients. Nystatin ointment is no longer available as vaginal tablets, so the ointment can be inserted, 100 000 units once or twice a day for 1-2 weeks. Or, nystatin vaginal suppositories can be compounded. With these topical preparations, the creams and ointments can be applied to the involved vulvar skin as well twice a day until the patient is comfortable.

Oral therapy has the advantage of avoiding irritation from the alcohols, preservatives, and stabilizers in topical creams, and it also has the benefit of treating both the vulva and vagina simultaneously, although many providers add a topical agent when there is marked vulvar involvement. Until recently, fluconazole was the only oral medication with FDA approval for vaginal candidiasis, although is itraconazole is known to be effective, as is ketoconazole. However, ketoconazole is no longer used for this condition, since it has specifically been withdrawn by the FDA for the indication of superficial fungal infections because of the risk of idiosyncratic hepatotoxicity, and the fact that fluconazole is equally effective but safer. The dose for an uncomplicated vulvovaginal *C albicans* infection is 150 mg once, although a repeat in 3 days is commonly prescribed. When larger numbers of tablets are prescribed, such as for suppression for frequently recurrent infection, the 200 mg size generally is inexplicably less expensive per tablet. The most common side effects of fluconazole are headache, occurring in about 13% of patients (as compared with 7% of those receiving placebo), and nausea, occurring in 7% of patients. Itraconazole is another oral azole that has similar efficacy to one fluconazole tablet in uncomplicated vaginal candidiasis at a dose of two 100-mg capsules twice in 1 day, but it does not have indication approval for vulvovaginal candidiasis.[10]

The average patient with *C albicans* vaginitis experiences resolution of symptoms within 2 or 3 days. Patients who have had severe vulvovaginal candidiasis can require longer time for their symptoms to resolve.

Patients who do not clear with these standard therapies most often do not have resistant *candidiasis* but rather have symptoms that are not due to yeast. In immunocompetent patients, symptoms of *C albicans* that do not clear are most often associated with vulvodynia or dermatoses such as lichen simplex chronicus or lichen sclerosus. Despite the frequent use of empiric anticandidal therapy and long-term suppressive use of fluconazole, resistant *C albicans* is not a common clinical issue in the usual outpatient setting.[5]

However, some patients have complicated vaginal candidiasis, defined as three or more episodes of vaginal yeast per year, an unusually severe episode of vulvovaginal yeast with vulvar redness, fissures, and erosions, candidiasis in an immunosuppressed patient, or a non-*albicans Candida* infection. These patients generally require therapy beyond the standard discussed above, and the reader is again referred to the CDC site regarding complicated yeast therapy, and in more detail on the Vulvovaginal Yeast App. Patients who simply experience frequent *C albicans* infections generally experience suppression of yeast with weekly fluconazole 150 mg, rarely requiring twice weekly dosing. Again, the use of fluconazole 200 mg rather than 150 mg is less expensive. Also, because fluconazole is only FDA approved as a one-time dose for uncomplicated candidiasis, the use of the 200 mg preparation avoids the issue of pre-authorization for off-label use of multiple doses. When symptoms persist despite weekly dosing, cultures should be performed to ensure that persistence of yeast is the cause of the patients' symptoms. When cultures are positive despite twice-weekly dosing of fluconazole, both cultures and sensitivities should be obtained. Whereas ongoing weekly fluconazole generally suppresses candidiasis, it is not curative, and discontinuation usually results in recurrence of yeast.[11] For patients whom fluconazole is not an option, either because of allergy, side effects, or potential medication reactions, a topical medication to clear the infection, when inserted two or three times a week is usually equally efficacious.

*In vitro* sensitivities do not correlate directly to clinical responses to antifungal therapy and should not be obtained routinely in clinical practice, but only for those patients with *C albicans* who do not respond to aggressive routine therapy. The pH of the vagina is different than that used during laboratory testing, which is one reason that clinical response may not mirror that expected from *in vitro* sensitivities. However, if the *in vitro* testing shows resistance to a medication, that medication will not be useful.

Women who exhibit severe vulvar candidiasis with extensive redness and fissuring should receive a topical vulvar antifungal therapy as well as vaginal therapy. Nystatin ointment applied three or four times a day is arguably the most soothing preparation. These patients may require longer than usual standard therapy.

Patients who are immunosuppressed, especially those with HIV disease, are more likely to require longer antifungal therapy, chronic suppression, and more likely to experience resistant *Candida* infection. Therefore, immunosuppressed patients who remain symptomatic following therapy lasting 2 weeks rather than 1 week should be re-evaluated with cultures and sensitivities. The standard next step when oral or topical azoles are not sufficient is the use of vaginal boric acid 600-mg capsules inserted once or twice a day for 2 or more weeks. These are poisonous if swallowed. A recently approved oral anticandidal therapy unrelated to fluconazole is ibrexafungerp; *in vitro* studies suggest that it may prove useful for resistant *C albicans* in immunosuppressed patients, as well as non-*albicans* yeast forms.[12]

The role of lactobacilli (probiotics) in the treatment is controversial with no definitive data at this time.[13]

**UNCOMPLICATED *C ALBICANS* VULVOVAGINITIS — Management**

- Fluconazole 150 or 200 mg once (90% cure), often repeated in 3 days
- Any topical azole suppository or cream, per package insert
- Topical azole or nystatin twice daily also to vulva when vulvar involvement

**FREQUENTLY RECURRENT *C ALBICANS* — Management**

- Fluconazole 150-200 mg weekly for 3-6 months; rarely needed q3d (confirm persistent yeast with a culture).
- Vaginal azole or boric acid 600 mg per vagina 2-3 times a week for 3-6 months if fluconazole is contraindicated.
- May continue longer than 6 months when needed.
- Probiotics and diet generally have not been shown beneficial, although there is some conflicting evidence for probiotics.

Unfortunately, most non-*albicans Candida* infections are clinically resistant to usual therapies, especially those caused by *C glabrata*, *C krusei*, and *S cerevisiae*, despite *in vitro*

TABLE 14-1

Therapies for Recalcitrant Non-*albicans Candida* Vaginal Infections

| Medication | Dosing | Advantages | Disadvantages[a,b] |
|---|---|---|---|
| Boric acid vaginal capsules | 600 mg inserted bid ×2-4 wk | Primary medication used for azole-resistant infection; inexpensive, usually effective | Sometimes irritating, poisonous if ingested orally |
| Nystatin vaginal suppositories or ointment | Insert bid ×1 mo | Inexpensive, nonirritating | Modestly effective |
| Gentian violet | 1% solution painted in the office weekly, or 0.5 cc onto tampon inserted for 3-4 h twice a day up to 12 d | Often effective medication | Can produce erosive contact dermatitis, stains skin, clothing, bathroom fixtures, exam tables |
| Flucytosine fourteen 500-mg capsules dissolved in 45 g of hydrophilic cream base | 6.4 g inserted hs × 1-2 wk | Well tolerated, effective | Very expensive |
| Amphotericin suppositories 50 mg | Insert hs for 2-4 wk | — | Expensive, can be irritating |
| Amphotericin/flucytosine vaginal suppositories | Insert hs | — | Expensive, can be irritating |

[a]All are often ineffective, and often several in sequence or together must be used for the best chance of success.
[b]All except nystatin are unavailable commercially and must be compounded, and nystatin suppositories must be compounded.

sensitivities that may indicate sensitivity to these medications. These yeast forms sometimes are extraordinarily difficult to eradicate (Table 14-1). Although an azole can be tried first for these non-*albicans Candida* infections (except *C krusei*, which is always resistant to azoles), patients should be advised that their infection likely will not clear. The occurrence of resistant non-*albicans Candida* organisms is related to characteristics of the organism rather than the presence of immunosuppression in the host.

First-line treatment for non-*albicans Candida* infections resistant to azole therapy is boric acid capsules, which are prescribed by instructing a pharmacist to place 600 mg of boric acid in a gelatin capsule.[14] This capsule is inserted in the vagina daily for 2 weeks. Boric acid capsules are irritating in some patients, particularly those who are already irritated by their infection. Most women experience significant improvement but not necessarily cure, with symptoms recurring off therapy, requiring maintenance therapy with boric acid. Nystatin vaginal tablets or ointment are sometimes more beneficial than azoles.

Also used is intravaginal flucytosine. Fourteen 500-mg capsules of flucytosine are dissolved in 45 g of a hydrophilic cream base, and a 6.4-g vaginal applicator filled with cream is inserted in the vagina daily for a week. This can be extremely expensive but the price fluctuates. Resistance occurs quickly.

Compounded 50 mg amphotericin vaginal suppositories inserted nightly represent still another alternative, but there are no data on the effectiveness of intravaginal amphotericin. There are several recipes for these suppositories, and these are generally available from any compounding pharmacy.

Gentian violet is a traditional potent fungicidal substance that is rarely used for practical reasons. This is an extreme irritant in some patients, occasionally producing even blisters and erosions. It is also extremely messy and causes permanent purple staining of clothes, furniture, and bathroom fixtures. One regimen consists of a weekly application of a 1% solution painted onto the vaginal walls with a saturated gauze swab in the office. However, to avoid the occasional blistering reaction to the 1% concentration of gentian violet, I use a 0.25% solution for the first treatment, followed by 0.5% a few days later, and then 0.75% solution before graduating to a full 1.0% solution. Medication is applied weekly in the office for 4-6 weeks. Far less burdensome for the provider's office, is the use of tampons as a delivery system. Gentian violet 1%, 0.5 cc, is applied to a tampon, which is inserted and left in place for 3-4 hours once or twice a day for up to 12 days.

Combinations of therapies may logically be useful, but there are no confirmatory data. Also, there are few data on these alternative therapies even singly for complicated yeast infections.[15]

In addition, ibrexafungerp, as noted above, is a novel oral triterpenoid antifungal therapy, the first of a new class of anticandidal agents to received FDA approval in decades. This medication shows promise against *C glabrata in vitro*, but it remains to be seen if this translates into a useful medication in vaginal non-*albicans Candida* infections.[16]

**NON-*ALBICANS CANDIDA* — Management**

- Usually, no symptoms, no need to treat
- Any azole or nystatin (except no fluconazole for *C krusei*)
- Boric acid 600-mg capsules ***per vagina*** once or twice a day, 2-4 weeks
- Nystatin ointment or vaginal suppository once or twice a day for 2-4 weeks
- Flucytosine per vagina hs for 7-14 days
- Gentian violet

## Trichomonas Vaginitis

Trichomoniasis is the most common nonviral sexually transmitted disease worldwide, more common in women than in men, with 2.1% of women in the United States affected, and the highest rate of 9.6% being in Black women.[17]

### *Clinical Presentation*

*Trichomonas* vaginitis produces extreme itching and irritation. Dysuria and lower abdominal pain are common, and most patients experience a copious yellow or green vaginal discharge.

Bright red erythema of the vestibule is usual on physical examination. The vagina is inflamed as well, and although a "strawberry" cervix with discrete, punctate, bright red, and hemorrhagic macules and papules is classic, this appearance is by no means sensitive or specific. A copious, yellow or greenish, vaginal discharge is typical. The vaginal pH is higher than normal, as occurs with most extremely inflammatory vaginal diseases and cervicitis characterized by an absence of lactobacilli.

Trichomonas can occur in men, where it remains a reservoir for infection, but it is generally asymptomatic. A purulent urethral discharge occurs in some patients.

Risk factors include the presence of bacterial vaginosis, poverty, multiple sex partners, and a history of incarceration.[17]

In the past few years, the *Trichomonas vaginalis* virus has been described and reported discovered in 40% of 355 isolates of archived frozen *T vaginalis* in Birmingham, AL.[18] However, this did not correlate with symptoms, clinical course, or resistance, suggesting that the virus is commensal.

### *Diagnosis*

This diagnosis often is made on a wet mount if it is examined immediately under high power. When identified, the trichomonads are obvious and the specificity is 100%.

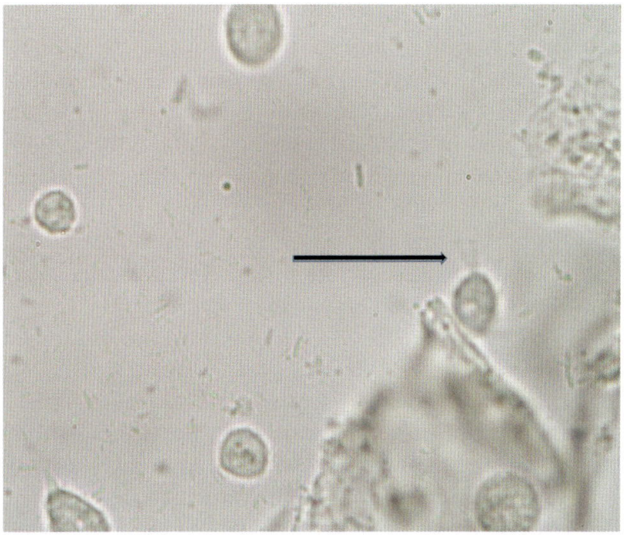

Fig. 14-6. Trichomonads are oval or teardrop-shaped protozoa with irregular jerky movements as they are pulled by faintly seen flagella (*arrow*).

These flagellate organisms are teardrop shaped, and they are extremely active, so their motion is not missed easily, and neutrophils are abundant (**Fig. 14-6**). However, the absence of trichomonads in no way rules out the diagnosis. As trichomonads cool, they lose their characteristic teardrop shape, becoming round and still, making differentiation from lymphocytes very difficult. The sensitivity of a microscopic examination varies from about 44% to 68%.[19] Therefore, when there is a high index of suspicion, cultures or DNA probes are indicated in the absence of a positive wet mount, with molecular studies being the most sensitive.[20] Although less sensitive, a thin prep Papanicolaou test showing the presence of trichomonads generally correlates with the presence of infection, although the accuracy is dependent upon the expertise of the examiner.[21] There are no specific histologic findings on biopsy.

The differential diagnosis of *Trichomonas* vaginitis includes all causes of a purulent vaginitis, including desquamative inflammatory vaginitis (DIV) and inflammation associated with an atrophic vaginal epithelium, an intravaginal foreign body, or any erosive vaginal skin disease.

***TRICHOMONAS* VAGINITIS — Diagnosis**

- Discharge, irritation, itching, burning.
- Red mucous membranes and modified mucous membranes; sometimes a classic "strawberry cervix."
- White or yellow copious vaginal secretions.
- pH higher than 5.
- Wet mount showing motile trichomonads; if negative, nucleic acid amplification testing is essential for diagnosis.

*Pathophysiology*

Trichomoniasis is caused by the protozoan *T vaginalis*. This disease is always sexually transmitted. The vagina is the primary area of involvement, but the organism is sequestered in other areas in both men and women, including the paraurethral ducts, the urethra, and Skene glands. Circumcision reduces infection rate with trichomonads in men, and this disease can be prevented by the use of condoms. Risk factors include the presence of an intrauterine device and older age in women.[22]

*Management*

Trichomoniasis should be treated orally because topical therapies do not eliminate organisms sequestered within the urethra and paraurethral ducts. In addition, sex partners must be treated to prevent immediate reinfection. Oral metronidazole, at a dose of 500 mg twice a day for 1 week is the treatment of choice and is superior to the single 2-g dose, which is also advocated.[23] The widely held belief in the disulfiramlike effect of metronidazole with alcohol consumption is erroneous, based on no scientific or theoretic data considering the mechanism of action of both metronidazole and tinidazole.[24] Individual case reports of this can be ascribed to effects of the alcohol or metronidazole alone, so there is no need to avoid alcohol with these medications, in some patients, although this is actually uncommon and poorly documented. Tinidazole is better tolerated with slightly higher cure rates.

Although treatment failure is discussed as an increasing issue, this is actually uncommon, with most "resistant" trichomonas due to reinfection. A large survey recently did not find prospective studies that confirm high levels of drug resistance, and very little in the way of high level *in vitro* resistance, although clinical resistance was widely reported.[25]

Old studies showed that resistance to metronidazole is present in 4%-10% of cases and to tinidazole in 1% of patients.[17] Often, high-dose therapy overcomes this resistance, and first-line therapy consists of high-dose metronidazole or tinidazole.[26,27] Other therapies include combination therapies, including high-dose tinidazole with intravaginal paromomycin cream, intravaginal boric acid, and intravaginal metronidazole/miconazole.[27]

An occasional patient is allergic to metronidazole, and if alternative therapies are not useful, desensitization can be used.

**TRICHOMONAS VAGINITIS — Management**

- STD screen.
- Metronidazole 500 mg bid for 1 week, or metronidazole or tinidazole 2 g once.
- Topical azoles can provide some comfort but not cure.
- Nucleic acid amplification testing in 3 months for test of cure and evaluation of reinfection.

## Bacterial Vaginosis

Bacterial vaginosis (BV) is the most common cause of vaginal discharge in premenopausal women,[28] but 84% of women with BV have no symptoms.[29] This is an unpleasant, but generally benign, disruption in the population of common premenopausal vaginal flora.

*Clinical Presentation*

Women with bacterial vaginosis report an increased volume of vaginal secretions and an unpleasant fishy odor, especially after contact with alkaline semen during intercourse. In spite of the increased volume of theoretically irritating alkaline secretions, itching and burning are generally absent or mild, and there is no vaginal or introital redness. This lack of clinical inflammation and the lack of inflammatory cells on wet mount are the reason for the term "vaginosis" rather than "vaginitis." Complications of symptomatic bacterial vaginosis include an increased risk of preterm labor and acquisition of sexually transmitted diseases including HIV, gonorrhea, chlamydia, and trichomonas, as well as pelvic inflammatory disease.[30] Herpes simplex virus 1 and 2 and human papillomavirus infection rates are higher as well.[31]

*Diagnosis*

The diagnosis of bacterial vaginosis is very easy and does not require laboratory testing beyond that provided by a microscope. A very quick, high-power scan of a wet mount shows clue cells and loss of lactobacilli, and the diagnosis is confirmed by a positive whiff test. For a formal diagnosis, the vaginal fluid should show at least three of the following Amsel criteria; a profuse, milky vaginal discharge; a vaginal pH >5 due to loss of lactobacilli; the presence of a fishy odor when secretions are exposed to 10% or 20% potassium hydroxide (positive whiff test); and the presence of clue cells on microscopic examination of vaginal smears **(Fig. 14-7)**. Clue cells are squamous epithelial cells covered by coccobacilli that give the cytoplasm a ground-glass appearance and obscure the crisp margins of the cell, leaving ragged borders. Bacterial vaginosis is also characterized by no increase in white blood cells.

For practical purposes, a vaginal pH > 5 and the milky nature of the vaginal discharge are nonspecific, and the diagnosis should not be made without the presence of clue cells and the absence of lactobacilli. The diagnosis can be suggested but not be made by molecular studies that show the presence of vaginal microbiota associated with bacterial vaginosis. In addition, bacterial vaginosis exists on a spectrum, from a few to very many clue cells, etc.

Vaginal biopsies are not performed for this disease, but they are presumably normal. Poor hygiene producing odor and a heavy but normal physiologic discharge can mimic bacterial vaginosis, but the relatively high pH and characteristic microscopic findings are diagnostic.

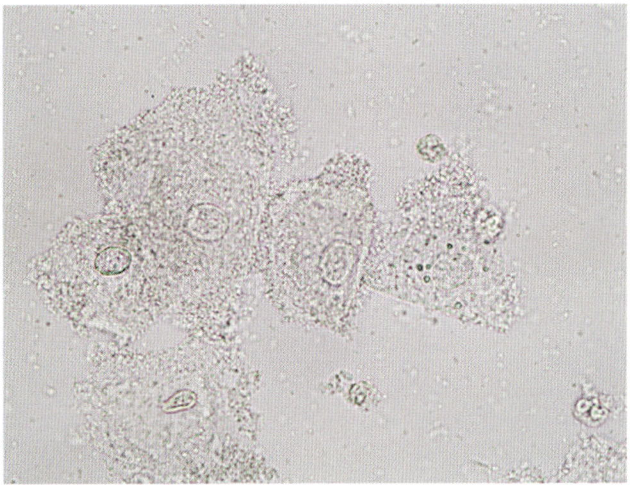

Fig. 14-7. Clue cells, pathognomonic for bacterial vaginosis, are cells that are covered with small bacteria that confer a ground-glass appearance to the cell, and overhang the borders, producing poorly demarcated ragged borders.

*Trichomonas* can produce a heavy discharge and pH >5, as can DIV, but these conditions exhibit an increase in white blood cells on wet mount, no clue cells, and a negative whiff test.

**BACTERIAL VAGINOSIS** — **Diagnosis**

- Discharge and odor, especially following sexual intercourse; occasional itching, irritation
- pH of 5 or higher
- Wet mount showing clue cells, lack of lactobacilli, lack of increased white blood cells
- Positive whiff test

*Pathophysiology*

Bacterial vaginosis is produced by shift in the proportion of organisms often present as part of the normal vaginal flora, a polybacterial dysbiosis. The usual predominance of lactobacilli is replaced by *Gardnerella vaginalis*, *Prevotella* species, *Mobiluncus* species, *Atopobium vaginae*, among others.[29] The characteristic odor of bacterial vaginosis is produced by the release of bacterial amines following exposure to an alkaline substance such as potassium hydroxide or semen.

Although bacterial vaginosis occurs primarily in women who are sexually active, the role of sexual activity is not clear, and this does not appear to be a sexually transmitted disease. Women who have never been sexually active are rarely affected.[32] However, multiple male sex partners, female partners, and sexual relationships with more than one person are risk factors.[33] A new sex partner and lack of condom use are risk factors,[29] as is regular douching,[34] and perhaps alcohol consumption.[35] Male circumcision decreases the risk of BV in female partners.[36]

*Management*

Metronidazole 500 mg twice daily for 7 days or 2 g in one dose usually clears these symptoms, although the single-dose therapy is slightly less effective. As noted above, the disulfiramlike effect of metronidazole with alcohol consumption does not occur as previously believed, so patients can be told that alcohol can be used in moderation with both metronidazole and tinidazole.[24] Topical metronidazole, inserted twice daily for 5 days, and clindamycin 2% vaginal cream, inserted at bedtime for 3-7 days, are equally beneficial, with fewer side effects compared to oral metronidazole. Oral clindamycin has not only been studied widely but also is effective at 300 mg twice daily for 1 week.[29] Clindamycin ovules 100 mg intravaginally once at bedtime for 3 days, secnidazole 2 g oral granules in a single dose, tinidazole 2 g orally once daily for 2 days, and tinidazole 1 g orally once daily for 5 days have all been listed by the CDC as alternative therapies.[29]

However, recurrence is very common, occurring in about three-quarters of patients.[30] Patients should be counseled regarding the risk factors for BV, including douching, condom use, etc. Probiotics are sometimes used as a means to enhance the repopulation of normal lactobacilli to prevent recurrence, primarily without compelling evidence for benefit.[29,37] Recent evidence suggests that use of probiotics for 1-3 months may be useful in minimizing recurrences.[38]

Another intervention often discussed to prevent recurrence is the wisdom of treating partners. BV-associated bacteria have been identified on the penis of males, but older studies did not show benefit with treatment.[39,40] A new study concludes that their data suggest that further study may be worthwhile.[41]

Although higher doses and longer courses of current medication have been suggested as means of decreasing recurrences, these have thus far not been especially useful. Borrowing from standard of care for the management of recurrent candidiasis, I use chronic suppressive doses of medication. Clindamycin 300 mg twice a day for 1 week followed by 150 twice a day ongoing has been uniformly successful in my office, with careful education regarding the risk of *Clostridium difficile*. Most patients have remained clear when clindamycin is discontinued after several months. Oral metronidazole is unpleasant, so other suppressive medications I have used are vaginal metronidazole gel and clindamycin cream, inserted several times weekly after initial clearing.

Because bacterial vaginosis is associated with a significant increased risk of acquisition of sexually transmitted disease, pelvic inflammatory disease, tendency toward future infertility, and complications with pregnancy, treatment should be considered even for those with asymptomatic disease.

**BACTERIAL VAGINOSIS** **Management**

- Metronidazole or tinidazole 2 g once, or 500 mg bid for 7 days.
- Metronidazole, 1 g inserted per vagina bid for 5 days.
- Clindamycin cream, one applicatorful per vagina hs for 3-7 days.
- Clindamycin 300 mg bid for 1 week (not FDA approved for this indication).
- Clindamycin ovules 100 mg intravaginally once at bedtime for 3 days, secnidazole 2 g oral granules in a single dose, tinidazole 2 g orally once daily for 2 days, and tinidazole 1 g orally once daily for 5 days.
- For recurrent BV, consider ongoing suppressive medication, at whatever dosing/frequency controls disease.

## Bacterial Vaginitis

Bacterial vaginitis, unlike bacterial vaginosis, is a rare specific infection with a bacterial organism that produces inflammation. Cultured organisms are much more often innocent bystanders rather than the cause of an infection.

### *Clinical Presentation*

Vulvovaginal redness, irritation, rawness, and soreness, associated with a yellow or yellow-green vaginal secretions, are typical complaints of women with bacterial vaginitis. Dyspareunia is common.

On physical examination, vulvar erythema is common, often associated with a slightly glazed texture to the vulvar skin. Although scale and fissures within skinfolds are common, the vulva occasionally appears entirely normal. The vaginal epithelium is generally red, and vaginal secretions are grossly and microscopically purulent, with a remarkable increase in neutrophils on wet mount **(Fig. 14-8)**. Often, many epithelial cells are immature parabasal cells, signifying erosions or the increased turnover of epithelial cells that would be manifested as scale on dry, keratinized epithelium. Also usual are a decrease in lactobacilli and a resulting pH of >5. Sometimes, especially when the organism is group A *Streptococcus*, or, less often group B *Streptococcus*, chains of cocci are seen.

### *Diagnosis*

The diagnosis is made by clinical suspicion and a bacterial culture showing a pure growth of a pathogen, but confirmation requires response to therapy. Most often, especially when *Streptococcus agalactiae* (GBS) is the identified organism, appropriate antibiotic therapy does not resolve signs or symptoms, because nearly always the organism is a coincidental colonizer of inflamed, compromised epithelium.[42] However, occasionally, inflammation resolves promptly with therapy, although immediate recurrence of antibiotics is common. Histology has not been described, but a biopsy would presumably exhibit an acute inflammatory infiltrate with stromal and epidermal edema.

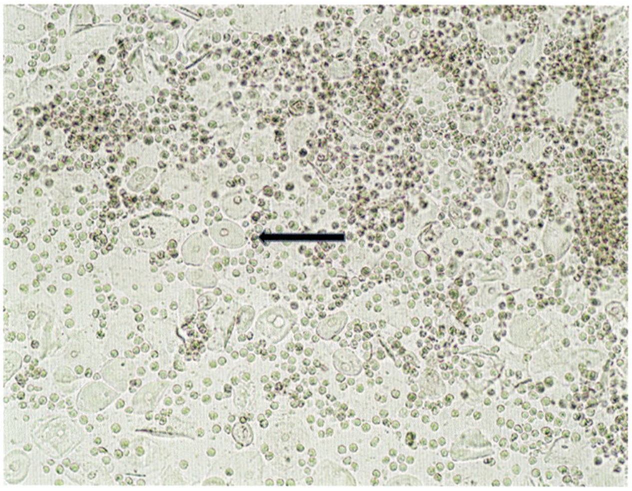

Fig. 14-8. Nearly always, a culture that yields bacteria is not a sign of infection, but only colonizing local organisms. Treating these usually does not eliminate symptoms, even when the result is a known pathogen such as *S aureus*. However, occasionally bacterial vaginitis does occur and can be considered when the culture is obtained in the setting of an inflammatory wet mount with increased white blood cells (*the small dark cells*) and sometimes parabasal cells (*arrow*). This wet mount is indistinguishable from erosive vaginitis, desquamative inflammatory vaginitis, and atrophic vaginitis. The setting, a clinical evaluation of vaginal walls and other mucous membranes, and molecular studies to rule out infection aid in diagnosis.

The signs and symptoms of symptomatic bacterial vaginitis can be identical to those associated with atrophic vaginitis due to age, pregnancy, or breastfeeding; with DIV; and with an inflammatory erosive dermatosis such as lichen planus. These diseases are distinguished by their setting, negative cultures, and response to appropriate therapy for each individual disease. As noted earlier, these diseases not only resemble bacterial vaginitis but also can be complicated by bacterial colonization or a secondary bacterial infection.

### *Pathophysiology*

Bacterial vaginitis is an infection with a specific bacterial organism. Group A β-hemolytic *Streptococcus* (GAS) infection is relatively common in children but rarely found in adult women as well.[43] Asymptomatic carriage from male partners has been implicated as a cause of recurrent GAS vaginitis.[43,44] Although the existence of vaginitis produced by GBS is controversial, many clinicians are confident that this entity exists, although it is uncommon.[45] Clinicians who care for vaginitis report the occasional patient who exhibits purulent vaginal secretions, symptoms of irritation, a culture yielding GBS, and immediate remarkable improvement with antibiotics. However, the overwhelming majority cultures that yield GBS represent colonization only. *Staphylococcus aureus* usually occurs in a predisposing setting (such as a retained tampon), vulvar lichen simplex chronicus/eczema that is secondarily infected or adjacent staphylococcal folliculitis. Cultures commonly yield *Escherichia coli* or other enterics, but in my experience, patients do not improve symptomatically or clinically with antibiotics, showing that these are contaminants rather than pathogens.

#### Management

The treatment of bacterial vaginitis includes amelioration of predisposing conditions including atrophic vaginitis or erosive vaginal disease and identification and removal of any foreign body. The patient should be treated with an antibiotic known to be active against the organism identified on culture. Often, prolonged therapy may be required while any underlying condition is adequately treated. GBS is recognized as extremely difficult to eradicate, and treatment with penicillin V potassium or oral clindamycin is often followed by immediate recurrence. Theoretically, the use of newer probiotics may help to minimize this recurrence.

A topical corticosteroid such as triamcinolone ointment applied twice a day to modified mucous membranes of an irritated vulva can improve comfort more quickly because this is a nonspecific anti-inflammatory medication.

Because some women tend to develop candidiasis with antibiotic use, particularly in combination with topical steroids, I treat with fluconazole once weekly to prevent intercurrent yeast while they are taking an antibiotic and topical corticosteroid. This oral medication avoids the irritation of a topical antifungal in an already irritated vulva and vagina.

### Aerobic Vaginitis

Aerobic vaginitis is a poorly understood vaginitis described by Donders.[46] Descriptions vary among scientists, with many Chinese authors reporting this as an infection produced by specific commensal pathogens. Donders, however, describes this as an inflammatory dysbiotic condition.

#### Clinical Presentation

Donders finds this to be a very common condition, occurring in 2.0%-25.8% of nonpregnant women and fewer pregnant women.[47] Patients experience variable degrees of dyspareunia and, sometimes, itching. Physical findings show variable degrees of redness and edema of the vagina, with yellow to green vaginal secretions that can have a rotten odor in more severe disease. A wet mount shows parabasal cells, leukocytes, no clue cells, and absent lactobacilli. The presence of aerobic vaginitis predisposes to preterm labor, premature rupture of membranes, and fetal infection.[47]

#### Diagnosis

The diagnosis is made by clinical findings and microscopy showing leukorrhea, parabasal cells, and loss of lactobacilli, with a pH > 5. Also required is the exclusion of atrophic vaginitis, infections, especially trichomoniasis, erosive dermatoses causing inflammatory vaginitis, and bacterial vaginitis. A culture showing organisms such as group B streptococci, *S aureus*, or *E coli* in no way proves a diagnosis of bacterial vaginitis, as these are common nonpathogens in aerobic vaginitis as well. This condition often coexists with other infections and causes of vaginitis. Phase microscopy is important in making the diagnosis by determining an AV score calculated according to lactobacillary grade, presence of inflammation, proportion of toxic leucocytes, and characteristics of the microflora.[46] This makes diagnosis in a private practice office difficult.

#### Pathophysiology

Like bacterial vaginosis, aerobic vaginitis is associated with the replacement of dominant lactobacilli microbiota by other bacilli or cocci, but in this case, aerobic bacteria rather than the anaerobic organisms replace lactobacilli as seen in bacterial vaginosis. Whether this occurs as a result of abnormal mucosa or whether the abnormal bacteria cause the changes in the mucosa is not known. Some have postulated that this is an immunologic disease.[48] Others believe that severe aerobic vaginitis represents desquamative inflammatory vaginitis. Produced by a disruption of the normal vaginal flora, there is overlap with bacterial vaginitis, and this may well represent the same process on those usual occasions when antibiotics do not clear the symptoms, the physical findings, and the microscopic appearance of vaginal fluid. Some feel that the severe end of the spectrum overlaps with desquamative inflammatory vaginitis.

Like bacterial vaginosis, aerobic vaginitis results from shift in the proportion of organisms often present as part of the normal vaginal flora. Lactobacilli are absent, and cultures often yield one or two enteric commensal organisms such as group B streptococci, *S aureus*, and *E coli*. In addition to the microbial component, there is a component of atrophy and inflammation.

#### Management

There is no specific treatment, and further research is needed to investigate the roles of estrogen, corticosteroids, antibiotics, and probiotics for the management of this condition.

### Cytolytic Vaginosis (Döderlein Cytolysis)

Cytologic vaginosis is a controversial vaginal condition said to be produced by an overgrowth of lactobacilli. The existence of this vaginal condition remains in debate, a recent review of 1152 wet mounts in patients with symptoms of candidiasis described 3.8% as having cytolytic vaginosis based on cytologic criteria.[37]

#### Clinical Presentation

Cibley and Cibley reported that patients present with symptoms similar to those of a yeast infection, with itching, irritation, and a thick, clumped, white vaginal discharge.[49] On physical examination, the skin appears normal without redness. There is a normally acid vaginal pH < 4.5.

#### Diagnosis

The diagnosis of cytolytic vaginosis is made by the constellation of symptoms in a setting of an acid vaginal pH and by characteristic findings on a cytologic examination of vaginal secretions.[33] Microscopically, there are large numbers of epithelial cells, many that are fragmented or exhibit nuclei that have been stripped of surrounding cytoplasm, "naked nuclei."[50] These nuclei can be difficult to distinguish from lymphocytes without phase microscopy or a Gram stain, incorrectly suggesting an inflammatory wet mount. In addition, lactobacilli are extremely abundant, yeast forms are absent, and white blood cells are not increased in number. There are no specific histologic findings, and a biopsy is not indicated.

*Candida* vaginitis is the major disease to be differentiated from cytolytic vaginosis, and *Lactobacillus* vaginosis also produces the same symptoms and characteristic discharge. However, these entities can be differentiated by the respective absence of yeast forms.

#### Pathophysiology

The cause of cytolytic vaginosis is postulated by some physicians to be an abnormal increase in lactobacilli and resulting lactic acid. However, a recent thoughtful review of the recent scant literature showed that reported patients were diagnosed without adequate exclusion of other causes of vaginitis, and there were inadequacies of sampling sites and techniques, and unreliable evidence of lactobacilli overgrowth, so that this disease cannot be characterized or confirmed as an entity.[51]

#### Management

The treatment for cytolytic vaginosis consists of alkaline douches with a dilute solution of sodium bicarbonate. Thirty to sixty grams of baking soda is mixed with 1 L of warm water. Patients douche two or three times a week, until they are comfortable. This therapy does not eliminate cytolytic vaginosis, and douching once or twice a week may be needed to control symptoms. As noted by Voytik and Nyirjesy, management for this condition has been stagnant, without reports of further treatments or response to this initial suggestion for treatment.[51]

### Vaginal Lactobacillosis (Lactobacillosis)

Like cytolytic vaginosis, vaginal lactobacillosis is a vaginal condition reported to be caused by an overgrowth of lactobacilli.[52] Also, like cytolytic vaginosis, the existence of this condition as a cause of symptoms is controversial.

#### Clinical Presentation

Women with *Lactobacillus* vaginosis report itching and irritation, which they generally assume to be caused by yeast. In addition, these patients often describe a yeastlike, white, thick, cheesy discharge. Physical examination reveals a normal vulva and vagina. A curdlike white discharge is often present, and the pH of these vaginal secretions is normally acid.

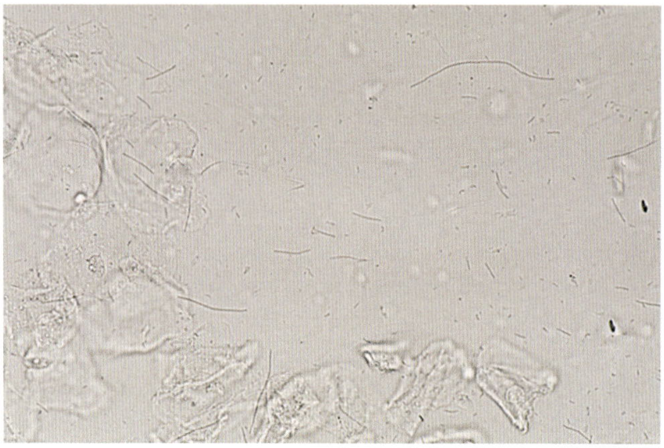

Fig. 14-9. Lactobacillosis is a controversial cause of vulvovaginal itching and irritation and is associated with long strands of lactobacilli formed by short lactobacilli that line up end-to-end. These are differentiated from yeast by their smaller caliber and nonbranching morphology.

#### Diagnosis

The diagnosis of this condition is based on the symptoms of itching and irritation in combination with characteristic microscopic findings of vaginal secretions. These reveal very elongated lactobacilli, once believed to represent leptothrix, and formerly thought to be a sign of trichomonas. There is no increase in white blood cells microscopically, and there are no yeast forms (**Fig. 14-9**). The histopathology of the vagina has not been described and is not important in the diagnosis. A normal biopsy would be expected.

The diseases most often confused with *Lactobacillus vaginosis* are vaginal candidiasis and cytolytic vaginosis. However, the microscopic appearance of the elongated lactobacilli is distinctive, and yeast forms are absent, as is cytolysis.

#### Pathophysiology

An increase in numbers of lactobacilli is believed to produce this controversial condition, and antifungal therapy was postulated to be a cause of this condition. Whether the therapy for yeast is causative or whether empiric anticandidal therapy is inevitable as first-line treatment for women with these symptoms is not known.

#### Management

Both eradication of symptoms and elimination of elongated lactobacilli can be achieved with either doxycycline (100 mg twice daily for 2 weeks), amoxicillin/clavulanic acid (500 mg twice daily), or ciprofloxacin 250 mg twice daily for a week. I have treated women with these microscopic findings in the setting of itching or irritation/burning on multiple occasions with elimination of the elongated lactobacilli but continuation of symptoms. I no longer believe lactobacillus vaginosis to be a cause of symptoms.

## Noninfectious Inflammatory Vaginal Diseases

Although the most common cause of acute vaginitis is an infection, chronic symptoms of vaginitis usually are not infectious in nature.

### Atrophic Vagina and Vaginitis (Genitourinary Syndrome of Menopause)

An atrophic vagina is part of the genitourinary syndrome of menopause (GSM) spectrum that generally occurs several years following menopause. With traditional menopause, this is chronic and progressive. However, this can also occur in other states that result in low estrogen, such as during breastfeeding, and with medications administered during breast cancer therapy that block the effects of estrogen. With the loss of estrogen, the vaginal epithelium becomes thin and dry; if friction produces erosions, inflammation can occur, resulting in atrophic vaginitis. GSM includes urinary symptoms of dysuria, urgency, stress incontinence, and recurrent urinary tract infections, as well as sexual symptoms of decreased libido, difficulty in arousal, and decreased orgasm in addition to the symptoms of vaginal atrophy are discussed here.

#### *Clinical Presentation*

The atrophic vagina has become extremely common since the routine use of systemic estrogen after menopause has become less common over the past 20 years. Although an atrophic vagina is often asymptomatic, especially in women who are not sexually active, about half of women develop sensations of dryness discomfort, and dyspareunia is common. Atrophic vaginitis, in which atrophy is accompanied by inflammation, is characterized by not only frequent sensations of dryness but sometimes irritation, rawness, and occasionally itching. Sexual intercourse is painful and exacerbates symptoms. An examination of the atrophic vulva and vagina shows pallor and smooth texture of the modified mucous membranes of the vulva. The normal wet, pink rugae of the vagina are replaced by pale, flat, inelastic, relatively dry mucosa **(Fig. 14-10)**. Occasionally, grossly purulent, although generally scant, vaginal secretions are present, representing actual atrophic vaginitis, and these women often exhibit erythema of mucous membranes. Rarely, there may even be erosions, in which fragile epithelium has been abraded by friction from intercourse or pressure from a vaginal wall that has been distended by a cystocele or a rectocele. Symptomatic atrophic vaginitis occurs when symptoms or signs of inflammation, such as vaginal erythema and white blood cells in vaginal secretions, develop as a result of erosions or, much less often, secondary infection.

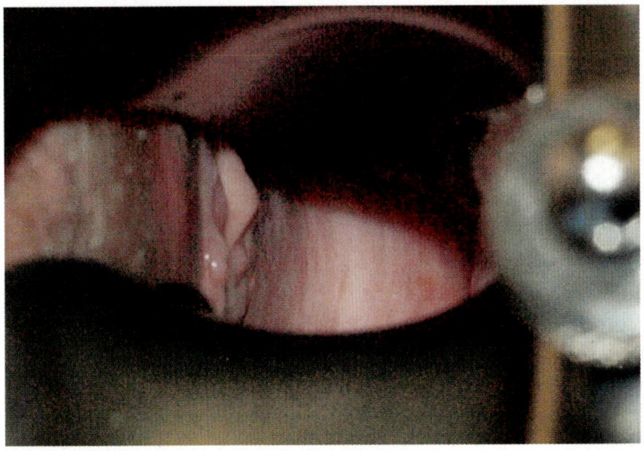

Fig. 14-10. The atrophic vaginal walls are pale, dry, and smooth instead of pink with prominent, wet rugae.

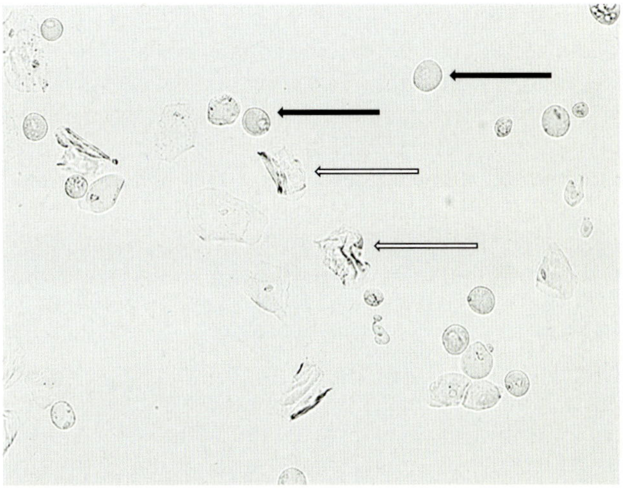

Fig. 14-11. An atrophic vagina is an expected development when estrogen levels diminish. When the vaginal walls thin, a wet mount is characterized by large numbers of round parabasal cells that represent immature epithelial cells (*black arrows*). These small, round squamous cells are shed from an epithelium only a few cell layers thick, so that all cells do not develop into the normal large flat mature cells before being shed into the vaginal fluid (*white arrows*).

#### *Diagnosis*

The diagnosis of an atrophic vagina is made by the above findings in a setting of estrogen deficiency and a typical wet mount that shows an increased proportion of parabasal cells and absent lactobacilli. Parabasal cells represent immature squamous cells, which are small, round, cells that have been shed from thinned, atrophic epithelium, rather than the mature, large, flat epithelial cells that are shed from the surface of well-estrogenized vaginal skin **(Fig. 14-11)**. Because lactobacilli are not present, the vaginal pH measures >5. Atrophic vaginitis occurs when significant inflammation from frictions or erosions occurs, and white cells are abundant on wet mount **(Fig. 14-12)**. The diagnoses of an atrophic vagina and atrophic vaginitis are confirmed by normalization of symptoms and signs promptly with estrogen therapy. A vaginal biopsy is performed for the diagnosis of atrophic vaginitis. Histologically, however, the tissue shows epithelial thinning. In addition, the absence of normal maturation with progressive flattening of epithelial cells closer to the surface is characteristic.

DIV presents similarly to atrophic vaginitis, with parabasal cells, purulent vaginal secretions, and a negative culture. However, the history of a woman with atrophic vaginitis should reveal a setting of estrogen deficiency, and

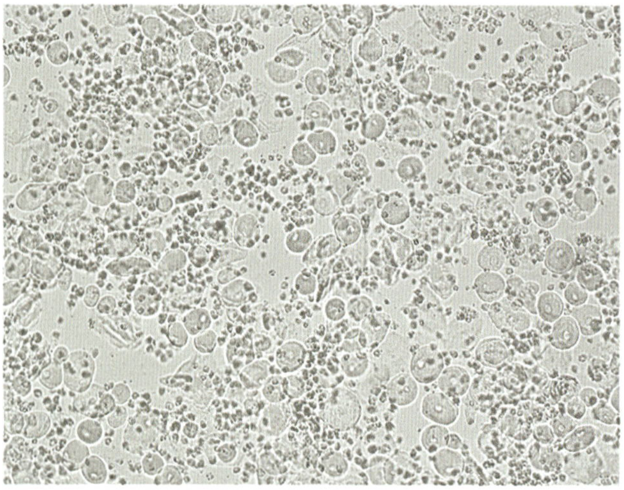

Fig. 14-12. The vaginal walls are so thin, that friction from rubbing against a cystocele or rectocele can produce erosions that lead to inflammation and atrophic vaginitis, with resulting erythema of vaginal walls, yellow vaginal secretions, and abundant white blood cells as well as parabasal cells. Again, this wet mount is indistinguishable from desquamative inflammatory vaginitis and other causes of vaginal erosions such as lichen planus.

estrogen should quickly correct the abnormalities. Bacterial vaginitis presents with this picture, but a positive culture with prompt response to antibiotic therapy rules out this entity. Aerobic vaginitis is also identical on presentation, but this often occurs in premenopausal women, and topical estrogen does not clear the process of aerobic vaginitis. Erosive mucosal skin disease such as lichen planus, pemphigus vulgaris, and mucous membrane pemphigoid can mimic atrophic vaginitis, but erosions should be prominent, nearly always occur on other mucosal surfaces, show characteristic histologic findings, and fail to respond to estrogen.

### ATROPHIC VAGINA/VAGINITIS — Diagnosis

- Sometimes asymptomatic, sometimes burning, dryness, dyspareunia
- Setting of low estrogen
- No specific other etiologies for inflammatory vaginitis; DIV, skin diseases
- Pale, smooth, dry vagina (atrophic vagina); red, smooth vagina (atrophic vaginitis)
- No discharge (atrophic vagina), or yellow discharge (atrophic vaginitis)
- pH > 5
- Wet mount showing parabasal cells, decreased lactobacilli (atrophic vagina); parabasal cells, absent lactobacilli, and increased white blood cells (atrophic vaginitis)
- Rapid response to therapy

#### *Pathophysiology*

The vaginal epithelium requires estrogen for normal maturation of squamous cells. In the absence of estrogen, there are fewer cell layers in the epithelium, and the epithelium becomes fragile. The atrophic vagina is at higher risk of erosions and secondary bacterial infection, with resulting inflammation producing pain and irritation. Risk factors for an atrophic vagina, in addition to traditional menopause itself, include the lack of vaginal childbirth, alcohol abuse, lack of sexual activity, and cigarette smoking.[53] Lower education levels, lower perceived income status, poorer marital satisfaction, and chronic disease, especially urogynecologic, are risk factors, although body weight is not.[54] Other causes of low estrogen to include cancer treatment such as pelvic radiation, chemotherapy, and endocrinologic therapies are associated with atrophic vagina and vaginitis.

#### *Management*

Although topical or systemic estrogen reverses most of the clinical abnormalities of estrogen deficiency, many women do not require estrogen. Those with only mild or occasional discomfort or dyspareunia may do well with simply using a vaginal lubricant with sexual activity or a moisturizer when uncomfortable with vaginal dryness. Lubricants are silicone, water, or oil-based products that are applied generously only before sexual activity. A vaginal moisturizer is for ongoing sensations of dryness, and these are bioadhesives that are inserted regularly.

When these are inadequate, estrogen is generally required when there are no contraindications. Unlike moisturizers, estrogens also increase blood flow, elasticity, and vaginal wall thickness. This therapy also can normalize pH levels due to restoration of a healthy lactobacilli-based flora and decrease the frequency of recurrent urinary tract infection when this is an issue. Local replacement can be accomplished by cream, vaginal tablet, or ring. Although the FDA-approved dosing is from 2-4 g daily for 1 or 2 weeks and then 1 g from one to three times a week long-term, experience has shown that much less is generally required. This author uses ½ g of estradiol (Estrace) inserted in the vagina two or three nights a week. Conjugated equine estrogen (Premarin) is equally effective, but this preparation is not available as a generic, is much more expensive, involves the suffering and deaths of animals, and some clinicians believe it is somewhat more irritating than estradiol cream. I reevaluate patients in 1 month by symptoms, the appearance of the vulva and vagina, and a wet mount, expecting to see a comfortable patient if this was the correct diagnosis without other issues. A healthy vaginal epithelium can be maintained with one to three intravaginal applications of estrogen, ½ g per dose, each week. Just as a good result is seen with far less medication than is reported in the package insert, the package insert reports side effects of systemic estrogen replacement as though they occur with this topical therapy, so patients should be reassured that these do not occur at the low doses of estrogen cream. Because Medicare does not cover estrogen for women over 65 years of age, insurance generally also does not cover these medications. However, medication plans such as goodrx.com makes estradiol cream, but not conjugated equine estrogen, quite affordable.

Less messy and more expensive are the estradiol vaginal tablets 10 μg, also inserted with an applicator thrice weekly, or via estradiol released slowly from an inert, nonirritating ring inserted into the upper vagina every 3-4 months (Estring). These methods produce a lower delivery of estradiol than the official dosing recommendations of cream.[55] Despite manufacturer's data reporting the benefit of estradiol 10 μg as equivalent to the 25 μg preparation when the 25 μg formulation was discontinued, many providers find the 10 μg preparation to be less effective, requiring ongoing thrice weekly or more insertion for adequate response.

A significant minority of patients develop candidiasis in the first few weeks of reestrogenization. They should be at least advised of this possibility and at most given fluconazole 150-200 mg weekly or an intravaginal azole suppository or cream two or three times a week for the first 2 weeks of estrogen therapy.

There are several barriers to the management of the atrophic vagina and atrophic vaginitis. Package inserts discuss the risk of breast and endometrial cancer, and an increased risk of stroke and heart disease. Women can be reassured that topical estrogen is nearly free of systemic side effects at the doses discussed above, although daily doses of several grams do indeed often result in breast tenderness, etc. The applicator for estradiol is unpopular with patients, with the shape being both uncomfortable and difficult to clean. Some patients use topical estrogen cream only on the vulva or use a small amount on the finger in the vagina, which often is insufficient. Many patients forget to use their estrogen, and others discontinued medication when symptoms persisted.

Therefore, the clinician should perform a follow-up wet mount if symptoms persist to ensure that the medication is being used as directed and that there are no additional factors in the patient's symptoms. Estrogen therapy should not be considered a failure unless the wet mount returns to normal and symptoms persist.

Although topical estrogen is generally found to be safe in breast cancer survivors, many oncologists do not allow this in their patients. These women, those with endometrial cancer, and women who for any other reasons are afraid of estrogen therapy have other options. Obviously, the above-mentioned lubricants and moisturizers are important, and those with atrophic vaginitis may improve with the addition of hydrocortisone acetate 25 mg rectal suppositories inserted into the vagina for the inflammatory component. Lifestyle changes to minimize the factors associated with worsened atrophic vagina risk can be useful—discontinuation of smoking, addition of exercise, for example. There is evidence that vitamin D can improve the atrophic vagina.[56] Recently, high-dose vaginal testosterone was reported to have beneficial effects.[57] Pelvic floor physical therapy can improve blood supply and improve the symptoms of the atrophic vagina.

Another topical option available is prasterone (dehydroepiandrosterone, or DHEA), also called Intrarosa. One of its metabolites is estrogen, so although it is promoted as a nonestrogen, it is not guaranteed as safe for those with breast cancer. However, the effects are felt to be strictly local.[58] This is inserted nightly. A nonestrogen systemic therapy for estrogen-deficient women is ospemifene (Osphena). This medication is a selective estrogen receptor modulator, so may produce the same side effects/effects as estrogen. The North American Menopause Society has stated that there is insufficient safety data to recommend its use in patients with breast or endometrial cancer.[59]

A popular, but unapproved, therapy for the atrophic vagina that completely bypasses the breast and endometrial cancer issue is vaginal rejuvenation. In 2020 and 2021, reviews of all trials revealed that there were three types of rejuvenation; fractional $CO_2$ laser (such as the MonaLisa Touch and FemTouch) and temperature controlled radiofrequency; none was controlled, all used different protocols and outcome measures, and there were more data for the fractional $CO_2$ laser than the other two treatments. All appeared safe, and there was a suggestion of benefit.[60,61] The fractional $CO_2$ laser produces a grid of very superficial holes in the epidermis, stimulating new collagen formation. From the natural course of this chronic, progressive condition, and the mechanism of action of the laser, regular treatments are expected to maintain improvement. The cost and uncovered nature of this treatment is a major drawback.

Patients with atrophic vaginitis do very well with long-term or intermittent estrogen replacement therapy. However, some patients do not require ongoing therapy to remain comfortable, particularly those who may have had a specific, correctable event such as an infection or local erosion that precipitated symptoms, and those who are not sexually active.

### ATROPHIC VAGINA/VAGINITIS — Management

- Topical estrogen replacement:
  - Estradiol vaginal cream or conjugated equine estrogen ½ g per vagina three times a week, then titrate to least frequent dosing of smallest quantity that controls symptoms
  - Estradiol vaginal tablets per vagina three times a week, then titrate to least frequent dosing of smallest quantity that controls symptoms
  - Estradiol ring changed every 3-4 months
- Systemic estrogen replacement:
  - Oral
  - Patch
- Consider oral fluconazole weekly or vaginal azole cream two to three times a week the first 2 weeks to prevent secondary candidiasis.

## Desquamative Inflammatory Vaginitis

Desquamative inflammatory vaginitis (DIV) is an arguably common inflammatory vaginitis not explained by infection, known erosive skin disease, or estrogen deficiency. First described by Herman Gardner in 1968, it has been better characterized by Jack Sobel in the years since.[62,63]

### *Clinical Presentation*

The symptoms of DIV consist of irritation, burning, dyspareunia, and, sometimes, itching. Patients often describe a yellow or green vaginal discharge. Inflammation of other mucosae, such as the oral mucosa and gingivae, are absent.

DIV occurs in both pre- and postmenopausal women. On physical examination, these women exhibit a variably red vestibule, probably as a result of an irritant contact dermatitis from purulent vaginal secretions **(Figs. 14-13 and 14-14)** and sometimes even redness of more of the modified mucous membranes. The vagina is red; sometimes this is striking, sometimes mild, but erosions are not present. The vaginal epithelium sometimes exhibits small, red macules similar to the classic "strawberry cervix" of trichomoniasis **(Fig. 14-15)**. At other times, the vagina is uniformly red **(Fig. 14-16)**. There is no scarring of the vulva or vagina as occurs with lichen planus and immunobullous diseases.

More severe cases exhibit poorly demarcated, mild erythema of the entire modified mucous membranes of the vulva and edema of the labia minora. However, these vulvar abnormalities are nonspecific.

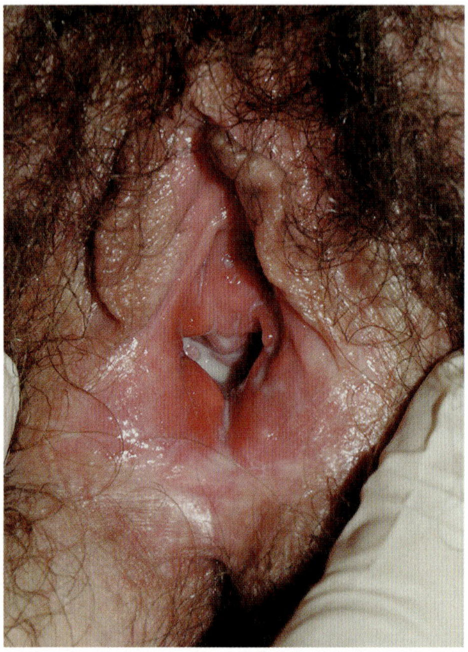

Fig. 14-13. Women with desquamative inflammatory vaginitis often demonstrate erythema of the vestibule and modified mucous membranes; the epithelium sometimes is unusually smooth due to edema, but there is never scarring with loss of architecture. The usually copious purulent discharge is often visible at the introitus.

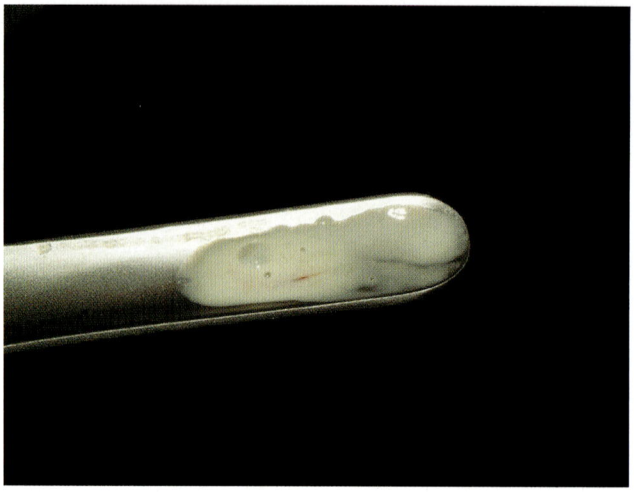

Fig. 14-14. Vaginal secretions from desquamative inflammatory vaginitis, as for erosive vaginal dermatoses and atrophic vaginitis, are purulent, showing various colors of yellow, green, or sometimes off-white.

A wet mount of vaginal secretions of DIV are characteristic but not specific, being identical to those of atrophic vaginitis, bacterial vaginitis, aerobic vaginitis, and erosive vaginitis such as that caused by lichen planus and mucous membrane (cicatricial) pemphigoid **(Figs. 14-8, 14-12, 14-17)**. Some of the epithelial cells seen with DIV are parabasal cells; these are round, small, and immature, having been shed from an epithelium that is too rapidly proliferating for maturation of the upper layer into the usual large, flattened cells. Inflammation usually recruits multiple white blood cells as well, and lactobacilli are absent, with a vaginal pH > 5.

### *Diagnosis*

DIV is diagnosed by the findings of vaginal erythema and characteristic secretions in the setting of adequate estrogen,

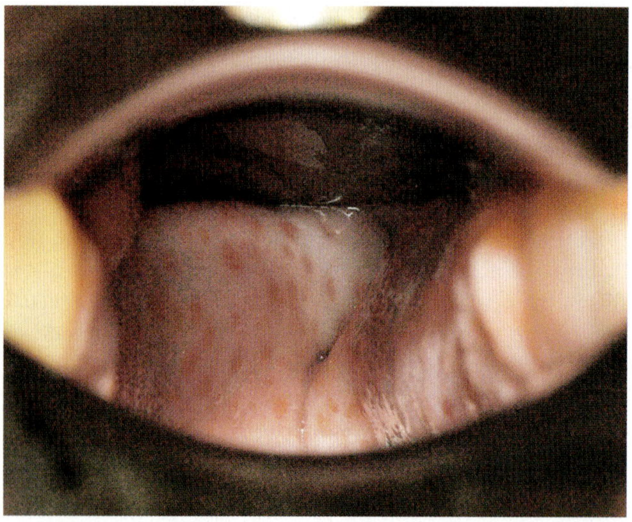

Fig. 14-15. The vagina of desquamative inflammatory vaginitis classically shows small discrete red macules that resemble the "strawberry cervix" said to distinguish trichomonas.

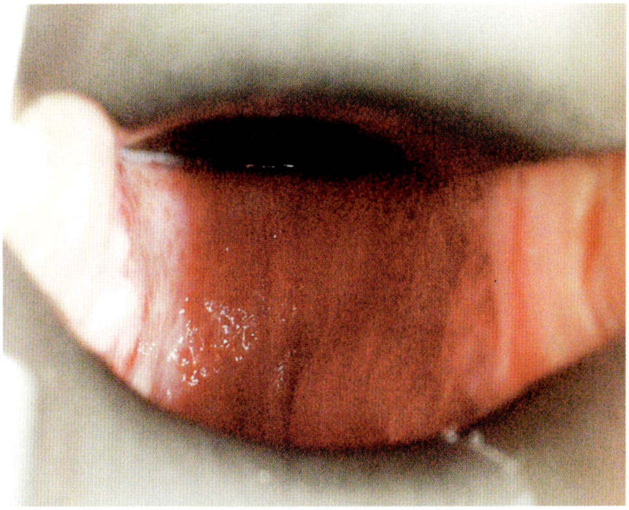

Fig. 14-16. Desquamative inflammatory vaginitis is most often characterized by a vagina that is variably and diffusely red, ranging from mild erythema to deep redness.

absence of other skin and mucous membrane disease, and negative cultures. For the most part, biopsies of DIV have not been reported. An older report found remarkably mild inflammation, with the histologic findings of DIV falling into one of two groups, either a lichenoid infiltrate without basement membrane changes or a nonspecific mixed inflammatory infiltrate with lymphocytes, eosinophils, and plasma cells.[64] A few of these patients revealed direct immunofluorescent biopsies showing nonspecific but distinct fine, granular C3 along the basement membrane. Whether these nonspecific findings are variants of the same process or represent two processes is not known. The lichenoid findings probably are only a common nonspecific reaction pattern characteristic of any inflammation on genital mucous membrane and modified mucous membrane skin. A recent survey of patients with DIV and plasma cell vulvitis compared biopsies and clinical findings and suggested that these conditions show overlap.[65]

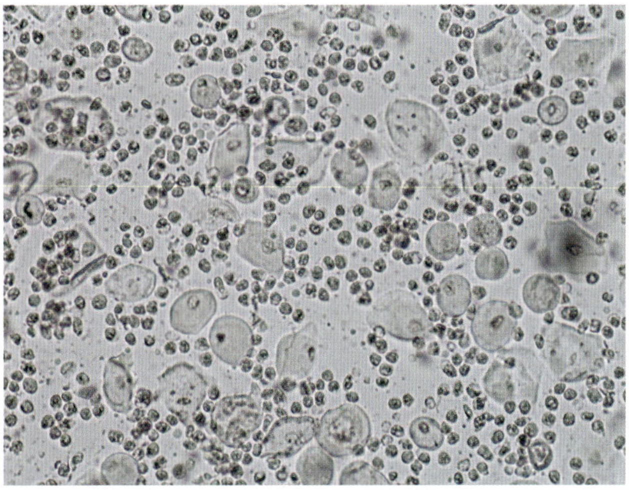

Fig. 14-17. This classic but nonspecific wet mount shows a marked increase in white blood cells and parabasal cells, with loss of lactobacilli. This wet mount is identical to those seen with atrophic vaginitis and erosive vaginal dermatoses such as lichen planus and mucous membrane pemphigoid.

The differential diagnosis includes atrophic vaginitis, erosive vaginitis of lichen planus or another erosive/bullous dermatosis, anaerobic vaginitis, bacterial vaginitis, and inflammation or infection associated with a retained foreign body. In addition, many women, both symptomatic and asymptomatic, exhibit an inflammatory wet mount that shows only an increase in white blood cells, without the presence of parabasal cells and absence of lactobacilli. When testing for infection is negative, this picture does not fall into any diagnostic category. Many vulvologists call this picture DIV for lack of another diagnostic possibility.

**DESQUAMATIVE INFLAMMATORY VAGINITIS — Diagnosis**

- Introital irritation, burning, dyspareunia
- Variably red vagina, often red, puffy vestibule, sometimes puffy labia minora
- Yellow/green discharge
- pH usually higher than 5
- Wet mount showing parabasal cells, increased white blood cells, decreased lactobacilli
- Negative molecular studies for trichomonas, gonorrhea, chlamydia
- Negative fungal and routine culture
- Adequate estrogen, no erosive skin disease of the vagina, vulva, or mouth

### *Pathophysiology*

The cause of DIV is not known. Most believe that DIV is an immune-mediated condition because it responds best to topical corticosteroids and clindamycin, which exhibits anti-inflammatory properties.[63] However, some believe that it may exist on a spectrum with aerobic vaginitis, representing a severe form of aerobic vaginitis.[66]

### *Management*

First, any estrogen deficiency should be corrected, and any accompanying infection should be treated. When there is doubt, these should be treated and the patient reevaluated.

First-line reported specific therapies for DIV are topical clindamycin cream[66] or 10% hydrocortisone cream inserted per vagina.[67] There are no controlled studies for the management of this condition and very little even in open trials and anecdotal reports. As a result of informally shared experiences with other vulvologists, I either instruct patients to insert an applicatorful of clindamycin cream nightly and I reevaluate in 1 month or I begin with a corticosteroid more potent than the 1% hydrocortisone cream. Theoretically, oral clindamycin would be a better choice than clindamycin cream, lacking the potentially irritating properties of a topical medication, but I have never had a patient improve with oral clindamycin or with other anti-inflammatory oral antibiotics (doxycycline or trimethoprim-sulfamethoxazole). When patients respond well, the frequency of application can be tapered to the least frequent use that controls the process, since recurrence is the rule. I provide these patients with clobetasol or halobetasol ointment to apply to the introitus daily as well.

For those patients who do not respond, I either use a compounded hydrocortisone acetate vaginal suppository, 100-300 g inserted at bedtime, or I have the patient insert 1-2 g of a superpotent corticosteroid ointment such as clobetasol at bedtime. When the ointment sticks to the end of the applicator rather than being delivered to the vagina, I have the patient warm the tube of medication in the sink first. Again, I reevaluate the patient, no longer than 1 month later. When disease remains unresponsive, I use clindamycin and a topical corticosteroid together. I have not had success with oral corticosteroids. The provider should be aware that there are no corticosteroids formulated for the vagina and that we know nothing about absorption of the topical corticosteroid from this area, and long-term use should be followed carefully. I obtain cortisol stimulation testing if a patient requires intravaginal corticosteroids more often than twice weekly long-term to control their DIV.

Both vaginal clindamycin and corticosteroids increase the risk of candidiasis, and I prescribe oral weekly fluconazole to prevent this infection, at least initially.

**DESQUAMATIVE INFLAMMATORY VAGINITIS — Management**

- Topical clindamycin cream, ½ to 1 applicatorful in vagina hs for 2-4 weeks.
- Ten percent hydrocortisone cream, 1 applicatorful in vagina/compounded hydrocortisone acetate 100-300 mg vaginal suppository per vagina hs for 2-4 weeks and reevaluate the patient and a wet mount.
- If uncontrolled with either, then both hydrocortisone suppositories and clindamycin cream hs for 2-4 weeks.
- Taper frequency to lowest frequency that controls the condition.
- Discontinue and wait for recurrence.
- Consider weekly fluconazole to prevent secondary candidiasis.

### Erosive Vaginitis due to Specific Skin Disease

Several erosive and blistering skin diseases show a predilection for mucous membranes, to include the vagina and, often, the mucous membranes and modified mucous membranes of the vulva. These are primarily discussed in Chapters 10 and 11.

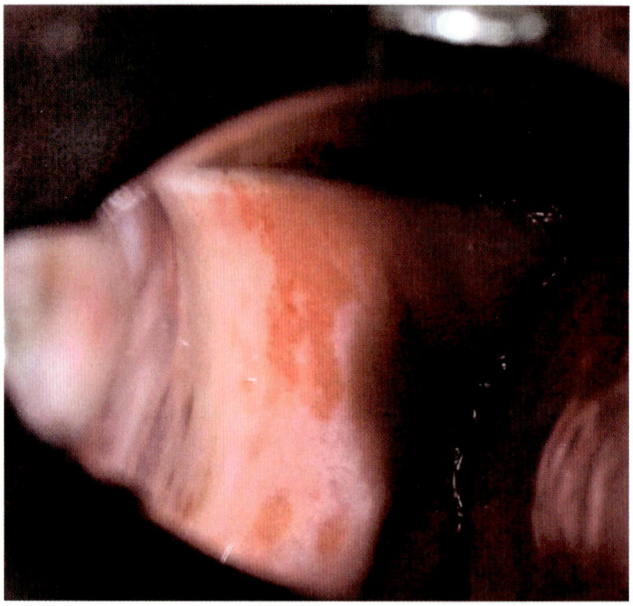

Fig. 14-18. Erosive and blistering vaginal dermatoses all show patchy vaginal erosions; this woman has lichen planus, by far the most common of the erosive mucous membrane diseases.

Lichen planus is far and away the most common of these diseases. Other mucosal erosive diseases include mucous membrane (cicatricial) pemphigoid, pemphigoid vulgaris, and erythema multiforme. These diseases exhibit frank erosions and also regularly affect other mucous membranes, especially the oral mucosa (Fig. 14-18). In addition, most of these diseases exhibit lesions of extragenital dry, keratinized skin surfaces as well, so that well-established disease is not difficult diagnostically.

The diagnosis is made by the constellation of findings, and by both routine histology from the edge, or an erosion, and direct immunofluorescent biopsies from nearby but unaffected epithelium.

### Vestibulodynia (Vulvar Vestibulitis Syndrome, Localized Provoked Vulvodynia)

Vulvar vestibulitis is not a vaginal disease, but it is often mistaken for vaginitis because of introital redness and symptoms of irritation and burning (see Chapter 13 for primary discussion) (Fig. 14-19).

### Physiologic Vaginal Discharge

A common complaint of premenopausal women is that of excess discharge, sometimes associated with odor. These patients occasionally report irritation manifested by itching or rawness, but more often the presence of the unpleasant discharge is the primary feature. Generally, the patient is convinced that infection is the cause of the secretions, and she often has been diagnosed with infections by previous providers.

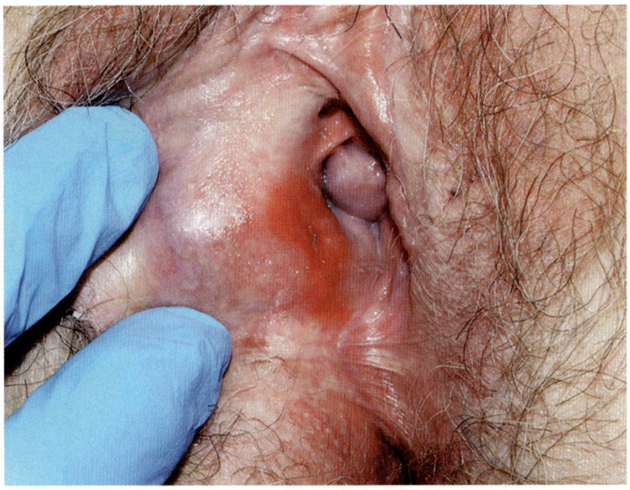

Fig. 14-19. Vestibulodynia (previously called vulvar vestibulitis syndrome) is sometimes mistaken for vaginitis. This vestibular erythema surrounding the pit that is the ostium of a vestibular gland, just medial to the hymeneal caruncles, exists on a spectrum of normal redness, but wet mounts and cultures are normal.

A physical examination is unremarkable, except, at times, vaginal secretions are copious but normal in color and consistency. The pH is normal, and a wet mount shows no evidence of yeast, clue cells, trichomonads, or increased white blood cells. Lactobacilli are present. A whiff test is negative, and vaginal secretions produce normal odor.

The "diagnosis" of physiologic discharge is made by the complaint of increased secretions, a normal wet mount, and a negative culture. The differential diagnosis includes all other vaginitis, especially bacterial vaginosis. In addition, an occasional patient experiences "discharge" and odor on the basis of excessive sweating from the groin area. This can be diagnosed by response to antiperspirant with a deodorant.

The management of physiologic secretions rests in patient education (see patient handout). Either patients accept the results of the evaluation, sometimes with relief, or, more often, with annoyance that there is no answer, or they refuse to believe that their secretions are normal. Some women have truly copious secretions that are troublesome. A menstrual cup or tampons changed frequently can make this less troublesome. At times, a morning douche with a weak vinegar and water douche can also be useful. However, she should be counseled regarding the small risks of douching and tampon use.

Some women are remarkably distressed by their secretions and perceived odor and continue to request reevaluation and empiric treatment. Occasionally, patients are crippled by their symptoms, believing that others can smell them; they avoid work and social activities. These women experience a body dysmorphic disorder and are best treated with psychiatric care and psychotropic medications, but they generally are resistant to this route.

**PHYSIOLOGIC DISCHARGE — Diagnosis**

- Complaints of copious vaginal discharge, sometimes with odor, with or without irritation/itching
- Normal color, consistency, odor
- Negative fungal culture/molecular vaginitis panel
- Normal wet mount without excess inflammatory cells, parabasal cells, normal pH

**PHYSIOLOGIC DISCHARGE — Management**

- Patient education (see patient handout).
- Reassurance.
- Reevaluate for flares once or twice for reassurance.
- Consider tampons changed frequently for management, or menstrual cups.
- Consider AM douching for management with patient education regarding adverse reactions.
- Try referral when psychologically distressed.

## Balanitis

Balanitis refers to inflammation of the glans penis. The term *balanoposthitis* is used when inflammation includes the prepuce. Because an intact prepuce provides a damp, occluded, warm space that is a favorable environment for some organisms, balanitis of all kinds is far more common in men who are uncircumcised.

### Infectious Balanitis/Balanoposthitis

Balanoposthitis is often an infectious condition, whereas balanitis in a circumcised male is usually not an infection. However, as often occurs in women, fungal infection is often blamed for chronic genital complaints of any cause.

#### *Candida* Balanitis

*Clinical Presentation*

*Candida* balanitis presents most often as red patches, primarily in uncircumcised males, although more severe involvement produces superficial erosions or even white papules (**Fig. 14-20**). Erosions are discrete and round, but these can become more confluent and less well demarcated as a result of the very fragile, occluded nature of this skin and resulting maceration. White papules representative of a yeast infection, like those of oral thrush, can be removed by gentle scraping. Unless the patient is incontinent or obese, the dry external prepuce and shaft of the penis are spared, but the moist crural creases and gluteal cleft may be affected. Gluteal cleft involvement often is characterized by fissuring.

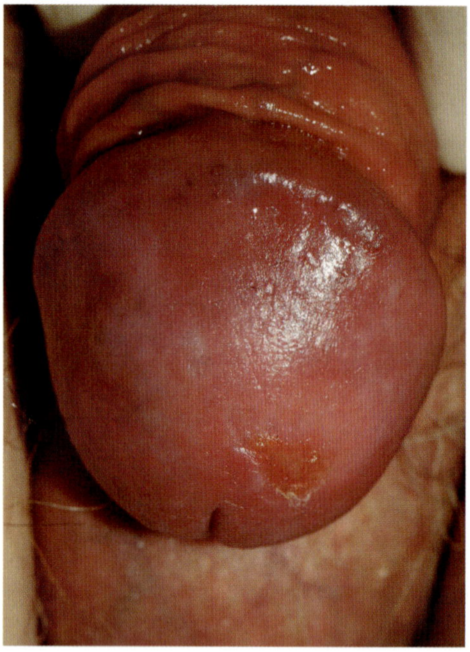

Fig. 14-20. Uncircumcised men are at higher risk for candidiasis, which usually presents as nonspecific patchy redness. A fungal preparation or culture should be performed for those not otherwise at risk or who are resistant to therapy.

*Diagnosis*

The diagnosis is confirmed by the identification of fungal elements from white material scraped from the skin or from the edge of an erosion. This can be accomplished either by culture or by examination of a microscopic smear. Biopsies are not indicated but are occasionally performed when the diagnosis is not suspected. A subcorneal pustule with infiltration of the stratum corneum by hyphae and pseudohyphae is usual. A circumcised man sometimes experiences irritation from yeast following sexual intercourse with an infected partner but usually does not show skin findings beyond subtle, patchy, evanescent erythema.

*Candida* balanitis should be included in the differential diagnosis of any inflammation of the glans penis. Not only is it a very common cause in uncircumcised men, it also complicates inflammation of other causes, such as psoriasis or herpes simplex virus infection. Lichen planus and penile intraepithelial neoplasia (erythroplasia of Queyrat, Bowen disease) can mimic *Candida* balanitis.

*CANDIDA* BALANITIS — **Management**

- Irritation and itching.
- Redness, erosion, white papules and plaques removed with a cotton-tipped applicator, in uncircumcised man.
- Fungal preparation of white material shows yeast forms.
- Otherwise, culture showing *Candida*.

*Pathophysiology*

Penile candidiasis is limited almost entirely to uncircumcised men. Colonization is fairly high, occurring in 26.2% of 478 men attending a sexually transmitted disease clinic, and over 18% exhibited *Candida* balanitis.[68] *C albicans* from the bowel or from a sexual partner provides the organisms, and risk factors include an age >60 years, diabetes, immunosuppression, and incontinence.[68] Newer medications for diabetes, sodium-glucose cotransporter 2-inhibitors, function by producing glycosuria, adding another very strong risk factor for genital *candidiasis*.[69]

*Management*

Topical therapy with an azole cream such as clotrimazole, miconazole, econazole, or ketoconazole applied twice a day is usually curative. Men with extreme erosive disease may experience burning with a cream. Nystatin ointment can be used for those patients, but it is sometimes macerating. An alternative treatment is oral therapy, using fluconazole.

*CANDIDA* BALANITIS — **Diagnosis**

- Topical azole cream once or twice a day if not eroded.
- Nystatin ointment one to four times a day if eroded or painful.
- Fluconazole 100-200 mg daily until clear.
- Treat any yeast in partner; manage, when possible, diabetes, incontinence, obesity, etc.
- Use medication of choice with the first onset of recurrence, or daily ongoing application to suppress recurrence.

### Bacterial Balanitis/Balanoposthitis

Again occurring primarily in uncircumcised men, bacterial infection is a very uncommon condition that can cause inflammation of the glans and prepuce. Bacterial balanitis can be accompanied by perianal infection as well. Erythema, purulence, and pain of the glans and foreskin are common clinical findings, particularly in a setting of *Streptococcus pyogenes*. Other bacteria found on culture include *S agalactiae* and *S aureus*.

The diagnosis is made by culture and response to therapy. Management includes oral antibiotics according to sensitivities reported on culture, and the avoidance of known contactants.

## Noninfectious Balanitis/Balanoposthitis

### Circinate Balanitis (Reactive Arthritis, Previous Called Reiter Syndrome)

Lesions of reactive arthritis syndrome on the glans penis are called circinate balanitis (see Chapters 5 and 10). These lesions are indistinguishable clinically and histologically from those of the closely related disease, pustular psoriasis. Uncircumcised men exhibit white, annular pap-

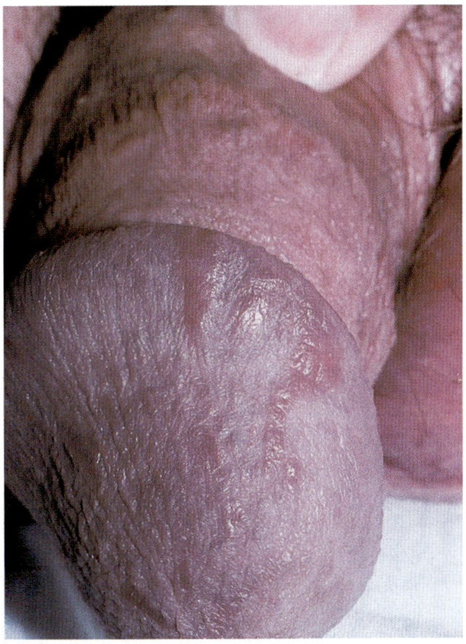

Fig. 14-21. The skin findings of reactive arthritis in an uncircumcised man characteristically shows annular, sometimes coalescing white papules, resulting in the term circinate ("circular") balanitis. This is sometimes accompanied by scale/crust or pustules of the palms and soles.

ules that sometimes coalesce into arcuate plaques, hence the term circinate balanitis (**Fig. 14-21**). Circumcised men generally experience relatively well-demarcated scaling, crusted papules, and plaques that are indistinguishable from psoriasis (**Fig. 14-22**). Patients with reactive arthritis and those with pustular psoriasis often have associated circumscribed crusted plaques on the palms and feet, and sometimes these are generalize to cover larger areas.

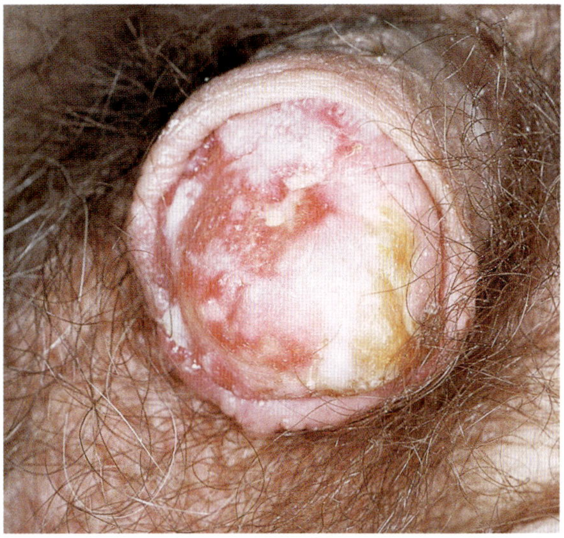

Fig. 14-23. Pseudoepitheliomatous, micaceous, and keratotic balanitis most often displays thick, adherent scale, which, in the uncircumcised male, appears thickened and white.

Treatment includes topical corticosteroids, oral acitretin, oral methotrexate, and biologics.

## Pseudoepitheliomatous, Micaceous, and Keratotic Balanitis

### *Clinical Presentation*

Pseudoepitheliomatous, micaceous, and keratotic balanitis presents as indolent, relatively asymptomatic, hyperkeratotic, and sometimes crusted plaques on the glans (**Figs. 14-23 and 14-24**). This condition is found most frequently in older men, often who have been circumcised late in life.[70]

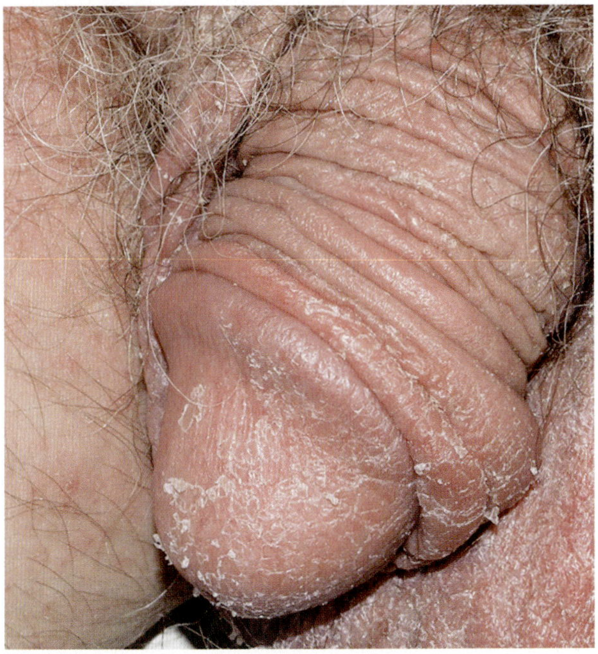

Fig. 14-22. The circumcised penis with reactive arthritis displays skin findings indistinguishable from psoriasis of the glans, showing flaking and scaling papules and plaques of scale.

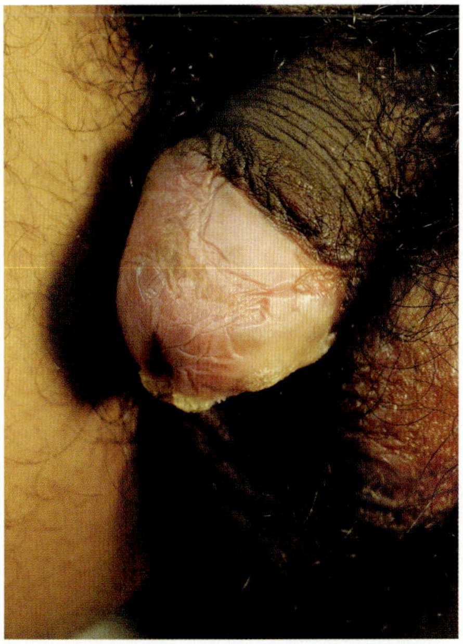

Fig. 14-24. Hyperkeratosis and crusting of the glans is characteristic of pseudoepitheliomatous, keratotic, and micaceous balanitis, a rare condition that can mimic squamous cell carcinoma and may exhibit malignant potential.

#### Diagnosis

The diagnosis is made by the clinical appearance and is confirmed by biopsy. A skin biopsy shows a moderately well-differentiated epithelium, with pseudoepitheliomatous hyperplasia, and a normal dermis with a mild chronic inflammatory infiltrate.

The main and most dangerous disease in the differential diagnosis is squamous cell carcinoma, which usually is distinguishable on biopsy.

#### Pathophysiology

The origin of this disease is not known, but it is postulated to be a premalignant condition with an observation of progression into invasive squamous cell carcinoma in the absence of HPV infection.[71] However, recently, low-risk HPV types have been detected in two patients.[72]

#### Management

Although the lesion can be followed carefully, removal by excision is preferred, both to prevent possible malignant transformation and to ensure adequate tissue for histology. Topical fluorouracil has also been used successfully, as has photodynamic therapy.[73]

### Plasma Cell Balanitis (Zoon Balanitis)

Plasma cell balanitis is an uncommon, distinctive dermatosis of unknown etiology. This condition is discussed primarily in Chapter 5. Plasma cell balanitis presents as a well-demarcated, red, purpuric, glistening plaque **(Fig. 14-25)**. Although it is largely asymptomatic, mild pruritus or tenderness may occur.

The diagnosis is made by correlating the clinical and histologic presentations and by ruling out diseases similar in appearance, including lichen planus, candidiasis, Bowen disease, and psoriasis. The histology of plasma cell balanitis is characteristic, showing a dense plasma cell infiltrate in the upper dermis. Plasma cell balanitis can mimic many inflammatory processes, especially in uncircumcised men. Lichen planus, candidiasis, Bowen disease, and psoriasis are the most common processes to exclude.

Although the cause of this inflammatory disease is unknown, plasma cell balanitis does not appear to be infectious or neoplastic, and some believe it to be related to lichen planus. Topical corticosteroids, topical retinoids, and laser therapy have all been reported useful. However, this is a chronic process that tends to recur if ablated and only improve but not clear with topical therapy.

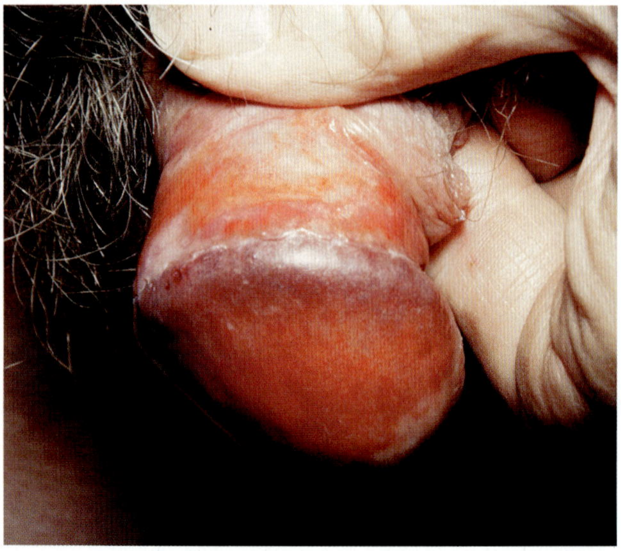

Fig. 14-25. Plasma cell balanitis (Zoon balanitis) presents as papules of deep red, sometimes purpuric, or red/brown/orange patches from the hemosiderin of previous purpura.

### Other Noninfectious Causes of Balanitis: Lichen Planus, Psoriasis, Penile Intraepithelial Neoplasia (Bowen Disease, Erythroplasia of Queyrat)

Other diseases can preferentially affect the glans penis. Common benign skin diseases are psoriasis and lichen planus **(Figs. 14-26 and 14-27)**. These diseases are red, usually well-demarcated papules and plaques that show a predilection for the glans on uncircumcised men (discussed primarily in Chapter 5). These often appear nonspecific and can be confused with red papules of intraepithelial neoplasia (Bowen disease, erythroplasia of Queyrat),

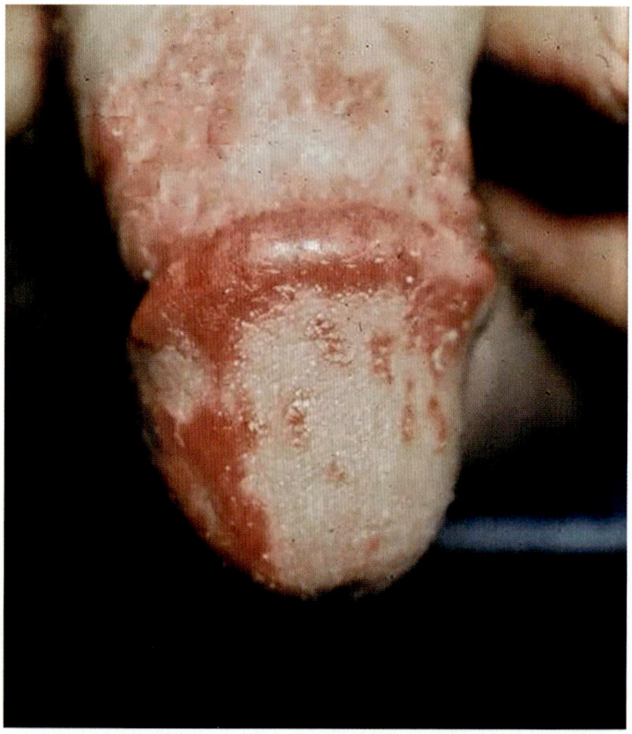

Fig. 14-26. Psoriasis of the uncircumcised penis shows red, glazed papules or plaques indistinguishable from squamous cell carcinoma *in situ*/high-grade squamous cell intraepithelial neoplasia/differentiated epithelial neoplasia. Often, an examination of other skin surfaces shows more typical psoriasis, but often a biopsy is needed.

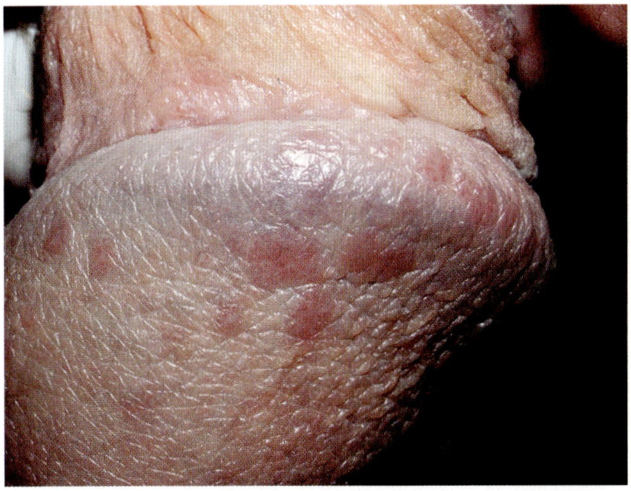

Fig. 14-27. Superficial, nonspecific red papules of erosive lichen planus. The diagnosis must be made by correlation with pathognomonic mucous membrane disease at other sites or by biopsy of a papule.

plasma cell balanitis, and candidiasis. An examination of other skin surfaces often shows more specific morphology of psoriasis or lichen planus, but a biopsy is often required.

Penile intraepithelial neoplasia (also called squamous cell carcinoma *in situ*, Bowen disease, erythroplasia of Queyrat, differentiated penile intraepithelial neoplasia, or high-grade squamous intraepithelial lesions) can produce red papules on the glans as well.

Chronic, unresponsive red papules or plaques on the glans should be examined by biopsy to ensure that neoplastic processes do not go undetected and untreated.

## REFERENCES


1. Barnes P, Vieira R, Harwood J, Chauhan M. Self-taken vaginal swabs versus clinician-taken for detection of candida and bacterial vaginosis: a case-control study in primary care. *Br J Gen Pract*. 2017;67(665):e824-e829.
2. *Vulvovaginal Candidiasis—2021 STD Treatment Guidelines*. https://www.cdc.gov/std/treatment-guidelines/candidiasis.htm
3. Achkar JM, Fries BC. Candida infections of the genitourinary tract. *Clin Microbiol Rev*. 2010;23:253-273.
4. Shi Y, Zhu Y, Fan S, Liu X, Liang Y, Shan Y. Molecular identification and antifungal susceptibility profile of yeast from vulvovaginal candidiasis. *BMC Infect Dis*. 2020;20:287. doi:10.1186/s12879-020-04985-w
5. Farr A, Effendy I, Frey Tirri B, et al. Guideline: vulvovaginal candidosis (AWMF 015/072, level S2k). *Mycoses*. 2021;64:583-602.
6. Shukla A, Sobel JD. Vulvovaginitis caused by Candida species following antibiotic exposure. *Curr Infect Dis Rep*. 2019;21:44.
7. McClelland RS, Richardson BA, Hassan WM, et al. Prospective study of vaginal bacterial flora and other risk factors for vulvovaginal candidiasis. *J Infect Dis*. 2009;199:1883-1890.
8. Mohammadi F, Hemmat N, Bajalan Z, Javadi A. Analysis of biofilm-related genes and antifungal susceptibility pattern of vaginal *Candida albicans* and non-*Candida albicans* species. *Biomed Res Int*. 2021;2021:5598907.
9. Available at: https://www.cdc.gov/std/treatment-guidelines/candidiasis.htm
10. Pitsouni E, Iavazzo C, Falagas ME. Itraconazole vs fluconazole for the treatment of uncomplicated acute vaginal and vulvovaginal candidiasis in nonpregnant women: a metaanalysis of randomized controlled trials. *Am J Obstet Gynecol*. 2008;198:153-160.
11. Collins LM, Moore R, Sobel JD. Prognosis and long-term outcome of women with idiopathic recurrent vulvovaginal candidiasis caused by *Candida albicans*. *J Low Genit Tract Dis*. 2020;24:48-52.
12. Sobel JD, Borroto-Esoda K, Azie N, Angulo D. In vitro pH activity of ibrexafungerp against fluconazole-susceptible and -resistant *Candida* isolates from women with vulvovaginal candidiasis. *Antimicrob Agents Chemother*. 2021;65:e0056221.
13. Xie HY, Feng D, Wei DM, et al. Probiotics for vulvovaginal candidiasis in non-pregnant women. *Cochrane Database Syst Rev*. 2017;(11):CD010496. doi:10.1002/14651858.CD010496.pub2
14. Iavazzo C, Gkegkes ID, Zarkada IM, Falagas ME. Boric acid for recurrent vulvovaginal candidiasis: the clinical evidence. *J Womens Health (Larchmt)*. 2011;20:1245-1255.
15. Watson C, Calabretto H. Comprehensive review of conventional and non-conventional methods of management of recurrent vulvovaginal candidiasis. *Aust N Z J Obstet Gynaecol*. 2007;47:262-272.
16. Gamal A, Chu S, McCormick TS, Borroto-Esoda K, Angulo D, Ghannoum MA. Ibrexafungerp, a novel oral triterpenoid antifungal in development: overview of antifungal activity against *Candida glabrata*. *Front Cell Infect Microbiol*. 2021;11:642358.
17. Available at: https://www.cdc.gov/std/treatment-guidelines/trichomoniasis.htm
18. Graves KJ, Ghosh AP, Schmidt N, et al. *Trichomonas vaginalis* virus among women with trichomoniasis and associations with demographics, clinical outcomes, and metronidazole resistance. *Clin Infect Dis*. 2019;69:2170-2176.
19. Šoba B, Skvarč M, Matičič M. Trichomoniasis: a brief review of diagnostic methods and our experience with real-time PCR for detecting infection. *Acta Dermatovenerol Alp Pannonica Adriat*. 2015;24:7-10.
20. Danby CS, Althouse AD, Hillier SL, Wiesenfeld HC. Nucleic acid amplification testing compared with cultures, gram stain, and microscopy in the diagnosis of Vaginitis. *J Low Genit Tract Dis*. 2021;25:76-80.
21. Heller DS, Pitsos M, Skurnick J. Does the presence of vaginitis on a Pap smear correlate with clinical symptoms in the patient? *J Reprod Med*. 2008;53:429-434.
22. Güdücü N, Gönenç G, Işçi H, Yiğiter AB, Başsüllü N, Dünder I. Clinical importance of detection of bacterial vaginosis, *Trichomonas vaginalis*, *Candida albicans* and actinomyces in Papanicolaou smears. *Clin Exp Obstet Gynecol*. 2012;39:333-336.
23. Muzny CA, Van Gerwen OT, Kissinger P. Updates in trichomonas treatment including persistent infection and 5-nitroimidazole hypersensitivity. *Curr Opin Infect Dis*. 2020;33:73-77.
24. Fjeld H, Raknes G. Is combining metronidazole and alcohol really hazardous? [Norwegian]. *Tidsskr Nor Laegeforen*. 2014;134:1661-1663.
25. Marques-Silva M, Lisboa C, Gomes N, Rodrigues AG. *Trichomonas vaginalis* and growing concern over drug resistance: a systematic review. *J Eur Acad Dermatol Venereol*. 2021;35:2007-2021.
26. Keating MA, Nyirjesy P. *Trichomonas vaginalis* infection in a tertiary care vaginitis center. *Sex Transm Dis*. 2015;42:482-485.
27. Alessio C, Nyirjesy P. Management of resistant trichomoniasis. *Curr Infect Dis Rep*. 2019;21:31.
28. Abou Chacra L, Fenollar F, Diop K. Bacterial vaginosis: what do we currently know? *Front Cell Infect Microbiol*. 2022;11:672429.

29. Available at: https://www.cdc.gov/std/treatment-guidelines/bv.htm
30. Abbai NS, Reddy T, Ramjee G. Prevalent bacterial vaginosis infection—a risk factor for incident sexually transmitted infections in women in Durban, South Africa. *Int J STD AIDS*. 2016;27:1283-1288.
31. Javed A, Parvaiz F, Manzoor S. Bacterial vaginosis: an insight into the prevalence, alternative treatments regimen and it's associated resistance patterns. *Microb Pathog*. 2019;127:21-30.
32. Fethers KA, Fairley CK, Morton A, et al. Early sexual experiences and risk factors for bacterial vaginosis. *J Infect Dis*. 2009;200:1662-1670.
33. Kenyon CR, Buyze J, Klebanoff M, Brotman RM. Association between bacterial vaginosis and partner concurrency: a longitudinal study. *Sex Transm Infect*. 2018;94:75-77. https://doi.org/10.1136/sextrans-2016-052652
34. Bautista CT, Wurapa E, Sateren WB, Morris S, Hollingsworth B, Sanchez JL. Bacterial vaginosis: a synthesis of the literature on etiology, prevalence, risk factors, and relationship with chlamydia and gonorrhea infections. *Mil Med Res*. 2016;3:4. https://doi.org/10.1186/s40779-016-0074-5
35. Froehle L, Ghanem KG, Page K, et al. Bacterial vaginosis and alcohol consumption: a cross-sectional retrospective study in Baltimore, *Maryland Sex Transm Dis*. 2021;48:986-990.
36. Morris BJ, Hankins CA, Banerjee J, et al. Does male circumcision reduce women's risk of sexually transmitted infections, cervical cancer, and associated conditions? *Front Public Health*. 2019;7:4. https://doi.org/10.3389/fpubh.2019.00004
37. Senok AC, Verstraelen H, Temmerman M, Botta GA. Probiotics for the treatment of bacterial vaginosis. *Cochrane Database Syst Rev*. 2009;(4):CD006289.
38. Liu HF, Yi N. A systematic review and meta-analysis on the efficacy of probiotics for bacterial vaginosis. *Eur Rev Med Pharmacol Sci*. 2022;26:90-98.
39. Amaya-Guio J, Martinez-Velasquez MY, Viveros-Carreño DA, Sierra-Barrios EM, Grillo-Ardila CF. Antibiotic treatment for the sexual partners of women with bacterial vaginosis. *Cochrane Database Syst Rev*. 2016;(10):CD011701.
40. Mehta SD. Systematic review of randomized trials of treatment of male sexual partners for improved bacteria vaginosis outcomes in women. *Sex Transm Dis*. 2012;39:822-830.
41. Plummer EL, Vodstrcil LA, Doyle M, et al. A prospective, open-label pilot study of concurrent male partner treatment for bacterial vaginosis. *MBio*. 2021;12:e0232321.
42. Sonnex C. Genital streptococcal infection in non-pregnant women: a case-note review. *Int J STD AIDS*. 2013;24:447-448.
43. Verstraelen H, Verhelst R, Vaneechoutte M, Temmerman M. Group A streptococcal vaginitis: an unrecognized cause of vaginal symptoms in adult women. *Arch Gynecol Obstet*. 2011;284:95-98.
44. Sobel JD, Funaro D, Kaplan EL. Recurrent group A streptococcal vulvovaginitis in adult women: family epidemiology. *Clin Infect Dis*. 2007;44:e43-e45.
45. Clark LR, Atendido M. Group B streptococcal vaginitis in postpubertal adolescent girls. *J Adolesc Health*. 2005;36:437-440.
46. Donders GGG, Bellen G, Grinceviciene S, et al. Aerobic vaginitis: no longer a stranger. *Res Microbiol*. 2017;168(9-10):845-858.
47. Lev-Sagie A, De Seta F, Verstraelen H, Ventolini G, Lonnee-Hoffmann R, Vieira-Baptista P. The vaginal microbiome: II. Vaginal dysbiotic conditions. *J Low Genit Tract Dis*. 2022;26:79-84.
48. Mendling W. Vaginal microbiota. *Adv Exp Med Biol*. 2016;902:83-93.
49. Cibley LJ, Cibley LJ. Cytolytic vaginosis. *Am J Obstet Gynecol*. 1991;165:1245-1249.
50. Shopova E, Tiufekchieva E, Karag'ozov I, et al. Cytolytic vaginosis—clinical and microbiological study. *Akush Ginekol (Sofiia)*. 2006;45(Suppl 2):12-13.
51. Voytik M, Nyirjesy P. Cytolytic vaginosis: a critical appraisal of a controversial condition. *Curr Infect Dis Rep*. 2020;22:1-6.
52. Horowitz BJ, Mårdh PA, Nagy E, et al. Vaginal lactobacillosis. *Am J Obstet Gynecol*. 1994;170:857-861.
53. Angelou K, Grigoriadis T, Diakosavvas M, Zacharakis D, Athanasiou S. The genitourinary syndrome of menopause: an overview of the recent data. *Cureus*. 2020;12:e7586. doi:10.7759/cureus.7586
54. Karakoç H, Uçtu AK, Özerdoğan N. Genitourinary syndrome of menopause: effects on related factors, quality of life, and self-care power. *Prz Menopauzalny*. 2019;18:15-22.
55. Phillips NA, Bachmann GA. Genitourinary syndrome of menopause: common problem, effective treatments. *Cleve Clin J Med*. 2018;85:390-398.
56. Kamronrithisorn T, Manonai J, Vallibhakara SA, Sophonsritsuk A, Vallibhakara O. Effect of vitamin D supplement on vulvovaginal atrophy of the menopause. *Nutrients*. 2020;12:2876.
57. Simon JA, Goldstein I, Kim NN, et al. The role of androgens in the treatment of genitourinary syndrome of menopause (GSM): International Society for the Study of Women's Sexual Health (ISSWSH) expert consensus panel review. *Menopause*. 2018;25:837-847.
58. Labrie F, Archer DF, Koltun W, et al.; Members of the VVA Prasterone Research Group. Efficacy of intravaginal dehydroepiandrosterone (DHEA) on moderate to severe dyspareunia and vaginal dryness, symptoms of vulvovaginal atrophy, and of the genitourinary syndrome of menopause. *Menopause*. 2018;25:1339-1353.
59. The 2020 genitourinary syndrome of menopause position statement of The North American Menopause Society. *Menopause*. 2020;27:976-992.
60. Photiou L, Lin MJ, Dubin DP, Lenskaya V, Khorasani H. Review of non-invasive vulvovaginal rejuvenation *J Eur Acad Dermatol Venereol*. 2020;34:716-726.
61. D'Oria O, Giannini A, Prata G, et al. Non-invasive treatment of vulvovaginal atrophy in menopause with CO2 laser. *Minerva Obstet Gynecol*. 2021;73:127-134.
62. Gardner HL. Desquamative inflammatory vaginitis: a newly defined entity. *Am J Obstet Gynecol*. 1968;102:1102-1105.
63. Reichman O, Sobel J. Desquamative inflammatory vaginitis. *Best Pract Res Clin Obstet Gynaecol*. 2014;28:1042-1050.
64. Murphy R, Edwards L. Desquamative inflammatory vaginitis: what is it? *J Reprod Med*. 2008;53:124-128.
65. Song M, Day T, Kliman L, et al. Desquamative inflammatory vaginitis and plasma cell vulvitis represent a spectrum of hemorrhagic vestibulovaginitis. *J Low Genit Tract Dis*. 2022;26:60-67.
66. Sonthalia S, Aggarwal P, Das S, Sharma P, Sharma R, Singh S. Aerobic vaginitis—an underdiagnosed cause of vaginal discharge—narrative review. *Int J STD AIDS*. 2020;31:1018-1027.
67. Sobel JD, Reichman O, Misra D, Yoo W. Prognosis and treatment of desquamative inflammatory vaginitis. *Obstet Gynecol*. 2011;117:850-855.
68. Lisboa C, Santos A, Dias C, Azevedo F, Pina-Vaz C, Rodrigues A. *Candida* balanitis: risk factors. *J Eur Acad Dermatol Venereol*. 2010;24:820-826.
69. Bartolo C, Hall V, Friedman ND, et al. Bittersweet: infective complications of drug-induced glycosuria in patients with

diabetes mellitus on SGLT2-inhibitors: two case reports. *BMC Infect Dis*. 2021;21:284.

70. Perry D, Lynch PJ, Fazel N. Pseudoepitheliomatous, keratotic, and micaceous balanitis: case report and review of the literature. *Dermatol Nurs*. 2008;20:117-120.
71. Child FJ, Kim BK, Ganesan R, et al. Verrucous carcinoma arising in pseudoepitheliomatous keratotic and micaceous balanitis, without evidence of human papillomavirus. *Br J Dermatol*. 2000;143:183-187.
72. Corbeddu M, Pilloni L, Satta R, Atzori L, Rongioletti F. Pseudoepitheliomatous keratotic and micaceous balanitis: low-risk human papilloma virus detection in two further cases. *Int J STD AIDS*. 2021;32:209-212.
73. Zhu H, Jiang Y, Watts M, Kong F. Treatment of pseudoepitheliomatous, keratotic, and micaceous balanitis with topical photodynamic therapy. *Int J Dermatol*. 2015;54:245-247.

## SUGGESTED READINGS

Abou Chacra L, Fenollar F, Diop K. Bacterial vaginosis: what do we currently know? *Front Cell Infect Microbiol*. 2022;11:672429. doi: 10.3389/fcimb.2021.672429. eCollection 2021.

Alessio C, Nyirjesy P. Management of resistant trichomoniasis. *Curr Infect Dis Rep*. 2019;21(9):31. doi:10.1007/s11908-019-0687-4

Coudray MS, Madhivanan P. Bacterial vaginosis—a brief synopsis of the literature. *Eur J Obstet Gynecol Reprod Biol*. 2020;245:143-148. doi:10.1016/j.ejogrb.2019.12.035. Review.

Farr A, Effendy I, Frey Tirri B, et al. Guideline: vulvovaginal candidosis (AWMF 015/072, level S2k). *Mycoses*. 2021;64:583-602.

Garzon S, Apostolopoulos V, Stojanovska L, Ferrari F, Mathyk BA, Laganà AS. Non-oestrogenic modalities to reverse urogenital aging. *Prz Menopauzalny*. 2021;20:140-147.

Sonthalia S, Aggarwal P, Das S, Sharma P, Sharma R, Singh S. Aerobic vaginitis—an underdiagnosed cause of vaginal discharge—narrative review. *Int J STD AIDS*. 2020;31:1018-1027.

Van Gerwen OT, Muzny CA. Recent advances in the epidemiology, diagnosis, and management of *Trichomonas vaginalis* infection. *F1000Res*. 2019;8:F1000 Faculty Rev-1666. doi:10.12688/f1000research.19972.1. eCollection 2019.

Workowski KA, Bachmann LH, Chan PA, et al. Sexually transmitted infections treatment guidelines, 2021. *MMWR Recomm Rep*. 2021;70(4):1-187. doi:10.15585/mmwr.rr7004a1.

Wu X, Zhang S, Li H, et al. Biofilm formation of *Candida albicans* facilitates fungal infiltration and persister cell formation in vaginal candidiasis. *Front Microbiol*. 2020;11:1117.

# Special Issues in Genital Dermatology 15

PETER J. LYNCH AND LIBBY EDWARDS

## Psychological Aspects

Clinical discussions about genital disorders and their role in the patient's psychological, social, and sexual function have historically been indirect, played down, or even avoided completely. In order to maximize the quality of care offered, these aspects need to be explored with virtually every patient presenting with a genital problem. There are two ways of doing so. One is to offer patients a chance to express these concerns indirectly by way of a computerized questionnaire filled out privately by the patient prior to a face-to-face interaction with the clinician. The other is for the clinician to take the initiative in bringing up this discussion at the time of the examination. Rarely, with individuals who by culture or temperament are very shy, it may be appropriate to defer this discussion until the second or third visit. Because of space limitations, only a few aspects or psychosocial and sexual function related to genital disease can be covered in this chapter.

Psychological factors obviously can play some role in the pathophysiology of all diseases and the degree to which they do so probably exists on a spectrum. Unfortunately, for most diseases, there is no consensus as to what these factors are and how important a role they play in the etiology of the disorder. Information is needed about the extent, severity, and duration of the psychosexual aspects that may be playing a part in the patient's problem. Also unfortunately, even when this information is available, there is always controversy over the degree to which psychological factors cause the disease vs the degree to which they are the consequence of the disease. Essentially, this presents a "chicken and egg" situation that, while it can be discussed, can never be resolved to the satisfaction of all participants. With this in mind, we have divided this section into three segments: (1) psychosocial and sexual dysfunction may cause the disease, (2) psychosocial and sexual dysfunction may influence the course of the disease, and (3) psychosocial and sexual dysfunction may occur as a result of the disease.

### Psychosocial Dysfunction May Cause Disease

The major genital disorders for which one of us (PJL) believes psychosocial and sexual dysfunction plays a significant etiologic role are (1) chronic idiopathic genital pain; (2) chronic itching and scratching in the absence of a recognizable disease; (3) fixed ideation that some aspect of the genitalia, although normal on clinical examination, is in fact abnormal (body dysmorphic disorder [BDD]); and (4) intentional or unintentional self-mutilation (dermatitis artefacta).

#### Chronic Idiopathic Genital Pain

Mucocutaneous pain can arise secondary to an underlying cutaneous or neurologic disorder or can occur as an idiopathic problem. The main idiopathic mucocutaneous pain disorders include unexplained pain involving the head (tongue, lips, face, and scalp) and the anogenital area (vulva, penis, scrotum, and anus). Idiopathic pain that occurs at these latter four sites is generally termed vulvodynia, penodynia, scrotodynia, and anodynia. Of these, only vulvodynia has been studied sufficiently to warrant discussion here. Nevertheless, one of us (PJL) believes that the information regarding vulvodynia, as cited below, can be generalized to pain occurring at the three other anogenital sites of involvement.

Nearly all patients with vulvodynia have psychological, social, and sexual dysfunction, although the degree to which this occurs is quite variable.[1,2] The major question, of course, is whether the presence of pain causes this dysfunction or whether the dysfunction causes the pain. While the majority of clinicians currently favors the former explanation, the minority including one of us (PJL) favors the latter. Support for this latter point of view is perhaps best established by examination of the data suggesting that psychosocial and/or sexual dysfunction precedes the development of the pain. In that regard, there is arguably acceptable evidence that significant depression, anxiety, somatization, relationship dysfunction, and painful physical, sexual, or psychological trauma precede the development of vulvar pain.

Regardless of whether psychosocial and sexual dysfunction causes the pain or arises from it, all agree that vulvodynia is a very debilitating condition and that it has a dramatic adverse effect on quality of life (QoL).[3] In fact, it appears that women with this condition have significantly poorer QoL than do women with most other general dermatologic disease and also worse than women with other vulvar disorders.[4] Finally, while both medical and procedural therapy can lead to good results for most patients with vulvodynia, it is clear that these individuals can also benefit from a variety of psychological approaches to therapy.[5,6] A generally ignored aspect of chronic vulvovaginal symptoms, especially vulvodynia, is the impact on the partner, which can be enormous.[7]

### Chronic Itching and/or Scratching in the Absence of Recognizable Disease

As is true for cutaneous pain, pruritus can arise either as an idiopathic process (psychogenic pruritus) or develop secondary to an underlying systemic, cutaneous, or neurologic (neuropathic) disorder (see Chapter 13). Psychogenic pruritus (including such disorders as neurotic excoriation, prurigo nodularis and pruritus with delusions of parasitosis) is associated with a variety of psychogenic problems, notably obsessive-compulsive behavior, anxiety, and depression.[8-10]

Psychogenic excoriation ("neurotic excoriation") and prurigo nodularis are the terms used for those patients who chronically scratch, gouge, or pick at skin that is otherwise visibly normal.[11,12] These conditions differ from the scratching and rubbing that occurs in pruritic skin disease such as atopic dermatitis and lichen simplex chronicus in several ways. First, there is no atopy or other recognizable underlying disorder. Second, the excoriations are appreciably deeper and thus usually appear as ulcers rather than erosions. And, third, individual gouge marks are separated one from another by areas of intervening normal skin.

On the other hand, patients with the more severe form of psychogenic excoriation, those who believe that their skin contains "bugs" (delusions of parasitosis) or fibers (Morgellons disease), are almost always delusional. These latter two conditions (which are essentially identical from a psychological viewpoint) only occur in the anogenital region when other parts of the body are also involved.

The fact that psychogenic pruritus responds well to psychotropic medications such as the tricyclics, benzodiazepines, SSRIs (selective serotonin reuptake inhibitors), and antipsychotic agents support the supposition that this form of itching is primarily related to psychological dysfunction.

### Body Dysmorphic Disorder

Body dysmorphic disorder is defined as preoccupation with some slight, or nonexistent, defect in appearance that causes significant distress resulting in psychosocial or sexual dysfunction. BDD is quite common with an overall prevalence of about 2% of the general adult population, ranging up to about 20% of individuals presenting for rhinoplasty.[13] In the fifth edition of the Diagnostic and Statistical Manual of Mental Disorders (DSM 5), BDD is classified under the category of obsessive-compulsive disorder (OCD), disorders with an extremely high comorbidity existing between BDD and OCD. Recent data suggest that OCD and BDD share common genetic and environmental risk factors, clinical features, and sociodemographic profiles.[13] Patients with both have higher rates of anxiety, schizotypal features, and suicidal ideation than with either alone. There is also comorbidity between BDD and other mental disorders such as depression, anxiety disorder, and social phobia.[14,15] Patients with real but slight anatomical abnormalities may only be preoccupied at the OCD level of severity, whereas in patients in whom no abnormalities can be detected may be delusional.[14]

Not surprisingly, preoccupation with minor or imagined defects most often involves the face, head, and hair but it can also involve the genitalia.[16,17] The level of preoccupation may be relatively mild and only obsessive in nature or it may be more severe, representing fully developed BDD. Preoccupation regarding the genitalia most often revolves around size or color.

In terms of preoccupation with size, men not surprisingly, most often focus on the penis perceiving that their normal size penis is too small.[18] On the other hand, in women it is usually the misperception that their labia minora are too large or too asymmetric.[19] Penile concerns in men have resulted in a huge industry involving the use of nonprescription medications advertised as "guaranteed" to result in penile enlargement. Similarly, misperception about labia size or asymmetry has resulted in a booming business for female genital cosmetic surgery.

There is very little published about preoccupation with genital color. However, a search of the internet reveals a considerable level of concern on the part of women regarding the perception that their external genitalia (primarily the labia majora) or perianal area are too darkly pigmented. Because of this concern, many products and services are offered for genital and anal bleaching. In addition, many women who develop vestibular pain examine the vulvar vestibule and perceive that the color is abnormally red. This perception may be reinforced by clinicians who on examination confirm the presence of "excessive" redness. This "excessive" redness is then perceived as an inflammatory process responsible for the occurrence of vestibular pain. This led to use of the term "vulvar vestibulitis." However, several studies have demonstrated that normal, asymptomatic women, with entirely normal biopsies, frequently have a similar degree of vestibular redness and, in any event, no form of anti-inflammatory therapy has led to a decrease in redness nor an improvement in pain. On the other hand, some studies support the presence of inflammation but these studies are not convincing, leaving the subject unresolved.[20] We believe that the red color is a normal finding unrelated to inflammation and the development of pain and thus support the consensus classification of vulvodynia that continues the elimination of the word "vestibulitis."[21]

A similar situation also occurs in men. A small number of men develop idiopathic scrotal skin pain and on self-examination, they perceive that excessive redness is present. They then believe that the redness is abnormal and that it is directly related to the development of their pain. This association may be supported by clinicians who are unfamiliar with genital skin color. The severity of preoccupation with this redness often reaches the level of BDD. However, invariably, examination by experienced clinicians reveals that the redness is within the normal variability of scrotal wall color and that there is no local pathology present. Very little has been written about this "red scrotum syndrome"[22] but we have seen nearly 50 such patients, and an informal show of hands at dermatology meetings suggesting that it is appreciably more common than the medical literature would suggest. Management is discussed in Chapter 13.

#### Self-mutilation (Dermatitis Artefacta, Factitial Dermatitis, Nonsuicidal Self-injury)

Self-mutilation involving the skin is an uncommon condition in which individuals knowingly and repeatedly damage the skin through burning, cutting, abrasion, chemical application, or other similar behaviors.[23,24] We exclude damage due to fingernails and those conditions that occur on a one-time basis such as tattooing and skin piercing. Self-mutilation can occur at any age, but most instances occur in adolescents and young adults. Characteristically, patients strenuously deny that they are doing anything injurious to the skin, and they may show an irrational lack of concern, considering the severity of the injuries.[23] Women are over represented,[23] and suicide ideation and even suicide sometimes occurs.[24]

Self-mutilation occurs in two major settings: with malingering, where secondary gain is the driving factor, and in those individuals with moderate to severe psychological impairment, where the behavior is carried out to satisfy an internal and unrecognized emotional need. The underlying psychiatric abnormalities present in these individuals are variable but include anxiety, depressive, bipolar, and personality disorders.[25] In fact, personality disorders are so common, nonsuicidal self-injury is a diagnostic criterion for borderline personality disorder.[25]

These traumatically self-induced lesions are fairly easy to recognize although it is extremely difficult to prove that they occur directly as a result of self-induction. A major clue is the observation that they develop only where the patient can reach. The most common sites are the face, arms, and legs, but the genitalia may be involved in a small percentage of cases.[26,27] There are very few publications in the medical literature about genital self-mutilation, but a short search on the internet suggests that the problem is much more common than physicians believe. Based mostly on anecdotal information, one of us (PJL) has concluded that major forms of mutilation (such as penile self-amputation) are more common in men, whereas less damaging behaviors such as genital cutting are more likely to occur in young women. A dramatic and disturbing example of nonsuicidal self-injury takes place in the 2010 movie, The Black Swan, and genital cutting figured prominently in the 2001 movie, The Piano Teacher.

Female genital mutilation (FGM) as a cultural ritual is not self-induced and does not lie within this area of self injury.

### Psychosocial Dysfunction Influences the Course of Disease

Psychosocial problems play an important, but not causative, role for many genital disorders. Since this is true of numerous genital diseases, this section will focus on only two examples, atopic dermatitis and psoriasis, wherein psychological factors may play an important role regarding the time of onset, extent, severity, and duration of the disease. The published literature on these two disorders relates almost entirely to generalized forms of the disease, but it is reasonable to expect that when the genital area is involved, there will be even greater psychosocial dysfunction than is described for generalized involvement.

#### Atopic Dermatitis and Lichen Simplex Chronicus

As indicated in Chapter 5, we believe that lichen simplex chronicus represents the localized form of atopic dermatitis, and these two conditions will be treated as a single entity in this section. Atopic dermatitis occurs in only a portion of patients who are biologically predisposed to develop the disease because of underlying atopy or through defects (such as filaggrin mutations) in the differentiation of epithelial keratinocytes. Psychological dysfunction appears to be one of the major factors influencing which of these predisposed individuals develop the disease. Often these psychological aspects are present very early in life and frequently occur as a result of a dysfunctional family relationship.[28] Moreover, infants and children with atopic dermatitis have an increased risk of developing attention-deficit hyperactivity disorder, major depression, anxiety, oppositional defiant disorder, and autistic spectrum disorder.[29]

For adults, several studies of patients with atopic dermatitis reveal increased levels of anxiety and depression.[30,31] The presence of these two disorders leads to increased itching that in turn leads to incessant scratching. This then is responsible for the development of the "itch-scratch cycle," which characterizes the disorder. In addition, there is evidence that patients with atopic dermatitis and lichen simplex have increased levels of somatization, obsession-compulsion, and suicidal ideation.[32-35] In more psychoanalytic terms, atopic dermatitis patients are often described as irritable, resentful, guilt-ridden, and hostile. Improved outcomes with psychological and educational intervention demonstrate the high level of importance that psychological factors play in the development of atopic dermatitis and lichen simplex chronicus.[36]

### Psoriasis

It is clear that there is a genetic, biologic predisposition for the development of psoriasis. But, as for atopic dermatitis, psychological factors appear to influence the time of lesion development, severity of disease, and response to therapy. There is some consensus that high stress levels, at least for some patients, precede the development and exacerbation of psoriasis.[37,38] Patients with psoriasis have significantly higher levels of anxiety and depression than control populations and it seems reasonable to believe that their presence is caused at least in part by stress.[33,39] Moreover, men with psoriasis consume more alcohol and patients of both genders, but especially women are more likely to smoke than do controls.[40] These behavioral aspects may also be associated with the noted anxiety and depression.

Patients with psoriasis are also appreciably more likely to exhibit alexithymia (an inability to understand, process, or describe emotions), and it is possible that this personality trait plays a role in the development of their disease.[41] Lastly, psoriatic patients are found to have higher than normal levels of stigmatization and social avoidance/attachment and tend to perceive that social support is lacking.[42]

## Psychosocial Dysfunction Occurs as a Result of Disease

Poor health always has a detrimental effect on patients' QoL and measurement of QoL by way of validated questionnaire surveys is probably the best approach to use in measuring psychosocial dysfunction.[43] These surveys have been carried out for a very large number of dermatologic diseases but because of space limitations, only psoriasis and atopic dermatitis will be considered here. Five aspects regarding the results of these QoL studies are worth exploring.

First, chronic dermatologic disorders when compared to significant systemic medical disease appear to have a disproportionably large detrimental effect on overall QoL. This is not surprising given the adverse social reaction to those with visible disease compared to those with "invisible" diseases such as hypertension and diabetes. Moreover, there is an unwarranted fear in many the general population that skin diseases are contagious.

Second the magnitude of effect that the presence of our two sample diseases, psoriasis and atopic dermatitis, has on QoL is not trivial but instead is quite significant.[44,45]

Third, the detrimental effect on QoL of patients with psoriasis and atopic dermatitis increases with cutaneous disease severity. This too is to be expected because as severity increases, social and intimate interactions are likely to become more troublesome to the patient.

Fourth, a distribution of psoriasis and atopic dermatitis that involves the face and/or anogenital region increases the detrimental effect that these two diseases have on QoL in general and on intimacy in particular.[46,47]

Fifth, the assessment of disease severity and its impact on QoL is quite different between patients and clinicians. Clinicians very frequently believe that the decrement in QoL is much less than that perceived by patients. This is largely related to the fact that clinicians base their estimate of disease effect on QoL almost entirely on their observation of the extent and severity of the disease without taking into account what even trivial disease may mean to individual patients. The use of patient-completed QoL questionnaires would alleviate this discrepancy between the viewpoint of the patient and the clinician, but, unfortunately, such surveys have almost only been used in a clinical research setting rather than for individual patient encounters. This needs to change as such underestimation of a patient's perception of disease effect on QoL is demeaning to the patient and will inevitably have an adverse effect on the clinician-patient relationship and possibly also on the patient's response to therapy.

## Genital Disease in Childhood

Some genital conditions occur only in children or are more common in prepubertal children. Also, many skin diseases that affect both children and adults present unique questions or management when occurring in children.

Genital complaints produce anxiety in patients generally, with fears of malignancy, sexual functioning, fertility, and sexually transmitted diseases. Genital symptoms and abnormalities in children are fraught with even more anxiety in parents, who feel responsibility for their child's disease, while being unable to alleviate it. Often, providers have investigated the possibility of sexually transmitted disease, or have broached the subject of sexual abuse, producing even more anxiety, defensiveness, and anger. Or, a parent's overattention to the child's symptoms can lead to either anxiety on the part of the child or enjoyment of the attention with subsequent manipulation.

The primary therapy for parents of children with genital complaints is reassurance, and words of caution regarding information they will find in social media. Printed handouts are supportive, as the written word is perceived as authoritative, and assures the parent that the problem is one recognized and shared by others. Their child is not alone, and both information and treatment of the condition are available. Specific reassurance that their condition is not the parent's fault, and that it will not affect fertility, sexual functioning, or the development of malignancy, is crucial to many families.

## Normal Genitalia

The appearance of the prepubertal external genitalia varies with the age of the child and with the normal differences among individuals. The range of normal is often not appreciated, since the genitalia are generally not examined closely on routine childhood examinations. And, except for the hymen, there is little information on the normal variants and changes in the external genitalia.

### Females

Newborn female genitalia reflect the effects of maternal hormones. The presence of estrogen produces generous labia minora, which extend beyond puffy labia majora **(Fig. 15-1)**. Symmetrical physiologic hyperpigmentation can occur. The mucosa is pink, resilient, and moist, with thick hymenal folds covering the small vaginal and urethral openings. Milky, physiologic secretions are often present.

When the effects of maternal estrogen disappear, the fat pads of the labia majora diminish, and the underlying labia minora become vestigial, and generally represent only anterior remnants of the clitoral frenulum **(Fig. 15-2)**. The thin hymenal ring is present within the vaginal opening. There are several normal variations of the appearance and shape of the hymen. The mucosa is now thin and atrophic, often with erythema that worries parents. Friction, urine, stool, overwashing, soaps, etc. produce irritation in this atrophic, fragile skin. Tissues lack elasticity in early childhood, and this contributes to tearing with trauma. Many children also experience adhesions of the clitoral hood to the clitoris simply as a result of this mild vulvar irritation, just as midline labial adhesions occur. Both processes generally reverse in later childhood. However, a recent study has reported that a third of college women exhibit synechiae of variable severity of the clitoris to the clitoral hood,[48] and these actually often persist into adulthood.[49]

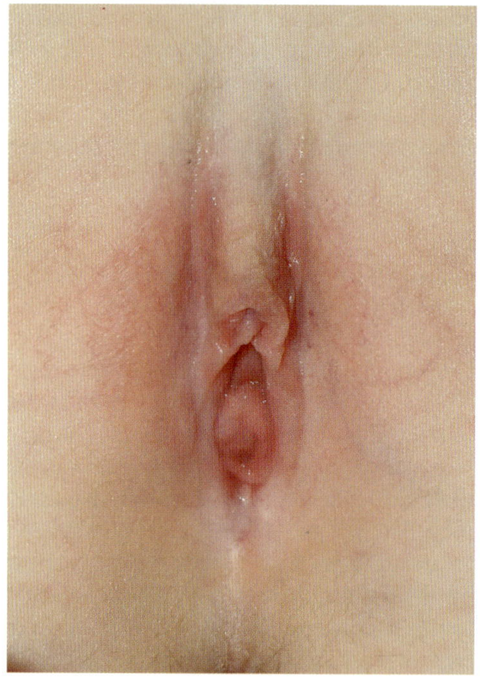

Fig. 15-2. The prepubertal vulva shows only vestigial labia minora that consist of only the clitoral frenulum; the labia minora begin to enlarge when estrogen appears. The labia majora have lost their fat pad and are nearly flat.

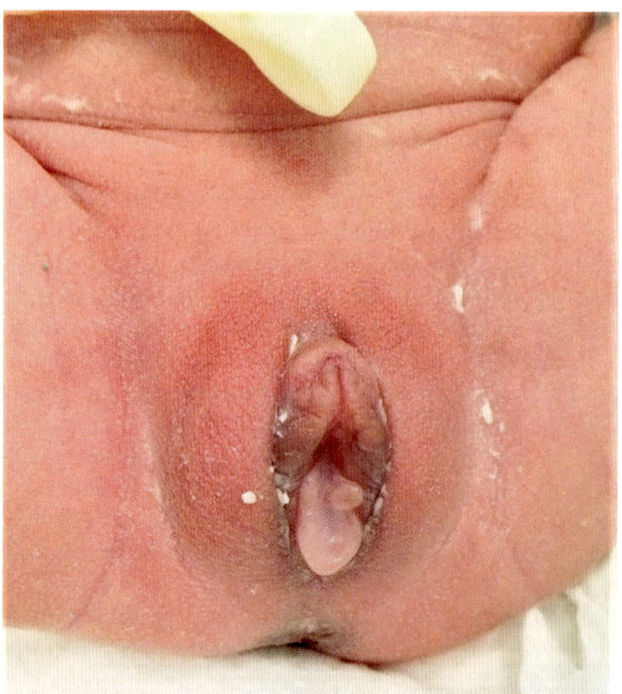

Fig. 15-1. This newborn girl shows a vulva with a strong maternal estrogen effect, with puffy labia minora that extend beyond the large labia majora, and the hymen is pink, thick and protrudes as well.

With the onset of puberty, there is thickening of all vulvar and vaginal tissues, and midline hair growth is noted. The labia majora again produce more prominent fat pads, and the labia minora elongate and thicken to variable degrees. The clitoris enlarges, and the hymen thickens with enlargement of the central opening. As in infancy, the mucosa becomes pink, soft, elastic, and moist. White discharge is common as endogenous estrogens stimulate vaginal secretions, and pruritus occurs in some girls as a result of the constant and unaccustomed wetness.

### Males

The influence of maternal hormones on male genitalia is less pronounced. Newborn boys often exhibit swelling of the scrotum resulting from fluid collection in the tunica vaginalis during the birthing process or a hydrocele.

Hyperpigmentation of the scrotum and penile shaft may be more prominent at birth, especially in those with darker natural skin colors. Nearly all newborns exhibit phimosis, but by adolescence, only 6.8% of boys could not retract the foreskin.[50] By adulthood, only 3.4% were found to have phimosis in a later review of the literature.[51]

The debate regarding the risks, benefits, and ethics of routine newborn circumcision rages on. Some point to the medical benefits of decreased penile cancer and skin diseases occurring on the glans in those who have been circumcised. Others strongly feel that circumcision for anything but a specific medical indication in a person below the age of consent is unethical. In fact, childhood circumcision was criminalized in Germany in 2012, although the outcry from the Jewish and Muslim communities resulted in recension of this law. The American Academy of Pediatrics policy statement reports that there are health benefits to circumcision, but not great enough to recommend this to all boys. However, with the complications being lower with newborn rather than later circumcision as well as the known health benefits, the American Academy of Pediatrics writes that parental decisions should be honored. The Canadian Pediatric Society also does not recommend routine newborn circumcision, and rates of circumcision are falling in both the United States and Canada.

Before puberty, the phallus is short and thin. Pigmentation is similar to the general body pigment. The scrotum is less pendulous, and the skin is soft, thin, and pink, with few rugae. Both testes are palpable as soft masses within the scrotal sac. Premature infants are more likely to exhibit undescended testes, which are usually unilateral. Generally, these will descend by age 9 months. Surgical correction is sometimes required, and those that do not descend are at greater risk of malignancy, even when corrected. Small milia may be present on the scrotum.

At puberty, there is enlargement of the penis, both in length and circumference, with thickening and development of the glans. The scrotal sac and testes also enlarge and become more pendulous. The skin of the scrotum darkens and thickens, developing a coarse texture and folding into rugae in most but not all males. Pubic hair is noted first along the base of the shaft and then extending into the inguinal creases and onto the medial thighs as it becomes darker, coarser, and curlier.

## Labial Adhesions

### *Clinical Presentation*

Labial adhesions are a fairly common occurrence, occurring in up to 3% of girls.[52] These are seen primarily under the age of 3 years.[53] These appear as midline fusion of the labia majora, resulting in variable narrowing of the introitus (**Fig. 15-3**). A survey of 108 girls showed that adhesions were posterior in 79%-93% of affected girls, sometimes with mid or anterior adhesions forming.[53]

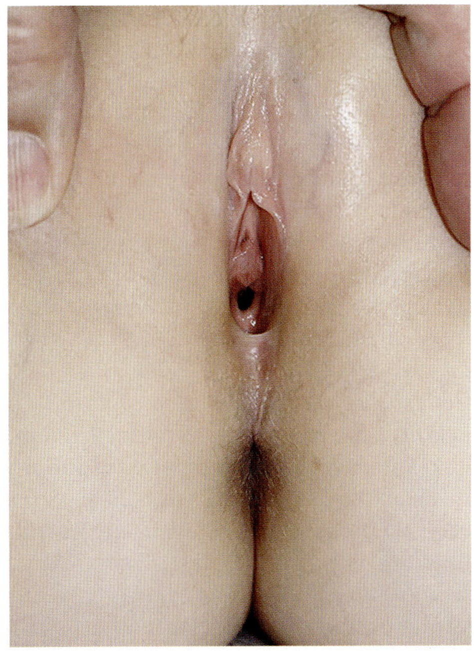

Fig. 15-3. Posterior labial agglutination and very mild anterior labial agglutination have occurred in this child with lichen sclerosus, a known association.

Uncommonly, the vulvar vestibule fuses entirely, covering the urethra (**Fig. 15-4**). Girls with labial agglutination are usually asymptomatic unless urinary retention or infection occurs behind the adhesions. In a series of 425 girls with labial adhesions, over 82% were asymptomatic, although 4% experienced urinary tract infections

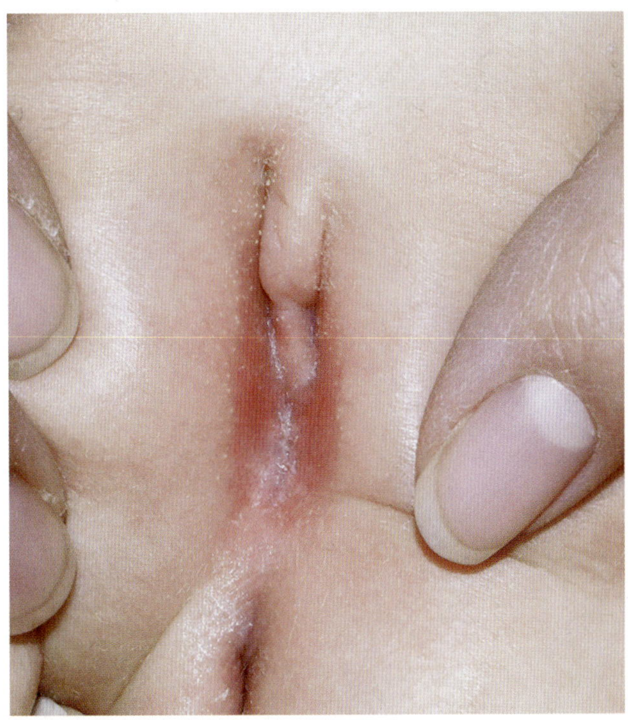

Fig. 15-4. This child has experienced near complete labial agglutination, although there is still no functional disruption in urine flow.

(UTIs).[54] Occasionally, even incomplete adhesions are bothersome as urine can become partially trapped above the synechiae, with dribbling when the child stands.

#### Diagnosis

The diagnosis is made by the clinical appearance. The smooth, flat surface that overlies the introitus can suggest absence of the vagina, but it is distinguished by the presence of a central thin translucent line of fibrous tissue at the site of fusion.

#### Pathophysiology

Synechiae usually occur as a result of mild chronic inflammation of the vulvar skin, resulting from mechanical trauma, infection, or skin disease, including lichen sclerosus or irritant dermatitis (**Fig. 15-5**). Some have suggested that, because topical estrogen generally lyses labial adhesions, low estrogen levels may play a role in the formation of these adhesions. However, serum levels of estrogen in girls with labial adhesions are the same as those in girls without adhesions. Still, the normal infantile estrogen-deficient (compared to postpubertal girls) vulvar epithelium is thin, easily irritated, and more likely to scar compared to well estrogenized vulvar skin. Vulvar epithelium scars easily in general, and even more so in atrophic prepubertal skin.

#### Management

Generally, no treatment beyond robust reassurance is required, as adhesions regularly resolve by puberty.

The traditional therapy for complete or symptomatic adhesions is the local application of estrogen cream combined with gentle massage and good hygiene. A survey of the literature shows 50%-90% of those treated with estrogen cream and massage cleared, with recurrence of 30%, and 68%-80% of girls receiving topical corticoids cleared with 23% of recurrences.[52] Surgical intervention has a success rate of 100% and recurrence of 0.[55] However, no series divide out the girls with primary adhesions (idiopathic) from those with adhesions due to lichen sclerosus. The use of a topical corticosteroid is crucial for the treatment management of girls with adhesions on the basis of skin disease, especially lichen sclerosus, which can cause permanent scarring of other structures if not treated appropriately.

Most vulvologists treat symptomatic labial adhesion with a superpotent topical corticosteroid ointment (much less irritating than a cream) such as clobetasol propionate 0.05% or betamethasone dipropionate ointment in augmented or optimized vehicle 0.05% applied very, very sparingly twice a day, with monthly follow-up. Those children with skin disease should be maintained on a lower potency corticosteroid ointment such as desonide ointment 0.05% daily or thrice weekly superpotent medication for several weeks beyond lysis of adhesions, or at least through puberty in the case of lichen sclerosus.

Rarely, surgical separation is required because of pain, infection, or urinary retention. In a cooperative child, this can be done using topical anesthesia with lidocaine/prilocaine; the frightened child is best treated under general anesthesia/conscious sedation. A well-lubricated cotton swab sometimes can be used to separate the labia. Estrogen cream or a corticosteroid ointment should be applied daily afterward until healed to prevent reformation of the adhesions. The area should be re-evaluated every few days initially by the clinician to detect early recurrence during healing.

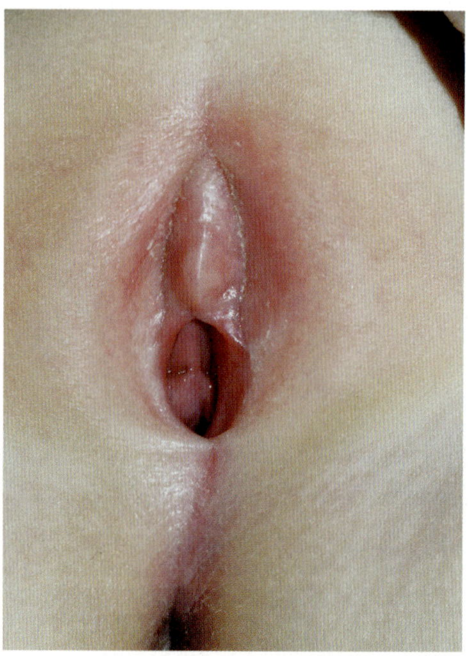

Fig. 15-5. Very slight posterior labial agglutination has formed, again in a setting of lichen sclerosus, but resolved with a topical corticosteroid.

## Red Plaques and Papules

### Diaper Dermatitis (Napkin Dermatitis)

Although diaper dermatitis is discussed as though this is a specific skin disease, this is actually any rash that occurs under a diaper. These rashes occur as a result of the unique environment of the diaper area and consist mostly of irritant contact dermatitis, friction, and, sometimes, Candidiasis. Modern diapers have rendered recalcitrant diaper dermatitis much, much more uncommon event.

#### Clinical Presentation

Diaper dermatitis is characterized by red plaques that show various degrees of scaling that may be somewhat obscured by moisture. This is covered by the diaper and sometimes exhibits maceration and erosion when severe. The morphology depends upon what factors are producing the dermatitis.

The most common issue causing diaper dermatitis is irritant contact dermatitis produced by urine and feces held against the skin. This appears as a rash occurring on the more convex surfaces that directly contact urine

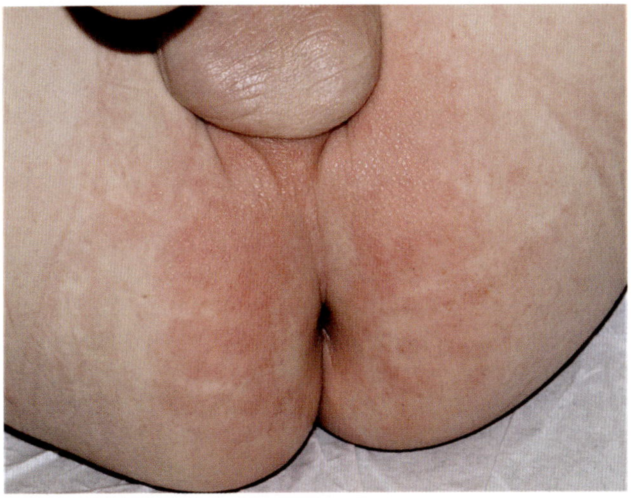

Fig. 15-6. Diaper dermatitis most often occurs as an irritant contact dermatitis as a result of urine and feces held against the skin by the diaper.

and stool, and relative sparing of the skin creases (Figs. 15-6 and 15-7). The perineum, buttocks, mons, and upper thighs are most commonly involved. Sharp margination where the diaper ends can occur. The skin is pink to bright red with a shiny, glazed appearance, occasionally with edema and sometimes even blisters or superficial erosions (Fig. 5-30). Eroded skin is tender and painful, especially when it is in contact with irritating substances such as diarrhea, alcohols, or propylene glycol that is contained in diaper wipes.

A severe form of irritant dermatitis is termed diaper dermatitis of Jacquet, granuloma gluteale infantum, or pseudowarts (see section "Granuloma Gluteale Infantum"). This is characterized by sharply marginated, red nodules, often with overlying erosion that confers an umbilicated appearance. These typically affect the labia majora, perianal skin, and perineum (Figs. 15-8 and 15-9).

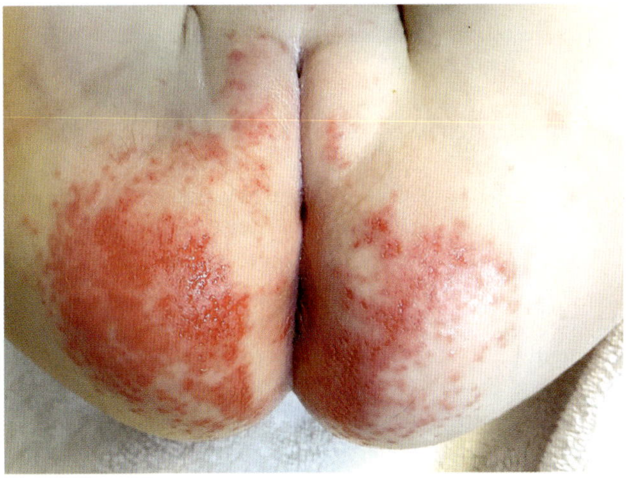

Fig. 15-7. Diarrheal stool is incredibly irritating, producing not only redness on the convex surfaces of the buttocks while sparing the relatively protected skinfold but even causing coalescing erosions.

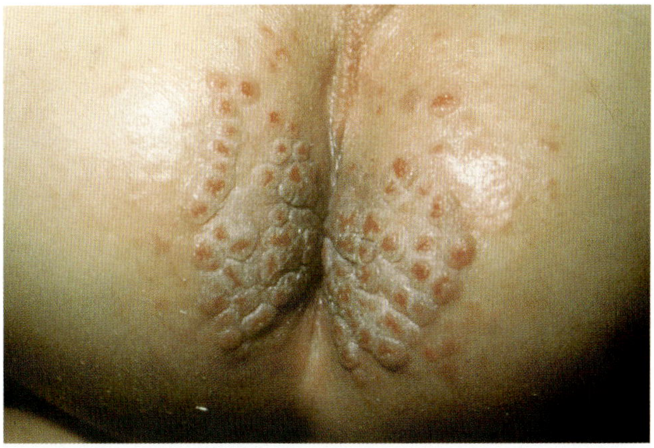

Fig. 15-8. Genital skin sometimes demonstrates an unusual reaction pattern of discrete, infiltrated, monomorphous, usually eroded papules in response to chronic inflammation, in this case to long-lasting diarrhea. This pattern is called Jacquet diaper dermatitis, pseudowarts, or granuloma gluteale infantum.

Frictional dermatitis is most pronounced on the inner thighs, under the fastening tabs and waistband of the diaper, and on other surfaces that rub against the diaper. It consists of mild erythema and papules that wax and wane and respond quickly to diapering more often so that moisture is minimized.

Intertrigo from moisture and friction occurs within the skinfolds of the diaper area but also can occur in the neck creases, under the axilla, and between the fat rolls on the thighs. A relatively sharp cutoff where the dry skin begins is noted. Affected areas may be oozing, macerated, and red. Superficial sloughing of white hydrated skin is common.

When *Candida albicans* complicates diaper dermatitis, the infection preferentially affects the skinfolds, with deep, bright erythema showing surrounding peripheral scale (Fig. 15-10). Satellite collarettes or round erosions are characteristic.

The shiny, glazed appearance of buttocks and the coalescing satellite papules and pustules are characteristic

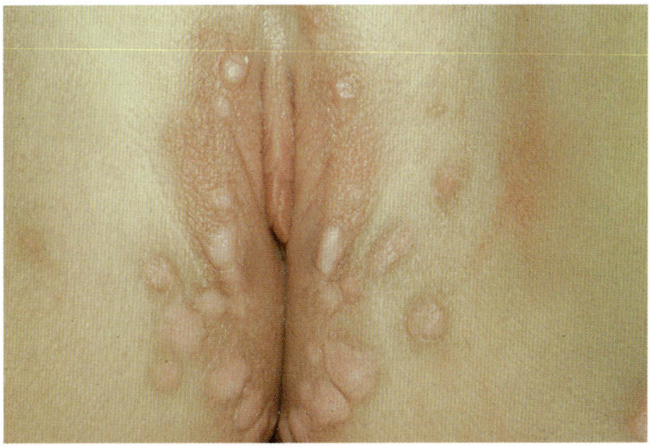

Fig. 15-9. These flat-topped papules in a symmetrical pattern are typical of Jacquet diaper dermatitis.

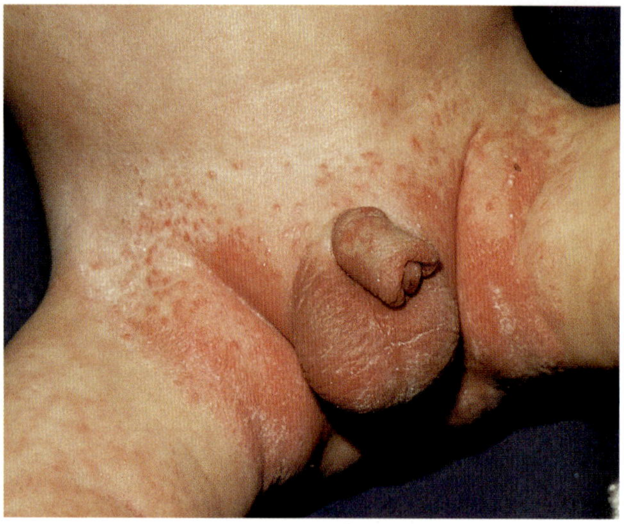

Fig. 15-10. When yeast plays a role in diaper dermatitis, the wet skinfolds are prominently involved, and classically with satellite lesions.

of *Candida* diaper dermatitis. This is confirmed by microscopic examination, culture, or response to therapy.

Psoriasis is another skin disease that less often contributes to diaper dermatitis, because psoriasis is a skin disease that is precipitated by irritation and injury, as occurs from the irritant diaper dermatitis. Often, psoriasis in the diaper area is unaccompanied, at least initially, by extragenital psoriasis.

### Diagnosis

The diagnosis of diaper dermatitis is made by the presence of erythema and scale, with or without erosions and maceration in the diaper area.

Specific diseases that preferentially affect the diaper area and can mimic routine diaper dermatitis include acrodermatitis enteropathica and Langerhans cell histiocytosis (see below). Patients with Kawasaki disease typically exhibit accentuation of their rash in the diaper area with desquamation late in the course of their disease.

### Pathophysiology

Diaper dermatitis is multifactorial but primarily irritant contact, sometimes with candidiasis. The irritants include wetness and friction of a diaper over skin exposed to urine and stool. Occasionally, atopic dermatitis or psoriasis plays a role.

### Management

The prevention and treatment of diaper dermatitis is primarily aimed at changing the environment to eliminate common irritants and re-evaluating the dermatitis that remains. With the advent of gel-containing disposable diapers, diaper rashes have become much less problematic. For the past 30-40 years, these disposable diapers have been the preferred option for diapering infants and toddlers. Disposable diapers were advertised as more convenient, hygienic, and less likely to cause diaper dermatitis than a cotton diaper with a vinyl or rubber pant covering. This cotton core and vapor impermeable outer layer was a set up for causing irritant contact dermatitis and many families gladly welcomed a readily disposable solution. However, the cost is high, and diapers can be left on for prolonged periods. In the last 15 years, cloth diapers have received a makeover to create a modern reusable option that can be cost effective, less likely to produce diaper rash than traditional cloth diapers, and more environmentally conscious. Data regarding comparisons between disposable diapers and current reusable diapers in regard to the frequency of diaper rash are generally lacking. There are suggestions that disposable diapers are superior, but all cloth diapers are not identical, nor are all disposable diapers.[56] There are a number of reports of increased numbers of infants with severe papulo-erosive Jacquet diaper dermatitis in those using reusable diapers, however.[57,58]

In addition to high-quality diapers and frequent diaper changes, the application of barrier cream to the involved areas is useful to protect from urine and feces, and supplying lipids to the epidermis; these should be applied at least twice weekly to the healthy diaper area.[59] When diaper dermatitis is present, large amounts should be applied to the skin with each diaper change, and avoidance of further irritation from cleansing soaps and some diaper wipes. Most wipes are not problematic.[59] However, care should be taken to ensure that the pH is appropriate to counteract the alkaline effects of faces and urine and maintain the slight acidity of the area, and that the chosen wipes are free of potential irritants such as alcohol, nonallergy screened fragrances, essential oils, soap, suboptimal surfactants, and harsh detergents (eg, sodium lauryl sulfate).[59] Allergens to be avoided include methylisothiazolinone (MI), methylchloroisothiazolinone (MCI), bronopol (2-bromo-2-nitropropane-1,3-diol), and iodopropynyl butylcarbamate.[59] Or, Water Wipes can be used. These contain only water and a trivial amount of grapeseed oil. These lack pH adjustment and antibacterial agents, but studies have shown wipes to be equivalent to washcloths, which also lack these features, and both avoid the potential irritating additives.

However, adherent stool is best removed by gently rinsing the perianal area with warm water and patting the skin dry. The application of a barrier cream to anogenital skin is more effective than the aggressive removal of feces by rubbing or the use of harsh cleansers. Mild corticosteroid preparations such as 1% or 2.5% hydrocortisone ointment (not cream) hastens resolution of inflammation when applied twice daily and covered with barrier cream or ointment. Potent corticosteroids should not be applied under diaper occlusion, which enhances the effect of the medication. Adrenal suppression and deaths due to immunosuppression have been reported in several infants treated with ultra potent corticosteroids under diaper occlusion.[60] Anticandidal agents should be added if there is a question of yeast. Nystatin is available in an ointment base and is less irritating than the azole creams. When disease is severe and erosions are present, antifungal medication should be administered orally until healing begins.

Persistence of dermatitis when these measures are taken usually indicates an ongoing irritant process or an alternative diagnosis. Chronic diarrhea is a common cause for persistence of dermatitis, and this predisposes to yeast. An evaluation of the child's diet and growth parameters and a search for underlying disease such as infection or malabsorption are indicated. In the absence of diarrhea, a skin biopsy may be helpful to identify other primary cutaneous disease.

### Seborrheic Dermatitis

Seborrheic dermatitis is a common form of dermatitis of the scalp infants but only affects anogenital skin when very severe, as part of a generalized eruption that preferentially affects other skinfolds as well, to include the axillae and neck.

First occurring at about 4-6 weeks of life but rarely after a year of age. The scalp is usually involved first, with greasy, yellow scales with minimal inflammation. The diaper area is the second most common area to develop a rash. Seborrheic diaper dermatitis consists of erythematous, sharply marginated scaling plaques with greasy, macerated scales **(Fig. 15-11)**. *Candida* frequently superinfects the area. The inguinal creases are more severely affected, but in many cases, the groin and perineum are confluently involved. Spread to other flexural areas and even onto the trunk as isolated scaly plaques can occur. Unlike atopic dermatitis, seborrheic dermatitis is nonpruritic, although newborns do not have the ability to rub and scratch.

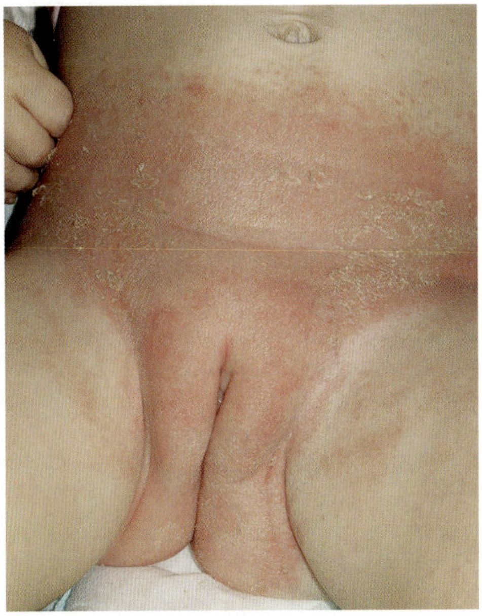

Fig. 15-11. The yellow scale with a somewhat greasy feel, and accompanying cradle cap and rash on other areas of the body demonstrate the diagnosis of seborrheic dermatitis.

The diagnosis of seborrheic dermatitis is usually made on a clinical basis in an infant with scalp and intertriginous erythema and yellowish scale.

The treatment of seborrhea of the diaper area consists of low-potency hydrocortisone ointment and barrier creams or ointments. Antifungal therapy can be helpful in the event of secondary candidiasis. The scalp should be treated for maximal improvement; this can be achieved by removing scale with mineral or baby oil. Antiseborrheic shampoos or mild baby shampoos, and mild topical steroid scalp solutions, such as hydrocortisone 1% or 2.5% to reduce recurrent inflammation, are also helpful. Scrubbing and shampoos with acids and other keratolytic agents should be discouraged.

### Atopic Dermatitis (Eczema)

Atopic dermatitis is an extremely pruritic eruption that occurs when irritation precipitates rubbing and scratching, which, in turn, cause erythema, lichenification, and excoriation **(Figs. 15-12 and 15-13)** (see Chapters 5 and 13). The diaper area is relatively spared in infants because the skin is covered and remains moist, and the diaper helps to protect the skin from rubbing and scratching. Treatment consists of a topical corticosteroid and avoidance of irritants.

### Psoriasis

Psoriasis is a skin condition that is relatively uncommon in children in the genital area (see Chapter 5). This is a skin disease characterized by increased turnover of epidermal

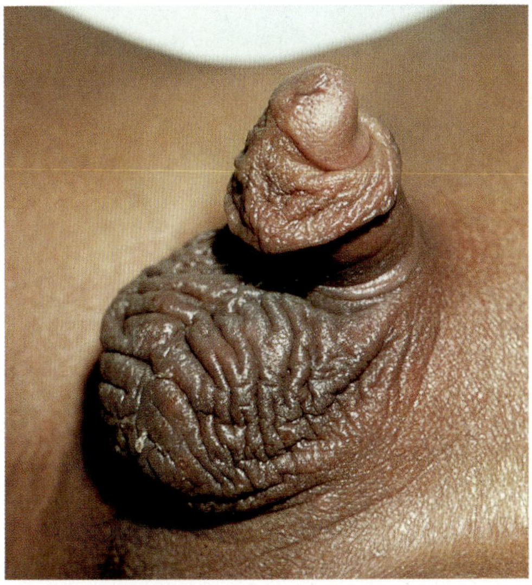

Fig. 15-12. Lichenification of the scrotum and penis are signs of the rubbing of atopic dermatitis.

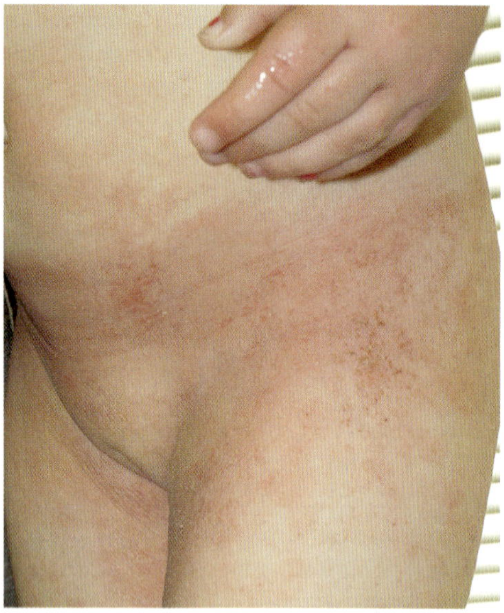

Fig. 15-13. Chronic scratching of atopic dermatitis has produced this poorly demarcated red plaque with scale and crusting.

cells, so the skin becomes thickened and covered by dense scale. It preferentially affects irritated or injured skin, so the genitalia and diaper area are often affected.

Plaques are red, well demarcated, and thickened **(Figs. 15-14 and 15-15)**. Often, psoriasis also affects the umbilicus, scalp, and gluteal cleft, and the fingernails may exhibit small pits. Often, however, there are no extragenital, pathognomonic signs of psoriasis. Psoriasis of the skinfolds and diaper area can mimic seborrheic dermatitis as well as cutaneous candidiasis, which is often a secondary factor. Even a biopsy is characteristic but often not diagnostic. In unclear cases, the course of the disease eventually provides a diagnosis, because psoriasis is chronic and other areas of the skin nearly always become involved eventually, showing typical psoriatic lesions.

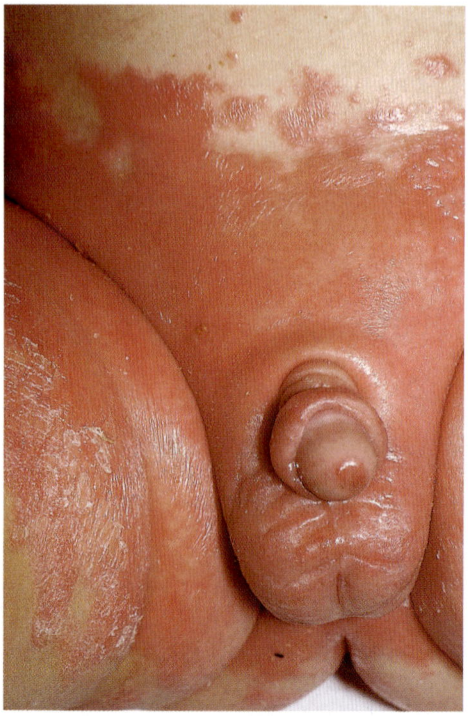

Fig. 15-14. Psoriasis exhibits sharply demarcated red plaques that, in the genital area, may show a glazed surface appearance rather than typical white scale.

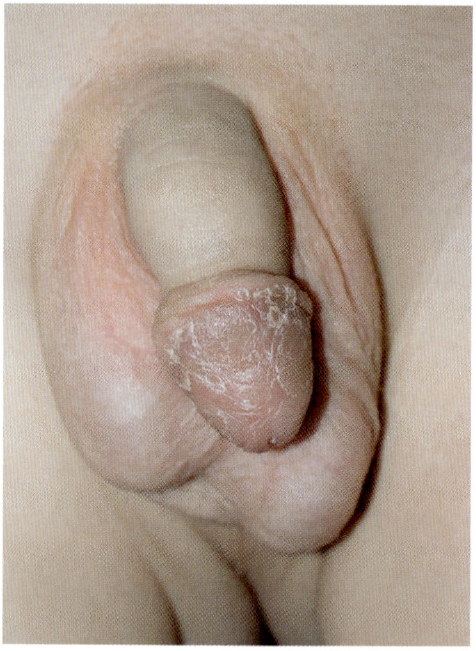

Fig. 15-15. The prominent flaking scale of the glans is classic for psoriasis.

Treatment consists of careful local care and topical corticosteroids. For the occasional unfortunate child with severe or widespread disease, systemic therapy may be required.

## Perianal Streptococcal Dermatitis (Perianal Bacterial Dermatitis, Perianal Streptococcal Cellulitis)

Perianal streptococcal dermatitis is a superficial bacterial infection that produces redness, scale and irritation of perianal skin. See also Chapter 5.

### *Clinical Presentation*

Perianal streptococcal dermatitis typically occurs in 3- to 5-year-old children, and it is more common in boys than in girls. Most often, 2 to 3 cm of erythema extends outward around the anus with minimal induration **(Figs. 15-16 to 15-18)**. In other individuals, this erythema is accompanied by painful anal fissuring and a mucoid discharge that makes defecation painful. Constipation and withholding of stool are common, and it is often unclear whether the fissure was produced by the primary disease or by passage of hard stool. Finally, well-demarcated, scaly, beefy red, crusted dermatitis with maceration of the anal verge can occur. In addition, induration of the perianal skin

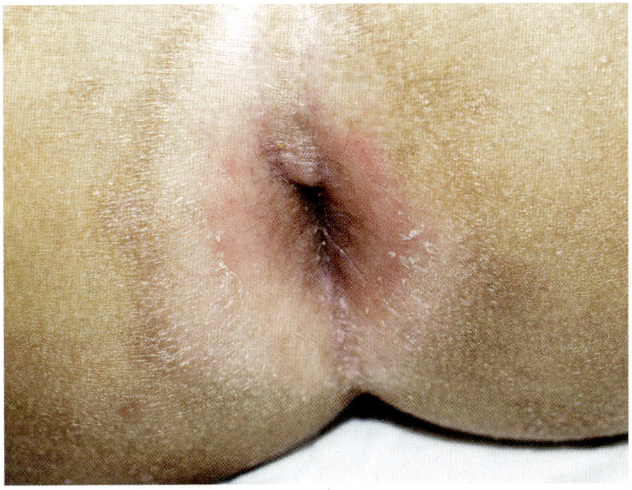

Fig. 15-16. Perianal redness and scale, sometimes with painful fissuring, are characteristic of perianal streptococcal dermatitis

and satellite-crusted plaques can be seen. Bleeding from the area is common. Girls can exhibit vulvar and vaginal involvement, and boys can experience penile involvement.

In all forms of anogenital bacterial dermatitis, pruritus, excoriations, and lichenification from scratching and rubbing are common. These superimposed eczematous changes can delay the diagnosis.

### *Diagnosis*

The diagnosis of perianal bacterial dermatitis is made on clinical grounds and is confirmed by a routine culture that yields *Streptococcus*, most often group A β-hemolytic *Streptococcus* and sometimes group B β-hemolytic *Streptococcus*. It is important to ask the laboratory to culture for these organisms because many laboratories select for enteric pathogens from perianal swabs.

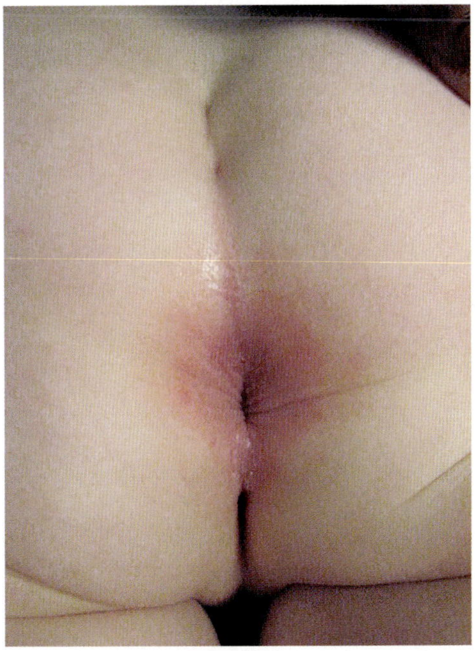

Fig. 15-17. The perianal redness of perianal streptococcal dermatitis mimics psoriasis, pinworms, irritant dermatitis, and Candidiasis.

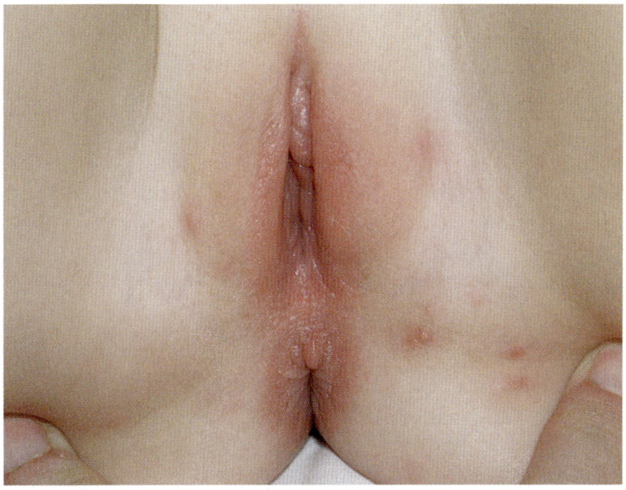

Fig. 15-18. Occasionally, the infection of perianal streptococcal dermatitis can affect the vagina producing a purulent vaginal discharge with vulvitis, and this child also has an accompanying folliculitis confirmed on culture.

The differential diagnosis of perianal bacterial dermatitis includes pinworm infestation, irritant or *Candida* dermatitis, atopic dermatitis, psoriasis, inflammatory bowel disease, and sexual abuse. Scratching and rubbing of the skin resulting from pruritus are common and can confuse the diagnosis. All perianal dermatitis should be cultured to rule out a bacterial component.

### *Pathophysiology*

Bacterial skin infection of the perianal skin, nearly always with group A and sometimes group B β-hemolytic *Streptococcus*, produces this distinctive dermatitis in children. Many patients diagnosed with perianal streptococcus have throat cultures positive for the organism without symptoms of pharyngitis. Presumably, digital contamination of the anus from the infected pharynx or other body site is the source of the infection.

### *Management*

The treatment of choice for perianal bacterial dermatitis consists of oral antibiotic therapy with concomitant mupirocin ointment several times a day. Beta-lactamase–resistant antibiotics, such as cephalosporines, amoxicillin-clavulanate, macrolides and clindamycin, appear to be less associated with recurrence than penicillin and amoxicillin, which have about a 32% recurrence rate.[61,62] Because recurrences are common, some clinicians support antibiotic therapy for as long as 21 days to allow for the skin to heal before discontinuation of medication. Mupirocin ointment applied two to four times a day may minimize recurrences as well. Stool softeners can be useful in children with painful defecation due to perianal inflammation and fissures, and hydrocortisone 1% or 2.5% ointment can minimize pain while awaiting improvement with the antibiotic.

## Pinworm

Pinworms infection is a common cause of perianal pruritus in small children.

### *Clinical Presentation*

The only symptoms of a pinworm infestation usually are dermatitis and pruritus of the perianal skin and/or vulva. Excoriations are often more prominent than obvious redness and scaling. Complaints of nighttime pruritus are the greatest complaint and may be severe enough to wake the child. Occasionally, a child describes pain rather than itching. Uncommonly, the worms migrate to the vagina in girls and cause vulvar dermatitis and a vaginal discharge or produce balanitis in boys. An uncommon complication is involvement of the appendix with pinworms, a cause of concomitant pinworms and abdominal pain.[63]

### *Diagnosis*

The diagnosis of pinworms is made in the setting of an unexplained perianal or vulvar pruritus, with or without a mild dermatitis, and is confirmed by response to therapy. Pinworms are usually difficult to find for diagnostic evaluation. At night, adult worms are occasionally seen on the perineum or in the anal canal when it is gently everted. Eggs can usually be collected using clear tape placed over the anus first thing in the morning before the eggs are disturbed. The eggs can be viewed adherent to the tape as thick-walled, ovoid structures most easily seen by light microscopy under low power.

The differential diagnosis of pinworm infection includes perianal bacterial dermatitis, atopic dermatitis, irritant dermatitis, and candidiasis. The presence of severe nighttime symptoms of perianal pruritus with minimal inflammation can help to distinguish this disorder from other forms of dermatitis.

### *Pathophysiology*

Pinworm infestation is the most common form of helminth infestation seen in humans and is produced by infestation with *Enterobius vermicularis*. Pinworms are much common in children than in adults, with more than 20% of school-aged children acquiring this ubiquitous infestation.

Pinworm infestation begins by ingestion of eggs, usually on fingers that have contacted perianal skin or dirt with eggs. Eggs hatch in the duodenum and mature during passage through the intestines. Migration to the perianal skin occurs, and gravid females deposit their eggs on the anal verge, causing pruritus. Four to six hours after the eggs are deposited, they become infectious, and when the eggs are swallowed, the cycle begins again.

### *Management*

Time honored treatment of pinworms has been with mebendazole 100 mg in a single dose, and application of a mild topical steroid ointment for any dermatitis that is present. For unexplained reasons, mebendazole is no longer available commercially, but it can be obtained through compounding pharmacies. Pyrantel pamoate, in a single dose of 11 mg/kg, can also be used. Treatment of adults and children with albendazole is 400 mg orally, repeated once in 2 weeks.

Multiple family members are often affected at the same time, necessitating widespread simultaneous treatment to cure the infestation. Reinfection is common in school-aged children.

Retreatment in 2-3 weeks is recommended because medication is ineffective against ova that may have been ingested at the time of the first treatment.

## Acrodermatitis Enteropathica and Acrodermatitislike Eruptions

Acrodermatitis enteropathica is a rare skin disease produced by zinc deficiency, showing characteristic findings. Similar findings are associated with other nutritional deficiencies.

### *Clinical Presentation*

The classic presentation of acrodermatitis enteropathica is a triad of periorificial dermatitis, diarrhea, and alopecia. Infants are irritable and have severe failure to thrive.

The dermatitis consists of periorificial erythematous, well-demarcated, and scaling plaques. At times, the skin may exhibit vesicopustular plaques and crusting **(Figs. 15-19 and 15-20)**. It is most pronounced around the mouth, eyes, and genital area. Neck folds are often involved in infants, and the acral extremities may have similar scaly, erythematous, well-marginated plaques, especially in older children and adults. The diaper dermatitis is usually severe and refractory to standard therapy. Secondary infections with *Staphylococcus* and *Candida* are common. Nail dystrophy and paronychia are also common, as is stomatitis.

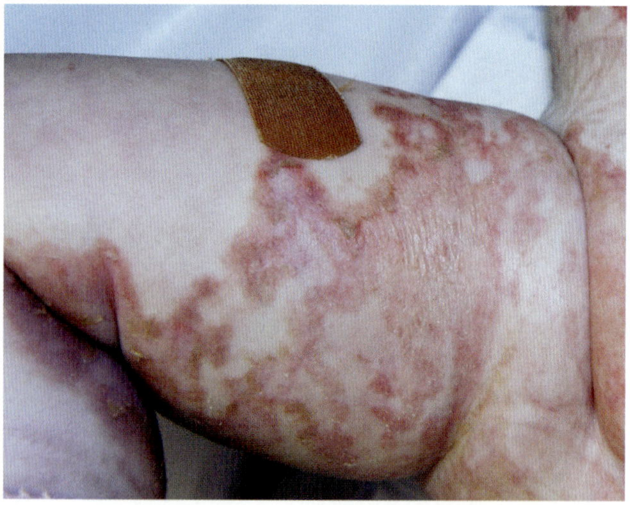

Fig. 15-19. These well-demarcated, annular, eroded plaques with crusted borders are characteristic of acrodermatitis enteropathica.

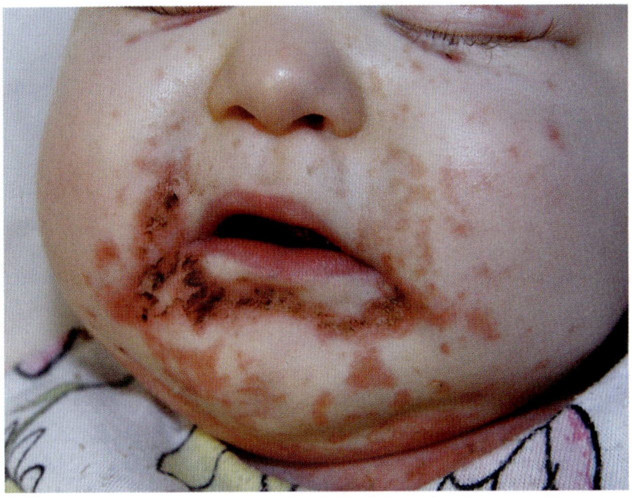

Fig. 15-20. Acrodermatitis enteropathica affects the perioral skin as well, again showing eroded and crusted plaques.

### Diagnosis

The diagnosis of acrodermatitis enteropathica is suspected based on the classical triad of dermatitis in a periorificial and acral distribution, alopecia, and diarrhea, and it is confirmed by low serum levels of zinc, alkaline phosphatase, and lipids. A skin biopsy is characteristic but not diagnostic; the upper part of the epidermis appears pale because of the presence of clear cells with balloonlike cytoplasm and loss of normal basophilia in early lesions. Subcorneal vesicles may be present in the upper epidermis, and there is diffuse parakeratosis. Hyperplasia of the epidermis and parakeratosis are seen in older lesions in a nonspecific pattern.

Severe cases of seborrheic dermatitis or psoriasis, especially those complicated by superinfection with *Candida*, can have a similar appearance, but accompanying extragenital skin is often pathognomonic. The presence of scalp dermatitis suggests seborrhea, and normal laboratory findings rule out acrodermatitis enteropathica.

### Pathophysiology

Acrodermatitis enteropathica is the classic manifestation of zinc deficiency. There are two pathways, both involving inherited mutations of zinc transporters; one is a transient neonatal zinc deficiency, the other is classic acrodermatitis enteropathica.[64] However, the skin findings can occur also in acquired nutritional deficiency states. All patients with acrodermatitis enteropathica have low levels of plasma zinc and other zinc-dependent metalloproteins such as alkaline phosphatase.

Symptoms of acrodermatitis enteropathica usually do not appear in breast-fed infants until weaning. A zinc-binding ligand that may be absent from the newborn's intestine appears to be present in breast milk, thus accounting for this observation.

Similar acral dermatitis is seen in other nutritional-deficiency states including biotin, protein, and essential fatty acid deficiency. These occur with cystic fibrosis, short bowel syndrome, anorexia nervosa, chronic illness, and Crohn disease. Organic acidemias also produce these skin findings, including maple syrup urine disease, methylmalonic acidemia, and phenylketonuria. When screening for zinc deficiency is normal, serum metabolic screening can differentiate among these diseases. In Middle Eastern adolescents, the defect develops as a result of ingestion of high quantities of phytate, which binds zinc and prevents intestinal absorption.

### Management

Treatment for acrodermatitis enteropathica consists of supplementation of zinc. Oral supplementation using zinc gluconate, acetate, or sulfate in doses of 5 mg/kg/d is recommended. Symptoms improve within 1-2 days of supplementation, and a response is noted in the dermatitis by 3-4 days. Hair growth begins in 2-4 weeks. After resolution of the disease symptoms, supplementation should be continued in the inherited form of the disease, with measurement of serum zinc levels once or twice yearly. The acrodermatitislike eruptions produced by other nutritional deficiencies are managed by identification of the cause of the deficiencies, and correction of these, just as the therapy of each metabolic disorders, requires its unique management.

## Langerhans Cell Histiocytosis, Letterer-Siwe Disease Type

Langerhans cell histiocytosis, formerly called histiocytosis X, is a group of diseases produced by proliferation of Langerhans cells, antigen presenting cells of the immune system that reside primarily in the skin. Generally, this is a rare, multisystem disease that occurs primarily in children, favoring boys slightly over girls.

### Clinical Presentation

Letterer-Siwe disease usually manifests in children aged 2 years or younger and affects internal structures as well as skin. Skin features are the presenting signs in most children, and systemic manifestations typically occur in weeks to months after the onset of the cutaneous disease.

Affected infants develop an erythematous, scaly rash on the scalp that mimicks seborrheic dermatitis. This also affects the intertriginous areas, including the inguinal creases and diaper area. Unlike seborrheic dermatitis or other inflammatory genital skin rashes, the scaling papules are infiltrated and firm (**Fig. 15-21**). The posterior auricular area and axilla are generally affected as well. Moist scale and crust often cover the papules, but the reddish brown or purpuric nature of the lesions can usually be appreciated. Ulcerations are common and may be present on the oral mucous membranes. Purpuric nodules on the palms and soles are a poor prognostic sign.

Letterer-Siwe disease is a systemic process, with dissemination of abnormal Langerhans cells into the skin and extracutaneous locations including the liver, bone marrow, lymph nodes, and central nervous system. This fulminant process can be fatal, even with early treatment.

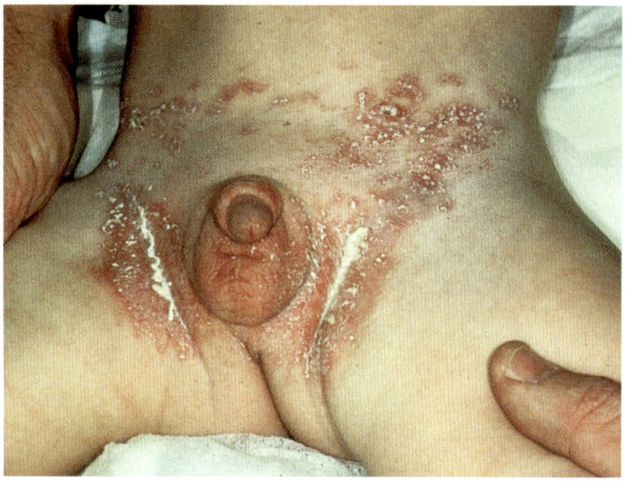

Fig. 15-21. Letterer-Siwe form of histiocytosis X superficially resembles seborrheic dermatitis or yeast, with papules within the crural creases. However, the papules are infiltrated and do not respond to treatment for yeast or seborrhea.

Infiltration into the pituitary gland can lead to diabetes insipidus, and orbital infiltrates produce exophthalmos. Fever, anemia, thrombocytopenia, hepatosplenomegaly, and adenopathy are typical. Bony tumors may be hard to appreciate clinically. Some infants have a typical histologic appearance and never develop extracutaneous manifestations. These patients retrospectively have what is called self-healing reticulohistiocytosis.

The prognosis depends on the age of onset, the duration of symptoms, and the degree of systemic involvement. Onset after 6 months of age, the absence of thrombocytopenia and lung involvement, the lack of extensive systemic involvement, and the lack of purpuric skin lesions are all good prognostic signs.

### Diagnosis

The diagnosis of Letterer-Siwe disease is made with skin biopsy. Immunohistochemistry and occasionally electron microscopy can be used to confirm the diagnosis.

The rash of Letterer-Siwe disease most closely resembles severe seborrheic dermatitis. Any infant with a seborrheiclike rash that is purpuric, ulcerated, indurated, or poorly responsive to topical therapy should be examined by biopsy to rule out this disease. Intertrigo can also be seen in this distribution, but lack of involvement of the scalp, trunk, or extremities allows distinction from Langerhans cell histiocytosis. The presence of nodular and ulcerated lesions in the groin also suggests scabies. The absence of a history of scabies or other lesions suggestive of this diagnosis should warrant a skin biopsy.

### Pathophysiology

Letterer-Siwe disease is produced by infiltration of the skin and other organs with histiocytes displaying Langerhans cell markers. The pathogenesis and origin of this disease remain obscure, although studies have demonstrated that lesions in Letterer-Siwe disease comprise cells that are clonal. The reasons for localization of the disease process in the other forms of Langerhans cell histiocytosis are also unknown.

### Management

Langerhans cell histiocytosis is evaluated and, when systemic, managed by an oncologist, but the skin disease can be treated with topical steroids, emollients, antibiotic ointments, and good local care. Topical nitrogen mustard has also been used in patients with severe skin involvement with good success. Spontaneous resolution of skin lesions occurs over time in many of these patients.

## Scabies

Scabies is a fairly common mite infection that is extraordinarily itchy and preferentially affects skinfolds and the penis and scrotum.

### Clinical Presentation

Scabies manifests as an excruciatingly pruritic dermatitis that is widespread in infants and young children but comes to the attention of the genital examiner by the inflammatory papules and nodules that occur preferentially on genital skin, particularly the penis and scrotum (**Fig. 15-22**). The rubbing and scratching of the generalized disease produce eczema in most patients. And, most of the pathognomonic skin burrows that house the mite are obscured by the eczema and excoriations. Other primary lesions include vesicles and papules that are often obliterated by scratching also. Tiny papules on the lateral fingers, hands, and ventral wrists are common. The most characteristic genital lesion is the firm nodule of the penis and scrotum; these can be red, skin-colored, or reddish brown in light complexioned children, and hyperpigmented in

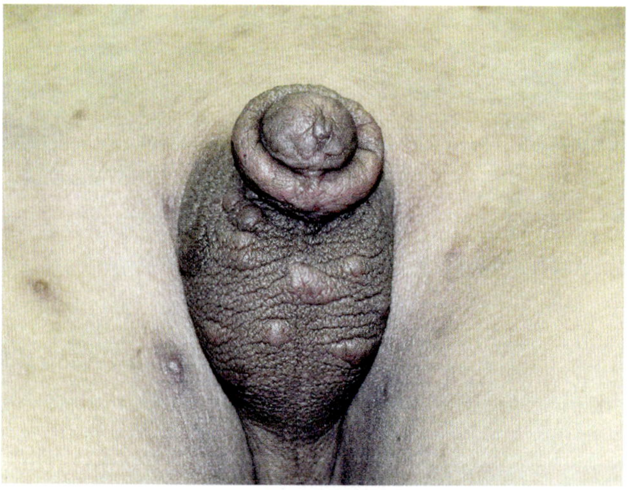

Fig. 15-22. Nodular scabies occurs primarily on the scrotum and penis of males, and in the axillae of babies, appearing as infiltrated excruciatingly pruritic nodules. There is lichenification of the glans and edema of the corona from rubbing.

those with naturally darker skin tones. Infants sometimes develop these nodules in the axillae as well, whereas older children and adolescents experience them only on the scrotum and penis. These lesions represent hypersensitivity reactions to retained dead mite and have a very atypical appearance on biopsy that can be mistaken for histiocytosis or lymphoma. These nodules can persist for months after treatment.

Scabies is often complicated by a prolonged course as a result of misdiagnosis. Administration of topical corticosteroids can mask the infestation and can contribute to the spread of the mites by suppressing the immune hypersensitivity reaction that produces symptoms. Superinfection of the excoriated, eczematized lesions with *Staphylococcus aureus* produces crusting and pustules.

#### *Diagnosis*

The diagnosis of scabies is made with the combination of clinical features in the typical distribution and microscopic evidence of infestation on mineral oil examination. Hand lesions, burrows, and nodular lesions are quite pathognomonic when present in infants and young children. Sometimes a presumptive diagnosis must be made and the diagnosis confirmed by response to therapy.

Scrapings of skin lesions and nail debris viewed microscopically in mineral oil are used for diagnosis. Mites and mite parts, eggs, and scybala (feces) are identified under 10× to 40× magnification. Ova are egg shaped and translucent centrally. Scybala are much smaller and are clusters of tiny round or oval lumps. Dermoscopy shows a brown triangular structure in the shape of a hang glider, followed by a white linear structure, a "jet with a contrail."[65] This helps to aid in identification of a site for scraping as well as making the diagnosis. This is also useful for evaluation of nodular scabies.[66]

On biopsy, histology reveals a nondiagnostic spongiotic dermatitis. Occasionally, a burrow or mite may be identified, but this is rare. Nodular lesions demonstrate intense inflammation with atypical histiocytes and lymphocytes. These can be mistaken for Langerhans cell histiocytosis or lymphoma in young children. It is important to consider scabies as a cause of nodular lesions in infants, even when there is little else clinically to suggest the diagnosis.

The differential diagnosis of scabies includes other eczematous dermatoses, especially such as seborrheic dermatitis, and atopic dermatitis. Multiple skin scrapings, a strong clinical suspicion, and, on occasion, a skin biopsy may be required to establish a diagnosis. Questioning and examining other family members for symptoms and signs of the infestation can often be helpful. Although the symptoms of scabies may lessen with topical corticosteroid application, gradual worsening as well as resurgence with withdrawal of this treatment is usual.

#### *Pathophysiology*

Scabies is caused by infestation of the skin by *Sarcoptes scabiei*. This minute mite is unique to humans and endemic in the population. Intimate contact is necessary for spread of the mite, but it is usual for most family members to acquire the infestation once it is present and undiagnosed in the household.

The adult mite is ~0.5 mm in length with eight legs and an oval, translucent, gray body when viewed with the naked eye. Children are infested with large numbers of mites compared with adults, a finding perhaps relating to the immune reaction to the parasite. Symptoms of scabies infestation typically occur in 4 weeks to 4 months after acquiring the mite because sensitization of the host must occur before clinical symptoms develop.

#### *Management*

The literature is replete with comparisons of different therapies such as variable concentrations and dosing schedules of topical permethrin, benzyl benzoate, and sulfur ointment, and oral ivermectin, but the highest cure rates are two doses of permethrin 5% cream and oral ivermectin 200 µg/kg given 1-2 weeks apart. Ivermectin is the least expensive of these two options and delivers medication to all areas of the body.

In the case of permethrin cream, care must be taken to cover all body areas, including the scalp in infants younger than 2 years old. The cream must be left in place overnight. Bathing before application is discouraged because this may increase percutaneous absorption. Fingernails should be cut and cleaned. Clothing and bedding that have been in contact with the patient or family members in the previous several days should be washed. Treatment of all family members at once is essential to avoid reinfestation. Persistence of symptoms relates more commonly to inadequate treatment or reinfestation than to resistance.

Oral ivermectin in a single dose has been shown to be highly effective against scabies, although it is used off-label. Larger series have shown this agent to be safe in children. Use of this oral treatment may replace topical treatment in the future.

The pruritus from scabies results from an immunological reaction to the mite, so that itching does not resolve promptly as long as dead mites are retained in the stratum corneum. A topical corticosteroid such as triamcinolone ointment 0.1% helps itching and control of any eczema precipitated by the scratching. The nodular lesions can persist for months. The most effective treatment for this, following specific antiscabetic therapy, is intralesional triamcinolone acetonide 10 mg/mL, ~0.1 mL into each nodule; in children, after pretreatment with a potent topical anesthetic such as lidocaine/prilocaine cream or lidocaine 4% or 5% cream.

### Granuloma Gluteale Infantum (Pseudowarts, Jacquet Diaper Dermatitis)

Granuloma gluteale infantum is an uncommon, unique reaction to a strong and chronic irritant in the anogenital area. Most common in infants, this has been recognized occasionally in adults as well, with the tentative name of granuloma gluteale adultorum.

### Clinical Presentation

Granuloma gluteale infantum is a nodular, skin-colored to red-brown eruption that develops in the diaper area (**Figs. 15-8, 15-9, and 15-23**). The individual lesions are indurated, flat-topped papules that may exhibit central erosion and are usually monomorphous in appearance and distribution. The papules are multiple and occur primarily on the anterior surface of the genital area, mons, and perineum. The buttocks are usually spared, although perianal skin can be involved. Classically, granuloma gluteale infantum is preceded by irritant diaper dermatitis that was treated with a potent topical corticosteroid.

### Diagnosis

The diagnosis is by the appearance, usually with a history of chronic diarrhea or the application of medications, such as anesthetics or antibacterial/antiseptic agents. When needed, the diagnosis can be confirmed with a skin biopsy. Histology of granuloma gluteale infantum reveals intensely infiltrated nodules with a hyperplastic epidermis with parakeratosis. There is exocytosis of neutrophils. The dermis is composed of a dense infiltrate of neutrophils, lymphocytes, histiocytes, plasma cells, eosinophils, giant cells, and hemorrhage. Fibrous spindle cells and mitoses are rare.

The differential diagnosis of granuloma gluteale infantum includes granulomatous processes such as infectious granulomas, talc or zirconium granulomas, or foreign body reactions. Scabetic nodules can have a similar appearance but are usually fewer in number and less monomorphous. Kaposi sarcoma, lymphomas, and histiocytic infiltrates such as those seen in Langerhans cell histiocytosis can present in a similar manner in the diaper area.

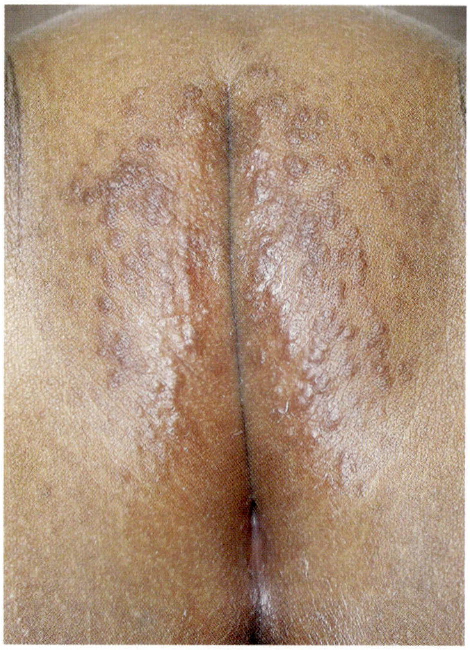

Fig. 15-23. Mild granuloma gluteale infantum, or Jacquet diaper dermatitis, consists of small infiltrated papules that are often, especially in patients of color, brown or dusky red.

The clinical picture of a healthy infant with a diaper rash that progresses to nodules is usually adequate for diagnosis. If any uncertainty exists, a skin biopsy can be performed.

### Pathophysiology

Granuloma gluteale infantum is believed to be an irritant dermatitis unique to the moisture, incontinence, and maceration of the local environment. This is especially likely to occur in the setting of chronic diarrhea in infants but can occur as a response to other irritants and allergens, especially in adults. Some believe that the use of potent topical steroids in the setting of an infection may play a role in the pathogenesis; I strongly believe that topical corticosteroids are not important in the pathogenesis, but rather most recalcitrant diaper rashes have been treated with corticosteroids, which are unhelpful.

### Management

Lesions of granuloma gluteale infantum resolve spontaneously over several weeks or months once the local environment of diarrhea or application of irritating medications have ceased.

## Infantile Perianal Pyramidal Protrusion

Infantile perianal pyramidal protrusions are puffy protrusions, usually in young girls, and usually located in the midline anterior to the anus. They generally appear on the median raphe as a pyramidal soft tissue swelling, covered by smooth, sometimes slightly erythematous skin (**Figs. 15-24 to 15-26**). Most are noted in the first 2 years of life and are asymptomatic.

Infantile perianal pyramidal protrusion occurs in normal children, in a setting of constipation, and in association with lichen sclerosus. This configuration can be seen with any irritation, and mechanical irritation from wiping after defecation is presumed to be a cause of an increase in the size or swelling of the protrusion. Biopsy of these lesions demonstrates an acanthotic epidermis with marked edema of the upper dermis and an inflammatory infiltrate in the lower dermis.

These lesions can be confused with and sometimes actually represent perianal skin tags.

Spontaneous resolution of these protrusions can occur without any treatment over several years. There is no need for treatment, as these are asymptomatic beyond that associated with any underlying cause. It is important to recognize this entity, to avoid concern that this represents a sign of sexual abuse.

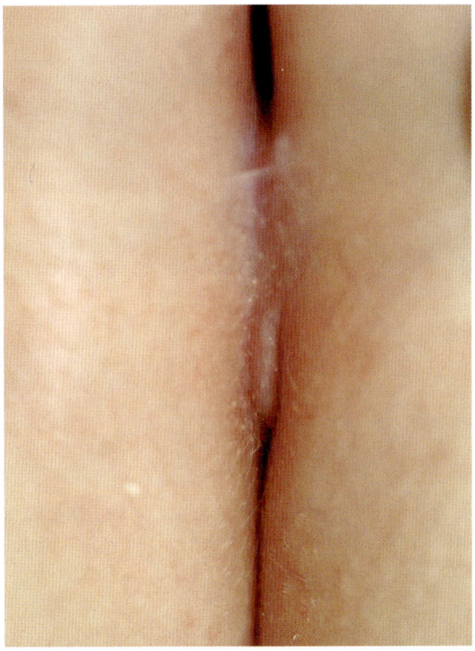

Fig. 15-24. A pink pyramidal protrusion is a linear or pyramidal swelling in the midline extending from the perianal skin at 12 o'clock to the perineal body.

## Urethral Prolapse

Urethral prolapse consists of extrusion of the distal urethral mucosa. This condition occurs most commonly in black prepubertal girls and postmenopausal women. Symptoms are often mild and include a sensation of a mass, dysuria, bleeding, and constipation.

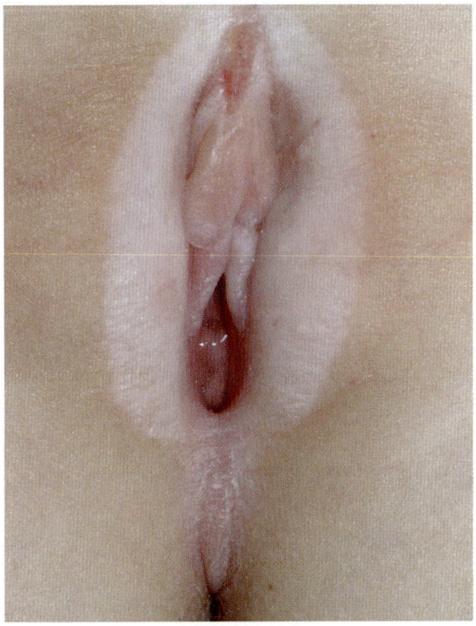

Fig. 15-25. Lichen sclerosus is associated with the occurrence of pyramidal protrusions, probably because of the atrophic skin and inflammation producing edema.

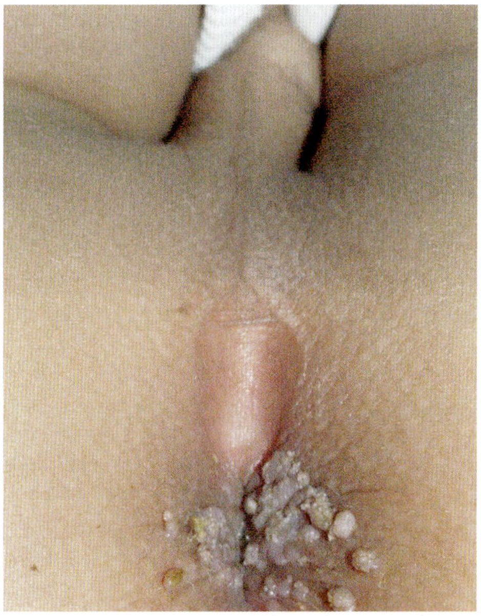

Fig. 15-26. This very prominent pink pyramidal protrusion is an incidental finding in this young boy with perianal warts.

The diagnosis is made can visually, where the mucosa is red, friable, and annular around the meatus.

The prolapse occurs in estrogen deficient tissue, primarily in the setting of increased intra-abdominal pressure, such as occurs with straining to defecate, crying, or coughing, but spontaneous occurrence also occurs. The distal urethra is structurally dependent on the surrounding tissue for support. Before puberty, these estrogen-dependent tissues are diminutive and atrophic with poor support **(Fig. 15-27)**. Urethral prolapse can be mistaken for vaginal bleeding or trauma, as well as tumor or a urethral caruncle, which are unlikely in this age group.

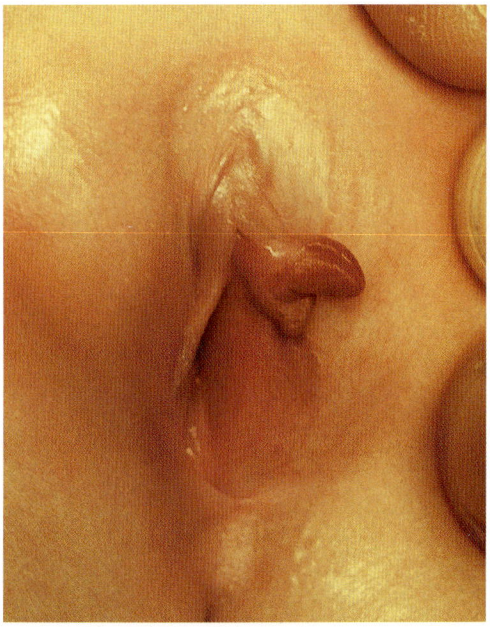

Fig. 15-27. Urethral prolapse in children occurs most often in children of African genetic background.

Most cases of prolapse resolve spontaneously with puberty and the onset of endogenous hormone production. Sitz baths can help to reduce swelling so the prolapse can be manually corrected, and topical estrogen may help to strengthen the tissue to minimize the risk of recurrence. Complications are rare. If conservative management does not resolve the prolapse, and if symptoms dictate, surgical reduction under general anesthesia is often useful, and excision is curative.[30,31] If vulvar bleeding is recurrent, surgical excision with re-approximation of the mucosal edges is curative.

## Infantile Hemangiomas

Hemangiomas are benign, proliferative vascular tumors that occur in infancy. They are more common in girls and in premature infants. The cause of these lesions is unknown. Most are absent at birth or are noted as a faint pink flush on the skin until 2-3 weeks of life. Rapid growth then commences, usually lasting about 4 months. Slower growth can continue up until 1 year of age, and then gradual involution begins. Half of hemangiomas resolve by 5 years of age. Most of the remainder continue to involute up until 9 years of age.

Although the most common sites for hemangiomas are on the face and scalp, these are fairly common on the genitalia, especially the vulva **(Figs. 15-28 and 15-29)**. Established hemangiomas are bright red, well-demarcated nodules or plaques. Hemangiomas can be both superficial and deep in the skin.

Complications of hemangiomas generally relate to their location on the body and their size. Ulcerations are a common complication of genital hemangiomas, producing pain. Ulcerated hemangiomas are often very painful, and they are easily infected, resulting in residual scarring

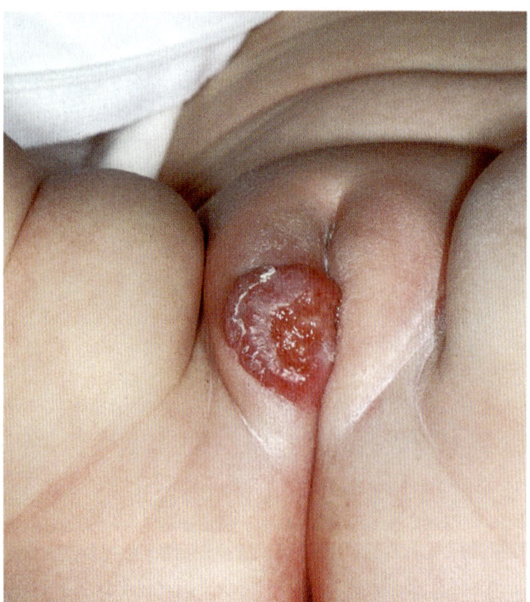

Fig. 15-28. The vulva is a common place for a hemangioma, and this rather large hemangioma has ulcerated, causing pain with friction against the diaper and contact with urine and feces.

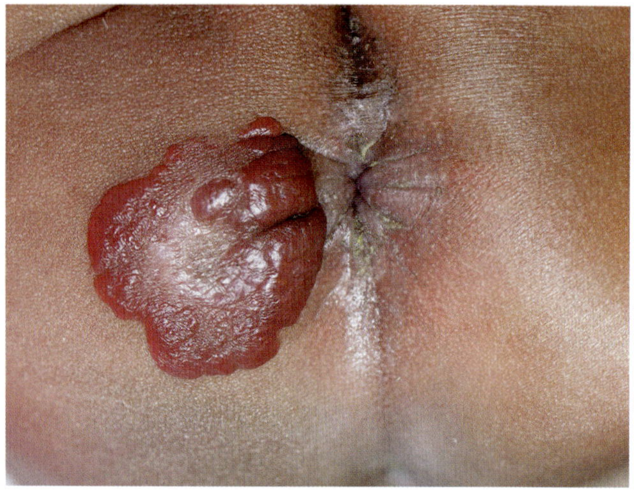

Fig. 15-29. This perianal hemangioma was at risk for ulceration and pain from contact with feces, but central regression from treatment with propranolol is visible in the center.

with involution. Withholding of stool and urine can occur as a response to severe pain.

If a genital hemangioma does not obstruct an orifice, ulceration is absent, and lesions are reasonably sized, observation rather than active therapy is the usual therapy. Complicated hemangiomas have been treated with oral propranolol, which prompts involution, avoiding the complications of past standard therapies of systemic and intralesional corticosteroids and surgery, to include laser. Side effects are uncommon but can be dangerous and require monitoring initially. Bradycardia, hypotension, and hypoglycemia are the more important adverse reactions. Recently, trials with atenolol and nadolol have been shown to be equally efficacious, and these medications circumvent the potential adverse reactions of bradycardia, hypotension, sleep disturbance, cognitive effects, and hypoglycemia with propranolol.[67,68] However, there has been one infant death with nadolol.[69]

Timolol maleate 0.5%, a nonselective β-blocker, represents a well-tolerated, safe, and efficacious treatment for thin superficial infant hemangiomas. It has been shown to be as effective as oral propranolol for treating superficial IH, with a lower rate of systemic adverse events and it is superior to topical corticosteroids.[70] However, use of this medication in the wrong patient population can lead to undertreatment and loss of the window of opportunity of benefit with systemic therapies.

There is also weak evidence to suggest that early treatment of superficial IH with laser, primarily pulsed dye and long-pulse Nd:YAG, may arrest growth and help treat ulcerated hemangiomas.[70]

When larger hemangiomas involute, permanent skin changes often remain. Especially in the case of deep hemangiomas, the overlying skin can be atrophic, telangiectatic, and baggy, with abnormal texture. Fibrofatty tissue may be deposited during the resolution phase of the hemangioma, so the deep component appears to resolve incompletely.

## Skin-Colored Lesions

### Anogenital Warts (Genital Warts, Condylomata Acuminata, Venereal Warts, Human Papilloma Virus Infection)

Genital warts are relatively common infections in young children. The primary issues are concerns regarding childhood sexual abuse, and the least painful and stressful means of management. For the primary discussion of anogenital wart infection, see Chapter 7.

Genital warts in infants and children usually present in a perianal location **(Fig. 15-26)**. Less frequently, the vulva and the penis are affected. Warts uncommonly develop on other mucous membranes such as the oral cavity, the nasopharynx, and the conjunctiva.

There are several methods of acquiring genital warts in childhood, although teenagers and adults almost always acquire these by sexual contact. Warts occur in young infants as a result of passive transfer of the virus during birth though an infected birth canal, or even by upstream contamination of amniotic fluid in infants born by cesarean section to infected mothers. In addition, innocent transmission from mother or caregiver to child of both genital wart types and common hand wart viruses can occur during routine diaper changing and bathing. Although genital warts can be acquired by innocent contact, the presence of condylomata acuminata in a child should alert the caregiver to the possibility of sexual abuse. For infants who develop lesions by the age of 3 years, nonsexual transmission is common.

The incubation period of the virus acquired perinatally is not known, but it can be up to several years. Laryngeal papillomatosis, infection of the airway by human papillomavirus (HPV) acquired at birth, typically does not manifest until the age of 2-4 years with stridor, hoarseness, and a weak cry. A possibility of sexual abuse should be considered in a child older than 3 years with new onset of anogenital warts. HPV typing does not determine the mode of transmission of the virus and cannot be used to determine sexual abuse. Any virus type can be transmitted by abuse, innocent contact, or vertical transmission.

The differential diagnosis of condyloma acuminatum includes condylomata lata, mollusca contagiosa, and acrochorda. Condylomata lata are generally flat topped, and other manifestations of syphilis are usually present, especially in infants. Pseudowarts, or granuloma gluteale infantum, can also resemble warts. If any doubt, a biopsy can confirm the diagnosis.

Spontaneous resolution of genital warts occurs in more than half of affected children within 5 years of age.[71] Treatment of warts by the various destructive modalities often is followed by recurrence. Morbidity, from pain with defecation and with repeated treatment, is considerable. More gentle, conservative treatment or expectant observation of the warts in children is recommended. The most important aspect of therapy is education of the parent. The difficulties of therapy, the frequency of recurrences, modes of transmission, and the phenomenon of latency should be discussed.

I prefer treating genital warts in children with the least painful method available. I use imiquimod applied topically overnight three times a week, titrating the frequency to the degree of inflammation. In resistant children, this can be applied while asleep at night. Otherwise, podofilox is another minimally invasive therapy whose frequency of application can be adjusted to the severity of inflammation. I do not use painful genital therapies without the use of topical anesthetics. Otherwise, the same treatments can be used for children as are used for adults.

### Molluscum Contagiosum

Molluscum contagiosum is a very common childhood infectious dermatosis caused by a DNA pox virus and discussed primarily in Chapter 7. Preschool and elementary school children are most frequently infected, but unlike HPV infection on anogenital skin in this age group, these are not markers for sexual contact.

Mollusca appear as skin colored or pink shiny, dome-shaped papules that often appear vesicular, lending the name "water wart" **(Figs. 15-30 and 15-31)**. In children, Mollusca occur almost exclusively in a setting of atopic dermatitis, which can be subtle.

Lesions rarely last longer than 2 years in healthy children. Therefore, avoidance of scarring or very painful procedures as well as parent education are the most important aspects of therapy. Although cryotherapy and curettage are quick and effective, these are painful and frightening

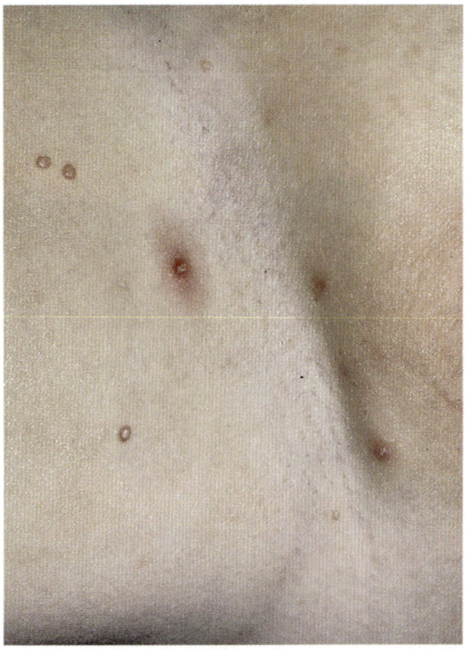

Fig. 15-30. These shiny dome-shaped papules are characteristic of mollusca contagiosa; the inflammation around one of her lesions suggests that she may be hosting an immune response that will eliminate the virus.

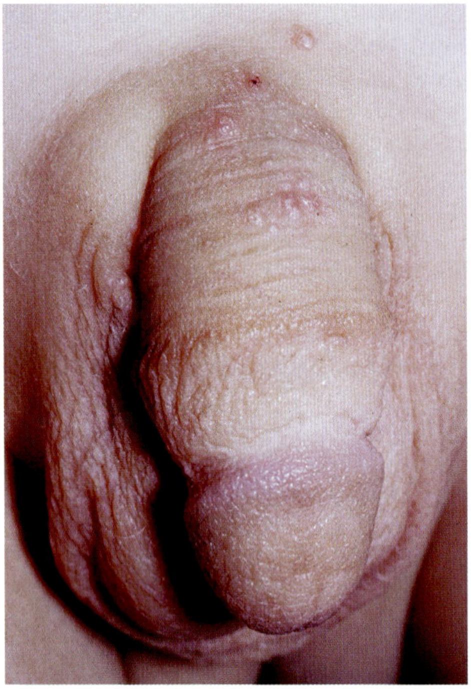

Fig. 15-31. Although this little boy has mollusca contagiosa on the penis, this in no way suggests sexual abuse.

modalities for children. Nonsurgical management is preferred, but there are no medical therapies that are approved by the United States Food and Drug Administration.

Cantharidin is an effective medication that is applied painlessly to the surface to create a superficial blister that night or the next morning.[72] This is not to say that the blister is painless. A very tiny amount of medication should be applied. Care must be taken to remove the cantharidin if pain or burning develop later, and some providers advise bathing the area several hours after application. The advantage is that the medication is applied in the office, usually requiring only two or three treatments, 1-2 weeks apart. This medication is not commercially available in the United States at this time and must be obtained from a compounding pharmacy as a 0.7% mixture in collodion. Imiquimod 5% cream applied overnight from nightly to two or three times weekly at home has been used for years, with open label studies showing benefit. However, large placebo controlled studies have shown no statistical difference compared to placebo.[73] Ten percent potassium hydroxide has been shown effective in controlled trials but must be compounded in the United States, although 5% and 10% potassium hydroxide are available in many other countries.[74] Open-label trials of oral cimetidine have suggested that this agent may be effective, but double blind controlled studies show no benefit.

## White Lesions

### Lichen Sclerosus

Lichen sclerosus (LS) is discussed primarily in Chapter 8. This genital skin disease characterized by white, crinkled, fragile, pruritic skin is found most often in postmenopausal women but occurs with regularity also in prepubertal girls and, less often, in uncircumcised boys.

Lichen sclerosus of childhood usually begins before the age of 7 years. Usually, lichen sclerosus affects only the genitalia, but extragenital lesions sometimes develop in both sexes. Misdiagnosis as sexual abuse sometimes occurs because purpura is common due to fragility of affected skin. Although many children with lichen sclerosus have no symptoms, others experience itching or irritation. Constipation has been reported in 57.9% of girls with lichen sclerosus, who regularly experience perianal involvement that produces splitting and pain with defecation that can result in retention of feces.[75] A review of my prepubertal girls with lichen sclerosus who were specifically asked about constipation has not confirmed this as a common occurrence. Constipation does not occur in boys as a result of perianal lichen sclerosus, as they almost never experience perianal involvement. UTIs have also been reported as a common occurrence, with 62.3% of 19 girls presenting with a UTI.[75] This uncharacteristically high number suggests contamination by secondarily infected/colonized lichen sclerosus in girls with vulvar dysuria.

Lichen sclerosus can be difficult to diagnose in pale girls who already exhibit light, thin, smooth skin compared to adults. The outline of the plaque, which encompasses the vulva and perianal skin connected by a narrower area of involvement on the perineal body, is often described as an hourglass or figure-of-eight configuration around the vulva and perianal skin. Atrophy of the skin, manifested by a shiny texture or crinkling, is typical. Hemorrhage, erosions, and fissuring occur as a result of fragility that allows for tearing and bruising with scratching (**Figs. 15-3, 15-25, 15-32, and 15-33**). The resorption of vulvar architecture that typically occurs with LS can be subtle; prepubertal girls normally have only vestigial labia minora, and at least minor midline agglutination of the clitoral hood is common. Bacterial superinfection is especially common in girls and is responsible for some of the associated irritation. Vaginal discharge from secondary bacterial vaginitis superimposed on the normally atrophic vagina may be present.

Genital lichen sclerosus generally affects only the glans penis and prepuce of boys, and it does not involve the perianal skin. This disease is a prominent cause of phimosis in boys, accounting for about 40% of phimosis requiring circumcision (**Fig. 15-34**).[76]

The differential diagnosis in the genital area includes irritant dermatitis with postinflammatory pigment loss, pinworm infestation, and sexual abuse. Lichenification from lichen simplex chronicus can appear white at times. Vitiligo can produce similar whitening but lacks the atrophy and hemorrhage seen in lichen sclerosus.

Treatment of childhood lichen sclerosus is the same as for adults with lichen sclerosus. Circumcision is the definitive therapy for boys with lichen sclerosus,[77] but this is not always curative, and meatal stenosis occurs in a significant minority of boys. Concomitant therapy with a corticosteroid or tacrolimus may further improve lichen sclerosus and also prevent meatal stenosis.[78,79] A recent study showed that the use of topical corticosteroids alone may relieve symptoms and phimosis, but the follow-up was short.[80]

The very clear treatment of choice in girls is the daily application of an ultrapotent topical steroid. This usually results in dramatic improvement in symptoms in a few days, and the clearing of lesions over several months. Vulvologists have long observed that discontinuation of medication regularly results in recurrence and scarring, but recent data confirm this observation.[81] Maintenance with an ultra-potent steroid applied one to three times a week or the regular use of a less potent topical steroid is crucial to prevent recurrence and scarring, but in practice, families seem to find this difficult and require support and careful follow-up. There is no benefit to topical testosterone, progesterone, or estrogen therapy in this disease beyond their lubricating effects.

Vulvar lichen sclerosus is more superinfected than occurs in adults, and this superinfection is sometimes the immediate cause of itching and pain associated with lichen sclerosus. A 1-week course of an antistaphylococcal/antistreptococcal antibiotic at the onset of a topical corticosteroid is warranted in girls with very inflamed or exudative skin.

Although lichen sclerosus was once believed to resolve at puberty in girls, a recent review showed that LS persisted in 20%-97% of girls.[82] The appearance of estrogen and resulting thickening of genital skin may account for the symptomatic improvement despite ongoing disease. Although malignancy as a sequela of lichen sclerosus is extremely rare in childhood, there appears to be an increased risk of vulvar carcinoma in adults with lichen sclerosus who experienced onset as a child compared to women with onset as adults[82]; one wonders if this correlates to adherence with medication, as is true with adult LS.

## Miscellaneous

### Phimosis

Phimosis is defined as tightening of the foreskin so that it cannot be retracted. Paraphimosis occurs when the foreskin is retracted and then entrapped behind the glans, unable to be replaced.

Physiologic phimosis is present at birth, when the foreskin is actually fused to the glans. Over time, with the production of smegma and physiologic erections, this fusion is broke, so that half of boys can retract their prepuce by age 7, and 90% by age 10.[83] Phimosis from disease is uncommon, occurring in only about 2% of boys.[84] Lichen sclerosus may be the most common specific diagnosable cause of phimosis in boys, but nonspecific inflammation and edema in general are often seen.

Care of the foreskin can minimize inflammation and perhaps help prevent pathologic phimosis. Boys should be taught to retract the prepuce during urination to prevent pooling of urine, and the foreskin should also be retracted and carefully cleaned during bathing.

For boys with phimosis producing pain, difficulty with urination or UTIs, treatment of phimosis is indicated. Historically, the management of phimosis has been circumcision. However, recent studies have shown that topical corticosteroids are effective for relieving phimosis, frequently avoiding the need for surgery.[85]

### Prepubertal Vaginitis

Vaginitis in prepubertal girls is uncommon, and any yellow panty stains, including those from vulvar skin diseases, are often lumped together as "vulvovaginitis." These are generally different processes, although the modified mucous membranes of the vulva can be secondarily irritated by irritating vagina secretions.

The vagina of prepubertal girls is, of course, estrogen deficient. Therefore, the causes of vaginitis differ from those of premenopausal women. Vaginal candidiasis and bacterial vaginosis basically do not occur. This discussion relates only to causes of vaginal inflammation.

Infection is usually the first consideration and the most common cause of acute vaginitis. The introitus is often very red, and a yellow discharge may be seen, primarily on panties. The most common infectious causes are group A β-hemolytic *Streptococcus* and pinworms. Other bacteria can be causative, including *S aureus*, and *H influenza*. Before varicella vaccination, varicella was a cause of purulent vaginitis.

Evaluation includes an examination of perianal skin for signs of perianal bacterial (streptococcal) dermatitis, a routine culture of the introitus, and a first morning scotch tape test for pinworms are indicated. Sometimes, a bacterial pathogen is identified on culture, with improvement on oral antibiotic therapy, but with prompt recurrence. These girls may have a foreign body acting as a nidus of infection. Sexually transmitted diseases can occur, so that children who seem at risk and who have no other causes for vaginitis should be evaluated for gonorrhea and chlamydia.

Rarely, a profuse, yellow, watery discharge can occur due to fistula that allows urine to enter the vagina.

By far the most common cause of a chronic vaginal discharge and vaginitis is a retained foreign body. Although the most common foreign body is toilet paper that has migrated into the vagina, the variety of foreign bodies can be interesting. Alkaline batteries are becoming increasingly reported as a cause of vaginal discharge associated with a foreign body and should be especially suspected when the discharge is gray and watery and accompanied

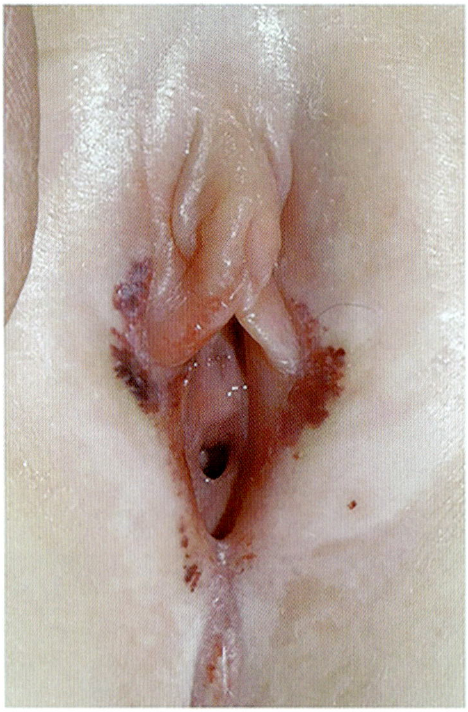

Fig. 15-32. Lichen sclerosus is far more common in girls than in boys and often manifested by smooth white skin rather than the classic crinkled texture; purpura is common in this rubbed and scratched fragile skin, erroneously suggesting sexual abuse, and a pink pyramidal protrusion is visible between the perineum and perianal skin.

by pain.[86] A plain film may be useful in some children for radiopaque objects, such as these batteries. Children with chronic vaginal discharge and no obvious cause on examination and culture should be examined under general anesthesia, although some older children may be able to be examined vaginally with a hysteroscope.[87]

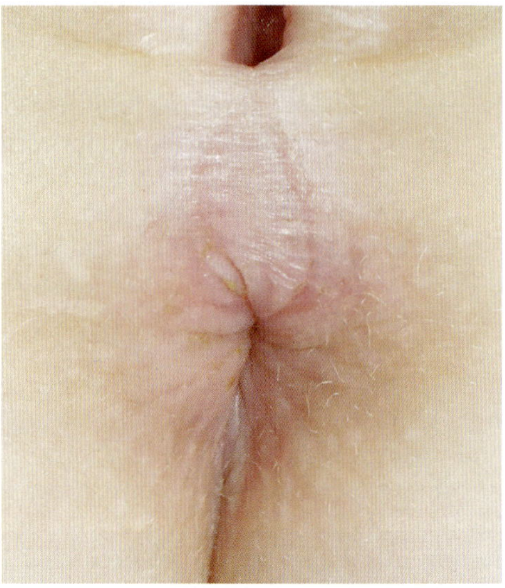

Fig. 15-33. Perianal involvement is extremely common in girls, and almost never occurs in boys; the skin here shows the nearly pathognomonic crinkled texture.

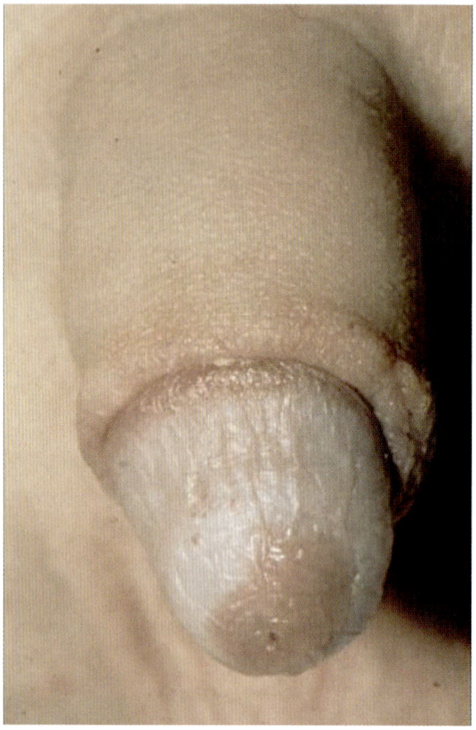

Fig. 15-34. Lichen sclerosus is one of the most common causes of phimosis in boys, and this diagnosis was only made after surgery for phimosis.

### Aphthae (Ulcus Vulvae Acutum, Lipshutz Ulcers, Nonsexually Acquired Genital Ulcerations)

These are rarely recognized but fairly common, very painful, nonsexually transmitted vulvar ulcers that primarily occur in the 11-20 years old range of young girls. These are primarily discussed in Chapter 11. The onset and description are so very typical that this diagnosis generally can be made provisionally by telephone.

Aphthae occur almost exclusively in females. They generally present as vulvar pain after a prodrome of a sore throat and malaise. Lesions are most often multiple, located primarily on the modified mucous membranes, although dry keratinized skin is sometimes affected. Initially, the surface is purple and then evolves to form a necrotic, black surface that sloughs and leaves a well-demarcated, "punched out," ulcer, usually with a white coagulum base (**Figs. 15-35 to 15-37**). Occasionally surrounding redness and swelling erroneously suggest accompanying cellulitis.

The disease most often confused with an aphthous ulcer is herpes simplex virus (HSV) infection, but HSV generally begins as blisters, expanding into superficial erosions rather than ulceration. In unclear cases, molecular studies to rule out HSV are indicated. If there is concern about childhood sexual abuse, the girl should be referred. Otherwise, this picture of vulvar ulcerations following a viral syndrome is classic for aphthae, and the diagnosis is presumptive, not requiring a biopsy or other painful and frightening studies.

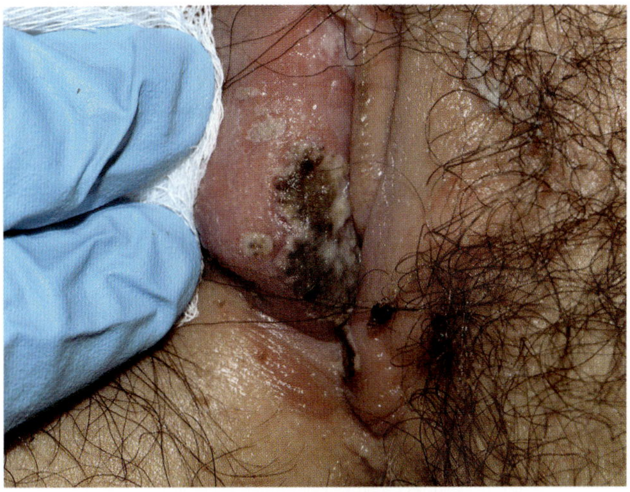

Fig. 15-35. The initial lesion of an aphthous ulcer is a purple plaque or papule that rapidly evolves into a necrotic eschar, as has occurred in this 14 year old.

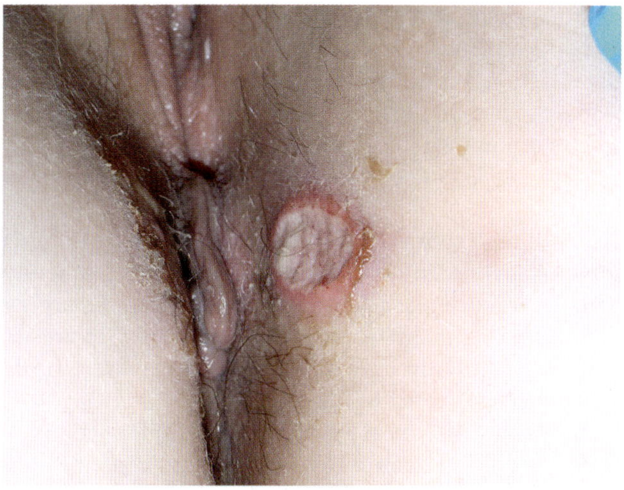

Fig. 15-37. Although aphthae are most often found on mucous membranes or modified mucous membranes, they occasionally occur on keratinized skin.

Although some providers treat these ulcers with superpotent topical corticosteroids or intralesional steroids, touching this skin is painful. Therefore, oral prednisone, at a dose of 1 mg/kg each morning up to 40 mg/day, or, 60 mg for larger teens, is more compassionate and effective. This medication is continued until pain subsides, usually 4 or 5 days, but occasionally much longer. Cool bathtub soaks, barriers such as petroleum jelly, and oral narcotics can improve discomfort while in the meantime. Some girls experience severe dysuria; urinating in a tub of tepid water or heavy barrier creams can minimize this discomfort.

Usually, this is a one-time event that does not signify Behçet disease or another dangerous underlying conditions. Some girls, however, experience recurrences. Frequent recurrences indicate a need for an ophthalmologic evaluation for signs of inflammatory eye disease, and a review of systems for signs of inflammatory arthritis, neurologic disease, or bowel disease.

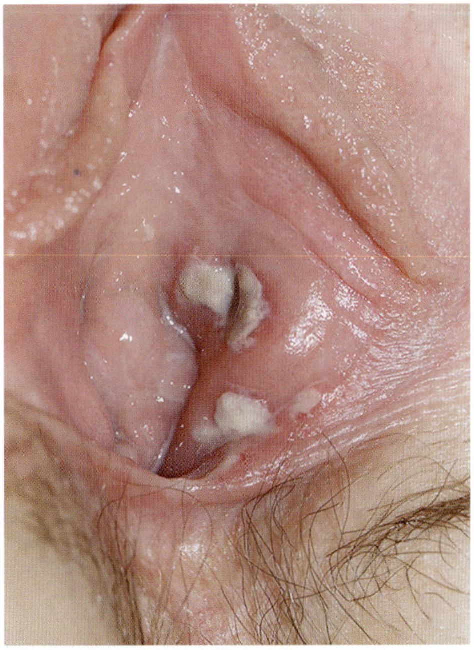

Fig. 15-36. When the necrotic surface of the aphthous ulcers desquamates, left behind is an ulcer with sharp margins and, usually, a white base.

Frequently recurrent vulvar aphthae can usually be suppressed with oral dapsone 25-100 mg daily. Colchicine is sometimes used, but diarrhea can be limiting at the doses required. The tumor necrosis factor blockers adalimumab and etanercept are effective in the suppression of recurrent aphthae.

## Immunosuppression

Both the presentation of some skin diseases and their management are changed when they occur in immunosuppressed individual. Infections and malignancies in particular are both more common and more likely to present atypically and more severely in patients who are immunosuppressed, either by virtue of medication or disease. In addition, patients who are immunosuppressed due to human immunodeficiency virus (HIV) infection are at increased risk of developing several inflammatory but noninfectious skin diseases, most notably psoriasis, reactive arthritis (Reiter disease), Steven-Johnson syndrome/toxic epidermal necrolysis (TEN), and aphthae. In the past, skin diseases, infectious, neoplastic, and autoimmune were remarkable in frequency and severity in individuals with HIV disease. It is a grateful tribute to researchers that these are now vanishingly rare in patients treated for HIV.

### Infections

#### Herpes Simplex Virus Infection (Discussed Primarily in Chapter 10)

Herpes simplex virus infection is a common complication of immunosuppression, sometimes manifested by chronic, enlarging ulcers rather than short-lived vesicles and erosions, as the immune system is not able to contain the infection. Fortunately, HIV has become a disease that is manageable, so the horrific skin diseases of the past are rarely seen in treated patients in industrialized countries.

*Clinical Manifestations*

Herpes simplex virus in an immunosuppressed patient is more likely than in other individuals to recur frequently and to produce persistent and progressively enlarging ulcerations rather than self-limited erosions. However, HSV is particularly problematic in patients with poorly controlled HIV infection.

As occurs in typical HSV, HSV in immunocompromised people is painful. However, chronic nonhealing erosions sometimes occur, gradually enlarging into ulcerations that are atypical and can produce diagnostic difficulties **(Figs. 15-38 and 15-39)**. However, the fact that genital ulcers in immunosuppressed patients are usually produced by HSV and the fact that careful questioning usually reveals prior, more typical recurrent HSV infection outbreaks usually suggests this diagnosis. The most common cause of a genital ulcer in an immunosuppressed patient is an HSV infection.

The infection begins as the typical grouped vesicles on an erythematous base, disintegrating almost immediately into well-demarcated, discrete erosions. Unlike immunocompetent patients, immunosuppressed patients often experience nonhealing erosions with scalloped borders that hint at the original blistering nature. These can then coalesce and deepen to form large, well-demarcated, painful ulcers that become poorly demarcated if untreated or secondarily infected. Cytomegalovirus infection can occur with HSV infections or can mimic HSV ulcers in immunosuppressed patients. Coinfection with Candida or HPV is common and can change the clinical appearance.

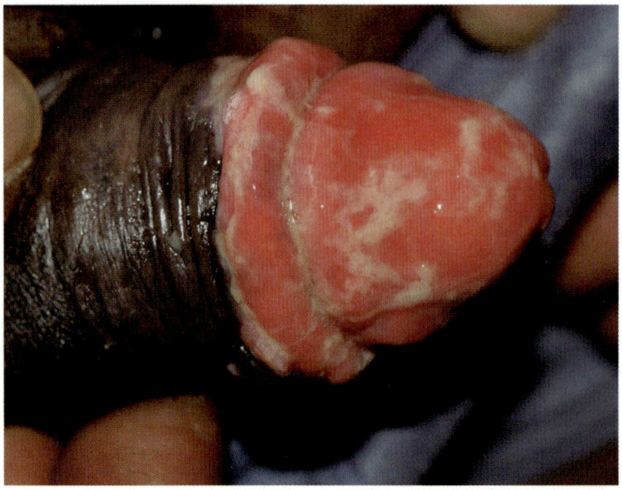

Fig. 15-38. Herpes simplex virus infection in this immunosuppressed man has, rather than healing within a week or two, inexorably enlarged to cover the entire glans and has deepened into an ulcer.

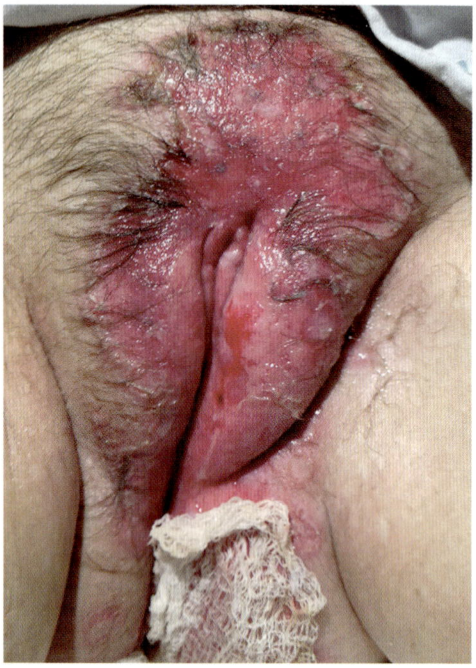

Fig. 15-39. This woman who is immunosuppressed due to a renal transplant has developed a herpes simplex virus infection unchecked by her immune system, and one that has become resistant to antiviral medications.

Men most often experience chronic HSV ulcers in a perianal and gluteal cleft distribution as well as on the penis, scrotum, or groin. In the female patient, ulcers may involve the mucous membrane portion of the vulva and may extend to the labia majora, lateral labia minora, and even to the crural creases or inner thighs. As in the male patient, HSV infection also often extends to a perianal location and gluteal cleft. Any chronic nonhealing ulcer located on or near a mucocutaneous surface in an immunosuppressed patient is statistically an HSV infection until proven otherwise.

Herpes simplex virus infection in immunosuppressed patients occasionally is exophytic, also called papular HSV infection, herpes pseudotumor, or hypertrophic herpes **(Fig. 15-40)**.

*Diagnosis*

A presumptive, but far from definitive, diagnosis is made by the presence of any genital ulcer in a setting of immunosuppression. The diagnosis should be proven while therapy is initiated. This can be done very quickly, depending upon the laboratory testing that is available. Molecular studies (polymerase chain reaction, nucleic acid amplification testing) is far and away the treatment of choice, although a biopsy from the edge of an erosion or ulcer is very sensitive, and fluorescent antibody testing of a swab is also fairly sensitive. Cultures show poor sensitivity, and Tzanck smears have poor specificity. A biopsy has the advantage of investigating for concomitant cytomegalovirus infection and the disadvantage of not

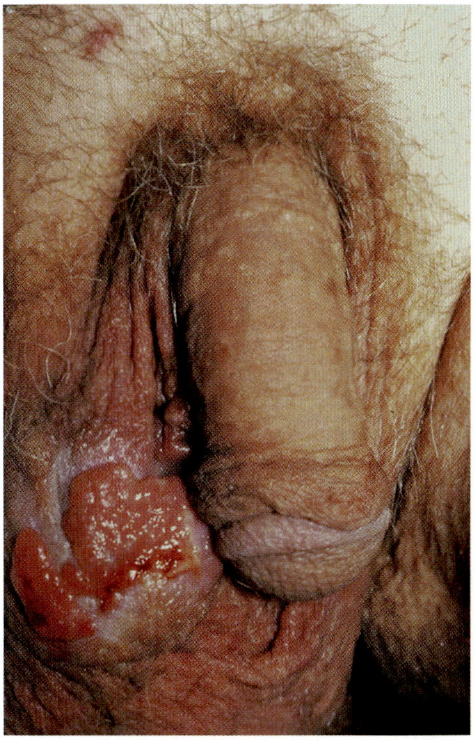

Fig. 15-40. Immunosuppressed individuals who experience HSV infections sometimes develop moist exophytic plaques, variably called papular herpes or hypertrophic herpes.

distinguishing between HSV and varicella zoster virus infection, usually a distinction easily made clinically by the location and distribution.

A biopsy from the edge of a chronic herpes ulcer shows the same histologic features as that of herpes in an immunocompetent person.

Syphilis and CMV should be seriously considered, especially in those with the acquired immunodeficiency syndrome (AIDS) with negative HSV testing or that are unresponsive to medication for HSV. Chancroid, lymphogranuloma venereum, granuloma inguinale, tuberculosis, atypical mycobacterial infections, and deep fungal infection (blastomycosis, coccidioidomycosis, and sporotrichosis) can cause ulcers but are extraordinarily uncommon in industrialized countries, and do not generally deserve extensive evaluation. These fungal infections do not, in general, show a predisposition for the genitalia. Patients with poorly controlled HIV occasionally exhibit unusually large aphthae, or "canker sores," which are indistinguishable morphologically from chronic HSV ulcers. These aphthae can occur in the mouth but may be extensive and produce impressively large and destructive genital ulcers as well.

### Pathophysiology

Herpes simplex virus ulcers in immunosuppressed patients most often arise from reactivation of preexisting recurrent disease, rather than from a primary outbreak. Patients who have altered cellular immunity, such as HIV infection, or patients receiving immunosuppressive agents are at increased risk of more severe herpes infections. HSV infection, usually type 2, becomes chronic and ulcerative rather than recurrent, because it is unchecked by the host's incompetent immune system. In addition, some HSV ulcerations are coinfected with CMV. The papular pseudotumor herpetic morphology likely occurs as a result of an ineffectual immunological reaction to a HSV infection.[88]

### Management

Herpes simplex ulcers should be treated with oral acyclovir, famciclovir, or valacyclovir. Ill patients who require hospitalization and HIV patients with malabsorption should receive intravenous acyclovir. Oral doses include acyclovir 400 mg three times a day, valacyclovir 1 g twice a day, or famciclovir 500 mg twice daily for 5-10 days. Once healing occurs, long-term suppressive oral antiviral therapy is generally required because recurrence rates are high, and chronic ulceration increases the risk of transmission of both HSV and other infections—including HIV—to others. Also, HSV and HIV are synergistic, with the presence and activity of HSV accelerating the transmission and progression of HIV.[89,90] Suggested doses for suppression, rather than treatment, of HSV infection include acyclovir 400-800 mg two to three times daily, famciclovir 500 mg twice daily, or valacyclovir 500 twice daily. Immunosuppressed patients are more likely to experience recurrences at standard doses, so higher doses are often used.

Interestingly, patients with HIV treated with effective antiretroviral therapy continue to have frequent HSV outbreaks and shedding, so logically would benefit from ongoing HSV suppression. Also, patients with HIV and HSV who are begun on antiretroviral therapy have an increased risk of HSV-associated ulcers in at the beginning of therapy, as well as transient increase in viral shedding.[91,92]

Hypertrophic or papular HSV infection is often difficult to treat, sometimes because the condition is due to the immunologic reaction to the HSV rather than the virus itself. Therefore, the addition of the immunosuppressant thalidomide orally or topical imiquimod as adjuvant therapy have been reported useful.[88,93,94]

Publications suggest that viral resistance to acyclovir and, by extension, valacyclovir and usually famciclovir may be becoming more common in immunosuppressed patients.[95] However, the numbers presented are old, and I find no recent data that support the contention that resistance is increasing. A French study found 3.8% of immunocompromised individuals with HSV exhibiting disease resistant to acyclovir in those studied between 2002 and 2006, increasing to 15.7% in those studied between 2007 and 2011.[96] Normal individuals continued to experience no more than 0.5% of HSV infections resistant to acyclovir during this time. This increase was especially represented in those with allogeneic hematopoietic stem cell transplants. Ongoing suppression is less associated with the emergence of resistance than episodic treatment.[97]

A viral culture should be obtained for phenotypic sensitivity testing in a patient with known HSV infection not responding to therapy, but these are difficult arrange and slow to obtain. Those found to have resistant HSV should be followed with an infectious disease consultant. Intravenous foscarnet and cidofovir are first-line therapies, and both topical imiquimod 5% and cidofovir gel (compounded) applied daily can be useful (CDC guidelines 2021).

## Genital Warts (See Also Chapter 7)

Very large anogential warts should raise the suspicious of immunosuppression. In addition to large size and numbers of genital warts in immunocompromised patients, there is also an increased risk for high-risk HPV types.

### *Clinical Manifestations*

In the immunosuppressed host, wart infections on all skin surfaces tend to be more severe. Warts are more numerous, larger, and more recalcitrant to treatment. Occasionally, they can be unusually hyperkeratotic.

Genital warts of all morphologies are seen in immunosuppressed individuals: lobular, papular, flat, and filiform. The warts often are larger, may coalesce to form plaques, and are highly recalcitrant to therapy (**Fig. 15-41**). The warts may become so large or numerous that they obstruct an orifice. Genital warts often extend into the anal canal and may cause difficulty with defecation (**Fig. 15-42**). Sometimes, these can be unusually keratotic for anogential warts (**Fig. 15-43**). When the warts enlarge to form plaques, they may fissure and crack, become painful, and develop secondary infections, especially *Staphylococcus aureus*, *Streptococcus* sp., or yeast. There is also an increased proportion of potentially oncogenic HPV serotypes found in warts in the immunosuppressed patient (HPV 16, 18, 31, 33).[98,99] This finding, as well as the ineffective immune system, explains the increased incidence of anogenital squamous cell carcinoma (SCC) in immunosuppressed patients, especially those with AIDS.

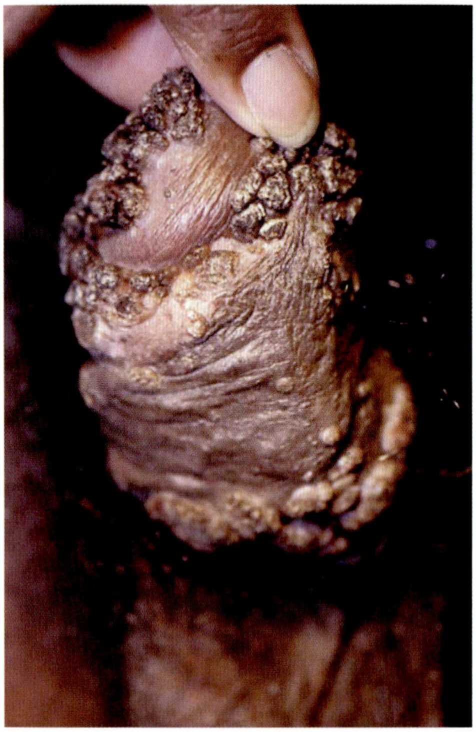

Fig. 15-42. Normally, genital warts are not hard and keratinized, but rather soft and moist; however, at times anogenital warts in immunosuppressed patients can be keratotic.

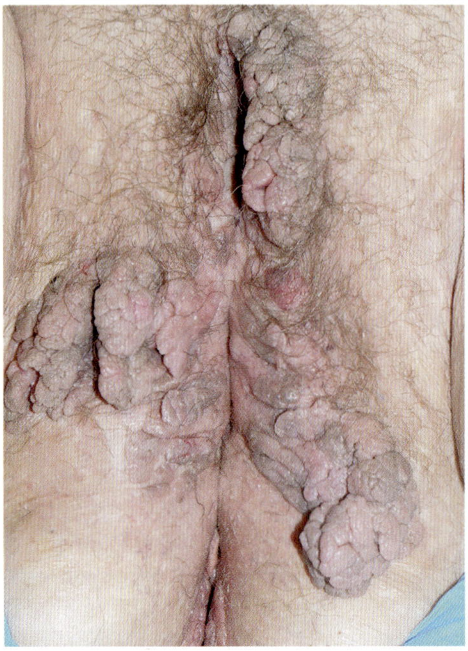

Fig. 15-41. Unusually large warts should raise a suspicion for immunosuppression.

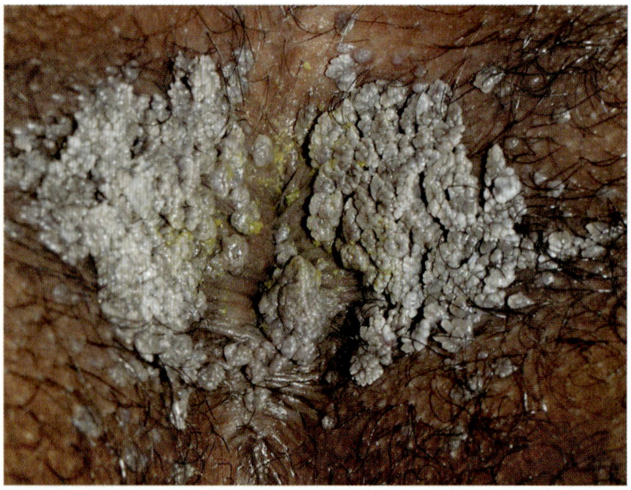

Fig. 15-43. This large plaque of warts with obstruction in the rectal canal suggests immunosuppression.

### Diagnosis

The diagnosis of genital HPV infection usually can be made by clinical impression. However, a biopsy of the lesion can and should be performed for confirmation and to evaluate for dysplasia, especially if warts are flat, very bulky, or hyperpigmented (except in patients with a naturally dark complexion).

### Pathophysiology

Human papillomavirus infection that is uncontrolled by a compromised immune system results in infection that is more recalcitrant and often more florid than the usual HPV infection.

### Management

Anogenital warts do not clear spontaneously in immunosuppressed patients. See Chapter 7 for the primary discussion of treatment. The lack of adequately functioning immunity translates into a condition that can be somewhat controlled only, requiring ongoing therapy. One alternative therapy is the removal of the largest lesions, particularly plaques that are obstructing orifices or are becoming secondarily infected. The higher risk of malignant transformation on the transitional epithelium of the cervix and within the anal canal as compared with squamous epithelium should be remembered so that these areas can be reevaluated frequently in high-risk patients.

Traditional therapies used for immunocompetent patients are also the standard of care for immunocompromised patients. Liquid nitrogen treatment, podophyllin resin, home application of podofilox, cantharidin, cold steel surgery, and laser surgery can all be used, either singly or in combination. The home use of imiquimod, a topical immune enhancer, although less effective in patients with an incompetent immune system, can be somewhat helpful in some patients. Topical cidofovir has also been shown to be beneficial.

## Molluscum Contagiosum (See Also Chapter 7 for Primary Discussion)

Molluscum contagiosum infection in the adult, when it is severe or extragenital, is now recognized as a cutaneous marker for possible immunodeficiency. It has been seen in many clinical settings, including HIV infection, mycosis fungoides, sarcoidosis, lymphoma, and leukemia. In the immunosuppressed host, molluscum contagiosum is characterized by numerous lesions that are often recalcitrant to therapy, or large lesions **(Fig. 15-44)**. The lesions are not self-limited, as in the immunologically normal host, and occur not only on the face, beard area, abdomen, and genitalia, but also over the entire body. Genital molluscum lesions in patients with AIDS are quite common.

Mollusca may be morphologically atypical in immunosuppressed patients **(Fig. 15-44)**. Lesions in these patients often coalesce to form plaques, and they may individually be much larger than the usual 2 to 3 mm.

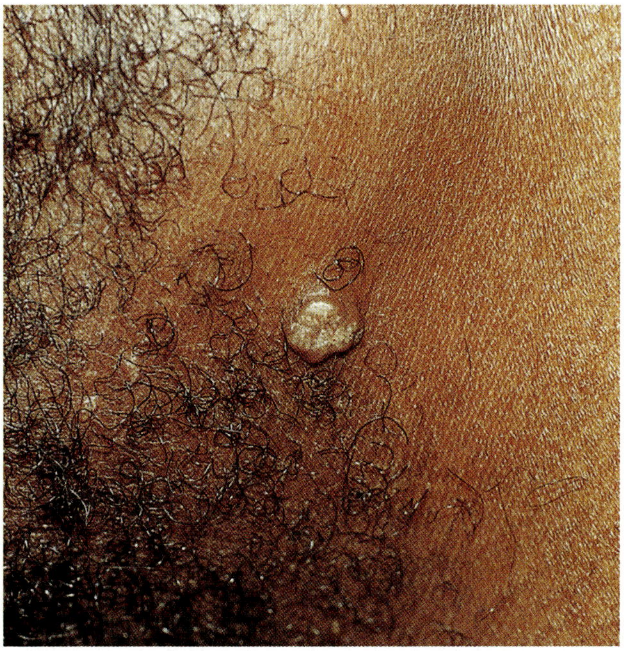

Fig. 15-44. Mollusca contagiosa in an immunosuppressed patient can be large and atypical.

When a lesion is not classic, a biopsy should be performed to confirm the diagnosis and ensure there is not an alternative infection. Deep fungal infection or even tumor can sometimes mimic mollusca. If the biopsy does not show the pathognomonic intracytoplasmic eosinophilic inclusion bodies or if a different infectious origin is strongly suspected, tissue should also be sent for culture because the fungal or other pathogenic organism may not always be seen on routine staining. Mollusca contagiosa in the immunosuppressed host can mimic a number of different infections. Disseminated cryptococcosis, histoplasmosis, coccidioidomycosis, and *Penicillium marneffei* have all been described as clinically resembling mollusca **(Fig. 15-45)**. Mollusca also may have a shiny, umbilicated appearance resembling vesicles, so HSV infections also should be considered at times in the differential diagnosis. Occasionally, warts, nevi, and basal cell carcinomas can resemble mollusca contagiosa.

Although immunocompetent hosts eventually clear the virus irrespective of therapy, molluscum contagiosum in immunosuppressed patients can be very resistant to therapy. Treating the largest, most bothersome lesions is more practical than the widespread destruction of affected skin. Many therapies have been tried, but light liquid nitrogen treatment is a mainstay of therapy. Cantharidin can also be used, but in the United States, this must be compounded because it is not commercially available. Occasionally, cantharidin can cause marked blistering, particularly in the genital region, so care should be used to apply this sparingly until tolerance is ascertained.

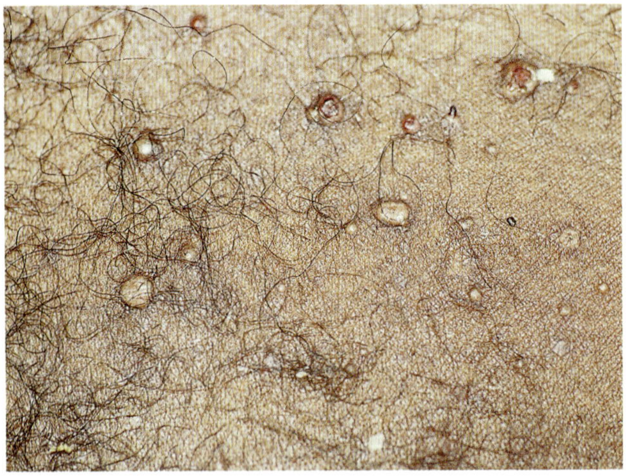

Fig. 15-45. Cryptococcal infection (among other infections), as seen here, can be indistinguishable from mollusca contagiosa in an immunosuppressed patient. These lesions should be sampled if not classic.

Cryotherapy and cantharidin have the advantage of minimal pain and irritation, with little bleeding. Curettage is effective but painful and bloody. Topical tretinoin has been used to decrease the occurrence of new lesions, but it is extremely irritating when used in the genital region. Topical cidofovir has been beneficial in some immunosuppressed patients with mollusca contagiosa. Mollusca exhibit no malignant potential and generally do not obstruct orifices.

## Tinea Cruris (See Also Chapter 5)

Immunosuppressed patients experience tinea cruris more often than other people, and their fungus infections may exhibit atypical morphology. Although tinea cruris usually shows typical inflamed plaques with peripheral accentuation, this infection occurring in immunosuppressed individuals often is more extensive with lack of the prominence of the borders (**Fig. 15-46**). The penis and scrotum are sometimes affected; this is extraordinarily uncommon in the immunocompetent patient. Tinea cruris is more likely to spread to the buttocks and occasionally extends to the abdomen in immunosuppressed patients. Although tinea cruris occurs much less often in women, when it is present, it can extend from the medial thighs to the hair-bearing labia majora. In addition, follicular involvement is common and is manifested by papules or pustules of fungal folliculitis within the plaques. Tinea cruris in immunosuppressed individuals rarely presents as hyperkeratotic, scaly plaques (**Fig. 15-47**).

Dermatophyte infections involving the skin usually are easily diagnosed by a dermatologist by a microscopic examination of scale from the periphery of the patch or plaque in a potassium hydroxide preparation. A biopsy also shows the organism.

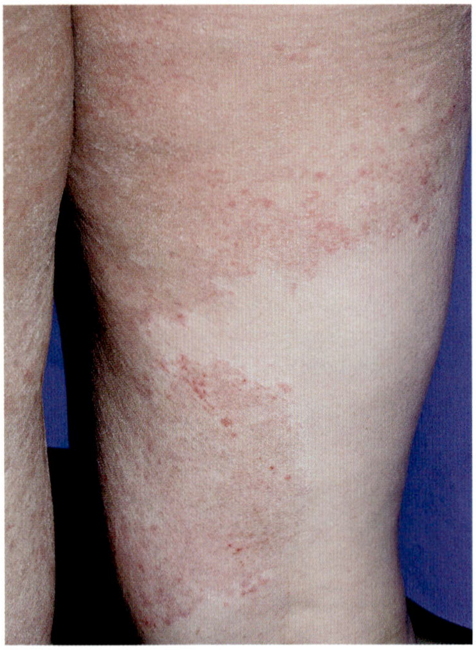

Fig. 15-46. This patient with tinea cruris is immunosuppressed by virtue of chronic oral corticosteroids. The plaques are extensive, without obvious accentuation of the periphery, and small red papules indicate follicular involvement.

Tinea cruris must be differentiated from inverse psoriasis, Candidiasis, and erythrasma.

Tinea cruris in immunosuppressed patients generally requires more aggressive therapy that that required for immunocompetent patients (see Chapter 5 for details). Immunosuppressed hosts have more extensive disease or have follicular involvement that often requires oral therapy. Combination oral and topical medication produce more rapid and complete clearing.

Topical antifungal therapy is helpful for immunosuppressed patients to use early when the eruption recurs,

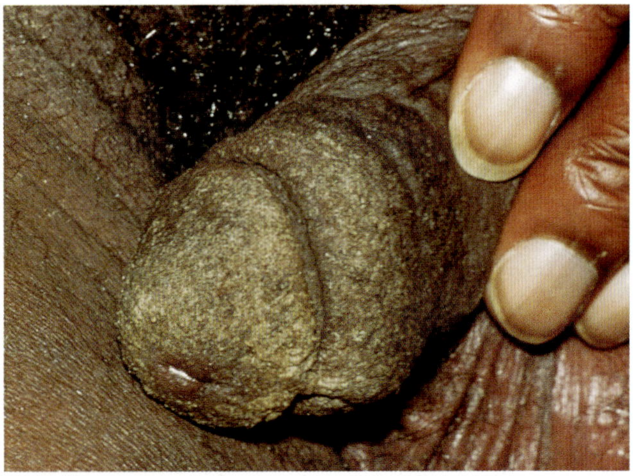

Fig. 15-47. Both the atypical location of tinea on the penis and the nearly hyperkeratotic appearance indicate the immunosuppressed status of this patient.

as is common. There are many effective topical antifungal medications, which include any of the azoles, such as clotrimazole, econazole, and ketoconazole, or the nonazole, terbinefine. Ongoing suppression is generally useful to prevent recurrent tinea.

### Crusted (Norwegian) Scabies

Norwegian scabies is defined as scabies occurring in an immunosuppressed person, resulting in a much higher parasite load. The patient can be immunosuppressed by disease or medication, or a rash misdiagnosed as eczema and treated with a topical corticosteroid can eventuate into Norwegian scabies.

Normally, scabies is characterized by intense pruritus and excoriations, with occasional tiny, linear, edematous papules called "burrows" concentrated in finger web spaces and skinfold areas. Usually, there is no involvement above the neck, except in infants and very ill people.

However, crusted scabies classically is manifested by thick, yellow, hyperkeratotic papules and plaques, rather than discrete excoriated and crusted papules **(Fig. 15-48)**. Itching may be mild or absent due to the relative absence of an immune response. The hyperkeratotic plaques commonly occur on hands, feet, scalp, ears, buttocks, and genitalia, but they can occur on any skin surface. This does not occur on genital skin without accompanying extragenital disease. The nails may be thickened with subungual and periungual crusting, which contain numerous mites. In the immunosuppressed host, hyperkeratotic, yellow, scaling plaques involving the scrotum, glans, or shaft of the penis may occur.

A suspected diagnosis is confirmed by microscopic examination of material scraped from a scaling plaque. In Norwegian scabies, mites, eggs, and feces are abundant and easily visualized because of the abundance of mites. When needed, however, a biopsy reveals epidermal spongiosis and a mixed perivascular inflammatory infiltrate, prominent with eosinophils, often with mites, ova, eggshells, or fecal deposits seen. Persistent nodules of scabies show a dense, inflammatory infiltrate in which eosinophils are prominent.

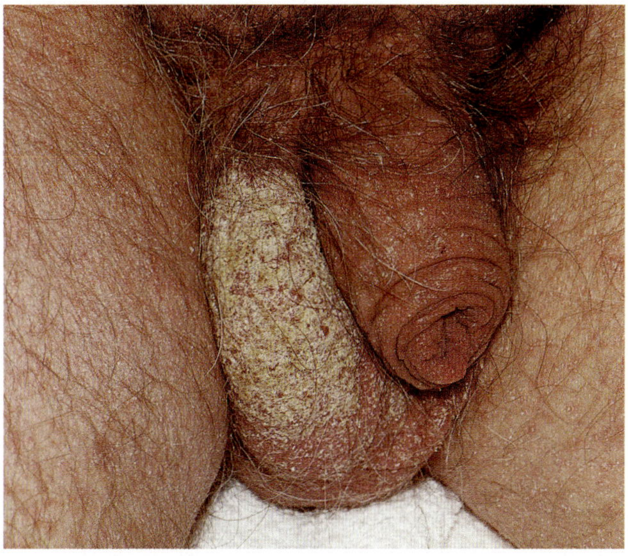

Fig. 15-48. Crusted scabies presents as plaques of scale/crust that, on microscopy, shows large numbers of mites.

Because scabies presents with marked secondary eczematous changes and occasional vesicles, the differential diagnosis of genital Norwegian scabies includes eczema or atopic dermatitis and allergic contact dermatitis. Nondescript excoriated papules also suggest a differential diagnosis of any bite reaction. Intense itching, worse at night, and abrupt onset of an eruption in a patient with no history of eczema should make scabies high in the differential diagnosis.

Because Norwegian scabies presents with hyperkeratotic plaques, rather than discrete excoriated papules, it may elicit a differential diagnosis that includes unusual psoriasis, tinea cruris, and even seborrheic dermatitis, when it occurs on the genitalia or scalp. Impetiginized eczema may also appear similar to scabies.

*Sarcoptes scabiei* var. *hominis* is the mite responsible for the infestation known as scabies. The severity of the infestation is entirely the result of the host's poor immunity, not a more virulent millions.[100]

The severity of Norwegian scabies, together with its crusted, relatively impenetrable skin results in a condition best treated both topically and orally with ivermectin 200 μg/kg. Permethrin cream daily for 1 week and then twice weekly till healing can be used, and ivermectin tablets (eg, on days 1, 2, 8, 9, and 15, and possibly also on days 22 and 29) is recommended.[101,102] Also, topically applied agents that debride the hyperkeratotic skin can enhance penetration of the permethrin; these medications include salicylic acid, lactic acid, or urea. However, these can be extremely irritating on the genitalia. Heavy hyperkeratoses may need to be mechanically removed after soaking or the use of these keratolytics. Permethrin is applied from the neck to the toes, is left on for 8-10 hours, and then is washed off. Those immunosuppressed patients with head and scalp involvement should treat these areas also, and care should be taken to treat under the fingernails as well as possible. All other household members and close contacts are treated. Recently worn clothing and bed linens should be washed in hot water. Although some advocate bagging clothing or linens for several days in lieu of washing, I (LE) have watched mites in scale/crust from an immunosuppressed patient still alive and moving more than a week after collection.

## Noninfectious Inflammatory Diseases Associated With HIV

### HIV-Associated Psoriasis (See Also Chapter 5)

Psoriasis can be triggered by sunburn, a streptococcal infection, and HIV disease. It is not more common in other types of immunosuppression.

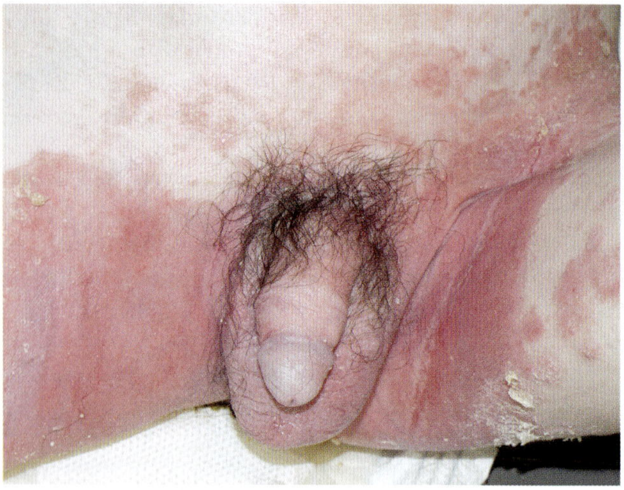

Fig. 15-49. Sudden onset of psoriasis, or sudden severe worsening of psoriasis, should raise a suspicion for AIDS; inverse psoriasis is especially common.

The sudden onset or remarkable worsening of psoriasis can occur in the setting of HIV disease and this should prompt a consideration of HIV testing. This occurs in patients with advanced rather than early HIV.

Psoriasis occurring in these patients is usually typical in appearance, showing well-demarcated, erythematous papules or plaques covered with silvery scale, but there is an increased incidence of inverse psoriasis, which preferentially affects the anogenital skin **(Fig. 15-49)**. AIDS-associated psoriasis is much more extensive and recalcitrant to treatment than in the immunologically normal host.

Well-demarcated plaques may involve the inguinal creases, suprapubic region, intergluteal cleft, axillae, inframammary skin, and umbilicus. Scale is less dense than the silvery scale that is classic for psoriasis on drier skin surfaces. Psoriasis may affect the labia majora and occasionally occurs on the scrotum and the shaft of the penis.

Severe psoriasis can become generalized. This generalized erythema and scale, called exfoliative erythroderma, are seen more commonly in the HIV-affected patient than in others, and they involve the genitalia incidentally. However, exfoliative erythroderma can also result from other severe dermatoses such as atopic dermatitis and from medication reactions, also both more common in HIV-infected patients than in noninfected individuals.

Although the diagnosis of psoriasis is often not difficult, the recognition of HIV requires a high index of suspicion based on the knowledge of the association of the sudden onset of psoriasis with HIV disease. When psoriasis is atypical, as in generalized, exfoliative erythroderma or inverse psoriasis, the biopsy also is often atypical, and a presumptive diagnosis must be made.

Psoriasis occurring in the inguinal creases and intergluteal cleft may mimic or coexist with tinea cruris, candidiasis, erythrasma, seborrheic dermatitis, or eczema. Although psoriasis classically presents with well-demarcated erythematous plaques with white scale, genital psoriasis generally does not exhibit prominent scale, but rather red skin that often displays maceration in skinfolds or a glazed surface on more convex areas. As long as infection is ruled out, topical corticosteroids are the mainstay in therapy for psoriasis, eczema, and seborrhea so that absolute differentiation is not always crucial.

Most important for the improvement of psoriasis in these patients is antiviral therapy for HIV, which usually results in substantial improvement in their psoriasis. Otherwise, usual first-line therapy for genital psoriasis occurring in the immunosuppressed host is the same as for that occurring in immunocompetent individuals (Chapter 5). Aggressive therapy including systemic retinoids and immunosuppressive agents such as methotrexate, cyclosporine, and tumor necrosis-alpha blockers such as adalimumab and etanercept can be used with care. Supportive care, including treatment of secondary infection, most often with *S aureus*, *Streptococcus* sp., or *C albicans*, is often needed and crucial to comfort.

## Reactive Arthritis (Reiter syndrome) (See Chapter 10 for Primary Discussion)

Reactive arthritis is a reactive skin condition related to psoriasis and defined by the presence of arthritis, urethritis, and conjunctivitis for >3 months. This condition, like psoriasis, is more common in men with HIV, but it is not more common in other forms of immunosuppression. Various organisms have been thought to act as triggering agents including *Chlamydia*, *Salmonella*, *Shigella*, *Yersinia*, and *Ureaplasma*. Many patients with reactive arthritis are found to have a human leukocyte antigen (HLA)-B27 genotype or closely related genotypes.

Reactive arthritis occurring in men with HIV disease presents in the same fashion as that in the immunologically normal host. About two-thirds of patients exhibit cutaneous lesions, primarily on the genitalia, palms, and soles. Genital lesions are most common on the penis, especially on the glans or the prepuce, and much less often on the vulva, where the hair-bearing labia majora are the usual involved area. The lesions closely resemble those of pustular psoriasis but may sometimes show more classic psoriatic lesions of redness and scale. In uncircumcised men, lesions most often are white, annular, "circinate" papules or plaques usually occurring on the glans (balanitis circinata) **(Figs. 14-21 and 15-50)**. These lesions may also be seen on the mucous membrane and modified mucous membrane portion of the vulva, vagina, or cervix. In circumcised men and on the hair-bearing portion of the vulva, the plaques are erythematous and scaly, often with crust **(Fig. 15-51)**. These skin findings are indistinguishable clinically and histologically from those of psoriasis. Lesions on the palms and soles exhibit pustules

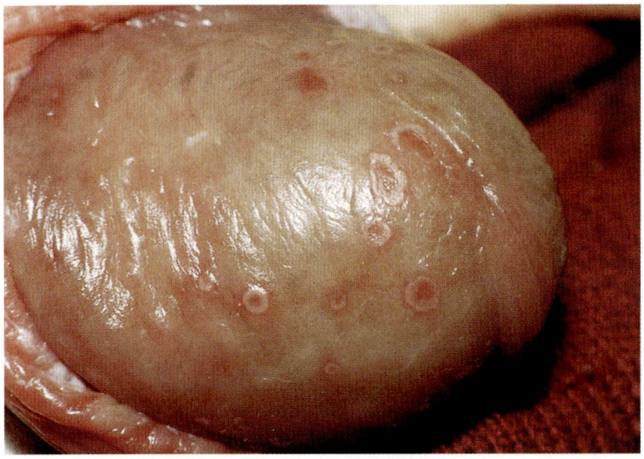

Fig. 15-50. Reactive arthritis classically shows, on the uncircumcised glans, small round or arcuate white papules.

that evolve into thick, hyperkeratotic plaques, a condition termed keratoderma blenorrhagica **(Fig. 15-52)**. Occasionally, there are pustular or crusted hyperkeratotic lesions elsewhere on the skin. Conjunctivitis and urethritis also occur in most patients. Arthritis affecting the large joints in an asymmetric distribution is common.

The diagnosis of reactive arthritis is made by a combination of clinical findings. Urethritis often precedes skin findings, and evaluation for gonorrhea or Chlamydia infection is often performed. Asymmetric arthritis, conjunctivitis, and dermatitis follow, but patients with this condition very often do not develop all aspects of the disease. Circinate balanitis and keratoderma blennorrhagica are classic, as in Chapter 10. Reactive arthritis and psoriasis with arthritis exist on a spectrum. Therefore, the differentiation sometimes cannot be made with certainty, since "incomplete reactive arthritis" lacks conjunctivitis and/or urethritis, the hallmarks that differentiate the two diseases.

Topical steroids are somewhat useful for the skin disease of reactive arthritis. Patients with arthritis often benefit from nonsteroidal anti-inflammatory agents, analgesics, and/or rest. As for psoriasis, patients with either severe skin disease or arthritis require methotrexate or antitumor necrosis factor medications with careful monitoring. The skin disease is sometimes improved remarkably by oral retinoids such as acitretin or isotretinoin, but these medications often aggravate joint disease. The conjunctivitis is self-limited.

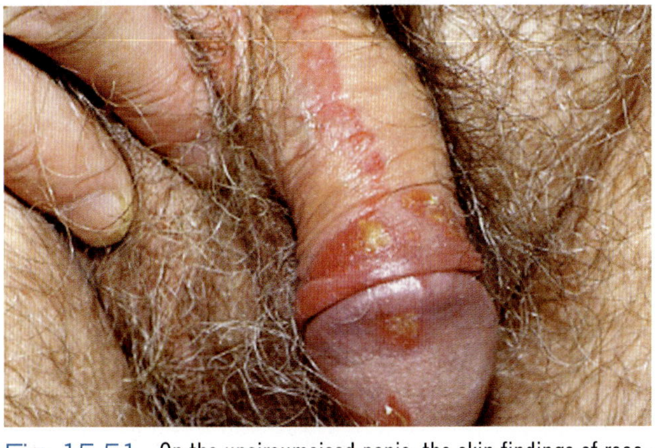

Fig. 15-51. On the uncircumcised penis, the skin findings of reactive arthritis are the same as psoriasis, with red, scaling plaques.

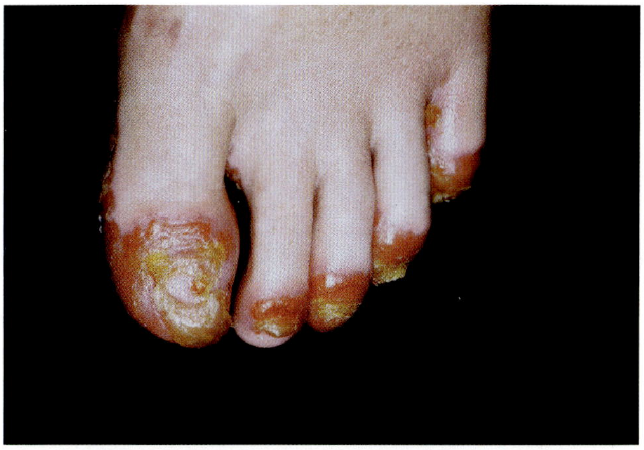

Fig. 15-52. The term keratoderma blenorrhagica is given to the plaques on the palms and soles of those with reactive arthritis; these are plaques of pustules that evolve into red, thickened plaques of scale/crust.

## Stevens-Johnson Syndrome/Toxic Epidermal Necrolysis (Discussed Primarily in Chapter 10)

Patients with HIV disease are at a marked increase in risk for the development of Stevens-Johnson syndrome (SJS) and TEN, blistering hypersensitivity reactions nearly always to medications. Not only are these patients at higher risk, but SJS and TEN are more severe in the setting of HIV disease.

These diseases begin with flat red papules with central blisters (SJS) or painful red sloughing skin (TEN) and mucosal erosions (Figs. 10-39, 10-42, and 10-43).

The most common medications that cause these skin findings are the antibiotics penicillin, sulfonamides, fluoroquinolones; the anticonvulsant medications carbamazepine, barbiturates, phenytoin, lamotrigine; the cardiovascular medications, hydrochlorothiazide, furosemide, procainamide; and allopurinol and nonsteroidal anti-inflammatory medications. Recurrent HSV also produces generalized blistering reactions, and some patients have no identifiable cause.

The treatment is primarily discontinuation of the inciting cause and supportive care. Other therapy is controversial and includes intravenous gamma globulin and cyclosporin.

## Aphthae (See Also Chapter 11)

Oral and genital aphthae associated with HIV are vanishingly rare as uncontrolled HIV disappears in industrialized

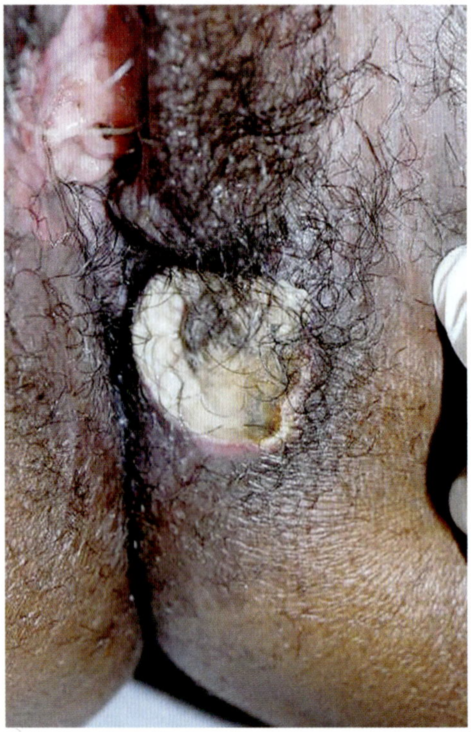

Fig. 15-53. Patients with HIV are known to develop large aphthous ulcers as part of their syndrome. However, these are indistinguishable from ulcerative HSV, and CMV should be excluded as well.

Western countries. These ulcers are usually unusually large, deep, and recalcitrant aphthae that are probably immune complex mediated. Aphthae are no more common in other forms of immunosuppression than in immunocompetent individuals.

Although typical, small aphthae are round, 1- to 3-mm erosions with a white fibrin base and a surrounding red flare, aphthae associated with HIV are deep, large, and often indistinguishable from ulcerative HSV in an immunosuppressive person **(Fig. 15-53)**. These can be several centimeters in diameter with usually, well-demarcated, clean borders. There is often significant scarring following healing.

Ulcerative HSV infection is the primary disease in the differential diagnosis, although any cause of infectious or neoplastic ulcers should be considered and ruled out with a biopsy. Topical and intralesional therapies are generally inadequate for these ulcers, and systemic corticosteroids may be required to initiate healing. Dapsone and colchicine can be tried, but thalidomide is the treatment of choice in these patients, producing remission in about half of patients; however, neuropathy occurs in about 40% of patients, but this is most often subclinical.[103]

## Neoplastic Diseases

Malignancy is more common in chronically immunosuppressed patients in general, as immune surveillance is poor. Skin lymphoreticular cancers are the most common of these malignancies. However, HIV is associated with Kaposi sarcoma, lymphomas, and SCC.

### Squamous Cell Carcinoma (Discussed Primarily in Chapter 7)

All chronically immunosuppressed patients are at higher risk than others for the development of this common malignancy. Most often, anogenital SCCs are associated with HPV infection, although patients with other at-risk diseases such as lichen sclerosus should be followed especially carefully as well. Immunosuppressed patients also have a higher risk of ultraviolet light–induced skin cancers, but not in the anogenital area. Anogenital SCC, HSIL, and differentiated intraepithelial neoplasia are also discussed in Chapters 6, 7, and 8.

Not only are anogenital SCCs more common in the immunosuppressed host, but tumors often are larger and more aggressive than in immunocompetent patients. The earliest clinical presentation usually is that of a genital wart, with lesions often multifocal or coalescent. These classically are either flat warts or are exuberant lobular warts (Bushke-Lowenstein wart). Growth is often more rapid, and response to wart therapy is poor. The plaques or nodules often become hyperkeratotic or impressively large, occasionally with ulceration **(Figs. 7-64 and 15-54)**. Penile SCC occurs on the prepuce, glans, or coronal sulcus, but it may occur elsewhere.

Anorectal SCC classically is seen in HIV-infected men who engage in receptive anal intercourse, but by no means is limited to these patients. It is found also in the setting of

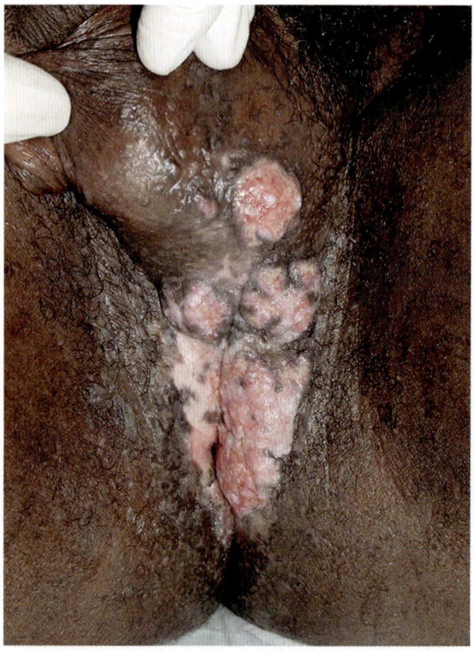

Fig. 15-54. HPV in patients who are immunosuppressed grow unchecked, and oncogenic types are highly likely to transform into SCC as has occurred here.

multiple genital warts, even in the absence of anal sexual activity. SCC presents as an indurated ulcerated plaque or as large, hyperkeratotic, verrucous nodules or plaques.

The diagnosis is by biopsy, which shows the same features as in immunocompetent patients. In contradistinction, verrucous, hyperkeratotic anogenital SCCs can be indistinguishable from large genital warts, with no evidence of malignancy on biopsy. This does not rule out SCC. Any remarkably large wart (in both immunosuppressed and immunocompetent patients) that yields a biopsy showing no signs of malignancy on biopsy should be re-evaluated in toto and sectioned for foci of malignancy.

In addition to other tumors, SCC mimics infectious processes, such as deep fungal infections, unusual atypical mycobacterial infection including tuberculosis, viral infections such as those produced by HSV or CMV, ecthyma, and even parasitic infections, including cutaneous *Acanthamoeba* infection.

Therapy for anogenital SCC is by surgical excision. Local radiation may or may not be used in conjunction with surgery, depending on the staging of the SCC.

### AIDS-Associated Kaposi Sarcoma (See Also Chapter 9)

Kaposi sarcoma is an unusual tumor strongly associated with HIV and herpesvirus 8 in the male homosexual patient, although classically found in older men from the Mediterranean gene pool. This lesion is seen most commonly in the male homosexual patient with AIDS. Kaposi sarcoma occurring in the HIV-affected patient usually begins as a pink or red papule, which becomes violaceous (Fig. 15-55). Lesions often enlarge to form plaques, and older lesions are red brown, as hemosiderin is deposited in the skin. Occasionally, early lesions may be flat and resemble a bruise. Kaposi sarcoma in patients who are naturally dark complexioned often is nearly black.

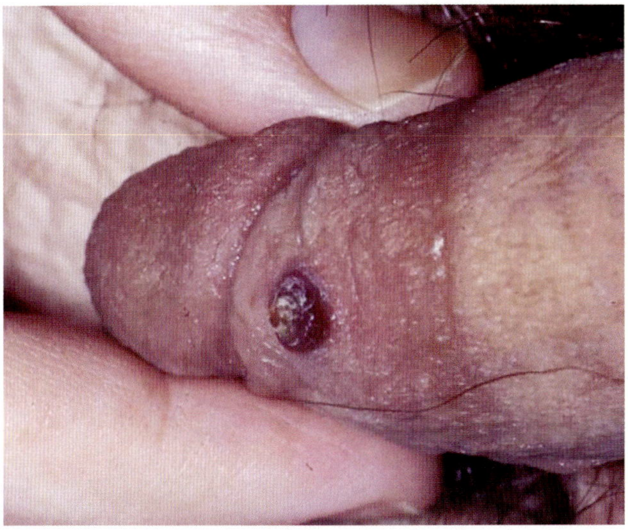

Fig. 15-55. AIDS-associated Kaposi sarcoma is generally a dusky red and almost appears vascular.

The initial lesions of AIDS-associated Kaposi sarcoma frequently occur on the face and ears, and 10% to 15% of patients experience oral mucosal lesions as the first site of involvement. Genital lesions occasionally occur and, when present, are most common on the shaft of the penis, but they may also be found in the suprapubic region. When plaques evolve, there is often associated lymphedema of the penis. As the plaques enlarge, they may ulcerate, becoming a source of recurrent infection, particularly with *S aureus*, *Streptococcus* sp., or *C albicans*. Because Kaposi sarcoma occurs almost exclusively in homosexual or bisexual men, few reports exist of female genital involvement.

The diagnosis is made on biopsy, which is always indicated, because bacillary angiomatosis may be indistinguishable clinically. A biopsy may also rule out concomitant infection, such as deep fungal (histoplasmosis, cryptococcosis) or viral (CMV) infections, which have been reported to occur in Kaposi lesions.

Kaposi sarcoma associated with HIV is due to herpesvirus 8. CMV, HPV, and even hepatitis B virus also have been described as associated with Kaposi sarcoma.

The therapy of Kaposi sarcoma depends on the clinical stage and location of the lesion. Control of underlying HIV is a mainstay in therapy. Otherwise, small lesions do not require therapy other than for psychological or cosmetic reasons, but these can be treated successfully with liquid nitrogen or surgical removal. Larger patches or plaques may be treated with chemotherapy or radiation therapy. Therapies include alitretinoin gel for topical administration and liposomal daunorubicin, liposomal doxorubicin, paclitaxel, and interferon-α for systemic administration.

## Transgender Issues

According to its discussion regarding gender dysphoria, the American Psychiatric Association (APA) defines gender diversity as an umbrella term that refers to individuals with gender identities and/or expressions that vary from expected developmental norms. The Diagnostic and Statistical Manual of Mental Disorders, Fifth Edition, reports that gender dysphoria consists of clinically significant distress or impairment resulting from a strong desire to be of another gender, which may include desire to change primary and/or secondary sex characteristics. They go on to say that not all transgender or gender diverse people experience dysphoria, and removed gender diversity from its list of psychiatric diseases in 2012.

Gender diversity has become much more recognized and much more accepted since it was considered a sexual perversion by the APA almost a century ago. As increasing numbers of people with gender dysphoria become transgender, some seeking gender affirming surgery, providers should become more educated about these transgender patients who will present in our offices, and about their care. There are several review articles on this subject.[104,105]

Much of the following discussion is obtained from Dr. Dev Gurjala, an experienced gender confirmation surgeon at Align Surgical Associates in San Francisco and speaker on the subject.

Gender disharmony between the brain and body is common; about 0.6% of the population is transgender, which translates into 1.4 million American adults and 150 000 teenagers. These individuals have remarkable obstacles, despite the increasing acceptance of gender diversity; 62% experience depression, with 45% having attempted suicide. They are more likely to be victims of homicide, and 47% have suffered sexual assault. In addition, the average annual income is $10 000 per year, so the tribulations of poverty are a major obstacle to comfortable existence. These are all issues that should be remembered when caring for patients with gender diversity.

Many who are cisgender, meaning individuals who identify with the gender they were assigned at birth, especially those who are older, are flummoxed by the terminology that has arisen. There are four axes of gender: (1) identity, or how a person thinks of himself; (2) expression, or how the person dresses and behaves based according to traditional roles; (3) biology, or genetic sex; and (4) orientation, or who the person is attracted to physically, emotionally, and spiritually. Each of these exists on a spectrum, and there are many, many different combinations. Patients may not identify as male or female; they may be parts of each, or on a spectrum. Terms for these individuals include nonbinary, gender queer, gender fluid, gender nonconforming, gender diverse, and gender expansive.

Trangender surgery, sex change surgery, and sex reassignment surgery are outdated terms which are offensive to many. Gender-affirming and gender-confirming surgery are the preferred terms. Chest surgery is referred to as top surgery, and genital surgery as bottom surgery. Pronouns have become a sensitive issue. Often, the best way to manage this is to ask the patient for their preferred pronoun. There are different techniques among centers, especially for FtM surgery, and different methods of outcome measurements. However, patient satisfaction is high, and regret very low, <1%.[106,107]

Before sex-confirming surgery, patients should have met rigorous criteria of the World Professional Association for Transgender Health. These include referral from two professionals, the persistent presence of gender dysphoria, having used hormones for at least a year, lived and dressed as the intended gender for at least a year, age of majority, the ability to give consent, and any medical and mental health concerns managed.

## Transgender Women

For transwomen, patients who were assigned male sex at birth and transition to female (MtF), surgery consists of use of the shaft of the phallus to fashion a vagina, the glans to form the clitoris, and conversion of the scrotum into the labia majora. The penile skin is degloved and used to produce a neovagina, so that the vagina is lined with keratinized epithelium rather than mucosa. The complications of this bottom surgery are generally minor and manageable; about a quarter develop granulation tissue, 20% experience vaginal narrowing, 19% reported prolonged pain, and 15% had incontinence or a disrupted urinary stream.[108] Major complications include 17% with necrosis requiring dressing changes, 10% with a hematoma, and 7% with a UTI.[108] Postoperative care includes douching daily for 2 weeks, then twice weekly for 3 months, and use of dilators three times a day for 3 months, then increasing the caliber of the dilators. A commitment to dilation is crucial, as vaginal narrowing is a common sequela.

The final appearance of the vulva and vagina is stunningly indistinguishable from a genetic female vulva (Fig. 15-56). Nine to twelve months are required for the final appearance of the new vulva and vagina, but dilation should continue, perhaps life-long. Late complications include those issues that occur with other women whose vaginas are lined with mucosa rather than keratinized epithelium; vaginal candidiasis, bacterial vaginosis, UTIs, and sexually transmitted diseases. The late care of the vaginoplasty is remarkably similar to the care of the vagina of ciswomen. Interesting, there is even a case report of lichen sclerosus occurring on the vulva of a transgender man following gender affirming surgery.[109] Like genetic females, and unlike genetic males, the perianal skin was affected.

However, there are some late problems that are specific to those who have undergone gender-confirming surgery. Vaginal tightness and difficulty with vaginal dilation can be an issue. Management includes decreasing the caliber of the dilator temporarily while increasing frequency and duration. Insertion of topical estrogen and injections of botulinum toxin to paralyze muscles and triamcinolone acetonide (Kenalog) 10 mg/mL to relax scar tissue can be

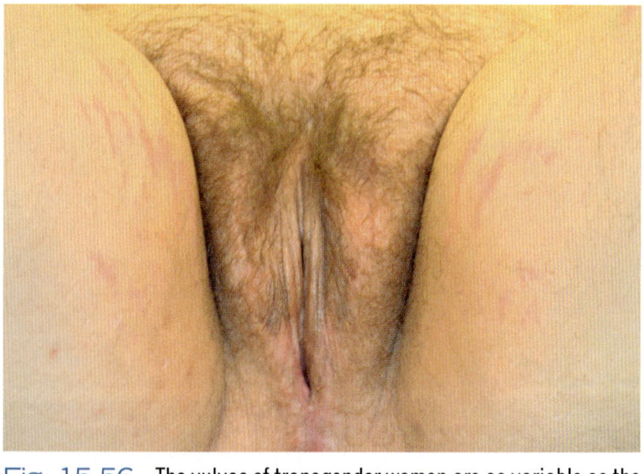

Fig. 15-56. The vulvas of transgender women are as variable as the vulvas of genetically females, with the cosmetic outcome of bottom gender affirming surgery stunningly ordinary. (Courtesy of Dr. Dev Gurjala.)

useful (see Chapter 4). Pelvic floor physical therapy can be beneficial and, finally, surgery. Because there is no cervix, Papanicolaou smears are not needed since there is no cervix, but surveillance for prostate cancer is. In addition, the traumas, emotional, and financial hurdles of these women are facets that should factor in to all aspects of their care.

Studies show differing levels of depression and sexual satisfaction following gender affirming surgery in transwoman. One shows the same rates of depression, but dyspareunia occurring in about half or women, and another shows improvement in depression, anxiety, and suicidal ideation following surgery, but still higher than the background population.[110,111] There is evidence that anxiety and depression correlate with the appearance of the genitalia as to conforming to the appearance of the natural vulva and vagina, and the psychological effects of surgery on young adults can improve them to the levels or better than age-matched general population.[112,113] Reports of sexual function vary, but are generally high, with 70%-80% of women reporting to be orgasmic.[114,115]

### Transgender Men

For transmen, patients assigned female sex at birth and transitioning to men, testosterone administered during the time before surgery affects the vagina and produces symptoms in about one of ten patients. These symptoms consist of a purulent vaginitis with irritation, burning, and dyspareunia, accompanied by redness of the modified mucous membranes and vagina. Due to the testosterone, estrogen levels decrease but not to the levels seen in postmenopausal women. There is thinning of the vaginal walls, with fewer cell layers of the epithelium and comprising immature epithelial cells with decreased glycogen. As a result, the microbiome changes, and lactobacilli decrease, and other bacteria increase.[116] These changes of an atrophic vagina are seen on wet mount as parabasal cells and absent lactobacilli, and there is a pH of >5. When erosions occur due to the fragility of the vagina, secondary inflammation can occur, and vaginal secretions become yellow, and sheets of white blood cells appear on the wet mount. Patients can be treated with topical estrogen cream, a gram three times a week, which may partially the changes. The use of topical estrogen does not change their testosterone requirements or affect masculinization.

There are some transmen using testosterone who, despite the use of topical estrogen, do not improve significantly, and therefore display a picture consistent with desquamative inflammatory vaginitis (DIV), that is, inflammatory vaginitis exhibiting parabasal cells, white blood cells, and absent lactobacilli on wet mount in the absence of infection, erosive skin disease, and estrogen deficiency (see Chapter 14). This may be because testosterone appears to produce changes beyond those related to estrogen deficiency. One study showed that high doses of testosterone produced loss of architecture, decreased glycogen, loss of estrogen receptors, and decreased proliferation of epithelium and stroma compared to both premenopausal women and postmenopausal women not given testosterone.[117] These patients can be treated as for DIV, with either clindamycin cream, an applicatorful per vagina at bedtime for 2 weeks at bedtime initially, and/or hydrocortisone acetate 200-300 mg compounded as per vagina. However, not all patients respond to DIV management, and some continue to have symptoms.

Some transmen go on to have bottom surgery, either metoidioplasty or phalloplasty. A metoidioplasty includes the creation of the neophallus from a hormonally enlarged clitoris, urethral lengthening, and scrotoplasty, which gives the appearance of male genitalia, allows for voiding while standing, and sexual arousal, but the penis is too short for penetrative intercourse. There are several techniques for a phalloplasty, which results in a longer penis, allowing for penetrative intercourse; these include free radial forearm flap, anterolateral thigh flap, and superficial circumflex iliac artery perforator flap surgeries. Unlike the fashioning of a vagina and clitoris, these surgeries are more fraught with major complications of strictures, fistulas, and even worsened mental health.[118,119] One study found 73% of patients required further surgery to correct these issues.[119] At times, transmen who are dissatisfied with the results of their metoidioplasty, either because of the appearance of the small penis, the inability to have intercourse, or difficulty with voiding while standing, elect later to undergo a secondary phalloplasty. This and this can be done with complication rates similar to those that occur with a primary phalloplasty.[120]

The effects of gender affirming surgery on the sexual functioning of transmen is less well understood as there are more different procedures used in this surgery. Most reports describe return on sensation in the phallus within several months, with orgasmic function ranging from 2/3 of patients to "the ability to orgasm, is present in nearly all patients after several months" although there is slightly less sensation in the neophallus.[121]

There are newer emerging gender expansive, or nonbinary, surgeries. These include a phallus-preserving neovagina, where the penis is preserved while a vagina is created, a vagina preserving neophallus, where a penis is fashioned while preserving the vagina, and nullification surgery, for those who identify as asexual and want no sexual structures.

## Geriatric Issues

Older people have difficulties that differ from and compound those of younger patients, especially in the arena of genital dermatology. There are multiple interrelated issues that produce problems when individuals age.

Attention to these confounding factors is important for maximal alleviation of the patient's genital symptoms.

## Normal Genital Aging

### The Aging Female Genitalia

Hair loss on the labia majora and mons is an early and obvious change of the vulva in the aging female. Often, this is most obvious in the center of the mons. Some women lose almost all genital hair. This is accompanied by loss of subcutaneous fat of the labia majora and mons in many women.

Estrogen deficiency and loss of pelvic floor muscle tone with resulting incontinence produce visual changes in the vulva as well. The modified mucous membranes of the vulva become pale, thin, and smooth compared to the thicker, more elastic pink epithelium of premenopausal women, who also generally exhibit Fordyce spots and, often, some degree of vulvar papillomatosis with a slight cobblestoned texture to the surface. The labia minora shrink, occasionally disappearing altogether, so that differentiation from resorption due to lichen sclerosus and lichen planus can be difficult. Urethral caruncles, bright red, asymptomatic, fleshy urethral meatal excrescences commonly occur. Less frequent are the urethral prolapse, an annular protrusion of urethral mucosa.

The vaginal epithelium becomes smooth and pale, with loss of the estrogenized rugae. The vagina also becomes dry and thin, often producing dyspareunia. Microscopically, epithelial cells are small and round (parabasal cells) rather than large, flat, and folded. Lactobacilli are absent and the pH increases to >5. With long-standing loss of estrogen, vaginal secretions are nearly acellular microscopically. Obese women may experience peripheral conversion of estrogen in fat and exhibit fewer signs of estrogen deficiency. As the pelvic floor muscles lose tone, cystoceles and rectoceles occur.

### The Aging Male Genitalia

The normal changes of the male genitalia with age are less obvious. Like women, men experience a decrease in genital hair. The skin of the penis and scrotum becomes more lax. Enlargement of the prostate produces urinary frequency, and prostate surgery sometimes results in incontinence and sexual dysfunction.

## Factors That Exacerbate Genital Symptoms in the Elderly

### Incontinence

Incontinence is a common factor in chronic anogenital irritation as patients age. Most elderly women experience some degree of urinary incontinence as a natural sequela of child birth, waning estrogen levels, and loss of muscle tone from aging. Partially due to this, many use potentially irritating over the counter products for cleaning and treatment. Men also experience loss of muscle tone, and prostate disease can require surgery that can contribute to incontinence. Neurologic disease interferes with normal bowel and bladder function in both genders. Urine and, especially, feces are irritating, particularly when held against the skin, producing an irritant diaper dermatitis characterized by poorly demarcated, edematous red plaques.

Constant moisture produces maceration of skin, promotes the growth of yeast, and increases friction between skinfolds. This results in intertriginous dermatitis, either as a primary disease or as a factor in other skin conditions (see Chapter 5).

The vulva and perianal skin exhibit an unusual morphology of irritant contact dermatitis that is seen most often in a setting of incontinence with diaper occlusion. Originally called granuloma inguinale infantum, Jacquet diaper dermatitis, or pseudowarts, this is now recognized in adults, primarily the elderly, and sometimes termed granuloma inguinale adultorum.[122,123] This can also occur with other caustic chemicals, notably benzocaine,[124] The appearance is that of eroded nodules. The management of this contact dermatitis and other forms of intertriginous dermatitis consists of strict avoidance of the offending chemicals, urine, and feces, and keeping the areas as dry as possible, using adult diapers, soft cloths placed between skinfolds and changed frequently, and, when skin is only slightly wet, powders. Barrier pastes applied heavily to irritated skin helps to protect from feces and urine. Topical corticosteroids are not useful.

### Obesity

Overweight, especially common in older individuals, complicates genital symptoms in several manners. Obesity compounds the irritation of incontinence by trapping both urine and sweat in skinfolds, and increasing friction between skin surfaces. Obesity also predisposes to diabetes mellitus, increasing the risk of Candidiasis.

When genital symptoms occur, treatment is more challenging for the obese patient. Application of medication is difficult, in part because the areas to be treated are difficult to visualize. Skinfolds can be difficult to both separate and treat with only two hands. This sometimes is achieved most easily by the application of medications when the patient is sitting on the toilet, where skinfolds can be separated by positioning on the seat. Also, excess weight interferes with adequate removal of feces, sweat, and smegma/desquamated epithelial cells from skinfolds.

Obesity interferes with sexual function in many people; positioning can be difficult and body image can suffer. This is especially problematic for individuals who already experience compromised sexual functioning due to chronic genital pain or itching, and for older individuals who may have loss of libido and natural lubrication. A good sex therapist can offer useful suggestions for these individuals.

### Arthritis

Joint pain and stiffness, like obesity, interferes with hygiene, application of medications, and sexual functioning. The addition of a nonsteroidal anti-inflammatory medication with meals may be useful, or a suggestion for the patient to consult his or her primary care provider may prove beneficial.

### Psychological Factors

Depression from declining health, loss of friends and family by death or dementia, pain of arthritis, waning strength, diminished intellectual capacity, decreased body image, and fear of incapacity and malignancy are common emotional stresses for the elderly. These all affect the patient's ability to treat and tolerate genital disease, and depression and anxiety escalate pain and itching. When possible, counseling can give the patient a badly needed emotional outlet, and an antidepressant adds immensely to the QoL.

### Declining Sexual Capability

Sexual function diminishes in the elderly. Falling hormone levels; effects of diabetes mellitus, cardiovascular disease, and neurologic disease; adverse effects to medication; depression; loss of a partner; pain; declining muscle strength and endurance; prostate surgery; and decreasing self-confidence in one's appearance and sexual ability are factors that interfere with sexual ability and pleasure. For many patients with these issues, genital itching and pain can be the final factors that end sexual activity. Emotional support, referral for counseling, and understanding of the patient and her/his partner's wishes and expectations for future sexual functioning can minimize the impact of chronic genital disease while conveying a realistic outlook. Simply helping the patient to acknowledge his/her desires and expectations for future sexual function can be a significant help for planning therapy. For example, the elderly woman with scarring associated with lichen sclerosus may be unable to engage in sexual intercourse. A frank discussion of her and her partner's wishes help to make the decision of whether to lyse her adhesions.

## Anogenital Diseases Most Common in the Elderly

Specific genital diseases associated with aging occur primarily in women and include lichen sclerosus and lichen planus. The only skin diseases that occur more commonly in older men are malignancies, particularly SCC. Extramammary Paget disease, basal cell carcinoma, and malignant melanoma occur more often in older men as well but are quite uncommon.

### Atrophic Vaginitis (See Chapter 14 for Primary Discussion)

Until the information from the Women's Health Initiative were widely publicized, postmenopausal women regularly received systemic estrogen replacement unless there was a compelling contraindication. Symptoms of an atrophic vagina or atrophic vaginitis were uncommon for many years, and the index of suspicion for this diagnosis has decreased. Now, an atrophic vagina is a common cause of dyspareunia and vulvovaginal irritation, rawness, and burning.

Nearly all women experience an atrophic vagina when the ovaries cease estrogen production. The vagina becomes dry, and the epithelium thin. Women who are not sexually active are usually comfortable and unaware of these changes. However, women who are sexually active often experience irritation and pain with intercourse because of the lack of lubrication. The fragility of skin and mucosa may result in erosions from friction between vaginal walls pressed together by a cystocele or rectocele, or with sexual activity. The presence of erosions causes secondary inflammation, and the patient develops atrophic vaginitis manifested by erythema and yellow vaginal secretions. A wet mount exhibits increased white blood cells and parabasal cells, with a loss of lactobacilli.

The diagnosis of atrophic vaginitis is made by the setting of low estrogen, a characteristic wet mount, and resolution with estrogen replacement.

The management of atrophic vaginitis is primarily estrogen replacement. This can be achieved with topical estrogen or systemic estrogen replacement. A discussion of systemic estrogen replacement is beyond the scope of this book but can be achieved by estrogens administered orally or by patch, with concomitant progesterone provided to women who have not undergone a hysterectomy. This, of course, provides additional benefits and risks compared to topical therapy.

The management of the atrophic vagina and atrophic vaginitis is discussed in Chapter 14.

### Lichen Sclerosus and Lichen Planus (See Chapters 8 and 11 for Primary Discussions)

These conditions are most common in postmenopausal women, and in the very elderly present additional issues, some discussed above. The application of medication can be challenging, and older women now no longer see gynecologists, so that the vulva is not monitored for control of the disease, side effects of medication, or early neoplastic changes. There is no provider to remind them of the importance of continuing to use medication.

Elderly individuals experience remarkable life and health changes. Specific issues such as incontinence and genital diseases that occur most often in older patients should be investigated and treated, and the issues of depression and loss of body image addressed with compassion.

### Female Genital Mutilation (Female Genital Cutting)

Female genital mutilation is defined as removal of part or all of the external female genitalia, stitching closed, or pricking of the clitoris for nonmedical purposes. As FGM interferes with healthy genital tissue in the absence of medical necessity and can lead to severe consequences for a girl's and woman's physical, mental, and sexual health, the Member States of the United Nations have agreed to declare FGM a violation of the human rights of girls and women. The affected girls and women have often undergone an extremely painful and mutilating procedure with permanent physical and emotional scarring, and these patients need and deserve thoughtful, compassionate, and knowledgeable care. The World Health Organization (WHO) has excellent material on FGM, including information on the physical and psychological care of these women and children. This section is garnered from the publication, The Care of Girls and Women Living With Female Genital Mutilation: A Clinical Handbook, which is available online at no cost from the WHO.[125] This handbook also has many links for additional support.

Approximately 200 million women have experienced this procedure, which is practiced in Africa, a few countries in Asia and the Middle East, and some ethnic groups in Central and South America and Eastern Europe. With international migration, other areas of the world, including North America, are seeing this procedure spread. About 513 000 women and girls in the United States have undergone FGM, but this is often unrecognized until the patient becomes pregnant. Cited reasons for this procedure include tradition, rite of passage, to enhance fertility, assure marriageability, social convention, ensure virginity and chastity, enhance cleanliness and beauty, and religious purposes (although this is not found in major religious texts). In actuality, there are no benefits to FGM, and there are multiple risks and adverse events.

There are four types of FGM. Type I consists of removal of the clitoral hood (1a) or the clitoris and clitoral hood (1b). Type 2 involves removal of the labia minora (labia minora only—IIa, labia minora, all or part of the clitoris, with or without the clitoral hood—IIb, and IIc when the labia majora are removed as well). Type III consists of cutting the labia minora or majora and appositioning them to create a seal; the clitoris and clitoris may or may not be removed. Suturing the vulva closed is referred to as infibulation. Type IV involves pricking, piercing, incising, scraping, and cauterization of the clitoris or any other nonmedically indicated injury to the vulva.

The care of these women includes opening lines of communication, and understanding when and how to ask about FGM, how to work with interpreters and cultural mediators, and understanding the providers' role when discussing FGM. Some women may not be aware of the part that their FGM has played in symptoms they have, and other women may delay seeking care due to embarrassment. The term "female genital mutilation" was coined by the World Health Organization to reflect the fact that this is a serious violation of girl's and women's rights. However, as such, it is judgmental, and other terms such as female genital cutting, excision, and genital cutting may be preferable when discussing this with the patient. Asking her what language she prefers can make her more comfortable. The provider should not assume that the patient finds FGM violation of her rights, or that the procedure has caused medical issues, and the patient should be the leader in both the discussion and attitude.

The medical history in a woman from a region where cutting is common should include questions regarding FGM. This is often best inserted casually into other questions regarding surgeries. Some women may have been cut at such an early age that they may have no memory of this and may be unaware, and some women need so special attention to the issue.

However, other women need education regarding FGM. For example, women who have symptoms, physical or psychological, as sequelae of their procedure, women planning a wedding or who have come for information, women with type III FGM who are or plan to become pregnant, and women with a daughter.

Immediate postprocedural complications of FGM include, obviously, pain. Bleeding, shock, septicemia, edema, and urinary retention are additional possible sequelae. Clearly, all aspects must be documented in the medical record, and in many areas this is actually the law.

Long-term sequalae include chronic vulvar pain, neuroma, genital and UTIs, dysmenorrhea and difficulty with elimination of menstrual flow, epidermal inclusion cysts, and keloid scarring. Vulvar pain should be evaluated by a careful examination for structural causes, with the realization that psychological issues may be operative. Neuromas, especially clitoral neuromas, may occur but may not be visible. These are best detected by careful touching with a cotton-tipped applicator for a painful area. And, vulvodynia is common in any population.

An increased risk of reproductive tract infection occurs due to obstruction from scarring or infibulation. Not only are these infections uncomfortable but some leaves the patient at higher risk for pelvic inflammatory disease, infertility, ectopic pregnancy, stillbirth, and congenital fetal infection. These women should be counseled on vulvar hygiene, and some may require deinfibulation.

Menstrual difficulties can occur, in addition to those of women who have not undergone FGM, as a result of obstruction of menstrual flow, leading to hematocolpos. Some women may experience a suprapubic mass, but often an ultrasound is needed to detect this. Deinfibulation may be required. Obstruction to urinary output can produce painful urination, or resulting stasis and stagnation can lead to UTIs. When scarring of the urethral meatus or infibulation is present, surgery may be required.

Epidermal inclusion cysts and keloids need no therapy if they do not cause pain or obstruction, although some women require therapy for cosmetic and psychological reasons. Importantly, some women experience changes in sexual function following surgery, especially if these structures were near the clitoris or clitoral remnant.

Screening for cervical dysplasia can be uncomfortable or impossible in women who have undergone type III FGM. If using a small speculum with lubrication is not possible, deinfibulation may be necessary. Likewise, these women have an increase in obstetrical complications. All forms of FGM result in narrowing of the introitus due to scarring to variable degrees, so that examinations may be difficult and painful. Women with types I, II, and IV FGM and those with type III who undergo deinfibulation are likely to be able to labor normally. However, those with significant narrowing from scarring from their procedures or infibulation have higher risk; during labor, progression is difficult to gauge, and lack of progression may not be detected early. If deinfibulation was not performed earlier, it should be performed early in labor so that progression can be followed, and absolutely before an episiotomy. Complications in these women include hemorrhage, injury to surrounding structures, rectovaginal and vesicovaginal fistulae, infection, and psychological problems, especially if there was loss of her baby.

Indications for deinfibulation include, in addition to childbirth, the patient's personal choice, the use of some contraceptive methods, urinary retention, recurrent UTIs, menstrual problems, dyspareunia, incomplete abortion, and need for treatment of cervical dysplasia or carcinoma. Contraindications include patient refusal and scar tissue that cannot be removed or cut. Before deinfibulation, counseling should be careful and complete regarding benefits, risk, and expectations. The World Health Organization publication The Care of Girls and Women Living With Female Genital Mutilation: A Clinical Handbook has an excellent section on the importance and specifics of discussion, as well as the procedure itself.

Women who have experienced FGM have a high risk of emotional repercussions, and because their trauma is sexually related, they are often ashamed and unwilling to share their feeling, leading to a sense of isolation. Anxiety, depression, and posttraumatic stress disorder are common and should be addressed. Not surprisingly, sexual dysfunction is common, but, surprisingly, some women who have been cut, and who have even undergone removal of the visible portion of the clitoris, have fulfilling sex lives. There is a substantial portion of the clitoris that remains intact, so that the female sexual response may remain intact. Sexual care and support can maximize this for women. Again, this WHO handbook is an excellent resource for the provider who wants to provide care for these women.

The health care provider has a legal duty to report any child under the age of 18 who had undergone FGM or who the provider is concerned is at risk for this procedure, even though this cannot be proven, or the provider is wrong.

FGM is life changing, with repercussions on a woman's health, self-image, and sexuality, and her provider should become familiar with her health and psychological risks and means of minimizing both the physical and emotional damage.

## REFERENCES


1. Barnabei VM. Vulvodynia. *Clin Obstet Gynecol.* 2020;63:752-769.
2. Bergeron S, Reed BD, Wesselmann U, Bohm-Starke N. Vulvodynia. *Nat Rev Dis Primers.* 2020;6:36.
3. Chisari C, Monajemi MB, Scott W, Moss-Morris R, McCracken LM. Psychosocial factors associated with pain and sexual function in women with Vulvodynia: a systematic review. *Eur J Pain.* 2021;25:39-50.
4. Ponte M, Klemperer E, Sahay A, Chren MM. Effects of vulvodynia on quality of life. *J Am Acad Dermatol.* 2009;60:70-76.
5. Brotto LA, Bergeron S, Zdaniuk B, Basson R. Mindfulness and cognitive behavior therapy for provoked vestibulodynia: mediators of treatment outcome and long-term effects. *J Consult Clin Psychol.* 2020;88:48-64.
6. Dunkley CR, Brotto LA. Psychological treatments for provoked vestibulodynia: integration of mindfulness-based and cognitive behavioral therapies. *J Clin Psychol.* 2016;72:637-650.
7. Pâquet M, Rosen NO, Steben M, Mayrand MH, Santerre-Baillargeon M, Bergeron S. Daily anxiety and depressive symptoms in couples coping with vulvodynia: associations with women's pain, women's sexual function, and both partners' sexual distress. *J Pain.* 2018;19:552-561.
8. Oliveira EC, Leppink EW, Derbyshie KL, Grant JE. Excoriation disorder: impulsivity and its clinical associations. *J Anxiety Disord.* 2015;30:19-22.
9. Caccavale S, Bove D, Bove RM, La Montagna M. Skin and brain: itch and psychiatric disorders. *G Ital Dermatol Venereol.* 2016;151:525-529.
10. Pereira MP, Kremer AE, Mettang T, Ständer S. Chronic pruritus in the absence of skin disease: pathophysiology, diagnosis and treatment. *Am J Clin Dermatol.* 2016;17:337-348.
11. Koblenzer CS, Gupta R. Neurotic excoriations and dermatitis artifacta. *Semin Cutan Med Surg.* 2013;32:95-100.
12. Zeidler C, Ständer S. The pathogenesis of prurigo nodularis—'super-itch' in exploration. *Eur J Pain.* 2016;20:37-40.
13. Eskander N, Limbana T, Khan F. Psychiatric comorbidities and the risk of suicide in obsessive-compulsive and body dysmorphic disorder. *Cureus.* 2020;12:e9805.
14. Mufaddel A, Osman OT, Almugaddam F, Jafferany M. A review of body dysmorphic disorder and its presentation in different clinical settings. *Prim Care Companion CNS Disord.* 2013;15. Pii: PCC. 12r01464L.
15. Frias A, Palma C, Farrois N, González L. Comorbidity between obsessive-compulsive disorder and body dysmorphic disorder:

prevalence, explanatory theories, and clinical characterization. *Neuropsychiatr Dis Treat.* 2015;11:2233-2244.
16. Pastoor H, Gregory A. Penile size dissatisfaction. *J Sex Med.* 2020;17:1400-1404.
17. Springgs M, Gillam L. Body dysmorphic disorder: contraindication or ethical justification for female genital cosmetic surgery in adolescents. *Bioethics.* 2016;30:706-713.
18. Soubra A, Natale C, Brimley S, Hellstrom WJG. Revelations on men who seek penile augmentation surgery: a review. *Sex Med Rev.* 2022;10:460–467. doi: 10.1016/j.sxmr.2021.10.003.
19. Veale D, Eshkevari E, Ellison N, et al. Psychological characteristics and motivation of women seeking labiaplasty. *Psychol Med.* 2014;44:555-556.
20. Zanotta N, Campisciano G, Scrimin F, et al. Cytokine profiles of women with vulvodynia: identification of a panel of pro-inflammatory molecular targets. *Eur J Obstet Gynecol Reprod Biol.* 2018;226:66-70.
21. Bornstein J, Goldstein AT, Stockdale CK, et al. 2015 ISSVD, ISSWSH, and IPPS consensus terminology and classification of persistent vulvar pain and vulvodynia. *Obstet Gynecol.* 2016;127:745-751.
22. Cardenas-de la Garza JA, Villarreal-Villarreal CD, Cuellar-Barboza A, et al. Red scrotum syndrome treatment with pregabalin: a case series. *Ann Dermatol.* 2019;31:320-324.
23. Shivakumar S, Jafferany M, Kumar SV, Sood S. A brief review of dermatitis artefacta and management strategies for physicians. *Prim Care Companion CNS Disord.* 2021;23:20nr02858.
24. Chandran V, Kurien G. Dermatitis artefacta. In: *StatPearls* [Internet]. StatPearls Publishing; 2022.
25. Horner G. Nonsuicidal self-injury. *J Pediatr Health Care.* 2016;30:261-267.
26. Rasian M, Donaldson J, Royle J. Penile self-harm: a case report and concise clinical review. *Scand J Urol.* 2015;49:341-343.
27. Farahani F, Gentry A, Lara-Torre E, McCuin E. Self-attempted labioplasty with elastic bands resulting in severe necrosis. *J Low Genit Tract Dis.* 2015;19:e35-e37.
28. Mitchell AE, Fraser JA, Ramsbotham J, et al. Childhood atopic dermatitis: a cross-sectional study of relationships between child and parent factors, atopic dermatitis management, and disease severity. *Int J Nurs Stud.* 2015;52:216-228.
29. Silverberg JI. Selected comorbidities of atopic dermatitis: atopy, neuropsychiatric, and musculoskeletal disorders. *Clin Dermatol.* 2017;35:360-366.
30. Patel KR, Immaneni S, Singam V, Rastogi S, Silverberg JI. Association between atopic dermatitis, depression, and suicidal ideation: a systematic review and meta-analysis. *J Am Acad Dermatol.* 2019;80:402-410.
31. Silverberg JI, Gelfand JM, Margolis DJ, et al. Symptoms and diagnosis of anxiety and depression in atopic dermatitis in U.S. adults. *Br J Dermatol* 2019;181:554-565.
32. Kim SH, Hur J, Jang JY, et al. Psychological distress in young males with atopic dermatitis: a cross-sectional study. *Medicine (Baltimore).* 2015;94:e49.
33. Dalgard FJ, Gieler U, Tomas-Aragones L, et al. The psychological burden of skin diseases: a cross-sectional multicenter study among dermatological out-patients in 13 European countries. *J Invest Dermatol.* 2015;135:984-991.
34. Liao YH, Lin CC, Tsai PP, et al. Increased risk of lichen simplex chronicus in people with anxiety disorder: a nationwide population-based retrospective cohort study. *Br J Dermatol.* 2014;170:890-894.
35. Kouris A, Christodoulou C, Efstathiou V, et al. Comparative study of quality of life and obsessive-compulsive tendencies in patients with chronic hand eczema and lichen simplex chronicus. *Dermatitis.* 2016;27:127-130.
36. Ersser SJ, Cowdell F, Latter S, et al. Psychological and educational interventions for atopic eczema in children. *Cochrane Database Syst Rev.* 2014;(1):CD004054.
37. Purzycka-Bohdan D, Kisielnicka A, Zabłotna M, et al. Chronic plaque psoriasis in Poland: disease severity, prevalence of comorbidities, and quality of life. *J Clin Med.* 2022;11:1254.
38. Kowalewska B, Krajewska-Kułak E, Sobolewski M. The impact of stress-coping strategies and the severity of psoriasis on self-esteem, illness acceptance and life satisfaction. *Dermatol Ther (Heidelb).* 2022;12:529-543.
39. Molina-Leyva A, Almodovar-Real A, Carrascosa JC, et al. Distribution pattern of psoriasis, anxiety and depression as possible causes of sexual dysfunction in patients with moderate to severe psoriasis. *An Bras Dermatol.* 2015;90:338-345.
40. Schielein MC, Tizek L, Knobloch L, Maaßen D, Biedermann T, Zink A. Psoriasis and addiction: assessing mental health based on a cross-sectional study in Germany. *Eur J Dermatol.* 2021;31:722-729.
41. Panasiti MS, Ponsi G, Violani C. Emotions, alexithymia, and emotion regulation in patients with psoriasis. *Front Psychol.* 2020;11:836.
42. Bolotna L, Sarian O. Psychopathological disorders as comorbidity in psoriasis (review). *Georgian Med News.* 2020;(301):143-147.
43. Prinsen CA, de Korte J, Augustin M, et al. Measurement of health-related quality of life in dermatological research and practice: outcome of the EADV Taskforce on Quality of Life. *J Eur Acad Dermatol Venereol.* 2013;27:1195-1203.
44. Armstrong A, Bohannan B, Mburu S, et al. Impact of psoriatic disease on quality of life: interim results of a global survey. *Dermatol Ther (Heidelb).* 2022;12:1055-1064.
45. Lugović-Mihić L, Meštrović-Štefekov J, Ferček I, Pondeljak N, Lazić-Mosler E, Gašić A. Atopic dermatitis severity, patient perception of the disease, and personality characteristics: how are they related to quality of life? *Life (Basel).* 2021;11:1434.
46. Duarte GV, Calmon H, Radel G, de Fátima Paim de Oliveira M. Psoriasis and sexual dysfunction: links, risks, and management challenges. *Psoriasis (Auckl).* 2018;8:93-99.
47. Linares-Gonzalez L, Lozano-Lozano I, Gutierrez-Rojas L, Lozano-Lozano M, Rodenas-Herranz T, Ruiz-Villaverde R. Sexual dysfunction and atopic dermatitis: a systematic review. *Life (Basel).* 2021;11:1314.
48. Wiesmeier E, Masongsong EV, Wiley DJ. The prevalence of examiner-diagnosed clitoral hood adhesions in a population of college-aged women. *J Low Genit Tract Dis.* 2008;12:307-310.
49. Aerts L, Rubin RS, Randazzo M, Goldstein SW, Goldstein I. Retrospective study of the prevalence and risk factors of clitoral adhesions: women's health providers should routinely examine the glans clitoris. *Sex Med.* 2018;6:115-122.
50. Yang C, Liu X, Wei GH. Foreskin development in 10 421 Chinese boys aged 0–18 years. *World J Pediatr.* 2009;5:312-315.
51. Morris BJ, Matthews JG, Krieger JN. Prevalence of phimosis in males of all ages: systematic review. *Urology.* 2020;135:124-132.
52. Ardila SDB, Baró AIT, Vargas JMS. [Labial adhesions: review of the literature]. *Arch Argent Pediatr.* 2017;115:597-601.
53. Jaresová V, Hrochová V, Sottner O, et al. [Synechia vulvae infantum—incidence on Department of Obstetric/Gynaecol-

ogy, Teaching Hospital Na Bulovce, the First Medical Faculty of Charles University in Prague, Czech Republic from 2001 through 2005]. *Ceska Gynekol.* 2007;72:131-135.

54. Rubinstein A, Rahman G, Risso P, Ocampo D. Labial adhesions: experience in a children's hospital. *Arch Argent Pediatr.* 2018;116:65-68.
55. Rahman Dhaiban MA, Chaudhary MA. Manual separation of labial synechiae: a cost-effective method in prepubertal girls. *Afr J Paediatr Surg.* 2021;18:139-142.
56. Babu MC, Tandur B, Sharma D, Murki S. Disposable diapers decrease the incidence of neonatal infections compared to cloth diapers in a level II neonatal intensive care unit. *J Trop Pediatr.* 2015;61:250-254.
57. Maruani A, Lorette G, Barbarot S, et al.; Groupe de Recherche de la Société Française de Dermatologie Pédiatrique. Re-emergence of papulonodular napkin dermatitis with use of reusable diapers: report of 5 cases. *Eur J Dermatol.* 2013;23:246-249.
58. Dithurbide-Hernández M, Del Río-Martínez CJ, Serrano-Vázquez IC, Rodríguez-Patiño G. [Sevestre-Jacquet posterosive syphilitic dermatitis associated with the use of reusable diapers: a clinical case]. *Rev Med Inst Mex Seguro Soc.* 2021;59:242-247.
59. Blume-Peytavi U, Kanti V. Prevention and treatment of diaper dermatitis. *Pediatr Dermatol.* 2018;35(Suppl 1):s19-s23.
60. Alkhuder L, Mawlawi H. Infantile iatrogenic Cushing syndrome due to topical steroids. *Case Rep Pediatr.* 2019;2019:2652961.
61. Olson D, Edmonson MB. Outcomes in children treated for perineal group A beta-hemolytic streptococcal dermatitis. *Pediatr Infect Dis J.* 2011;30:933-936.
62. Serban ED. Perianal infectious dermatitis: an underdiagnosed, unremitting and stubborn condition. *World J Clin Pediatr* 2018;7:89-104.
63. Gümüş S, Söğütçü N. Parasitic appendicitis in 14.797 cases: a retrospective cohort study. *Turkiye Parazitol Derg.* 2021;45: 113-116.
64. Kambe TY, Fukue K, Ishida R, Miyazaki S. Overview of inherited zinc deficiency in infants and children. *J Nutr Sci Vitaminol (Tokyo).* 2015;61(Suppl):S44-S46.
65. Bakos RM, Reinehr C, Escobar GF, Leite LL. Dermoscopy of skin infestations and infections (entomodermoscopy)—Part I: dermatozoonoses and bacterial infections. *An Bras Dermatol.* 2021;96:735-745.
66. Ma Y, Hu W, Wang P, Bian K, Liu Z. Dermoscopy combined with ink staining as one more method to diagnose nodular scabies. *Indian J Dermatol Venereol Leprol.* 2019;85:324-325.
67. Bayart CB, Tamburro JE, Vidimos AT, Wang L, Golden AB. Atenolol versus propranolol for treatment of infantile hemangiomas during the proliferative phase: a retrospective noninferiority study. *Pediatr Dermatol.* 2017;34:413-421.
68. Pope E, Lara-Corrales I, Sibbald C, et al. Noninferiority and safety of nadolol vs propranolol in infants with infantile hemangioma: a randomized clinical trial. *JAMA Pediatr.* 2022;176:34-41.
69. McGillis E, Baumann T, LeRoy J. Death associated with nadolol for infantile hemangioma: a case for improving safety. *Pediatrics.* 2020;145:e20191035. https://doi.org/10.1542/peds.2019-1035
70. Sebaratnam DF, Rodríguez Bandera AL, Wong LF, Wargon O. Infantile hemangioma. Part 2: management. *J Am Acad Dermatol.* 2021;85:1395-1404.
71. Allen AL, Siegfried EC. The natural history of condyloma in children. *J Am Acad Dermatol.* 1998;39:951-955.
72. Eichenfield LF, McFalda W, Brabec B, et al. Safety and efficacy of VP-102, a proprietary, drug-device combination product containing cantharidin, 0.7% (w/v), in children and adults with molluscum contagiosum: two phase 3 randomized clinical trials. *JAMA Dermatol.* 2020;156:1315-1323.
73. Papadopoulos EJ. Clinical review. Accessed March 3, 2022. https://www.fda.gov/files/drugs/published/N20-723S020-Imiquimod-Clinical-BPCA.pdf
74. Giner-Soriano M, Teixidó C, Marsal JR, et al.; Working Group for the Clinical Trial IJG-KOH-2014. Randomized placebo-controlled clinical trial on efficacy and safety of topical 10% Potassium hydroxide for molluscum contagiosum treatment in children. *J Dermatolog Treat.* 2019;30:750-756.
75. Wang M, Arlen AM, Vash-Margita A. Characteristics among premenarchal girls with lichen sclerosus. *J Low Genit Tract Dis* 2021;25:152-157.
76. Kiss A, Király L, Kutasy B, et al. High incidence of balanitis xerotica obliterans in boys with phimosis: prospective 10-year study. *Pediatr Dermatol.* 2005;22:305-308.
77. Nguyen ATM, Holland AJA. Balanitis xerotica obliterans: an update for clinicians. *Eur J Pediatr.* 2020;179:9-16.
78. Homer L, Buchanan KJ, Nasr B, Losty PD, Corbett HJ. Meatal stenosis in boys following circumcision for lichen sclerosus (balanitis xerotica obliterans). *J Urol.* 2014;192:1784-1788.
79. Ebert AK, Rösch WH, Vogt T. Safety and tolerability of adjuvant topical tacrolimus treatment in boys with lichen sclerosus: a prospective phase 2 study. *Eur Urol.* 2008;54:932-937.
80. Folaranmi SE, Corbett HJ, Losty PD. Does application of topical steroids for lichen sclerosus (balanitis xerotica obliterans) affect the rate of circumcision? A systematic review. *J Pediatr Surg.* 2018;53:2225-2227.
81. Kherlopian A, Fischer G. Does compliance to topical corticosteroid therapy reduce the risk of development of permanent vulvar structural abnormalities in pediatric vulvar lichen sclerosus? A retrospective cohort study. *Pediatr Dermatol.* 2022;39:22-30.
82. Morrel B, van Eersel R, Burger CW, et al. The long-term clinical consequences of juvenile vulvar lichen sclerosus, a systematic review. *J Am Acad Dermatol.* 2020;82:469-477.
83. Hsieh TF, Chang CH, Chang SS. Foreskin development before adolescence in 2149 schoolboys. *Int J Urol.* 2006;13:968-970.
84. Dave S, Afshar K, Braga LH, et al. Canadian Urologic Association guideline on the care of the normal foreskin and neonatal circumcision in Canadian infants. *Can Urol Assoc J.* 2017;12:E76-E99.
85. Moreno G, Corbalán J, Peñaloza B, Pantoja T. Topical corticosteroids for treating phimosis in boys. *Cochrane Database Syst Rev.* 2014;(9):CD008973.
86. Laufer M, Emans SJ. Overview of vulvovaginal complaints in the prepubertal child. 2019. Accessed March 3, 2022. www.uptodate.com/contents/overview-of-vulvovaginal-complaints-in-the-prepubertal child
87. Johary J, Xue M, Xu B, et al. Use of hysteroscope for vaginoscopy or hysteroscopy in adolescents for the diagnosis and therapeutic management of gynecologic disorders: a systemic review. *J Pediatr Adolesc Gynecol.* 2015;28:29-37.
88. Sbidian E, Battistella M, Legoff J, et al. Recalcitrant pseudotumoral anogenital herpes simplex virus type 2 in HIV-infected patients: evidence for predominant B-lymphoplasmocytic infiltration and immunomodulators as effective therapeutic strategy. *Clin Infect Dis.* 2013;57:1648-1655.

89. Munawwar A, Singh S. Human herpesviruses as copathogens of HIV infection, their role in HIV transmission, and disease progression. *J Lab Physicians.* 2016;8:5-18.
90. Desai DV, Kulkarni SS. Herpes simplex virus: the interplay between HSV, Host, and HIV-1. *Viral Immunol.* 2015;28: 546-555.
91. Fife KH, Mugwanya K, Thomas KK, et al.; Partners in Prevention HSV/HIV Transmission Study Team. Transient increase in herpes simplex virus type 2 (HSV-2)-associated genital ulcers following initiation of antiretroviral therapy in HIV/HSV-2-coinfected individuals. *J Infect Dis.* 2016;213:1573-1578.
92. Ford ES, Magaret AS, Spak CW, et al. Increase in HSV shedding at initiation of antiretroviral therapy and decrease in shedding over time on antiretroviral therapy in HIV and HSV-2 infected persons. *AIDS.* 2018;32:2525-2531.
93. Hu J, Krauss JC, Moyal-Barracco M, Washer LL, Haefner HK, Parker-Featherstone E. Vulvar pseudotumoral acyclovir-resistant herpes in an HIV-negative, non-immunosuppressed patient: a therapeutic challenge. *Int J Womens Dermatol.* 2021;7(5Part B):731-736.
94. Barroso dos Reis HL, Tosato Boldrini NA, da Silva Campos LC, et al. Hypertrophic genital herpes in an HIV-infected female patient: Imiquimod as an alternative treatment. *Int J Infect Dis.* 2020;95:153-156.
95. Jiang YC, Feng H, Lin YC, Guo XR. New strategies against drug resistance to herpes simplex virus. *Int J Oral Sci.* 2016;8:1-6.
96. Frobert E, Burrel S, Ducastelle-Lepretre S, et al. Resistance of herpes simplex viruses to acyclovir: an update from a ten-year survey in France. *Antiviral Res.* 2014;111:36-41. https://www.cdc.gov/std/treatment-guidelines/herpes.htm#AntiviralResistant
97. Erard V, Wald A, Corey L, Leisenring WM, Boeckh M. Use of long-term suppressive acyclovir after hematopoietic stem-cell transplantation: impact on herpes simplex virus (HSV) disease and drug-resistant HSV disease. *J Infect Dis.* 2007;196:266-270.
98. Massad LS, Xie X, Burk RD, et al. Association of cervical precancer with human papillomavirus types other than 16 among HIV co-infected women. *Am J Obstet Gynecol.* 2016;214:354.e1-354.e6.
99. Boudes M, Venard V, Routiot T, Buzzi M, Maillot F. Prevalence and distribution of HPV genotypes in immunosuppressed patients in lorraine region. *Viruses.* 2021;13:2454.
100. Sunderkötter C, Wohlrab J, Hamm H. Scabies: epidemiology, diagnosis, and treatment. *Dtsch Arztebl Int.* 2021;118:695-704.
101. Sunderkötter C, Feldmeier H, Fölster-Holst R, et al. S1 guidelines on the diagnosis and treatment of scabies—short version. *J Dtsch Dermatol Ges.* 2016;14:1155-1167.
102. Salavastru CM, Chosidow O, Boffa MJ, et al. European guideline for the management of scabies. *J Eur Acad Dermatol Venereol.* 2017;31:1248-1253.
103. Harte MC, Saunsbury TA, Hodgson TA. Thalidomide use in the management of oromucosal disease: a 10-year review of safety and efficacy in 12 patients. *Oral Surg Oral Med Oral Pathol Oral Radiol.* 2020;130:398-401.
104. Haseen B, Kahn A, Belton A, Bayer CR. Health care for transgender men: what is missing in OB/GYN care? *J Low Genit Tract Dis.* 2020;24:232-233.
105. Grimstad F, McLaren H, Gray M. The gynecologic examination of the transfeminine person after penile inversion vaginoplasty. *Am J Obstet Gynecol.* 2021;224:266-273.
106. Oles N, Darrach H, Landford W, et al. Gender affirming surgery: a comprehensive, systematic review of all peer-reviewed literature and methods of assessing patient-centered outcomes (part 2: genital reconstruction). *Ann Surg.* 2022;275:e67-e74.
107. Bustos VP, Bustos SS, Mascaro A, et al. Regret after gender-affirmation surgery: a systematic review and meta-analysis of prevalence. *Plast Reconstr Surg Glob Open.* 2021;9:e3477.
108. Massie JP, Morrison SD, Van Maasdam J, Satterwhite T. Predictors of patient satisfaction and postoperative complications in penile inversion vaginoplasty. *Plast Reconstr Surg.* 2018;141:911e-921e.
109. McMurray SL, Overholser E, Patel T. A transgender woman with anogenital lichen sclerosus. *JAMA Dermatol.* 2017;153:1334-1335.
110. Vedovo F, Di Blas L, Aretusi F, et al. Physical, mental and sexual health among transgender women: a comparative study among operated transgender and cisgender women in a national tertiary referral network. *J Sex Med.* 2021;18:982-989.
111. Meier AC, Papadopulos N. [Quality of life after gender reassignment surgery: an overview]. *Handchir Mikrochir Plast Chir.* 2021;53:556-563.
112. To M, Zhang Q, Bradlyn A, et al. Visual conformity with affirmed gender or "passing": its distribution and association with depression and anxiety in a cohort of transgender people. *J Sex Med.* 2020;17:2084-2092.
113. de Vries AL, McGuire JK, Steensma TD, Wagenaar EC, Doreleijers TA, Cohen-Kettenis PT. Young adult psychological outcome after puberty suppression and gender reassignment. *Pediatrics.* 2014;134:696-704.
114. LeBreton M, Courtois F, Journel NM, et al. Genital sensory detection thresholds and patient satisfaction with vaginoplasty in male-to-female transgender women. *J Sex Med.* 2017;14:274-281.
115. Manrique OJ, Adabi K, Martinez-Jorge J, Ciudad P, Nicoli F, Kiranantawat K. Complications and patient-reported outcomes in male-to-female vaginoplasty-where we are today: a systematic review and meta-analysis. *Ann Plast Surg.* 2018;80:684-691.
116. McPherson GW, Long T, Salipante SJ, et al. The vaginal microbiome of transgender men. *Clin Chem.* 2019;65:199-207.
117. Baldassarre M, Giannone FA, Foschini MP, et al. Effects of long-term high dose testosterone administration on vaginal epithelium structure and estrogen receptor-α and -β expression of young women. *Int J Impot Res.* 2013;25:172-177.
118. Robinson IS, Blasdel G, Cohen O, Zhao LC, Bluebond-Langner R. Surgical outcomes following gender affirming penile reconstruction: patient-reported outcomes from a multi-center, international survey of 129 transmasculine patients. *J Sex Med.* 2021;18:800-811.
119. Veerman H, de Rooij FPW, Al-Tamimi M. Functional outcomes and urological complications after genital gender affirming surgery with urethral lengthening in transgender men. *J Urol.* 2020;204:104-109.
120. Al-Tamimi M, Pigot GL, van der Sluis WB, et al. The surgical techniques and outcomes of secondary phalloplasty after metoidioplasty in transgender men: an international, multicenter case series. *J Sex Med.* 2019;16:1849-1859.
121. Calotta NA, Kuzon W, Dellon AL, Monstrey S, Coon D. Sensibility, sensation, and nerve regeneration after reconstructive genital surgery: evolving concepts in neurobiology. *Plast Reconstr Surg.* 2021;147:995e-1003e.

122. Kaushik A, Bakshi S, Bishnoi A. Jacquet's erosive diaper dermatitis in an adult female. *Indian Dermatol Online J.* 2021;12:957.
123. Isogai R, Yamada H. Factors involved in the development of diaper-area granuloma of the aged. *J Dermatol.* 2013;40:1038-1041.
124. Robson KJ, Maughan JA, Purcell SD, Petersen MJ, Haefner HK, Lowe L. Erosive papulonodular dermatosis associated with topical benzocaine: a report of two cases and evidence that granuloma gluteale, pseudoverrucous papules, and Jacquet's erosive dermatitis are a disease spectrum. *J Am Acad Dermatol.* 2006;55(5 Suppl):S74-S80.
125. The Care of Girls and Women Living with Female Genital Mutilation: A Clinical Handbook. 2018, printed in France. https://iris.who.int/bitstream/handle/10665/272429/9789241513913-eng.pdf?sequence=1

## SUGGESTED READINGS

Blume-Peytavi U, Kanti V. Prevention and treatment of diaper dermatitis. *Pediatr Dermatol.* 2018;35(Suppl 1):s19-s23.

Chandran V, Kurien G. Dermatitis artefacta. In: *StatPearls* [Internet]. StatPearls Publishing; 2022.

Chisari C, Monajemi MB, Scott W, Moss-Morris R, McCracken LM. Psychosocial factors associated with pain and sexual function in women with Vulvodynia: a systematic review. *Eur J Pain.* 2021;25:39-50.

Grimstad F, McLaren H, Gray M. The gynecologic examination of the transfeminine person after penile inversion vaginoplasty. *Am J Obstet Gynecol.* 2021;224:266-273.

Gualtieri R, Bronz G, Bianchetti MG, et al. Perianal streptococcal disease in childhood: systematic literature review. *Eur J Pediatr.* 2021;180:1867-1874.

Harte MC, Saunsbury TA, Hodgson TA. Thalidomide use in the management of oromucosal disease: a 10-year review of safety and efficacy in 12 patients. *Oral Surg Oral Med Oral Pathol Oral Radiol.* 2020;130:398-401.

Haseen B, Kahn A, Belton A, Bayer CR. Health care for transgender men: what is missing in OB/GYN care? *J Low Genit Tract Dis.* 2020;24:232-233.

Kherlopian A, Fischer G. Does compliance to topical corticosteroid therapy reduce the risk of development of permanent vulvar structural abnormalities in pediatric vulvar lichen sclerosus? A retrospective cohort study. *Pediatr Dermatol.* 2022; 39:22-30.

Morrel B, van Eersel R, Burger CW, et al. The long-term clinical consequences of juvenile vulvar lichen sclerosus, a systematic review. *J Am Acad Dermatol.* 2020;82:469-477.

Reusser NM, Downing C, Guidry J, Tyring SK. HPV carcinomas in immunocompromised patients. *J Clin Med.* 2015;4:260-281.

Nguyen ATM, Holland AJA. Balanitis xerotica obliterans: an update for clinicians. *Eur J Pediatr.* 2020;179:9-16.

Oles N, Darrach H, Landford W, et al. Gender affirming surgery: a comprehensive, systematic review of all peer-reviewed literature and methods of assessing patient-centered outcomes (Part 2: Genital Reconstruction). *Ann Surg.* 2022;275:e67-e74.

Pope E, Lara-Corrales I, Sibbald C, et al. Noninferiority and safety of nadolol vs propranolol in infants with infantile hemangioma: a randomized clinical trial. *JAMA Pediatr.* 2022;176:34-41.

Sebaratnam DF, Rodríguez Bandera AL, Wong LF, Wargon O. Infantile hemangioma. Part 2: management. *J Am Acad Dermatol.* 2021;85:1395-1404.

Sridharan K, Sivaramakrishnan G. Topical corticosteroids for phimosis in children: a network meta-analysis of randomized clinical trials. *Pediatr Surg Int.* 2021;37:1117-1125.

Šterbenc A, Točkova O, Lah LL, et al. A retrospective analysis of clinical characteristics and management of perianal streptococcal dermatitis in children and adults. *Acta Dermatovenerol Alp Pannonica Adriat.* 2021;30:99-104.

Sunderkotter C, Wohlrab J, Hamm H. Scabies: epidemiology, diagnosis, and treatment. *Dtsch Arztebl Int.* 2021;118:695-704.

*The Care of Girls and Women Living with Female Genital Mutilation: A Clinical Handbook.* 2018, printed in France. https://iris.who.int/bitstream/handle/10665/272429/9789241513913-eng.pdf?sequence=1

# APPENDIX A
# Patient Handouts

**Spanish language versions of the patient handouts below can be downloaded from the VitalSource eBook.**

## Lichen Sclerosus

Lichen sclerosus (LS) (sometimes called lichen sclerosus et atrophicus, or LS&A) is a skin condition that is most common on the vulva of older women who have gone through menopause. However, lichen sclerosus sometimes affects girls before puberty, as well as younger adult women, and the penis of uncircumcised boys and men. In females, lichen sclerosus often affects rectal skin also. Only about 1 in 30 women with vulvar LS experience LS on other areas of the body, and when this occurs, it is most often on the back, chest, or abdomen. Lichen sclerosus almost never appears on the face or hands.

Lichen sclerosus of the vulva, rectal skin, or penis typically appears as white skin that is itchy. The skin is also fragile, so that rubbing and scratching can cause tearing, cracks, and bruises that hurt. Sexual activity is often painful or may be impossible. Untreated lichen sclerosus eventually can scar and, occasionally, narrow the opening to the vagina. In boys and men, the foreskin can scar over the head of the penis. Also, untreated lichen sclerosus is associated with skin cancer of the vulva in about 1 in 20-30 women, and there is an increased risk of skin cancer of the penis with untreated lichen sclerosus also. Lichen sclerosus that is well controlled and managed with ongoing treatment shows much less scarring and much less threat for cancer. Lichen sclerosus of dry skin away from the genital area does not scar or develop cancer and usually does not itch.

The causes of lichen sclerosus are not completely understood, but a main cause is a confused immune system. The immune system, that part of the body that normally fights off infection, attacks the skin by mistake. Why this happens is not known. Other immune conditions can occur in patients with lichen sclerosus as well. Older women with lichen sclerosus generally also have an underactive thyroid, so thyroid tests should be performed yearly. Psoriasis seems to be more common in women with LS. Vitiligo, symptom-free milk-white patches also is associated with LS at times. Another cause of lichen sclerosus is genetics. This conditions sometimes—but not often—runs in some families. We know that lichen sclerosus is not an infection that can be passed to another person, and it is not caused by diet. There are no lifestyle issues that cause lichen sclerosus.

Lichen sclerosus improves tremendously in nearly all patients with topical corticosteroid ointments, and sometimes the skin even returns to a completely normal appearance, although scarring does not go away. The overwhelming first-line therapy, proven in clinical studies for LS, is topical corticosteroids (also called a cortisone or steroid but not the same kind of steroid that some athletes use illegally). But, lichen sclerosus is not cured by this or any treatment. The corticosteroid ointment (most often used is clobetasol, halobetasol, or betamethasone dipropionate in augmented vehicle) is applied sparingly once or twice a day, far, far *less* than a pea-sized amount. If the skin feels greasy after medication is applied, too much is being used. After it has been on the skin for 30 minutes, it is not easily removed, so that reapplication is not needed after urination or bowel movements and wiping. When too much medication is used, or when medication accidently spreads to surrounding skin such as the groin or inner thighs, corticosteroids can cause thinning, acne, redness, stretch marks, and irritation over time. Therefore, a health care provider should examine the area every couple of months until the skin disease is controlled and frequency or strength of the medication is decreased. Fortunately, because of the very small area of the genitals, there is no concern about absorption of medication into the bloodstream and affecting the internal organs. The package insert often advises against using strong steroids on genital skin or for longer than 2 weeks. However, those instructions were formulated decades ago, and experience since that time has taught us that long-term use on genital skin is safe and necessary when used in tiny amounts and with careful follow-up with a provider. At the beginning, a touch of petroleum jelly (plain Vaseline) applied over the steroid helps the skin to heal and helps symptoms of itching and irritation by covering tiny breaks and cracks in the skin.

After several months, when the skin disease is controlled, either the medication is decreased to once, two, or three times a week, or a milder cortisone is prescribed for daily use. If therapy is stopped, the lichen sclerosus eventually returns and so does the risk of scarring and cancer. With ongoing use of medication, the risk of scarring and cancer is very low. Even when there are no symptoms, it is important that treatment is not stopped, since LS can be active with an increased risk of silent scarring and cancer. Medication should never be used only "when needed."

For boys and men whose lichen sclerosus is not controlled with superpotent steroid ointments, circumcision is the treatment of choice and is often curative. For areas of recurrence, topical steroids can be used.

Most often, women whose discomfort with lichen sclerosus does not improve enough with the clobetasol or halobetasol ointments have problems other than resistant lichen sclerosus that make them uncomfortable. Common problems include low estrogen or irritation from things that touch the area. Examples include irritating creams, unnecessary medications, some panty liners, wet wipes, soaps, and overwashing. Some irritants, such as sweat in overweight people and urine in incontinent people, can be hard to avoid. Otherwise, the most common irritant is rubbing and scratching. Many people can keep from scratching during the day, but much rubbing and scratching occur during normal sleeping hours, when people do not realize they are scratching. Although there are no effective anti-itch pills, any medication that produces a very deep sleep can stop nighttime scratching and allow the skin to heal. Finally, lichen sclerosus sometimes triggers vulvodynia, a pain syndrome most often described as burning, irritation, or rawness, even though the skin appears normal.

About 1 in 10 people have lichen sclerosus that does not clear with cortisone ointments. The white plaques of lichen sclerosus are still visible on the skin in spite of using a strong steroid ointment, so other medications are added. These medications include tacrolimus ointment or pimecrolimus cream, nonsteroid medications that have been shown to be useful for lichen sclerosus, but are only approved by the U.S. Food and Drug Administration (FDA) for eczema. These medications are not as beneficial as steroids, but sometimes they improve lichen sclerosus when added to the steroid, and sometimes these are used to keep lichen sclerosus controlled once a steroid has cleared the skin. Newer nonablative lasers (such as the MonaLisa Touch or the Femtouch) are showing early promise for the treatment of lichen sclerosus that shows persistent white skin after treatment with topical steroids. These are not approved for LS, and there are no good studies showing benefit, so they should be used only in patients who have failed treatments like topical steroids that have been shown in studies to be safe and effective. The laser therapies, like topical steroids, do not cure LS, so that either repeat treatments or topical steroids are necessary to maintain control of the condition. Popular among lay patients is platelet-rich plasma. There are a few enthusiastic providers who use this therapy, but studies do not provide convincing evidence of benefit. There is weak evidence that methotrexate pills may be useful for some patients with resistant lichen sclerosus.

Nearly all patients do extremely well following treatment for lichen sclerosus. Even when lichen sclerosus is completely controlled, patients should be followed every 6 months to be sure that the disease remains controlled, to detect side effects of the medication, and to examine for very early skin cancers. Patients should let family members know of this diagnosis, so that they can inform their providers if they also have genital itching or irritation.

## Genital Lichen Simplex Chronicus (Eczema, Neurodermatitis, Dermatitis)

Lichen simplex chronicus (LSC), also called eczema, is a common skin condition that is very itchy. Although not dangerous in any way, both the itching and the pain from rubbing and scratching can be miserable. Eczema/LSC of the genital area most often affects the scrotum of men, the vulva of women, or the rectal skin of both. Many people with eczema/LSC have had sensitive skin or eczema/LSC on other areas of the skin at some point, and many have a tendency toward allergies, especially hay fever or asthma.

The skin usually appears red or darker brown than surrounding skin, and thick from rubbing and scratching, sometimes with sores from scratching. Less often, the skin is lighter in color than nearby, normal skin. Sometimes hair is broken off from rubbing. However and strangely, sometimes the skin can look almost normal, in spite of rubbing and scratching.

The cause of eczema/LSC is not entirely clear. Eczema/LSC often starts with some irritation that triggers itching. Then rubbing and scratching feels really good, but all of that rubbing irritates the skin even more, causing more itching, that ends up with more scratching, what is called the "itch-cycle." At the office visit with the health care provider, the cause of the original irritation often is no longer present. Common triggers include a yeast or fungus infection, an irritating medication, moisturizer or lubricant, anxiety or depression, overwashing, panty liners, sweat, heat, urine, contraceptive jelly, an irritating condom, or any other activity or substance that can irritate the skin and start the itching. Lichen simplex/eczema is not an infection, it cannot be passed to another person by sexual contact, it does not scar, and it does not cause cancer.

Treatment is very effective. First is avoidance of irritation. Common irritants are listed above and include irritating creams, unnecessary medications, some lubricants, some panty liners, wet wipes, soaps, and overwashing. Washing should be limited to once a day with clear water only. Some irritants, such as sweat in overweight people and urine in incontinent people, can be hard to avoid. Otherwise, the most common irritant is rubbing and scratching. Many people can keep from scratching during the day, but much rubbing and scratching occur during normal sleeping hours, when people do not realize they are scratching. Although there are no effective anti-itch pills, any medication that produces a very deep sleep can stop nighttime scratching and allow the skin to heal.

Lichen simplex chronicus usually improves with a very strong cortisone (or "steroid," although not the same kind of steroid that some athletes use illegally) ointment. The corticosteroid ointment (most often used is clobetasol, halobetasol, or betamethasone dipropionate in augmented vehicle) is applied sparingly once or twice a day, far, far *less* than a pea-sized amount. If the skin feels greasy after medication is applied, too much is being used. After it has been on the skin for 30 minutes, it is not easily removed, so that reapplication is not needed after urination or bowel movements and wiping. When too much medication is used, or when medication accidently spreads to surrounding skin such as the groin or inner thighs, corticosteroids can cause thinning, acne, redness, stretch marks, and irritation over time. Therefore, a health care provider should examine the area every couple of months until the skin disease is controlled and frequency or strength of the medication is decreased. Fortunately, because of the very small area of the genitals, there is no concern about absorption of medication into the bloodstream and affecting the internal organs. The package insert often advises against using strong steroids on genital skin or for longer than 2 weeks. However, those instructions were formulated decades ago, and experience since that time has taught us that long-term use on genital skin is safe and necessary when used in tiny amounts and with careful follow-up with a provider. At the beginning, a touch of petroleum jelly (plain Vaseline) applied over the steroid helps the skin to heal and helps symptoms of itching and irritation by covering tiny breaks and cracks in the skin.

Lichen simplex chronicus recurs when the superpotent corticosteroid is stopped too quickly. Medication should be continued not only until itching stops but also until the skin has normal appearance and thickness. Generally, gradually tapering the frequency of application is the best way to prevent immediate recurrence of itching and LSC.

Occasionally, LSC is not completely controlled with a superpotent steroid, so other medications are added. These medications include tacrolimus ointment or pimecrolimus cream. These are not used first, before corticosteroids, because their benefit is slower and less predictable, they are sometimes not covered by insurance, and because they often cause burning when they are applied.

After the treatment has been discontinued, a patient with LSC/eczema remains at risk for recurrence of itching, because the genital skin is an area with unavoidable irritation from normal sweat, friction, sexual activity, etc., that can restart itching. A patient with eczema/LSC should not be surprised when itching returns, but immediate treatment can prevent the return of the itch-scratch cycle and LSC/eczema.

## Hidradenitis Suppurativa (Inverse Acne)

Hidradenitis suppurativa (HS) is a skin condition that forms tender bumps and boils, which sometimes enlarge until they drain pus. These are found mostly in or around the groin or underarm areas but sometimes can affect the buttocks, inner thighs, abdomen, and breasts. Although the boils look like infection, they are not, and they cannot be passed from one person to another. Instead, this condition actually is cystic acne and begins when hair pores are clogged by dead skin and become inflamed when they become so large that they burst. HS is not caused by germs or dirt. Often, genetics plays a role, so many people with HS have family members with this condition.

Like acne, HS most often begins after puberty. It occurs in men and women, and it is often more severe in men, because it is worsened by testosterone. HS is more common in people of African descent as well. People who are very overweight and those who smoke are at risk for worse hidradenitis.

HS can be mild, where a person gets one small sore nodule every few years, or it can be a very severe form with many deep, painful boils that connect under the skin and make tunnels with several openings to the surface, continuously drain pus and scarring. Hidradenitis does not spread outside the groin, armpits, buttocks, breasts, and abdomen to the lower legs, feet, forearms, or hands. However, since HS is a form of cystic acne, people with HS sometimes develop painful red cysts of acne on the face, back, and chest.

Hidradenitis suppurativa is not just a disease of the skin. People with HS also have a higher risk of obesity, diabetes, high blood pressure, and high cholesterol. When these are not controlled, there is a higher risk of heart disease, stroke, and kidney disease, especially if the person is a smoker. Rarely, HS is associated with Crohn disease.

The treatment of HS starts with the hardest thing—weight loss in people who are overweight. Weight loss alone can make a tremendous improvement in the boils of hidradenitis. Not only that but weight loss, tobacco avoidance, and very careful attention to blood sugar and cholesterol help to prevent diabetes, heart disease, stroke, and kidney disease. A plan and medical help for losing weight and stopping smoking is important for all of these reasons.

For those people who only get a boil every few months, they may choose not to treat it at all, or these can be treated with an injection of a few drops of a cortisone into the cyst when it starts to feel sore and appear. When treated very early, sometimes the bump is nearly gone in a day. Some patients can even inject themselves or have a family member do this at home, after covering the area with numbing medication.

If bumps and boils appear often, ongoing daily pills can decrease the number of new boils that appear. First-line medication is antibiotics by mouth, even though HS is not an infection. Some antibiotics improve inflammation, even when the cause is not infection. Doxycycline, minocycline, clindamycin, and trimethoprim-sulfamethoxazole are the most often ones used. Unlike treating an infection, the antibiotics do not cure the problem, and they take about a month to begin to slow down the appearance of new bumps and about 3 months to reach peak effectiveness. Then, the medication must be continued, because the hidradenitis is not cured, but only controlled. A common mistake is stopping the antibiotic after only a few weeks because it does not seem to be working, when it has actually been too soon to see improvement. Oral contraceptive pills and spironolactone pills in women are believed to be useful by some, by decreasing the effects of testosterone.

Besides weight loss in those who are very overweight, the most useful medication available for HS is adalimumab (Humira). Adalimumab is an injection given at home just under the skin weekly. It decreases inflammation and weakens the immune system very slightly. It has been used for years for rheumatoid arthritis, psoriasis, and inflammatory bowel disease. Infliximab (Remicade) is a similar, somewhat stronger medication sometimes used as well, but because this is not yet approved by the Food and Drug Administration for HS, this expensive intravenous infusion is generally not covered by insurance. There are other new medications in development that are showing promise for HS as well.

When the boils of HS form only in small areas, the skin in that area can be surgically removed. Underarm skin is loose and the area is small, so underarm HS is usually cured by surgery, but boils sometimes appear at the edge of the removed skin. But, in the genital area, the areas of involvement can be too large to entirely take out, although the worst areas can be removed. Even if medical treatment keeps new boils from appearing, old draining cysts generally do not completely heal. These areas either can be cut out, or the top removed so that the draining area can heal from the underneath, without trapping the pus under the surface, called an "unroofing procedure."

Washing frequently and scrubbing are not helpful, and simply irritate the skin, since infection and dirt do not cause HS. Diet is not usually helpful; junk food, chocolate, and fatty food do not cause acne, although these contribute to weight gain, which worsens HS. Some providers believe that dairy products can worsen HS. Shaving the area can cause ingrown hairs and small bumps but does not cause the large, deep boils. Topical medications such as benzoyl peroxide or tretinoin normally used for acne are too irritating to put on sensitive underarm and groin skin. You may find milder topical antibiotics such as clindamycin solution useful, and antiperspirants can help the area feel better by decreasing sweat and friction. Isotretinoin (Accutane) is a wonderful medication for acne of the face and trunk, but for some reason, it is not as useful for HS.

Although HS is a chronic skin problem, the combination of weight loss, medical therapies, patience, and, when needed, surgeries improve skin enormously.

## Lichen Planus

Lichen planus (LP) is a fairly common skin condition that sometimes affects the genital skin. Genital LP is especially common on the vulva and in the vagina of older women who have gone through menopause. However, lichen planus occasionally affects the genital area of men, mostly the head of the penis of uncircumcised men. Lichen planus sometimes occurs on the rectal skin of both men and women with genital lichen planus. LP does not affect the genital area of children. Patients with lichen planus of genital skin usually have lichen planus of the mouth also, especially in the insides of the cheeks, or sometimes the gums and tongue. Other skin surfaces are generally not affected in patients with genital LP, but sometimes lichen planus occurs in the esophagus and cause difficulty with swallowing or heartburn. Very uncommonly, people with genital lichen planus have red or brown flat spots on the dry skin areas outside the genital area or a scalp rash of LP with hair loss.

Lichen planus of genital skin usually looks like thin red patches, but sometimes there is white skin, or white streaks and interlacing white lines. The genital skin is often itchy, but soreness and burning are usual as well. Sexual activity is frequently painful. Untreated lichen planus usually causes scarring. In women, the inner lips can disappear, the clitoris can become buried under the skin and, occasionally, there is narrowing of the opening to the vagina. At times, the vagina actually scars closed. In men, the foreskin can scar to the head of the penis.

Lichen planus is caused by a confused immune system. The immune system is that part of the body that fights off infection, but in this case, it attacks the skin by mistake. Why this happens is not known. We know that lichen planus is not an infection that can be passed to another person, and it is not caused by diet. It does not usually occur in families. There are no lifestyle issues that cause lichen planus.

Lichen planus usually improves quite a lot with treatment, but it is not cured by medication. First is the avoidance of irritating products such as creams, overwashing, unnecessary topical medications, and soaps. Then, for men, circumcision is the best treatment if strong corticosteroid ointments do not control the problem. Corticosteroids are also called cortisones or steroids (but not the same kind of steroid as used illegally by some athletes). The corticosteroid ointment (generally clobetasol, halobetasol, or betamethasone dipropionate in augmented vehicle) is applied very sparingly once or twice a day until the discomfort is controlled and the skin has improved or cleared. Far, far *less* than a pea-sized amount is used for the entire area to prevent any extra medication from spreading to surrounding dry skin such as the inner thighs or groin area, where side effects occur more easily. If the skin feels greasy after medication is applied, too much is being used. This is very safe medication when used in the correct amount and for the correct length of time. Although package inserts often report that these strong corticosteroids should not be used in the genital area, or should only be used for 2 weeks, these instructions were developed 40 years ago. Experience has shown us that strong corticosteroids can be used safely on genital skin for very long periods of time or even forever—but carefully. And, fortunately, side effects are visible. When too much medication is used, or when medication is used for too long on surrounding skin, corticosteroids can cause thinning, redness, acne, stretch marks, and irritation. Therefore, a health care provider should examine the area frequently initially.

Corticosteroids usually improve itching and irritation within a few days. When discomfort and the skin have improved or cleared, your provider will either decrease the frequency of the strong medication, usually to two or three times a week, or a milder cortisone daily. But the corticosteroid should not be discontinued or used only when symptoms recur. Medication should be used continuously to prevent scarring and cancer, which can occur even when there is no pain or itching. Mild lichen planus sometimes clears altogether, whereas severe lichen planus may only improve a moderate amount, and additional medications may be needed.

Because lichen planus often affects the inside of the vagina, many women need to use a corticosteroid inside the vagina, and use a vaginal dilator several days a week to prevent the vagina from narrowing and scarring closed. And, because most women with lichen planus are usually postmenopausal with thinning from low estrogen levels, estrogen can be useful as well, with a cream, vaginal tablets, oral tablets, or a patch.

The mouth is often affected and painful, so those patients benefit from clobetasol gel, dexamethasone elixir, or other corticosteroid medications in the mouth several times a day. More than twice a day usually is needed since medications do not stick to the wet surface of the mouth. Both the vagina and the mouth are at risk for yeast infection, since cortisones work by lowering the immune system. If sudden vaginal itching occurs, or the mouth becomes more tender, yeast should be suspected. Some providers add regular antiyeast medications with the cortisones, to prevent yeast.

When the corticosteroid ointment does not improve the skin enough, other medications are added. These medications include tacrolimus ointment or pimecrolimus cream, and oral methotrexate, mycophenolate mofetil, azathioprine, griseofulvin, hydroxychloroquine, or cyclophosphamide pills. The medication tofacitinib (Xeljanz) and other JAK inhibitors have shown promise and are being evaluated for effectiveness in lichen planus.

Often, a patient needs a dentist, a dermatologist, and a gynecologist to care for lichen planus in these different areas. Lichen planus is not cured with treatment. However, it improves, and most patients become generally comfortable. Patients should be followed carefully to evaluate for scarring as well as for side effects to medications. Although skin cancers caused by lichen planus are uncommon, cancer occasionally occurs and should be diagnosed early. Therefore, the genital skin should be evaluated at least twice a year, even when doing well, to ensure that the skin is not developing early signs of skin cancer, side effects from the medication, silent scarring, or return of the lichen planus.

Although lichen planus improves with corticosteroids, it is not cured. Therefore, medications are stopped, itching and irritation reappear. And when the LP recurs, even when symptom-free, scarring continues, and the risk of cancer increases. Because of this, medications should be used ongoing, rather than as-needed.

Occasionally, after vulvar lichen planus is improved or cleared with therapy, discomfort remains. A pain syndrome called vulvodynia can be triggered by any injury or inflammation of the vulva, including lichen planus, and this should be addressed in those women.

## Vaginal Atrophy (Estrogen Deficiency)

Estrogen is a hormone that maintains the elastic, moist, and supple skin of the vagina. The ovaries produce estrogen from puberty to menopause, but after a woman goes through menopause, estrogen levels decline, and the internal vaginal skin often becomes thin, dry, and fragile. This is called vaginal atrophy. Some women remain comfortable, although many need to use a lubricant with sexual activity. Others experience dryness, irritation, rawness, painful sexual activity, and burning of the opening to the vagina despite using a moisturizer. This is a common and normal—but uncomfortable and fixable—experience for women as they age. This can occur in women who have other reasons for low estrogen levels, such as when ovaries are surgically removed, when a woman is breastfeeding, or when taking some medications for breast cancer that block the effects of estrogen.

Fortunately, the treatment of vaginal atrophy is easy and extremely effective for most women. Estrogen can be inserted in the vagina, with minimal side effects to the body as a whole. Or, estrogen can be taken orally or by patch ("systemic" estrogen replacement), if other symptoms of low estrogen are a problem, such as hot flashes, bone loss, or psychological symptoms. When estrogen is given by pill or patch, care must be taken to monitor for breast cancer. Although estrogen does not cause breast cancer, estrogen can allow breast cancer to grow faster. Like birth control pills, estrogen by pill or patch is also a risk factor for an increased risk of blood clots that cause heart attack and stroke. The risk is very small in some women and higher in others, depending upon the woman's family history and whether or not she smokes.

Estrogen inserted in the vagina is absorbed into the bloodstream to a trivial degree when used correctly, so that these risks are minor, despite the package insert warnings. Estrogen can be inserted in the vagina in several forms, with differing degrees of comfort, convenience, and cost. Estrogen cream is a treatment that has been used for many years. Either conjugated equine estrogen cream (Premarin—collected from **pre**gnant **mar**e ur**in**e) or estradiol (Estrace) cream can be inserted into the vagina, ½ g three times a week, for several weeks, and then frequency decreased to once or twice weekly. Some believe that estradiol may be less irritating.

Alternatives to estrogen creams include a small estradiol tablet (Vagifem) inserted into the vagina about three nights a week. Also, a flexible ring containing estradiol (Estring) can be inserted into the vagina, where the hormone is released gradually over 3 months, when it should be replaced. The amount of estrogen that is absorbed with all of these forms of local estrogen replacement is very small.

These local forms of estrogen have become expensive at drug stores in the United States, and despite their safety, Medicare does not approve them for women aged 65 years and over, so insurance often does not cover them. However, estradiol cream and vaginal tablets are now generic, and with local pharmacy "clubs" and medication plans such as goodrx.com or singlecare.com, these are now affordable for the astute consumer. There are no generic forms of the estrogen ring as of this writing.

Estrogen by pill or patch (systemic estrogen) is less expensive, but women who have not had a hysterectomy and still have a uterus must take progesterone to prevent the uterine lining from building up and risking uterine bleeding and cancer. Estrogen by pill or patch is absorbed and has greater risks than estrogen used locally, but it also has greater benefits. Systemic estrogen use should be discussed with the person's provider to decide if she is a good candidate for this treatment.

After only a week or two of estrogen, most women notice a significant increase in vaginal moisture, which can be mistaken for a discharge from infection, rather than a return of normal vaginal secretions. However, there is a slightly increased risk of a yeast infection during the first month of estrogen replacement, so new itching or irritation could signal a yeast infection that is easily treatable with over-the-counter or prescription medications.

Once estrogen has been replaced and the woman is comfortable, the frequency of use of the local estrogen can be adjusted to that needed to remain comfortable. Occasionally, the estrogen can be stopped altogether when she is comfortable, and just restarted when and if symptoms recur. Most of the time, however, without this added estrogen, the vaginal skin again thins and dries.

The management of an atrophic vagina in a woman who has had estrogen receptor–positive breast cancer, whose cancer doctor is not comfortable with her using vaginal estrogen is trickier. Some women do well simply with a moisturizer such as a dot of petroleum jelly at the opening. Replens is a moisturizer that is inserted with an applicator and provides more moisturizing effect that lasts longer. Lubrication with sexual activity is important, with Jo Premium, Slippery Stuff (must be obtained online), Astroglide, or any vegetable oil being very soothing choices. Sometimes, when there is redness and irritation, a mild cortisone ointment or rectal suppository (there are none formulated for the vagina) inserted into the vagina can be soothing. A nonestrogen hormone vaginal insert, prasterone (Intrarosa), is sometimes cleared by oncologists. However, this medication is converted into estrogen. The fractional $CO_2$ laser (such as the MonaLisa Touch) has shown promise in improving the appearance of atrophic vaginal walls, but the effect is temporary, use is controversial for this problem, and there is no FDA approval for this treatment for the vagina.

## Bacterial Vaginosis

Bacterial vaginosis (BV) is the most common vaginal condition in women between ages of 15 and 44 years. This is a strange disorder; and although it sounds like an infection, it is not exactly that. It is caused when the numbers of bacteria that can be found normally in the vagina change. Like the mouth and intestines, a healthy vagina is supposed to be a germy place. But, at times, too many of some bacteria and too few of another can cause bacterial vaginosis.

We do not know what exactly causes the numbers of these bacteria to change and cause BV. Bacterial vaginosis occurs almost only in people who are sexually active, either sexually active with men or with women, and even those who only masturbate. We know that men do not get BV, and treating men does not keep women from getting BV, but women can pass this back and forth. We know that BV is more common in women with higher numbers of lifetime sex partners. We know that BV is more common when condoms are not used, and that douching, or vaginal washing, increases the chance of developing BV.

Most women have no symptoms at all. Other women experience a discharge, often with a fishy odor that is especially strong after intercourse. Occasionally, there may be itching or irritation at the opening of the vagina. Usually, there is no redness or signs of inflammation.

BV cannot be diagnosed by simply the presence of a discharge and odor. BV can only be diagnosed absolutely by examining vaginal fluid under the microscope, measuring the acidity of the vaginal fluid, and performing a "whiff test," where a fishy odor is released when a drop of potassium hydroxide is added to a drop of vaginal secretion.

If most women have no symptoms at all, then why bother to treat BV? There are several reasons. First, sexually transmitted diseases such as HIV and gonorrhea are easier to catch if someone has BV. Second, women with BV are more likely to develop an infection in the uterus and fallopian tubes (pelvic inflammatory disease). Third, unborn babies of pregnant women with BV are at higher risk of being born prematurely and having a lower birth weight, but it is not known if treating BV prevents these complications.

BV is treated with antibiotics that eliminate the overgrowth of bacteria; either metronidazole or clindamycin either by mouth or inserted into the vagina are routinely used. Recurrence is common but can be minimized by use of a condom, avoiding douching, and limiting the number of sex partners. Occasionally, when recurrences are a problem, either ongoing oral or vaginal antibiotics can keep BV clear.

More information is available at the CDC site: https://www.cdc.gov/std/bv/stdfact-bacterial-vaginosis.htm.

## Yeast Infections (Candidiasis)

Yeast infections are very common infections that occur in the vagina almost entirely between the ages of puberty and menopause, but postmenopausal women who use estrogen also have vaginal yeast infections. Yeast inside the vagina is more common in premenopausal women who are sexually active, taking birth control pills, antibiotics, have poorly controlled diabetes, are pregnant, or who have immune systems that are not working well, either because of medications they are taking or because of underlying medical illnesses. Yeast is also likely to occur in the groin, skinfolds, and around rectal skin of diapered infants and both men and women who are overweight, incontinent, immunosuppressed, or have diabetes.

Most yeast infections are caused by the common yeast called *Candida albicans*, and the main symptom of vulvovaginal yeast is itching. Sometimes, the scratching and rubbing cause irritation, burning, and painful sex, and more severe vaginal yeast infections may have redness and swelling of the vulva as well. Although discharge is often discussed as a sign of yeast, many women have no abnormal discharge. Yeast in skinfolds shows up as a red rash, often with scaling and rawness. Only uncircumcised men get yeast of the penis, with redness of the head of the penis under the foreskin. In the past, some health care providers believe that chronic yeast caused depression, bloating, constipation, fatigue, and headaches. Now, we know that this is not true.

Vaginal yeast infections caused by *C albicans* are easily treated with any of several types of medication. Over-the-counter vaginal creams and suppositories such as miconazole and clotrimazole are very effective, although the 1-day and 3-day preparations can be irritating to raw skin. Terconazole and butoconazole are equally effective prescription medications inserted into the vagina. Nystatin ointment is a very soothing and old medication that is effective and available by prescription. A fluconazole (Diflucan) tablet by mouth is also effective and avoids the risk of irritation with topical creams.

Research does not clearly prove that probiotics in the form of pills, yogurt, or acidophilus are useful in the treatment or prevention of yeast infections, nor does diet seem important, except for people with poorly controlled diabetes. Yeast is not associated with poor hygiene, so washing more is not useful.

Some women experience recurrent yeast infections. This is not an early sign of immunosuppression or a mark of a dangerously aggressive yeast infection. But, newer research suggests that some yeast forms have characteristics that are more likely to allow recurrence. Frequently, recurrent yeast has been shown to respond well to ongoing medication, such as weekly fluconazole for 3-6 months. *C albicans* is rarely resistant to medications, except in patients who are immunosuppressed.

There are other types of yeast besides *C albicans*, and some of the most common are *Candida glabrata*, *Candida parapsilosis*, *Candida krusei*, and *Saccharomyces cerevisiae*. These yeasts almost never cause symptoms of itching or burning, which is fortunate since they can be much harder to cure. Usually, there is no real need to treat these infections.

Most of the time, when women still have itching or irritation immediately after treatment of a yeast infection, the problem is not a resistant yeast infection. Usually, the symptoms are a different problem, such as LSC (eczema) or vulvodynia, a pain syndrome. Whereas yeast is the most common cause of itching that has just recently occurred, long-standing itching and irritation, rawness, or pain with sex is nearly always caused by a different or additional problem. Therefore, any troublesome ongoing issues with yeast should be proved by a culture or a molecular study in a provider's office.

## Penodynia/Scrotodynia

Penodynia is defined as sensations of penile discomfort, including irritation, burning, painful sex, stinging, soreness, or discomfort that has been present for at least 6 months, when there is no infection or skin disease causing the discomfort. Scrotodynia is less common and occurs when the scrotum is affected. Some men have anal discomfort also, called anodynia. Patients with penodynia or scrotodynia often find that redness, swelling, or texture changes of the skin occur, or even a stickiness. These do not necessarily mean that there is skin disease or infection; redness and texture change can be caused by the nerve pain of penodynia or scrotodynia.

There is very little research on scrotodynia and penodynia. However, vulvodynia, a similar pain syndrome in women, is well researched and we believe that this is the female equivalent of penodynia and scrotodynia. So, most of our knowledge about genital discomfort in men without infection or skin disease is based on this research and experience in women.

In women, vulvodynia is a symptom most often caused by several problems occurring at the same time. First is abnormalities of the pelvic floor muscles, those muscles a person uses to stop urinating midstream. These muscles should be very relaxed but strong. However, some people have tightness of these muscles. Abnormal pelvic floor muscles sometimes lead to symptoms of constipation, diarrhea, irritable bowel syndrome, frequent urination, or burning with urination.

Second is nerve discomfort (also called neuropathy, neuritis, neuralgia). People with pelvic floor muscle abnormalities are at risk for the development of neuropathic discomfort, which often is set off by any irritation or injury, such as an infection or zipper burn.

Third, anxiety and depression are factors in genital discomfort and in pain in general. Depression regularly worsens discomfort of any kind, and anxiety increases the tenseness of the pelvic floor muscles and intensifies discomfort. In addition, fear of sexually transmitted disease, malignancy, and infertility worsen symptoms and tend to make those with genital discomfort focus on this condition.

Penodynia/scrotodynia is not associated with dangerous illnesses. Penodynia/scrotodynia is not caused by sexually transmitted diseases, cancer, diabetes, or other dangerous conditions. Penodynia/scrotodynia is not associated with infertility. However, the discomfort of penodynia/scrotodynia seriously interferes with normal activities of daily life and disrupts enjoyment of life and relationships.

There is no cure for penodynia, but there are treatments that make the discomfort much better. The goal for the treatment of penodynia/scrotodynia is to relieve discomfort so that daily activities, including sexual activity, exercise, and sitting, are comfortable.

Treatment begins with the avoidance of irritation. Common irritants include medicated creams, moisturizers and some lubricants, overwashing, contraceptive jelly, irritating condom, or any other activity or substance that can irritate the skin.

Also important are medications for nerve pain. These medications were originally developed for either depression or seizures but have been found to be useful for neuropathic discomfort. Those from the antidepressant class include amitriptyline, desipramine, imipramine, duloxetine (Cymbalta), and venlafaxine (Effexor), whereas those from the antiseizure class include gabapentin (Neurontin) and pregabalin (Lyrica). An advantage of the medications from the antidepressant class is the once a day rather than twice or thrice a day dosing schedule, and the fact that they affect both neuropathy and anxiety, two causes of genital discomfort. These are not pain medications that immediately produce short-term relief, but rather help to regulate the nerve pain long-term. Normally, these medications are begun at very low doses and gradually increased to minimize side effects, since we know that women with vulvodynia are often very sensitive to medications. Some health care providers use topical medications as well, including topical lidocaine, gabapentin, or amitriptyline/baclofen combination.

If these medications alone do not make patients comfortable, another therapy for penodynia/scrotodynia targets pelvic floor muscle abnormalities with a pelvic floor evaluation and physical therapy. This strengthens the pelvic floor muscles while retraining the muscles to relax. Cognitive-behavioral therapy has been shown in women to improve vulvovaginal pain as well. Also, counseling improves quality of life by helping patients avoid the isolation that accompanies genital pain.

Many people find that, after a long period of discomfort with sexual activity, reestablishing comfortable and enjoyable sexual activity is difficult. Fear and the psychological effects of this chronic genital discomfort very often require counseling, to include couple counseling.

With proper therapy, the discomfort of penodynia/scrotodynia usually is controlled, and men are able to lead a normal life.

## Physiologic Discharge

Vaginal secretions are a normal part of vaginal health. When these secretions are heavy, we call it a discharge. We usually think of a vaginal discharge as a sign of infection, especially yeast or bacterial vaginosis. However, many women have a heavy discharge normally without an infection or any other disease as a cause. We call this a physiologic discharge; heavy but otherwise normal. This is a very common complaint, and sometimes women also describe odor. Even though this is often not a sign of disease, a heavy discharge can be annoying or even upsetting to some women.

Vaginal secretions normally are made mainly of mucous from the vagina and cervix, skin cells from the lining of the vagina, and many kinds of normal bacteria. The amount of vaginal secretions changes with hormone levels and with factors that are not well understood. The amount, color, and odor can suddenly change, even when there is no obvious cause. Abundant vaginal secretions can be either caused by infection or disease, or they can even be a sign of a healthy vagina. Estrogen increases vaginal secretions.

To make a diagnosis of physiologic (normal) discharge, the provider must find no signs of low estrogen, infection, or inflammation in vaginal secretions examined under a microscope, as well as negative infection testing. Also, an examination of the vaginal walls is normal, without redness, thinning, or sores.

A vaginal discharge is a common complaint by women who do not like the messy, constant wetness, and this helps to explain the large number of panty liners in stores. Although panty liners are sometimes irritating, most women find this a partially acceptable answer for controlling the effects of a vaginal discharge. Some women, once they are diagnosed with a physiologic discharge rather than an infection, are less bothered because they know there is not a medical problem.

Because a physiologic discharge is not a disease, there are no good treatments. Although douching is never needed for vaginal health, an occasional patient with physiologic discharge may find that a weak vinegar and water douche flushes excess discharge in the morning and allows for some discharge-free time. A half teaspoon vinegar in a pint of warm water is an acceptable fragrance-free and preservative-free mixture that is also inexpensive. Douching slightly increases the risk of bacterial vaginosis, a condition where the numbers of different bacteria change and can actually cause a discharge and odor. Douching also increases the risk of sexually transmitted disease and infections of the uterus and fallopian tubes. Another way of managing a physiologic discharge is the use of tampons, changed very frequently. Tampon use was associated in the past with toxic shock syndrome, a now very rare but dangerous bacterial infection that causes diarrhea, shock, and rash, so you should ensure that you change the tampon very frequently.

As mysteriously as a heavy physiologic discharge can appear, it can just as mysteriously disappear. Unfortunately, there are no medications, creams, or pills, that eliminate a physiologic discharge.

## Vulvar Care

The vulva needs little special care over usual skin care. When a woman is comfortable, her vulvar care in unimportant. However, if itching, rawness, or pain with sex become an issue, then taking care to avoid irritating the vulvar skin becomes important.

Despite all of the products available for vulvar care, the vulva needs no special cleaning or medications. Many women believe that frequent washing prevents infections and skin disease. Actually, overwashing with soap produces more irritation than poor hygiene.

Panty liners help to prevent the wet feeling from vaginal secretions, but many have fragrances, deodorants, or additives that sometimes cause irritation or allergy. Also, even baby wet wipes have preservatives and fragrances that occasionally cause allergy or irritation. Water Wipes are the exception and have no irritating additives. Douching is not needed for vaginal health and even increases the risk of some infections. Also, commercial douches contain fragrances, preservatives, deodorants, etc., which sometimes irritate the skin. Other feminine hygiene products have no advantage over mild soaps and even simply water. "Unscented" or "natural" products are not necessarily "safer."

Unscented does not mean fragrance-free; unscented products have a masking fragrance added. Products without fragrances are labeled as "fragrance-free." Although these products are unnecessary, they are well tolerated by most women.

Many health care providers believe that only white cotton underwear should be worn. However, there is no evidence that colored fabric or synthetic fabric cause skin problems or infection, but "breathable" fabric may be more comfortable for some women. Fabric softeners and detergents are not the cause of vulvovaginal problems unless other areas of skin covered by clothing are affected as well.

Diet does not play a role in the development of infection, even yeast infections, so avoidance of yeast breads or sugars is not useful unless you are diabetic. Research to evaluate the benefit of yogurt or acidophilus in preventing yeast is not convincing.

Guidelines for vulvar care to reduce irritation include the following:

- Wash only once a day, with clear water. Avoid soap when irritated. Pat dry, do not use a hairdryer.
- Use tampons if tolerated rather than pads.
- Douching is not needed and does not promote vaginal health; if necessary for psychological reasons, avoid commercial douches with additives, and use a homemade recipe of a half teaspoon of vinegar per cup of water.
- Nonirritating vaginal lubricants include vegetable oils; commercial products such as Slippery Stuff (slipperystuff.com), Jo Premium, and Astroglide among others are good choices. Traditional K-Y Jelly is irritating to many, and lubricants that are "warming" or flavored should be avoided.
- Wear loose fitting clothing if constricting clothing is uncomfortable.

## Vulvodynia/Vestibulodynia/Vulvar Vestibulitis/Anodynia

Vulvodynia is defined as feelings of vulvovaginal irritation, burning, painful sex, rawness, stinging, soreness, or pain that has been present for at least 6 months, when there is no infection or skin disease causing the discomfort. Vulvodynia is a very common problem, experienced by about one woman in six at some point in her life. About 1 in 14 women walking around today has vulvodynia.

Vulvodynia is never associated with dangerous illness. Vulvodynia is not caused by sexually transmitted diseases, cancer, diabetes, or other medical conditions. Vulvodynia is not associated with infertility. However, the effects of the discomfort of vulvodynia seriously interfere with normal activities of daily life and disrupt enjoyment of life and relationships.

Vulvodynia is a symptom most often caused by several problems occurring together, as well as other issues under investigation by researchers. First is tightness of pelvic floor muscles. Pelvic floor muscles are those muscles a person uses to stop urinating midstream. These muscles should be relaxed normally, but strong when needed. However, these muscles are tight in some women, and this puts those women at higher risk for vulvar discomfort. An abnormal pelvic floor sometimes also leads to symptoms of constipation, diarrhea, cramping, and symptoms of a urinary tract infection such a frequent urination and burning with urination, when there is no infection.

The second factor is nerve pain (also called neuropathic pain, neuritis, neuralgia). This nerve pain can be triggered by any irritation or injury, such as a vaginal infection, skin condition, or injury, or it can occur without any obvious cause. Although there are many kinds of nerve pain, from peripheral neuropathy as is seen with diabetes to nerve pain with sciatica, we believe that the nerve pain of vulvodynia is most often a "central processing disorder." This nerve discomfort starts in the brain, where the brain recognizes normal touch and movement as painful.

Third, anxiety and depression are understandable factors in vulvar and vaginal pain. Depression regularly worsens pain of any kind, and anxiety increases the tenseness of the pelvic floor muscles and intensifies pain.

Research on the causes of vulvodynia has increased dramatically in the past 25 years. Other possible factors that are emerging include increased numbers of nerve fibers in the vulvar skin of some women with localized vulvodynia, and substances in the painful skin that are sometimes associated with inflammation. As more information surfaces and further understanding of vulvodynia occurs, treatment will improve.

In addition, most women with vulvodynia also have other annoying issues, such as headaches, joint or muscle pain as in fibromyalgia, sleep problems, irritable bowel syndrome, temporomandibular joint disorder, chronic fatigue syndrome, or interstitial cystitis.

There is no cure for vulvodynia, but there are treatments that make the discomfort much better. The goal for the treatment of vulvodynia is to relieve discomfort so that daily activities, including sexual activity, exercise, and sitting are comfortable.

Treatment begins with the avoidance of irritation. This includes avoidance of irritating medications, moisturizers and some lubricants, overwashing, panty liners, contraceptive jelly, condoms, or any other activity or substance that can irritate the skin. Women with low estrogen due to menopause, breastfeeding, or some hormonal contraceptives should have this corrected.

A first-line therapy for vulvodynia targets pelvic floor muscle abnormalities with a pelvic floor evaluation and physical therapy. This strengthens the pelvic floor muscles while retraining them to relax.

Also important are medications for nerve pain. These medications were originally developed for either depression or seizures but were found to be useful for neuropathic discomfort.

Those from the antidepressant class include amitriptyline, desipramine, imipramine, duloxetine (Cymbalta), and venlafaxine (Effexor), whereas those most often used from the anti-seizure class include gabapentin (Neurontin) and pregabalin (Lyrica). An advantage of the medications from the antidepressant class is the once a day rather than twice or thrice a day dosing schedule, and the fact that they affect both neuropathy and anxiety, two causes of genital discomfort. These are not pain medications that immediately produce short-term relief, but rather help to regulate the nerve pain long-term. Normally, these medications are begun at very low doses and gradually increased to minimize side effects, since we know that women with vulvodynia are often very sensitive to medications. Some health care providers use topical medications as well, including topical estrogen, lidocaine, gabapentin, or amitriptyline/baclofen combination.

Cognitive-behavioral therapy and, to a lesser degree, psychotherapy have been shown to improve pain as well. Also, counseling improves quality of life by helping women avoid the isolation that accompanies genital pain.

There are two main types of vulvodynia. Most common is vestibulodynia, formerly called vulvar vestibulitis syndrome or vestibulitis, where burning, stinging, or stabbing pain occurs only at the opening or just inside the vagina, mostly with sexual activity, tampons, tight clothing—anything that touches or rubs the area. Some women experience pain occurring in a larger area; this type is called generalized vulvodynia. The treatment for these types of vulvodynia are the same for the most part. However, women with the very localized pain of vestibulodynia have the option of an additional therapy; surgical removal of the painful area if medications and physical therapy do not provide adequate relief. This surgery, called a vestibulectomy, is extremely beneficial, especially when the pelvic floor muscle abnormalities have been corrected before the procedure.

Many women find that, after pain is controlled, reestablishing comfortable and enjoyable sexual activity is difficult. Fear and the psychological effects of this chronic genital pain very often require counseling, to include couple counseling, or sex therapy. With proper therapy, the discomfort of vulvodynia usually is controlled and women are able to lead a normal life.

The National Vulvodynia Association (NVA.org) is a superb clearing house for information on this condition.

# Index

*Note*: Page numbers ending in "*f*" refer to figures. Page numbers ending in "*t*" refer to tables.

## Q



## R